ESSENTIALS OF Exercise Physiology

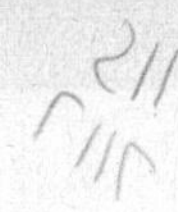

FIFTH EDITION

ESSENTIALS OF Exercise Physiology

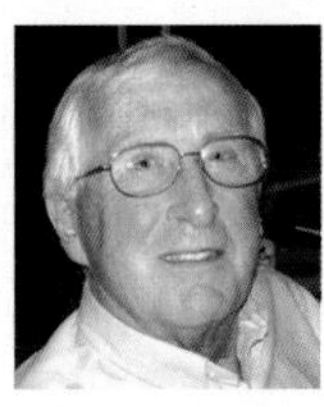

William D. McArdle

Professor Emeritus
Department of Family, Nutrition, and Exercise Science
Queens College of the City University of New York
Flushing, New York

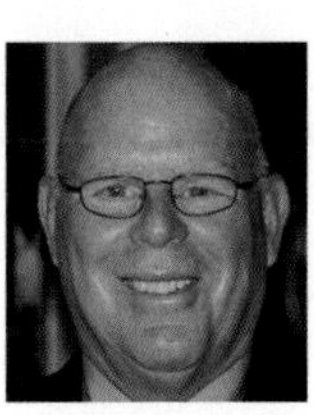

Frank I. Katch

Former Professor and Chair of
Exercise Science
University of Massachusetts
Amherst, Massachusetts

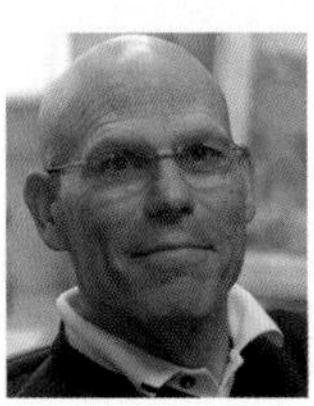

Victor L. Katch

Professor Emeritus
Department of Movement Science
School of Kinesiology
University of Michigan
Ann Arbor, Michigan

Wolters Kluwer

Philadelphia • Baltimore • New York • London
Buenos Aires • Hong Kong • Sydney • Tokyo

Acquisitions Editor: Michael Nobel
Supervising Product Development Editor: Eve Malakoff-Klein
Editorial Assistant: Tish Rogers
Marketing Manager: Shauna Kelley
Production Project Manager: David Orzechowski
Design Coordinator: Stephen Druding
Art Director: Jennifer Clements
Artist/Illustrators: Jonathan Dimes and Dragonfly Media Group
Manufacturing Coordinator: Margie Orzech
Prepress Vendor: SPi Global

Fifth Edition

9 8 7 6 5 4 3 2 1

Printed in China

Library of Congress Cataloging-in-Publication Data
McArdle, William D., author.
Essentials of exercise physiology / William D. McArdle, Frank I. Katch, Victor L. Katch. — Fifth edition.
p. ; cm.
Victor L. Katch's name appears first in the previous edition.
Includes bibliographical references and index.
ISBN 978-1-4963-0909-9
I. Katch, Frank I., author. II. Katch, Victor L., author. III. Title.
[DNLM: 1. Exercise—physiology. 2. Physical Fitness—physiology. 3. Sports Medicine. QT 256]
QP301
612'.044—dc23

2015008837

LWW.com

CCS0915

To my wife Kathleen, my children Theresa, Amy, Kevin, and Jennifer, and my grandchildren, Liam, Aiden, Quinn, Dylan, Kelly Rose, Owen, Henry, Kathleen (Kate), Grace, Elizabeth, Claire, Elise, Charlotte, and Sophia. Keep your eye on the ball, your skis together, and go for the gold. All my love, Grandpa, and to the late Guido F. Foglia, my mentor, my "brother," and my unbelievably good and loyal friend.

—Bill McArdle

To my beautiful wife Kerry, who has been there for me from the beginning, and our great children, David, Kevin, and Ellen, and Ellen's husband Sean and grandson James.

—Frank I. Katch

To my lovely wife Heather, my children Erika, Leslie, and Jesse, and my grandchildren, Ryan, Cameron, Ella, Emery, and Jude. You all light up my life.

—Victor L. Katch

In Memoriam

We are each saddened by the loss of the following friends and colleagues whom we had the privilege of their close association, friendship, and support over the past four decades.

Barbara Campaigne: Barbara Campaigne, a dedicated and accomplished student of exercise physiology, passed away following a brief illness at age 63. Her Master's and PhD research at Michigan with Author VK was innovative and unique and resulted in several first-authored papers prior to graduation. Barbara did post-doctoral research at Children's Hospital in Cincinnati, OH. Barbara moved on to contribute to the body of knowledge in glucose regulation, diabetes and physical activity, and nutrition. Her career included a faculty position at Children's Hospital in Cincinnati, OH; director of research for the ACSM; and a researcher and writer for Elli Lilly Co. Barbara was a lifelong friend, athlete, and teacher, particularly in tennis. Her infectious smile, compassion, and empathy for all people will be remembered and missed.

Priscilla Clarkson: Author FK hired Priscilla Clarkson to her first teaching position in 1977 as an Assistant Professor of Exercise Science at the University of Massachusetts, Amherst, and watched her grow into the "star" she became in our field well after she achieved full professor. Priscilla was caring and dedicated; she was a wonderfully supportive faculty member, and she mentored a cadre of outstanding undergraduate, Master's, and PhD students. She developed an internationally known Muscle Biology and Imaging lab, and published hundreds of articles and abstracts related to the field, including studies of DOMS, genomics, nutrition, and exercise biochemistry related to physical activity. Members of the Board of Trustees of ACSM in the early 1980s knew from her interactions then she would go on to achieve distinction within ACSM in future years, which she did—culminating as 2000–2001 ACSM President. She also took time for one of her first nonacademic loves—ballet—dancing as the mother in the annual Nutcracker ballet each Christmas. Priscilla continued to prosper both scientifically and academically to the time of her passing in 2013, serving as Associate Dean for the School of Public Health and Health Sciences; in her honor as the first Dean of the Commonwealth Honors College, the courtyard of the building was named after her. In 2008 she was appointed Distinguished Professor in the Department of Kinesiology. She also was honored in 2014 by having an ongoing kinesiology fellowship award named in her behalf. Priscilla's life was one well lived and cut short far too early.

Jack H. Wilmore: Authors VK and FK first met Jack as graduate students when he was an Assistant Professor of Physical Education at UC Berkeley in the late 1960s. We enrolled in classes that he taught, we worked in the exercise physiology laboratory he created, and we engaged in many spirited discussions concerning relevant topics in exercise physiology in our graduate seminars. Jack was the consummate gentleman, whether a visitor to our homes after our children were born, at the nearly 40 years of attending the annual ACSM meetings, and in his dedicated and unwavering service to ACSM (including serving as 1978–1979 ACSM President). We shared many jogging sessions together, and he always was so considerate to run with us, although we knew he wanted to go much faster. A little known fact about Jack was his athletic prowess—while a graduate student at the University of California at Santa Barbara, Jack was the all-around intramurals champion in many sports—2 years in a row!

VK worked closely with Jack, completing his MS thesis under his direction. Jack was one of the first exercise scientists to elegantly design theoretical studies on the effects of jogging/running of different intensities and durations on aerobic capacity and cardiovascular function. These studies resulted in many publications by Jack and his students, as well as laying the foundation for future studies.

All of us consider Jack Wilmore a trusted friend and colleague. He too mentored a cadre of outstanding graduate students and made many contributions to physical education and exercise physiology research (including his competing exercise physiology textbook with co-author Dr. David Costill, and his book on body composition assessment techniques with Dr. Albert Behnke). Jack Wilmore will be sorely missed. God bless you Jack!

William D. McArdle
Frank I. Katch
Victor L. Katch

Reviewers

Heather Dillon Anderson, PT, DPT, NCS
Assistant Professor
Physical Therapy
Neumann University
Aston, Pennsylvania

Kyle Barnes, PhD
Visiting Professor
Department of Movement Science
Grand Valley State University
Allendale, Michigan

Julie Barnett, PT, DPT, MTC
Clinical Assistant Professor
School of Health Professions Physical Therapy
University of Texas Health Science Center San Antonio
San Antonio, Texas

Philip Buckenmeyer, PhD
Associate Professor, Department Chair
Kinesiology Department
State University of New York at Cortland
Cortland, New York

Patrick Carley, DHA, MS, PT
Professor
Physical Therapy Department
American International College
Springfield, Massachusetts

Ellen Glickman, PhD, FACSM
Professor
School of Health Sciences
Kent State University
Kent, Ohio

Alison Godwin, PhD
Assistant Professor
Human Kinetics Department
Laurentian University
Greater Sudbury, Ontario, Canada

Huang Guoyuan, PhD
Associate Professor
Kinesiology and Sport
University of Southern Indiana
Evansville, Indiana

Nicholas J. Hanson, PhD, CSCS
Lecturer
Human Sciences
The Ohio State University
Columbus, Ohio

Gina Kraft, PhD
Assistant Professor
Kinesiology Department
Oklahoma Baptist University
Shawnee, Oklahoma

John E. Lowry, MS
Assistant Professor
Kinesiology Department
Saginaw Valley State University
University Center, Michigan

Gary W. Mack, PhD
Professor
Department of Exercise Science
Brigham Young University
Provo, Utah

Laura Gray Malloy, PhD
Professor
Biology Department
Hartwick College
Oneonta, New York

Joel Martin, PhD
Assistant Professor
Kinesiology Department
George Mason University
Manassas, Virginia

Maurice Martin, PhD
Associate Professor
Community Health
University of Maine Farmington
Farmington, Maine

Steven E. Martin, PhD
Clinical Associate Professor
Department of Health & Kinesiology
Texas A&M University
College Station, Texas

Craig O. Mattern, PhD
Associate Professor and Program Director
School of Health and Human Performance
The College at Brockport—State University of New York
Brockport, New York

Matthew S. Palmer, PhD
Instructor
Kinesiology
University of Guelph-Humber
Toronto, Ontario, Canada

Paul A. Smith, PhD
Professor
Kinesiology Department
McMurry University
Abilene, Texas

Hirofumi Tanaka, PhD
Professor
Kinesiology Department
University of Texas at Austin
Austin, Texas

Rene Vandenboom, PhD
Professor
Kinesiology Department
Brock University
St. Catherines, Ontario, Canada

Eric Vlahov, PhD
Professor
Health Science and Human Performance
The University of Tampa
Tampa, Florida

Scott Waldeis, DC, MS
Lecturer
Physical and Life Sciences
State University of New York Alfred State College
Alfred, New York

Jay Williams, PhD
Professor
Human Nutrition, Foods and Exercise
Virginia Tech
Blacksburg, Virginia

Bradley Wilson, PhD
Professor
Health Promotion and Education
University of Cincinnati
Cincinnati, Ohio

Brian W. Witz, PhD
Professor
Biology Department
Nazareth College of Rochester
Rochester, New York

Karen Wonders, PhD, FACSM
Associate Professor
Kinesiology Department
Wright State University
Dayton, Ohio

Amanda J. Wooldridge, MS, ATC, CSCS
Instructor
Exercise Science and Wellness
Montgomery County Community College
Blue Bell, Pennsylvania

Stacey Zimmer, MS
Instructor
Exercise Physiology
Rowan University
Glassboro, New Jersey

Preface

The fifth edition of *Essentials of Exercise Physiology* represents an updated, compact version of the eighth edition of *Exercise Physiology: Nutrition, Energy, and Human Performance* and is ideally suited for an undergraduate introductory course in exercise physiology or health-related science. *Essentials of Exercise Physiology* maintains many of the features that have made *Exercise Physiology: Nutrition, Energy, and Human Performance* a leading textbook in the field since 1981 and the First Prize winner in medicine of the British Medical Association's 2002 Medical Book Competition. This *Essentials* text continues the same strong pedagogy, writing style, and graphics and flow charts of prior editions, with considerable added materials.

In preparing this edition, we incorporated feedback from students and faculty from a wide range of interests and disciplines. We are encouraged that all reviewers continue to embrace the major theme of the book: *"understanding interrelationships among energy intake, energy transfer during physical activity, and the physiologic systems that support that energy transfer."*

ORGANIZATION

We have rearranged material within and among chapters to make the information flow more logically. To improve readability, we have combined topic headings, incorporated common materials, and rearranged other materials necessary for an essentials text. This restructuring now makes it easier to cover most of the chapters in a one-semester course and adapt materials to diverse disciplines.

Section I, "Introduction to Exercise Physiology," introduces the historical roots of exercise physiology and discusses professional aspects of exercise physiology and the interrelationship between exercise physiology, sports medicine, and other health professions.

Section II, "Nutrition and Energy," consists of three chapters that emphasize the interrelationship between food energy and optimal nutrition for physical activity and exercise. A critical discussion includes the alleged benefits of commonly promoted nutritional (and pharmacologic) aids to enhance physical performance.

Section III, "Energy Transfer," has four chapters that focus on energy metabolism and how energy transfers from stored nutrients to muscle cells to produce movement during rest and various physical activities. We also include a discussion of the measurement and evaluation of the different capacities for human energy transfer.

Section IV, "The Physiologic Support Systems," contains four chapters that deal with the major physiologic systems (pulmonary, cardiovascular, neuromuscular, and endocrine) that interact to support the body's response to acute and chronic physical activity and exercise.

Section V, "Exercise Training and Adaptations," includes three chapters that describe application of the scientific principles of physical training, including the highly specific functional and structural adaptation responses to chronic overload. We discuss the body's response to resistance training and the effects of different environmental challenges on energy transfer and exercise performance. We also critique the purported performance-enhancing effects of various "physiologic" agents.

Section VI, "Optimizing Body Composition, Successful Aging, and Health-Related Physical Activity Benefits," contains three chapters that feature health-related aspects of regular physical activity. We include a discussion of body composition assessment; the important role physical activity plays in weight control, successful aging, and disease prevention; and clinical aspects of exercise physiology.

Highlights of New and Expanded Content

The following highlights new and expanded content of the fifth edition of *Essentials of Exercise Physiology*:

- Each section has undergone a major revision, incorporating the most recent research and information about the topic.
- We have included emerging topics within each chapter based on current research.
- We have included updated selected references at the end of every chapter.
- Where applicable, we have included relevant Internet sites related to exercise physiology. Additional useful Internet sites, including links to videos and animations, can be found online at **http://thePoint.lww.com/MKKESS5e.**
- We have expanded the number of *FYI For Your Information* boxes. These boxes highlight cutting-edge research. New and updated material has also been added to the *"A Closer Look" boxes.*
- Within each chapter, we color highlight key terms and concepts that are defined at the end of the chapters. These terms are also provided online with their definitions in the form of electronic flashcards.
- The full-color art program continues to be a stellar feature of the textbook. We have updated and expanded the art program and tables to maintain consistency with the 2015 eighth edition of *Exercise Physiology: Nutrition, Energy, and Human Performance.*

Special Features

- **A Closer Look.** This engaging feature focuses on timely and important physical activity, sport, and clinical topics in exercise physiology that relate to chapter content. Many of the boxes present practical applications to related topics of interest. This material, often showcased in a step-by-step, illustrated format, provides relevance to the practice of exercise physiology. Some of these boxes contain self-assessment or laboratory-type activities.

- **FYI For Your Information.** These boxes throughout the text highlight key up-to-date information about different exercise physiology areas. We designed these boxes to help bring topics to life and make them relevant to student learning.
- **Key Terms and Glossary.** Each chapter's color highlighted key terms and concepts are defined at the end of each chapter and in the online flashcards available as part of the student resources on thePoint (**http://thePoint.lww.com/MKKESS5e**).
- **Think It Through.** *Think It Through* questions at the end of each chapter section summary encourage integrative, critical thinking to help students apply information from the chapter. The instructor can use these questions to stimulate class discussion about chapter content and application of material to practical situations.
- **Appendices.** Appendices in the text and online at thePoint provide useful current information at the student's fingertips:

  Appendix A: The Metric System and Conversion Constants in Exercise Physiology

  Appendix B: Dietary Reference Intakes (DRIs): Recommended Vitamin and Mineral Intakes for Individuals

  Appendix C: Metabolic Computations in Open-Circuit Spirometry

  Appendix D: Evaluation of Body Composition—Girth Method

  Appendix E: Evaluation of Body Composition—Skinfold Method

Appendices A through E are available in the book and online. Supplemental Appendices SR-1 through SR-6, which include readings, reference materials, and links to supplemental animations and videos, may be accessed online at **http://thePoint.lww.com/MKKESS5e** using the code found on the inside front cover of this text.

User's Guide

FEATURES

Essentials of Exercise Physiology, fifth edition, was created and developed as a compact version of the popular *Exercise Physiology: Nutrition, Energy, and Human Performance*, eighth edition. This comprehensive package integrates the basic concepts and relevant scientific information to understand nutrition, energy transfer, and exercise training. Please take a few moments to look through this User's Guide, which will introduce you to the tools and features that will enhance your learning experience.

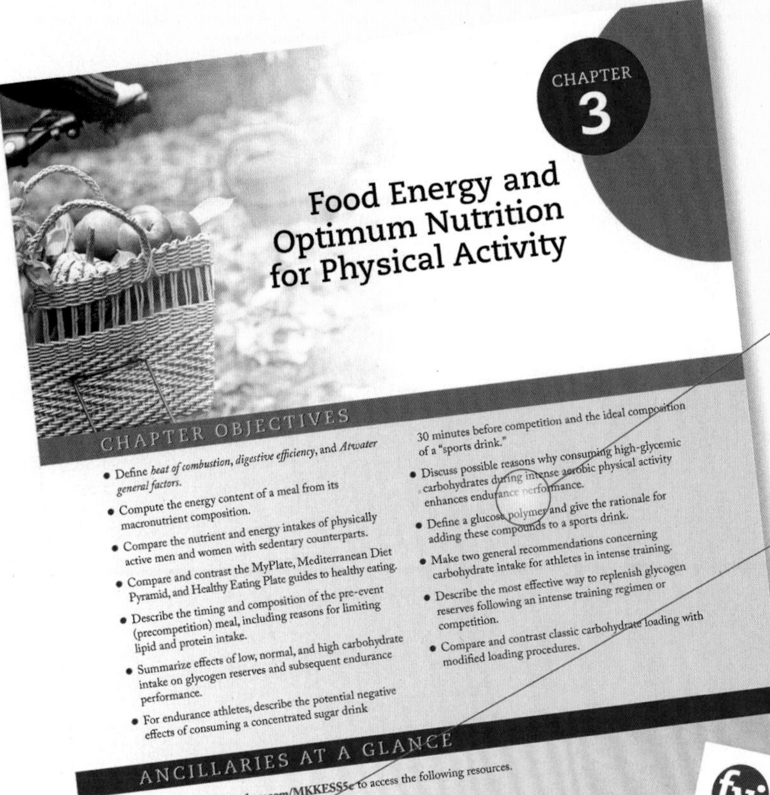

CHAPTER 3

Food Energy and Optimum Nutrition for Physical Activity

CHAPTER OBJECTIVES

- Define *heat of combustion*, *digestive efficiency*, and *Atwater general factors*.
- Compute the energy content of a meal from its macronutrient composition.
- Compare the nutrient and energy intakes of physically active men and women with sedentary counterparts.
- Compare and contrast the MyPlate, Mediterranean Diet Pyramid, and Healthy Eating Plate guides to healthy eating.
- Describe the timing and composition of the pre-event (precompetition) meal, including reasons for limiting lipid and protein intake.
- Summarize effects of low, normal, and high carbohydrate intake on glycogen reserves and subsequent endurance performance.
- For endurance athletes, describe the potential negative effects of consuming a concentrated sugar drink 30 minutes before competition and the ideal composition of a "sports drink."
- Discuss possible reasons why consuming high-glycemic carbohydrates during intense aerobic physical activity enhances endurance performance.
- Define a glucose polymer and give the rationale for adding these compounds to a sports drink.
- Make two general recommendations concerning carbohydrate intake for athletes in intense training.
- Describe the most effective way to replenish glycogen reserves following an intense training regimen or competition.
- Compare and contrast classic carbohydrate loading with modified loading procedures.

ANCILLARIES AT A GLANCE

Visit **http://thePoint.lww.com/MKKESS5e** to access the following resources.

- References: Chapter 3
- Interactive Question Bank
- Appendix A: The Metric System and Conversion Constants in Exercise Physiology
- Appendix B: Dietary Reference Intakes (DRIs): Recommended Vitamin and Mineral Intakes for Individuals
- Appendix SR-3: Nutritive Values for Common Foods, Alcoholic and Nonalcoholic Beverages, and Specialt Fast-Food Items
- Animation: Digestion of Carbohydrate
- Animation: Glycogen Synthesis

Chapter Objectives open each chapter and present learning goals to help you focus on and retain the crucial topics discussed in each chapter.

Ancillaries at a Glance provide a quick summary of the numerous resources available online at **http://thePoint.lww.com/MKKESS5e** to enhance your learning.

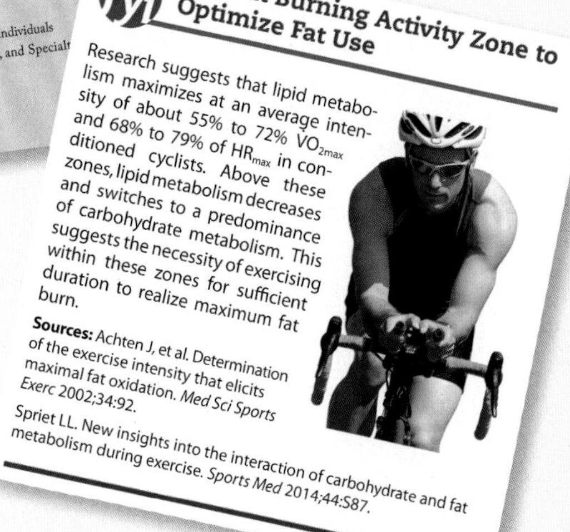

fyi

The Fat Burning Activity Zone to Optimize Fat Use

Research suggests that lipid metabolism maximizes at an average intensity of about 55% to 72% VO_{2max} and 68% to 79% of HR_{max} in conditioned cyclists. Above these zones, lipid metabolism decreases and switches to a predominance of carbohydrate metabolism. This suggests the necessity of exercising within these zones for sufficient duration to realize maximum fat burn.

Sources: Achten J, et al. Determination of the exercise intensity that elicits maximal fat oxidation. *Med Sci Sports Exerc* 2002;34:92.

Spriet LL. New insights into the interaction of carbohydrate and fat metabolism during exercise. *Sports Med* 2014;44:S87.

FYI For Your Information boxes highlight key information about different exercise physiology areas and help bring topics to life, making them exciting and relevant for all readers.

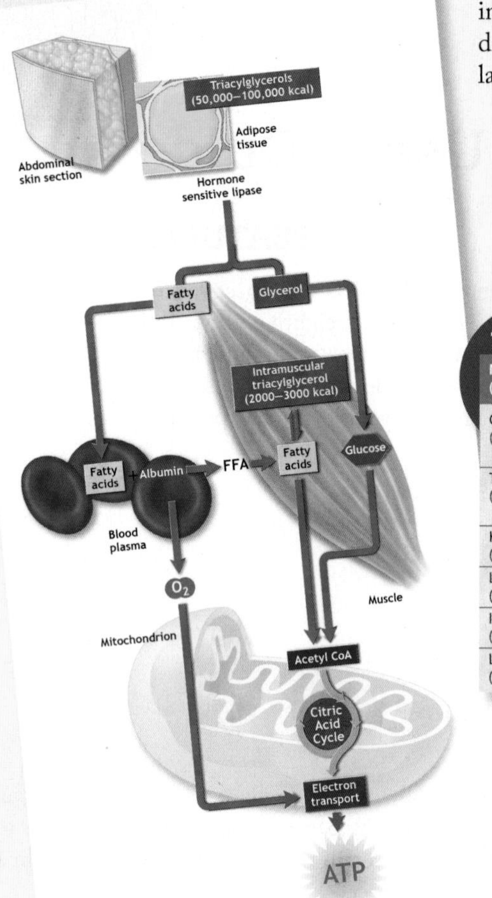

Illustrations throughout the text draw attention to important concepts in a visually stimulating and intriguing manner. Detailed, full-color drawings and photographs amplify and clarify the text and are particularly helpful for visual learners.

TABLE 5.1 Six Classifications of Enzymes

Name (Example)	Action
Oxidoreductases (lactate dehydrogenase)	Catalyze oxidation-reduction reactions where the substrate oxidized is regarded as hydrogen or electron donor; includes dehydrogenases, oxidates, oxygenases, reductases, peroxidases, and hydroxylases.
Transferases (hexokinase)	Catalyze the transfer of a group (e.g., the methyl group or a glycosyl group) from one compound regarded as donor to another compound regarded as acceptor; include kinases, transcarboxylases, and transaminases.
Hydrolases (lipase)	Catalyze reactions that add water; includes esterases, phosphatases, and peptidases.
Lyases (carbonic anhydrase)	Catalyze reactions that cleave C–C, C–O, C–N, and other bonds by different means than by hydrolysis or oxidation. Includes synthases, deaminases, and decarboxylases.
Isomerases (phosphoglycerate mutase)	Catalyze reactions that rearrange molecular structure; include isomerases and epimerases. These enzymes catalyze changes within one molecule.
Ligases (pyruvate carboxylase)	Catalyze bond formation between two substrate molecules with concomitant hydrolysis of the diphosphate bond in ATP or a similar triphosphate.

Tables organize complex concepts concisely and clearly.

A CLOSER LOOK

How to Measure Work on a Treadmill, Cycle Ergometer, and Step Bench

The most common ergometers to quantify work include treadmills, cycle and arm-crank ergometers, stair steppers, and rowers.

Work and Power

Work (*W*) represents application of force (*F*) through a distance (*D*):

$$W \times F \times D$$

Power (*P*) represents work (*W*) performed per unit time (*T*):

$$P = F \times D \div T$$

Units of measurement to express work include kg-m, foot-pounds (ft-lb), joules (J), Newton-meters (Nm), and kilocalories (kcal); units of measurement for power are kg-m · min⁻¹, Watts (1 W = 6.12 kg-m · min⁻¹), and kcal · min⁻¹.

For example, for a body mass of 70 kg and vertical jump score of 0.5 m, the work accomplished would equal 35 kilogram-meters (kg-m) (70 kg × 0.5 m). If the person were to accomplish work in the vertical jump of 35 kg-m in 500 milliseconds (0.500 seconds; 0.008 minutes), the power attained would equal 4375 kg-m · min⁻¹.

Calculation of Treadmill Work

The treadmill is a moving conveyor belt with variable angle of incline and speed. Work performed equals the product of the weight (mass) of the person (*F*) and the vertical distance (*D*) achieved walking or running up the incline. Vertical distance equals the sine of the treadmill angle (theta or θ) multiplied by the distance traveled along the incline (treadmill speed × time).

$$W = \text{Body mass } (F) \times \text{Vertical distance } (D)$$

Example

For an angle θ of 8 degrees (measured with an inclinometer or determined by knowing the percent grade of the treadmill), the sine of angle θ equals 0.1392 (see table). The vertical distance represents treadmill speed multiplied by exercise duration multiplied by sine θ. For example, vertical distance on the incline while walking at 5000 m · h⁻¹ for 1 hour equals 696 m (5000 × 0.1392). If a 50-kg person walked at an incline of 8 degrees (percent grade ~14%) for 60 minutes at 5000 m · h⁻¹, work accomplished computes as:

$$W = F \times \text{Vertical distance } (\sin\theta \times D)$$
$$= 50\text{ kg} \times (0.1392 \times 5000\text{ m})$$
$$= 34{,}800\text{ kg-m}$$

The value for power equals 34,800 kg-m ÷ 60 minutes or 580 kg-m · min⁻¹.

Degree θ	Sine θ	Tangent θ	Percent Grade (%)
1	0.0175	0.0175	1.75
2	0.0349	0.0349	3.49
3	0.0523	0.0523	5.23
4	0.0698	0.0698	6.98
5	0.0872	0.0872	8.72
6	0.1045	0.1051	10.51
7	0.1219	0.1228	12.28
8	0.1392	0.1405	14.05
9	0.1564	0.1584	15.84
10	0.1736	0.1763	17.63
15	0.2588	0.2680	26.80
20	0.3420	0.3640	36.40

A Closer Look boxes explore real-life cases and practical applications of exercise physiology to elite athletes and average people.

Summaries at the end of each chapter section provide a numbered list of the need-to-know facts and important information to help you review and remember what you have learned.

SUMMARY

1. Vitamins neither supply energy nor contribute to body mass.
2. Vitamins serve crucial functions in almost all bodily processes and must be obtained from food or dietary supplementation.
3. The 13 known vitamins are classified as either water soluble or fat soluble.
4. Vitamins A, D, E, and K comprise the fat-soluble vitamins; vitamin C and the B-complex vitamins constitute the water-soluble vitamins.
5. Excess fat-soluble vitamins accumulate in body tissues and can increase to toxic concentrations.
6. Excess water-soluble vitamins remain nontoxic and eventually pass in the urine.
7. Vitamins regulate metabolism, facilitate energy release, and serve important functions in bone formation and tissue synthesis.
8. Vitamins C and E and β-carotene serve key protective antioxidant functions by reducing the potential for free radical damage or oxidative stress, while potentially offering protective benefits against heart disease and cancer.
9. Excess vitamin supplementation does not improve performance or potential for sustaining hard, physical training.
10. Serious illness can occur from regularly consuming excess fat-soluble and, in some cases, water-soluble vitamins.
11. Approximately 4% of body mass consists of 22 elements called minerals distributed in all body tissues and fluids.
12. Minerals occur freely in nature; in the waters of rivers, lakes, and oceans; and in soil.
13. The root system of plants absorbs minerals; these minerals are eventually incorporated into the tissues of animals that consume plants.
14. Minerals function primarily in metabolism as important parts of enzymes, including providing structure to bones and teeth, and in synthesizing glycogen, fat, and protein.
15. A balanced diet provides adequate mineral intake except in geographic locations with poor soil and inadequate iodine.
16. Osteoporosis has reached epidemic proportions among older individuals, especially women; one strategy is to advocate for adequate calcium intake and regular weight-bearing exercise or resistance training to help protect against bone loss.

20. Excessive sweating during physical activity produces body water loss and related minerals, which should judiciously be replaced during and following the activity.

THINK IT THROUGH

1. Discuss two specific conditions that justify vitamin and mineral supplementation.
2. Discuss three factors that may contribute to gender-specific recommendations for vitamin and mineral intakes.
3. Outline the dynamics of bone loss and give two suggestions to high school females regarding protection against future osteoporosis.
4. Discuss the role played by physical activity and calcium intake on bone health.
5. Respond to an athlete who asks, "Is there anything wrong with taking megadoses of vitamin and mineral supplements to ensure getting an adequate intake on a daily basis?"
6. Why does resistance training for the body's major muscle groups offer unique benefits to bone mass compared with a typical weight-bearing program of brisk walking?

PART 3 **Water**

THE BODY'S WATER CONTENT

Age, gender, and body composition influence an individual's body water content, which can range from 40% to 70% of total body mass. Water constitutes 72% of muscle weight and approximately 20% to 50% of the weight of body fat or adipose tissue. Differences among individuals in relative percentage of total body water largely result from variations in body composition (i.e., differences in fat-free vs. fat tissue).

The body contains two fluid "compartments." The first, the **intracellular compartment**, refers to fluid inside cells; the second, the **extracellular compartment**, includes blood plasma (~20% of total extracellular fluid) and interstitial

Think It Through questions, located at the conclusion of each chapter section, encourage critical thinking and problem-solving skills to help you use and apply information learned throughout each chapter in a practical manner.

Key Terms are highlighted through the chapter and defined at the end of each chapter. An audio glossary of the key terms is available online.

● *KEY TERMS*

Active site: Groove, cleft, or cavity on an enzyme's protein surface that joins in a "perfect fit" with a specific substrate's active site.

Active transport: Molecular movement of a substance through a cell membrane in a direction against its concentration gradient; requires an input of ATP energy.

Adenosine 3′,5′-cyclic monophosphate (cyclic AMP): A second messenger important in ... cesses; used in ...

...iring oxygen.

β-Oxidation: Fatty acid molecules break down in mitochondria to generate acetyl-CoA, which then enters

in muscle moves to the liver for conversion to glucose, which then returns to muscle and metabolizes back to lactate.

Coupled reactions: Reactions that occur in pairs, such that breakdown of one compound provides energy for building another compound.

Creatine kinase (CK): Also known as creatine phosphokinase (CPK) or phosphocreatine kinase. An enzyme ...essed by various tissues and cell types; catalyzes the ...ersion of creatine and consumes ATP to create phos...reatine (PCr) and ADP.

...tine kinase reaction: Reaction in which creatine ... catalyzes the conversion of creatine + ATP to create ...DP, and free energy release.

...hrome oxidase: Last enzyme in the respiratory elec...nsport chain; receives an electron from each of four ...ome c molecules and transfers them to one oxygen ...e, converting molecular oxygen to two molecules of ...

...genase enzymes: Specific enzymes including ... NAD⁺ that catalyze hydrogen's release from ...ubstrates.

...: Passive net movement of atoms, ions, or ... from a region of higher concentration to lower ...ion.

...c: "Uphill" energy processes that store or absorb ...ch proceed with an increase in free energy for ...k.

...namic state related to change; the presence of ... emerges only when change occurs, and energy relates to the performance of work and occurrence of change.

Entropy: Degree of unpredictability or disorder in a closed thermodynamic system; when related to the system's total energy availability; it indicates little energy availability from the system to produce work.

Anabolism uses energy to synthesize new compounds. For example, many glucose molecules join together to form the larger, complex glycogen molecule; similarly, glycerol and fatty acids combine to synthesize **triacylglycerols (triglyceride)**, and amino acids bind together to create larger protein molecules. Each reaction starts with simple compounds and groups them as building blocks to form larger, more intricate compounds.

Catabolic reactions release energy to form ADP. During this hydrolytic process, adenosine triphosphatase catalyzes the reaction when ATP joins with water. For each mole of ATP degraded to ADP, the outermost phosphate bond divides and liberates approximately 7.3 kcal of **free energy**, making it available for further biological functions.

$$ATP + H_2O \xrightarrow{ATPase} ADP + Pi - \Delta G\ 7.3\ kcal \cdot mol^{-1}$$

The symbol ΔG refers to the standard free energy change measured under laboratory conditions, which ... from chemical reactions not

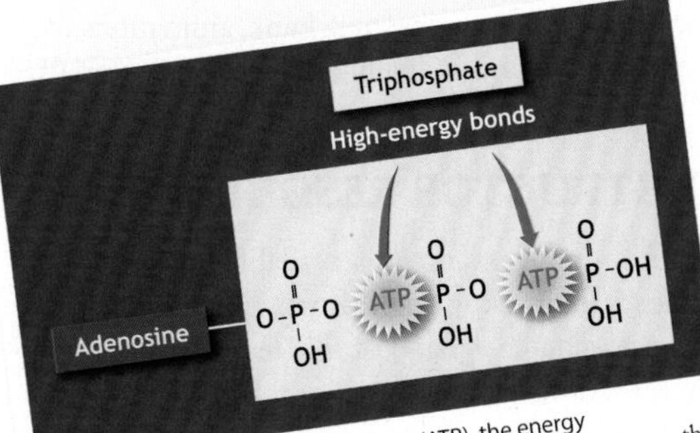

FIGURE 5.6 Adenosine triphosphate (ATP), the energy currency of the cell. The starbursts represents the high-energy bonds.

The enzyme accelerates hydrolysis to form a new compound, **adenosine diphosphate (ADP)**. In turn, these reactions couple to other reactions that incorporate the "freed" phosphate-bond chemical energy. The ATP molecules

References at the end of each chapter have been updated to provide students with the most current resources available. References are also searchable online at **http://thePoint.lww.com/MKKESS5e.**

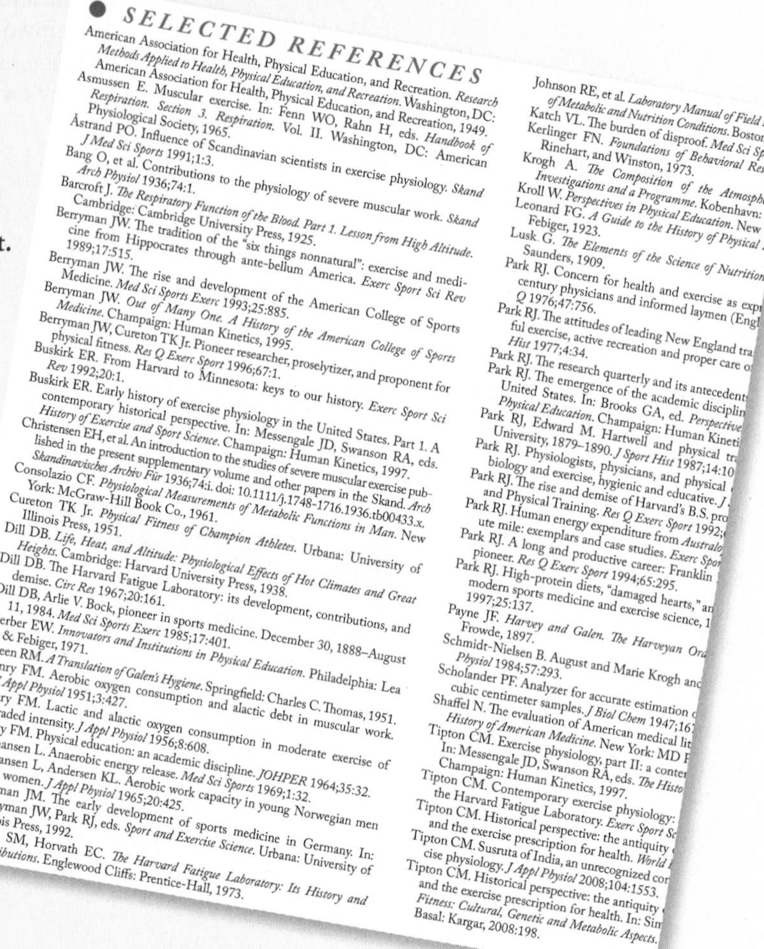

SELECTED REFERENCES

American Association for Health, Physical Education, and Recreation. *Research Methods Applied to Health, Physical Education, and Recreation.* Washington, DC: American Association for Health, Physical Education, and Recreation, 1949.

Asmussen E. Muscular exercise. In: Fenn WO, Rahn H, eds. *Handbook of Respiration. Section 3. Respiration.* Vol. II. Washington, DC: American Physiological Society, 1965.

Åstrand PO. Influence of Scandinavian scientists in exercise physiology. *Scand J Med Sci Sports* 1991;1:3.

Bang O, et al. Contributions to the physiology of severe muscular work. *Skand Arch Physiol* 1936;74:1.

Barcroft J. *The Respiratory Function of the Blood. Part 1. Lesson from High Altitude.* Cambridge: Cambridge University Press, 1925.

Berryman JW. The tradition of the "six things nonnatural": exercise and medicine from Hippocrates through ante-bellum America. *Exerc Sport Sci Rev* 1989;17:515.

Berryman JW. The rise and development of the American College of Sports Medicine. *Med Sci Sports Exerc* 1993;25:885.

Berryman JW. *Out of Many One. A History of the American College of Sports Medicine.* Champaign: Human Kinetics, 1995.

Berryman JW, Cureton TK Jr. Pioneer researcher, proselytizer, and proponent for physical fitness. *Res Q Exerc Sport* 1996;67:1.

Buskirk ER. From Harvard to Minnesota: keys to our history. *Exerc Sport Sci Rev* 1992;20:1.

Buskirk ER. Early history of exercise physiology in the United States. Part 1. A contemporary historical perspective. In: Messengale JD, Swanson RA, eds. *History of Exercise and Sport Science.* Champaign: Human Kinetics, 1997.

Christensen EH, et al. An introduction to the studies of severe muscular exercise published in the present supplementary volume and other papers in the Skand. *Arch Skandinavisches Archiv Für* 1936;74:i. doi: 10.1111/j.1748-1716.1936.tb00433.x.

Consolazio CF. *Physiological Measurements of Metabolic Functions in Man.* New York: McGraw-Hill Book Co., 1961.

Cureton TK Jr. *Physical Fitness of Champion Athletes.* Urbana: University of Illinois Press, 1951.

Dill DB. *Life, Heat, and Altitude: Physiological Effects of Hot Climates and Great Heights.* Cambridge: Harvard University Press, 1938.

Dill DB. The Harvard Fatigue Laboratory: its development, contributions, and demise. *Circ Res* 1967;20:161.

Dill DB, Arlie V. Bock, pioneer in sports medicine. December 30, 1888–August 11, 1984. *Med Sci Sports Exerc* 1985;17:401.

Gerber EW. *Innovators and Institutions in Physical Education.* Philadelphia: Lea & Febiger, 1971.

Green RM. *A Translation of Galen's Hygiene.* Springfield: Charles C. Thomas, 1951.

Henry FM. Aerobic oxygen consumption and alactic debt in muscular work. *J Appl Physiol* 1951;3:427.

Henry FM. Lactic and alactic oxygen consumption in moderate exercise of graded intensity. *J Appl Physiol* 1956;8:608.

Henry FM. Physical education: an academic discipline. *JOHPER* 1964;35:32.

Hermansen L. Anaerobic energy release. *Med Sci Sports* 1969;1:32.

Hermansen L, Andersen KL. Aerobic work capacity in young Norwegian men and women. *J Appl Physiol* 1965;20:425.

Hoberman JM. The early development of sports medicine in Germany. In: Berryman JW, Park RJ, eds. *Sport and Exercise Science.* Urbana: University of Illinois Press, 1992.

Horvath SM, Horvath EC. *The Harvard Fatigue Laboratory: Its History and Contributions.* Englewood Cliffs: Prentice-Hall, 1973.

Johnson RE, et al. *Laboratory Manual of Field Metho of Metabolic and Nutrition Conditions.* Boston: Ha

Katch VL. The burden of disproof. *Med Sci Sports*

Kerlinger FN. *Foundations of Behavioral Researc* Rinehart, and Winston, 1973.

Krogh A. *The Composition of the Atmosphere: Investigations and a Programme.* Kobenhavn: A.

Kroll W. *Perspectives in Physical Education.* New Yo

Leonard FG. *A Guide to the History of Physical E* Febiger, 1923.

Lusk G. *The Elements of the Science of Nutrition* Saunders, 1909.

Park RJ. Concern for health and exercise as expr century physicians and informed laymen (Engl Q 1976;47:756.

Park RJ. The attitudes of leading New England tra ful exercise, active recreation and proper care o *Hist* 1977;4:34.

Park RJ. The research quarterly and its antecedents

Park RJ. The emergence of the academic disciplin United States. In: Brooks GA, ed. *Perspective Physical Education.* Champaign: Human Kineti

Park RJ, Edward M. Hartwell and physical tr University, 1879–1890. *J Sport Hist* 1987;14:10

Park RJ. Physiologists, physicians, and physical biology and exercise, hygienic and educative. *J*

Park RJ. The rise and demise of Harvard's B.S. pro and Physical Training. *Res Q Exerc Sport* 1992;

Park RJ. Human energy expenditure from Australo ute mile: exemplars and case studies. *Exerc Spor*

Park RJ. A long and productive career: Franklin pioneer. *Res Q Exerc Sport* 1994;65:295.

Park RJ. High-protein diets, "damaged hearts," an modern sports medicine and exercise science, 1 1997;25:137.

Payne JF. *Harvey and Galen. The Harveyan Ora* Frowde, 1897.

Schmidt-Nielsen B. August and Marie Krogh and *Physiol* 1984;57:293.

Scholander PF. Analyzer for accurate estimation cubic centimeter samples. *J Biol Chem* 1947;16

Shaffel N. The evaluation of American medical lit *History of American Medicine.* New York: MD P

Tipton CM. Exercise physiology, part II: a conte In: Messengale JD, Swanson RA, eds. *The Histo* Champaign: Human Kinetics, 1997.

Tipton CM. Contemporary exercise physiology: the Harvard Fatigue Laboratory. *Exerc Sport Sc*

Tipton CM. Historical perspective: the antiquity and the exercise prescription for health. *World*

Tipton CM. Susruta of India, an unrecognized con cise physiology. *J Appl Physiol* 2008;104:1553.

Tipton CM. Historical perspective: the antiquity and the exercise prescription for health. In: Sim *Fitness: Cultural, Genetic and Metabolic Aspects.* Basal: Kargar, 2008:198.

thePoint®

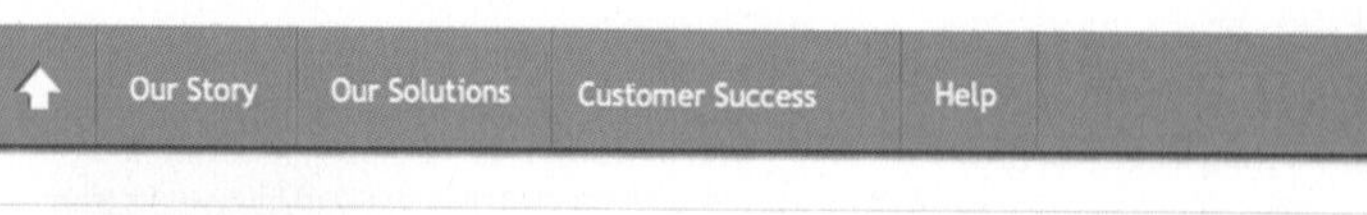

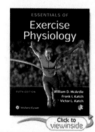

Essentials of Exercise Physiology, Fifth Edition

William D. McArdle
Frank I. Katch
Victor L. Katch

STUDENT RESOURCES

Inside the front cover of your textbook you will find your personal access code. Use it to log on to **http://thePoint.lww.com/MKKESS5e**, the companion Web site for this textbook. On the Web site, you can access various supplemental materials available to help enhance and further your learning, including an interactive quiz bank, animations of key concepts, and supplemental reading materials.

INSTRUCTOR RESOURCES

A full suite of resources is available online for all instructors adopting this text, including a fully searchable version of this text, PowerPoint presentations, a Test Generator, and a complete Image Bank.

Acknowledgments

The fifth edition of *Essentials of Exercise Physiology* represents a team effort. We are pleased to thank the many dedicated professionals at Wolters Kluwer. Many thanks to our publishing team members, including the expert talents of the following dedicated and resourceful individuals: Jennifer Clements, Art Director, who continues to inspire the hundreds of figures in this text with her expertise and constructive enhancements; Emily Lupash, Acquisitions Editor, for her many years of support for our projects, and our new editor Mike Nobel, who has been helpful and gracious and with whom we look forward to many years of working together; David Orzechowski, Production Product Manager; and Loftin Paul Montgomery, Permissions Editor, for their excellence. A special and most sincere thanks to Eve Malakoff-Klein, our extraordinarily gifted editor, resource person, mediator, and spokesperson, who consistently did everything in her power to keep the three of us focused on the tasks at hand and to ensure the highest quality of this endeavor. Eve, you are the best!

We also thank the many reviewers, colleagues, and adopters of the first four editions for their insightful comments and helpful and thoughtful suggestions for this revision. We also are grateful to our many undergraduate, master's, and PhD students who achieved the highest levels in their studies and laboratory and research work at Queens College of the City University of New York, University of Massachusetts at Amherst, and University of Michigan at Ann Arbor. Finally, we salute our steadfast golfing and fitness buddies who have been there for us from the very beginning. You didn't help our golf games or improve our flexibility as we tried to age gracefully over the past 45 years, but we sure have had fun along the way!

Contents

Appendix

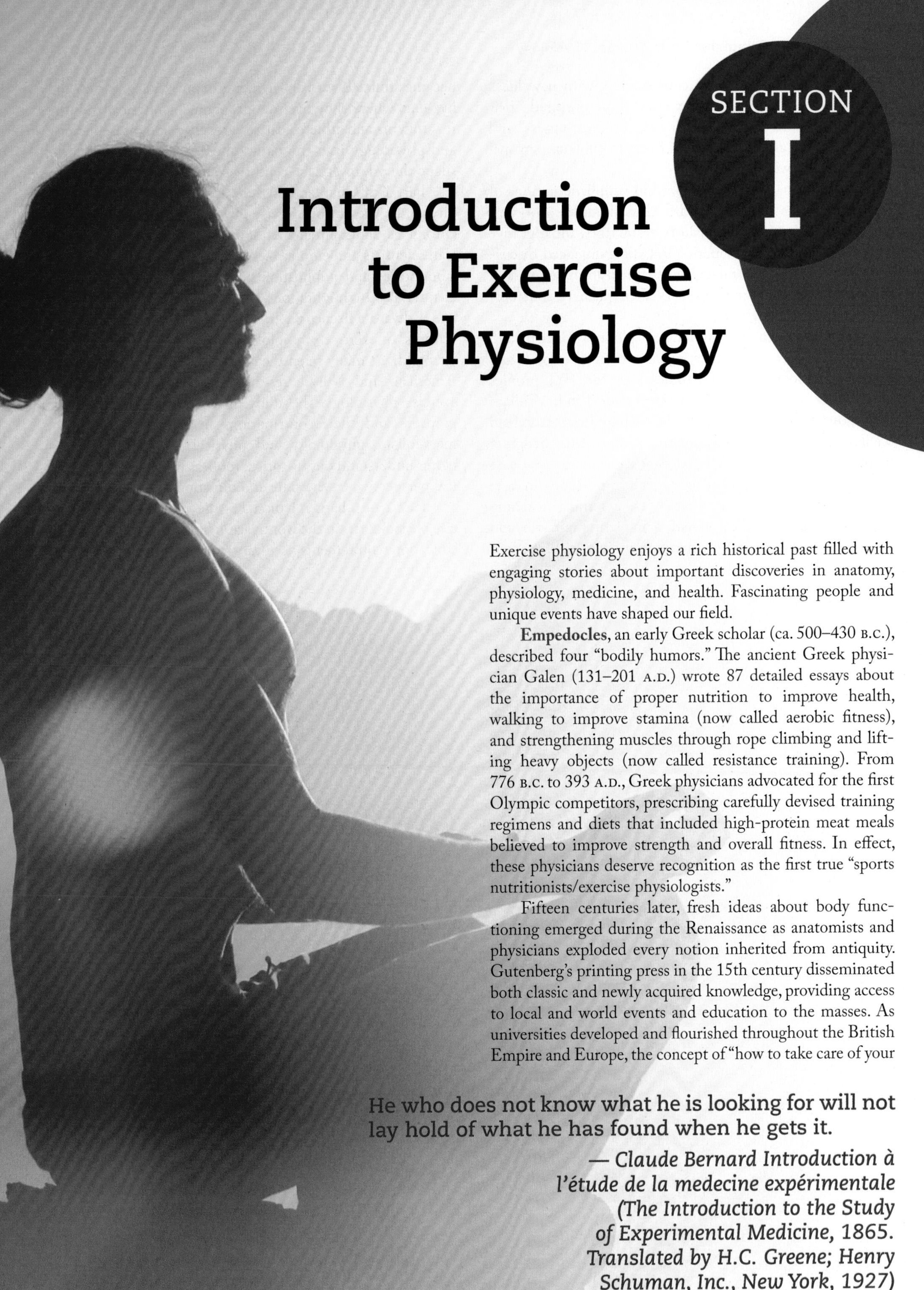

SECTION I

Introduction to Exercise Physiology

Exercise physiology enjoys a rich historical past filled with engaging stories about important discoveries in anatomy, physiology, medicine, and health. Fascinating people and unique events have shaped our field.

Empedocles, an early Greek scholar (ca. 500–430 B.C.), described four "bodily humors." The ancient Greek physician Galen (131–201 A.D.) wrote 87 detailed essays about the importance of proper nutrition to improve health, walking to improve stamina (now called aerobic fitness), and strengthening muscles through rope climbing and lifting heavy objects (now called resistance training). From 776 B.C. to 393 A.D., Greek physicians advocated for the first Olympic competitors, prescribing carefully devised training regimens and diets that included high-protein meat meals believed to improve strength and overall fitness. In effect, these physicians deserve recognition as the first true "sports nutritionists/exercise physiologists."

Fifteen centuries later, fresh ideas about body functioning emerged during the Renaissance as anatomists and physicians exploded every notion inherited from antiquity. Gutenberg's printing press in the 15th century disseminated both classic and newly acquired knowledge, providing access to local and world events and education to the masses. As universities developed and flourished throughout the British Empire and Europe, the concept of "how to take care of your

He who does not know what he is looking for will not lay hold of what he has found when he gets it.

— *Claude Bernard Introduction à l'étude de la medecine expérimentale (The Introduction to the Study of Experimental Medicine, 1865. Translated by H.C. Greene; Henry Schuman, Inc., New York, 1927)*

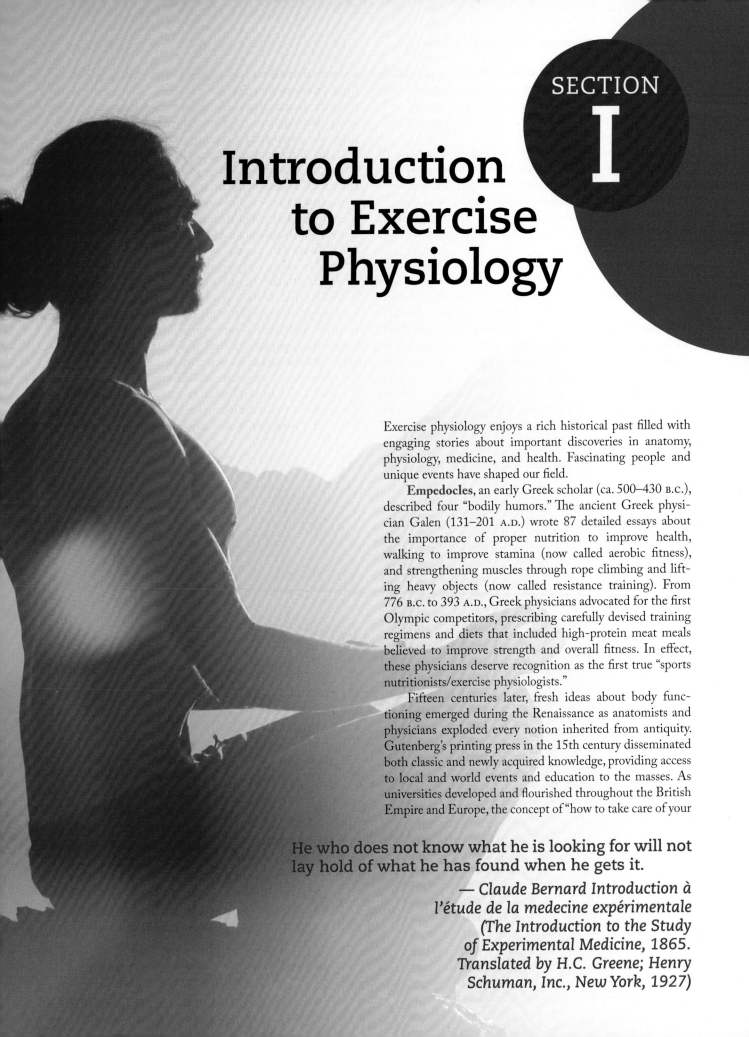

body" became a key topic of conversation, with new ideas from many self-designated "experts" who nurtured their personal opinions about how to best develop "fitness" and what kinds and amounts of foods to eat to enhance personal "nutrition" and well-being.

The new anatomists went beyond simplistic notions of the early Greeks and put forward ideas about the workings and complexities of the circulatory, respiratory, and digestive systems. Although the supernatural still influenced discussions of physical phenomena, many turned from dogma and superstition to experimentation as their primary source of newly acquired knowledge.

The early experimentation of pioneer British and European science researchers laid a cornerstone for future exercise physiology–related studies (see the FYI profiles in Chapter 1 of William Harvey, James Lind, William Beaumont, Claude Bernard, August Krogh, and Archibald Vivian Hill). By the middle of the 19th century, fledgling medical schools in the United States began to graduate students who would go on to leadership positions in academia and related medical sciences, assuming teaching responsibilities in medical schools, conducting research, and writing textbooks. Some of the more influential physicians became affiliated with departments of physical education and hygiene, where they oversaw programs of physical training for students and athletes. These early efforts to infuse biology and physiology into the basic school curriculum helped to shape the origin of 21st-century exercise physiology.

Part 1 of Chapter 1 highlights the genesis from antiquity to the present of exercise physiology worldwide. It also chronicles achievements of several early American physician scientists and emphasizes the growth of formal research laboratories and publication of textbooks in the field. The chapter also highlights the work of Drs. Edward Hitchcock and Edward Hitchcock, Jr., who could be considered the "fathers" of exercise physiology as we know it today. Finally, we highlight many scientific contributions of contemporary American and Nordic researchers who greatly impacted exercise physiology. The study of these exercise physiology pioneers and their contributions in chemistry, nutrition, metabolism, physiology, and physical fitness helps us to better understand our historical roots as well as give a historical perspective on the state and direction of our field today.

Part 2 of Chapter 1 discusses the various roles of exercise physiologists in the workplace, including certification and education requirements necessary to attain professional status.

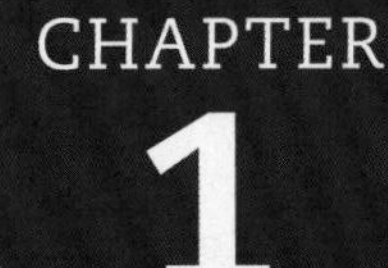

CHAPTER 1

Origins of Exercise Physiology: Foundations for the Field of Study

CHAPTER OBJECTIVES

- Briefly outline Galen's contributions to health and scientific hygiene.
- Discuss the beginnings of the development of exercise physiology in the United States.
- Discuss three contributions of George Wells Fitz to the evolution of the academic field of exercise physiology.
- List contributions of four Nordic scientists to the field of exercise physiology.
- Outline the course of study for the first academic 4-year program in the United States from the Department of Anatomy, Physiology, and Physical Training at Harvard University.
- Describe the creation of the Harvard Fatigue Laboratory, identify two of its major scientists, and detail five research contributions to the field of exercise physiology.
- Describe six different roles of the exercise physiologist.
- Discuss three roles of social networking and how they relate to exercise physiologists.
- List two of the most prominent exercise physiology professional organizations.

ANCILLARIES AT A GLANCE

Visit **http://thePoint.lww.com/MKKESS5e** to access the following resources.

- References: Chapter 1
- Interactive Question Bank
- Appendix SR-1: Physical Education: An Academic Discipline, by Franklin Henry
- Appendix SR-2: Frequently Cited Journals in Exercise Physiology

INTRODUCTION

The ability to effectively interact with the external environment depends on one's capacity for physical activity. Movement represents more than just a convenience; it represents a fundamental human evolutionary development—no less important than the complexities of intellect and emotion. Scientists have amassed considerable new knowledge about the role physical activity plays in our daily life, knowledge that exercise physiology now embraces as separate academic subfields of study and research.

The "big picture" view of exercise physiology as an academic discipline consists of three distinct, interrelated components illustrated in **Figure 1.1**:

1. Body of knowledge built on facts and theories derived from theoretical, clinical, and practical research
2. Formal course of study in accredited institutions of higher learning
3. Professional preparation and certification of practitioners and future investigators and leaders in the field

Academic Discipline Emerges

The current academic discipline of exercise physiology emerged from the influences of traditional academic fields of anatomy, physiology, and medicine, with contributions from 18th-century English and European physicians and researchers. Their influence on American university research endeavors started in the mid-1800s. Each of these disciplines uniquely contributed to understanding human structure and function along a continuum from optimal health to disease and infirmity.

Sharpening the Focus

Human physiology integrates aspects of chemistry, physics, biology, nutrition, genetics, and growth and development to explain biological events and their functions. The discipline of physiology compartmentalizes into subdisciplines, usually based on either a systems approach that includes pulmonary, cardiovascular, renal, endocrine, muscular, reproductive, and neuromuscular systems or a broad spectrum approach that studies cells, invertebrates, vertebrates, and humans. A key difference between the interests of the physiologist and the exercise physiologist, while often subtle, arises from their research focus. Both endeavor to systematically discover basic facts and laws, and establish new knowledge about a given topic, but exercise physiologists frame their research efforts with physical activity—acute or chronic—as the main focus, rather than using physical activity solely as an intervention strategy to study physiological processes.

In a presentation at the 67th annual conference of the National College Physical Education Association in 1964 (see Appendix SR-1 for Franklin Henry's classic paper Physical education. An academic discipline. *J Health Physical Education Recreation* 1964;35:32), **Franklin M. Henry** (1904–1993) laid out the rationale for the academic discipline of physical education with special emphasis in the areas of exercise physiology, neuromotor control, and biomechanics. In the 50 years since Henry's presentation, what once seemed like discreet content areas within the science-based domain of physical education have now emerged as more integrated areas of research, with many common connections to other established disciplines. In some cases, exercise physiology integrates into departments of physiology. Graduates of physiology from traditional physiology programs and exercise physiology graduates from kinesiology programs now share common interests and often work side-by-side in kinesiology or physiology departments.

Knowledge Explosion and Scientific Research

The knowledge explosion of the late 1950s greatly increased the number of citations in the research literature. Consider the terms *exercise* and *exertion*. In 1946, a hand search of resource manuals yielded just 12 citations in five journals. Only 16 years later in 1962, the number increased to 128 citations in 51 journals and by 1981, 655 citations appeared in 224 journals. The exponential explosion in new scientific knowledge in the exercise physiology-related fields during the past decade, however, has dwarfed these earlier increases. In early October, 2002, more than 6000 citation listings *exercise* and *exertion* appeared in more than 1400 journals. As of June 2, 2015, the term *exercise* yielded an almost 60% increase to 296,211 entries when searching PubMed (**www.ncbi.nlm.nih.gov/pubmed/?term=exercise**), with a further increase of 6274 entries to 60,972 for the term *exertion*. It is indeed fair to say that exercise physiology represents a mature field of study, with its research focus continuing to expand.

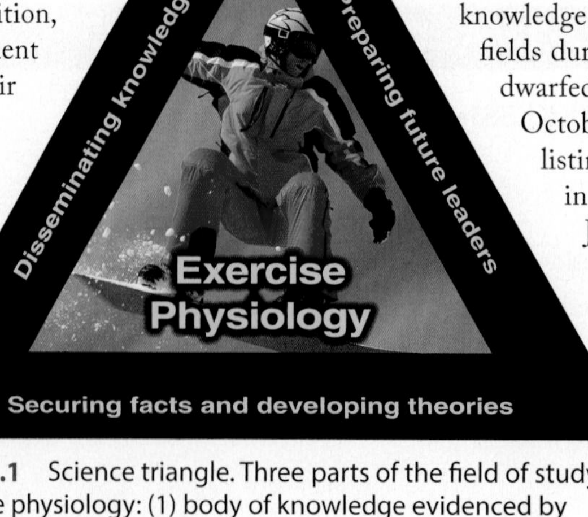

FIGURE 1.1 Science triangle. Three parts of the field of study of exercise physiology: (1) body of knowledge evidenced by experimental and field research engaged in the enterprise of securing facts and developing theories, (2) formal course of study in institutions of higher learning for the purpose of disseminating knowledge, and (3) preparation of future leaders in the field. (Adapted from Tipton CM. Contemporary exercise physiology: fifty years after the closure of the Harvard Fatigue Laboratory. *Exerc Sport Sci Rev* 1998;26:315.)

PART 1

Origins of Exercise Physiology: From Ancient Greece to the United States

EARLIEST DEVELOPMENT FROM ANTIQUITY

The roots of exercise physiology have many common links to antiquity. Exercise, sports, games, and health concerned the earliest civilizations, including the Minoan and Mycenaean cultures; the great biblical empires of David and Solomon, Assyria, Babylonia, Media, and Persia; and the empires of Alexander. The ancient civilizations of Syria, Egypt, Greece, Arabia, Mesopotamia, India, and China also recorded references to sports, games, and health practices that included personal hygiene, exercise, and training.

The doctrines and teachings of **Susruta**, a 6th century B.C. Indian physician, promoted the positive influence of different exercise modes on human health and disease. Susruta is remembered as the first plastic surgeon and as a scholar who produced the ancient treatise *Susruta Samhita* 150 years before Hippocrates lived (**http://archive.org/stream/englishtranslati00susruoft#page/n3/mode/2up**). This text is one of three foundational texts of Ayurveda (Indian traditional medicine). Susruta detailed 800 medical procedures and penned detailed accounts of hundreds of medical conditions relating to various disease states and organ deficiencies (**www.faqs.org/health/topics/50/Sushruta.html**), including the health-related benefits of exercise. Susruta considered obesity a disease and posited that a sedentary lifestyle contributed to this malady.

The earliest focus on the physiology of exercise can be seen in early Greece and Asia Minor. The greatest influence on Western Civilization came from the Greek physicians of antiquity—**Herodicus** (5th century B.C.), **Hippocrates** (460–377 B.C.), and Claudius Galenus or **Galen** (A.D. 131–201b). Herodicus, a physician and athlete, strongly advocated proper diet in physical training. His early writings influenced Hippocrates, considered the "father" of modern medicine, who first wrote about preventive medicine. Hippocrates produced 87 treatises on medicine, including several on health and hygiene, during the influential Golden Age of Greece. He espoused a profound understanding of human suffering, emphasizing a doctor's place at the patient's bedside. Today, physicians take either the classical or modern *Hippocratic Oath* (**www.nlm.nih.gov/hmd/greek/greek_oath.html**) based on Hippocrates' "**Corpus Hippocratum.**"

Five centuries after Hippocrates, during the early decline of the Roman Empire, Galen emerged as perhaps one of the most influential of the historical early physicians. The son of a wealthy architect, Galen was born in Pergamos, an ancient city on the Aegean Coast in Asia Minor (now Pergamo, Turkey), and educated by scholars of the time. He began studying medicine at approximately age 16. During the next 50 years, he enhanced current thinking about health and scientific hygiene, an area that some might consider "applied" exercise physiology. Throughout his life, Galen taught and practiced the "laws of health," ideas not uncommon today: breathe fresh air, eat proper foods, drink the right beverages, exercise, get adequate sleep, have a daily bowel movement, and control one's emotions.

A prolific writer, Galen produced at least 80 sophisticated treatises and perhaps 500 essays on numerous topics, many of which addressed human anatomy and physiology; nutrition, growth, and development; the beneficial effects of exercise; the deleterious consequences of sedentary living; and a variety of diseases and their treatment including obesity. Susruta's notions about obesity were undoubtedly influenced by Galen, who introduced the concept of *polisarkia*, now called morbid obesity. Galen proposed treatments commonly in use today—diet, exercise, and medications. As physician to the gladiators of Pergamos, Galen used various surgical procedures he invented to treat torn tendons and muscles ripped apart in combat. He formulated rehabilitation therapies and exercise regimens, including therapeutic treatment for a dislocated shoulder. He also wrote detailed descriptions about the forms, kinds, and varieties of "swift" vigorous exercises, including their proper quantity and duration. These writings about exercise and its effects might be considered the first formal "how to" treatise and remained influential for the next 15 centuries.

DAWN OF EXERCISE PHYSIOLOGY

The dawn of exercise physiology began in the periods of Renaissance, Enlightenment, and Scientific Discovery in Europe and the British Empire. During this time, Galen's ideas continued to influence the writings of the early physiologists, physicians, and teachers of hygiene and health. For example, in Venice in 1539, the Italian physician **Hieronymus Mercurialis** (1530–1606) published ***De Arte Gymnastica Apud Ancientes*** (*The Art of Gymnastics Among the Ancients*). This text, influenced by Galen and other Greek and Latin authors, profoundly affected subsequent writings about gymnastics (now called physical training and exercise) and health or hygiene in the 19th century in Europe and America. The panel in **Figure 1.2**, redrawn from *De Arte Gymnastica*, acknowledges the early Greek influence of one of Galen's well-known essays, "Exercise with the Small Ball." It illustrates his regimen of specific strengthening exercises featuring discus throwing and rope climbing.

Most of the credit for modern-day medicine has been attributed to the early Greek physicians, but other influential physicians contributed to knowledge about physiology, particularly the pulmonary circulation. The contribution of Arab physician **Ibn al-Nafis** (1213–1288) challenged the longstanding beliefs of Galen about how blood moved from the right to the left side of the heart. Ibn al-Nafis also predicted the existence of capillaries 400 years before Italian physician, biologist, and founder of microscopic

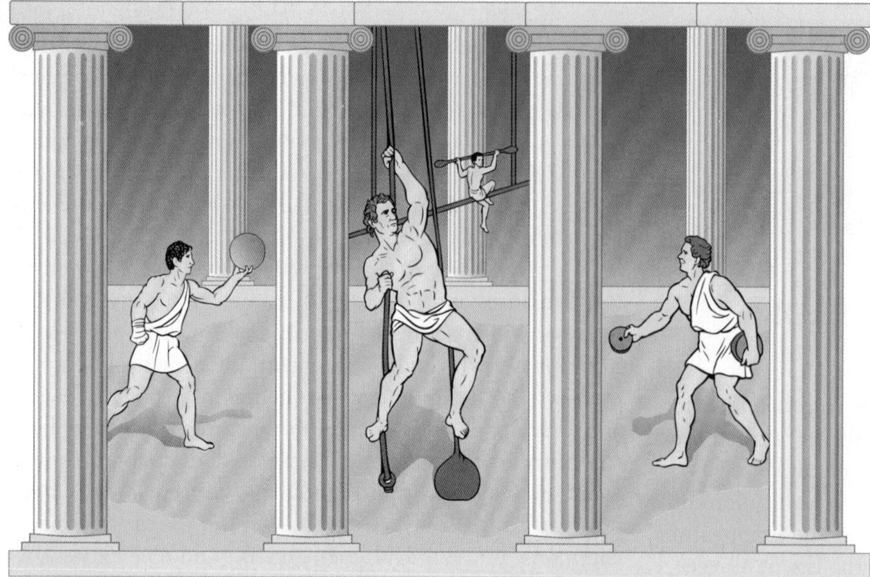

FIGURE 1.2 The early Greek influence of Galen's famous essay, "Exercise with the Small Ball" clearly appears in Mercurialis' *De Arte Gymnastica*, a treatise about the many uses of exercise for preventive and therapeutic medical and health benefits. The three panels represent the exercises as they might have been performed during Galen's time.

anatomy and histology Marcello Malpighi's discovery of pulmonary capillaries. The timeline in **Figure 1.3** shows the period of the Islamic Golden Age of Medicine. During this interval, interspaced between the Galenic era in 200 A.D. and the late 1400s and early 1500s, many physicians, including Persian physician **Ibn Sina** (Avicenna [ca. 980–1037]: **www.muslimphilosophy.com/sina/**), contributed their knowledge to 200 books (e.g., the influential Shifa [*The Book of Healing*] and Al Qanun fi Tibb [*The Canon of Medicine*; **https://archive.org/details/IbnSinasAl-qanunFiAl-tibbtheCanonOfMedicine**] about bodily functions).

William Harvey Proves Blood Flows One-Way in the Body

Renowned British physician **William Harvey's** (1578–1657) discovery that blood flowed continuously and in one direction throughout the body governed subsequent research on circulation for the next 100 years. Combining the new technique of experimentation on living creatures with mathematical logic, Harvey's epic discovery deduced that contrary to conventional wisdom, blood flowed in only one direction—from the heart to the arteries and from the veins to the lungs before reentering the heart. Harvey publicly demonstrated the one-way flow of blood by placing a tourniquet around a man's upper arm that constricted arterial blood flow to the forearm and stopped the pulse. By loosening the tourniquet, Harvey allowed some blood into the veins. Applying pressure to specific veins forced blood from a peripheral segment with little pressure into the previously empty veins. Thus, Harvey proved that the heart pumped blood through a closed, unidirectional (circular) system, from arteries to veins and back to the heart.

Harvey's monumental discovery overthrew 2000 years of ancient medical dogma that taught blood moved from the heart's right to the left side through pores in the heart's septum. His 72-page monograph, *On the Motion of the Heart and Blood in Animals; A Statement of the Discovery of the Circulation of the Blood*, published in 1894 three years after his 3-day public dissection/lecture before the Royal College of Physicians in London, represents one of the most important and famous contributions in the distinguished history of physiologic analysis.

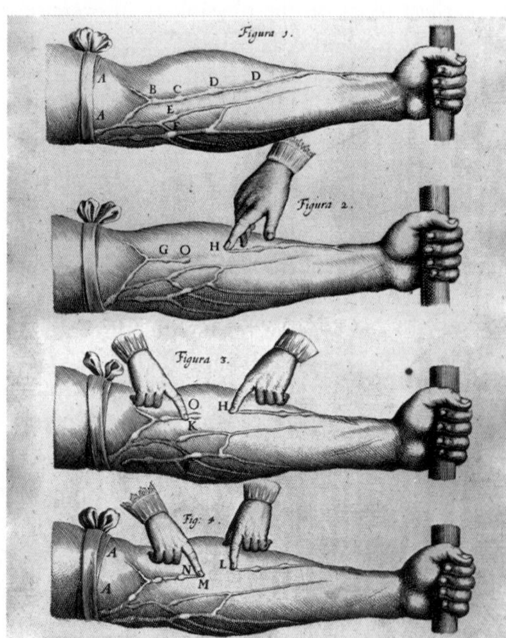

Harvey's demonstrated the one-way flow of the circulation. (Image courtesy National Library of Medicine.)

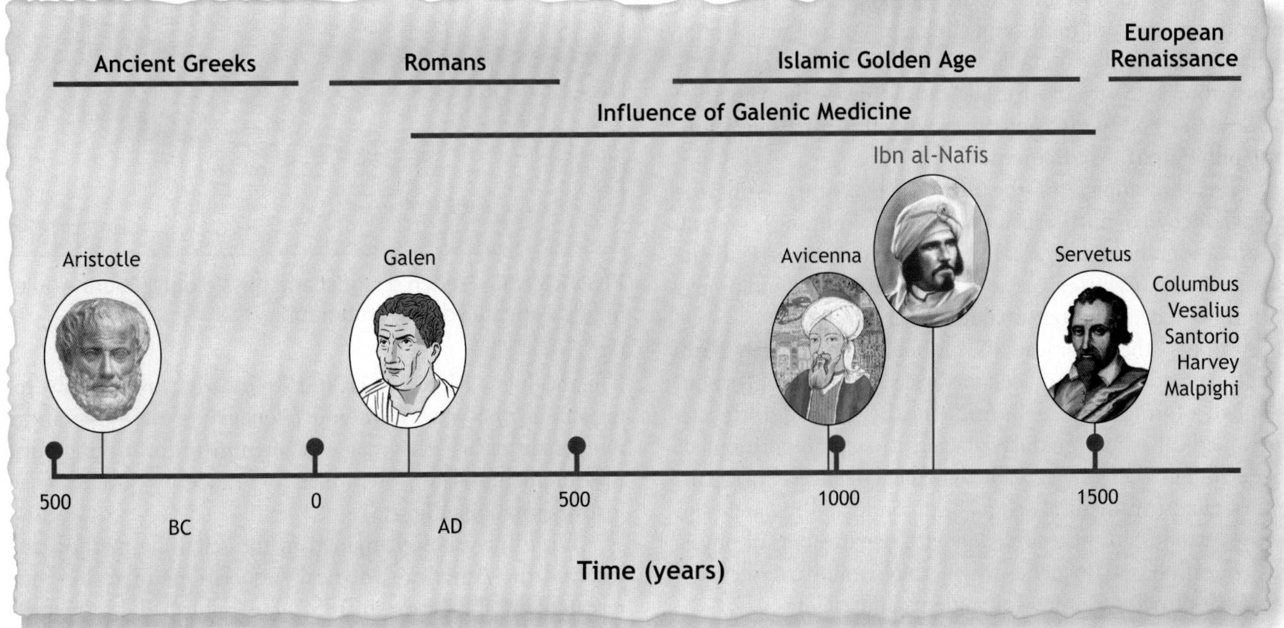

FIGURE 1.3 Timeline of the influence of Galenic medicine and the Islamic Golden Age. (Reprinted with permission from McArdle WD, Katch FI, Katch VL. *Exercise Physiology: Nutrition, Energy, and Human Performance*. 8th Ed. Baltimore: Wolters Kluwer Health, 2015.)

EARLY CONTRIBUTIONS FROM THE UNITED STATES

According to Ackerknecht's *A Short History of Medicine* (p. 219; Ronald Press Co, NY, 1955; see also **http://dittrickmuseumblog.com/2014/06/12/first-medical-publication-in-america-smallpox/**), the first medical publication in America appeared in 1677. Written by Thomas Thatcher (1670–1678), a minister, it had the long title "*A Brief Rule to Guide the Common People of New England How to Order Themselves and Theirs in the Small Pocks, of Measels*", (sometimes abbreviated to *A Brief Guide in The Small Pox and Measles*). The guide was published more than 100 years before the founding of the Harvard Medical School. By 1800, however, only 39 first edition American-authored medical books had been published; seven medical societies existed (the first was the **New Jersey State Medical Society** in 1766); and only one medical journal was available (*Medical Repository*, initially published on July 26, 1797). In contrast, in the same time period in Europe and England, 176 medical journals were published, mostly from Britain, France, Germany, and Italy. By 1850, the number of United States published medical journals increased to 117.

Medical journal publications in the United States increased tremendously during the first half of the 19th century as the steady growth in scientific contributions from France and Germany influenced the thinking and practice of American medicine.

To a large extent, however, scientific knowledge about health and disease was still in its infancy. Lack of knowledge and factual information about bodily system function spawned a new generation of "healers," who fostered quackery and primitive practices on a public that was all too eager to experiment with almost anything that offered a promise of cure. Many health faddists practiced "medicine" without a license, while some charlatans enrolled in newly created medical schools without entrance requirements, obtaining MD degrees in as little as 16 weeks.

For the average American, a not always accurate explosion of information was available through books, magazines,

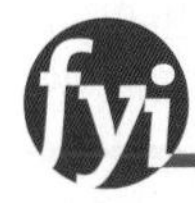

James Lind and the First Planned Controlled Clinical Trial

Trained in Edinburgh, **James Lind** (1716–1794) entered the British Navy as a Surgeon's Mate in 1739. During an extended trip in the English Channel in 1747, Lind carried out the first planned, controlled clinical trial, a decisive experiment that altered the course of naval medicine.

Lind knew that scurvy often killed two thirds of a ship's crew. The typical diet for British sailors comprised 1 lb daily of biscuits, 4 oz of cheese trice weekly, 2 lb of salt beef twice weekly, 2 oz each of dried fish and butter thrice weekly, 8 oz of peas 4 days per week, and 1 gallon of beer daily. Deprived of the then undiscovered vitamin C, sailors fell prey to scurvy ("the great sea plague"). By adding fresh fruit to their diet, Lind fortified their immune systems so that an unusually large number of British sailors no longer perished on extended voyages. Lind's landmark emphasis on the crucial importance of dietary supplements antedates modern practices. His treatment regimen defeated scurvy, but 50 years had to pass with thousands more lives lost before the British Admiralty changed its required "rules" and ordered fresh citrus fruit be carried on all naval vessels.

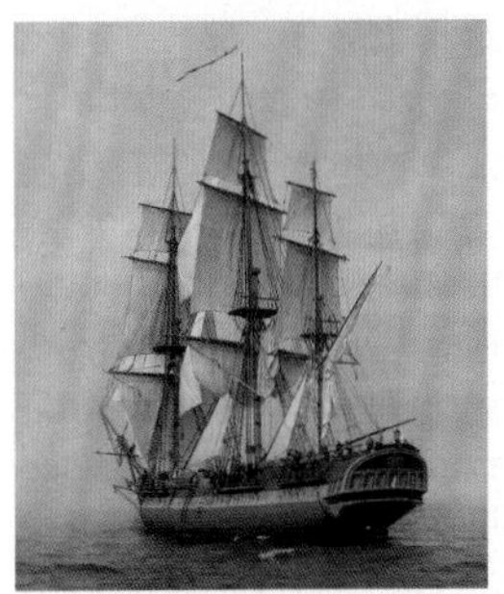

newspapers, and traveling "health salesmen"; the latter sold an endless variety of tonics and elixirs, promising to optimize health and cure disease. Many health reformers and physicians from 1800 to 1850 used "exotic" procedures to treat disease and bodily discomforts (**www.pilgrimhallmuseum.org/pdf/Patent_Medicine.pdf**).

The "hot topics" of the early 19th century (still true today) included nutrition and dieting (slimming), general information about exercise, how to best develop overall fitness, training (gymnastic) exercises for recreation and preparation for sports, and personal health and hygiene.

Prior to the American Revolution, approximately 3500 medical practitioners provided medical services, yet only about 400 had a formal "degree" in medicine. By the mid-19th century, medical school graduates began to assume positions of leadership in academia and allied medical sciences. Physicians either taught in medical school and conducted research and wrote textbooks or were affiliated with departments of physical education and hygiene, where they would oversee programs of physical training for students and athletes.

Austin Flint, Jr., MD: A Pioneering American Physician-Physiologist

Austin Flint, Jr., MD (1836–1915), contributed significantly to the burgeoning literature in physiology (**Fig. 1.4**). A respected American physician, physiologist, and successful textbook author, he fostered the belief among 19th-century American physical education teachers that muscular exercise should be taught from a strong foundation of science and experimentation, not personal opinion and anecdote. Flint, professor of physiology and microscopic anatomy at Bellevue Hospital Medical College of New York (founded in 1736, the oldest public hospital in the United States), chaired the Department of Physiology and Microbiology from 1861 to 1897 and also served as New York State's first surgeon general. In 1866, he published a series of five classic textbooks, beginning with *The Physiology of Man; Designed to Represent the Existing State of Physiological Science as Applied to the Functions of the Human Body*. Eleven years later, Flint published *The Principles and Practice of Medicine*, a synthesis of his first five textbooks comprising 987 pages of meticulously organized information with supporting documentation. This tome included illustrations of equipment used to record physiological phenomena, including

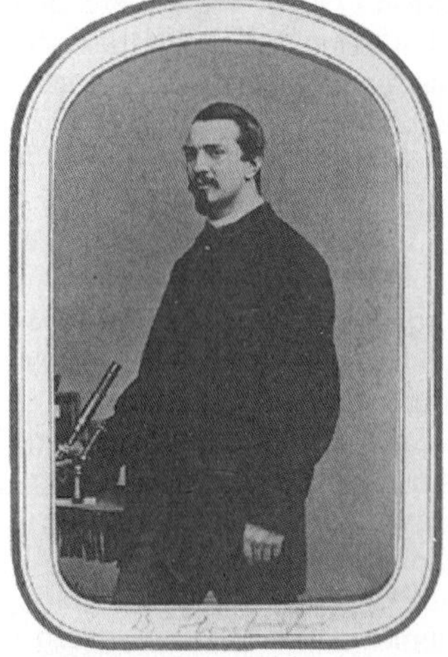

FIGURE 1.4 Austin Flint, Jr., MD, American physician-physiologist, taught that muscular exercise should be taught from a strong foundation of science and laboratory experimentation. (Image courtesy National Library of Medicine.)

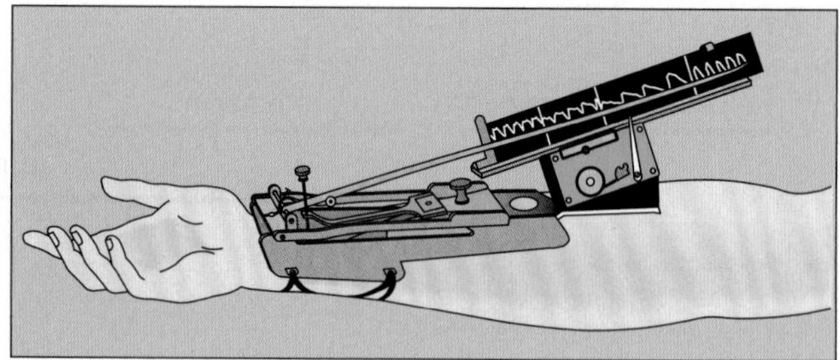

FIGURE 1.5 French scientist and physiologist Etienne-Jules Marey's advanced sphygmograph.

Etienne-Jules Marey's (1830–1904) early cardiograph for registering the wave form and frequency of the pulse and a refinement of his sphygmograph instrument for making pulse measurements—the forerunner of modern cardiovascular instrumentation (**Fig. 1.5**).

Dr. Flint was well trained in the scientific method and received the American Medical Association's prize for basic research on the heart in 1858. He published his medical school thesis, "*The Phenomena of Capillary Circulation*," in an 1878 issue of the *American Journal of the Medical Sciences*. His 1877 textbook included many exercise-related details about the influence of posture and exercise on pulse rate, the influence of muscular activity on respiration, and the influence of exercise on nitrogen elimination. Flint also published a well-known monograph in 1871 that influenced future work in the early science of exercise, "*On the Physiological Effects of Severe and Protracted Muscular Exercise, with Special Reference to its Influence Upon the Excretion of Nitrogen.*" Flint was well aware of scientific experimentation in France and England and cited the experimental works of leading European physiologists and physicians, including the incomparable **François Magendie** (1783–1855) and **Claude Bernard** (1813–1878) and the influential German physiologists **Justis von Liebig** (1803–1873), **Eduard Friedrich Wilhelm Pflüger** (1829–1910), and **Carl von Voit** (1831–1908). Flint also discussed the important contributions to metabolism of Frenchman **Antoine Lavoisier** (1743–1784) and to digestive physiology of pioneer American physician-physiologist **William Beaumont** (1785–1853).

Through his textbooks, Flint influenced **Edward Hitchcock, Jr.**, MD, the first medically trained and science-oriented professor of physical education (see next section). Hitchcock quoted Flint about the muscular system in his syllabus of *Health Lectures*, which became required reading for all students enrolled at Amherst College between 1861 and 1905.

Amherst College Connection

Two physicians, father and son, pioneered the American sports science movement (**Fig. 1.6**). Edward Hitchcock, DD, LL.D. (1793–1864), served as professor of chemistry and natural history at Amherst College and as president of the College from 1845 to 1854. He convinced the college president in 1861 to allow his son Edward (1828–1911), an Amherst graduate (1849) with a Harvard medical degree granted in 1853, to assume duties of his anatomy course. On August 15, 1861, Edward Hitchcock, Jr., became Professor of Hygiene and Physical Education with full academic rank in the Department

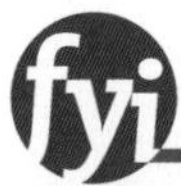

William Beaumont's Revolutionary Concepts About Digestion

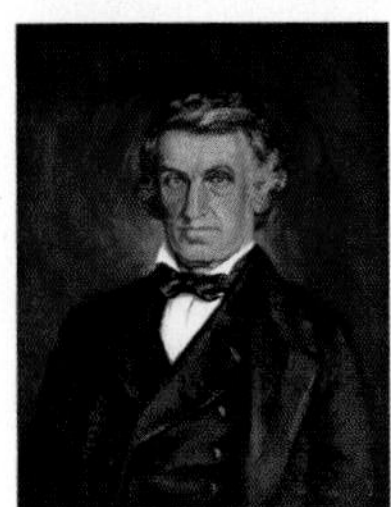

For centuries, the stomach was thought to produce heat that somehow cooked foods. Alternatively, the stomach was imaged as a mill, a fermenting vat, or a stew pan. A revolution in theories of digestion arose in the 19th century out of a fortuitous accident.

In June 1822 on the upper Michigan peninsula at Fort Mackinac, MI (**www.mackinacparks.com/parks-and-attractions/fort-mackinac/**), physician William Beaumont (1785–1853) tended the accidental shotgun wound that perforated the abdominal wall and stomach of Alexis St. Martin, a 19-year-old voyageur for the American Fur Company. From 1825 to 1833, Beaumont performed *in vivo* and *in vitro* experiments on the digestive processes.

Part of St. Martin's wound formed a small natural "valve" that led directly into the stomach. By turning St. Martin on his left side, Beaumont depressed the valve, then inserted a tube the size of a large quill 5 or 6 inches into the stomach. Beaumont observed the fluids discharged by the stomach when different foods were eaten (an *in vivo* experiment). Then, he extracted samples of the stomach's content and put them into glass tubes to determine the time required for "external" digestion (an *in vitro* experiment).

In 1825, Beaumont published the first results of his experiments on St. Martin in the *Philadelphia Medical Recorder;* he later published full details in his book *Experiments and Observations on the Gastric Juice and the Physiology of Digestion* (1833). Beaumont ends his treatise with a list of 51 inferences based on his 238 separate experiments. All of his work obeyed the scientific method, and his conclusions were based on direct experimentation. His findings quickly reached an international audience.

Beaumont, in essence a "backwoods physiologist," inspired future studies in exercise physiology of gastric emptying, intestinal absorption, electrolyte balance, rehydration, and nutritional supplementation. His accomplishment is even more remarkable because the United States, unlike England, France, and Germany, provided no research facilities for experimental medicine.

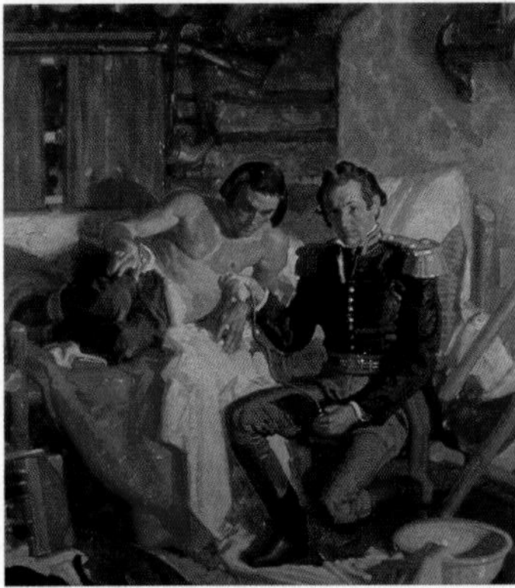

Beaumont attending Alexis St. Martin. (Reproduced with permission from McArdle WD, Katch FI, Katch VL. *Sports and Exercise Nutrition.* Baltimore: Lippincott Williams & Wilkins, 1999.)

of Physical Culture at an annual salary of $1000—a position he held almost continuously for 50 years until 1911. Hitchcock's professorship became the second such appointment in physical education in an American college. The first, to **John D. Hooker** 1 year earlier at Amherst College in 1860 was short lived because of his poor health. Hooker resigned in 1861, and Hitchcock, Jr., was appointed in his place.

The original idea of a Department of Physical Education with a professorship had been proposed in 1854 by William Augustus Stearns, DD, fourth president of Amherst College. Stearns considered physical education instruction essential for the health of students and useful to prepare them physically, spiritually, and intellectually. In 1860, the Barrett Gymnasium at Amherst College was completed; all students were required to perform systematic exercises at the facility for 30 minutes daily, 4 days a week (**Fig. 1.7**). A unique feature of the gymnasium was Hitchcock's scientific laboratory. It included strength and anthropometric equipment and a spirometer to measure respiratory function, which he used to obtain the vital statistics of all Amherst students. Dr. Hitchcock was the first to statistically record basic data on a large group of subjects on a yearly basis. These measurements provided solid information for his counseling duties concerning health, hygiene, and exercise training.

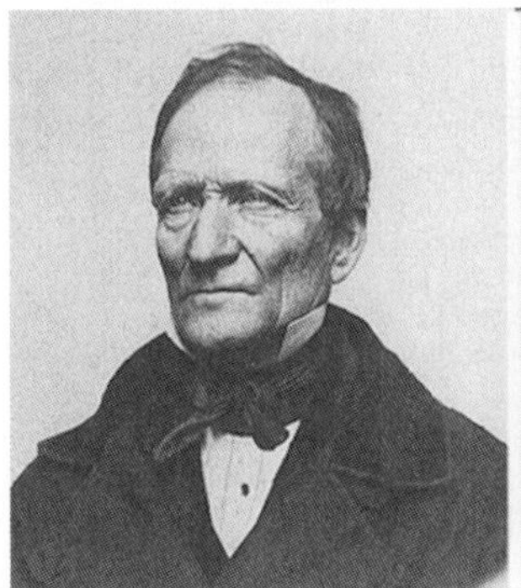

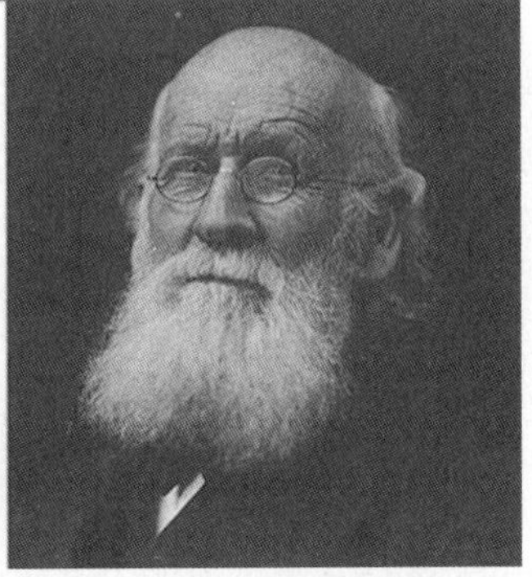

FIGURE 1.6 Drs. Edward Hitchcock (1793–1864) **(left)** and Edward Hitchcock, Jr. (1828–1911) **(right)**, father and son educators, authors, and scientists pioneered the early sports science movement in the United States.

In 1860, the Hitchcocks' coauthored *Elementary Anatomy and Physiology for Colleges, Academies, and Other Schools,* an anatomy and physiology textbook geared to college physical education; 29 years earlier, the father had published a science-oriented hygiene textbook. Interestingly, the anatomy and physiology book predated Flint's similar text by 6 years. This illustrated that an American-trained physician, with an allegiance to the implementation of health and hygiene in the university curriculum, helped set the stage for the study of exercise and training well before the medical establishment focused on this aspect of the discipline. A pedagogical aspect of the Hitchcocks' text included questions at the bottom of each page about topics

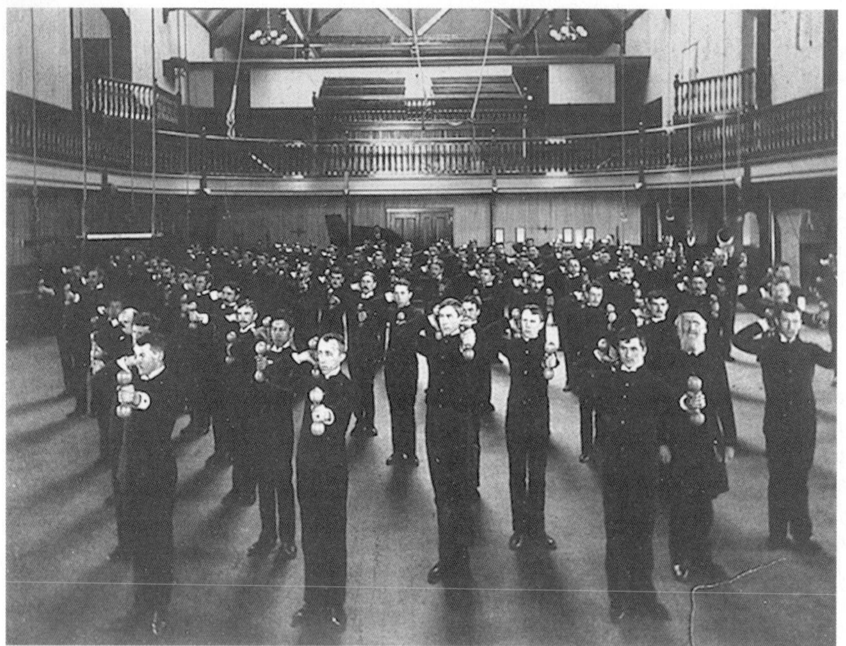

FIGURE 1.7 Dr. Edward Hitchcock, Jr. (*second from right with beard*) with the entire class of students perform regimented barbell exercises at Amherst College in the 1890s. In later years, the gymnasium served a dual purpose: a practice facility for baseball (the wood floor was replaced by a dirt infield with pitching mound), and a wooden-banked running track surrounding the inside circumference of the gym. (Photo courtesy of Amherst College Archives, and by permission of the Trustees of Amherst College, 1995.)

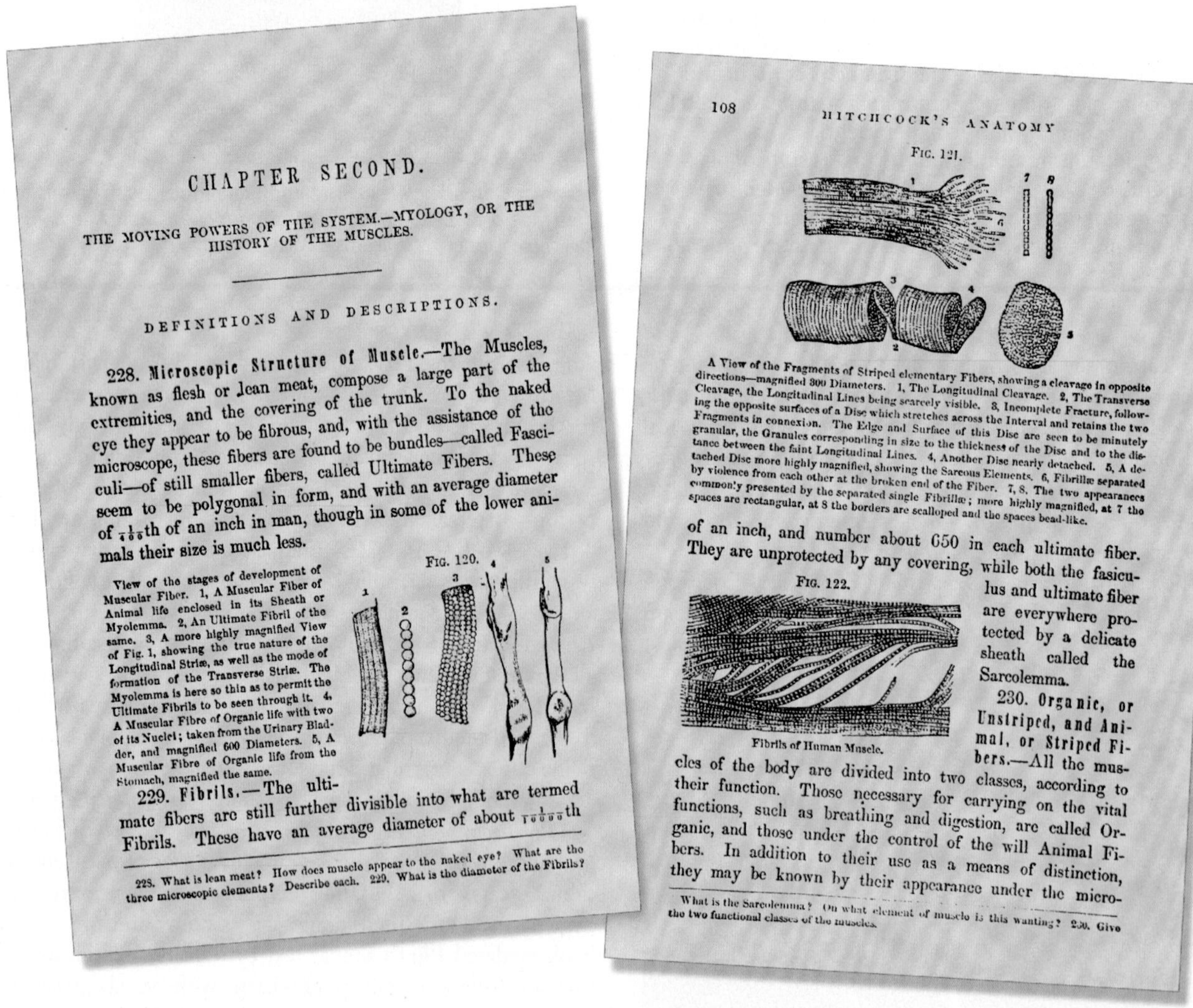

CHAPTER SECOND.

THE MOVING POWERS OF THE SYSTEM.—MYOLOGY, OR THE HISTORY OF THE MUSCLES.

DEFINITIONS AND DESCRIPTIONS.

228. **Microscopic Structure of Muscle.**—The Muscles, known as flesh or lean meat, compose a large part of the extremities, and the covering of the trunk. To the naked eye they appear to be fibrous, and, with the assistance of the microscope, these fibers are found to be bundles—called Fasciculi—of still smaller fibers, called Ultimate Fibers. These seem to be polygonal in form, and with an average diameter of $\frac{1}{400}$th of an inch in man, though in some of the lower animals their size is much less.

FIG. 120.

View of the stages of development of Muscular Fiber. 1, A Muscular Fiber of Animal life enclosed in its Sheath or Myolemma. 2, An Ultimate Fibril of the same. 3, A more highly magnified View of Fig. 1, showing the true nature of the Longitudinal Striæ, as well as the mode of formation of the Transverse Striæ. The Myolemma is here so thin as to permit the Ultimate Fibrils to be seen through it. 4, A Muscular Fibre of Organic life with two of its Nuclei; taken from the Urinary Bladder, and magnified 600 Diameters. 5, A Muscular Fibre of Organic life from the Stomach, magnified the same.

229. **Fibrils.**—The ultimate fibers are still further divisible into what are termed Fibrils. These have an average diameter of about $\frac{1}{10000}$th

228. What is lean meat? How does muscle appear to the naked eye? What are the three microscopic elements? Describe each. 229. What is the diameter of the Fibrils?

108 HITCHCOCK'S ANATOMY

FIG. 121.

A View of the Fragments of Striped elementary Fibers, showing a cleavage in opposite directions—magnified 300 Diameters. 1, The Longitudinal Cleavage. 2, The Transverse Cleavage, the Longitudinal Lines being scarcely visible. 3, Incomplete Fracture, following the opposite surfaces of a Disc which stretches across the Interval and retains the two Fragments in connexion. The Edge and Surface of this Disc are seen to be minutely granular, the Granules corresponding in size to the thickness of the Disc and to the distance between the faint Longitudinal Lines. 4, Another Disc nearly detached. 5, A detached Disc more highly magnified, showing the Sarcous Elements. 6, Fibrillæ separated by violence from each other at the broken end of the Fiber. 7, 8, The two appearances commonly presented by the separated single Fibrillæ; more highly magnified, at 7 the spaces are rectangular, at 8 the borders are scalloped and the spaces bead-like.

of an inch, and number about 650 in each ultimate fiber. They are unprotected by any covering, while both the fasiculus and ultimate fiber are everywhere protected by a delicate sheath called the Sarcolemma.

FIG. 122.

Fibrils of Human Muscle.

230. **Organic, or Unstriped, and Animal, or Striped Fibers.**—All the muscles of the body are divided into two classes, according to their function. Those necessary for carrying on the vital functions, such as breathing and digestion, are called Organic, and those under the control of the will Animal Fibers. In addition to their use as a means of distinction, they may be known by their appearance under the micro-

What is the Sarcolemma? On what element of muscle is this wanting? 230. Give the two functional classes of the muscles.

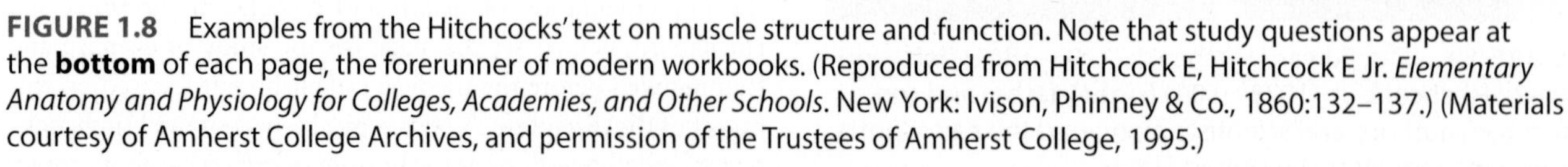

FIGURE 1.8 Examples from the Hitchcocks' text on muscle structure and function. Note that study questions appear at the **bottom** of each page, the forerunner of modern workbooks. (Reproduced from Hitchcock E, Hitchcock E Jr. *Elementary Anatomy and Physiology for Colleges, Academies, and Other Schools*. New York: Ivison, Phinney & Co., 1860:132–137.) (Materials courtesy of Amherst College Archives, and permission of the Trustees of Amherst College, 1995.)

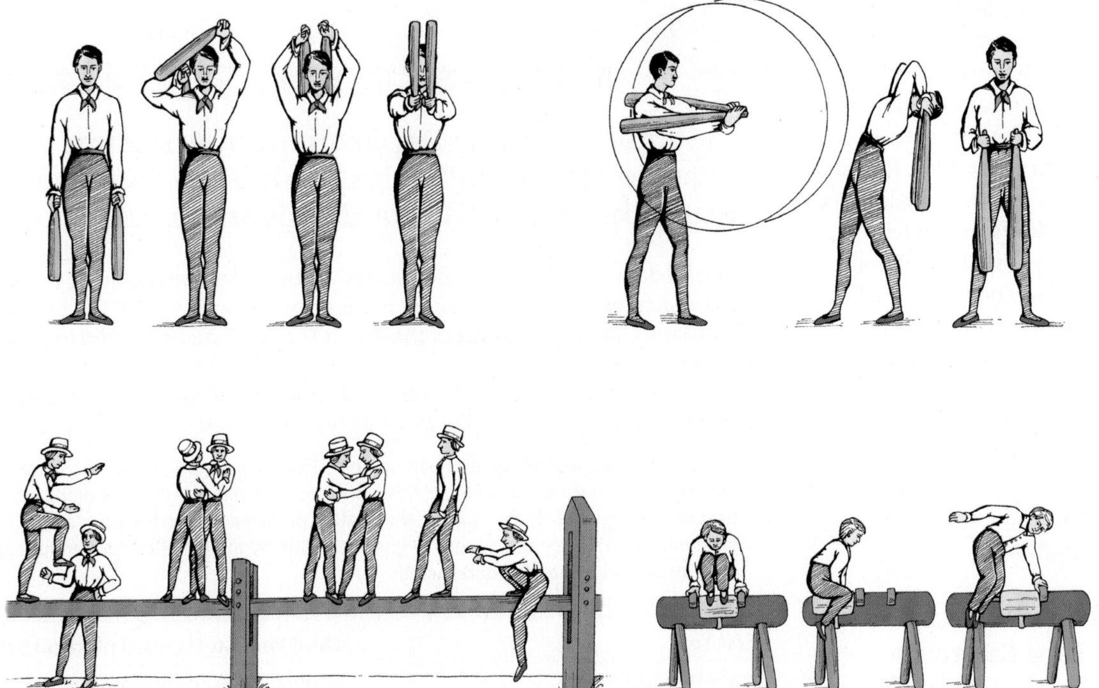

FIGURE 1.9 Exercise with Indian clubs **(top)**. Exercise on a balance beam and pommel horse **(bottom)**. Such exercises were performed routinely in physical activity classes at Amherst College from 1860 to 1920. Changes in girth anthropometric measurements taken by Dr. Hitchcock and his staff in their "exercise physiology" laboratory showed significant improvements in body dimensions, primarily upper arm and chest, from the daily workouts.

under consideration. In essence, the textbook also served as a "study guide" or "workbook." **Figure 1.8** shows sample pages from the 1860 book on muscle structure and function.

An 1880 reprint of the book contained 373 woodcut drawings about the body's physiological systems, including detailed drawings of exercise apparatus (bars, ladders, ropes, swings) and different exercises performed with Indian clubs or "scepters," one held in each hand. **Figure 1.9** shows examples of exercises with Indian clubs and those performed on a balance beam and pommel horse by Amherst College students from 1860 to the early 1890s.

Anthropometric Assessment of Body Build

From 1861 to 1888, Hitchcock, Jr., became interested in the influence of body measurements on overall health. The idea of physique assessment gained prominence in the physician's arsenal because of prevailing beliefs that such measurements would provide insights about health status. Hitchcock, Jr., measured all students enrolled at Amherst College for six segmental heights, 23 girths, six breadths, eight lengths, and eight indices of muscular strength, lung capacity, and pilosity (amount of body hair). In 1889, Hitchcock, Jr., and Hiram H. Seelye, MD (a colleague who also served as college physician from 1884 to 1896 in the Department of Physical Education and Hygiene) published a 37-page anthropometric manual that included five tables of anthropometric statistics based on measurements of students from 1861 to 1891. Hitchcock's measurement methods undoubtedly influenced European-trained anthropometrists in France and England in the early 1890s, notably the French biometrician Alphonese Bertillon (1853–1914), who developed a formal criminal identification system based on physical measurements.

Predating the work of Hitchcock, Jr., the American military made the first detailed anthropometric, spirometric, and muscular strength measurements on Civil War soldiers in the early 1860s. Trained military anthropometrists (practitioners with a specialty in taking body measurements according to strict standards) used a unique device, the **andrometer** (**Fig. 1.10**), to secure the physical dimensions of soldiers

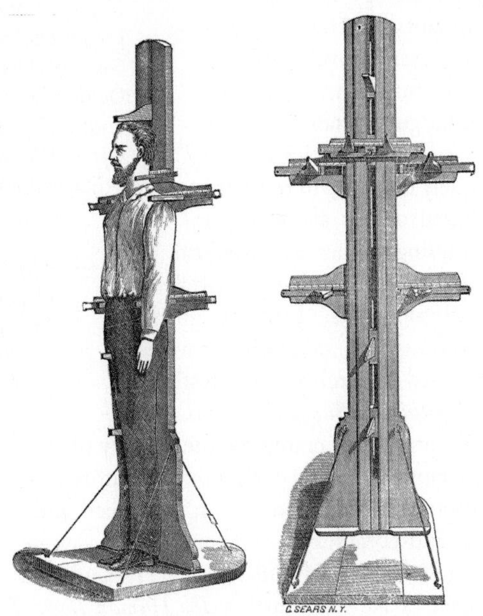

FIGURE 1.10 The United States Sanitary Commission first used the andrometer at numerous military installations along the Atlantic seaboard during the early 1860s to properly size soldiers for their military uniforms.

for purposes of fitting uniforms. The andrometer, originally devised in 1855 by a tailor in Edinburgh, Scotland, determined the proper clothing size for British soldiers. Special "sliders" measured total height; breadth of the neck, shoulders, and pelvis; and length of the legs and height to the knees and crotch.

Currently, most university exercise physiology research laboratories and numerous medical school, military, and ergonomic and exercise research laboratories include quantitative assessment procedures to routinely assess aspects of muscular strength, anthropometry, and body composition.

A CLOSER LOOK

Course of Study: Department of Anatomy, Physiology, and Physical Training, Lawrence Scientific School, Harvard University, 1893

Few of today's undergraduate physical education (exercise physiology) majors could match the strong science core required at Harvard in 1893. The table provides the core requirements of the 4-year course of study as listed in the school's 1893 course catalog.

Along with core courses, Professor Fitz established an exercise physiology laboratory. The catalog set out the laboratory's objectives:

> "A well-equipped laboratory has been organized for the experimental study of the physiology of exercise. The object of this work is to exemplify the hygiene of the muscles, the conditions under which they act, the relation of their action to the body as a whole affecting blood supply and general hygienic conditions, and the effects of various exercises on muscular growth and general health."

First Year

- Experimental Physics
- Elementary Zoology
- Morphology of Animals
- Morphology of Plants
- Elementary Physiology and Hygiene (taught by Fitz[a])
- General Descriptive Chemistry
- Rhetoric and English Composition
- Elementary German
- Elementary French
- Gymnastics and Athletics (taught by Sargent and Lathrop)

Second Year

- Comparative Anatomy of Vertebrates
- Geology
- Physical Geography and Meteorology
- Experimental Physics
- General Descriptive Physics
- Qualitative Analysis
- English Composition
- Gymnastics and Athletics (taught by Sargent and Lathrop)

Third Year (at Harvard Medical School)

- General Anatomy and Dissection
- General Physiology (taught by Bowditch and Porter)
- Histology (taught by Minot and Quincy)
- Hygiene
- Foods and Cooking [Nutrition] (at Boston Cooking School)
- Medical Chemistry
- Auscultation and Percussion
- Gymnastics and Athletics (taught by Sargent and Lathrop)

Fourth Year

- Psychology (taught by James)
- Anthropometry (Sargent[b])
- Applied Anatomy and Animal Mechanics [Kinesiology] (taught by Sargent[c])
- Physiology of Exercise (taught by Fitz[d])
- Remedial Exercise (taught by Fitz[e])
- History of Physical Education (taught by Sargent and Fitz[f])
- Forensics
- Gymnastics and Athletics (Sargent and Lathrop[g])

Course Explanation

[a]The Elementary Physiology of and Hygiene of Common Life, Personal Hygiene, Emergencies. Half-course. One lecture and one laboratory hour each week throughout the year (or three times a week, first half-year). Dr. G.W. Fitz. This is a general introductory course intended to give the knowledge of human

George Wells Fitz, MD: A Key Exercise Physiology Pioneer

George Wells Fitz, MD (1860–1934), physician and pioneer exercise physiology researcher (**Fig. 1.11**), helped establish the Department of Anatomy, Physiology, and Physical Training at Harvard University in 1891, shortly after he received his MD degree from Harvard Medical School in 1891. One year later, Fitz developed the first formal exercise physiology laboratory, where students investigated the effects of exercise on cardiorespiratory function, including muscular fatigue, metabolism, and nervous system functions. Fitz was uniquely qualified to teach this course based on his sound experimental training at Harvard's Medical School under the tutelage of well-known physiologists. Fitz designed new recording and measuring devices and published research in the prestigious *Boston Medical and Surgical Journal*, including studies on muscle cramping, the efficacy of protective clothing, spinal curvature, respiratory function, carbon dioxide measurement, and speed and accuracy of simple and complex movements. He also wrote a 1908 textbook (*Principles of Physiology and Hygiene*) and revised physiologist H Newell Martin's *The Human Body. Textbook of Anatomy, Physiology and Hygiene; with Practical Exercises.* Well-known researchers in the new program included distinguished Harvard Medical School physiologists Henry Pickering Bowditch (1840–1911), whose research produced the "all or none principle" of cardiac contraction and "treppe" (staircase phenomenon of muscle contraction), and William Townsand Porter (1862–1949), professor of comparative anatomy.

Fitz also taught a course in comparative physiology of muscle that included increased laboratory work. As the

anatomy, physiology, and hygiene, which should be possessed by every student; it is suitable also for those not intending to study medicine or physical training.

[b]Anthropometry. Measurements and Tests of the Human Body, Effects of Age, Nurture and Physical Training. Lectures and practical exercises. Half-course. Three times a week (first half-year). Dr. Sargent. This course affords systematic training in making measurements and tests of persons for the purpose of determining individual strength and health deficiencies. Practice is also given in classifying measurements, forming typical groups, etc., and in determining the relation of the individual to such groups. This course must be preceded by the course in General Anatomy at the Medical School, or its equivalent.

[c]Applied Anatomy and Animal Mechanics. Action of Muscles in Different Exercises. Lectures and Demonstrations. Half-course. Three times a week (second half-year). Dr. Sargent. The muscles taking part in the different exercises and the mechanical conditions under which they work are studied. The body is considered as a machine. The development of force, its utilization, and the adaptation of the different parts to these ends are made prominent in the work. This course must be preceded by the course in General Anatomy at the Medical School, or its equivalent.

[d]Physiology of Exercise. Experimental work, original work, and thesis. Laboratory work 6 hours a week. Dr. G.W. Fitz. This course is intended to introduce the student to the fundamental problems of physical education and to give him the training in use of apparatus for investigation and in the methods in such work. This course is preceded by the course in General Physiology at the Medical School, or its equivalent.

[e]Remedial Exercises. The Correction of Abnormal Conditions and Positions. Lectures and Demonstrations. Half-course. Twice a week (second half-year). Dr. G.W. Fitz. Deformities such as spinal curvature are studied and the corrective effects of different exercises observed. The students are trained in the selection and application of proper exercises and in the diagnosis of cases when exercise is unsuitable.

[f]History of Physical Education. Half-course. Lecture once a week and a large amount of reading. Drs. Sargent and G.W. Fitz. The student is made acquainted with the literature of physical training; the history of the various sports is traced and the artistic records (statuary, etc.) studied.

[g]Gymnastics and Athletics. Dr. Sargent and Mr. J.G. Lathrop. Systematic instruction is given throughout the 4 years in these subjects. The students attend the regular afternoon class in gymnastics conducted by Dr. Sargent, work with the developing appliances to remedy up their own deficiencies and take part in the preliminary training for the various athletic exercises under Mr. Lathrop's direction. Much work is also done with the regular apparatus of the gymnasium.

need for new equipment emerged, a joint venture between Harvard and Porter in 1901 created the *Harvard Apparatus, Inc.*, a company offering over 11,000 products worldwide for science research (**www.harvardapparatus.com/**). **Charles Sedgwick Minot** (1852–1914), a Massachusetts Institute of Technology–educated chemist with European training in physiology and biology at Leipzig, Paris, and Wurzburg, taught the histology course and served as the James Stillman Professor of comparative anatomy until his death.

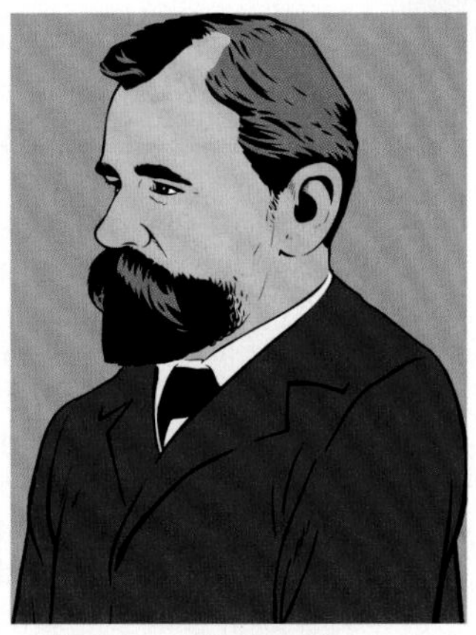

FIGURE 1.11 George Wells Fitz, MD, physician and pioneer exercise physiology researcher.

Acclaimed Harvard psychologist and philosopher William James (1842–1910), trained as a biologist and physician, the brother of novelist Henry James, taught Harvard's fourth year psychology course. Presumably, students were introduced to his newly published 1890 text, *The Principles of Psychology*, one of the most influential texts in modern psychology (**http://psychclassics.asu.edu/James/Principles/wozniak.htm**).

Harvard's pioneering 4-year course of study, well grounded in the basic sciences even by today's standards, provided students with a rigorous, challenging curriculum in what Fitz hoped would be a new science of physical education. A Closer Look: "Course of Study" provides details of all 4 years of the program.

Prelude to Exercise Science: Harvard's Department of Anatomy, Physiology, and Physical Training (BS Degree, 1891–1898)

Harvard's new physical education major and exercise physiology research laboratory focused on three objectives:

1. Prepare students, with or without subsequent training in medicine, to become directors of gymnasia or instructors in physical training.
2. Provide general knowledge about the science of exercise, including systematic training to maintain health and fitness.
3. Provide suitable academic preparation to enter medical school.

Physical education students took general anatomy and physiology courses in the medical school; after 4 years of study, graduates could enroll as second-year medical students and graduate in 3 years with an MD degree. Fitz taught the physiology of exercise course; thus, he deserves recognition as the "first" person to formally teach such a course. The new degree included experimental investigation and original work and a thesis, including 6 hours a week of laboratory study. The prerequisite for Fitz's Physiology of Exercise course included general physiology or its equivalent taken at the medical school. His Physiology of Exercise course introduced students to the fundamentals of physical education and provided training in experimental methods related to exercise physiology. In addition to the course in remedial

fyi The Greatest Physiologist Prior to 1900

Claude Bernard (1813–1878) is generally acclaimed as the greatest physiologist of all time prior to 1900. He discovered fundamental properties about physiology and participated in the explosion of scientific knowledge in the mid-19th century. His adherence to exact truth was absolute, and he was always willing to recognize the limitations or the error of what seemed like promising ideas until they were tested in the laboratory.

Claude Bernard

Bernard believed strongly in the need to always having a working hypothesis derived from perusal of the literature and observation of natural phenomena before starting on the experiment proper. He extracted from his results the most general and far-reaching conclusions that could be solidly supported by them; hence, his role as a progenitor in so many branches of the biological sciences.

Bernard conducted research on gastric juice and its role in nutrition and documented the presence of sugar in the hepatic vein of a dog whose diet lacked carbohydrate. In addition, his experiments changed medicine with the following seven discoveries:

1. The discovery of the role of the pancreatic secretion in the digestion of fats (1848)
2. The discovery of a new function of the liver—the "internal secretion" of glucose into the blood (1848)
3. Induction of diabetes by puncture of the floor of the fourth ventricle (1849)
4. Discovery of local skin temperature elevation upon section of the cervical sympathetic nerve (1851)
5. Production of sugar by washed excised liver (1855) and isolation of glycogen (1857)
6. Demonstration that curare specifically blocks transmission by motor nerve endings (1856)
7. Demonstration that carbon monoxide blocks the erythrocyte respiration (1857)

Upon Bernards's death, renowned French physiologist and "Father of Aviation Medicine" Paul Bert (1833–1886) offered as a eulogy, *"Bernard is not merely a physiologist, he is physiology. The light, which has just been extinguished, cannot be replaced."*

Exercise physiologists owe a debt of gratitude to Bernard's relentless pursuit of excellence in scientific discovery.

---

exercise, students took a required course in applied anatomy and animal mechanics. This thrice-weekly course, taught by Dr. **Dudley Allen Sargent** (1849–1924), was the forerunner of modern biomechanics courses. Its prerequisite was general anatomy or its equivalent taken at the medical school.

Before the program's dismantling in 1900, nine men graduated from it with a bachelor of science. The first graduate, James Francis Jones (1893), became instructor in physiology and hygiene and director of the gymnasium at Marietta College in Ohio.

One year after Fitz's untimely resignation from Harvard in 1899, the department changed its curricular emphasis to anatomy and physiology (dropping the term *physical training* from the department title). This terminated (at least temporarily) a unique experiment in higher education. For almost a decade before the turn of the century, the field of physical education was moving forward on a strong scientific foundation similar to other developed disciplines. Unfortunately, this opportunity to nurture the next generation of students in exercise physiology (and physical education) was momentarily stymied. Twenty years would pass before Fitz' visionary efforts to *"study the physiological and psychological effects of exercise"* and establish exercise physiology as a bona fide field of investigation would be revived, but outside of a formal physical education curriculum.

One of the legacies of the Fitz-directed "Harvard experience" from 1891 to 1899 was the mentoring it provided to specialists, who began their careers with a strong scientific basis in physical training and its relationship to health. They were taught that experimentation and the discovery of new knowledge about exercise and training furthered the development of a science-based curriculum. Unfortunately, it would take another 60 years before the next generation of science-oriented educators, led by physiologists such as **A.V. Hill** (1886–1977) and **D.B. Dill** (1891–1986), who were not trained educators, would again influence physical education curricula and propel exercise physiology to the forefront of scientific investigation.

By 1927, 135 institutions in the United States offered bachelor's degree programs in Physical Education with coursework in the basic sciences; this included four master's degree programs and two doctoral programs (Teachers College, Columbia University, and New York University). Since then, programs of study with differing emphasis in exercise physiology have proliferated. Currently, more than 86 recognized programs offer doctoral degrees and roughly 300 have master's level degree with specialization in a topic related to Kinesiology and Exercise Science with course work in exercise physiology (**www.gradschools.com/search-programs/kinesiology**).

Exercise Studies in Research Journals

In 1898, three articles on physical activity appeared in the first volume of the *American Journal of Physiology*. Other articles and reviews subsequently appeared in prestigious journals, including the first published review in *Physiological Reviews* (1922;2:310) on the mechanisms of muscular contraction by Nobel laureate A.V. Hill (1886–1977). The German applied physiology publication *Internationale Zeitschrift für angewandte Physiologie einschliesslich Arbeitsphysiologie* (1929–1940; now *European Journal of Applied Physiology and Occupational Physiology*; **www.springerlink.com/content/108306/**) became a significant journal for research about

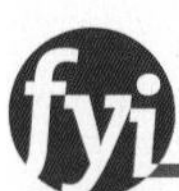

A.V. Hill, Exercise Physiology Nobel Laureate

A student at Trinity and Kings Colleges, Cambridge, England, Arcibald Vivian Hill (1886–1977), attracted the notice of two eminent physiologists, Sir Walter Morley Fletcher and **Sir Frederick Gowland Hopkins** (1929 Nobel Prize in Physiology or Medicine), who convinced Hill to pursue advanced studies in physiology rather than mathematics. An avid sportsman, Hill became interested in recovery from exercise after experiencing fatigue during track meets. He coined the term "oxygen debt" based on his field experiments, maintaining that the amount of oxygen consumed above resting in recovery represented the oxidation of approximately one-fifth of the lactic acid produced during exercise, providing the necessary energy to resynthesize the remaining lactic acid to glycogen.

Hill's early experiments focused on the effects of electrical stimulation on nerve function, the mechanical efficiency of muscle, energy processes in muscle during recovery, the interaction between oxygen and hemoglobin, and quantitative aspects of drug kinetics on muscle.

Hill devised mathematical models to describe heat production in muscle and applied kinetic analysis to explain the time course of oxygen uptake during both exercise and recovery. His important scientific achievements included discovery and measurement of heat production associated with the nerve impulse; improved analysis of heat development accompanying active shortening in muscle; application of thermoelectric methods to measure vapor pressure above minute fluid volumes; analysis of physical and chemical changes associated with nerve excitation; and excitation laws for animal tissue.

Hill combined aspects of physics and biology, a discipline which he championed and which we now call biophysics.

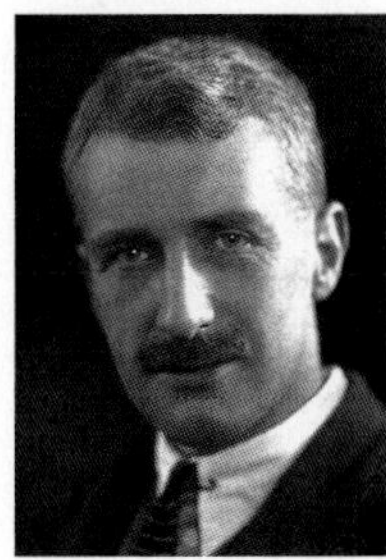

Hill achieved international acclaim for his research in muscle physiology. He shared the 1922 Nobel Prize in Physiology or Medicine with German chemist **Otto Fritz Meyerhof** for discoveries about the chemical and mechanical events in muscle contraction.

exercise physiology-related topics. The *Journal of Applied Physiology*, first published in 1948, contained the classic paper by British exercise physiologist and growth and development researcher **John Mourilyan Tanner** (1920–2010) of the Institute of Child Health at the University of London (**www.ucl.ac.uk/ich/homepage**). The paper dealt with ratio expressions of physiological data with reference to body size and function, a "must read" for all exercise physiologists (Fallacy of per-weight and per-surface area standards, and their relation to spurious correlation. *J Appl Physiol* 1949;2:1), including his numerous earlier exercise physiology-related studies (**www.ncbi.nlm.nih.gov/pubmed/?term=tanner+jm**). The official journal of the **American College of Sports Medicine** (**www.acsm.org/**) *Medicine and Science in Sports*, first appeared in 1969. The journal aimed to integrate both medical and physiological aspects of the emerging fields of sports medicine and exercise science. Note that in 1980, the journal's name changed to *Medicine and Science in Sports and Exercise*.

First Textbook in Exercise Physiology

Debate exists over the question; "What was the first textbook in exercise physiology?" Several exercise physiology textbook authors give the distinction of being "first" to the English translation of **Fernand Lagrange**'s 1888 French publication of *The Physiology of Bodily Exercise*. We disagree. To deserve such historical recognition, a textbook should meet the following three criteria:

1. Provide sound scientific rationale for major concepts
2. Provide summary information (based on experimentation) about important prior research in a particular topic area (e.g., contain scientific references to research in the area)
3. Provide sufficient "factual" information about a topic area to give it academic legitimacy

Lagrange, an accomplished writer, wrote extensively about exercise. Despite the titles of several of his books, Lagrange was not a scientist, but we believe a practicing "physical culturist." Bibliographic information about Lagrange is limited in the French and American archival records of the period—a further indication of his relative obscurity as a scholar of distinction. As far as we know, there were no citations to his work in any physiology text or scientific article of that era. In addition, his text contained fewer than 20 reference citations (based on observations of friends performing exercise). For these reasons, we contend the Lagrange book does not qualify as the first exercise physiology textbook.

If the Lagrange book is "disqualified" based on the above, what text then deserves the title as the first exercise physiology text? Possible candidates for "first" include these four choices published between 1843 and 1919:

1. Andrew Combe's 1843 text, *The Principles of Physiology Applied to the Preservation of Health, and to the Improvement of Physical and Mental Education*. New York: Harper & Brothers.
2. Edward Hitchcock and Edward Hitchcock Jr's 1860 book, *Elementary Anatomy and Physiology for Colleges, Academies, and Other Schools*. New York: Ivison, Phinney & Co.
3. H. Newell Martin's 1881 text, *The Human Body. An Account of its Structure and Activities and the Conditions of its Healthy Working*. New York: Holt & Co.
4. George Kolb's 1892 English Translation from the German Text, *Physiology of Sport*, 2nd Ed. London: Krohne and Sesemann.

CONTRIBUTIONS OF THE HARVARD FATIGUE LABORATORY (1927–1946)

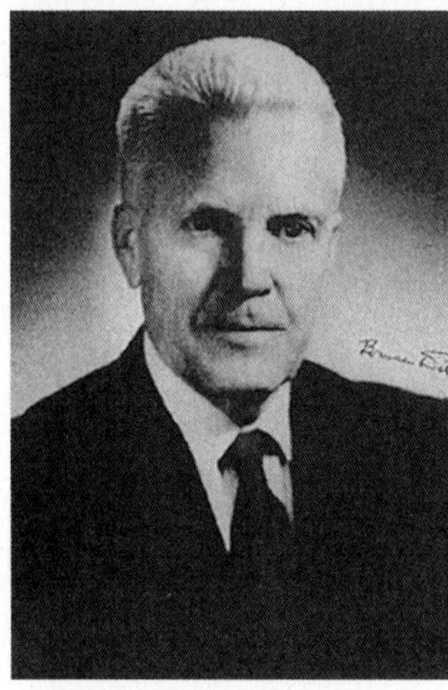

FIGURE 1.12 David Bruce Dill (1891–1986), prolific experimental exercise physiologist, helped to establish the highly acclaimed Harvard Fatigue Laboratory.

The real impact of laboratory research in exercise physiology (along with many other research specialties) occurred in 1927, again at Harvard University, 27 years after Harvard closed the first exercise physiology laboratory in the United States. The 800-square-foot **Harvard Fatigue Laboratory** in the basement of Morgan Hall of Harvard's Business School legitimized exercise physiology as an important area of research and study. Renowned Harvard chemist and professor of biochemistry **Lawrence Joseph Henderson**, MD, (1878–1942; **http://oasis.lib.harvard.edu/oasis/deliver/~bak00041**) established the laboratory.

Many of 20th century's great scientists with an interest in exercise affiliated with the Fatigue Laboratory. David Bruce Dill (1891–1986; **www.the-aps.org/fm/presidents/introdbd.html**; **Fig. 1.12**), a Stanford Ph.D. in physical chemistry, became the first and only scientific director of the laboratory. While at Harvard, Dill refocused his efforts from biochemistry to experimental physiology and became the driving force behind the laboratory's numerous scientific accomplishments. His early academic association with physician Arlie Bock [a student of British high-altitude physiologist **Sir Joseph F. Barcroft** (1872–1947) and Dill's closest friend for 59 years] and contact with 1922 Nobel laureate A.V. Hill provided Dill with the confidence to successfully coordinate the research efforts of dozens of scholars from 15 different countries. Hill convinced Bock to write a third edition of F.A. Bainbridge's 1919 text, *Physiology of Muscular Activity*, and Bock invited Dill to coauthor this 1931 book.

Similar to the legacy of the first exercise physiology laboratory established in 1891 at Harvard's Lawrence Scientific School 31 years earlier, the Harvard Fatigue Laboratory demanded excellence in research and scholarship. Cooperation among scientists from around the world fostered lasting collaborations. Many of its charter scientists influenced a new generation of exercise physiologists worldwide.

OTHER EARLY EXERCISE PHYSIOLOGY RESEARCH LABORATORIES

Other notable research laboratories helped exercise physiology become an established field of study at colleges and universities. The **Nutrition Laboratory at the Carnegie Institute in Washington, DC** (established 1904), initiated experiments in nutrition and energy metabolism (*Science* 1915;42:75). The first research laboratories established in a department of physical education in the United States originated at George Williams College (1923) (founded by the YMCA Training School in Chicago, Illinois, now merged with Aurora College, Aurora, Illinois); University of Illinois (1925), Springfield College, Massachusetts (1927); and Laboratory of Physiological Hygiene at the University of California, Berkeley (1934). In 1936, Franklin M. Henry (**Fig. 1.13**) assumed responsibility for the laboratory; shortly thereafter, his research appeared in various physiology and motor performance–oriented journals (120 articles in peer-reviewed journals; 1975 ACSM Honor Award).

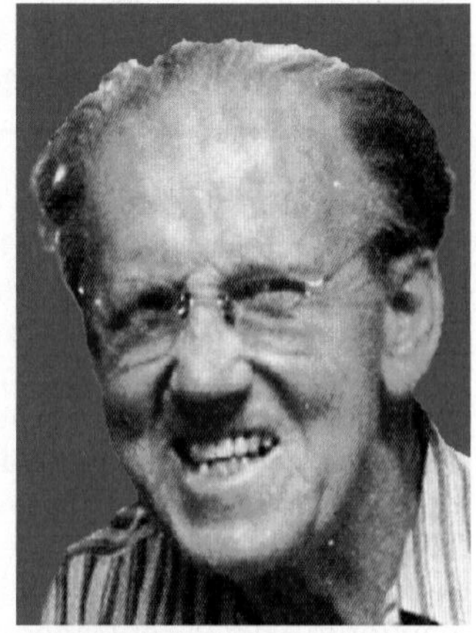

FIGURE 1.13 Franklin M. Henry (1904–1993), University of California, Berkeley, psychologist, physical educator, and researcher first proposed physical education as an academic discipline. He conducted basic experiments in oxygen uptake kinetics during exercise and recovery, muscular strength, and cardiorespiratory variability during steady-rate exercise, determinants of heavy-work endurance exercise, and neural control factors related to human motor performance.

NORDIC CONNECTION (DENMARK, SWEDEN, NORWAY, AND FINLAND)

Denmark and Sweden also were pioneers in the field of exercise physiology. In 1800, Denmark became the first European country to require physical training (military-style gymnastics) in the grade-school curriculum. Since then, Danish and Swedish scientists have continued to contribute significant research in both traditional physiology and the latest subdisciplines in exercise physiology and adaptations to physical training.

Danish Influence

In 1909, the University of Copenhagen endowed the equivalent of a Chair in Anatomy, Physiology, and Theory of Gymnastics. The first docent, Johannes Lindhard, MD (1870–1947), later teamed with future Nobel Laureate **August Krogh**, PhD (1874–1949; refer to FYI, "August Krogh, Nobel Laureate—An Ultimate Exercise Physiologist"), who specialized in physiological chemistry and research instrument design and construction, to conduct many of the classic experiments in exercise physiology (**Fig. 1.14**). Professors Lindhard and Krogh investigated

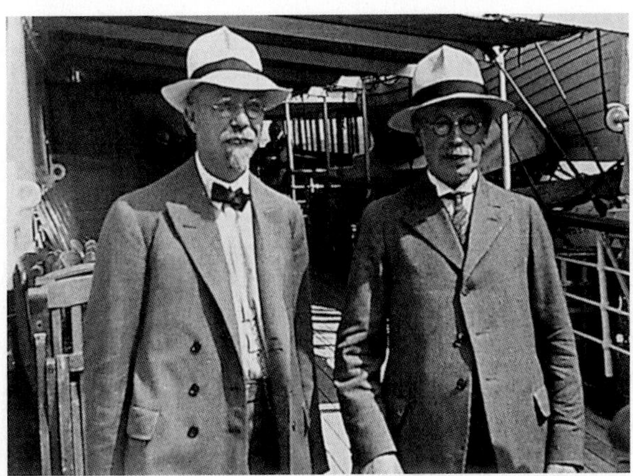

FIGURE 1.14 Professors August Krogh and Johannes Lindhard, early 1930s, pioneering exercise physiology experimental scientists.

gas exchange in the lungs, pioneered studies of the relative contribution of fat and carbohydrate oxidation during exercise, measured blood flow redistribution during different exercise intensities, and quantified cardiorespiratory dynamics in exercise.

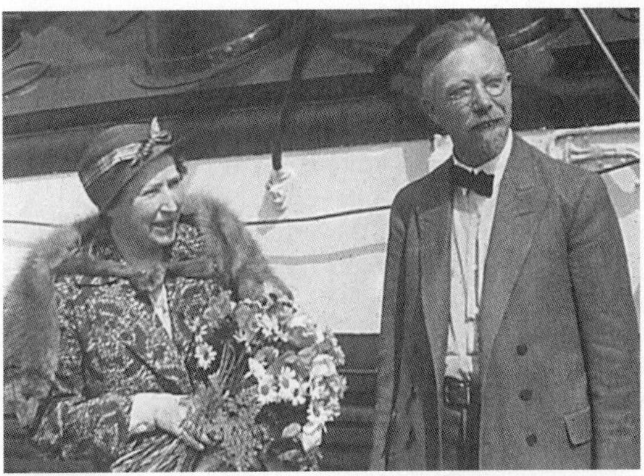

FIGURE 1.15 Marie (Jorgensen) Krogh (a physician and researcher) and August Krogh, 1920 Nobel Prize achievement in Physiology or Medicine that explained capillary control of blood flow in resting and exercising muscle. Dr. A. Krogh published more than 300 scientific papers in scientific journals on numerous topics in exercise physiology.

Three other Danish researchers—physiologists Erling Asmussen (1907–1991; ACSM Citation Award, 1976 and ACSM Honor Award, 1979), Erik Hohwü-Christensen

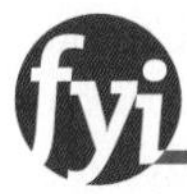

August Krogh, Nobel Laureate—An Ultimate Exercise Physiologist

August Krogh's research strongly influenced basic and applied experimentation in the biological sciences, including the emerging field of exercise physiology. Krogh and his wife **Marie (Jorgensen) Krogh (Fig. 1.15)**, herself a respected researcher, proved through a series of ingenious experiments that respiratory gases diffused rapidly through the thin pulmonary membranes, disproving the prevailing view that lungs were gland-type structure that secreted oxygen and carbon dioxide. Krogh's highly accurate equipment analyzed respiratory gases and established that pulmonary gas exchange occurred by the mechanism of diffusion, not secretion. Krogh solved the problem of whether or not free nitrogen or nitrogenous gases were released from the body as a normal by-product of metabolism. In 1906, he proved that gaseous nitrogen remained constant.

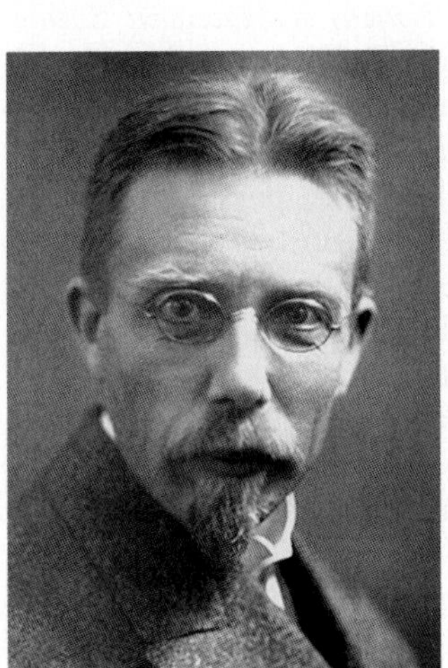

In 1905, the Kroghs' conducted experiments in three basic areas:

1. Carbon dioxide transport in the lungs using his invention of the microtonometer, indispensable for quantifying gas transport in blood
2. Field studies of Eskimo metabolism
3. Insulin's important physiological role in the body.

Krogh published nearly 300 research papers, many of which are considered "classics" in exercise physiology. The husband and wife team co-authored seven important papers known as the "seven little devils," and he teamed with other colleagues notably Johannes Lindhard (1870–1947), to investigate regulation of respiration and circulation during exercise and recovery. His other laboratory achievements included devising a bicycle ergometer with magnets and weights to determine exercise intensity, devising a method to estimate exercise cardiac output using nitrous oxide gas and quantifying capillary blood flow and oxygen's pressure and diffusing capacity through tissues.

Krogh won the 1920 Nobel Prize in Physiology or Medicine for discovering the mechanism that controlled capillary blood flow in resting and active muscle in frogs (**www.nobelprize.org/nobel_prizes/medicine/laureates/1920/**). August Krogh's research also linked exercise physiology with nutrition and metabolism. Krogh interacted with distinguished physiologists worldwide. He influenced the next generation of scientists in exercise physiology, particularly those in Nordic countries and the United States to investigate exercise physiology (and nutrition) during acute and chronic physical activity.

We highly recommend a biography by August Krogh's daughter that furnishes the most "up-close and personal" information about the lives of both August and Marie Krogh (Schmidt-Nielsen, B. *August and Marie Krogh. Lives in Science*. Published for the American Physiological Society by Oxford University Press. New York, 1995. ISBN 0-19-509099-3).

In Copenhagen, the **August Krogh Institute** (**http://akc.ku.dk/**) was established in recognition of his many achievements and contributions to exercise physiology research.

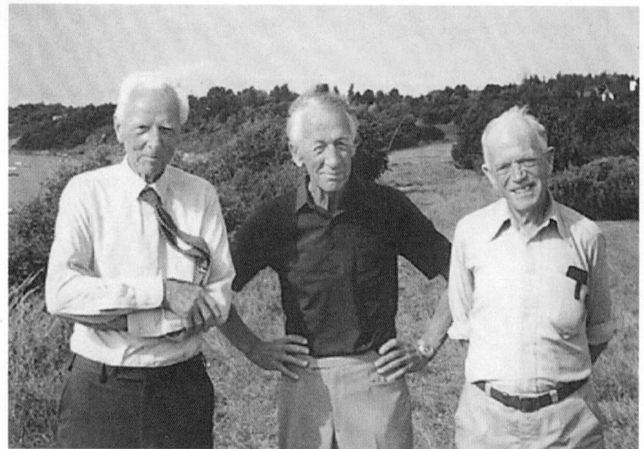

FIGURE 1.16 Drs. Erling Asmussen **(left)**, Erik Hohwü-Christensen **(center)**, and Marius Nielson **(right)**, 1988, acclaimed Swedish exercise physiology researchers.

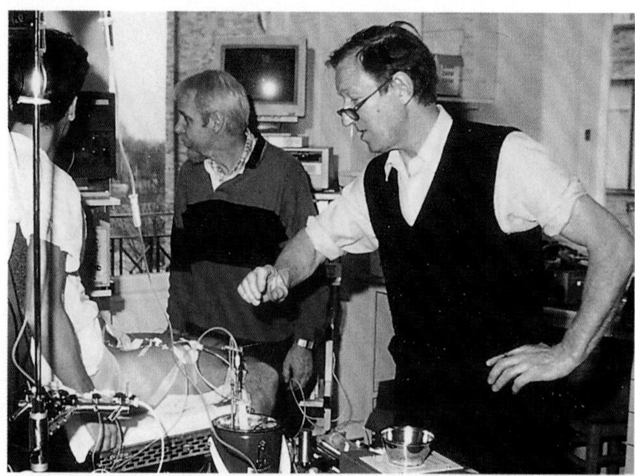

FIGURE 1.17 Swedish researcher Dr. Bengt Saltin (*hand on hip*) during an experiment at the August Krogh Institute, Copenhagen. (Photo courtesy of Dr. David Costill.)

(1904–1996; ACSM Honor Award, 1981), and Marius Nielsen (1903–2000)—conducted significant exercise physiology studies (**Fig. 1.16**). These "three musketeers," as Krogh called them, published voluminously from the 1930s to 1970s. Asmussen, initially an assistant in Lindhard's laboratory, became a prolific researcher, specializing in muscle fiber architecture and mechanics. He also published papers with Nielsen and Christensen on many applied topics, including muscular strength and performance, ventilatory and cardiovascular response to changes in posture and exercise intensity, maximum working capacity during arm and leg exercise, changes in oxidative response of muscle during exercise, comparisons of positive and negative work, hormonal and core temperature response during different intensities of exercise, and respiratory function in response to decreased ambient oxygen levels.

Christensen became Lindhard's student in Copenhagen in 1925. In his 1931 doctoral thesis, Christensen reported studies of cardiac output, body temperature, and blood sugar concentration during intense exercise on a cycle ergometer, compared arm versus leg exercise, and quantified the effects of training. Together with Krogh and Lindhard, Christensen published an important 1936 review article describing physiological dynamics during maximal exercise (Christensen EH, et al. An introduction to the studies of severe muscular exercise published in the present supplementary volume and other papers in *Arch Skandinavisches Archiv Für Physiologie* 1936;74:i.Doi:10.1111/j.1748-1716.1936.tb00433.x).With J.W. Hansen, he used oxygen uptake and the respiratory quotient to describe how diet, state of training, and exercise intensity and duration affected carbohydrate and fat utilization. Discovery of the "carbohydrate loading" concept actually occurred in 1939. Experiments by physician Olé Bang in 1936, inspired by his mentor Ejar Lundsgaard, described the fate of blood lactate during exercise of different intensities and durations. The research of Christensen, Asmussen, Nielsen, and Hansen took place at the Laboratory for the Theory of Gymnastics at the University of Copenhagen.

Since 1973, the late Swedish-trained scientist **Bengt Saltin** (1935–2014) (**Fig. 1.17**; the only Nordic researcher besides Erling Asmussen to receive the ACSM Citation Award [1980] and ACSM Honor Award [1990]; former student of Per-Olof Åstrand, discussed in the next section) continued his noteworthy scientific studies at the Muscle Research Institute in Copenhagen until his death in 2014.

Swedish Influence

Modern exercise physiology in Sweden can be traced to **Per Henrik Ling** (1776–1839), who in 1813 became the first director of Stockholm's Royal Central Institute of Gymnastics (RCIG). Ling, in addition to his expertise in exercise and movement and as a fencing master, developed a system of "medical gymnastics" that incorporated his studies of anatomy and physiology, which became integral to Sweden's school curriculum in 1820. Ling's son, **Hjalmar Ling** (1820–1886), published an important textbook about the "kinesiology of body movements" in 1866 (from a translation in Swedish: *The First Notions of Movement Science. Outline Regarding the Teaching at RCIG and an Introduction with References to the Elementary Principles of Mechanics and Joint-Science*). As a result of Per Henrik and his son Hjalmar's philosophy and pioneering influences, physical education graduates from the RCIG were extremely well schooled in the basic biological sciences in addition to proficiency in many sports and games. The RCIG graduates were all men until 1864 when women were first admitted. Ling's early teachings and curriculum advances consisted of four branches of his System of Gymnastics—the most influential and long lasting being medical gymnastics that has evolved into the discipline of physiotherapy. Course work included anatomy and physiology, pathology with dissections, and basic study in movement science (*Rörelselära* in Swedish). One of Ling's lasting legacies was his steadfast insistence that RCIG graduates have a strong science background. This was carried out by Ling's disciples, who assumed positions of leadership in predominantly Germany, France, Denmark, Belgium, and England, with the influence extending to the United States beginning in the 1830s. Founded in 1813, the Gymnastik-Och Idrottshögskolan or **Swedish School of Sport and Health Sciences** (GIH; **www.gih.se/In-English/**) has the distinction as the oldest University College in the world within its field. GIH along with the Department of Physiology in the Karolinska Institute Medical School in Stockholm (**http://ki.se/en/fyfa/molecular-and-cellular-exercise-physiology**), the Royal Institute of Technology, Stockholm University (**www.kth.se/en/sth/forskning/2.23210**), and Örebro University, also in Stockholm (**www.oru.se/English/Research/Research-Environments/Research-environment/MH/Research-in-Sport-and-Physical-Activity-RISPA1/Research-teams/Research-team/?rdb=127**) conduct research in exercise physiology and musculoskeletal health and disease.

Per-Olof Åstrand, MD, PhD (b. 1922–; **Fig. 1.18**), is the most famous graduate of the Swedish College of Physical Education (1946); in 1952, he presented his doctoral thesis at the Karolinska Institute Medical School. Åstrand taught in the Department of Physiology in the College of Physical Education from 1946 to 1977; it then became a department at the Karolinska Institute, where he served as professor and department head from 1977 to 1987. Christensen, Åstrand's mentor, supervised his thesis, which evaluated physical working capacity of men and women ages 4 to 33. This important study, among others, established a line of research that propelled Åstrand to the forefront of experimental exercise physiology research for which he achieved worldwide fame. Four of his papers, published in 1960 with Christensen as coauthor, stimulated further studies on the physiological responses to intermittent exercise. Åstrand has mentored an impressive group of exercise physiologists, including the late "superstar" Dr. Bengt Saltin.

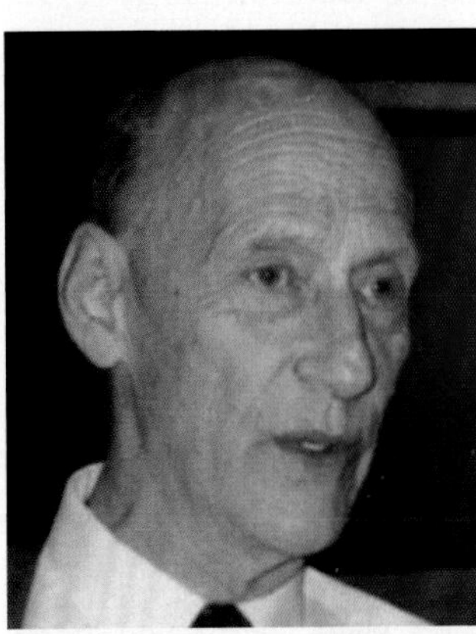

FIGURE 1.18 Dr. Per-Olof Åstrand, Department of Physiology, Karolinska Institute, Stockholm, was instrumental in charting the course of exercise physiology research and breaking new ground in testing and evaluation of fitness and human performance.

Two Swedish scientists from the Karolinska Institute, Drs. Jonas Bergström and Erik Hultman (**Fig. 1.19**), in the mid-1960s conducted some of the first needle biopsy experiments on humans before and after exercise. With this procedure, muscle could be studied under various conditions of exercise, training, and varying nutritional states. Collaborative work with other Scandinavian researchers (Saltin and Hultman from Sweden and Hermansen from Norway) and researchers in the United States (e.g., Phillip Gollnick [d. 1991], Washington State University) provided new vistas to view the physiology of exercise.

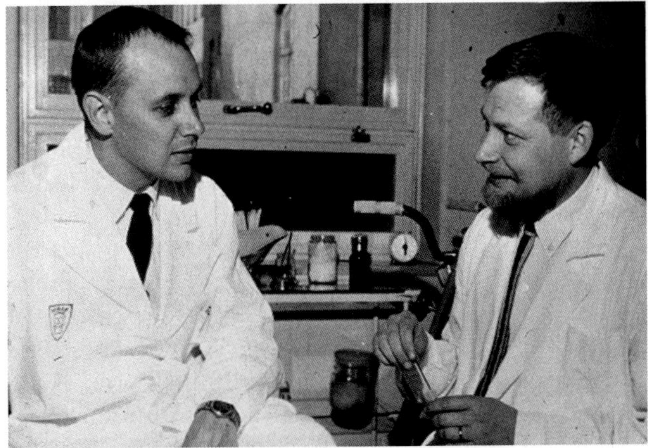

FIGURE 1.19 Drs. Jonas Bergström **(left)** and Eric Hultman **(right)**, Karolinska Institute, Stockholm, pioneered needle biopsy techniques to assess the ultrastructural architecture of muscle fibers and their biochemical functions.

Norwegian and Finnish Influence

The new generation of exercise physiologists trained in the late 1940s analyzed respiratory gases with a highly accurate sampling apparatus that measured minute quantities of carbon dioxide and oxygen in expired air. Norwegian physiologist Per Fredrik Scholander (1905–1980), noted for his field and experimental studies on animals and plants living in extreme ecological environments, developed a method in 1947 for determining gas concentrations in small samples of expired air (Scholander analyzer that bears his name), and establishing and directing the Physiological Research Laboratory at the Scripps Institute of Oceanography, La Jolla, California (**http://publishing.cdlib.org/ucpressebooks/view?docId=kt109nc2cj&chunk.id=ch08**).

Another prominent Norwegian researcher, Lars A. Hermansen (1933–1984: **Fig. 1.20**; ACSM Citation Award, 1985), from the Institute of Work Physiology made many contributions, including a classic 1969 article titled "Anaerobic Energy Release," which appeared in the initial volume of *Medicine and Science in Sports*.

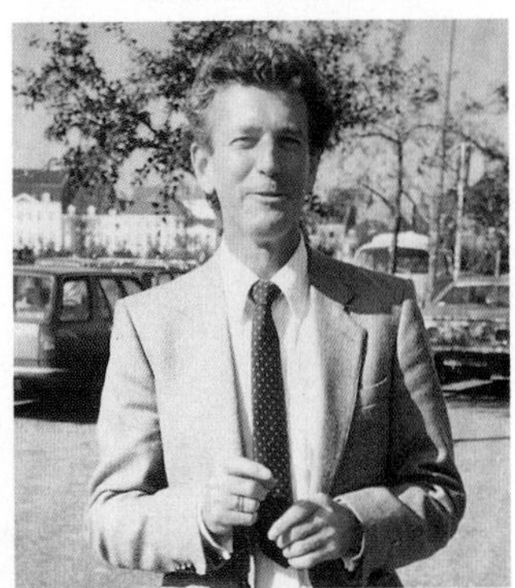

FIGURE 1.20 Dr. Lars A. Hermansen (1933–1984), Institute of Work Physiology, Oslo.

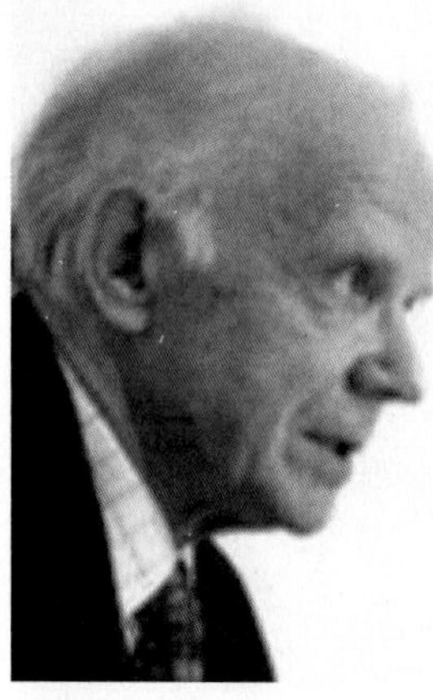

FIGURE 1.21 Dr. Paavo Komi (1940–), one of Finland's pioneer researchers in biomechanics, muscle mechanics, and exercise work physiology.

In Finland, Martti Karvonen, MD, PhD (ACSM Honor Award, 1991), from the Physiology Department of the Institute of Occupational Health, Helsinki, achieved notoriety for a method to predict optimal exercise training heart rate, now called the "Karvonen formula" (see Chapter 14). Paavo Komi (**Fig. 1.21**), Department of Biology of Physical Activity, University of Jyväskylä (**www.jyu.fi/sport/laitokset/liikuntabiologia/en**), has been one of Finland's most prolific researchers with numerous experiments published in the combined areas of exercise physiology and sport biomechanics. Prof. Keijo Häkkinen also deserves mention as a prolific exercise physiology scientist with over 300 peer-reviewed articles (**www.ncbi.nlm.nih.gov/pubmed/?term=Häkkinen+K**) dealing with neuromuscular, hormonal, and mechanical responses to resistance exercise.

OTHER CONTRIBUTORS TO EXERCISE PHYSIOLOGY

In addition to the American and Nordic scientists who achieved distinction as exercise scientists, many other "giants" in the fields of physiology and experimental science made monumental contributions that indirectly contributed to the knowledge base in exercise physiology. These include the physiologists shown in **Figure 1.22**: **Antoine Laurent Lavoisier** (1743–1794; fuel combustion); Sir Joseph Barcroft (1872–1947; altitude); Christian Bohr (1855–1911; oxygen-hemoglobin dissociation curve); John Scott Haldane (1860–1936; respiration); Otto Myerhoff (1884–1951; Nobel Prize, cellular metabolic pathways); **Nathan Zuntz** (1847–1920; portable metabolism apparatus); Carl von Voit (1831–1908) and his student, **Max Rubner** (1854–1932; direct and indirect calorimetry, and specific dynamic action of food); **Max Joseph von Pettenkofer** (1818–1901; nutrient metabolism); and Eduard F.W. Pflüger (1829–1910; tissue oxidation).

The field of exercise physiology also owes a debt of gratitude to the pioneers of the physical fitness movement in the United States, notably **Thomas K. Cureton** (1901–1993; ACSM charter member, 1969 ACSM Honor Award; **Fig. 1.23**) at the University of Illinois, Champaign. Cureton, a prolific and innovative physical educator/exercise physiologist and pioneer researcher, trained four generations of students beginning in 1941. Cureton's graduate

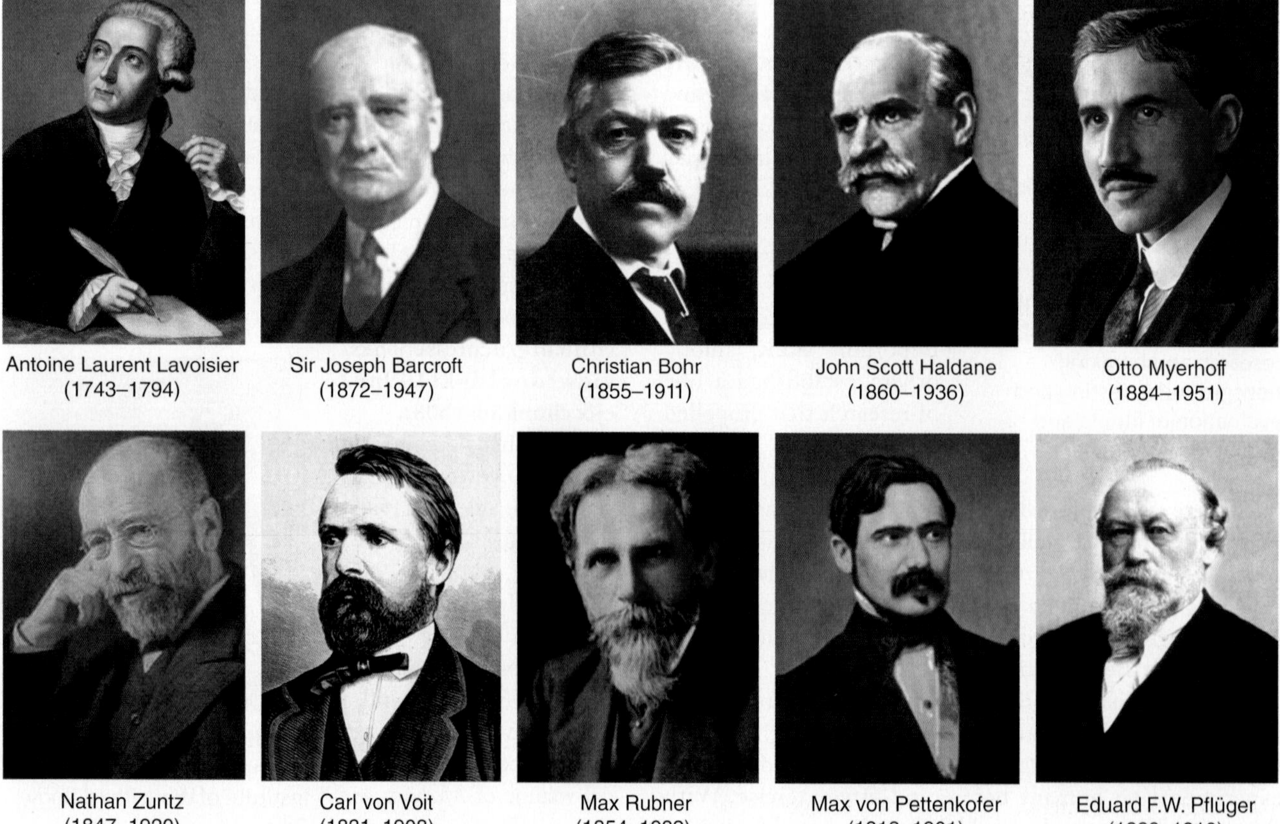

FIGURE 1.22 Ten prominent scientist-researchers paved the way in developing modern exercise physiology.

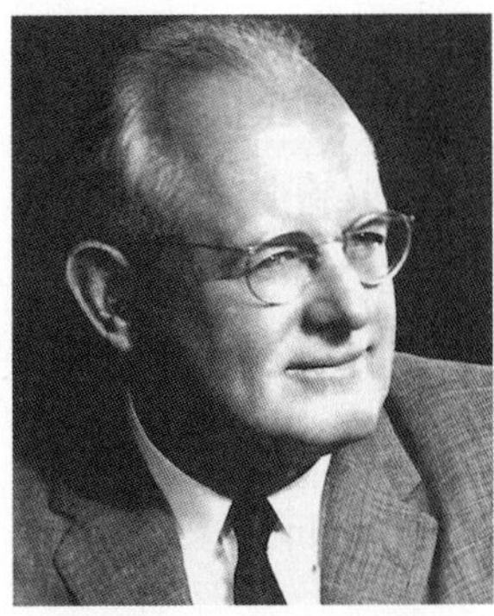

FIGURE 1.23 Dr. Thomas Kirk Cureton (1901–1993), prolific researcher and author, helped to establish the influential graduate program at the University of Illinois that mentored several generations of future exercise physiologists achieved distinction at colleges and universities in the United States and abroad for their innovative laboratory research and mentoring their own cadre of productive graduate student scholars.

students soon assumed leadership positions as professors of physical education/kinesiology with teaching and research responsibilities in exercise physiology at numerous colleges, universities, and military establishments in the United States and throughout the world. Dr. Cureton was author or coauthor of 50 textbooks about exercise, health, sport-specific training, and physical fitness and served on the President's Council on Physical Fitness and Sports (**www.fitness.gov**) under five presidents. Cureton, a champion masters swimmer, established 14 age-group world records, also tutored Sir Roger Bannister (b. 1929), who first shattered the sub-4-minute mile barrier on May 6, 1954.

CONTEMPORARY DEVELOPMENTS

Exercise Physiology, the Internet, and Online Social Networking

Since publication of the 4th edition of this textbook in 2011, topics related to exercise physiology on the Internet have expanded tremendously. Information about almost every topic area, no matter how seemingly remote, can quickly be obtained through popular search engines. In a Google search on June 4, 2015, there were 4,590,000 "hits" for the term *exercise physiology* (**www.google.com**). Adding the word *muscle* to that search yielded 1,660,000 hits. However, if we still wanted to pinpoint the search further because of an interest about *DNA*, *muscle*, and *twins*, the search on June 4, 2015 returned "only" 502,000 entries, still a sizable number. The point becomes clear—the Internet provides a wonderful repository of useful information to target a focus of inquiry—no matter how specific.

However, when you drill down into a particular topic area, you must make qualitative decisions about how to sift through the information to determine what is pertinent (and more importantly, reliable) for your needs. For the latest scientific research information about a particular topic, we recommend PubMed (**www.ncbi.nlm.nih.gov/pubmed**) to obtain the published and *In Press* articles about a specific topic. For example, in determining how many scientific articles the late Swedish researcher Bengt Saltin published throughout his illustrious career (entered into the PubMed search bar as Saltin B), the search returned a citation list of 445 publications from the latest 2014 entry to his first publication in 1960.

Online Social Networking

Online Social Networking refers to the common grouping of individuals into more specific groups.

The five most popular social networking sites based on unique visitors (UV), are listed in the table below.

Top ranked social media sites based on unique visitors, as of June 2015.

Rank	Site	Estimated Unique Monthly Visitors
1	Facebook (**facebook.com**)	900,000,000
2	Twitter (**twitter.com**)	310,000,000
3	Linkedin (**linkedin.com**)	250,000,000
4	Pinterest (**pinterest.com**)	250,000,000
5	Google Plus+ (**google.com**)	120,000,000

From: **http://www.ebizmba.com/articles/social-networking-websites**

These types of sites allow users to gather and share information or experiences about specific topics and develop friendships and continue professional relationships. Numerous electronic discussion groups and blogs exist in exercise physiology and related areas (e.g., **http://greatist.com/health/must-read-health-fitness-blogs** lists more than 60 Health, Fitness, and Happiness Blogs for 2015). Various electronic bulletin boards with specific areas of interest (e.g., pediatric exercise immunology, molecular biology, and exercise) enable subscribers to receive and reply to the same inquiry. Many of the field's top scientists routinely participate in discussion groups, which makes such interactions a productive pastime, and allow for shared experiences and common interests. Anyone with an Internet connection and e-mail address can participate in a discussion group. Appendix SR-2, available online at **http://thePoint.lww.com/MKKESS5e**, lists frequently cited journals in exercise physiology. Entering the journal name in an online search engine directs you to that site.

CONTEMPORARY PROFESSIONAL EXERCISE PHYSIOLOGY ORGANIZATIONS

Just as knowledge dissemination via publications in research and professional journals signals expansion of a field of study, development of professional organizations to certify and monitor professional activities becomes critical to continued growth.

The American Association for the Advancement of Physical Education (**AAAPE**), formed in 1885, represented the first professional organization in the United States to include topics related to exercise physiology. AAAPE changed its name to American Alliance for Health, Physical Education, Recreation and Dance (**AAHPERD**) in 1979, which in 2014 again changed its name to **ShapeAmerica** (Society of Health and Physical Educators—**www.shapeamerica.org/**). Until the early 1950s, this organization represented the predominant professional organization for exercise physiologists.

As the field expanded and diversified its focus, a separate professional organization was needed to more fully respond to professional needs. In 1954, Joseph Wolffe, MD

(1958 ACSM Honor Award), and 11 other physicians, physiologists, and physical educators founded the American College of Sports Medicine (ACSM). Presently, ACSM has more than 50,000 members in 90 countries. ACSM now represents the largest professional organization in the world for exercise physiology (including allied medical and health areas).

ACSM's mission "promotes and integrates scientific research, education, and practical applications of sports medicine and exercise science to maintain and enhance physical performance, fitness, health, and quality of life." It publishes the often-cited research journal *Medicine and Science in Sport and Exercise*, the *Health & Fitness Journal, Exercise and Sport Science Reviews, Guidelines for Exercise Testing and Prescription* (9th edition), *ACSM's Resources for Clinical Exercise Physiology* (2nd edition), *ACSM's Resource Manual for Guidelines for Exercise Testing and Prescription* (7th edition), and *ACSM's Certification Review* (4th edition) (see **www.ACSM.org** for a complete list of titles and journals).

Other important professional organizations related to exercise physiology include the **International Council of Sport Science and Physical Education (ICSSPE; www.icsspe.org/)**, founded in 1958 in Paris, France, originally under the name the International Council of Sport and Physical Education. ICSSPE serves as an international umbrella organization concerned with promoting and disseminating results and findings in the field of sport science. Its main professional publication, *Sport Science Review*, deals with thematic overviews of sport sciences research.

The Federation Internationale de Medicine Sportive (FIMS; www.fims.org), composed of the national sports medicine associations of more than 100 countries, originated in 1928 during a meeting of Olympic medical doctors in Switzerland. FIMS promotes the study and development of sports medicine throughout the world and hosts major international conferences in sports medicine every 3 years; it also produces position statements on topics related to health, physical activity, and sports medicine, which can be downloaded as PDFs from its Web site. The three most recent position statements include "Physical Activity and Cancer" (June, 2014), "Fluids in Sports" (June, 2012), and "Cardiovascular Adaptations and Exercise" (May, 2012). In conjunction with the 2018 Olympic Games, Rio de Janeiro will host the 2018 World Congress of Sports Medicine. A joint position statement with the World Health Organization (WHO; **www.who.int**) titled "Physical Activity and Health" represents one of FIMS's best-known documents.

Other organizations representing exercise physiologists include the following:

1. **European College of Sport Science** (ECSS; **www.ecss.de**) founded in 1995, whose purpose is to promote science and research, with emphasis on interdisciplinary cooperation among sports science and sports medicine.
2. **British Association of Sport and Exercise Sciences** (BASES; **www.bases.org.uk**), whose mission promotes excellence in sports and the exercise sciences, with emphasis on interdisciplinary cooperation among the subdisciplines of biomechanics, physiology, and psychology. BASES publishes expert statements about a variety of topics including recent documents about "Exercise, Immunity, and Infection" (**www.bases.org.uk/Exercise-Immunity-and-Infection**), "Exercise and Cancer" (**www.bases.org.uk/Exercise-Immunity-and-Infection**), and "Use of Music in Exercise" (**www.bases.org.uk/Music-in-Exercise**).
3. **American Physiological Association** (**www.the-aps.org**), publishes 16 scientific journals, including at least three that often feature exercise physiology–related research (e.g., *Journal of Applied Physiology* (**http://jap.physiology.org/front**), *Physiological Reviews* (**http://physrev.physiology.org**), and *Endocrinology and Metabolism* (**http://ajpendo.physiology.org**). One unique feature of APS is its Living History of Physiology Project. Since 2005, video interviews have been conducted with senior members of APS (e.g., Ellsworth Buskirk, John Faulkner, Charles Tipton, Peter Raven, John Greenleaf, G. Edgar Folk, Jr., Bodil Schmidt-Nielsen, Karlman Wasserman, John B. West, and Loring Rowell), many of whom are pioneers in exercise physiology . We encourage readers to view video interviews with these key researchers and scientists, who have played pivotal roles in basic and applied research specifically related to exercise physiology.
4. **American Society of Exercise Physiologists** (ASEP; **www.asep.org**) is a "professional organization representing and promoting the profession of exercise physiology, is committed to the professional development of exercise physiology, its advancement, and the credibility of exercise physiologists."
5. **Australian Sports Commission (Australian High Performance Sport Agency: www.ausport.gov.au)**. The Australian Sports Commission's Sports Science and Sports Medicine section includes all the service delivery departments of the Australian Institute of Sport (AIS), which was founded in 1981 to guide Australia's international sporting endeavors and organized into five categories:
   - Clinical Services: medicine, physical therapies (physiotherapy, massage, acupuncture, pilates), strength and conditioning, and performance psychology
   - Sport Sciences: nutrition; AIS movement science (biomechanics, performance analysis, skill acquisition); aquatic testing, training, and research; and physiology (incorporates fatigue and recovery)
   - Athlete and Career Education
   - Performance Research Centre: AIS applied sensors unit, sport interface unit, and AIS technical laboratory
   - National Sport Science Quality Assurance program

AIS offers postgraduate scholarships (honors, masters, PhD) and visiting scholar opportunities (**www.ausport.gov.au/ais/innovation/programs_and_projects**). The Clearinghouse for Sport (**https://secure.ausport.gov.au/clearinghouse/knowledge_base/high_performance_sport/dte**) provides searchable information about exercise and sport skill acquisition, sports biomechanics, sports performance analysis, psychology, and recovery, and sports nutrition and strength and conditioning.

A COMMON LINK

One theme unites the 2300-year history of exercise physiology—the value of mentoring by visionaries who spent an extraordinary amount of time "infecting" students with a passion for science. These demanding but inspiring relationships develop researchers who nurture the next generation of productive scholars. This nurturing process from mentor to student remains fundamental to the continued academic enhancement of exercise physiology. The connection between mentor and student remains the hallmark of most fields of inquiry—from antiquity to the present.

SUMMARY

1. Exercise physiology as an academic field of study consists of three distinct components: first, a body of knowledge built on facts and theories derived from research; second, a formal course of study at institutions of higher learning, and third, professional preparation of practitioners and future leaders in the field.
2. Exercise physiology has developed as a field separate from physiology because of its unique focus on the study of movement and physical activity.
3. Galen, one of the first "sports medicine" physicians, wrote prolifically, producing at least 80 treatises and perhaps 500 essays on topics related to human anatomy and physiology, nutrition, growth and development, the benefits of exercise and deleterious consequences of sedentary living, and diseases and their treatment.
4. Austin Flint, Jr., MD (1836–1915), one of the first American pioneer physician-scientists, incorporated studies about physiological responses to exercise in his influential medical physiology textbooks.
5. Edward Hitchcock, Jr. (1828–1911), Amherst College Professor of Hygiene and Physical Education, devoted his academic career to the scientific study of exercise and training and body size and shape. His 1860 text on anatomy and physiology, coauthored with his father, significantly impacted the sports science movement in the United States after 1860.
6. Hitchcock's insistence on the need for science applied to physical education undoubtedly influenced Harvard's commitment to create an academic Department of Anatomy, Physiology, and Physical Training in 1891.
7. George Wells Fitz, MD (1860–1934), created the first departmental major in Anatomy, Physiology, and Physical Training at Harvard University in 1891, and the first formal exercise physiology laboratory in the United States. Fitz may have been first to teach an exercise physiology course at the university level.
8. The onset of exercise physiology laboratory research along with many other research specialties occurred in 1927 with the creation of the Harvard Fatigue Laboratory at Harvard University's business school, legitimizing exercise physiology as a key area of research and study.
9. The Nordic countries (particularly Denmark and Sweden) played a historically important role in setting the stage for the nurturing of exercise physiology as a bona fide field of study.
10. Danish physiologist August Krogh (1874–1949) won the 1920 Nobel Prize in physiology or medicine for discovering the mechanism that controlled capillary blood flow in resting and active muscle. Krogh's basic experiments led him to conduct other experiments with exercise scientists worldwide.
11. Krogh's pioneering work in exercise physiology continues to inspire exercise physiology research in oxygen uptake kinetics and metabolism, muscle physiology, and nutritional biochemistry.
12. Publications of applied and basic exercise physiology research have increased as the field expands into different areas and with the explosive growth of online media, resources, and networking capabilities.
13. ACSM, with more than 50,000 members from North America and 90 other countries, is the largest professional organization in the world for those in exercise physiology, including allied medical and health areas.
14. One theme unites the 2300-year history of exercise physiology—the value of mentoring by professors and scientist/researchers who devoted an extraordinary amount of time "infecting" students and colleagues with a passion for science.

THINK IT THROUGH

1. Name your top five most influential persons from antiquity to the present and discuss the impact of each on the field of exercise physiology.
2. If the Greek physician Galen, Edward Hitchcock, Jr., and A.V. Hill could have a conversation about the importance of physical activity and health, what kinds of questions do you think each would ask the other?
3. Do you agree or disagree with the following statement: "William Harvey's discovery of the one-way circulation of blood was the single most important discovery in the history of medicine." If you agree, explain how that discovery impacted research in exercise physiology. If you disagree, what other discovery would you nominate as the most impactful?

PART 2 The Exercise Physiologist

WHAT DEFINES THE EXERCISE PHYSIOLOGIST?

Many individuals view exercise physiology as an undergraduate or graduate academic major or concentration completed at an accredited college or university. In this regard, only those who complete this academic major have the "right" to be called "exercise physiologist." However, many individuals complete undergraduate and graduate degrees in related fields with considerable coursework and practical experience in exercise physiology or related areas. Consequently, the title "exercise physiologist" might also apply to individuals with adequate academic preparation. Resolution of this dilemma becomes difficult because no national consensus exists as to what constitutes an acceptable or minimal academic program of course work in exercise physiology. In addition, no universal standards exist for hands-on laboratory experiences such as in anatomy, biomechanics, and exercise physiology and demonstrated level of competency and internship hours that would stand the test of national certification or licensure. Moreover, because areas of concentration within the field are so broad, consensus certification testing becomes challenging.

WHAT DO EXERCISE PHYSIOLOGISTS DO?

Exercise physiologists assume diverse careers. Some use their skills primarily in colleges, universities, and private industry settings. Others are employed in health, fitness, and rehabilitation centers; still others serve as educators, personal trainers, coaches, managers, and entrepreneurs in the health and fitness industry.

Exercise physiologists also own health and fitness companies or are hands-on practitioners who teach and serve

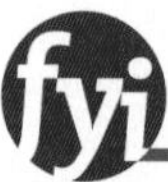

Help Wanted: The Exercise Physiologist in the Real World

A job posting by the Cleveland Clinic, one of the premier hospitals in the United States known worldwide for its medical excellence and leadership role in health care prevention (**http://my.clevelandclinic.org/services/heart/medical-professionals/careers/exercise-physiologist**), for an exercise physiologists in its Heart and Vascular Institute Stress Lab and Cardiac Rehab Department, provides an example of the type of opportunities available for prospective exercise physiologists:

> The Heart & Vascular Institute Stress Lab and Cardiac Rehab department offers an exciting setting for exercise physiologists. Performing over 12,000 stress tests, 8000 inpatient cardiac rehab visits, and 7000 outpatient cardiac rehab visits each year. A wide array of patients, including healthy preventive testing to more complicated cases involving many types of cardiac and pulmonary diseases, provide a challenging and educational experience. Exercise physiologists are employed in both the Stress Testing area and the Section of Preventive Cardiology and Rehabilitation. Exercise physiologists in the Stress Testing area perform a variety of exercise and pharmacologic stress tests.

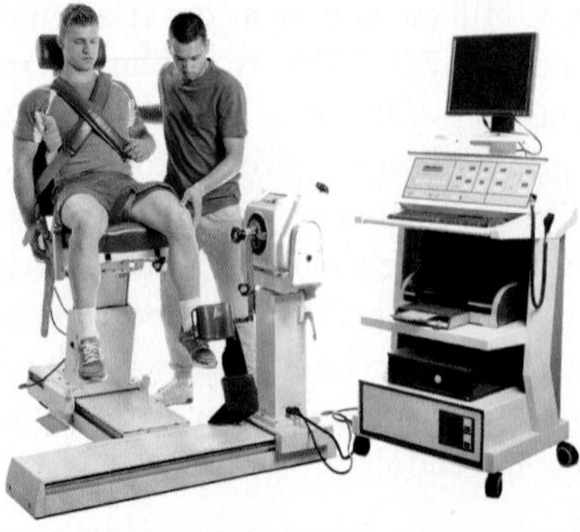

Responsibilities:

- Review and abstraction of patient medical records
- Exercise and pharmacologic stress test supervision and preliminary test interpretation
- Administration and interpretation of cardiopulmonary exercise tests
- Static and dynamic ECG monitoring and interpretation (12 lead and rhythm strips)
- Patient ECG hookup
- Rest and exercise blood pressure monitoring
- Equipment maintenance and calibration
- Research data collection
- Provision of technical support in emergency situations

Requirements include:

- Master's degree in exercise physiology, nursing, or similar science-based allied health curriculum to include a three 6-month clinical internship in stress testing or cardiac rehabilitation.
- Good communication and interpersonal skills as well as ability to provide physical assistance to patients when needed.
- BCLS certified and have completed ACSM Clinical Exercise Specialist or Registered Clinical Exercise Physiologist certification within 1 year of hire.
- Candidates need to demonstrate 12 Lead ECG interpretation and arrhythmia recognition skills.
- Previous work experience in stress testing or cardiac rehab is desirable.

This is one of many job descriptions now appearing with growing frequency, and we believe it's just the beginning of a wide open talent search to fill similar positions within the booming health care industry. For 2015, the latest Forbes summary of most desirable jobs in the health care industry in the United States listed exercise physiologist in the top ten (**www.forbes.com/pictures/mkl45ehjij/physiologist-2/**)!

TABLE 1.1 Partial List of Employment Opportunities for Qualified Exercise Physiologists

Sports	College University	Community	Clinical	Government Military	Business	Private
Sports director	Professor	Manage/direct health/wellness programs	Test/supervise cardiopulmonary patients	Fitness director/manager	Sports management	Personal health/fitness consultant
Strength/conditioning coach	Researcher	Community education	Evaluate/supervise special populations (diabetes, obesity, arthritis, dyslipidemia, cystic fibrosis, cancer, hypertension, children, low pregnancy)	Health fitness director in correctional institutions	Health/fitness promotion	Own business
Director, manager of state/national teams	Administrator	Occupational rehabilitation	Exercise technologist in cardiology practice	Sports nutrition programs	Sport psychologist	
Consultant	Teacher, Instructor		Researcher		Health/fitness club instructor	

the community or who work with employees of corporate, industrial, and governmental agencies. Some specialize in other types of professional work such as massage therapy; others go on to pursue professional degrees in physical therapy, occupational therapy, nursing, nutrition, medicine, and chiropractic.

Table 1.1 presents a partial list of different employment descriptions for a qualified exercise physiologist in one of six major areas.

EXERCISE PHYSIOLOGISTS AND HEALTH AND FITNESS PROFESSIONALS IN THE CLINICAL SETTING

The well-documented health benefits of regular physical activity have enhanced exercise physiologists' role beyond traditional lines. A clinical exercise physiologist becomes part of the health and fitness professional team. This approach to preventive and rehabilitative services requires different personnel depending on the program mission, population served, location, number of participants, space availability, and funding.

A comprehensive clinical program may include the following personnel in addition to an exercise physiologist:

- Physicians
- Dietitians
- Nurses
- Physical therapists
- Occupational therapists
- Social workers
- Respiratory therapists
- Psychologists
- Health educators

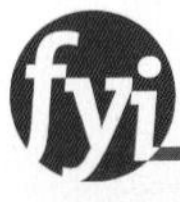

Sports Medicine and Exercise Physiology: A Vital Link

The traditional view of **sports medicine** involves rehabilitating athletes from sports-related injuries. *A more contemporary view relates sports medicine to a scientific and medical focus (preventive and rehabilitative aspects of physical activity, physical fitness, and exercise and sports performance).* Sports medicine closely links to clinical exercise physiology. Sports medicine professionals and exercise physiologists work hand in hand with similar populations. These include, at one extreme, sedentary people who need only a modest amount of regular exercise to reduce risk of degenerative diseases; at the other extreme, they may work with able-bodied and disabled athletes who strive to further enhance their performance and daily living skills.

Carefully prescribed physical activity significantly contributes to overall health and quality of life. In conjunction with sports medicine professionals, clinical exercise physiologists test, treat, and rehabilitate individuals with diverse diseases and physical disabilities. Prescription of physical activity and athletic competition for physically challenged individuals plays an important role in sports medicine and exercise physiology, providing unique opportunities for research, clinical practice, and professional advancement.

- Certified exercise leaders, health and fitness instructors, directors, exercise test technologists, preventive and rehabilitative exercise specialists, preventive and rehabilitative exercise directors

TRAINING AND CERTIFICATION BY PROFESSIONAL ORGANIZATIONS

To properly accomplish their responsibilities in the exercise setting, health and fitness professionals must integrate unique knowledge, skills, and abilities related to exercise, physical fitness, and health. Different professional organizations provide leadership in training and certifying health and fitness professionals at different levels. **Table 1.2** lists organizations offering training and certification programs with diverse emphases and specializations. The American College of Sports Medicine has emerged as the preeminent academic organization offering comprehensive programs in areas related to the health and fitness profession. The ACSM, since initiation of its certification programs in 1975, has certified more than 20,000 professionals worldwide and is used often as a de-facto requirement for hiring. ACSM certifications encompass cognitive and practical competencies evaluated by written and practical examinations. ACSM offers a wide variety of certification programs with ample print and online support resources throughout the United States and in other countries. A Closer Look: "ACSM Qualifications and Certifications" provides additional details.

A CLOSER LOOK

ACSM Qualifications and Certifications

Health and fitness professionals should be knowledgeable and competent in different areas, including first-aid and CPR certification, depending on personal interest. The table presents content areas for different ACSM certifications. Each has its own educational requirement, general and specific learning objectives, resources and qualifying experiences. See the ACSM web portal for more detailed information (**http://certification.acsm.org/get-certified**).

ACSM Certifications	
Health and Fitness Certifications	
Certified Personal Trainer (CPT)	The Certified Personal Trainer qualifies to plan and implement exercise programs for healthy individuals or those who have medical clearance to exercise. The CPT also facilitates motivation and adherence as well as develops and administers programs designed to enhance muscular strength, endurance, flexibility, cardiorespiratory fitness, body composition, and/or any of the motor skills related components of physical fitness.
Certified Group Exercise Instructor (GEI)	The Certified Group Exercise Instructors are familiar and flexible with various exercise techniques, and can supervise participants or lead instructional sessions. The GEI works in a group exercise setting with apparently healthy individuals and those with health challenges who are able to exercise independently to improve health-related physical fitness, manage health risk, and promote lasting health behavior change.
Certified Exercise Physiologist (EP-C)	The Certified Exercise Physiologist has a minimum of a bachelor's degree in exercise science. The EP-C is able to perform pre-participation health screenings, conduct physical fitness assessments, interpret results, develop exercise prescriptions, and apply behavioral and motivational strategies to apparently healthy individuals and individuals with medically controlled diseases and health conditions to support clients in adopting and maintaining healthy lifestyle behaviors. Academic preparation for an EP-C also includes fitness management, administration, and supervision. The EP-C is usually employed or self-employed in commercial, community, studio, corporate, university, and hospital settings.
Clinical Certifications	
Certified Clinical Exercise Physiologist (CEP)	The Certified Clinical Exercise Physiologist works with patients and clients challenged with cardiovascular, pulmonary, and metabolic diseases and disorders, as well as with apparently healthy populations in cooperation with other healthcare professionals. The goal of the CEP is to enhance quality of life, manage health risk, and promote lasting health behavior change. The CEP educates clients about testing, exercise program components, and self-care for the control of chronic disease and health conditions.

Registered Clinical Exercise Physiologist (RCEP)	The Registered Clinical Exercise Physiologist is an allied health professional that applies physical activity and behavioral interventions that are proven to provide therapeutic and/or functional benefit for those with chronic diseases or disabilities. The RCEP provides prevention and rehabilitative strategies designed to improve physical fitness and health across the lifespan. The practice and supervision of the RCEP is guided by published professional guidelines, standards, and applicable state and federal laws and regulations.
Specialty Certifications	
Exercise is Medicine Credential (EMI)	In 2007, ACSM's Exercise is Medicine (EIM) campaign was initiated to promote exercise as a health strategy for the general public and to promote a collaboration between health care providers and exercise professionals. The EIM initiative now includes a credential program that provides exercise professionals the opportunity to work closely with the medical community. The Exercise is Medicine Credential contains three levels, designed to serve clients and patients depending on health status. Eligibility requirements for the three credential levels vary, based on the patient population you work with. See the ACSM web materials for more information on this credential; **http://certification.acsm.org/exercise-is-medicine-credential**.
Certified Ringside Physician℠ (CRP)	The ACSM in collaboration with the Association for Ringside Physicians (ARP) certifies physicians who are involved in the care of boxers, mixed martial artists, and other competitors in the combat arts. The CRP are experienced in ringside protocol and are instrumental in the care before, during, and after the bout. The CRP has a basic understanding in various fields of medicine, which include, but are not limited to, wound care, orthopaedics, neurology, cardiology, dermatology, infectious disease, emergency medicine, and even psychology.
Certified Inclusive Fitness Trainer (CIFT)	The ACSM in collaboration with the National Center on Health, Physical Activity and Disability (NCHPAD) certifies fitness trainers to master an understanding of exercise precautions for people with disabilities, and utilize safe, effective, and adapted methods of exercise training to provide exercise recommendations. CIFTs provide services with an understanding of current ADA (Americans with Disabilities Act) policy specific to recreation facilities (U.S. Access Board Guidelines) and standards for accessible facility design.
Certified Cancer Exercise Trainer℠ (CET)	The ACSM in collaboration with the American Cancer Society (ACS) developed the Certified Cancer Exercise Trainers (CET) certification. A CET designs and administers fitness assessments and exercise programs specific to a client's cancer diagnosis, treatment, and current recovery status. The CET will utilize a basic understanding of cancer diagnoses, surgeries, treatments, related symptoms, and side-effects of the various therapies.
Certified Physical Activity in Public Health Specialist (PAPHS)	The ACSM in collaboration with the National Society of Physical Activity Practitioners in Public Health (NSPAPPH) developed the PAPHS certification. A PAPHS engages key decision makers at the national, state or local level; conducts needs assessments, plans, develops and coordinates physical activity interventions; is often called upon to provide leadership, develop partnerships and advise local, state, and federal health departments on all physical activity-related initiatives.
Legacy Certifications—ACSM has several certifications that are still active and renewable, but are no longer being offered.	
ACSM Program Director (PD)	This was the highest level of certification in the clinical track and was directed toward professionals whose primary responsibilities were to develop and direct clinical exercise programs. The PD certification requires significant increase in breadth and depth of knowledge and experience in graded exercise testing, exercise prescription, exercise leadership, patient counseling, and education in clinical exercise programs.
ACSM Health Fitness Director (HFD)	This was the highest level of certification in the fitness track. The HFD certification is for individuals with demonstrated competence as an administrative leader of health and fitness programs in the corporate, commercial, or community setting in which apparently healthy individuals and individuals with controlled disease participate in health promotion and fitness-related activities.

TABLE 1.2 Organizations Offering Training or Certification Programs Related to Physical Activity

Organization	Areas of Specialization and Certification	Website
Aerobics and Fitness Association of America (AFAA), 15250 Ventura Blvd., Suite 200, Sherman Oaks, CA 91403	AFP Fitness Practitioner, Primary Aerobics Instructor, Personal Trainer & Fitness Counselor, Step Reebok Certification, Weight Room/ Resistance Training Certification, Emergency Response Certification	**www.afaa.com**
American College of Sports Medicine (ACSM) 401 West Michigan St. Indianapolis, IN 46202	Exercise Leader, Exercise Physiologist, Exercise Test Technologist, Health/ Fitness Director, Clinical Exercise Physiologist, Program Director	**www.acsm.org**
American Council on Exercise (ACE) 5820 Oberlin Dr., Suite 102 San Diego, CA 92121	Group Fitness Instructor, Personal Trainer, Lifestyle & Weight Management Consultant	**www.acefitness.org/**
Canadian Personal Trainers Network (CPTN) Ontario Fitness Council (OFC) 1185 Eglington Ave. East, Suite 407 North York, ON M3C 3C6 Canada	CPTN/OFC Certified Personal Trainer, CPTN Certified Specialty PersonalTrainer, CPTN/OFC Assessor of Personal Trainers, CPTN/OFC Course Conductor for Personal Trainers	**www.cptn.com**
Canadian Society for Exercise Physiology 1600 James Naismith Dr., Suite 311 Gloucester, ON K1B 5N4	CFC (Certified Fitness Consultant), PFLC (Professional Fitness & Lifestyle Consultant), AFAC (Accredited Fitness Appraisal Center)	**www.csep.ca/**
Disabled Sports USA 451 Hungerford Dr., Suite 100 Rockville, MD 20850	Adapted Fitness Instructor	**www.disabledsportsusa.org**
International Society of Sports Nutrition 4511 NW 7th Street, Deerfield Beach, FL 33442	Sports Nutrition Certification, Body Composition Certification	**www.sportsnutritionsociety.org**
International Sports Sciences Association (ISSA) 1015 Mark Avenue, Carpinteria, California 93013	Master Trainer; Elite Trainer; Certified Fitness Trainer; Specialist in Fitness Nutrition; Specialist in Exercise Therapy; Specialist in Senior Fitness; Specialist in Strength and Conditioning; Youth Fitness Trainer	**www.issaonline.edu**
Jazzercise 2808 Roosevelt Blvd. Carlsbad, CA 92008	Certified Jazzercise Instructor	**www.jazzercise.com**
National Academy of Sports Medicine (NASM) 5845 E. Still Creek, Circle Suite 206 Mesa, AZ 85206	(CPT) Certified Personal Trainer	**www.nasm.org**
National Strength & Conditioning Association (NSCA) P.O. Box 38909 Colorado Springs, CO 80937	Certified Strength & Conditioning Specialist, Certified Personal Trainer	**www.nsca.com**
The Cooper Institute 12330 Preston Rd. Dallas, TX 75230	PFS (Physical Fitness Specialists; Personal Trainer), GEL (Group Exercise Leadership; Aerobic Instructor), ADV.PFS (Advanced Physical Fitness Specialist, Biomechanics of Strength Training, Health Promotion Director)	**www.cooperinstitute.org**

SUMMARY

1. A close link ties sports medicine to clinical exercise physiology.
2. Sports medicine professionals and exercise physiologists work side by side with similar populations.
3. Sports medicine professionals and exercise physiologists work with sedentary people who need only a modest amount of regular exercise to reduce degenerative disease risk, and patients recovering from surgery or requiring regular exercise to combat a decline in functional capacity brought on by serious illness.
4. Sports medicine professionals and exercise physiologists work with able-bodied and disabled athletes to enhance their sports performance.
5. In their clinical role, exercise physiologists work cooperatively with sports medicine professionals to test, treat, and rehabilitate individuals with diverse diseases and physical disabilities.
6. The ACSM has emerged as the preeminent academic organization offering comprehensive certification programs in several areas related to the health and fitness profession.
7. ACSM certifications encompass a wide range of entry level and advanced placement credentialing recognized as a preeminent certification program throughout the world.

THINK IT THROUGH

1. Discuss the advantages for personal trainers to become trained in exercise physiology and related areas and/or obtain a special certification from a recognized organization.
2. Explain why a personal trainer requires additional academic competencies and not just practical experience.
3. How would you explain the apparent differences in quality of certification requirements of different organizations?
4. Discuss whether professionals in the field should be required by their certifying organization to take continuing education courses and subscribe to professional research journals.

KEY TERMS

AAAPE: American Association for the Advancement of Physical Education formed in 1885; represented the first professional organization in the United States to include topics related to exercise physiology.

AAHPERD: American Alliance for Health, Physical Education, Recreation, and Dance (now Society of Health and Physical Educators or SHAPE; **www.shapeamerica.org**).

ACSM Clinical Certifications: Includes the Certified Clinical Exercise Physiologist and Registered Clinical Exercise Physiologist.

ACSM Health and Fitness Certifications: Includes the Certified Personal Trainer, Certified Group Exercise Instructor, and Certified Exercise Physiologist.

ACSM Specialty Certifications: Includes the Exercise is Medicine Credential, Certified Ringside Physician, Certified Inclusive Fitness Trainer, Certified Cancer Exercise Trainer, and Certified Physical Activity in Public Health Specialist.

American College of Sports Medicine (ACSM): Largest sports medicine and exercise science organization in the world with more than 50,000 members and certified professionals in 90 countries (**www.acsm.org**).

American Physiological Association: Professional organization that publishes 16 scientific journals, including *Journal of Applied Physiology* (**http://jap.physiology.org/front**), *Physiological Reviews* (**http://physrev.physiology.org**), and *Endocrinology and Metabolism* (**http://ajpendo.physiology.org**).

American Society of Exercise Physiologists (APA): Professional organization representing and promoting the profession of exercise physiology (**www.asep.org**).

Andrometer: Device devised in 1855 by a tailor in Edinburgh to secure the physical dimensions of soldiers for purposes of fitting uniforms.

August Krogh Institute: Research institute in Copenhagen (**www1.bio.ku.dk/English**) named to honor 1920 Nobel Laureate August Krogh for his innovative and pioneering exercise physiology research studies.

Barcroft, Sir Joseph F.: British research physiologist who pioneered fundamental concepts concerning hemoglobin function, and performed experiments to determine how cold temperature affected the central nervous system. For up to 1 hour, he would lie without clothing on a couch in subfreezing temperatures and record his subjective reactions to cold stress.

Beaumont, William: Nineteenth-century American physician—physiologist (1785–1853) whose decisive experiments in food digestion paved the way for future studies in exercise physiology of gastric emptying, intestinal absorption, electrolyte balance, rehydration, and nutritional supplementation.

Bernard, Claude: French physician and experimental scientist generally acknowledged as one of the greatest physiologists of his time. His medical experiments in the mid-1800s in chemical and regulatory physiology profoundly impacted medicine (e.g., documented role of pancreatic secretion in lipid digestion, liver function physiology, glucose regulation, and crucial role of experimentation and search for scientific truths) (**www.claude-bernard.co.uk/page2.htm**).

British Association of Sport and Exercise Sciences (BASES): Mission promotes excellence in sports and the exercise sciences, with emphasis on interdisciplinary cooperation among the subdisciplines of biomechanics, physiology, and psychology (**www.bases.org.uk**).

Corpus Hippocratum: During Greece's Golden Age, scholars collected medical books, lectures, research, notes, and philosophical essays on various medicine topics, including the solemn "Hippocratic Oath," which had as one of its main tenants that physicians consider the patient first, and provide excellent patient care at all times.

Cureton, Thomas K.: Remembered as the Father of Physical Fitness Research, ACSM charter member, 1969 ACSM Honor Award recipient, University of Illinois Professor of Physical Education, researcher, and prolific author who trained four generations of graduate students beginning in 1941.

***De Arte Gymnastica Apud Ancientes*:** Essay penned by Italian physician Hieronymus Mercurialis (1530–1606; "*The Art of Gymnastics Among the Ancients*"); influenced by Greek physician Galen, it discussed many uses of exercise for preventive and therapeutic medical and health benefits.

Dill, D.B.: Prolific experimental exercise physiologist who helped establish the Harvard Fatigue Laboratory from 1927 to 1946 in the basement of Morgan Hall of Harvard's Business School; legitimized exercise physiology as an important area of research and study.

Empedocles: Ancient Greek scholar (ca. 500–430 B.C.) who promoted the idea of four "bodily humors" and their role in the circulatory, respiratory, and digestive systems.

European College of Sport Science (ECSS): Founded in 1995 to promote science and research and interdisciplinary cooperation among sports science and sports medicine (**www.ecss.de**).

Fitz, George Wells, MD: Created the first departmental major in Anatomy, Physiology, and Physical Training at Harvard in 1891 and the following year started the first formal exercise physiology laboratory in the United States.

Flint, Austin Jr.: One of the first American pioneer physician-scientists who incorporated studies about physiological responses to exercise; his influential medical physiology textbooks fostered the belief among 19th-century American physical education teachers that muscular exercise should be taught from a strong foundation of science and experimentation.

Galen: Ancient Greek physician (131–201 A.D.) who wrote extensively about the importance of proper nutrition to improve health, walking to improve stamina, and strengthening muscles through rope climbing and lifting heavy objects.

Harvard Fatigue Laboratory: Founded at Harvard's Business School in 1927 to become one of the world's foremost research centers to study exercise physiology-related topics, thereby legitimizing exercise physiology as a valid area of research and study.

Henderson, Lawrence Joseph: Renowned Harvard chemist and professor of biochemistry who founded the Harvard Fatigue Laboratory, dedicated to study exercise and environmental physiology (**www.the-aps.org/fm/125th-APS-Anniversary/125th-Timeline/APS-Panel-5.pdf**).

Henry, Franklin M.: University of California professor of Physical Education who first proposed physical education as an academic discipline. He conducted basic experiments in exercise physiology and psychology, and is remembered for developing the "specificity principle" of motor coordination, learning, and performance (**http://senate.universityofcalifornia.edu/inmemoriam/rranklinmhenry.html**).

Herodicus: Fifth century B.C. Greek physician who advocated proper diet in physical training.

Hieronymus Mercurialis: Greek physician of antiquity (460–377 B.C.).

Hill, A.V.: Awarded the 1922 Nobel Prize in Physiology or Medicine for investigations concerning the mechanism involved in the activity of striated muscle contraction, and discovery that nerve impulses produced heat.

Hippocrates: Considered the "father" of modern medicine during the Golden Age of Greece; remembered for his writings about preventative medicine.

Hitchcock, Edward Jr.: Amherst College Professor of Hygiene and Physical Education who devoted his academic career to the scientific study of physical exercise and training and body size and shape. His 1860 text on anatomy and physiology, coauthored with his father, significantly influenced the sports science movement in the United States after 1860.

Hooker, John D.: First professor of physical education in an American college (Amherst College, Amherst, MA).

Ibn al-Nafis: Challenged the long-standing beliefs of Galen about how blood moved from the heart's right to left side; also predicted the existence of capillaries 400 years before eminent Italian microscopist Malpighi's discovery of the pulmonary capillaries.

Ibn Sina (Avicenna): Persian physician who contributed knowledge to 200 books, including the influential Shifa (*The Book of Healing*) and Al Qanun fi Tibb (*The Canon of Medicine)* (**https://archive.org/details/IbnSinasAl-qanunFiAl-tibbtheCanonOfMedicine**) about bodily functions.

Krogh, August: Awarded the 1920 Nobel Prize in Physiology or Medicine for discovering the mechanism that controlled capillary blood flow in resting and active muscle. Krogh's basic experiments resulted in more than 300 scientific papers in scientific journals on many topics in exercise physiology.

Krogh, Marie (Jorgensen): Physician and research collaborator with husband August Krogh (1920 Nobel Prize in Physiology or Medicine) on many exercise physiology research projects, including respiration at high altitude (**www.ncbi.nlm.nih.gov/pubmed/6381437**).

Lagrange, Fernand: Accomplished French "physical culturist" who wrote extensively on exercise, including the 1888 text, *The Physiology of Bodily Exercise*; the book is believed by some to be the first exercise physiology textbook (a viewpoint not shared by the current authors).

Lavoisier, Antoine Laurent: Eighteenth-century French scientist (1743–1784) remembered for his contributions to the metabolic role of oxygen uptake and carbon dioxide production.

Lind, James: Carried out the first planned, controlled clinical trial in 1747 aboard a sailing ship by proving that adding lemons and limes to the sailor's diets prevented almost sure death from scurvy, the "great sea plague." Lind's landmark experiment emphasized the crucial importance of dietary supplements (as yet undiscovered vitamin C) in preventing disease.

Ling, Hjalmar: Published an important textbook about the "kinesiology of body movements" in 1866 (from a translation in Swedish: *The First Notions of Movement Science. Outline Regarding the Teaching at RCIG and an Introduction with References to the Elementary Principles of Mechanics and Joint-Science*).

Ling, Per Henrik: Became the first director of Stockholm's Royal Central Institute of Gymnastics (RCIG) in 1913, and developed a system of "medical gymnastics" that incorporated studies of anatomy and physiology, and his steadfast insistence that RCIG graduates have a strong science background.

Magendie, François: French physiologist who contributed to the foundations of experimental physiology, neuroscience, and neurosurgery (**www.ncbi.nlm.nih.gov/pubmed/18447728**).

Meyerhoff, Otto Fritz: German physician and cell physiologist awarded the 1922 Nobel Prize in Physiology or Medicine for discovering the fixed relationship between a muscle's oxygen uptake and lactic acid metabolism.

Minot, Charles Sedgwick: Massachusetts Institute of Technology–educated chemist with European training in physiology who in 1891 taught the histology course at Harvard's Department of Anatomy, Physiology, and Physical Training.

New Jersey State Medical Society: Oldest medical professional society in the United States; it was founded in 1766 (**www.msnj.org/p/cm/ld/fid=25**).

Nutrition Laboratory at the Carnegie Institute in Washington, DC: Founded by Andrew Carnegie in 1904 as an organization for scientific discovery, including experiments in nutrition and energy metabolism (**http://carnegiescience.edu**).

Pflüger, Eduard Friedrich Wilhelm: German physiologist and professor at the Bonn Institute of Physiology from 1859 until the early 1900s who founded the scientific journal *Pflugers's Archiv* and pioneered physiological gas pumps and catheter instrumentation related to pulmonary medicine.

Rubner, Max: German physiologist remembered for studies with direct and indirect calorimetry, and determining food's specific dynamic action.

Saltin, Bengt: Swedish research physician and exercise physiologist (1935–2014) who published 445 scientific studies from 1960 to 2014 in exercise physiology and related fields; awarded the 2002 International Olympic Committee Medical Commission Olympic Prize on Sport Sciences for pioneering work on the effects of exercise and training on health, illness, and aging.

Sargent, Dudley Allen: Physician, educator, and director of physical training at Bowdoin College, Maine, in 1869, Director of the Hemenway Gymnasium at Harvard from 1879 to 1889, and from 1879 to 1916, director of the Normal School of Physical Training at Cambridge, Massachusetts. After his retirement, he became president of the Sargent School of Physical Education, which specialized in preparing teachers of physical education.

Sports medicine: Link between the scientific and medical preventive and rehabilitative aspects of physical activity, physical fitness, and exercise and sports performance.

Susruta: Sixth-century B.C. Indian physician who promoted the positive influence of different exercise modes on human health and disease; detailed 800 medical procedures and penned accounts of hundreds of physical conditions relating to various disease states and organ deficiencies including the health-related benefits of exercise. He considered obesity a disease and posited that a sedentary lifestyle contributed to this malady.

Tanner, John Mourilyan: British exercise physiologist and growth and development researcher who developed the Tanner scale to assess pubertal sexual development stages; also studied ratio expressions of physiological data with reference to body size and function (published in the first edition of *J Appl Physiol*), cardiac output, cholesterol and body build, physiological responses to exercise, and resistance training.

von Liebig, Justis: German physiologist remembered for his scientific contributions to agricultural and biological chemistry; considered the founder of organic chemistry.

von Pettenkofer, Max Joseph: German 19th-century theoretical and applied chemist who performed experiments related to hygiene, diet, and disease transmission, and also conducted studies on electrical and neural activity of muscle, and various factors affecting the velocity of blood flow.

von Voit, Carl: Discovered the isodynamic law and the calorific heat values of proteins, lipids, and carbohydrates. He disproved Liebig's assertion that protein was a primary energy fuel by showing that protein breakdown does not increase in proportion to exercise duration or intensity (**http://jn.nutrition.org/content/13/1/2.full.pdf**).

Zuntz, Nathan: Devised the first portable metabolic apparatus to assess respiratory exchange in animals and humans at different altitudes; proved that carbohydrates were precursors for lipid synthesis and maintained that dietary lipids and carbohydrates should not be consumed equally for proper nutrition (**www.ncbi.nlm.nih.gov/pubmed/7726783**).

SELECTED REFERENCES

American Association for Health, Physical Education, and Recreation. *Research Methods Applied to Health, Physical Education, and Recreation*. Washington, DC: American Association for Health, Physical Education, and Recreation, 1949.

Asmussen E. Muscular exercise. In: Fenn WO, Rahn H, eds. *Handbook of Respiration. Section 3. Respiration*. Vol. II. Washington, DC: American Physiological Society, 1965.

Åstrand PO. Influence of Scandinavian scientists in exercise physiology. *Skand J Med Sci Sports* 1991;1:3.

Bang O, et al. Contributions to the physiology of severe muscular work. *Skand Arch Physiol* 1936;74:1.

Barcroft J. *The Respiratory Function of the Blood. Part 1. Lesson from High Altitude*. Cambridge: Cambridge University Press, 1925.

Berryman JW. The tradition of the "six things nonnatural": exercise and medicine from Hippocrates through ante-bellum America. *Exerc Sport Sci Rev* 1989;17:515.

Berryman JW. The rise and development of the American College of Sports Medicine. *Med Sci Sports Exerc* 1993;25:885.

Berryman JW. *Out of Many One. A History of the American College of Sports Medicine*. Champaign: Human Kinetics, 1995.

Berryman JW, Cureton TK Jr. Pioneer researcher, proselytizer, and proponent for physical fitness. *Res Q Exerc Sport* 1996;67:1.

Buskirk ER. From Harvard to Minnesota: keys to our history. *Exerc Sport Sci Rev* 1992;20:1.

Buskirk ER. Early history of exercise physiology in the United States. Part 1. A contemporary historical perspective. In: Messengale JD, Swanson RA, eds. *History of Exercise and Sport Science*. Champaign: Human Kinetics, 1997.

Christensen EH, et al. An introduction to the studies of severe muscular exercise published in the present supplementary volume and other papers in the Skand. *Arch Skandinavisches Archiv Für* 1936;74:i. doi: 10.1111/j.1748-1716.1936.tb00433.x.

Consolazio CF. *Physiological Measurements of Metabolic Functions in Man*. New York: McGraw-Hill Book Co., 1961.

Cureton TK Jr. *Physical Fitness of Champion Athletes*. Urbana: University of Illinois Press, 1951.

Dill DB. *Life, Heat, and Altitude: Physiological Effects of Hot Climates and Great Heights*. Cambridge: Harvard University Press, 1938.

Dill DB. The Harvard Fatigue Laboratory: its development, contributions, and demise. *Circ Res* 1967;20:161.

Dill DB, Arlie V. Bock, pioneer in sports medicine. December 30, 1888–August 11, 1984. *Med Sci Sports Exerc* 1985;17:401.

Gerber EW. *Innovators and Institutions in Physical Education*. Philadelphia: Lea & Febiger, 1971.

Green RM. *A Translation of Galen's Hygiene*. Springfield: Charles C. Thomas, 1951.

Henry FM. Aerobic oxygen consumption and alactic debt in muscular work. *J Appl Physiol* 1951;3:427.

Henry FM. Lactic and alactic oxygen consumption in moderate exercise of graded intensity. *J Appl Physiol* 1956;8:608.

Henry FM. Physical education: an academic discipline. *JOHPER* 1964;35:32.

Hermansen L. Anaerobic energy release. *Med Sci Sports* 1969;1:32.

Hermansen L, Andersen KL. Aerobic work capacity in young Norwegian men and women. *J Appl Physiol* 1965;20:425.

Hoberman JM. The early development of sports medicine in Germany. In: Berryman JW, Park RJ, eds. *Sport and Exercise Science*. Urbana: University of Illinois Press, 1992.

Horvath SM, Horvath EC. *The Harvard Fatigue Laboratory: Its History and Contributions*. Englewood Cliffs: Prentice-Hall, 1973.

Johnson RE, et al. *Laboratory Manual of Field Methods for the Biochemical Assessment of Metabolic and Nutrition Conditions*. Boston: Harvard Fatigue Laboratory, 1946.

Katch VL. The burden of disproof. *Med Sci Sports Exerc* 1986;18:593.

Kerlinger FN. *Foundations of Behavioral Research*. 2nd Ed. New York: Holt, Rinehart, and Winston, 1973.

Krogh A. *The Composition of the Atmosphere: An Account of Preliminary Investigations and a Programme*. Kobenhavn: A.F. Host, 1919.

Kroll W. *Perspectives in Physical Education*. New York: Academic Press, 1971.

Leonard FG. *A Guide to the History of Physical Education*. Philadelphia: Lea & Febiger, 1923.

Lusk G. *The Elements of the Science of Nutrition*. 2nd Ed. Philadelphia: W.B. Saunders, 1909.

Park RJ. Concern for health and exercise as expressed in the writings of 18th century physicians and informed laymen (England, France, Switzerland). *Res Q* 1976;47:756.

Park RJ. The attitudes of leading New England transcendentalists toward healthful exercise, active recreation and proper care of the body: 1830–1860. *J Sport Hist* 1977;4:34.

Park RJ. The research quarterly and its antecedents. *Res Q Exerc Sport* 1980;51:1.

Park RJ. The emergence of the academic discipline of physical education in the United States. In: Brooks GA, ed. *Perspectives on the Academic Discipline of Physical Education*. Champaign: Human Kinetics, 1981.

Park RJ, Edward M. Hartwell and physical training at the Johns Hopkins University, 1879–1890. *J Sport Hist* 1987;14:108.

Park RJ. Physiologists, physicians, and physical educators: nineteenth century biology and exercise, hygienic and educative. *J Sport Hist* 1987;14:28.

Park RJ. The rise and demise of Harvard's B.S. program in Anatomy, Physiology, and Physical Training. *Res Q Exerc Sport* 1992;63:246.

Park RJ. Human energy expenditure from *Australopithecus afarensis* to the 4-minute mile: exemplars and case studies. *Exerc Sport Sci Rev* 1992;20:185.

Park RJ. A long and productive career: Franklin M. Henry—Scientist, mentor, pioneer. *Res Q Exerc Sport* 1994;65:295.

Park RJ. High-protein diets, "damaged hearts," and rowing men: antecedents of modern sports medicine and exercise science, 1867–1928. *Exerc Sport Sci Rev* 1997;25:137.

Payne JF. *Harvey and Galen. The Harveyan Oration, Oct. 19, 1896*. London: Frowde, 1897.

Schmidt-Nielsen B. August and Marie Krogh and respiratory physiology. *J Appl Physiol* 1984;57:293.

Scholander PF. Analyzer for accurate estimation of respiratory gases in one-half cubic centimeter samples. *J Biol Chem* 1947;167:235.

Shaffel N. The evaluation of American medical literature. In: MartiIbanez F, ed. *History of American Medicine*. New York: MD Publications, 1958.

Tipton CM. Exercise physiology, part II: a contemporary historical perspective. In: Messengale JD, Swanson RA, eds. *The History of Exercise and Sports Science*. Champaign: Human Kinetics, 1997.

Tipton CM. Contemporary exercise physiology: fifty years after the closure of the Harvard Fatigue Laboratory. *Exerc Sport Sci Rev* 1998;26:315.

Tipton CM. Historical perspective: the antiquity of exercise, exercise physiology and the exercise prescription for health. *World Rev Nutr Diet* 2008;98:198.

Tipton CM. Susruta of India, an unrecognized contributor to the history of exercise physiology. *J Appl Physiol* 2008;104:1553.

Tipton CM. Historical perspective: the antiquity of exercise, exercise physiology and the exercise prescription for health. In: Simopoulos AP, ed. *Nutrition and Fitness: Cultural, Genetic and Metabolic Aspects*. Vol. 98. *World Rev Nutr Diet*. Basal: Kargar, 2008:198.

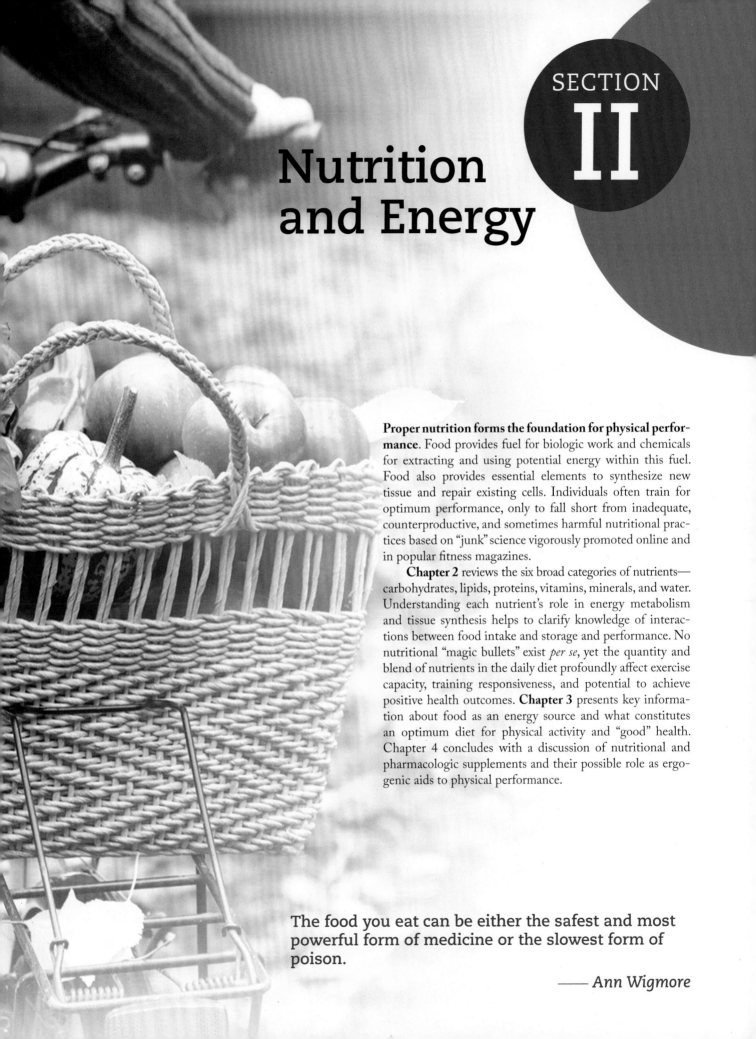

SECTION II

Nutrition and Energy

Proper nutrition forms the foundation for physical performance. Food provides fuel for biologic work and chemicals for extracting and using potential energy within this fuel. Food also provides essential elements to synthesize new tissue and repair existing cells. Individuals often train for optimum performance, only to fall short from inadequate, counterproductive, and sometimes harmful nutritional practices based on "junk" science vigorously promoted online and in popular fitness magazines.

Chapter 2 reviews the six broad categories of nutrients—carbohydrates, lipids, proteins, vitamins, minerals, and water. Understanding each nutrient's role in energy metabolism and tissue synthesis helps to clarify knowledge of interactions between food intake and storage and performance. No nutritional "magic bullets" exist *per se*, yet the quantity and blend of nutrients in the daily diet profoundly affect exercise capacity, training responsiveness, and potential to achieve positive health outcomes. **Chapter 3** presents key information about food as an energy source and what constitutes an optimum diet for physical activity and "good" health. Chapter 4 concludes with a discussion of nutritional and pharmacologic supplements and their possible role as ergogenic aids to physical performance.

The food you eat can be either the safest and most powerful form of medicine or the slowest form of poison.

—— *Ann Wigmore*

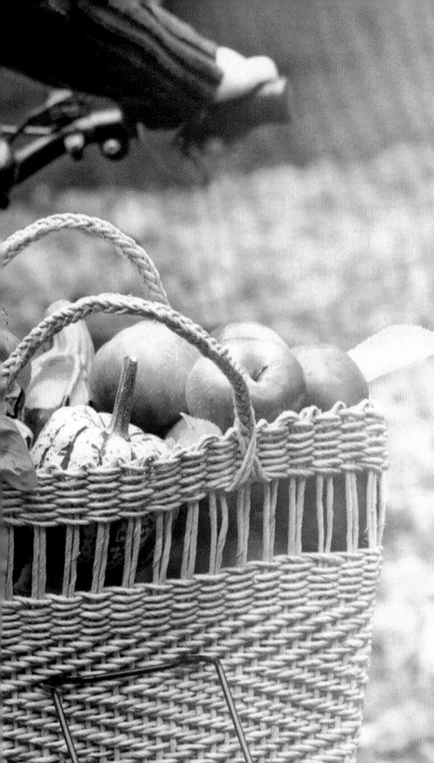

CHAPTER 2

Macronutrients and Micronutrients

CHAPTER OBJECTIVES

- Distinguish differences among monosaccharides, disaccharides, and polysaccharides.
- Discuss carbohydrates' role as an energy source, protein sparer, metabolic primer, and central nervous system fuel.
- Define and give an example for these terms: triacylglycerol, saturated fatty acid, polyunsaturated fatty acid, monounsaturated fatty acid, and *trans* fatty acid.
- List four major characteristics of high- and low-density lipoprotein cholesterol, and discuss their role in coronary heart disease.
- List four important functions of fat in the body.
- Contrast essential and nonessential amino acids and give food sources for each.
- List the fat- and water-soluble vitamins and explain potential risks of consuming these in excess.
- Outline three broad roles of minerals in the body.
- Define osteoporosis, exercise-induced anemia, and sodium-induced hypertension.
- Describe how regular physical activity affects bone mass and the body's iron stores.
- Outline four factors related to the female athlete triad.
- List four important functions of water in the body.
- Define heat cramps, heat exhaustion, and heat stroke.
- Explain four factors that affect gastric emptying and fluid replacement.
- List three predisposing factors to hyponatremia with long-duration ultraendurance physical activities.

ANCILLARIES AT A GLANCE

Visit **http://thePoint.lww.com/MKKESS5e** to access the following resources:

- References: Chapter 2
- Interactive Question Bank
- Appendix A: The Metric System and Conversion Constants in Exercise Physiology
- Animation: Biologic Function of Vitamins
- Animation: Bone Growth
- Animation: Calcium in Muscle
- Animation: Condensation
- Animation: Digestion of Carbohydrate
- Animation: Fat Mobilization and Use
- Animation: Glycogen Synthesis
- Animation: Hydrolysis
- Animation: Renal Function
- Animation: Transamination
- Animation: Vitamin C as an Antioxidant
- Animation: Water Balance

PART 1 Macronutrients: Energy Fuel and Building Blocks for Tissue Synthesis

The carbohydrate, lipid, and protein macronutrients consumed daily supply the energy to maintain bodily functions during rest and diverse physical activities. The macronutrients also help to maintain and enhance the organism's structural and functional integrity with training. **Part 1** discusses each macronutrient's general structure, function, and source in the diet and emphasizes their importance in sustaining physiologic function during rest and physical activity.

CARBOHYDRATES

All living cells contain **carbohydrates**. With the exception of lactose and a small amount of glycogen obtained in animal tissues, plant sources provide all of the dietary carbohydrate. Atoms of carbon, hydrogen, and oxygen combine to form a carbohydrate or sugar molecule, always in a ratio of 1 atom of carbon and 2 atoms of hydrogen for each oxygen atom. The general formula $(CH_2O)n$ represents a simple carbohydrate, where *n* equals from 3 to 7 carbon atoms.

Monosaccharides

*The **monosaccharide** molecule forms the basic unit of carbohydrates.* The molecule's number of carbon atoms determines its category. The Greek name for this number, ending with "ose," indicates sugars. For example, 3-carbon monosaccharides are **trioses**, 4-carbon sugars are **tetroses**, 5-carbon sugars are **pentoses**, 6-carbon sugars are **hexoses**, and 7-carbon sugars are **heptoses**. The hexose sugars glucose, fructose, and galactose represent the nutritionally important monosaccharides.

Glucose, also called *dextrose* or *blood sugar*, consists of 6 carbon, 12 hydrogen, and 6 oxygen atoms ($C_6H_{12}O_6$; **Fig. 2.1**). This sugar forms when energy from sunlight interacts with water, carbon dioxide, and chlorophyll. It occurs naturally in food or produced through digestion (**hydrolysis**) of more complex carbohydrates. After its absorption by the small intestine, glucose functions in one of four ways:

1. Used directly by the cell for energy
2. Stores as glycogen in muscles and liver
3. Converts to fat for energy storage
4. Provides carbon skeletons to synthesize nonessential amino acids

See the animation "Digestion of Carbohydrate" on **http://thePoint.lww.com/MKKESS5e** for a demonstration of this process.

Fructose (also called *levulose* or *fruit sugar*), the sweetest of the monosaccharides, occurs in honey, tree and vine fruits, flowers, berries, and most root vegetables. Fructose, like glucose, also serves as an energy source. It usually moves rapidly directly from the digestive tract into the blood to primarily convert to fat but also glucose in the liver.

Galactose does not exist freely in nature; rather, it forms milk sugar (**lactose**) in the mammary glands of lactating animals. In the body, galactose readily converts to glucose for energy metabolism.

See the animation "Hydrolysis" on **http://thePoint.lww.com/MKKESS5e** for a demonstration of this process.

Disaccharides

Combining two monosaccharide molecules forms a **disaccharide** or double sugar. The monosaccharides and disaccharides collectively make up the **simple sugars**.

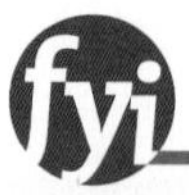

What's in a Name?

Simple sugars are packaged commercially under a variety of names. This figure illustrates simple sugars with their percentage content of glucose and fructose.

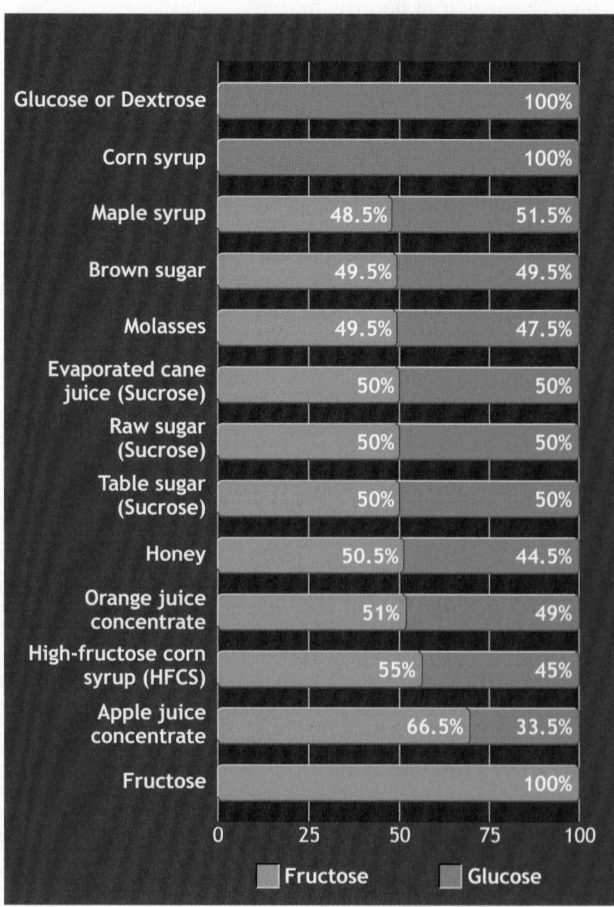

Source: Adapted with permission from McArdle WD, Katch FI, Katch VL. *Exercise Physiology: Nutrition, Energy, and Human Performance*. 8th Ed. Baltimore: Wolters Kluwer Health, 2015, based on U.S. Department of Agriculture data.

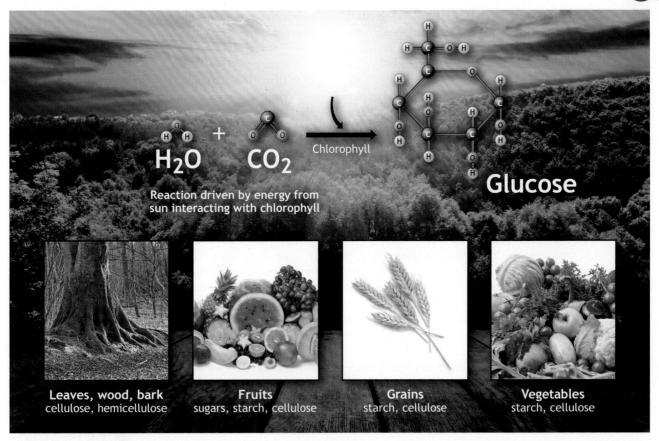

FIGURE 2.1 Three-dimensional ring structure of the simple sugar glucose molecule formed during photosynthesis when energy from sunlight interacts with water, carbon dioxide, and the green pigment chlorophyll. (Adapted with permission from McArdle WD, Katch FI, Katch VL. *Exercise Physiology: Nutrition, Energy, and Human Performance*. 8th Ed. Baltimore: Wolters Kluwer Health, 2015.)

Each of the disaccharides contains glucose as a principal component. The three disaccharides of nutritional importance include the following:

1. **Sucrose**: Glucose + fructose; the most common dietary disaccharide; composed of 12 atoms of carbon, 22 atoms of hydrogen, and 11 atoms of oxygen ($C_{12}H_{22}O_{11}$). It occurs naturally in most foods that contain carbohydrate, particularly beet sugar, cane sugar, brown sugar, maple syrup, and honey.
2. **Lactose**: Glucose + galactose; found in natural form only in milk and called *milk sugar*.
3. **Maltose**: Glucose + glucose; occurs in beer, cereals, and germinating seeds.

Polysaccharides

Polysaccharides include plant and animal carbohydrate categories.

Plant Polysaccharides

Starch and fiber represent the two most common plant polysaccharide forms.

Starch

Starch, the storage form of plant polysaccharide, forms from hundreds of individual sugar molecules joined together. It appears as large granules in seed and corn cells and in grains that constitute bread, cereal, pasta, and pastries. Large amounts also exist in peas, beans, potatoes, and roots, in which starch stores energy for the plant's future needs. The term **complex carbohydrates** refers to dietary starch.

Fiber

Fiber, classified as a nonstarch, structural polysaccharide, includes **cellulose**, the most abundant organic molecule on earth. Fibrous materials resist hydrolysis by human digestive enzymes in the oral cavity, stomach, and small intestine. Plants exclusively contain fiber, which constitutes the structure of leaves, stems, roots, seeds, and fruit coverings. Fibers differ in physical and chemical characteristics and physiologic action; they occur primarily within the cell wall as cellulose, gums, hemicellulose, pectin, and noncarbohydrate lignins. Other fibers—mucilage and the gums—serve as integral components of the plant cell itself. The term **functional fiber** refers to nondigestible carbohydrates with beneficial human physiologic effects. Adequate fiber intake ameliorates constipation and diverticular disease, provides fuel for colonic cells, reduces blood glucose and lipid levels, and provides a source of nutrient-rich, low–energy-dense foods that contribute to satiety.

Health Implications of Dietary Fiber

Americans typically consume about 12 to 15 g of fiber daily, far short of the recommendations of the Food and Nutrition Board of the National Academy of Sciences

(NAS) (**www.iom.edu/About-IOM/Leadership-Staff/Boards/Food-and-Nutrition-Board.aspx**). NAS recommends 38 g for men and 25 g for women up to age 50 years and 30 g for men and 21 g for women older than age 50 years.

Fibers hold considerable water and give "bulk" to food residues in the intestines, often increasing stool weight and volume by 40% to 100%. This bulking action may aid gastrointestinal functioning and reduce the chances of contracting colon cancer and other gastrointestinal diseases later in life. Increased fiber intake, particularly of **water-soluble fibers**, may modestly reduce serum cholesterol. Water-soluble fibers include pectin and guar gum and are present in oats (e.g., rolled oats, oat bran, oat flour), legumes, barley, brown rice, peas, beans, apples, carrots, and citrus fruits.

For men with elevated blood lipids, adding 100 g of oat bran to their daily diets reduced serum cholesterol levels by 13% and lowered the low-density lipoprotein (LDL) component of the cholesterol profile. In contrast, the **water-insoluble fibers**—cellulose, hemicellulose, lignin, and cellulose-rich products, such as wheat bran—did not reduce cholesterol levels.

Current consensus among health professionals maintains that a dietary fiber intake of between about 20 and 40 g daily (at a ratio of 3:1 for water-insoluble to soluble fiber), depending on age and gender, plays an important role in well-structured meal plans.

Animal Polysaccharides

During the process of **glycogenesis**, a few hundred to thousands of glucose molecules combine to form **glycogen**, the large storage polysaccharide residing in mammalian muscle and liver. A well-nourished 80-kg person stores approximately 500 g of carbohydrate (**Fig. 2.2**). Of this, approximately 400 g exists as muscle glycogen (largest reserve), and 90 to 110 g exists as liver glycogen (highest concentration representing between 3% and 7% of the liver's weight); only about 2 to 3 g exists as blood glucose. Each gram of carbohydrate, as either glycogen or glucose, contains about 4 kcal of energy (see Chapter 3). The average-size individual stores between 1500 and 2000 kcal as carbohydrate, enough total energy to power a continuous 20-mile round-trip run on relatively level terrain at a moderate intensity of effort.

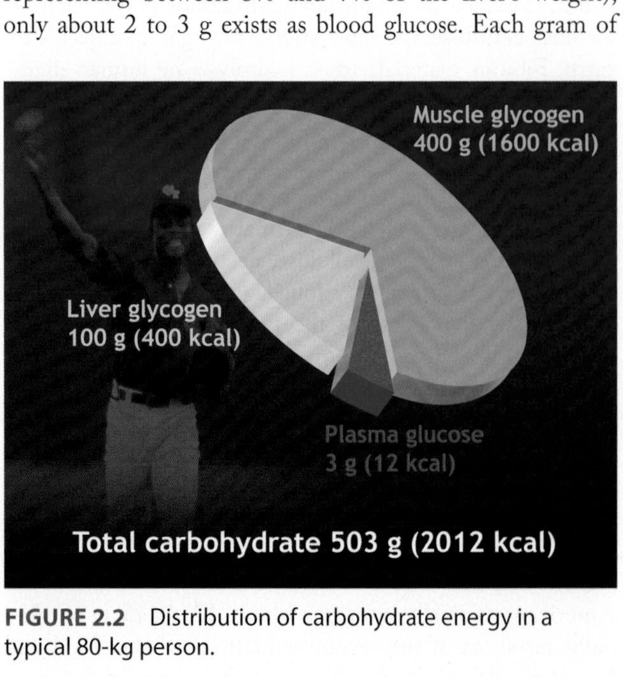

FIGURE 2.2 Distribution of carbohydrate energy in a typical 80-kg person.

thePoint® Appendix A: The Metric System and Conversion Constants in Exercise Physiology, available online at **http://thePoint.lww.com/MKKESS5e**, shows the relationship between metric units and US units, including common expressions of work, energy, and power.

Muscle glycogen serves as the major source of carbohydrate energy for active muscles during physical activity. In contrast to muscle glycogen, liver glycogen reconverts to glucose for transport in the blood to the working muscles. **Glycogenolysis** describes this reconversion process (glycogen → glucose); it provides a rapid extramuscular glucose supply. Unlike liver cells, muscle cells do not contain the enzyme to remake glucose from stored glycogen. Glucose or glycogen within a muscle cell cannot supply the carbohydrate needs of surrounding cells. Depleting liver and muscle glycogen through dietary restriction or intense activity stimulates glucose synthesis from the other macronutrients' structural components, principally protein's amino acids, through **gluconeogenesis** (glucose formation from nonglucose sources).

Hormones regulate liver and muscle glycogen stores by controlling circulating blood sugar level. Elevated blood sugar causes pancreatic beta (β) cells to secrete additional insulin that facilitates muscle uptake of the glucose excess, inhibiting further insulin secretion. This *feedback regulation* maintains blood glucose at an appropriate physiologic concentration. In contrast, if blood sugar decreases below normal, called **hypoglycemia**, the pancreas' alpha (α) cells immediately secrete **glucagon** to increase glucose availability and normalize the blood sugar level. When increases in blood glucose occur, glucagon (known as the insulin antagonist **hormone**) stimulates liver glycogenolysis and gluconeogenesis.

See the animation "Glycogen Synthesis" on **http://thePoint.lww.com/MKKESS5e** for a demonstration of this process.

Diet Affects Glycogen Stores

The body stores comparatively little glycogen, so dietary intake considerably impacts glycogen quantity. For example, a 24-hour fast or a low-carbohydrate, normal-calorie (**isocaloric**) diet dramatically reduces glycogen reserves. In contrast, maintaining a carbohydrate-rich isocaloric diet for several days doubles the body's carbohydrate stores compared with a normal, well-balanced diet. The body's upper limit for glycogen storage equals about 15 g per kilogram (kg) of body mass, equivalent to 1050 g for the average 70-kg man or 840 g for a typical 56-kg woman. To estimate the body's maximum glycogen storage capacity (in grams), multiply body weight in kilograms (lb ÷ 2.205 = kg) by 15. The contrast can be striking for people who vary considerably in body size. For example, the maximum glycogen storage for an All-Pro NFL defensive lineman who weighs 335 lb (152 kg) would equal 2280 g (152 kg × 15) or about 2.3 kg (5 lb). For a 134 lb (60 kg) world-class male marathoner, the maximum stored glycogen would equal 900 g, or only about 2 lb. Based on your body weight, what is your stored glycogen content?

Carbohydrates' Role in the Body

Carbohydrates serve four primary functions related to energy metabolism and exercise performance:

1. **Energy source**. Energy from blood-borne glucose and muscle glycogen breakdown ultimately powers muscle action (particularly intense activity) and other more "silent" forms of biologic work. For physically active people, adequate daily carbohydrate intake maintains the body's limited glycogen stores. However, more is not necessarily better; if dietary carbohydrate intake exceeds the cells' capacity to store glycogen, the carbohydrate excess readily converts to fat, triggering an increase in the body's total fat content.
2. **Protein sparer**. Adequate carbohydrate intake preserves tissue proteins. Normally, protein contributes to tissue maintenance, repair, and growth and serves as a minor nutrient energy source. With reduced glycogen reserves, gluconeogenesis synthesizes glucose from amino acids and the glycerol portion of the triacylglycerol molecule. This metabolic process increases carbohydrate availability and maintains plasma glucose levels under three conditions:
   (1) Dietary restriction
   (2) Prolonged physical activity
   (3) Repeated bouts of intense training
3. **Metabolic primer**. By-products of carbohydrate breakdown serve as a "primer" to facilitate the body's use of fat for energy, particularly in the liver. Insufficient carbohydrate metabolism, through either limitations in glucose transport into the cell as occurs in diabetes or glycogen depletion through inadequate diet or prolonged exertion, increases dependence on fat utilization for energy. When this happens, the body cannot generate a sustained high level of aerobic energy transfer from fat-only metabolism. This may reduce an individual's sustained maximum intensity by up to 50%.
4. **Fuel for the central nervous system**. The central nervous system requires carbohydrate for proper functioning. Under normal conditions, the brain almost exclusively uses blood glucose for fuel without maintaining a backup supply of this nutrient. In poorly regulated diabetes, during starvation, or with a low-carbohydrate intake, the brain adapts metabolically after about 8 days to use fat in the form of ketones as an alternative to glucose as a primary fuel source.

   At rest and physical activity, the liver serves as the main source to maintain normal blood glucose levels. In prolonged intense effort, blood glucose eventually decreases below normal levels because of liver glycogen depletion and active muscles' continual use of available blood glucose. Symptoms of a modest hypoglycemia include feelings of weakness, hunger, and dizziness. This ultimately impacts exercise performance and partially explains "central" or neurologic fatigue associated with prolonged physical activity or starvation.

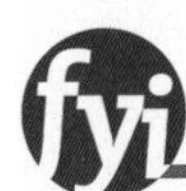

Important Carbohydrate Conversions

Glycogenesis—Glycogen synthesis from glucose (glucose → glycogen)
Gluconeogenesis—Glucose synthesis largely from structural components of noncarbohydrate nutrients (protein → glucose)
Glycogenolysis—Glucose formation from glycogen (glycogen → glucose)

Recommended Carbohydrate Intake

Figure 2.3 illustrates the carbohydrate content of selected foods. Rich carbohydrate sources include cereals, pasta, cookies, candies, breads, and cakes. Fruits and vegetables with a high water content contain less carbohydrate compared to those with low water content. This occurs because the food's total weight, including its water content, determines its carbohydrate percentage. Dried portions of fruits and vegetables exist as almost all carbohydrate; hikers and ultraendurance athletes often rely on dried apricots, pears, apples, bananas, and tomatoes to provide a ready but relatively lightweight carbohydrate source.

Carbohydrates account for between 40% and 55% of total calories in the typical American diet. For a sedentary 70-kg person, this translates to a daily carbohydrate intake of roughly 300 g. Average Americans consume about half of their carbohydrate as simple sugars, predominantly as sucrose and high-fructose corn syrup. This amount of simple sugar intake represents the yearly intake equivalent to 60 lb of table sugar or 16 ts of sucrose daily and 46 lb of corn syrup!

For physically active people and those involved in structured exercise training, carbohydrates should equal about 60% of daily calories or 400 to 600 g, predominantly as unrefined, fiber-rich fruits, grains, and vegetables. During periods of intense training over extended duration, carbohydrate intake should increase to 70% of total calories consumed, the equivalent of 8 to 10 g per kg of body mass. Note that this level of intake does not apply to "normal" dietary intake patterns for most Americans, where an excess intake of carbohydrate-rich foods leads to increased caloric intake, weight gain, and often, an increase in coronary risk.

All Carbohydrates Are Not Physiologically Equal

Digestion and absorption rates of different carbohydrate-containing foods might explain the carbohydrate intake–diabetes link. Whereas low-fiber processed starches and simple

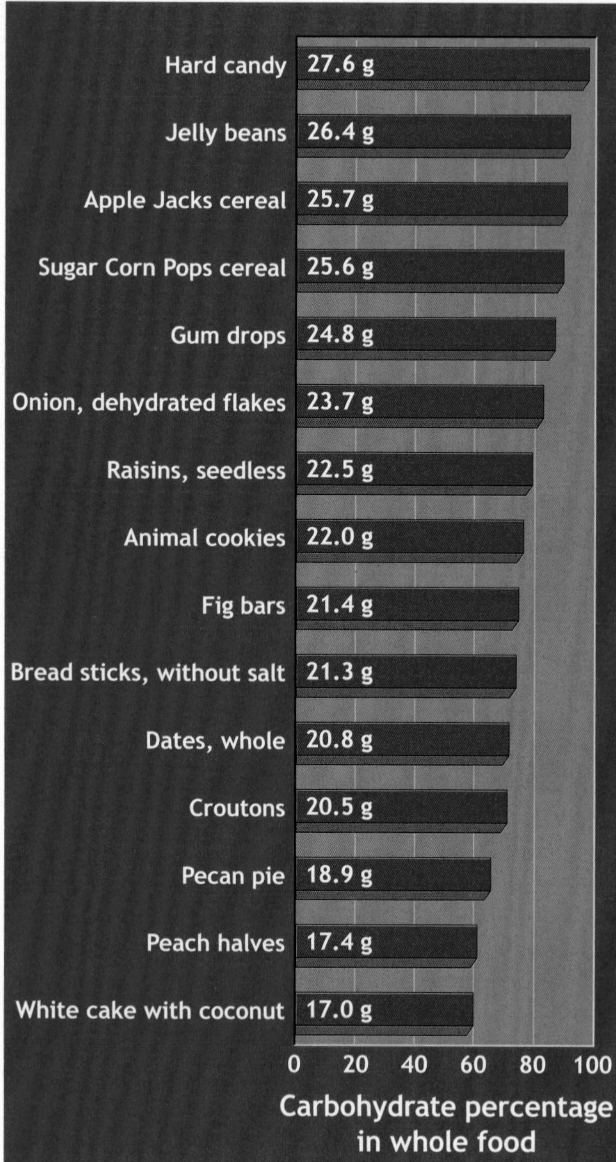

FIGURE 2.3 Percentage of carbohydrates in commonly served foods. The number in each bar displays the number of grams of carbohydrate per ounce (28.4 g) of food.

sugars in soft drinks digest quickly and enter the blood at a relatively rapid rate (i.e., have a high glycemic index), slow-release high-fiber foods, unrefined complex carbohydrates, and carbohydrate foods rich in lipids slow digestion to minimize surges in blood glucose. The rapid increase in blood glucose that accompanies refined processed starch and simple sugar intake increases insulin demand; stimulates the pancreas to overproduce insulin, which accentuates hyperinsulinemia; increases plasma triacylglycerol concentrations; and augments fat synthesis. Consistently eating high glycemic foods can reduce the body's sensitivity to insulin (i.e., the body resists insulin's effects), requiring progressively greater insulin output to control blood sugar levels. *Type 2 diabetes results when the pancreas cannot produce sufficient insulin to regulate blood glucose or becomes insensitive to the effects of insulin, causing blood glucose to rise.* In contrast, meals with fiber-rich, low-glycemic carbohydrates tend to lower blood glucose and the insulin response after eating, improve blood lipid profiles, and increase insulin sensitivity. Frequent bouts of physical activity also increase insulin sensitivity.

Glycemic Index

*The **glycemic index** serves as a relative or qualitative indicator of carbohydrate-containing foods' ability to increase blood glucose levels.* Blood sugar increase, termed the *glycemic response*, is quantified after the ingestion of a food containing 50 g of a carbohydrate or carbohydrate-containing food and comparing the increases over a 2-hour period with a "standard" for carbohydrate. This comparison, usually contrasted against white bread or glucose, is assigned a value of 100. The glycemic index expresses the percentage of total area under the blood glucose–response curve for a "specific food" compared with only glucose. A food with a glycemic index of 45, for example, indicates that ingesting 50 g of the food increases blood glucose concentrations to levels that reach 45% of that associated with 50 g of glucose.

The glycemic index provides a more useful physiologic concept than simply classifying a carbohydrate based on its chemical configuration as simple or complex, as a sugar or starch, or as available or unavailable. A high glycemic index rating does not necessarily indicate poor nutritional quality because carrots, brown rice, and corn, with their rich quantities of health-protective micronutrients, phytochemicals, and dietary fiber, have relatively high indices.

The **glycemic load** associates with consuming specified serving sizes of different foods. While the glycemic *index* compares equal quantities of a carbohydrate-containing food, the glycemic *load* quantifies the overall glycemic effect of a typical food portion. *In other words, the glycemic load represents the amount of available carbohydrate in that serving and the food's glycemic index.* A high glycemic load reflects a greater expected elevation in blood glucose and greater insulin release to that food. Consuming a diet with a high glycemic load on a regular basis associates with increased risk for type 2 diabetes and coronary heart disease.

Figure 2.4 lists the glycemic index for common items in various food groupings. For easy identification, foods are placed into high, medium, and low categories. Interestingly, a food's index rating does not depend simply on its classification as "simple" (monosaccharides and disaccharides) or "complex" (starch and fiber) carbohydrates. For example, the plant starch in white rice and potatoes has a higher glycemic index than the simple sugar fructose in apples and peaches. A food's fiber content slows digestion rate, so fiber-containing peas, beans, and other legumes have low glycemic indexes. Ingesting lipids and proteins also tends to slow food passage into the small intestine, thereby reducing the glycemic load of the meal's carbohydrate content.

High Glycemic Foods: A Possible Role in Obesity

About 25% of the adult population produces excessive insulin in response to a "challenge" of rapidly absorbed or high glycemic carbohydrates. These insulin-resistant individuals require more insulin to regulate blood glucose and increase

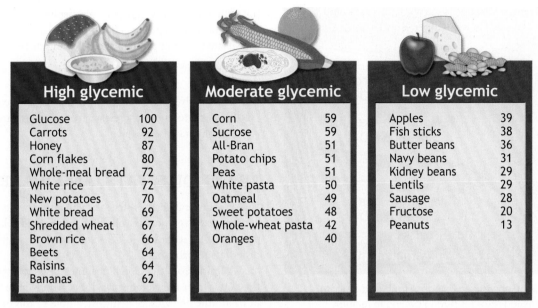

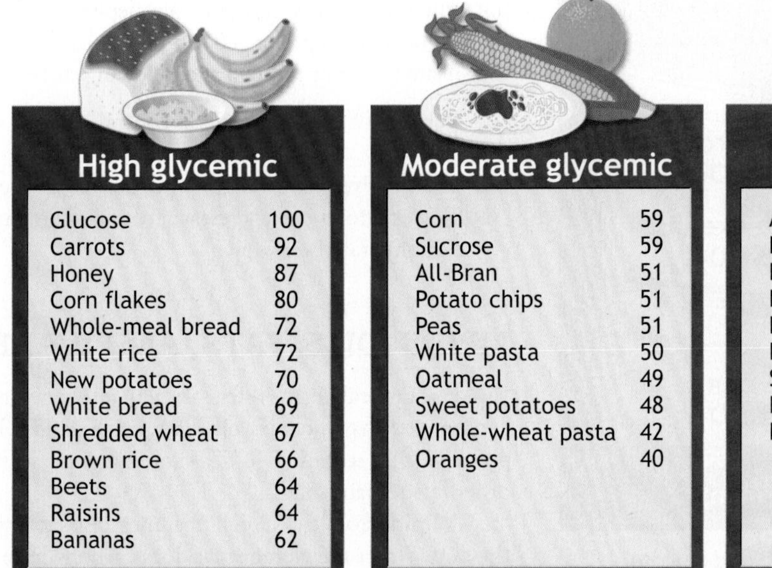

High glycemic
Glucose 100
Carrots 92
Honey 87
Corn flakes 80
Whole-meal bread 72
White rice 72
New potatoes 70
White bread 69
Shredded wheat 67
Brown rice 66
Beets 64
Raisins 64
Bananas 62
Moderate glycemic
Corn 59
Sucrose 59
All-Bran 51
Potato chips 51
Peas 51
White pasta 50
Oatmeal 49
Sweet potatoes 48
Whole-wheat pasta 42
Oranges 40
Low glycemic
Apples 39
Fish sticks 38
Butter beans 36
Navy beans 31
Kidney beans 29
Lentils 29
Sausage 28
Fructose 20
Peanuts 13

FIGURE 2.4 Categorization for glycemic index (GI) of common food sources of carbohydrates. (Adapted with permission from McArdle WD, Katch FI, Katch VL. *Exercise Physiology: Nutrition, Energy, and Human Performance*. 8th Ed. Baltimore: Wolters Kluwer Health, 2015.)

their obesity risk by consistently consuming a high glycemic food diet. Weight gain occurs because excessive insulin facilitates glucose oxidation at the expense of fatty acid oxidation; excessive insulin also stimulates fat storage in adipose tissue.

The insulin surge in response to high glycemic carbohydrate intake often abnormally decreases blood glucose. This "rebound hypoglycemia" sets off hunger signals to trigger overeating. A repetitive scenario of high blood sugar followed by low blood sugar exerts the most profound effect on sedentary obese individuals who present with the greatest insulin resistance and exaggerated insulin response to a blood glucose challenge. Regularly engaging in low to moderate intensity physical activity produces the following three beneficial effects:

1. Improves insulin sensitivity to reduce the insulin requirement for a given glucose uptake
2. Stimulates plasma-derived fatty acid oxidation to decrease the liver's fatty acid availability, thereby depressing any increase in plasma very low density lipoprotein (VLDL) cholesterol and triacylglycerol concentration
3. Exerts a potent positive calorie-burning influence for weight control

Insulin Index of Foods

The glycemic index ranks foods according to the extent they increase blood glucose concentration, but does not consider the concurrent insulin response. In general, insulin secretion largely assumes to be proportional to postprandial glycemia. In contrast, carbohydrate is not the only stimulus for insulin secretion. The **insulin index** explores the importance of dietary stimulus and postprandial insulinemia of different foods with different glycemic indices. Protein-rich foods or the addition of protein to a carbohydrate-rich meal stimulates a modest rise in insulin secretion in diabetic individuals without increasing blood glucose concentration. Similarly, adding a large amount of fat to a carbohydrate-rich meal modestly increases insulin secretion even though plasma glucose responses decrease.

The insulin index compares the insulin response of different foods administered as a standard 1000-kJ portion (metric equivalent of calories; 1 kJ = 0.239 kcal) with 220-mL water, with white bread as the reference food. In general, the glycemic index predicts the insulin index, with some notable exceptions. For example, brown rice with a glycemic index of 55 has a corresponding insulin index score of 62; a chocolate bar has a glycemic index score of 79 with a corresponding insulin index score of 122. Some protein- and fat-rich eggs, beef, fish, lentils, cheese, cake, and doughnuts induce as much insulin secretion as do some carbohydrate-rich foods (e.g., in terms of insulin secretion, beef equals brown rice and fish equals whole-grain bread).

Carbohydrate Use During Physical Activity

The fuel mixture used during physical activity depends on the intensity and duration of effort, including the exerciser's fitness and nutritional status.

Intense Physical Activity

Stored muscle glycogen and blood-borne glucose primarily contribute to the total energy required during intense physical activity and in the early minutes of movement when oxygen supply fails to meet aerobic metabolic demands.

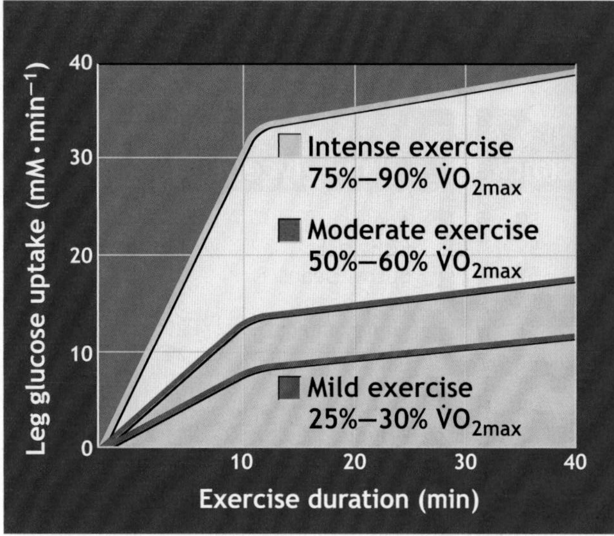

FIGURE 2.5 Generalized response for blood glucose uptake by the leg muscles during cycling in relation to exercise duration and intensity. Exercise intensity is expressed as a percentage of $\dot{V}O_{2max}$. (Adapted with permission from McArdle WD, Katch FI, Katch VL. *Exercise Physiology: Nutrition, Energy, and Human Performance*. 8th Ed. Baltimore: Wolters Kluwer Health, 2015.)

Figure 2.5 shows that early during intense activity, muscle uptake of circulating blood glucose increases sharply and continues to rise with continuing effort. After 40 minutes of activity, muscle's glucose uptake increases 7 to 20 times over resting uptake, with the highest use occurring at the most intense activity level. Carbohydrate's large energy contribution occurs because it is the only macronutrient that provides energy without oxygen (i.e., anaerobically). During intense aerobic activity, intramuscular glycogen becomes the preferential energy fuel. This provides an advantage because glycogen supplies energy for physical activity twice as rapidly as fat and protein (see Chapter 8).

Moderate and Prolonged Physical Activity

During the transition from rest to submaximal activity, almost all energy comes from glycogen stored in active muscles. Following this transition, liver and muscle glycogen provide about 40% to 50% of the energy requirement during the next 20 minutes, with the remainder from fat breakdown with minimal amounts from blood glucose. As physical activity continues but glycogen stores deplete, fat catabolism increases its percentage contribution to the total energy for muscular activity. Additionally, blood-borne glucose becomes the major source of the limited carbohydrate energy. Eventually, liver glucose output does not keep pace with its use, and blood glucose concentration declines toward hypoglycemic levels.

Inability to maintain a desired performance level, often referred to as fatigue, can occur if physical activity intensity progresses to the point where liver and muscle glycogen decrease severely. This occurs even if muscle has sufficient oxygen available to it and almost unlimited potential energy from stored fat. Endurance athletes commonly refer to fatigue under these conditions as "bonking" or **"hitting the wall."** Research does not fully explain why carbohydrate depletion coincides with the fatigue onset in prolonged submaximal activity. The answer may relate to one or more of the following three reasons:

1. Key role of blood glucose in central nervous system function
2. Muscle glycogen's role as a "primer" in fat breakdown
3. Slower rate of energy release from fat compared with carbohydrate breakdown

LIPIDS (OILS, FATS, AND WAXES)

Lipid, a general term, refers to a heterogeneous group of compounds that includes oils, fats, waxes, and related compounds. Oils remain liquid at room temperature, whereas other fats remain solid.

A **lipid** (from the Greek *lipos* meaning fat) molecule has the same structural elements as does carbohydrate but differs in its atomic linkages. Specifically, a lipid's ratio of hydrogen to oxygen considerably exceeds that for carbohydrate. For example, the formula $C_{57}H_{110}O_6$ describes the common lipid stearin with an H-to-O ratio of 18.3:1; for carbohydrate, the ratio equals 2:1. Lipids can be placed into one of three main groups: **simple lipids**, **compound lipids**, and **derived lipids**. Approximately 98% of dietary lipid exists as triacylglycerols.

Simple Lipids

The simple lipids or "neutral fats" consist primarily of **triacylglycerols.** They constitute the major storage form of fat; more than 90% of body fat exists as triacylglycerol, predominantly in adipose cells. Synthesis of a lipid molecule involves the union of two different atom clusters:

- A glycerol component consists of a 3-carbon molecule that itself does not qualify as a lipid because of its high water solubility.
- A component consisting of three clusters of carbon-chained atoms termed fatty acids that attach to the glycerol molecule unit. Fatty acids contain straight hydrocarbon chains with as few as 4 carbon atoms or more than 20; the most prevalent chain lengths have 16 and 18 carbons.

See the animation "Condensation" on **http://thePoint.lww.com/MKKESS5e** for a demonstration of this process.

Figure 2.6 illustrates the basic structure of saturated and unsaturated fatty acid molecules. All lipid-containing foods contain mixtures of different proportions of saturated and unsaturated fatty acids.

Saturated Fatty Acids

Saturated fatty acids contain only single bonds between carbon atoms, with hydrogen attaching to the remaining bonds. The fatty acid holds as many hydrogen atoms as chemically possible (i.e., saturated relative to hydrogen).

Saturated fatty acids occur plentifully in beef, lamb, pork, chicken, and egg yolk and in dairy fats found in cream, milk, butter, and cheese. Saturated fatty acids from plants include coconut and palm oil, vegetable shortening, and hydrogenated margarine; commercially prepared cakes, pies, and cookies rely heavily on saturated fatty acids. Owing to their molecular stability, saturated fats are resistant to oxidation by heat and so are suitable for high- and low-heat cooking.

Unsaturated Fatty Acids

Unsaturated fatty acids contain one or more double bonds along the main carbon backbone. Each double bond in the carbon chain reduces the number of potential hydrogen-binding sites. In this case, the molecule remains unsaturated relative to hydrogen. Monounsaturated fatty acids contain one double bond along the main carbon chain; examples include canola oil, olive oil, peanut oil, and oils in almond, and other tree nuts and avocado fruit. Polyunsaturated fatty acids contain two or more double bonds along the main carbon chain; examples include safflower, sunflower, soybean, and corn oils.

Fatty acids from plant sources are typically unsaturated and liquefy at room temperature. Lipids with more carbons in the fatty acid chain and containing more saturated fatty acids remain firmer at room temperature.

Chains of Fats

Most naturally occurring fatty acids form a chain of an even number of 4 to 28 carbon atoms, often categorized as short to very long. Fatty acids undergo different metabolic fates depending on chain length and degree of saturation.

- **Short-chain fatty acids (SCFA)** ≤6 carbons (e.g., butyric acid, acetic acid, and caprylic acid); found in butter and some tropical fats.
- **Medium-chain fatty acids (MCFA or MCT)** = 6 to 12 carbons (e.g., lauric and capric acid); found in coconut oil, palm kernel oil, and breast milk.
- **Long-chain fatty acids (LCFA)** = 13 to 21 carbons (e.g., palmitic, oleic, and stearic acid); found in animals, fish, cocoa, seeds, nuts, and vegetable oils.
- **Very long chain fatty acids (VLCFA)** ≥22 carbons (e.g., cerotic acid); too long for direct mitochondrial metabolism present in small amounts in foods and normally in all mammalian tissue, particularly the part of brain membranes, including myelin, the "insulation" around nerve fibers.

Saturated Fatty Acid

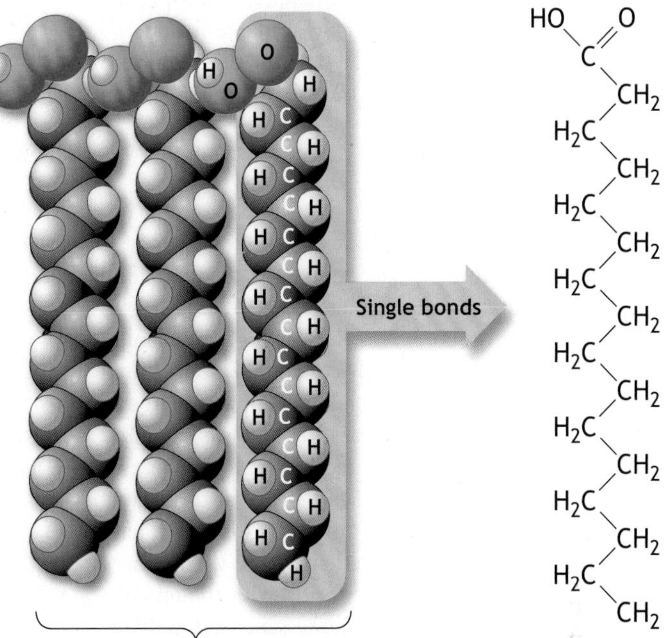

Ⓐ No double bonds; fatty acid chains fit close together

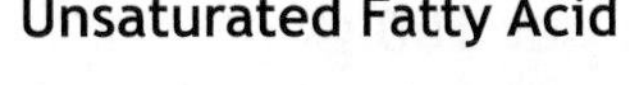

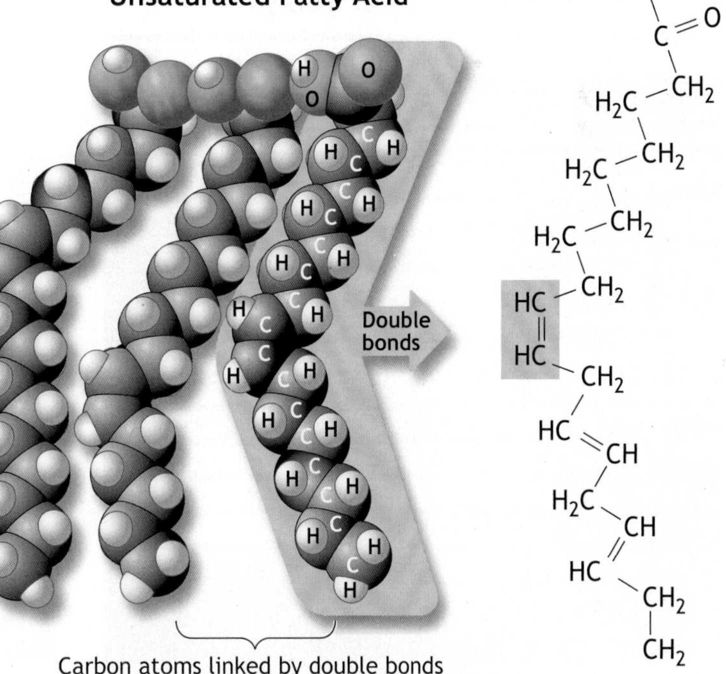

Ⓑ Double bonds present; fatty acid chains do not fit close together

FIGURE 2.6 The presence or absence of double bonds between the carbon atoms is the major structural difference between saturated and unsaturated fatty acids. **A.** The saturated fatty acid palmitic acid has no double bonds in its carbon chain and contains the maximum number of hydrogen atoms. Without double bonds, the three saturated fatty acid chains fit together closely to form a "hard" fat. **B.** The three double bonds in linoleic acid, an unsaturated fatty acid, reduce the number of hydrogen atoms along the carbon chain. Insertion of double bonds into the carbon chain prevents close association of the fatty acids; this produces a "softer" fat or an oil. (Adapted with permission from McArdle WD, Katch FI, Katch VL. *Exercise Physiology: Nutrition, Energy, and Human Performance*. 8th Ed. Baltimore: Wolters Kluwer Health, 2015.)

SCFA and MCFA diffuse directly from the gastrointestinal tract into the portal vein without requirement for modification like LCFA, becoming quickly available for energy use. In contrast, LCFA require bile salts for digestion and incorporate into chylomicrons for transport through lymph for deposit as fat.

Dietary Fatty Acids

The average person in the United States consumes about 15% of total calories as saturated fats, equivalent to more than 50 lb of saturated fat annually. This contrasts with some indigenous tribes in Mexico, whose diets are high in complex, unrefined carbohydrate and typically contain only 2% of total calories as saturated fat. The strong relationship between saturated fatty acid intake and coronary heart disease risk has prompted health professionals to recommend replacing at least a portion of dietary saturated fatty acids with unsaturated fatty acids. Monounsaturated fatty acids lower coronary risk even below average levels. Include no more than 10% of total energy intake as saturated fatty acids, with the remainder distributed in equal amounts among saturated, polyunsaturated, and monounsaturated fatty acids.

fyi Saturated, Monounsaturated, and Polyunsaturated Fatty Acid Content in Common Fats and Oils in Grams per 100 g

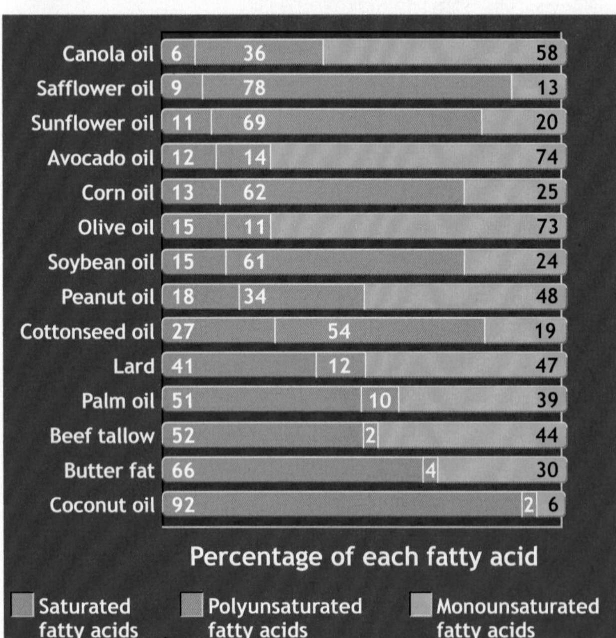

Source: Data from Food Composition Tables, U.S. Department of Agriculture; **www.ndb.nal.usda.gov.** Graph used with permission from McArdle WD, Katch FI, Katch VL. *Exercise Physiology: Nutrition, Energy, and Human Performance.* 8th Ed. Baltimore: Wolters Kluwer Health, 2015, based on U.S. Department of Agriculture data.

Compound Lipids

Compound lipids consist of neutral fat combined with phosphorus (phospholipids) or glucose (glucolipids). Another group of compound fats comprise the **lipoproteins.** These form primarily in the liver from the union of triacylglycerols, phospholipids, or cholesterol with protein. *Lipoproteins serve important functions because they constitute the main form for lipid transport in the blood.* If blood lipids did not bind to protein, they literally would float to the top like cream in nonhomogenized milk.

High- and Low-Density Lipoprotein Cholesterol

The four types of lipoproteins classify by their gravitational densities: chylomicrons, high density, low density, and very low density. Chylomicrons form after emulsified lipid droplets leave the small intestine and enter the lymphatic vasculature. Normally, the liver takes up chylomicrons, metabolizes them, and delivers them for storage to adipose tissue.

The liver and small intestine produce **high-density lipoprotein (HDL).** Of the lipoproteins, HDLs contain the greatest percentage of protein and the lowest total lipid and cholesterol. VLDL contains the greatest percentage of lipid. VLDLs transport triacylglycerols (formed in the liver from fats, carbohydrates, alcohol, and cholesterol) to muscle and adipose tissue. Degradation of a **very low density lipoprotein (VLDL)** produces a **low-density lipoprotein (LDL).** The enzyme lipoprotein lipase acts on VLDL to transform it to a denser LDL molecule with less lipid. LDL and VLDL contain the highest lipid and lowest protein content.

"Bad" Cholesterol (Low-Density Lipoprotein)

Among the lipoproteins, LDLs normally transport between 60% and 80% of total serum cholesterol. LDLs have the greatest affinity for cells located in the arterial wall. Here, the LDL oxidizes to ultimately participate in the proliferation of smooth muscle cells and other unfavorable changes that damage and narrow arteries. Three factors influence serum LDL concentration:

1. Regular physical activity
2. Visceral fat accumulation
3. Diet composition

"Good" Cholesterol (High-Density Lipoprotein): A Health Perspective

Unlike LDL, HDL operates as so-called "good" cholesterol to protect against heart disease. HDL, acting as a scavenger, facilitates the reverse transport of cholesterol, removing it from the arterial wall and transporting it to the liver where it joins in bile formation for excretion from the intestinal tract.

The amounts of LDL and HDL cholesterol and their specific ratios (e.g., HDL:total cholesterol) and subfractions provide more meaningful indicators of coronary artery disease risk than total blood cholesterol *per se.* Regular moderate- and high-intensity aerobic activity and abstinence from cigarette smoking increase HDL, lower LDL, and favorably alter the LDL:HDL ratio. The National Institutes of Health offers an online tool that calculates an adult's risk of having a heart attack, using total cholesterol and HDL cholesterol as input variables along with blood pressure, gender, and smoking status (**http://cvdrisk.nhlbi.nih.gov/calculator.asp**).

Derived Lipids

Derived lipids include substances formed from simple and compound lipids. **Cholesterol**, the most widely known derived lipid, exists *only* in animal tissue. Cholesterol does not contain fatty acids, yet shares some of the physical and chemical characteristics of lipids and, from a dietary viewpoint, is considered a lipid. Cholesterol, widespread in the plasma membrane of all animal cells, is obtained through either food intake (**exogenous cholesterol**) or synthesis within the body (**endogenous cholesterol**). Even if an individual attempts a "cholesterol-free" diet, endogenous cholesterol synthesis usually varies between 0.5 and 2.0 g (500 to 2000 mg · d^{-1}) daily. *The body forms more cholesterol with a high saturated fatty acid diet because saturated fat facilitates the liver's cholesterol synthesis.* Endogenous synthesis rate usually meets the body's needs; hence, severely reducing cholesterol intake, except in pregnant women and in infants who require exogenous cholesterol, causes little harm.

Cholesterol participates in many complex bodily processes, including the following five necessary functions:

1. Builds plasma membranes
2. Precursor in synthesizing vitamin D
3. Synthesizes adrenal gland hormones, including estrogen, androgen, and progesterone
4. Serves as a bile component (emulsifies lipids during digestion)
5. Helps tissues, organs, and body structures form during fetal development

Foods rich in cholesterol include egg yolks, red meats, organ meats (liver, kidney, brains), shellfish, and full-fat dairy products (ice cream, cream cheese, butter, whole milk). *Foods of plant origin contain no cholesterol.*

Figure 2.7 illustrates cholesterol dynamics in the body and highlights cholesterol transport via lipoproteins.

Trans Fatty Acids: The Unwanted Fat

The hydrogenation of unsaturated corn, soybean, or sunflower oil creates ***trans* fatty acids**. This fatty acid forms when one of the hydrogen atoms along the restructured carbon chain moves from its naturally occurring *cis* position to the opposite *trans* position side of the double bond that separates two carbon atoms. The richest *trans* fat sources include vegetable shortenings, some margarines, crackers, candies, cookies, snack foods, fried foods, baked goods, salad dressings, and other processed foods made with partially hydrogenated vegetable oils.

Health concern about *trans* fatty acids center on their possible detrimental effects on serum lipoproteins. A diet high in margarine and commercial baked goods like cookies, cakes, doughnuts, pies, and deep-fried foods prepared with hydrogenated vegetable oils increases LDL cholesterol concentration by a similar amount as a high saturated fatty acid diet. Unlike saturated fats, hydrogenated oils also decrease the concentration of beneficial HDL cholesterol. In light of the strong evidence that *trans* fatty acids place individuals at increased heart disease risk, the U.S. Food and Drug Administration (FDA; **www.fda.gov**) mandated that food producers, beginning in 2006, include the amount of *trans* fatty acid on their product nutrition labels.

In December, 2006, New York City became the nation's first city to enforce a ban on essentially all *trans* fats in foods prepared in its 24,000 eateries—from fast foods and delicatessens to five-star restaurants. A full statewide California ban on *trans* fat became law on January 1, 2010. Calgary, Canada, in June, 2008, was the first Canadian city to ban *trans* fats, requiring that *trans* fats in cooking oils cannot exceed 2% of the total fat content. Other European and Scandinavian countries have adopted strict rules for *trans* fat content in foods (**www.news-medical.net/health/Trans-Fat-Regulation.aspx**).

In March 2014, the FDA announced its preliminary determination that partially hydrogenated oils (PHOs), the primary dietary source of artificial *trans* fat in processed foods, are not "generally recognized as safe" for use in food, based on available scientific evidence and the findings of expert scientific panels. By 2020, the FDA plans to require the food industry to gradually phase out all *trans* fat from the food supply pending further investigation of the technical challenges to food suppliers to comply with this directive. Prior to the labeling requirement and limits placed on the use of *trans* fat, the FDA estimated that the average American had consumed approximately 2.2 kg of *trans* fats yearly.

fyi New U.S. Guidelines Lift Limits on Dietary Cholesterol

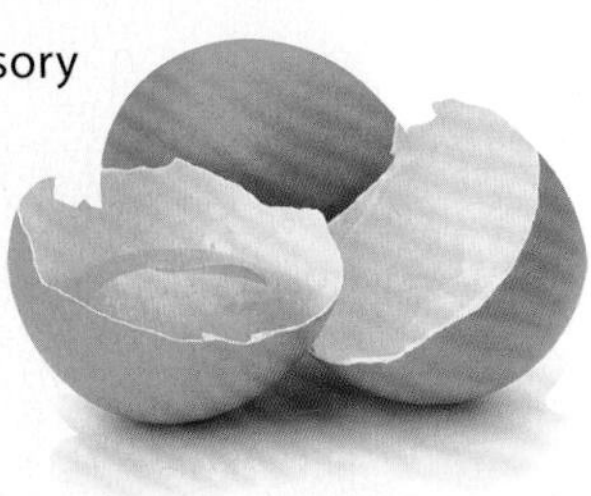

The Dietary Guidelines Advisory Committee (DGAC; **www.health.gov/dietaryguidelines/committee/**) has done a complete about-face regarding recommendations for dietary cholesterol intake by recommending that limits on dietary cholesterol be removed from the upcoming 2015 *Dietary Guidelines for Americans*. This represents a reversal of the cholesterol limitations that have been widely circulated since the 1960s. This is not to say that blood cholesterol level is unimportant as a health risk indicator. Rather, the scientific evidence indicates that only about 20% of your blood cholesterol level comes from dietary intake. The liver produces the rest of the body's cholesterol.

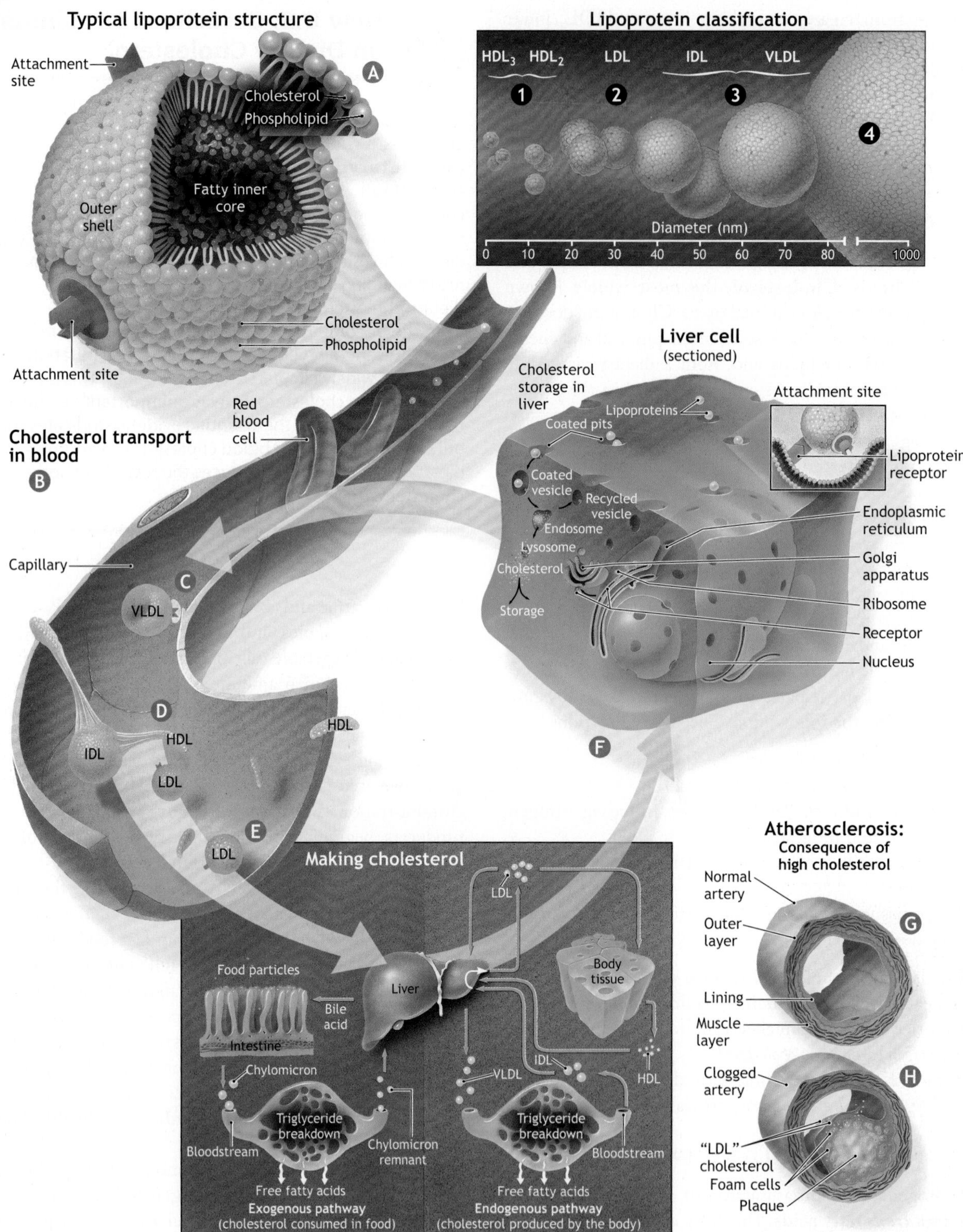

FIGURE 2.7 Cholesterol dynamics in the body. **A.** Lipoproteins are combined fat and protein particles that transport cholesterol throughout the body. **B.** Lipoproteins transport cholesterol via the bloodstream. **C.** The large VLDL particle attaches to the capillary lining where its cholesterol core is extracted. **D.** The smaller IDL particle remains in the blood for transport back to the liver for removal. **E.** LDL remains in the blood and travels back to the liver for removal. **F.** An excess of cholesterol reduces the lipoprotein receptor number on the liver cell surface. **G.** With normal blood cholesterol levels, arterial walls remain smooth and slippery. **H.** High blood cholesterol levels concentrate cholesterol in arterial walls, thereby reducing blood flow. Lipoprotein classification: 1, high-density lipoprotein (HDL); 2, low-density lipoprotein (LDL); 3, intermediate-density lipoprotein (IDL) and very low density lipoprotein (VLDL); 4, chylomicron, dietary cholesterol, and triacylglycerol particles absorbed by small intestine. (Adapted with permission from McArdle WD, Katch FI, Katch VL. *Exercise Physiology: Nutrition, Energy, and Human Performance*. 8th Ed. Baltimore: Wolters Kluwer Health, 2015, as adapted with permission from Anatomical Chart Company. © 2000 Anatomical Chart Company.)

Fish Consumption Is Healthful

Greenland Eskimos who consume lipids from fish, seal, and whale have a low incidence of coronary heart disease compared to other populations. Their general health profiles indicate that two long-chain polyunsaturated fatty acids, **eicosapentaenoic acid (EHA)** and **docosahexaenoic acid (DHA)**, confer health benefits. These oils belong to an omega-3 fatty acid family found primarily in the oils of shellfish and cold water herring, salmon, sardines, bluefish, mackerel, and sea mammals. **Omega-3 fatty acids**, particularly when consumed in fish, may prove beneficial in the treatment of diverse psychological disorders in addition to decreasing overall heart disease risk (chance of ventricular fibrillation and sudden death) and mortality rate, inflammatory disease risk, and, for smokers, the risk of contracting chronic obstructive pulmonary disease.

Several mechanisms explain how eating fish may protect against heart disease. The omega-3 fatty acids in fish may:

1. Serve as an antithrombogenic agent to prevent blood clot formation on arterial walls
2. Inhibit atherosclerotic plaque growth, reduce pulse pressure and total vascular resistance (increase arterial compliance), and stimulate endothelial-derived nitric oxide to facilitate myocardial perfusion (see Chapter 10)
3. Lower triacylglycerol and thus provide additional heart disease protection

Lipids in Food

Figure 2.8 shows the approximate percentage contribution of common food groups to the total lipid content of the typical American diet. Plant sources contribute about 34% to the daily lipid intake, and lipids of animal origin contribute the remaining 66%.

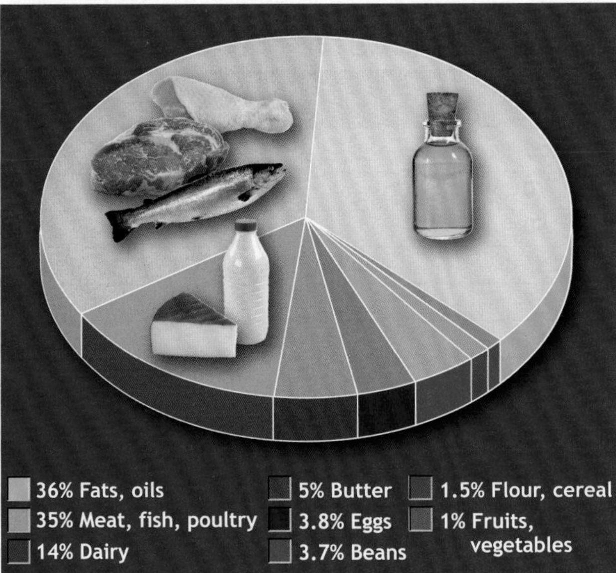

FIGURE 2.8 Contribution from the major food groups to the lipid content of the typical American diet. (Used with permission from McArdle WD, Katch FI, Katch VL. *Exercise Physiology: Nutrition, Energy, and Human Performance*. 8th Ed. Baltimore: Wolters Kluwer Health, 2015.)

Lipid's Role in the Body

Lipids serve four important functions in the body:

1. Energy reserve
2. Protect vital organs and promote thermal insulation
3. Transport medium for fat-soluble vitamins
4. Hunger suppressor

Energy Reserve

Fat constitutes the ideal cellular fuel for three reasons:

1. Each molecule carries large quantities of energy per unit weight.
2. Transports and stores easily
3. Provides a ready energy source

In well-nourished individuals at rest, fat can provide 80% to 90% of the body's energy requirements. Due to lipid's greater number of hydrogen atoms, 1 g of pure lipid contains about 9 kcal of energy, more than twice the energy available in 1 g of carbohydrate or protein.

Approximately 15% of the body mass for men and 25% for women consists of fat. **Figure 2.9** illustrates the total mass and energy content of fat in an 80-kg young adult man. The amount of fat in adipose tissue triacylglycerol translates to about 108,000 kcal. Most of this energy remains available for physical activity and would supply enough energy for a person to run the approximate 950-mile from Oklahoma City, OK to Tempe, AZ. This run assumes a theoretical energy expenditure of about 100 kcal per mile. Contrast this with the limited 2000 kcal reserve of stored glycogen that would provide only enough energy for a 20-mile run. Viewed from

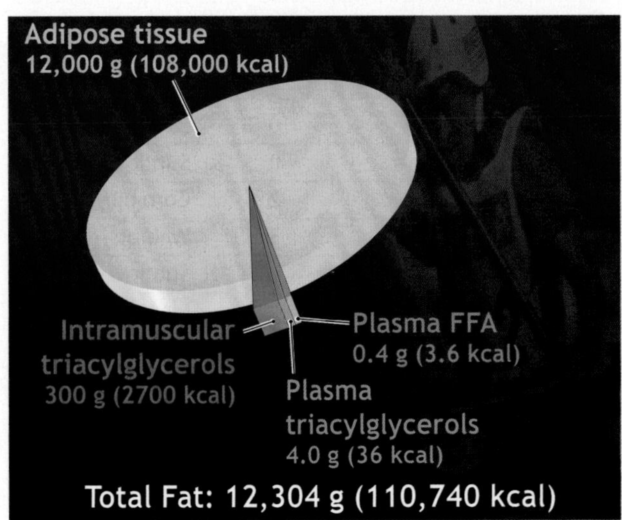

FIGURE 2.9 Distribution of the quantity and energy stored as fat within an average 80-kg man. FFA, free fatty acids. (Adapted with permission from McArdle WD, Katch FI, Katch VL. *Exercise Physiology: Nutrition, Energy, and Human Performance*. 8th Ed. Baltimore: Wolters Kluwer Health, 2015.)

a different perspective, the body's energy reserves from carbohydrate could power intense running for only about 1.6 hours, but the fat reserves would last 75 times longer or about 120 hours! As was the case for carbohydrates, fat as a fuel "spares" protein to carry out its important functions of tissue synthesis and repair.

Protection and Insulation

Up to 4% of the body's fat protects against trauma to the vital organs—heart, lungs, liver, kidneys, spleen, brain, and spinal cord. Fats stored just below the skin in the subcutaneous fat layer provide insulation, determining one's ability to tolerate exposure to cold extremes. This insulatory fat layer probably affords little protection except to deep-sea divers, or ocean swimmers, or others exposed to extremely cold environments. In contrast, excess body fat hinders temperature regulation during thermal stress, most notably during sustained physical activity in air, when the body's heat production can increase 20 times above resting levels. In this case, insulation from subcutaneous fat retards heat flow from the body.

Vitamin Carrier and Hunger Suppressor

Dietary lipid serves as a carrier and transport medium for the fat-soluble vitamins A, D, E, and K, which require about 20 g of dietary fat consumption daily. Voluntarily

TABLE 2.1 Examples of Foods High and Low in Saturated Fatty Acids, Foods High in Monounsaturated and Polyunsaturated Fatty Acids, and the Polyunsaturated to Saturated Fatty Acid (P/S) Ratio of Common Fats and Oils

High Saturated	%	High Monosaturated	%	Fats and Oils	P/S Ratio
Coconut oil	91	Olives, black	80	Coconut oil	0.2/1.0
Palm kernel oil	82	Olive oil	75	Palm oil	0.2/1.0
Butter	68	Almond oil	70	Butter	0.1/1.0
Cream cheese	57	Canola oil	61	Olive oil	0.6/1.0
Coconut	56	Almonds, dry	52	Lard	0.3/1.0
Hollandaise sauce	54	Avocados	51	Canola oil	5.3/1.0
Palm oil	51	Peanut oil	48	Peanut oil	1.9/1.0
Half and half	45	Cashews, dry roasted	42	Soybean oil	2.5/1.0
Cheese, Velveeta	43	Peanut butter	39	Sesame oil	3.0/1.0
Cheese, mozzarella	41	Bologna	39	Margarine, 100% corn oil	2.5/1.0
Ice cream, vanilla	38	Beef, cooked	33	Cottonseed oil	2.0/1.0
Cheesecake	32	Lamb, roasted	32	Mayonnaise	3.7/1.0
Chocolate almond bar	29	Veal, roasted	26	Safflower oil	13.3/1.0
Low Saturated	**%**	**High Polyunsaturated**	**%**		
Popcorn	0	Safflower oil	77		
Hard candy	0	Sunflower oil	70		
Yogurt, nonfat	2	Corn oil	58		
Crackerjacks	3	Walnuts, dry	51		
Milk, skim	4	Sunflower seeds	47		
Cookies, fig bars	4	Margarine, corn oil	45		
Graham crackers	5	Canola oil	32		
Chicken breast, roasted	6	Sesame seeds	31		
Pancakes	8	Pumpkin seeds	31		
Cottage cheese, 1%	8	Tofu	27		
Milk, chocolate, 1%	9	Lard	11		
Beef, dried	9	Butter	6		
Chocolate, mints	10	Coconut oil	2		

Data from the Science and Education Administration. *Home and Garden Bulletin 72, Nutritive Value of Foods*. Washington, DC: US Government Printing Office, 1985, 1986 (modified in 2009), **www.ars.usda.gov/Main/docs.htm?docid=6282**; Agricultural Research Service, United States Department of Agriculture. *Nutritive Value of American Foods in Common Units*. Agricultural Handbook no. 456. Washington, DC: US Government Printing Office, 1975.

reducing lipid intake concomitantly depresses these vitamin levels and may ultimately lead to vitamin deficiency. In addition, dietary lipid delays the onset of "hunger pangs" and contributes to satiety following meals because emptying lipid from the stomach takes about 3.5 hours after its ingestion. Thus, weight-loss diets that contain some lipid sometimes prove initially successful in blunting the urge to eat more than the heavily advertised extreme so-called "fat-free" diets.

Recommended Lipid Intake

In the United States, dietary lipid represents between 34% and 38% of total calorie intake. Most health professionals recommend that lipids should not exceed 30% of the diet's total energy content. Of this 30%, 70% should be in the form of unsaturated fatty acids.

For dietary cholesterol, the American Heart Association (**www.aha.org**) recommends that no more than 300 mg or 0.01 oz of cholesterol consumed daily, an intake equivalent to about 100 mg per 1000 kcal of consumed food or about 300 mg for the average person. The average American male consumes more than twice this amount.

Consume Lipids in Moderation

In the quest to achieve good health and optimal exercise performance, prudent practice entails cooking with and consuming lipids derived primarily from vegetable sources containing large amounts of unsaturated fatty acids. This approach may be too simplistic, however, because total fat intake, even unsaturated fatty acid intake, constitutes a diabetes and heart disease risk. If so, then one should reduce the intake of all lipids, *particularly* those high in saturated and *trans* fatty acids. Concerns also exist over the association of high-fat diets with ovarian, colon, endometrium, and other cancers.

Table 2.1 lists the saturated, monounsaturated, and polyunsaturated fatty acid content of various dietary lipids sources. All fats contain a mix of each fatty acid type, yet different fatty acids predominate in certain foods. Several polyunsaturated fatty acids, most prominently linoleic acid present in cooking and salad oils, must be consumed because they serve as precursors of *essential fatty acids* the body cannot synthesize. Humans require about 1% to 2% of total energy intake from linoleic acid, an omega-6 fatty acid. The best sources for alpha-linolenic acid or one of its related omega-3 fatty acids, EPA and DHA, include cold water salmon, tuna, or sardines; canola, soybean, safflower, sunflower, and sesame oils; and flax.

Contribution of Fat During Physical Activity

The contribution of fat to the energy requirements of physical activity depends on two factors:

1. Fatty acid release from triacylglycerols in fat storage sites

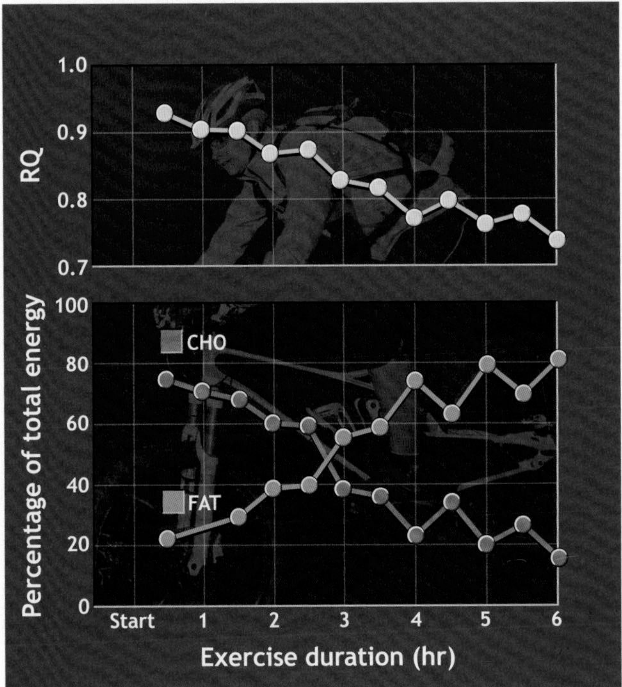

FIGURE 2.10 The relationship between respiratory quotient (RQ) and substrate use during long-duration, submaximal exercise. (**Top**) Progressive reduction in RQ during 6 hour of continuous exercise. (**Bottom**) Percentage of energy derived from carbohydrate and fat. (Used with permission from McArdle WD, Katch FI, Katch VL. *Exercise Physiology: Nutrition, Energy, and Human Performance*. 8th Ed. Baltimore: Wolters Kluwer Health, 2015, as adapted with permission from Edwards HT, et al. Metabolic rate, blood sugar and utilization of carbohydrate. *Am J Physiol* 1934;108:203.)

2. Delivery in the circulation to muscle tissue as free fatty acids (FFA) bound to blood albumin

Triacylglycerols stored within the muscle cell also contribute to exercise energy metabolism. **Figure 2.10** shows that FFA uptake by active muscle increases during hours 1 and 4 of moderate activity. In the first hour, fat (including intramuscular fat) supplies about 50% of the energy; by the 3rd hour, fat contributes up to 70% of the total energy requirement. *With greater dependence on fat catabolism (e.g., with carbohydrate depletion), intensity decreases to a level governed by the body's capacity to mobilize and oxidize fat.*

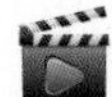 See the animation "Fat Mobilization and Use" on **http://thePoint.lww.com/MKKESS5e** for a demonstration of this process.

PROTEINS

A normal-size adult contains between 10 and 12 kg of protein, primarily within skeletal muscle. The caloric equivalent for this protein mass ranges between 18,160 and 21,792 kcal (1 kg = 454 g; 1 g protein = 4 kcal. Thus, 454 × 4 = 1816 kcal × 10 kg = 18,160 kcal). Structurally, proteins resemble carbohydrates and lipids because they contain atoms of carbon, oxygen, and hydrogen. They differ because they also contain nitrogen (~16% of the molecule) along with sulfur and occasionally phosphorus, cobalt, and iron.

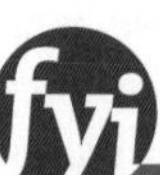

The Nine Essential Amino Acids and Common Food Sources

1. Histidine (breast milk; soybeans, fish, chicken breasts, beef, wheat germ)
2. Leucine (egg white, soy, seaweed, spirulina)
3. Lysine (chicken, turkey, tuna, black beans, lentils, garbanzo beans)
4. Isoleucine (egg white, soy, seaweed, spirulina, turkey)
5. Methionine (egg white, fish, chicken, sesame flour, turnips, sunflowers)
6. Phenylalanine (pork, beef, lamb, veal, fish, tofu, swiss chard)
7. Threonine (watercress, seaweed, spirulina, game meat, turkey, fish)
8. Tryptophan (fatty fish, game meat, seaweed, spirulina, soy protein isolate, spinach, egg white)
9. Valine (egg white, game meat, seaweed, spirulina, soy protein isolate, watercress)

Amino Acids

Protein forms from amino acid "building-block" linkages. Peptide bonds join amino acids in chains representing diverse forms and chemical combinations; combining two amino acids produces a dipeptide, and three amino acids linked together form a tripeptide. Combining more than 50 amino acids forms a polypeptide protein of which humans can synthesize about 80,000 different kinds. A **polypeptide** may contain a linear configuration of up to 1000 amino acids. Whereas single cells contain thousands of different protein molecules, the body contains approximately 50,000 different protein-containing compounds. The biochemical functions and properties of each protein depend on the sequencing of its specific amino acids.

Figure 2.11 shows the four common features that constitute the general structure of all amino acids. Of the 20 different amino acids required by the body, each contains a positively charged amine group at one end and a negatively charged organic acid group at the opposite end. The amine group combines 2 hydrogen atoms attached to nitrogen (NH_2). The organic acid group, technically termed a carboxylic acid group, joins 1 carbon atom, 2 oxygen atoms, and 1 atom of hydrogen; it is symbolized chemically as COOH. The remainder of the amino acid molecule contains a side chain specific to each amino acid. *The unique structure of the side chain dictates the amino acid's particular characteristics.*

Essential and Nonessential Amino Acids

Tens of thousands of the same amino acids may combine in a single protein compound. Of the different amino acids, the body cannot synthesize eight (nine in infants) at a sufficient rate to prevent impairment of normal cellular function. These make up the indispensable or **essential amino acids** because they must be ingested preformed in foods. The body manufactures the remaining 12 **nonessential amino acids**. This does not mean they are unimportant; rather, they form from compounds already existing in the body at a rate that meets demands for normal growth and tissue repair.

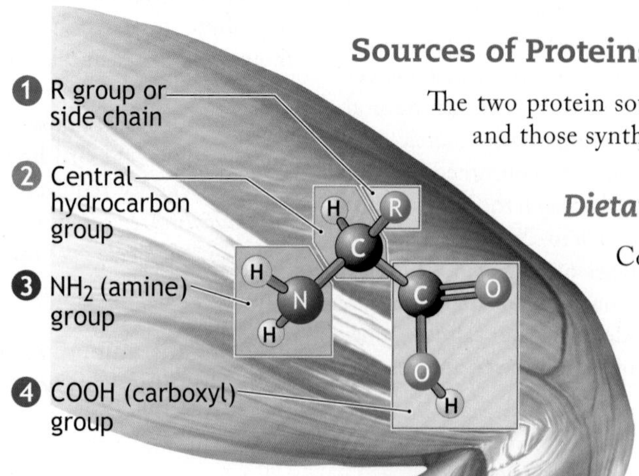

Animals and plants manufacture proteins that contain essential amino acids. *No health or physiological advantage comes from an amino acid derived from an animal compared with the same amino acid derived from vegetable origin.* Plants synthesize protein, and thus amino acids, by incorporating nitrogen from the soil along with carbon, oxygen, and hydrogen from air and water. In contrast, animals do not possess a broad capability for protein synthesis; they obtain much of their protein from ingested sources.

Constructing a body protein requires specific amino acid availability at the time of protein synthesis. **Complete proteins** come from foods with all of the essential amino acids in their correct ratio. This maintains protein balance and allows tissue growth and repair. An **incomplete protein** lacks one or more of the essential amino acids. Diets that contain mostly incomplete protein eventually produce protein malnutrition despite the food source's adequacy for energy and protein quantity.

Sources of Proteins

The two protein sources include those in the diet and those synthesized in the body.

Dietary Sources

Complete proteins are present in eggs, milk, meat, fish, and poultry. Eggs provide the optimal mixture of essential amino acids among food sources; hence, eggs receive the highest quality rating for protein compared with other foods. Presently, almost two thirds of dietary protein in the United States comes from animal sources, whereas a century ago, protein consumption occurred equally

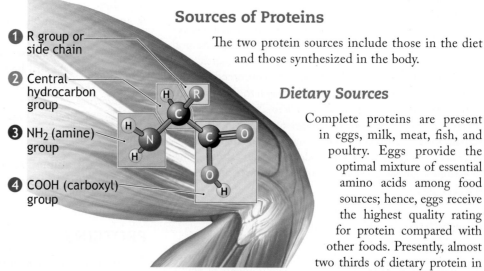

1 R group or side chain
2 Central hydrocarbon group
3 NH_2 (amine) group
4 COOH (carboxyl) group

FIGURE 2.11 Four common features of amino acids. (Adapted with permission from McArdle WD, Katch FI, Katch VL. *Exercise Physiology: Nutrition, Energy, and Human Performance*. 8th Ed. Baltimore: Wolters Kluwer Health, 2015.)

TABLE 2.2 Rating of Common Sources of Dietary Protein

Food	Protein Rating
Eggs	100
Fish	70
Lean beef	69
Cow's milk	60
Brown rice	57
White rice	56
Soybeans	47
Brewer's hash	45
Whole-grain wheat	44
Peanuts	43
Dry beans	34
White potato	34

from plants and animals. Reliance on animal sources for dietary protein accounts for the high current intake of cholesterol and saturated fatty acids.

The **"biologic value"** or protein rating of food refers to its completeness for supplying essential amino acids. Animal sources contribute high-quality protein, whereas lentils, dried beans and peas, nuts, and cereals remain incomplete in one or more of the essential amino acids; these rate lower in biologic value. Eating a variety of grains, fruits, and vegetables, each providing a different quality and quantity of amino acids, contributes all of the required essential amino acids. **Table 2.2** lists examples of common food sources of protein and their relative protein rating.

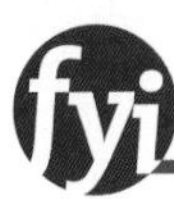

Egg White or Egg Yolks for Health?

Egg Whites

Low-calorie (17 kcal), fat-free food containing the bulk of the egg's protein (4 g); also contain 55 mg sodium, 53.8 mg potassium, 4.9 mg phosphorus, 3.6 mg magnesium, 2.3 mg calcium, 1.3 mcg folate, and 6.6 mcg selenium.

VS.

Egg Yolks

Contain the egg's cholesterol, saturated fat, fat-soluble vitamins, and essential fatty acids. One egg yolk contains about 55 kcal, 4.5 g total fat, 2.7 g protein, 1.6 g saturated fat, 210 mg cholesterol, and 8 mg sodium.

Synthesis in the Body

Enzymes in muscle facilitate nitrogen removal from certain amino acids and subsequently pass nitrogen to other compounds in the biochemical reactions of **transamination** (see **Fig. 2.12**). An amine group shifts from a donor amino acid to an acceptor acid, while the acceptor becomes a new amino acid. *This allows amino acids to form from non–nitrogen-carrying organic compounds generated in metabolism.*

Deamination represents the opposite process to transamination. It involves removing an amine group from the amino acid molecule, with the remaining carbon skeleton converting to a carbohydrate or lipid or being used for energy. The cleaved amine group forms urea in the liver for excretion by the kidneys. Urea must dissolve in water, so excessive protein catabolism involving increased deamination promotes fluid loss.

See the animation "Transamination" on **http://thePoint.lww.com/MKKESS5e** for a demonstration of this process.

For deamination and transamination, the remaining carbon skeleton of the nonnitrogenous amino acid residue further degrades during energy metabolism. In well-nourished individuals at rest, the breakdown or **catabolism** of protein contributes between 2% and 5% of the body's total energy requirement. During catabolism, protein first degrades into its amino acid components. The liver then strips the nitrogen from the amino acid molecule for excretion as urea via deamination.

Protein's Important Roles in the Body

No body "reservoirs" of protein exist; all protein contributes to tissue structures or exists as constituents of metabolic, transport, and hormonal systems. Protein constitutes between 12% and 15% of the body mass, but its content varies considerably in different cells. Brain cells, for example, contain only about 10% protein, but protein represents up to 20% of the mass of red blood cells and muscle cells. The systematic application of resistance training increases skeletal muscle's protein content, which represents about 65% of the body's total protein.

Fate of Amino Acids After Nitrogen Removal

Following deamination, the remaining carbon skeletons of the α-ketoacids such as pyruvate, oxaloacetate, or α-ketoglutarate follow one of three distinct biochemical routes:

1. *Gluconeogenesis*—18 of the 20 amino acids serve as a source for glucose synthesis.
2. *Energy source*—The carbon skeletons oxidize for energy because they form intermediates in citric acid cycle metabolism or related molecules.
3. *Fat synthesis*—All amino acids provide a potential source of acetyl-CoA to furnish substrate to synthesize fatty acids.

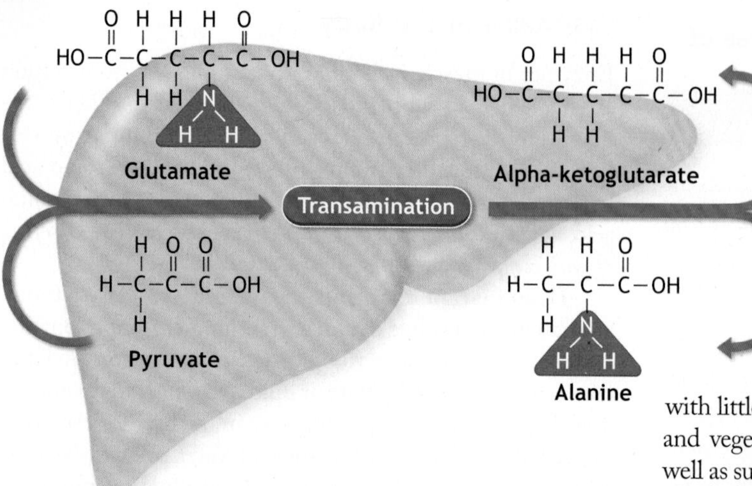

FIGURE 2.12 The biochemical process of transamination provides for the intramuscular synthesis of amino acids from nonprotein sources. An amine group from a donor group transfers to an acceptor, non-nitrogen-containing acid to form a new amino acid.

Amino acids provide the building blocks to synthesize:

- RNA and DNA
- The heme components of the oxygen-binding hemoglobin and myoglobin compounds
- The catecholamine hormones epinephrine and norepinephrine and the neurotransmitter serotonin

Amino acids also activate vitamins that play a key role in metabolic and physiologic regulation.

Tissue synthesis (anabolism) accounts for more than one third of the protein intake during rapid growth in infancy and childhood. As growth rate declines, so does the percentage of protein retained for anabolic processes. Continual turnover of tissue protein occurs when a person attains optimal body size and growth stabilizes. Adequate protein intake replaces the amino acids continually degraded in the turnover process.

Proteins serve as primary constituents for plasma membranes and internal cellular material. Proteins within cell nuclei called nucleoproteins "supervise" cellular protein synthesis and transmit hereditary characteristics. Structural proteins serve as key components in hair, skin, nails, bones, tendons, and ligaments; globular proteins constitute the nearly 2000 different enzymes that dramatically accelerate chemical reactions and regulate the catabolism of fats, carbohydrates, and proteins during energy release. Proteins also regulate the acid-base quality of body fluids, which contributes to neutralizing or buffering excess acid metabolites formed during vigorous physical exertion.

Vegetarian Approach to Sound Nutrition

True vegetarians (**vegans**) consume nutrients from only two sources—plants and dietary supplements. Nearly 10% of Americans consider themselves "almost" vegetarians, although true vegans represent fewer than 1% of the US population.

An increasing number of competitive and champion athletes consume diets consisting predominately of nutrients from varied plant sources. Considering the time required for training and competition, athletes often encounter difficulty in planning, selecting, and preparing nutritious meals from predominantly plant sources without relying on supplementation. The fact remains that two thirds of the world's population subsists on largely vegetarian diets with little reliance on animal protein. Well-balanced vegetarian and vegetarian-type diets provide abundant carbohydrates, as well as sufficient fat and protein, crucial when training intensely. Vegetarian-type diets demonstrate these five characteristics:

1. Usually low or devoid of cholesterol
2. Relatively high in fiber
3. Relatively high in plant protein
4. Relatively low in saturated and relatively high in unsaturated fatty acids
5. Relatively rich in fruit and vegetable sources of antioxidant vitamins and phytochemicals

A **lactovegetarian** diet includes milk and related dairy products—ice cream, cheese, and yogurt. The lactovegetarian approach increases calcium, phosphorus, and vitamin B_{12} intake; the latter produced by bacteria in the digestive tract of animals. An **ovolactovegetarian** diet includes eggs to the diet.

Good meatless iron sources include fortified ready-to-eat cereals, soybeans, and cooked farina (fine flour or meal from cereal grains or starch), and cereals and wheat germ contain a relatively high concentration of zinc.

Figure 2.13 displays the contribution of various food groups to the protein content of the American diet. By far, the greatest protein intake comes from animal sources, with only about 30% from the plant kingdom.

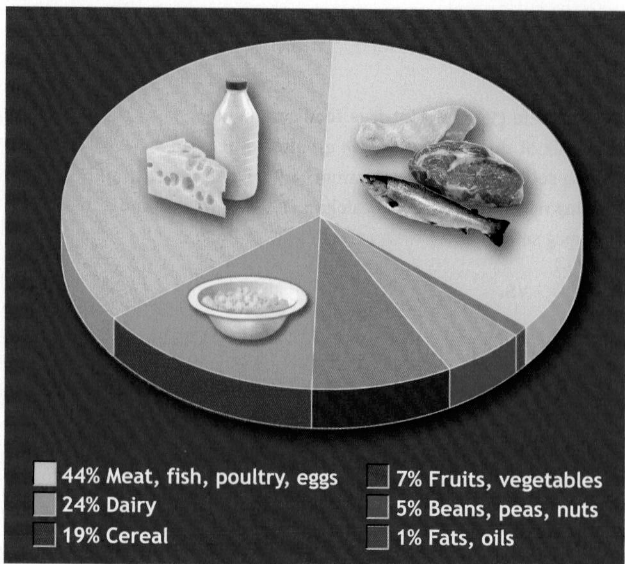

FIGURE 2.13 Contribution from the major food sources to the protein content of the typical American diet.

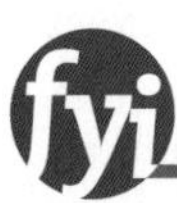

Do Vegetarians Consume Enough Protein?

In 2013, the largest study of its kind compared differences in nutrient profiles between nonvegetarians, semivegetarians, pescovegetarians, ovolactovegetarians, and strict vegetarians. Subjects included 71,751 participants (mean age 59). Nonvegetarians had the lowest intakes of plant proteins, fiber, β-carotene, and magnesium and the highest intakes of saturated, *trans*, arachidonic, and docosahexaenoic fatty acids compared with those following vegetarian dietary patterns. Vegetarians had the lowest caloric intake, yet their total daily protein intake was within 5% of the nonvegetarian group intake. All groups exceeded the recommended protein intake, averaging in excess of 70 g · d^{-1}, a value almost twice the recommended value.

Rizzo NS, et al. Nutrient profiles of vegetarian and nonvegetarian dietary patterns. *J Acad Nutr Diet* 2013;113:1610.

Recommended Protein Intake

Protein intake that exceeds three times the recommended level does not enhance physical activity capacity during intensive training or subsequent sports performance. *For athletes, muscle mass does not increase simply by eating high-protein foods.* If lean tissue synthesis resulted from all the extra protein intake consumed by the typical athlete, then muscle mass would increase tremendously. For example, eating an extra 100 g or 400 kcal of protein daily would translate to a daily 500-g (1.1-lb) increase in muscle mass. This obviously does not happen. Additional dietary protein, after deamination, provides for energy or recycles as components of other molecules including stored fat. Dietary protein intake substantially above recommended values can prove harmful because excessive protein breakdown strains liver and kidney function from production and elimination of urea and other solutes.

Table 2.3 lists the **recommended protein requirements** for adolescent and adult men and women. On average, 0.83 g protein per kg body mass represents the recommended daily intake. To determine the protein requirement for men and women ages 18 to 65, multiply body mass in kg by 0.83. For a 90-kg man, the total protein requirement equals 75 g (90 × 0.83). The protein requirement holds even for overweight people; it includes a reserve of about 25% to account for individual differences in protein requirements for about 98% of the population. Generally, aging decreases the protein requirement and quantity of the required essential amino acids. In contrast, the protein required for infants and growing children equals 2.0 to 4.0 g per kg body mass to facilitate growth and development. During pregnancy, women should increase their daily protein intake by 20 g · d^{-1}, and nursing mothers should increase intake by 10 g · d^{-1}. *A 10% increase in the calculated protein requirement, particularly for a vegetarian-type diet, accounts for dietary fiber's effect in reducing the digestibility of many plant-based protein sources.* Stress, disease, and injury also increase protein requirements.

Protein Requirements for Physically Active People

Any discussion of protein requirements must include the assumption of adequate energy intake to match the added physical activity needs. *If energy intake falls below the total energy expended during intense training, even augmented protein intake above recommended values may fail to maintain nitrogen balance.* This holds true because a disproportionate quantity of dietary protein catabolizes to balance an energy deficit rather than augment tissue maintenance and muscle development.

The common practice among weightlifters, bodybuilders, and other power athletes who consume liquids, powders, or pills made of predigested protein represents a waste of money and actually may be counterproductive to achieve the intended outcome. For example, many preparations contain proteins predigested to simple amino acids through chemical action in the laboratory. Simple amino acids do not absorb more easily or facilitate muscle growth. The small intestine absorbs amino acids rapidly when part of more complex dipeptide and tripeptide molecules. The intestinal tract handles proteins effectively in their more complex form. In contrast, a concentrated amino acid solution draws water into the small intestine, which in susceptible individuals can cause irritation, cramping, and diarrhea.

Researchers have questioned the necessity of advocating a larger protein requirement for these three athlete groups:

TABLE 2.3 Recommended Protein Intake for Adolescent and Adult Men and Women

Recommended Amount	Men		Women	
	Adolescent	Adult	Adolescent	Adult
Grams of protein per kg of body weight	0.9	0.8	0.9	0.8
Grams of protein per day based on average weight[a]	59.0	56.0	50.0	44.0

[a]Average weight is based on a "reference" man and woman. For adolescents (ages 14–18), the average weight equals 65.8 kg (145 lb) for young men and 55.7 kg (123 lb) for young women. For adult men, the average weight equals 70 kg (154 lb); for adult women, the average weight equals 56.8 kg (125 lb).

1. Growing and maturing adolescent athletes
2. Athletes involved in resistance training (to enhance muscle growth) and endurance training programs (to counter increased protein breakdown for energy)
3. Wrestlers and football players subjected to recurring muscle trauma

Inadequate protein intake can reduce body protein, particularly from muscle, with concomitant impaired performance. If athletes do require additional protein, then more than likely, their increased food intake would compensate for training's increased energy expenditure. Nonetheless, this may not occur in athletes with poor nutritional habits or who voluntarily restrict food consumption (dieting) and reduce their energy intake to hopefully gain a competitive advantage.

Do Athletes Require More Protein?

Much of the current understanding of protein dynamics and physical activity comes from studies that have expanded the classic method of determining protein breakdown through urea excretion. The output of "labeled" CO_2 from amino acids, either injected or ingested, increases during physical activity in proportion to the metabolic rate. As exertion level increases, plasma urea concentration also increases, coupled with a dramatic increase in nitrogen excretion in sweat without substantially altering urinary nitrogen excretion. The sweat mechanism helps to excrete nitrogen produced from protein breakdown during physical activity. Furthermore, plasma and intracellular amino acid oxidation increases significantly during moderate activity independent of changes in urea production. Protein use for energy reaches its highest level when subjects exercise in a glycogen-depleted state. This emphasizes the important role of carbohydrate as a protein sparer, meaning that carbohydrate availability impacts the demand on protein "reserves" during physical activity. Protein breakdown and accompanying gluconeogenesis undoubtedly become important factors in endurance activity and frequent intense training when glycogen reserves diminish. Eating a high-carbohydrate diet with adequate energy intake preserves muscle protein during intense training for protracted durations.

We *recommend that athletes who train intensely on a daily basis consume between 1.2 and 1.8 g of protein per kg of body mass, and not more than 2.0 g per kg of body mass.* This protein intake falls within the range typically consumed by physically active men and women, obviating the need to consume over-the-counter protein supplements. With adequate protein intake, consuming animal sources of protein does *not* facilitate muscle strength or size gains with resistance training compared with protein intake from plant sources.

SUMMARY

1. Carbon, hydrogen, oxygen, and nitrogen represent the primary structural units for most of the body's biologically active substances.
2. Proteins consist of combinations of carbon, oxygen, and hydrogen, including nitrogen and minerals.
3. Simple sugars consist of chains of from 3 to 7 carbon atoms with hydrogen and oxygen in a 2:1 ratio.
4. Glucose, the most common simple sugar, contains a 6-carbon chain, $C_6H_{12}O_6$.
5. Three classifications that define carbohydrates include monosaccharides, disaccharides, and polysaccharides.
6. Glycogenolysis reconverts glycogen to glucose.
7. Gluconeogenesis synthesizes glucose largely from the carbon skeletons of amino acids.
8. Fiber, a nonstarch, structural plant polysaccharide, provides resistance to human digestive enzymes.
9. Americans typically consume 40% to 50% of their total calories as carbohydrates, with about half as sucrose and high-fructose corn syrup.
10. Carbohydrates, stored in limited quantity in liver and muscle, serve four important functions: major source of energy, spares protein breakdown, metabolic primer for fat metabolism, and fuel for the central nervous system.
11. Muscle glycogen and blood glucose serve as primary fuels for intense physical activity.
12. The body's glycogen stores provide energy in sustained, intense aerobic marathon running, triathlon-type events, long-distance cycling, and endurance swimming.
13. A carbohydrate-deficient diet rapidly depletes muscle and liver glycogen, profoundly impacting capacity for both intense anaerobic activity and long-duration aerobic activity.
14. Individuals who exercise regularly should consume at least 60% of their daily calories as carbohydrates (400 to 600 g), predominantly in unrefined, fiber-rich complex forms.
15. A lipid contains carbon, hydrogen, and oxygen atoms and consists of one glycerol molecule with three fatty acid molecules.
16. Plants and animals synthesize lipids into one of three groups—simple lipids, compound lipids, and derived lipids.
17. Saturated fatty acids are considered saturated relative to hydrogen because they contain as many hydrogens as chemically possible.
18. Consistently consuming foods high in saturated fatty acids can elevate blood cholesterol and, over a lifetime, perhaps accelerate coronary heart disease.
19. Unsaturated fatty acids contain fewer hydrogen atoms attached to the carbon chain and exist as monounsaturated or polyunsaturated relative to hydrogen.
20. Dietary lipid represents 34% to 38% of the typical person's total caloric intake.
21. Prudent lipid recommendations suggest a 30% level or lower of total energy intake, of which 70% to 80% of these lipids should consist of unsaturated fatty acids.
22. Lipids provide the largest nutrient store of potential energy for biologic work. They protect vital organs, provide insulation from cold, transport fat-soluble vitamins, and depress hunger.

23. During light and moderate physical activity, fat contributes about 50% of the energy requirement. As activity continues, fat becomes more important, supplying more than 70% of the body's energy needs.
24. Proteins differ chemically from lipids and carbohydrates because they contain nitrogen in addition to sulfur, phosphorus, and iron.
25. The body requires 20 different amino acids to form proteins from specific amino acid subunits.
26. The body cannot synthesize all of the 20 amino acids and some must be consumed in the diet; for that reason, they are called essential amino acids.
27. Complete, higher-quality proteins contain all the essential amino acids; the other protein type represents incomplete or lower-quality proteins.
28. Consuming a variety of plant-based foods provides all the essential amino acids because each food source contains a different quality and quantity of amino acids.
29. For adults, the recommended protein intake equals 0.83 g per kg of body mass.
30. Protein breakdown above the resting level occurs during endurance and resistance-training exercise to a degree greater than previously believed.
31. Athletes who train intensely 2 to 6 $h \cdot d^{-1}$ should consume between 1.2 and 1.8 g of protein per kg of body mass.
32. Reduced carbohydrate reserves from either diet or exercise increase protein catabolism, making it imperative to maintain optimal levels of glycogen during strenuous training.

THINK IT THROUGH

1. Outline a presentation to a high school class about how to eat "well" for a physically active, healthy lifestyle.
2. Many college students do not eat well-balanced meals. Give three recommendations concerning macronutrient intake to ensure proper energy reserves for moderate and intense physical activities.
3. Explain the importance of regular carbohydrate intake when maintaining a high level of daily physical activity.
4. Discuss three "nonexercise" health benefits for a diet rich in food sources containing unrefined, complex carbohydrates.
5. Discuss a rationale for recommending adequate carbohydrate intake, rather than excess protein, for a person who wants to increase muscle mass through a structured resistance-training regimen.
6. What two benefits derive from storing excess calories as fat in adipose tissue compared to storing an equivalent caloric excess as glycogen?
7. Outline three reasons why exercise physiologists debate the adequacy of the current protein RDA for individuals involved in intense training.

PART 2 Micronutrients: Facilitators of Energy Transfer and Tissue Synthesis

VITAMINS

The Nature of Vitamins

The formal discovery of vitamins at the beginning of the 20th century revealed that the body requires essential organic substances in minute amounts to perform highly specific metabolic functions. Contrary to popular belief, vitamins do *not* supply energy, serve as basic building units for other compounds, or contribute substantially to the body's mass. Rather, humans require a steady stream of vitamins in the daily diet to maintain optimal physiological function. A prolonged inadequate intake of a particular vitamin can trigger vitamin deficiency symptoms and lead to severe medical complications. For example, symptoms of thiamin deficiency occur after only 2 weeks on a thiamin-free diet, and symptoms of vitamin C deficiency appear after 3 or 4 weeks. At the other extreme, consuming an excess of the fat-soluble vitamins A, D, E, and K can produce a toxic overdose manifested by hair loss, irregularities in bone formation, fetal malformation, hemorrhage, bone fractures, abnormal liver function, and ultimately death.

Vitamin Classification

Thirteen different vitamins have been isolated, analyzed, classified, and synthesized and recommended intake levels established. Vitamins classify as either fat soluble or water soluble. The fat-soluble vitamins are vitamins A, D, E, and K. The water-soluble vitamins are vitamin C, the B-complex vitamins (vitamin B_6 [pyridoxine], vitamin B_1 [thiamin], vitamin B_2 [riboflavin], niacin [nicotinic acid], pantothenic acid, biotin, folic acid, and vitamin B_{12} [cobalamin]).

Fat-Soluble Vitamins

Fat-soluble vitamins dissolve and are stored in the body's fatty tissues. In fact, symptoms of fat-soluble vitamin insufficiency may not appear for decades. Dietary lipid provides the source of fat-soluble vitamins. Whereas the liver stores vitamins A, D, and K, vitamin E distributes throughout the body's fatty tissues. Prolonged intake of a "fat-free" diet accelerates a fat-soluble vitamin insufficiency. **Table 2.4** lists the major bodily functions, dietary sources, and symptoms of a deficiency or excess for the fat-soluble vitamins for men and women ages 19 to 50 years. Chapter 3 discusses the dietary reference intakes (DRIs), including tolerable upper intake levels for all vitamins and minerals for different life-stage groups.

TABLE 2.4 Food Sources, Major Bodily Functions, and Symptoms of Deficiency or Excess of the Fat-Soluble Vitamins for Healthy Adults (Ages 19–50 Years)[a]

Vitamin	Dietary Sources	Major Bodily Functions	Deficiency	Excess
Vitamin A (retinol)	Provitamin A (beta-carotene) widely distributed in green vegetables; retinol present in milk, butter, cheese, fortified margarine	Constituent of rhodopsin (visual pigment); maintenance of epithelial tissues; role in mucopolysaccharide synthesis	Xerophthalmia (keratinization of ocular tissue), night blindness, permanent blindness	Headache, vomiting, peeling of skin, anorexia, swelling of long bones
Vitamin D	Cod liver oil, eggs, dairy products, fortified milk, and margarine	Promotes growth and mineralization of bones; increases absorption of calcium	Rickets (bone deformities) in children, osteomalacia in adults	Vomiting, diarrhea, weight loss, kidney damage
Vitamin E (tocopherol)	Seeds, green leafy vegetables, margarines, shortenings	Functions as an anti-oxidant to prevent cell damage	Possibly anemia	Relatively nontoxic
Vitamin K (phylloquinone)	Green leafy vegetables, small amount in cereals, fruits, and meats	Important in blood clotting (helps form active prothrombin)	Conditioned deficiencies associated with severe bleeding, internal hemorrhages	Relatively nontoxic; synthetic forms at high doses may cause jaundice

[a]Food and Nutrition Board, National Academy of Sciences. 2009. Available at **www.nal.usda.gov/fnic/etext/000105.html**. This website provides interactive dietary reference intakes for health professionals.

Water-Soluble Vitamins

Vitamin C (ascorbic acid) and the B-complex group constitute the nine **water-soluble vitamins**. They act largely as **coenzymes**—small molecules that combine with a larger protein compound (apoenzyme) to form an active enzyme that accelerates chemical compound interconversions. Coenzymes participate directly in chemical reactions; when the reaction runs its course, coenzymes remain intact and participate in yet further reactions. Water-soluble vitamins play a crucial role as part of coenzymes in the cells' energy-generating reactions.

Water-soluble vitamins disperse in the body fluids without appreciable storage because of their water solubility, with any excess voided in urine. If the diet regularly contains less than 50% of the recommended values for water-soluble vitamins, marginal deficiencies may develop within 4 weeks. **Table 2.5** summarizes food sources, major bodily functions, and symptoms from a water-soluble vitamin excess. The B-complex vitamins serve as coenzymes in energy-yielding reactions during carbohydrate, fat, and protein catabolism. They also contribute to hemoglobin synthesis and red blood cell formation.

Vitamin Toxicity

Excess vitamins function as potentially harmful chemicals once enzyme systems catalyzed by specific vitamins become saturated. A higher likelihood exists for "overdosing" with fat-soluble than water-soluble vitamins. Adverse reactions occur at a lower level with fat-soluble vitamins than with water-soluble vitamins. For this reason, fat-soluble vitamins should not be consumed in excess without medical supervision. Women who consume excess vitamin A early in pregnancy (as retinol but not in the provitamin carotene form) increase infant birth defect risk. Excessive vitamin A accumulation, called **hypervitaminosis A**, causes irritability, bone swelling, weight loss, and dry, itchy skin in young children. In adults, symptoms include nausea, headache, drowsiness, hair loss, diarrhea, and bone brittleness from calcium loss. Discontinuing excessive vitamin A consumption reverses these symptoms. Regular excess vitamin D can damage kidneys. An "overdose" from vitamins E and K rarely occurs, but intakes above the recommended level provide *no* health or fitness benefits.

Vitamins' Role in the Body

Vitamins contain no useful energy for the body; instead, they link and regulate the sequence of metabolic reactions that release energy within food molecules. They also play an intimate role in tissue synthesis and other biologic processes. A vitamin participates repeatedly in metabolic reactions regardless of the person's physical activity level. This means that the vitamin needs of athletes do not exceed those of sedentary counterparts. **Figure 2.14** summarizes the important biologic functions of vitamins in the body.

Physically active individuals need not consume special foods or supplements that increase the diet's vitamin content above established requirements. At high levels of daily physical activity, food intake usually increases to sustain the activity's added energy requirements. Additional food consumed through nutritious meals proportionately increases vitamin and mineral intake.

TABLE 2.5 Food Sources, Major Bodily Functions, and Symptoms of Deficiency or Excess of the Water-Soluble Vitamins for Healthy Adults (Ages 19–50 Years)[a]

Vitamin	Dietary Sources	Major Bodily Functions	Deficiency	Excess
Vitamin B_1 (thiamin)	Pork, organ meats, whole grains, legumes	Coenzyme (thiamin pyrophosphate) in reactions involving removal of carbon dioxide	Beriberi (peripheral nerve changes, edema, heart failure)	None reported
Vitamin B_2 (riboflavin)	Widely distributed in foods	Constituent of two flavin nucleotide coenzymes involved in energy metabolism (FAD and FMN)	Reddened lips, cracks at mouth corner(cheilosis), eye lesions	None reported
Vitamin B_3 (niacin-nicotinic acid)	Liver, lean meats, grains, legumes (can be formed from tryptophan)	Constituent of two coenzymes in oxidation-reduction reactions (NAD^+ and NADP)	Pellagra (skin and gastrointestinal lesions, nervous mental disorders)	Flushing, burning, and tingling around neck, face, and hands
Vitamin B_5 (pantothenic acid)	Widely distributed in foods	Constituent of coenzyme A, which plays a central role in energy metabolism	Fatigue, sleep disturbances, impaired coordination, nausea	None reported
Vitamin B_6 (pyridoxine)	Meats, vegetables, whole-grain cereals	Coenzyme (pyridoxal phosphate) involved in amino acid and glycogen metabolism	Irritability, convulsions, muscular twitching, dermatitis, kidney stones	None reported
Folate	Legumes, green vegetables, whole-wheat products	Coenzyme (reduced form) involved in transfer of single-carbon units in nucleic acid and amino acid metabolism	Anemia, gastrointestinal disturbances, diarrhea, red tongue	None reported
Vitamin B_7 (biotin)	Legumes, vegetables, meats	Coenzymes required for fat synthesis, amino acid metabolism, and glycogen (animal starch) formation	Fatigue, depression, nausea, dermatitis, muscular pains	None reported
Vitamin B_{12} (cobalamin)	Muscle meats, eggs, dairy products, (absent in plant foods)	Coenzyme involved in transfer of single-carbon units in nucleic acid metabolism	Pernicious anemia, neurologic disorders	None reported
Vitamin C (ascorbic acid)	Citrus fruits, tomatoes, green peppers, salad greens	Maintains intercellular matrix of cartilage, bone, and dentine, important in collagen synthesis, cofactor in enzymatic reactions, free radical scavenger	Scurvy (degeneration of skin, teeth, blood vessels, epithelial hemorrhages)	Relatively nontoxic, possibility of kidney stones

[a]Food and Nutrition Board, National Academy of Sciences. (2009). Available at **www.nal.usda.gov/fnic/etext/000105.html**. This website provides interactive dietary reference intakes for health professionals.

This general rule has several possible exceptions. First, vitamin C and folic acid exist in foods that usually comprise only a small part of most Americans' total caloric intake; the availability of these foods also varies by season. Second, some athletic groups consume relatively low amounts of vitamins B_1 and B_6. An adequate intake of these two vitamins occurs if the daily diet contains fresh fruit, grains, and uncooked or steamed vegetables. Individuals who only consume foods from the plant kingdom need to consume foods "fortified" with vitamin B_{12}, or take supplements, because plant-based diets do not supply B_{12}. Nonanimal sources of fortified vitamin B_{12} include plant milks like almond, soy, and coconut milk, nutritional yeast, tempeh (cooked slightly fermented soy product), and most ready-to-eat cereals. Also, many whole breads are vitamin B_{12} fortified.

See the animation "Biologic Function of Vitamins" on **http://thePoint.lww.com/MKKESS5e** for a demonstration of this process.

Free Radical Production and Antioxidant Role of Specific Vitamins

Most of the oxygen consumed in the mitochondria during energy metabolism combines with hydrogen to produce water. Normally, about 2% to 5% of oxygen forms the oxygen-containing free radicals superoxide (O_2^-), hydrogen peroxide (H_2O_2), and hydroxyl (OH^-) from electron "leakage" along the electron transport chain (see Chapter 5). A **free radical** represents a chemically reactive molecule or molecular fragment with at least one unpaired electron in its outer orbital or valence shell. Heat and ionizing radiation produce these same free radicals; cigarette smoke and environmental pollutants primarily carry them.

See the animation "Vitamin C as an Antioxidant" on **http://thePoint.lww.com/MKKESS5e** for a demonstration of this process.

Free radical buildup increases the potential for cellular damage, referred to as **oxidative stress**, to biologically important substances (see A Closer Look: *Increased Metabolism and Free Radical Production During Physical Activity*). Oxygen radicals exhibit strong affinity for the polyunsaturated fatty acids located in the cell membrane's lipid bilayer. During oxidative stress, deterioration occurs in the plasma membrane's fatty acids. Membrane damage occurs through a series of chain reactions termed **lipid peroxidation.** These undesirable reactions incorporate oxygen into lipids and increase the vulnerability of the cell and its constituents. Free radicals also facilitate LDL cholesterol oxidation and thus accelerate the atherosclerotic process. Oxidative stress ultimately increases the likelihood of cellular deterioration associated with advanced aging, cancer, diabetes, coronary artery disease, and a general decline in central nervous system and immune function.

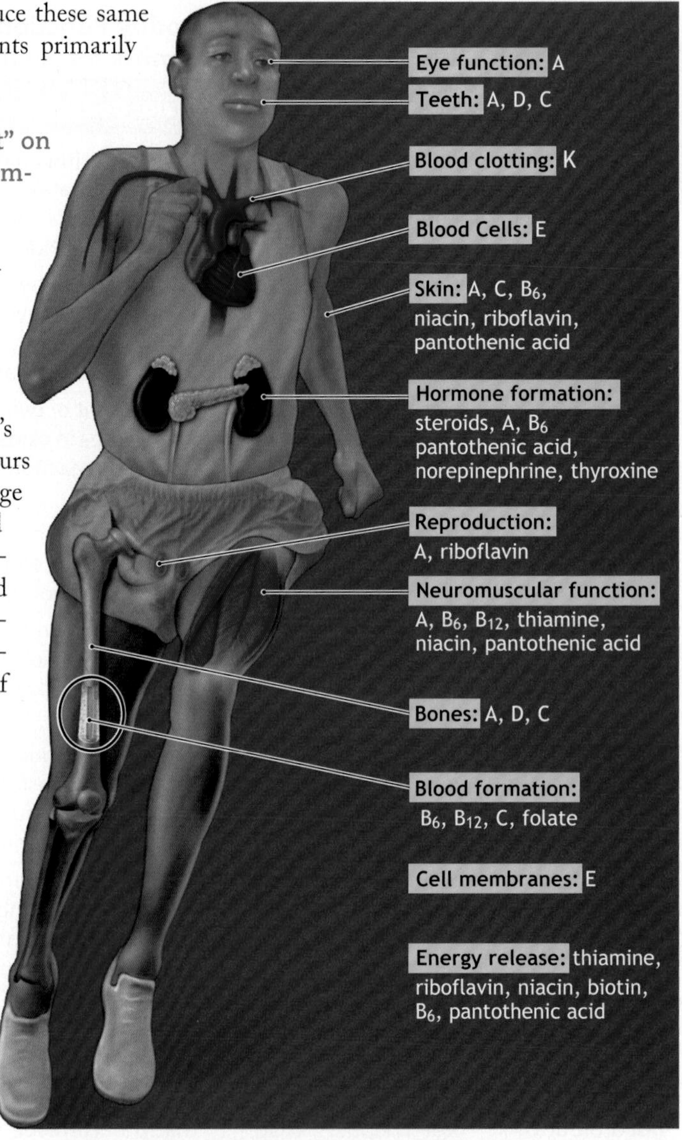

FIGURE 2.14 Biologic functions of vitamins.

Vitamins Behave as Chemicals

Current estimates from nationally representative data available on dietary supplement use for the 5-year period 2007–2011 indicate the percentage of respondents who regularly consumed a variety of supplements increased from 28% to 36%, with the increase from 2010 to 2011 reaching statistical significance. The percentage of respondents regularly using only a multivitamin declined from 24% to 17%. Detailed survey results confirmed that supplement use increases with age and is higher in women than men. Of all survey respondents in 2011, 67% used vitamin or mineral supplements, particularly specialty supplements (35%), botanicals (23%), and sports supplements (17%). Among supplement users, multivitamin use was the most common (71%), followed by omega-3 or fish oil (33%), calcium (32%), vitamin D (32%), and vitamin C (32%). The most common reasons for supplement use included overall health and wellness (58%) and to fill perceived nutrient gaps in the diet (42%). Over 90% of all nutrition counselors recommend supplement use, particularly multivitamins.

The supplement industry targets exercise enthusiasts, competitive athletes, and coaches and personal trainers. More than 50% of competitive athletes in some sports consume supplements on a regular basis, either to ensure adequate micronutrient intake or to achieve an excess with the hope of enhancing performance and training responsiveness. *More than 60 years of research data in healthy persons with nutritionally adequate diets* ***do not*** *provide evidence that consuming vitamin and mineral supplements above recommended levels improves performance, hormonal and metabolic responses to activity, or the ability to train arduously and recover from such training.*

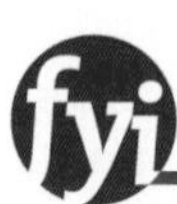

Rich Dietary Sources of Antioxidant Vitamins

- **β-carotene** (best known of the pigmented compounds or carotenoids that give color to yellow, orange, and green leafy vegetables and fruits): Carrots; dark-green leafy vegetables such as spinach, broccoli, turnips, beet, and collard greens; sweet potatoes; winter squash; and apricots, cantaloupe, mangos, and papaya
- **Vitamin C:** Citrus fruits and juices; cabbage, broccoli, and turnip greens; cantaloupe; green and red sweet peppers; and berries
- **Vitamin E:** Poultry, seafood, vegetable oils, wheat germ, fish liver oils, whole-grain breads and fortified cereals, nuts and seeds, dried beans, green leafy vegetables, and eggs

When vitamin-mineral deficiencies appear in physically active people, they often occur among three groups:

1. Individuals with low energy intake—dancers, gymnasts, and weight-class sport athletes—who strive to maintain or reduce body weight
2. Individuals who eliminate one or more food groups from their diet
3. Endurance athletes who consume large amounts of processed foods and simple sugars with low micronutrient density

Any significant excess of vitamins functions as chemicals or essentially drugs in the body. For example, a megadose of water-soluble vitamin C increases serum uric acid levels, which precipitate gout in people predisposed to this disease. At intakes greater than 1000 mg daily, urinary oxalate excretion (a breakdown product of vitamin C) increases, thereby accelerating kidney stone formation in susceptible individuals. For those with iron deficiency, megadoses of vitamin C can destroy concentrations of vitamin B_{12}. In healthy people, vitamin C supplements frequently irritate the bowel and cause diarrhea.

Excess vitamin B_6 may induce liver and nerve damage. Excessive riboflavin (B_2) intake can impair vision, and a megadose of nicotinic acid (niacin) serves as a potent vasodilator and inhibits fatty acid mobilization during physical activity, rapidly depleting liver and muscle glycogen. Folic acid concentrated in supplement form can trigger an allergic response, producing hives, light-headedness, and breathing difficulties. Vitamin A megadoses can induce toxicity to the nervous system, and excess vitamin D intake can damage kidneys.

A CLOSER LOOK

Increased Metabolism and Free Radical Production During Physical Activity

Physical activity produces reactive oxygen in at least two ways:

1. From an electron leak in the mitochondria, probably at the cytochrome level, which produces superoxide radicals
2. During alterations in blood flow and oxygen supply—underperfusion during intense physical activity followed by substantial reperfusion in recovery—which trigger excessive free radical generation

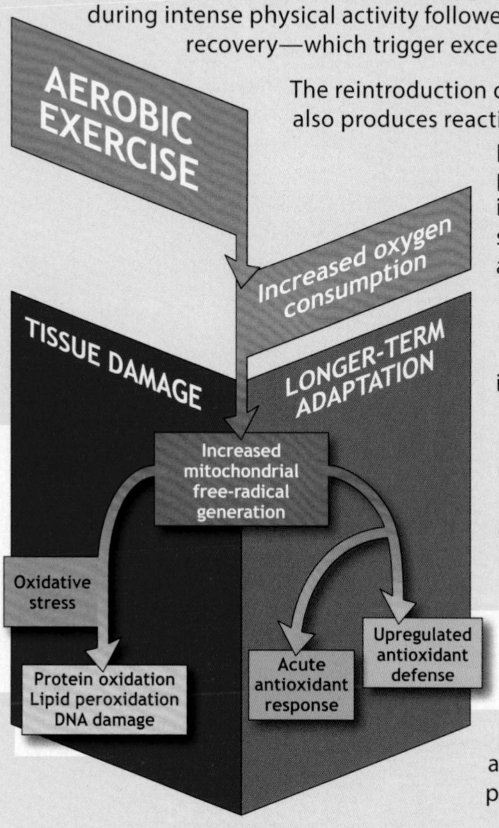

The reintroduction of molecular oxygen in recovery also produces reactive oxygen species that precipitates oxidative stress. The potential for free radical damage increases during trauma, general stress, and muscle damage and from the environmental pollutant smog (**www.epa.gov/groundlevelozone/**).

The risk of oxidative stress increases with intense effort. Exhaustive endurance activity by untrained persons produces oxidative damage in active muscle. Intense resistance exercise also increases free radical production, indirectly measured by malondialdehyde, a lipid peroxidation by-product. Variations in estrogen levels during the menstrual cycle do not affect the mild oxidative stress that accompanies moderate-intensity physical activity. The figure illustrates how regular aerobic physical activity affects oxidative response and potential for tissue damage, including protective adaptive responses.

Cascade of events and adaptations produced by regular aerobic physical activity that lessen the likelihood of tissue damage from intense activity.

Nothing can stop oxygen reduction and free radical production, but an elaborate natural defense exists within the cell and extracellular space against its damaging effects. This defense includes enzymatic and nonenzymatic mechanisms that work synchronously to immediately counter potential oxidative damage. The three major antioxidant enzymes are **superoxide dismutase**, **catalase**, and **glutathione peroxidase**. The nutritive-reducing vitamins A, C, and E and the vitamin A precursor β-carotene also serve important protective functions. These antioxidant vitamins protect the plasma membrane by reacting with and removing free radicals to terminate the chain reaction.

Vitamins and Exercise Performance

Figure 2.15 illustrates how the water-soluble B-complex vitamins play key roles as coenzymes to regulate energy-yielding reactions during carbohydrate, fat, and protein catabolism. These vitamins also contribute to hemoglobin synthesis and red blood cell production. The belief that "if a little is good, more must be better" has led many coaches, athletes, fitness enthusiasts, and even some scientists to advocate using vitamin supplements above recommended

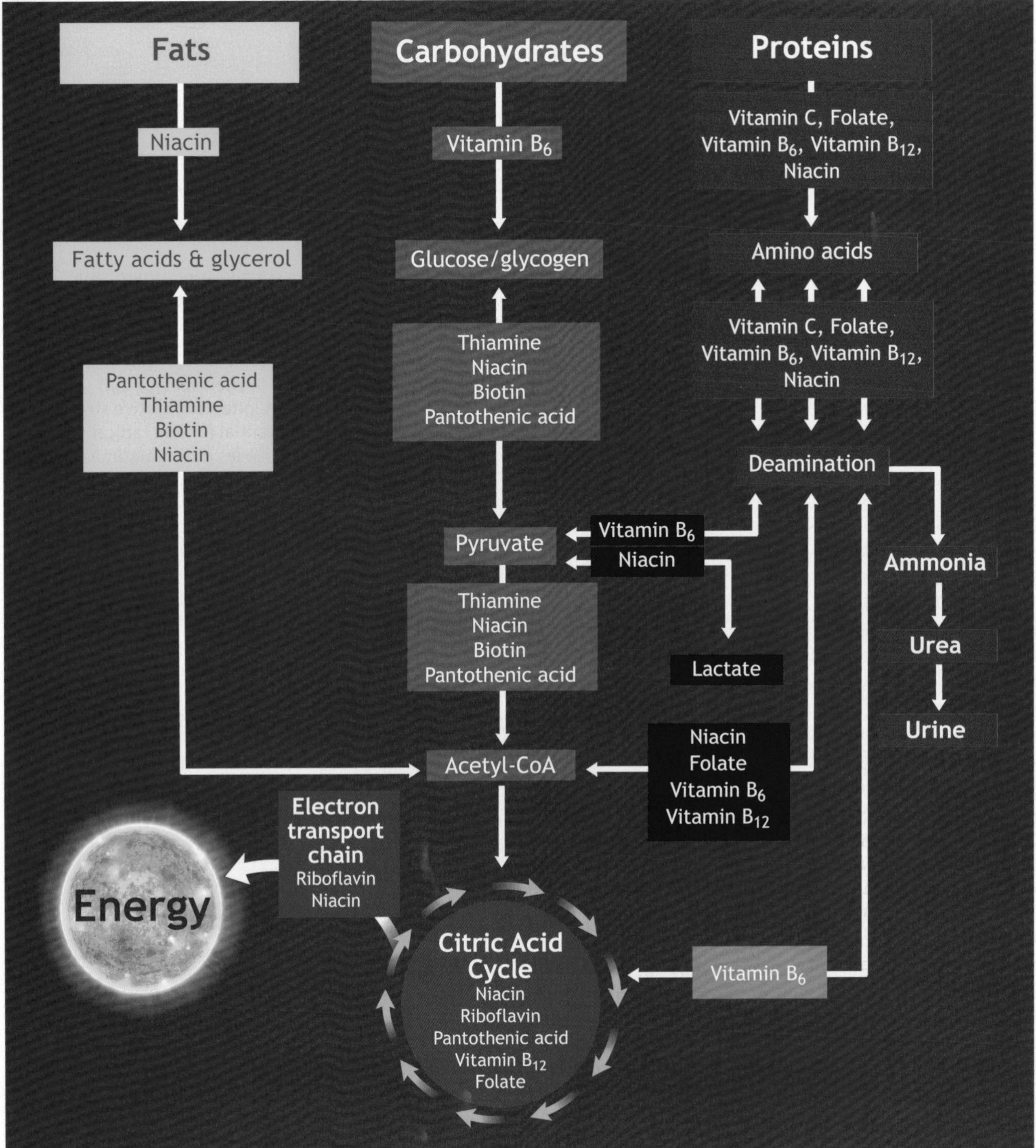

FIGURE 2.15 General schema for the role of water-soluble vitamins in carbohydrate, fat, and protein metabolism. (Adapted with permission from McArdle WD, Katch FI, Katch VL. *Sports and Exercise Nutrition*. 4th Ed. Philadelphia: Wolters Kluwer Health, 2013.)

levels. The facts *do not* support such advice for individuals who consume an adequate diet.

Supplementing with vitamin B_6, an essential cofactor in glycogen and amino acid metabolism, did not benefit the metabolic mixture metabolized by women during intense aerobic physical activity. In general, athletes' status for this vitamin equals reference standards for the population and does not decrease with strenuous activity to a level warranting supplementation. For endurance-trained men, 9 days of vitamin B_6 supplementation of 20 mg daily provided no ergogenic effect on cycling to exhaustion performed at 70% of aerobic capacity.

Chronic high-potency, multivitamin-mineral supplementation for well-nourished, healthy individuals does not augment aerobic fitness, muscular strength, neuromuscular performance after prolonged running, and general athletic performance. In addition to the B-complex group, consuming excess vitamins C and E confers no benefits on stamina, circulatory function, or energy metabolism. Short-term daily supplementation with 400 IU of vitamin E produced no effect on normal neuroendocrine and metabolic responses to strenuous exertion or performance time to exhaustion. Vitamin C status in trained athletes, assessed by serum concentrations and urinary ascorbate levels, does not differ from that in untrained individuals despite large differences in daily physical activity level. Active persons typically increase their daily energy intake to match an increased energy requirement; thus, a proportionate increase occurs in micronutrient intake, often in amounts that exceed recommended levels.

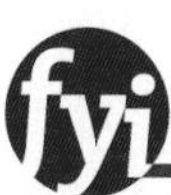

Consuming Supplements May Not Impact Disease

Think again if you are counting on your daily multivitamin-multimineral (MVM) pill to ward off the chronic diseases cancer or heart disease. The latest two systematic reviews of the worldwide literature reported that MVM supplementation in healthy populations had only a *modest protective effect* on all-cause mortality, cancer incidence or mortality, or cardiovascular disease incidence or mortality. The duration of supplementation made no difference in disease status. Unfortunately, Americans spend over $30 billion annually on these supplements with little or no chance of affecting change in health status.

References: Alexander DD, et al. A systematic review of multivitamin-multimineral use and cardiovascular disease and cancer incidence and total mortality. *J Am Coll Nutr* 2013;32:339.

Fortmann SP. *Vitamin, Mineral, and Multivitamin Supplements for the Primary Prevention of Cardiovascular Disease and Cancer: A systematic Evidence Review for the U.S. Preventive Services Task Force [Internet]*. Rockville: Agency for Healthcare Research and Quality (US), 2013. Report No.: 14-05199-EF-1.

MINERALS

The Nature of Minerals

Approximately 4% of the body's mass consists of 22 mostly metallic elements collectively called **minerals**. Minerals serve as constituents of enzymes, hormones, and vitamins; they combine with other chemicals (e.g., calcium phosphate in bone and iron in the heme of hemoglobin) or exist singularly (e.g., free calcium in body fluids). In the body, **trace minerals** are those required in amounts of 100 mg a day or less, and **major minerals** are required in amounts of 100 mg daily or more. Excess minerals serve no useful physiologic purpose yet can precipitate serious toxic side effects.

Kinds, Sources, and Mineral Functions

Most major and trace minerals occur freely in nature, mainly in the waters of rivers, lakes, and oceans, in topsoil, and beneath the earth's surface. Minerals exist in the root systems of plants and in the body structure of animals that consume plants and water containing minerals. **Table 2.6** lists the major bodily functions, dietary sources, and symptoms of a deficiency and excess for important major and trace minerals.

Minerals often become part of the body's structures and existing chemicals. They serve three broad roles:

1. Provide structure in bone and teeth formation
2. Help maintain normal heart rhythm, muscle contractility, neural conductivity, and acid-base balance
3. Help regulate cellular metabolism by becoming part of enzymes and hormones that modulate cellular activity

Figure 2.16 lists minerals that participate in catabolic and anabolic cellular processes. Minerals activate numerous reactions, releasing energy during carbohydrate, fat, and protein catabolism. Minerals help to synthesize biologic nutrients—glycogen from glucose, triacylglycerols from fatty acids and glycerol, and proteins from amino acids. Without essential minerals, the fine balance would be disrupted between catabolism and anabolism. Minerals also form important hormone constituents. An inadequate thyroxine production from iodine deficiency, for example, slows resting metabolism. In extreme cases, this predisposes a person to obesity. The synthesis of insulin, the hormone that facilitates cellular glucose uptake, requires zinc, as do approximately 100 enzymes; the mineral chlorine forms the digestive acid hydrochloric acid.

Minerals and Physical Activity

Food sources in a well-balanced diet provide the body's mineral requirements. The next sections describe specific functions for key minerals related to physical activity.

Calcium

Calcium, the body's most abundant mineral, combines with phosphorus to form bones and teeth. These two minerals represent about 75% of the body's total mineral content of about 2.5% of body mass. Approximately 1% of the body's 1200 mg of calcium exists in ionized form and participates in these six important functions:

1. Muscle action
2. Blood clotting
3. Nerve impulse transmission
4. Enzymes activation (e.g., tissue transglutaminase, mitochondrial glycerol phosphate dehydrogenase [mGPD])
5. Synthesis of calciferol (active vitamin D form)
6. Fluid transport across cell membranes

TABLE 2.6 Important Major and Trace Minerals for Healthy Adults (Ages 19–50 Years): Their Food Sources, Functions, and Effects of Deficiencies and Excesses[a]

Mineral	Dietary Sources	Major Bodily Functions	Effects of Deficiency	Effects of Excess
Major				
Calcium	Milk, cheese, dark green vegetables, dried legumes	Bone and tooth formation, blood clotting, nerve transmission	Stunted growth, rickets, osteoporosis, convulsions	Not reported in humans
Phosphorus	Milk, cheese, yogurt, meat, poultry, grains, fish	Bone and tooth formation, acid-base balance	Weakness, demineralization of bone, loss of calcium	Erosion of jaw (phossy jaw)
Potassium	Leafy vegetables, cantaloupe, lima beans, potatoes, bananas, milk, meats, coffee, tea	Fluid balance, nerve transmission, acid-base balance	Muscle cramps, irregular cardiac rhythm, mental confusion, loss of appetite, can be life-threatening	None if kidneys function normally; poor kidney function causes potassium buildup and cardiac arrhythmias
Sulfur	Obtained as part of dietary protein and present in food preservatives	Acid-base balance, liver function	Unlikely to occur with adequate dietary intake	Unknown
Sodium	Common salt	Acid-base balance, body water balance, nerve function	Muscle cramps, mental apathy, reduced	High blood pressure
Chlorine (chloride)	Part of salt-containing food; some vegetables and fruits	Important part of extracellular fluids	Unlikely to occur with adequate dietary intake	With sodium, contributes to high blood pressure
Magnesium	Whole grains, green leafy vegetables	Activates enzymes in protein synthesis weakness, spasms	Growth failure, behavioral disturbances	Diarrhea
Trace				
Iron	Eggs, lean meats, legumes, whole grains, green leafy vegetables	Constituent of hemoglobin and enzymes involved in energy metabolism	Iron deficiency anemia (weakness, reduced resistance to infection)	Siderosis; cirrhosis of liver
Fluorine	Drinking water, tea, seafood	May be important to maintain bone structure	Higher frequency of tooth decay	Mottling of teeth; increased bone density, neurologic disturbances
Zinc	Widely distributed in foods	Constituent of digestive enzymes	Growth failure, small sex glands	Fever, nausea, vomiting, diarrhea
Copper	Meats, drinking water	Constituent of enzymes associated with iron	Anemia, bone changes (rare in humans)	Rare metabolic condition (Wilson disease)
Selenium	Seafood, meat, grains	Functions in close association with vitamin E	Anemia (rare)	Gastrointestinal disorders; lung irritation
Iodine (iodide)	Marine fish and shellfish dairy products, vegetables, iodized salt	Constituent of thyroid hormones	Goiter (enlarged thyroid)	Very high intakes depress thyroid activity
Chromium	Legumes, cereals, organ meats, fats, vegetable oils, meats, whole grains	Constituent of some enzymes; involved in glucose and energy metabolism	Rarely reported in humans; impaired glucose metabolism	Inhibition of enzymes; skin and kidney damage

[a]Food and Nutrition Board, National Academy of Sciences. (2009). Available at **www.nal.usda.gov/fnic/etext/000105.html**.

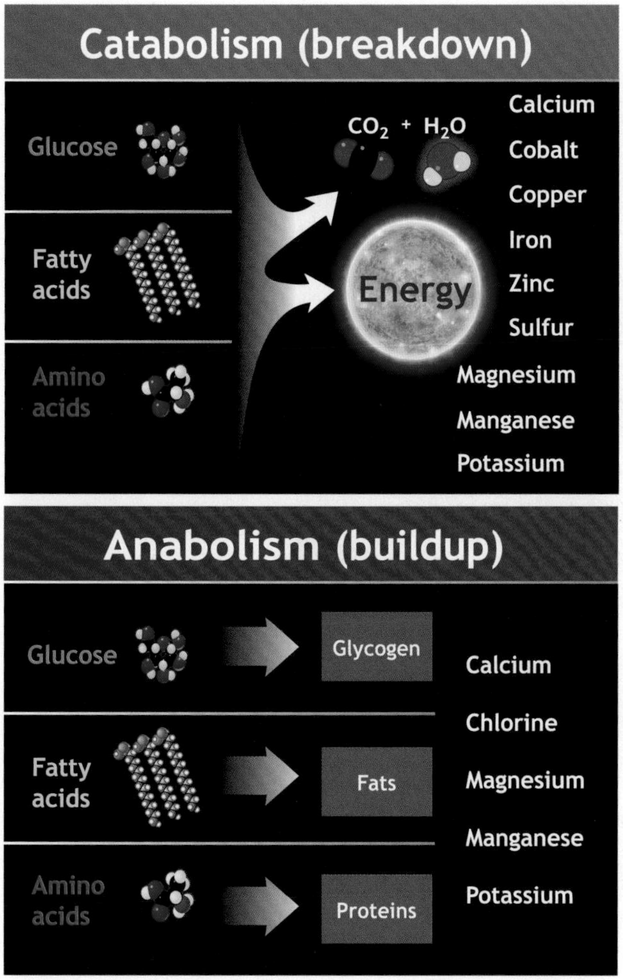

Catabolism (breakdown)

Glucose
Fatty acids
Amino acids
CO_2 + H_2O
Energy
Calcium
Cobalt
Copper
Iron
Zinc
Sulfur
Magnesium
Manganese
Potassium

Anabolism (buildup)

Glucose → Glycogen
Fatty acids → Fats
Amino acids → Proteins
Calcium
Chlorine
Magnesium
Manganese
Potassium

FIGURE 2.16 Minerals that function in macronutrient catabolism and anabolism. (Adapted with permission from McArdle WD, Katch FI, Katch VL. *Sports and Exercise Nutrition*. 4th Ed. Philadelphia: Wolters Kluwer Health, 2013.)

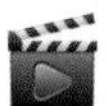

See the animation "Calcium in Muscle" on **http://thePoint.lww.com/MKKESS5e** for a demonstration of this process.

Osteoporosis: Calcium Intake, Estrogen, and Physical Activity

The skeleton contains more than 99% of the body's total calcium. When calcium deficiency is present, the body draws on its calcium reserves in bone to restore the deficit. With prolonged negative imbalance, **osteoporosis** (literally, "porous bones") eventually develops as bones lose calcium mass (mineral content) and calcium concentration (diminished mineral density) and progressively become porous, fenestrated, hollow, and brittle. **Figure 2.17** illustrates two opposing processes:

1. Calcium buildup by its efficient transport from the small intestine for storage in the bone matrix (note that the blue arrowhead points into the bone)
2. Inadequate calcium intake or ineffective calcium absorption by intestinal mucosa, where calcium travels opposite from bone into bodily fluids called *calcium resorption*, an insidious and destructive process that negatively impacts males and females of all ages

Osteoporosis, a silent disease, often goes undetected for years until a bone fracture occurs. Current worldwide statistics for osteoporosis are frightening (**www.iofbonehealth.org/facts-statistics#category-23**):

- Osteoporosis causes more than 8.9 million fractures annually, resulting in an osteoporotic fracture every 3 seconds.
- Osteoporosis affects an estimated 200 million women worldwide—approximately one tenth of women aged 60, one fifth of women aged 70, two fifths of women aged 80, and two thirds of women aged 90.
- Osteoporosis affects an estimated 75 million people in Europe, United States, and Japan.
- Europe and the Americas account for 51% of all osteoporotic fractures.
- One in three women over age 50 will experience osteoporotic fractures, as well as one in five men.
- Nearly 75% of hip, spine, and distal forearm fractures occur among individuals beyond age 65.
- Men are not immune to osteoporosis; by 2050, the worldwide hip fracture incidence of men is projected to increase by 310%; in women, it will increase by 240%.

Dietary Calcium Crucial. As a general guideline, adolescent boys and girls ages 9 to 13 and young adult men and women ages 14 to 18 require 1300 mg of calcium daily or about as much calcium in six 8-oz glasses of milk. For adults ages

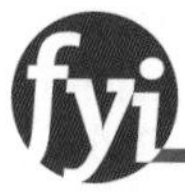

Fourteen Risk Factors for Osteoporosis

1. Advancing age
2. History of fracture as an adult, independent of cause
3. Fracture history in parent/sibling
4. Cigarette smoking
5. Slight build or tendency toward being underweight
6. White or Asian female
7. Sedentary lifestyle
8. Early menopause
9. Eating disorder
10. High protein intake, mainly animal protein
11. Excess sodium intake
12. Alcohol abuse
13. Low calcium diet before/after menopause
14. Vitamin D deficiency

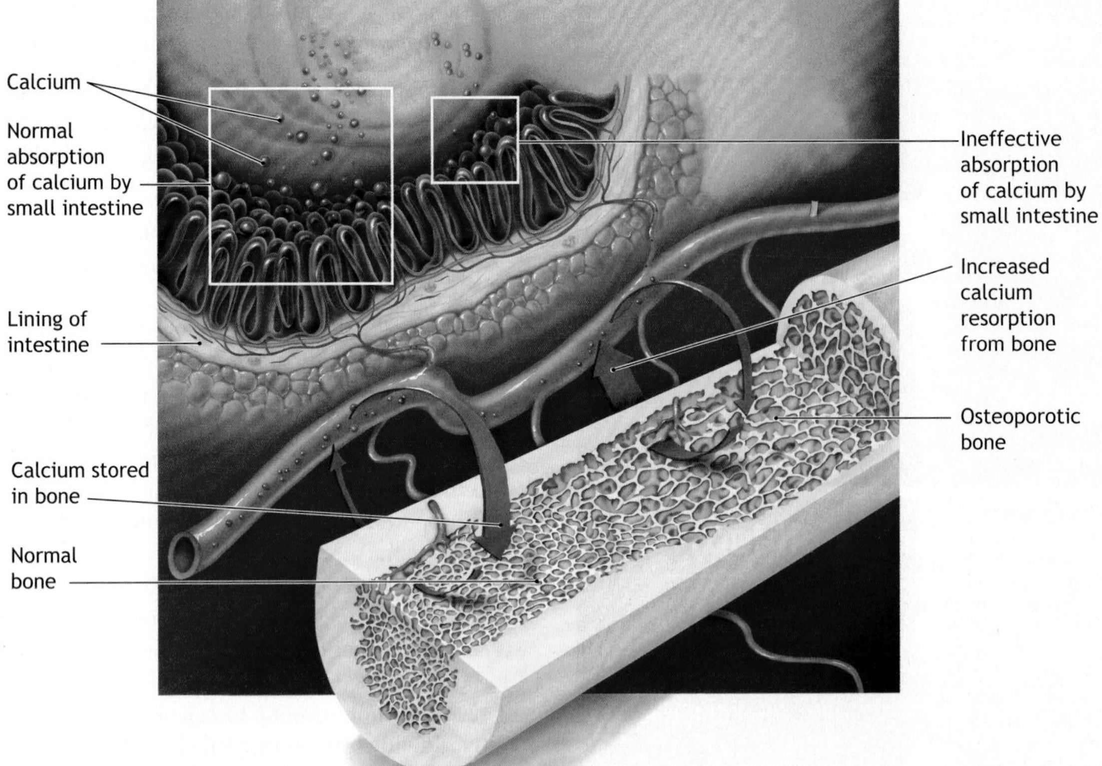

FIGURE 2.17 (1) Calcium buildup by its efficient transport from the small intestine for storage in the bone matrix (note that the *large blue arrowhead* points into the bone) and (2) the opposing process of ineffective calcium intestinal absorption, where calcium leaches from the bones (*large blue arrowhead* points into blood stream), leaving them brittle and likely to fracture.

19 to 50, the daily requirement decreases to 1000 mg. Growing children require more calcium per unit body mass on a daily basis than adults, yet many adults remain calcium deficient. For example, the typical adult's daily calcium intake ranges between 500 and 700 mg. More than 75% of adults consume less than the recommended amount, and about 25% of American women consume less than 300 mg of calcium daily. The segment of the female athletic population most prone to calcium dietary insufficiency comprises dancers, gymnasts, and endurance track and field and swim competitors.

 See the animation "Bone Growth" on **http://thePoint.lww.com/MKKESS5e** for a demonstration of this process.

Physical Activity Helps Slow Skeletal Aging. *Regular physical activity participation slows the rate of skeletal aging regardless of age or gender*. The decline in vigorous activity as one ages closely parallels the age-related loss of bone mass. Moderately intense activity provides a safe and potent stimulus to maintain or increase bone mass. Weight-bearing activity represents a particularly desirable form of physical activity; examples include walking, running, dancing, and rope skipping. Resistance training, which generates considerable muscular force against the body's long bones, also proves beneficial.

Female Athlete Triad: An Unexpected Problem for Women Who Train Intensely

A paradox exists between vigorous physical activity and bone dynamics for athletic premenopausal women. Women who train intensely and emphasize weight loss often engage in disordered eating behaviors. This results in low energy intake, which in the extreme, cause life-threatening complications

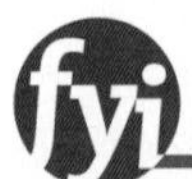

Six Principles to Promote Bone Health

1. *Specificity:* Physical activity provides a local osteogenic effect
2. *Overload:* Progressively increasing exercise intensity promotes continued improvement.
3. *Initial values:* Individuals with the smallest total bone mass exhibit greatest improvement potential.
4. *Diminishing returns:* As the bone density biologic ceiling is approached, further gains require greater effort
5. *More is not necessarily better:* Bone cells desensitize with prolonged mechanical loading
6. *Reversibility:* Discontinuing exercise overload reverses positive osteogenic exercise effects

(see *How to Recognize Warning Signs of Disordered Eating* in Chapter 16). Reducing body weight and body fat eventually results in menstrual cycle irregularity (oligomenorrhea) or cessation (secondary amenorrhea). The tightly integrated continuum illustrated in **Figure 2.18** reflects the clinical condition known as **female athlete triad**, which begins with disordered eating and ends with energy drain, amenorrhea, and eventual osteoporosis.

Many girls and young women who participate in sports have at least one of the triad's disorders, particularly disordered eating behavior from low-energy availability. Amenorrhea prevalence among female athletes in body weight–related distance running, gymnastics, ballet, cheerleading, figure skating, and bodybuilding ranges between 25% and 65%, while no more than 5% of the general population suffer from this medical condition.

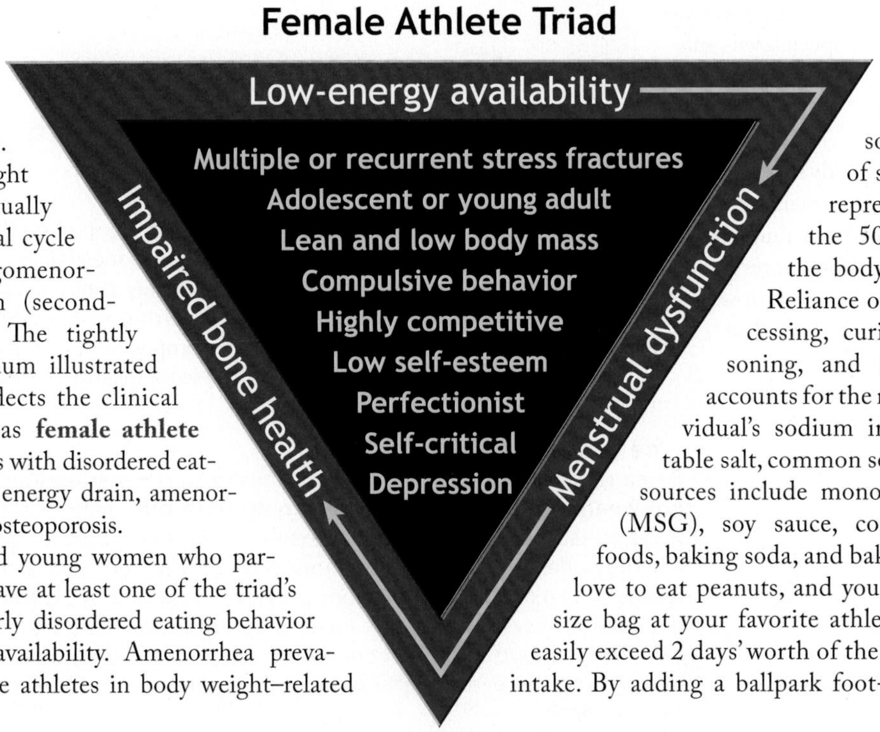

Female Athlete Triad

FIGURE 2.18 The female athlete triad: low-energy availability, menstrual dysfunction, and impaired bone health. (Adapted with permission from American College of Sports. Medicine Position Stand. The female athlete triad. *Med Sci Sports Exerc* 2007;39:1867.)

Sodium, Potassium, and Chlorine

The minerals sodium, potassium, and chlorine, collectively termed **electrolytes**, dissolve in the body as electrically charged ion particles. Sodium and chlorine represent the chief minerals contained in blood plasma and extracellular fluid. Electrolytes modulate fluid movement within the body's various fluid compartments. This allows for a constant, well-regulated exchange of nutrients and waste products between the cell and its external fluid environment. Potassium represents the chief intracellular mineral.

The most important function of sodium and potassium ions establishes proper electrical gradients across cell membranes. A difference in electrical balance between the cell's interior and exterior allows nerve impulse transmission, muscle stimulation and contraction, and proper gland functioning. Electrolytes maintain plasma membrane permeability and tightly regulate the acidic and basic qualities of body fluids, particularly blood.

Sodium: How Much Is Enough?

The widespread availability of sodium in foods, particularly that added in the manufacturing process, makes it easy to obtain the daily requirement without adding salt to foods. In the United States, sodium intake regularly exceeds the adult daily level recommended of 2400 mg or 1 tbsp of table salt. The typical Western diet contains about 4500 mg of sodium (8 to 12 g of salt) each day. This represents 10 times the 500 mg of sodium the body actually requires. Reliance on table salt in processing, curing, cooking, seasoning, and food preservation accounts for the majority of an individual's sodium intake. Aside from table salt, common sodium-rich dietary sources include monosodium glutamate (MSG), soy sauce, condiments, canned foods, baking soda, and baking powder. If you love to eat peanuts, and you consume a small-size bag at your favorite athletic event, you will easily exceed 2 days' worth of the recommended salt intake. By adding a ballpark foot-long hotdog with condiments, the new total just for those foods now exceeds 3 days' worth of the recommended sodium intake.

The body's normal sodium balance usually occurs throughout a range of dietary intakes. For some "salt-sensitive" individuals, excessive sodium intake is inadequately excreted from the body. A chronic excess of dietary sodium increases fluid volume and possibly increases peripheral vascular resistance; both factors result in elevated blood pressure to levels that may pose a serious health risk. **Sodium-induced hypertension** occurs in about one third of hypertensive individuals in the United States.

For decades, the first strategy in treating high blood pressure relied on attempts to minimize excess dietary sodium. Conventional wisdom maintained that reducing sodium intake would reduce the body's sodium and fluid levels, thereby lowering blood pressure. Unfortunately, sodium restriction per se does not lower blood pressure in people with normal blood pressure. For the salt-sensitive individual, reducing dietary sodium decreases blood pressure and thus provides a prudent, nonpharmacologic first line of defense to attenuate hypertension.

Iron

The body normally contains between 3 and 5 g of iron (about one sixth of an ounce). Of this amount, approximately 80% exists in functionally active compounds, predominantly combined with hemoglobin in red blood cells. This iron-protein compound increases the oxygen-carrying capacity of blood approximately 65 times. Iron also serves as a structural component of myoglobin (~5% of total iron), a compound similar to hemoglobin that stores oxygen for release within muscle cells. Small amounts of iron exist in cytochromes, the specialized substances that transfer cellular energy.

Iron Stores

About 20% of the body's iron does not combine in functionally active compounds. **Hemosiderin and ferritin** constitute the iron stores in the liver, spleen, and bone marrow. These stores replenish iron lost from the functional compounds to provide an iron reserve during periods of insufficient dietary iron intake. The plasma protein **transferrin** transports iron from ingested food and damaged red blood cells to tissues in need. Transferrin plasma levels often reflect the adequacy of current iron intake.

Athletes should include iron-rich foods in their daily diets. People with inadequate iron intake, or with limited iron absorption rates or high rates of iron loss, often develop a reduced hemoglobin concentration in red blood cells. This extreme condition of iron insufficiency, commonly called **iron deficiency anemia**, produces general sluggishness, loss of appetite, and reduced capacity to sustain even mild physical activity. "Iron therapy" normalizes the hemoglobin content of the blood and exercise capacity. **Table 2.7** lists recommendations for iron intake for children and adults.

Females: A Population at Risk

Inadequate iron intake frequently occurs among young children, teenagers, and females of childbearing age, including physically active women.

Iron loss between 5 and 45 mg occurs during a menstrual cycle. This produces an additional 5-mg dietary iron requirement daily for premenopausal females, increasing the average monthly dietary iron intake need by about 150 mg. The small intestine absorbs only about 15% of ingested iron, depending on current iron status, iron form ingested, and meal composition. An additional 20 to 25 mg of iron becomes available each month from the additional 150-mg monthly dietary requirement for synthesizing red blood cells lost during menstruation. Not surprisingly, 30% to 50% of

A CLOSER LOOK

Lowering High Blood Pressure With Dietary Intervention: The DASH Diet

Nearly 50 million Americans have hypertension, a condition that if left untreated, increases stroke and heart attack risk, including kidney failure. Fifty percent of people with hypertension seek treatment, but only about half achieve long-term success. One reason for poor compliance concerns possible side effects of readily available antihypertensive medication. For example, fatigue and impotence often discourage patients from maintaining a chronic medication schedule required by pharmacologic hypertension treatment.

The DASH Approach

Research using DASH (Dietary Approaches to Stop Hypertension; **www.nhlbi.nih.gov/health/public/heart/hbp/dash/new_dash.pdf**) demonstrates this diet lowers blood pressure to almost the same extent as pharmacologic therapy and often more than other lifestyle changes. Two months on the diet reduced systolic pressure an average of 11.4 mm Hg and diastolic pressure decreased by 5.5 mm Hg. Every 2 mm Hg reduction in systolic pressure lowers heart disease risk by 5% and stroke risk by 8%. The standard DASH diet combined with reduced daily dietary salt intake of 1500 mg produces even greater blood pressure reductions than achieved with the DASH diet only.

Nutrient Goals for the DASH Diet

The table shows daily nutrient goals for the DASH approach for a 2100-kcal intake for a typical 70-kg person. More physically active and heavier individuals should boost their portion size or number of individual items to maintain their weight. Individuals desiring to lose weight or who are lighter or sedentary should eat less, but not less than the minimum number of servings for each food group (**http://dashdiet.org/what_is_the_dash_diet.asp**).

Daily Nutrient Goals Used in the Dash Studies for a 2100-Calorie Eating Plan

Total fat	27% of calories	Sodium	2300 mg
Saturated fat	6% of calories	Potassium	4700 mg
Protein	18% of calories	Calcium	1250 mg
Carbohydrate	55% of calories	Magnesium	500 mg
Cholesterol	150 mg	Fiber	30 g

From: US Department of Health and Human Services, National Institutes of Health, National Heart, Lung, and Blood Institute; **www.nhlbi.nih.gov/files/docs/public/heart/hbp_low.pdf**

References

Calton JB. Prevalence of micronutrient deficiency in popular diet plans. *J Int Soc Sports Nutr* 2010;10:24.

Miller PE, et al. Comparison of four established DASH diet indexes: examining associations of index scores and colorectal cancer. *Am J Clin Nutr* 2013;98:794.

Smith PJ, et al. Effects of the dietary approaches to stop hypertension diet, exercise, and caloric restriction on neurocognition in overweight adults with high blood pressure. *Hypertension* 2010;55:1331.

Troyer JL, et al. The effect of home-delivered Dietary Approach to Stop Hypertension (DASH) meals on the diets of older adults with cardiovascular disease. *Am J Clin Nutr* 2010;91:1204.

TABLE 2.7 **Recommended Dietary Allowances for Iron**[a]

	Age (y)	Iron (mg/d)
Children	1–3	7
	4–8	10
Men	9–13	8
	14–18	11
	19–70	8
Women	9–13	8
	14–18	15
	19–50	18
	51–70	8
Pregnant	<19	27
	≥19	27
Lactating	<19	10
	≥19	9

[a]Food and Nutrition Board, Institute of Medicine. *Dietary Reference Intakes: Recommended Intakes for Individuals*. Washington, DC: National Academy Press, 2002. Available at **www.iom.edu**.

American women experience dietary iron insufficiencies from menstrual blood loss, including an insufficient dietary iron intake.

Functional Anemia: Normal Hemoglobin but Low Iron Reserves

A high prevalence of nonanemic iron depletion exists among athletes in diverse sports including recreationally active women and men. Low values for hemoglobin within the "normal" range often reflect **functional anemia** or marginal iron deficiency. Depleted iron reserves and reduced iron-dependent protein production (e.g., oxidative enzymes) with a relatively normal, nonanemic hemoglobin concentration characterize this condition. Iron-deficient athletes benefit from the ergogenic effects of iron supplementation on aerobic exercise performance and training responsiveness. Current recommendations support iron supplementation for nonanemic physically active women with low serum ferritin levels, a measure of iron reserves. Supplementation in this case exerts little effect on hemoglobin concentration and red blood cell volume. Any improved exercise capacity likely occurs from increased muscle oxidative capacity, not the blood's increased oxygen transport capacity.

Athletes and Iron Supplements

If an individual's meals contain the recommended iron intake, supplementing with iron does not increase hemoglobin, hematocrit, or other iron status measures. Any increase in iron loss with physical training coupled with poor dietary habits in adolescent and premenopausal women could strain an already limited iron reserve. This does not mean that individuals involved in strenuous training should take supplementary iron or that indicators of sports anemia result from dietary iron deficiency or exercise-induced iron loss. Iron overconsumption or overabsorption could potentially contribute to diabetes, liver disease, and heart and joint and ligament damage. Thus, over-the-counter supplements containing high iron levels should not be used indiscriminately. Iron excess even may facilitate growth of latent cancers and infectious organisms. At-risk athletes' iron status should be monitored by systematic evaluation of hematologic characteristics and iron reserves.

Minerals and Exercise Performance

Consuming mineral supplements above recommended levels on an acute or chronic basis does not benefit exercise performance or enhance training responsiveness. Loss of water and sodium chloride and potassium chloride salts in sweat does pose an important challenge in prolonged, hot weather physical activity. Excessive water and electrolyte loss impairs heat tolerance and performance and can trigger heat cramps, heat exhaustion, or heat stroke. The yearly number of heat-related deaths during spring and summer football practice provides a tragic illustration of the importance of replacing fluids and electrolytes. Data from the National Center for Catastrophic Sport Injury Research reported that of 243 football deaths recorded between July 1990 and June 2010, 38 were from heat-related causes. Many of those deaths happened in more southern states during preseason play, including at two-a-day practices. During practice or competition, an athlete may sweat up to 5 kg of water. This corresponds to about 8.0 g of salt depletion because each kilogram (1 L) of sweat contains about 1.5 g of salt (of which 40% represents sodium). Immediate replacement of water lost through sweating should become the overriding consideration.

Defense Against Mineral Loss During Physical Activity

Vigorous physical activity triggers a rapid and coordinated release of the hormones **arginine vasopressin** and aldosterone, and the enzyme renin, to minimize sodium and water loss through the kidneys and sweat. An increase in sodium conservation by the kidneys occurs even under extreme marathon running in warm, humid weather, during which sweat output often reaches 2 L an hour. Adding a "pinch" of salt to fluid ingested or food consumed usually replenishes electrolytes lost in sweat. For runners during a 20-day road race in Hawaii, plasma minerals remained normal when the athletes consumed an unrestricted diet *without* mineral supplements. This finding (and the findings of others) indicates that ingesting a "sports drink" (e.g., Gatorade) provides no special benefit in replacing the minerals lost through sweating compared with ingesting the same minerals in a well-balanced diet. Taking extra salt may prove beneficial for prolonged physical activity in the heat when fluid loss exceeds 4 or 5 kg. This can be achieved by drinking a 0.1% to 0.2% salt solution (adding 0.3 ts of table salt per L of water). Intense physical activity during heat stress can produce a mild potassium deficiency. A diet that contains the recommended amount of potassium corrects any deficiencies. Drinking an 8-oz glass of orange or tomato juice replaces the calcium, potassium, and magnesium lost in 3 L (7 lb) of sweat, an amount not likely to occur if an individual performs less than 60 minutes of vigorous physical activity. Older age Master's athletes and other older recreational enthusiasts who take blood pressure medications should remain vigilant against dehydration symptoms of dizziness, light-headedness, and nausea during physical activity from the medication's effect to lower blood pressure, coupled with water and fluid losses from environmental and physical activity effects.

SUMMARY

1. Vitamins neither supply energy nor contribute to body mass.
2. Vitamins serve crucial functions in almost all bodily processes and must be obtained from food or dietary supplementation.
3. The 13 known vitamins are classified as either water soluble or fat soluble.
4. Vitamins A, D, E, and K comprise the fat-soluble vitamins; vitamin C and the B-complex vitamins constitute the water-soluble vitamins.
5. Excess fat-soluble vitamins accumulate in body tissues and can increase to toxic concentrations.
6. Excess water-soluble vitamins remain nontoxic and eventually pass in the urine.
7. Vitamins regulate metabolism, facilitate energy release, and serve important functions in bone formation and tissue synthesis.
8. Vitamins C and E and β-carotene serve key protective antioxidant functions by reducing the potential for free radical damage or oxidative stress, while potentially offering protective benefits against heart disease and cancer.
9. Excess vitamin supplementation does not improve performance or potential for sustaining hard, physical training.
10. Serious illness can occur from regularly consuming excess fat-soluble and, in some cases, water-soluble vitamins.
11. Approximately 4% of body mass consists of 22 elements called minerals distributed in all body tissues and fluids.
12. Minerals occur freely in nature; in the waters of rivers, lakes, and oceans; and in soil.
13. The root system of plants absorbs minerals; these minerals are eventually incorporated into the tissues of animals that consume plants.
14. Minerals function primarily in metabolism as important parts of enzymes, including providing structure to bones and teeth, and in synthesizing glycogen, fat, and protein.
15. A balanced diet provides adequate mineral intake except in geographic locations with poor soil and inadequate iodine.
16. Osteoporosis has reached epidemic proportions among older individuals, especially women; one strategy is to advocate for adequate calcium intake and regular weight-bearing exercise or resistance training to help protect against bone loss.
17. Women who train vigorously often do not match energy intake to energy output.
18. Reduced body weight and body fat can adversely affect menstruation and cause advanced bone loss at an early age.
19. Approximately 40% of American women of childbearing age have dietary iron insufficiency, which could lead to iron-deficiency anemia and negatively impact aerobic exercise performance and ability to train intensely.
20. Excessive sweating during physical activity produces body water loss and related minerals, which should judiciously be replaced during and following the activity.

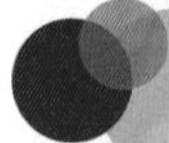

THINK IT THROUGH

1. Discuss two specific conditions that justify vitamin and mineral supplementation.
2. Discuss three factors that may contribute to gender-specific recommendations for vitamin and mineral intakes.
3. Outline the dynamics of bone loss and give two suggestions to high school females regarding protection against future osteoporosis.
4. Discuss the role played by physical activity and calcium intake on bone health.
5. Respond to an athlete who asks, "Is there anything wrong with taking megadoses of vitamin and mineral supplements to ensure getting an adequate intake on a daily basis?"
6. Why does resistance training for the body's major muscle groups offer unique benefits to bone mass compared with a typical weight-bearing program of brisk walking?

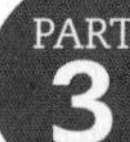

PART 3 Water

THE BODY'S WATER CONTENT

Age, gender, and body composition influence an individual's body water content, which can range from 40% to 70% of total body mass. Water constitutes 72% of muscle weight and approximately 20% to 50% of the weight of body fat or adipose tissue. Differences among individuals in relative percentage of total body water largely result from variations in body composition (i.e., differences in fat-free vs. fat tissue).

The body contains two fluid "compartments." The first, the **intracellular compartment**, refers to fluid inside cells; the second, the **extracellular compartment**, includes blood plasma (~20% of total extracellular fluid) and interstitial fluids, which primarily comprise fluid flowing in the microscopic spaces between cells. The six sources of interstitial fluid include:

1. Lymph
2. Saliva
3. Eye fluids
4. Fluids secreted by glands and the digestive tract
5. Fluids that bathe spinal cord nerves
6. Fluids excreted from skin and kidneys

Much of the fluid lost through sweating comes from extracellular fluid, predominantly blood plasma.

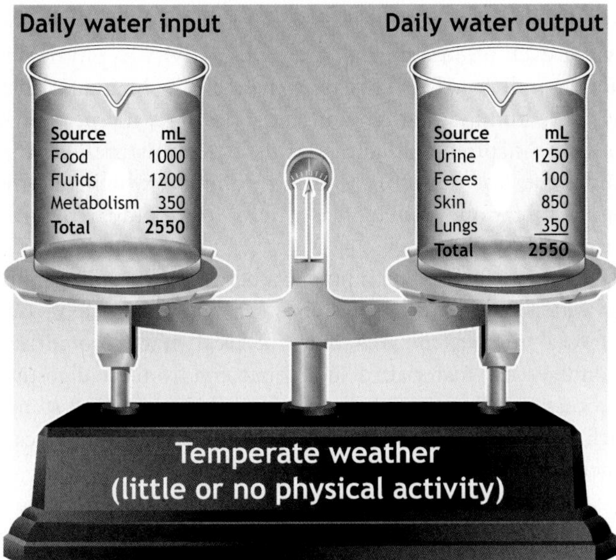

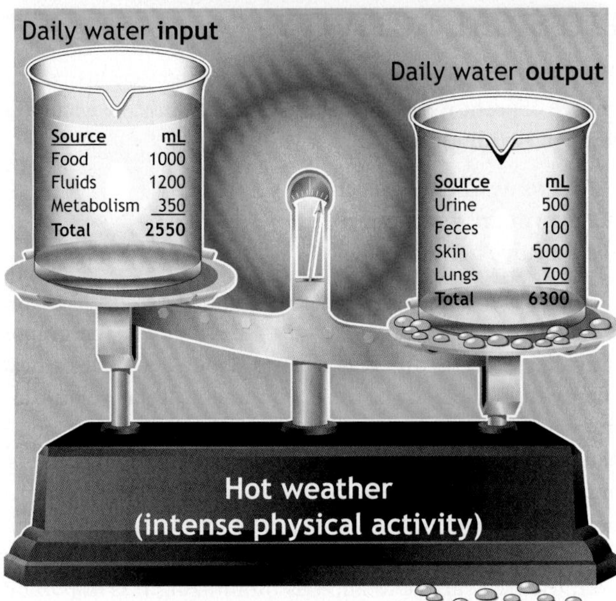

FIGURE 2.19 Water balance in the body. **Top**. Little or no exercise with thermoneutral ambient temperature and humidity. **Bottom**. Moderate-to-intense exercise in a hot, humid environment. (Adapted with permission from McArdle WD, Katch FI, Katch VL. *Exercise Physiology: Nutrition, Energy, and Human Performance*. 8th Ed. Baltimore: Wolters Kluwer Health, 2015.)

Functions of Body Water

Water serves six important functions:

1. Provides the body's transport and reactive medium.
2. Diffusion of gases occurs across moist body surfaces.
3. Waste products leave the body through the water in urine and feces.
4. Water absorbs considerable heat with only minimal changes in temperature from its heat-stabilizing qualities.
5. Watery fluids lubricate joints, keeping bony surfaces from grinding against each other.
6. Being noncompressible, water provides structure and form through the turgor it imparts to the body's tissues.

Water Balance: Intake Versus Output

The body's water content remains relatively stable over time. Appropriate fluid intake rapidly restores any imbalance. **Figure 2.19** displays the sources of water intake and water output. The bottom panel illustrates that fluid balance can change dramatically during physical activity, particularly in a hot, humid environment.

See the animation "Water Balance" on **http://thePoint.lww.com/MKKESS5e** for a demonstration of this process.

Water Intake

In a normal environment, a sedentary adult requires about 2.5 L (2.64 qt) of water daily. For an active person in a warm environment, the water requirement often increases to between 5 and 10 L daily. Three sources provide this water:

1. Liquids
2. Foods
3. Metabolic processes

The average individual living in a thermoneutral environment normally consumes about 1.2 L (1.26 qt) of water daily. Fluid intake can increase five or six times above normal during physical activity and thermal stress. A decline in body weight of 0.9 kg (2 lb) during physical activity represents approximately 1.0 L (1.06 qt) of fluid. At the extreme, an individual lost 13.6 kg (30 lb) of water weight during a

fyi The Hidden Water in Food

Most fruits and vegetables contain considerable water—more than 90% (e.g., lettuce, celery, cucumber, red and green tomatoes, spinach, zucchini, watermelon, cantaloupe, eggplant, sweet peppers, cabbage, and broccoli); in contrast, butter, oils, dried meats and chocolate, cookies, and cakes contain relatively little water (<20%).

2-day, 17-hour, 55-mile run across the desert in Death Valley, California. Proper fluid ingestion with salt supplements kept the body weight loss to only 1.4 kg (3.1 lb). In this example, fluid loss and replenishment represented between 14 and 16 qt of liquid!

Metabolizing food molecules for energy forms carbon dioxide and water. For sedentary persons, this **metabolic water** provides about 25% of their daily water requirement. This includes 55 g of water from the complete breakdown of 100 g of carbohydrate, 100 g of water from 100 g of protein breakdown, and 107 g of water from 100 g of fat catabolism. Additionally, each gram of glycogen joins with 2.7 g of water as the glucose unit's link together, thus making glycogen a heavy energy fuel. Glycogen subsequently releases this water during catabolism. For runners and other endurance athletes who consume additional carbohydrates to "overstock" their muscles' glycogen content, this practice provides a double-edged sword. On the one hand, additional glycogen is essential for elite performance in prolonged effort, yet the additional water storage decreases exercise economy because extra body mass increases energy expenditure.

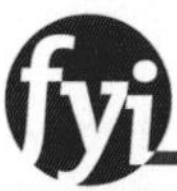

Hydration Terminology

- *Euhydration:* Normal daily water variation
- *Hyperhydration:* New steady-state condition of increased water content
- *Hypohydration:* New steady-state condition of decreased water content
- *Rehydration:* Process of gaining water from hypohydrated state toward euhydration

Water Output

The body loses water in four ways:

1. In urine
2. Through the skin
3. As water vapor in expired air
4. In feces

The kidneys normally reabsorb about 99% of the 140 to 160 L of filtrate formed daily, leaving from 1 to 1.5 L of urine or about 1.5 qt for daily excretion. Every gram of solute (e.g., the urea end product of protein breakdown) eliminated by the kidneys requires about 15 mL of water. From a practical standpoint, consuming large quantities of protein for energy via a high-protein diet *accelerates* dehydration during physical activity.

See the animation "Renal Function" on **http://thePoint.lww.com/MKKESS5e** for a demonstration of this process.

A small amount of water (perhaps 350 mL), termed **insensible perspiration**, continually seeps from the deeper tissues through the skin to the body's surface. Subcutaneous sweat glands also produce water loss through the skin. Evaporation of sweat's water component provides the refrigeration mechanism to cool the body. The daily sweat rate under most conditions amounts to between 500 and 700 mL. This by no means reflects sweating capacity; for example, a well-trained, acclimatized person produces up to 12 L of sweat (equivalent of 12 kg) at a rate of 1 L per hour during prolonged exertion in a hot environment.

Insensible water loss of 250 to 350 mL per day occurs through small water droplets in exhaled air. The complete moistening of all inspired air passing down the pulmonary airways accounts for this loss. Physical activity affects this source of water loss. Depending on climatic conditions, the respiratory passages release 2 to 5 mL of water each minute during strenuous activity in physically active individuals. Ventilatory water loss happens least in hot, humid weather and most in cold temperatures because inspired cold air contains little moisture. At altitude, the less dense inspired air volumes, which require humidification, also increase fluid loss compared with sea-level conditions.

Intestinal elimination produces between 100 and 200 mL of water loss because water constitutes approximately 70% of fecal matter; the remainder of fecal matter comprises nondigestible material, including bacteria from the digestive process and digestive juice residues from the intestine, stomach, and pancreas. With diarrhea or vomiting, water loss can increase to between 1500 and 5000 mL.

WATER REQUIREMENT DURING PHYSICAL ACTIVITY

The loss of body water represents the most serious consequence of profuse sweating. Three factors determine water loss through sweating:

1. Severity of physical activity
2. Environmental temperature
3. Relative humidity

The major physiologic defense against overheating comes from evaporation of sweat from the skin's surface. The evaporative loss of 1 L of sweat releases about 600 kcal of heat energy from the body to the environment. **Relative humidity**, which refers to water content of the ambient air compared to what the air can contain at that temperature, impacts the efficiency of the sweating mechanism in temperature regulation. At 100% relative humidity, ambient air fully saturates with water vapor. This blocks fluid evaporation from the skin surface to air, thus minimizing this important avenue for body cooling. When this happens, sweat beads on the skin and eventually rolls off without generating any cooling effect.

Dry air can hold considerable moisture, and in dry conditions, fluid evaporates rapidly from the skin. In dry air, the sweat mechanism functions at optimal efficiency to regulate body temperature.

Sweat loss equal to 2% to 3% of body mass decreases plasma volume. This amount of fluid loss strains circulatory functions and ultimately diminishes thermoregulatory control, diminishing exercise capacity. Chapter 15 presents a comprehensive discussion of thermoregulatory dynamics during physical activity in hot climates.

Exertional Heat Stroke

Heat stroke, the most serious and complex heat stress malady, requires immediate medical attention. **Heat stroke syndrome** reflects a failure of heat-regulating mechanisms triggered by excessively high body temperatures. Thermoregulatory failure strains the circulatory system, causing sweating to cease, the skin to become dry and hot, and body temperature to rise to 105.8°F (41°C) or higher. Unfortunately, subtle symptoms often confound the complexity of **exertional hyperthermia**. Instead of ceasing, sweating can occur during intense aerobic activity (e.g., 10-km running race) in young, hydrated, and highly motivated individuals. With high metabolic heat production from the intense activity, the body's heat gain greatly exceeds avenues for heat loss. If left untreated, circulatory collapse and damage to the central nervous system and other organs lead to death.

Heat stroke represents a medical emergency. While awaiting medical treatment, only aggressive treatment to rapidly lower elevated core temperature can avert death; the magnitude and duration of hyperthermia determine organ damage and mortality. Immediate treatment includes alcohol rubs and ice packs. Whole-body cold or ice water immersion remains the *most effective* treatment for a collapsed hyperthermic athlete.

Practical Recommendations for Fluid Replacement in Physical Activity

Depending on environmental conditions, total sweat loss during a marathon run in elite athletes at world record pace averages about 5.3 L (12 lb). The fluid loss corresponds to a 6% to 8% body mass loss.

Optimal fluid replacement maintains plasma volume to optimize the circulatory and sweating response. Ingesting "extra" water before exercising in the heat provides some thermoregulatory protection. Pre-exercise hyperhydration helps to:

- Delay dehydration
- Increase sweating during physical activity
- Blunt the increase in body temperature compared with exercising without prior fluids

As a practical step, a person can consume 400 to 600 mL (13 to 20 oz) of cold water 10 to 20 minutes before exercising. This prudent practice should be combined with judicious fluid replacement during the activity.

Gastric Emptying

As fluids exit the stomach, they first enter the small intestine to begin the nutrient absorption journey through the digestive tract. The following seven factors influence gastric emptying:

1. **Fluid temperature**. Cold fluids (5°C or 41°F) empty from the stomach at a faster rate than fluids at body temperature.
2. **Fluid volume**. Keeping stomach fluid volume at a relatively high level speeds gastric emptying and may compensate for any inhibitory effects of a beverage's carbohydrate or electrolyte content. Optimizing stomach volume effects on gastric emptying occurs by consuming 400 to 600 mL of fluid 10 to 20 minutes before physical activity. Ingesting fluids throughout physical activity can replenish the fluid passed into the intestine and maintains a large gastric volume during physical activity.
3. **Caloric content**. Increased energy content decreases gastric emptying rate.
4. **Fluid osmolarity**. Gastric emptying slows when the ingested fluid contains concentrated electrolytes or simple sugars glucose, fructose, or sucrose. For example, a 40% sugar solution empties from the stomach at a rate 20% slower than plain water. *As a general rule, a 5% and 8% carbohydrate-electrolyte beverage consumed during physical activity in the heat contributes to temperature regulation and fluid balance as effectively as plain water.* As an added bonus in prolonged physical activity, this drink helps to stabilize glucose metabolism and glycogen reserves.
5. **Physical activity intensity**. Physical activity up to an intensity of about 75% of maximum does not negatively affect gastric emptying; the stomach's emptying rate becomes restricted above this point.
6. **pH**. Marked deviations from a pH of 7.0 decrease emptying rate.
7. **Hydration level**. Dehydration decreases gastric emptying and increases gastrointestinal distress risk.

The trade-off between ingested fluid composition and gastric emptying rate must be evaluated based on environmental stress and energy demands. Physical activity in a cold environment does not stimulate much fluid loss from sweating. In cold environments, reduced gastric emptying and subsequent water absorption are tolerated, and a more concentrated sugar solution (15 to 20 g per 100 mL of water) may prove beneficial. Chapter 4 addresses the desirable composition of "sports drinks" and their fluid replacement effects.

Adequacy of Rehydration

Preventing dehydration and its consequences, especially a dangerously elevated body temperature (**hyperthermia**), requires adherence to an adequate water replacement schedule. This often is "easier said than done" because some individuals mistakenly believe ingesting water hinders performance. For some athletes, chronic dehydration remains a way of life during the competitive season. Competitors intentionally lose considerable fluid to compete in a lower wrestling weight class—often with fatal outcomes if dehydration becomes severe enough from electrolyte imbalances to precipitate cardiovascular abnormalities. Chronic dehydration also occurs in ballet, in which dancers focus on body weight to appear thin. Many individuals on weight loss programs incorrectly believe that restricting fluid intake in some way accelerates body fat loss.

At the extreme, some fanatics and new-age, self-help proclaimed gurus advocate abstinence of food and fluids for several days while participating in spiritual ceremonies and other "mind and body cleansing" activities while enclosed in sealed heat chambers. These harsh environmental enclosures, essentially saunas covered with plastic tarps called sweat lodges, often exceed 115°F. In October 2009, three people died as part of a group crowded into one of these structures which lacked air circulation, for purposes of "cleansing their bodies of toxins."

Monitoring changes in body weight provides a convenient method to assess fluid loss during physical activity or heat stress and the adequacy of rehydration in recovery. In addition to having athletes "weigh in" before and after practice, coaches can minimize weight loss by providing scheduled water breaks during practice or training sessions and unrestricted access to water during competition. Each 0.45 kg (1 lb) of body weight loss corresponds to 450 mL (15 oz) of dehydration. Following physical activity, the thirst mechanism can provide a "rough and imprecise" guide to water needs. If full rehydration depended entirely on a person's thirst, it could take several days to reestablish fluid balance following severe dehydration.

A CLOSER LOOK

Distinguishing Heat Cramps, Heat Exhaustion, and Heat Stroke

Human heat dissipation occurs by the following two mechanisms:

1. Blood redistribution to the periphery from deeper tissues
2. Activation of the refrigeration mechanism provided by evaporation of sweat from the surface of the skin and respiratory passages

During heat stress, cardiac output increases, vasoconstriction and vasodilation move central blood volume toward the skin, and thousands of previously dormant capillaries threading through the upper skin layer open to accommodate blood flow. Heat conduction away from warm blood at the skin's cooled surface provides about 75% of the body's heat-dissipating functions. Heat production during physical activity often strains heat-dissipating mechanisms, especially under high ambient temperature and humidity. This triggers a broad array of physical signs and symptoms collectively termed *heat illness*, ranging in severity from mild to life threatening.

Condition	Causes	Signs and Symptoms	Prevention
Heat cramps	Intense, prolonged physical activity in the heat; negative Na^+ balance	Tightening cramps, involuntary active muscle spasms, low serum Na^+	Replenish salt loss; ensure acclimatization
Heat syncope	Peripheral vasodilation and pooling of venous blood, hypotension, hypohydration	Giddiness; syncope, mostly in upright position during rest or physical activity; pallor; high rectal temperature	Ensure acclimatization and fluid replenishment; reduce exertion on hot days; avoid standing
Heat exhaustion	Cumulative negative water balance	Exhaustion, hypohydration, flushed skin, reduced sweating in extreme dehydration, syncope, high rectal temperature	Proper hydration before physical activity and adequate replenishment during physical activity; ensure acclimatization
Heat stroke	Extreme hyperthermia leading to thermoregulatory failure; aggravated by dehydration	Acute medical emergency; includes hyperpyrexia (rectal temperature > 41°C), lack of sweating, and neurologic deficit (disorientation, twitching, seizures, coma)	Ensure acclimatization; identify and exclude individuals at risk; adapt activities to climatic constraints

Hyponatremia: Water Intoxication

Under normal conditions, one can consume a maximum of about 9.5 L (10 qt) of water daily without unduly straining kidneys or diluting chemical concentrations of body fluids. Consuming more than 9.5 L can produce hyponatremia or water intoxication, a condition that dilutes the body's normal sodium concentration. In general, mild hyponatremia exists when serum sodium concentration decreases below 135 $mEq \cdot L^{-1}$; serum sodium below 125 $mEq \cdot L^{-1}$ usually triggers severe symptoms.

A sustained low–plasma sodium concentration creates an osmotic imbalance across the blood-brain barrier that forces rapid water influx into the brain. The swelling of brain tissue leads to a cascade of mild symptoms that range from headache, confusion, malaise, nausea, and cramping to medically severe symptoms that include seizures, coma, pulmonary edema, cardiac arrest, and death. The five most important predisposing factors to hyponatremia include:

1. Prolonged intense physical activity in hot weather
2. Poorly conditioned individuals who experience excessive sweat loss with high sodium concentration
3. Physical activity performed in a sodium-depleted state because of a "salt-free" or "low-sodium" diet
4. Diuretic medication for hypertension
5. Frequent consumption of excessive sodium-free fluids during prolonged physical activity

A CLOSER LOOK

Reducing Overhydration Risk During Extended-Duration Endurance Physical Activities: A Divergence From Existing Dogma Worth Considering

The International Marathon Medical Director's Association (IMMDA; **http://aims-association.org/guidelines_fluid_replacement.htm**; USA Track and Field; [USATF; **www.usatf.org/Home.aspx**] and many governing bodies of marathon and ultraendurance events (i.e., Boston Marathon, South African Ironman Triathlons, South African Comrades ultramarathon [**www.comrades.com**] and about 50 New Zealand walking, minimarathons, marathons, and ultramarathons; **www.runningcalendar.co.nz**) provides guidance for runners and walkers at all levels in their training and competitive events. These IMMDA guidelines are congruent with guidelines adopted at an International Consensus Conference on **exercise-associated hyponatremia (EAH)**.

Ten Convenient Guidelines:

1. Do **not** load up on fluids (water or sports drinks) 2 to 3 hours before the event.
2. If you feel thirsty before the event, drink 5 to 10 oz of plain water 10 to 15 minutes prior to its start. Too much fluid in the gut does not immediately absorb.
3. During the event, drink **only** when thirsty, not necessarily at every water station. Do **not** load up on fluids at the water stations. It is acceptable to drink water from cups along the way (300 to 400 mL an hour equivalent to a normal soda can, but no more than 600 mL an hour), but not repeated multiple, large gulps equivalent to 2 to 4 cans of soda every few miles. This will add to weight gain, a predictor of potential maladies with EAH and particularly exercise-associated hyponatremic encephalopathy (EAHE). A 2% increase in total body water produces generalized edema that can precipitate deterioration in athletic and mental performance; increased levels of overhydration or "waterlogging" result in EAHE—severe cerebral edema that produces confusion, seizures, coma, and ultimately death from respiratory arrest.
4. Despite heavy advertising and promotion by the soft drink industry, do **not** consume commercially prepared "sports drinks" (particularly those containing added sodium, sodium chloride, and potassium) during the event.
5. Following the event, do **not** voluntarily consume large fluid quantities, attempting to immediately replace all fluids lost during the event.
6. To reduce dehydration and EAH and EAHE risk, drink **only** when you truly feel thirsty. In other words, let thirst dictate how much you drink. Refrain from drinking if you do not feel thirsty.
7. Do **not** consume "salt tablets" during the event or days before the event, even under hot weather conditions.
8. Do **not** add "extra" salt to your meals or fluids in the days prior to the event. Meals consumed following the event will replace any electrolyte deficits.
9. Do **not** load up on sports drinks in the days before the event believing it will "build up" electrolyte reserves.

As with any endurance endeavor, do **not** participate if you have not devoted weeks or months to a structured, endurance training regimen. If you plan to participate in a hot weather event, train under similar hot weather conditions of temperature and relative humidity, using a replacement water strategy you have come to rely on during training and which you can replicate during the event.

References

American College of Sports Medicine. American College of Sports Medicine position stand. Exercise and fluid replacement. *Med Sci Sports Exer* 2007;39:377.

Hew-Butler T, et al. Consensus statement of the 1st International Exercise-Associated Hyponatremia Consensus Development Conference, Cape Town, South Africa 2005. *Clin J Sport Med* 2005;15:208.

Noakes TD. *Waterlogged: The Serious Problem of Overhydration in Endurance Sports*. Champaign: Human Kinetics, 2012.

Hyponatremia results from extreme sodium loss through prolonged sweating, coupled with diluted extracellular sodium including reduced osmolality from drinking low or no sodium fluids. Hyponatremia can occur in experienced athletes. The likely scenario includes intense, ultramarathon-type, continuous exertion lasting 6 to 8 hours or more, although it can occur in only 4 hours. Nearly 30% of athletes who competed in an Ironman triathlon experienced hyponatremic symptoms; these occurred most frequently late in the race or in the recovery following competition. In a large study of more than 18,000 ultraendurance athletes including triathletes, approximately 9% of collapsed athletes during or after competition presented with symptoms of hyponatremia.

SUMMARY

1. Water constitutes 40% to 70% of an individual's total body mass.
2. Muscle contains 72% water by weight; in contrast, water represents only 20% to 50% of the weight of body fat.
3. Approximately 62% of total body water occurs intracellularly; the remaining 38% occurs extracellularly in the plasma, lymph, and other fluids.
4. Aqueous solutions supply food and oxygen to cells, and waste products always leave via a watery medium.
5. The normal average daily water intake of 2.5 L comes from liquid intake (1.2 L), food (1.0 L), and metabolic water produced during energy-yielding reactions (0.3 L).
6. Daily water loss occurs through urine (1.0 to 1.5 L), through the skin as insensible perspiration (0.35 L) and sweat (500 to 700 mL), as water vapor in expired air (0.25 to 0.35 L), and in feces (0.10 L).
7. Hot weather physical activity greatly increases the body's water requirement from fluid loss via sweating; in extreme thermal conditions, fluid needs increase five or six times above normal.
8. The three major forms of heat illness include heat cramps, heat exhaustion, and heat stroke.
9. Heat stroke represents the most serious and complex heat illness malady.
10. Factors affecting gastric emptying rate include keeping fluid volume in the stomach at a relatively high level, avoiding concentrated sugar solutions, and consuming cold fluids.
11. The primary aim of fluid replacement is to maintain plasma volume.
12. The ideal fluid replacement schedule during physical activity should match fluid loss.
13. Monitoring change in body weight during and following workouts indicates the effectiveness of fluid replacement strategies.
14. Drinking concentrated sugar-containing beverages slows gastric emptying rate.
15. The ideal oral rehydration solution (between 5% and 8% carbohydrates) attempts to replenish carbohydrate without adversely affecting fluid balance and thermoregulation.
16. Excessive sweating and ingesting large volumes of plain water during prolonged physical activity decrease extracellular sodium concentration and set the stage for the potentially dangerous condition hyponatremia or water intoxication.

THINK IT THROUGH

1. What two specific approaches can a coach establish for athletes to guard against dehydration and possible heat injury? Include two factors that optimize fluid replenishment.
2. In what way would knowledge about hyponatremia modify your recommendations concerning fluid intake prior to, during, and in recovery from longer-duration endurance physical activity?

KEY TERMS

Arginine vasopressin: Amino acid peptide secreted from the posterior pituitary gland, whose function helps to minimize water loss in urine; also known as antidiuretic hormone (ADH).

Biologic value: Food rating that ranks its completeness for supplying essential amino acids.

Carbohydrates: A large biological molecule or macromolecule consisting of carbon (C), hydrogen (H), and oxygen (O) atoms, usually with a 2:1 hydrogen-to-oxygen atom ratio (e.g., glucose = $C_6H_{12}O_6$).

Catabolism: Enzyme-mediated metabolic pathways that degrade molecules in processes that release energy.

Catalase: Antioxidant enzyme found in nearly all living organisms exposed to oxygen; catalyzes the decomposition of hydrogen peroxide to water and oxygen.

Cellulose: Nonstarch, structural polysaccharide found exclusively in plants.

Cholesterol: Derived lipid with numerous functions found only in animal tissues and widespread in the cell's plasma membrane and obtained through food intake (exogenous cholesterol) or synthesized within the body (endogenous cholesterol).

Coenzymes: Nonprotein organic substances facilitate enzyme action by binding the substrate with a specific enzyme.

Complete proteins: Foods containing all of the essential amino acids in their proper ratio to support normal body functions.

Complex carbohydrates: Term used to classify polysaccharides.

Compound lipids: Neutral fat combined with phosphorus (phospholipid) or glucose (glucolipid).

Deamination: Opposite process of transamination; involves removal of an amine group from an amino acid molecule, with the remaining carbon skeleton converting to a carbohydrate or lipid or used as an energy source.

Derived lipid: Substances formed from simple and compound lipids; an example is cholesterol.

Disaccharide: Combination of two monosaccharide molecules forms a double sugar. Examples include sucrose, lactose, and maltose.

Docosahexaenoic acid (DHA): Omega-3 fatty acid with a 22-carbon chain and six *cis* double bonds; primary structural component of brain, cerebral cortex, skin, sperm, testicles, and retina.

Eicosapentaenoic acid (EHA): Omega-3 fatty acid with a 20-caron chain and five *cis* double bonds; serves as a precursor for prostaglandins.

Electrolytes: Substances that dissociate into ions in ionizing solvents such as water; include most soluble salts, acids, and bases.

Endogenous cholesterol: Cholesterol synthesized in the body.

Essential amino acids: Indispensable amino acids the body cannot synthesize at a sufficient rate to prevent impaired, normal cellular function, so they must be ingested preformed in foods.

Exercise-associated hyponatremia (EAH): Potentially fatal fluid retention imbalance ("overdrinking" or water intoxication) during prolonged endurance-type exercise, congruent with poor brain regulation of posterior pituitary arginine vasopressin hormone secretion; sustained fluid intake beyond fluid excretion capacity, which can induce vomiting, altered mental status, seizures, and ultimately death.

Exertional hyperthermia: Elevated core temperature caused by physical activity.

Exogenous cholesterol: Cholesterol obtained through food intake.

Extracellular compartment: Fluids outside cells (blood plasma, interstitial fluids, microscopic spaces between cells); about 17 L in 70-kg man and 14 L in woman.

Fat-soluble vitamins: Vitamins A, D, K, and E dissolve and store in the body's fatty tissues.

Female athlete triad: Condition of low energy intake from disordered eating, menstrual cycle irregularities, and eventual osteoporosis.

Fiber: Nondigestible carbohydrates and lignin intrinsic and intact in plants, which includes functional fiber consisting of isolated nondigestible carbohydrates with beneficial physiologic effects.

Free radical: Chemically reactive molecule, or molecular fragment with at least one unpaired electron in its outer orbital or valence shell; examples include superoxide (O_2^-), hydrogen peroxide (H_2O_2), and hydroxyl (OH^-).

Fructose: The sweetest sugar monosaccharide found in honey, tree and vine fruits, flowers, berries, and most root vegetables.

Functional anemia: Low values for hemoglobin within the "normal" range but with low iron reserves; individual with this exhibits poor exercise performance.

Functional fiber: Nondigestible carbohydrates with beneficial human physiologic outcomes.

Galactose: Forms milk sugar in lactating animal's mammary glands.

Glucagon: Known as the insulin antagonist hormone; glucagon stimulates liver glycogenolysis and gluconeogenesis.

Gluconeogenesis: Glucose formed from nonglucose sources, mostly protein.

Glucose: Six-carbon monosaccharide in plants, and one of three dietary monosaccharides along with fructose and galactose; absorbed directly during digestion.

Glutathione peroxidase: Peroxidase-containing "protective" enzyme helps to reduce lipid hydroperoxides to alcohols and hydrogen peroxide to water.

Glycemic index: Relative index of a food's carbohydrate content to increase blood glucose levels; quantified after ingesting a food containing 50 g of carbohydrate and comparing it over a 2-hour period with a "standard" for carbohydrate, usually white bread or glucose with an assigned value of 100.

Glycemic load: Quantifies the overall glycemic effect of a typical portion of food, and represents the amount of available carbohydrate in that serving and the food's glycemic index.

Glycogen: Stored polysaccharide mainly in muscle tissue.

Glycogenesis: Intracellular process that transforms glucose molecules into glycogen.

Glycogenolysis: Liver glycogen converted to glucose.

Heat stroke syndrome: Failure of heat-regulating mechanisms, where skin surface becomes dry and hot and core temperature increases to 105.8°F (41°C) or higher.

Hemosiderin and ferritin: Iron stores in the liver, spleen, and bone marrow.

High-density lipoprotein (HDL): Contains greatest percentage of protein and least total lipid and cholesterol.

Hitting the wall: Severe depletion of liver and muscle glycogen, making the athlete wanting to "quit" further participation in an activity.

Hormone: Internally secreted, regulatory chemical messenger released from a host gland (e.g., pituitary), which circulates in body fluids to target specific cells or tissues remote from the host to produce a particular physiologic action.

Hydrolysis: Complex carbohydrate degrades into its component sugar molecules (e.g., sucrose breaks down to glucose and fructose) by cleavage of chemical bonds and addition of water.

Hyperthermia: Elevated core temperature.

Hypervitaminosis A: Condition of high storage levels of vitamins, which can lead to toxic symptoms.

Hypoglycemia: Blood sugar below normal blood levels; $<45\ mg \cdot dL^{-1}$.

Incomplete protein: Foods that lack one or more essential amino acids.

Insensible perspiration: Perspiration that seeps from deeper tissues through skin to the body's surface.

Insulin index: Measure to quantify the typical insulin response to various foods by comparing the insulin response of different foods administered as a standard 1000 kJ portion with water to white bread.

Intracellular compartment: Fluids within body cells; about 28 L in 70-kg man and 23 L in woman.

Iron deficiency anemia: Low red blood cell or hemoglobin levels caused by insufficient dietary intake and absorption of iron and/or bodily iron loss.

Isocaloric: Nutrient-balanced "normal" diet for an individual; energy intake balances energy expenditure.

Lactose: Glucose + galactose present in natural form only in milk (often called milk sugar).

Lactovegetarians: Individuals who consume nutrients mainly from plants; their diet may include dairy products but not eggs.

Lipid: Category of complex molecules that include fatty acids, neutral fats, waxes, and steroids.

Lipid peroxidation: Oxidative degradation of lipids; free radicals "steal" electrons from lipids in cell membranes resulting in cell damage.

Lipoproteins: Formed in the liver from joining protein with triacylglycerols, phospholipids, or cholesterol, each defined by their gravitational densities as chylomicrons, high density, low density, and very low density.

Low-density lipoprotein (LDL): Carries between 60% and 80% of total serum cholesterol and greatest affinity for cells in the arterial wall. LDL delivers cholesterol to arterial tissue, where LDL oxidizes to participate in smooth muscle cell proliferation and other unfavorable changes that damage and narrow arteries.

Major minerals: Minerals required in amounts above $100\ mg \cdot d^{-1}$.

Maltose: Glucose + glucose present in beer, cereals, and germinating seeds.

Metabolic water: Water created inside a living organism through metabolism by oxidizing energy-containing substances in their food.

Minerals: Twenty-two mostly metallic elements ingested and found in the body; serve as constituents of enzymes, hormones, and vitamins.

Monosaccharide: The simplest form of sugar, usually colorless, water soluble, and a crystalline solid. Examples include glucose (dextrose or blood sugar), fructose (levulose), and galactose.

Nonessential amino acids: Amino acids formed from compounds in the body at a rate that meets demands for normal growth and tissue repair.

Omega-3 fatty acids: Fatty acid family found primarily in the oils of shellfish and cold water herring, salmon, sardines, bluefish, mackerel, and sea mammals; currently considered a healthful form of fat.

Osteoporosis: Skeletal disease characterized by loss of bone mineral density that leaves bones hollow, fenestrated, and susceptible to fracture.

Ovolactovegetarians: Individuals who consume nutrients only from plants, but their diet may include dairy products including eggs.

Oxidative stress: Free radical buildup, increasing the potential for cellular damage including inflammation.

Polypeptide: Amino acid chain chemically linked together by peptide bonds.

Polysaccharides: Carbohydrate molecules composed of long chains of monosaccharide units bound together by glycosidic linkages; in digestion, undergoes hydrolysis to yield constituent monosaccharides or oligosaccharides. Examples include starch (plants) and glycogen (animals), and structural polysaccharides (cellulose and chitin).

Recommended protein requirements: How much protein needed to remain healthy based on age. For men and women ages 18 to 65, multiply 0.83 g protein per kg body mass. Requirement may increase with regular intense physical activity.

Relative humidity: Ambient air's water content compared to what it could contain at that temperature.

Saturated fatty acids: Contain only single bonds between carbon atoms, with the remaining bonds attached to hydrogen, holding as many hydrogen atoms as chemically possible (i.e., saturated relative to hydrogen).

Simple lipids: Referred to as neutral fat; triacylglycerols consist of a glycerol component and three clusters of carbon-chained fatty acids attached to the glycerol molecule.

Simple sugars: Monosaccharides (glucose, fructose, galactose) and disaccharides (sucrose, lactose, maltose) are referred to as simple sugars.

Sodium-induced hypertension: Chronic excess of dietary sodium that increases fluid volume and possibly increased peripheral vascular resistance, which can undesirably elevate blood pressure and pose a health risk.

Starch: Storage form of plant polysaccharide formed from hundreds of bound sugar molecules.

Sucrose: Joining of glucose and fructose, which occurs naturally in most foods that contain carbohydrate, particularly beet sugar, cane sugar, brown sugar, maple syrup, and honey.

Superoxide dismutase: Enzyme that catalyzes the dismutation of superoxide (O_2^-) into oxygen and hydrogen peroxide; important antioxidant defense in nearly all cells exposed to oxygen.

Trace minerals: Minerals required in amounts below $100\ mg \cdot dL^{-1}$.

Transamination: Process of nitrogen removal from an amino acid, when an amine group shifts from a donor amino acid to an acceptor acid, with the acceptor becoming a new amino acid.

***Trans* fatty acids:** Compound formed during hydrogenation of unsaturated corn, soybean, or sunflower oil when one hydrogen atom along the carbon chain moves from its naturally occurring position to the opposite side of the double bond that separates two carbon atoms. Currently considered an unhealthful compound, *trans* fat sources include vegetable shortenings, some margarines, crackers, candies, cookies, snack foods, fried foods, baked goods, salad dressings, and other processed foods made with partially hydrogenated vegetable oils.

Transferrin: Iron-binding blood plasma glycoproteins, which control the free iron level in biological fluids.

Triacylglycerols: Most prevalent lipid in body; neutral fat consisting of glycerol + 3-carbon cluster of fatty acids.

Unsaturated fatty acids: Contain one or more double bonds along the main carbon chain; each double bond along the chain reduces the potential number of hydrogen-binding sites (i.e., molecule remains unsaturated relative to hydrogen).

Vegans: According to the Vegetarian Society founded in 1847 (**www.vegsoc.org**), a vegan "lives on a diet of grains, legumes, nuts, seeds, vegetables and fruits with or without the use of dairy products and eggs. They do not eat any meat, poultry, game, fish, shellfish or crustacea, or slaughter by-products."

Very low density lipoprotein (VLDL): Contains greatest percentage of lipid; transports triacylglycerols formed in the liver from fats, carbohydrates, alcohol, and cholesterol to muscle and adipose tissue.

Water-insoluble fibers: Insoluble fibers in water; includes cellulose, hemicellulose, lignin, and wheat bran.

Water-soluble fibers: Soluble fibers in water; includes pectin and guar gum present in oats, legumes, barley, brown rice, peas, and carrots.

Water-soluble vitamins: Vitamin C and the B-complex vitamin group soluble in the body's watery compartments.

SELECTED REFERENCES

Adams-Hillard PJ, Deitch HR. Menstrual disorders in the college age female. *Pediatr Clin North Am* 2005;52:179.

Alexander DD, et al. A systematic review of multivitamin-multimineral use and cardiovascular disease and cancer incidence and total mortality. *J Am Coll Nutr* 2013;32(5):339.

American College of Sports Medicine, American Dietetic Association, and Dietitians of Canada. Joint Position Statement. Nutrition and athletic performance. *Med Sci Sports Exerc* 2000;32:2130.

American College of Sports Medicine. American College of Sports Medicine Position Stand. Osteoporosis and exercise. *Med Sci Sports Exerc* 1995;27:i.

American College of Sports Medicine. Position stand on physical activity and bone health. *Med Sci Sports Exerc* 2004;36:1985.

American Dietetic Association; Dietitians of Canada; American College of Sports Medicine. American College of Sports Medicine position stand. Nutrition and athletic performance. *Med Sci Sports Exerc* 2009;41:709. Review.

Aoi W. Exercise and food factors. *Forum Nutr* 2009;61:147.

Astrup A. Yogurt and dairy product consumption to prevent cardiometabolic diseases: epidemiologic and experimental studies. *Am J Clin Nutr* 2014;99(5 Suppl):1235S.

Barberger-Gateau P, et al. Dietary patterns and risk of dementia: the Three-City cohort study. *Neurology* 2007;69:1921.

Bartali B, et al. Serum micronutrient concentrations and decline in physical function among older persons. *JAMA* 2008;299:3208.

Bartoszewska M, et al. Vitamin D, muscle function, and exercise performance. *Pediatr Clin North Am* 2010;57:849.

Berkulo MA, et al. Ad-libitum drinking and performance during a 40-km cycling time trial in the heat. *Eur J Sport Sci* 2015;12:1.

Boon H, et al. Substrate source use in older, trained males after decades of endurance training. *Med Sci Sports Exerc* 2007;39:2160.

Bratland-Sanda S, Sundgot-Borgen J. "I'm concerned—What Do I Do?" recognition and management of disordered eating in fitness center settings. *Int J Eat Disord* 2015;48:415.

Cases N, et al. Differential response of plasma and immune cell's vitamin E levels to physical activity and antioxidant vitamin supplementation. *Eur J Clin Nutr* 2005;59:781.

Chlíbková D, et al. The prevalence of exercise-associated hyponatremia in 24-hour ultra-mountain bikers, 24-hour ultra-runners and multi-stage ultra-mountain bikers in the Czech Republic. *J Int Soc Sports Nutr* 2014;11:3.

Cox GR, et al. Daily training with high carbohydrate availability increases exogenous carbohydrate oxidation during endurance cycling. *J Appl Physiol* 2010;109:126.

Coyle EF. Improved muscular efficiency displayed as Tour de France champion matures. *J Appl Physiol* 2005;98:2191.

Davies JH, et al. Bone mass acquisition in healthy children. *Arch Dis Child* 2005;90:373.

Davis JK, Green JM. Caffeine and anaerobic performance: ergogenic value and mechanisms of action. *Sports Med* 2009;39:813.

Demark-Wahnefried W, et al. Lifestyle intervention development study to improve physical function in older adults with cancer: outcomes from Project LEAD. *J Clin Oncol* 2006;24:3465.

Dickinson A, et al. Consumer usage and reasons for using dietary supplements: report of a series of surveys. *J Am Coll Nutr* 2014;33:176.

Donsmark M, et al. Hormone-sensitive lipase as mediator of lipolysis in contracting skeletal muscle. *Exerc Sport Sci Rev* 2005;33:127.

Draper SB, et al. Overdrinking-induced hyponatraemia in the 2007 London Marathon. *BMJ Case Rep* 2009;2009.

Erdman KA, et al. Influence of performance level on dietary supplementation in elite Canadian athletes. *Med Sci Sports Exerc* 2006;38:349.

Fairey AS, et al. Randomized controlled trial of exercise and blood immune function in postmenopausal breast cancer survivors. *J Appl Physiol* 2005;98:1534.

Feiereisen P, et al. Is strength training the more efficient training modality in chronic heart failure? *Med Sci Sports Exerc* 2007;39:1910.

Food and Nutrition Board, Institute of Medicine. *Dietary Reference Intakes for Energy, Carbohydrates, Fiber, Fat, Protein and Amino Acids.* Washington, DC: National Academy Press, 2002.

Fortmann SP, et al., eds. *Vitamin, Mineral, and Multivitamin Supplements for the Primary Prevention of Cardiovascular Disease and Cancer: A Systematic Evidence Review for the U.S. Preventive Services Task Force [Internet].* Rockville: Agency for Healthcare Research and Quality (US), 2013. Report No.: 14-05199-EF-1. U.S. Preventive Services Task Force Evidence Syntheses, formerly Systematic Evidence Reviews.

Foskett A, et al. Carbohydrate availability and muscle energy metabolism during intermittent running. *Med Sci Sports Exerc* 2008;401:96.

Gaine PC, et al. Postexercise whole-body protein turnover response to three levels of protein intake. *Med Sci Sports Exerc* 2007;39:480.

Ganio MS, et al. Effect of various carbohydrate-electrolyte fluids on cycling performance and maximal voluntary contraction. *Int J Sport Nutr Exerc Metab* 2010;20:104.

Geleijnse JM, et al. Effect of low doses of n-3 fatty acids on cardiovascular diseases in 4,837 post-myocardial infarction patients: design and baseline characteristics of the Alpha Omega Trial. *Am Heart J* 2010;159:539.

Godek SF, et al. Sweat rate and fluid turnover in American football players compared with runners in a hot and humid environment. *Br J Sports Med* 2005;39:205.

Green HJ, et al. Mechanical and metabolic responses with exercise and dietary carbohydrate manipulation. *Med Sci Sports Exerc* 2007;391:139.

Greydanus DE, et al. The adolescent female athlete: current concepts and conundrums. *Pediatr Clin North Am* 2010;57:697.

Gropper SS, et al. Iron status of female collegiate athletes involved in different sorts. *Biol Trace Elem Res* 2006;109:1.

Guadalupe-Grau A, et al. Exercise and bone mass in adults. *Sports Med* 2009; 39:439.

Hamilton KL. Antioxidants and cardioprotection. *Med Sci Sports Exerc* 2007; 39:1544.

Hew-Butler, et al. Practical management of exercise-associated hyponatremic encephalopathy: the sodium paradox of non-osmotic vasopressin secretion. *Clin J Sport Med* 2008;18:350.

Holt SH, Miller JC, Petocz P. An insulin index of foods: the insulin demand generated by 1000-kJ portions of common foods. *Am J Clin Nutr* 1997;66(5):1264.

Irwin ML. Randomized controlled trials of physical activity and breast cancer prevention. *Exerc Sport Sci Rev* 2006;34:182.

Jentjens RL, Jeukendrup AE. High rates of exogenous carbohydrate oxidation from a mixture of glucose and fructose ingested during prolonged cycling exercise. *Br J Nutr* 2005;93:485.

Jeukendrup AE, et al. Nutritional considerations in triathlon. *Sports Med* 2005;35:163.

Jeukendrup AE, Wallis GA. Measurement of substrate oxidation during exercise by means of gas exchange measurements. *Int J Sports Med* 2005;26 (Suppl 1):S28.

Jeukendrup AE. Carbohydrate and exercise performance: the role of multiple transportable carbohydrates. *Curr Opin Clin Nutr Metab Care* 2010;13:452.

Jeukendrup AE. Carbohydrate intake during exercise and performance. *Nutrition* 2004;20:669.

Klungland Torstveit M, Sundgot-Borgen J. The female athlete triad: are elite athletes at increased risk. *Med Sci Sports Exerc* 2005;37:184.

Kobayashi IH, et al. Intake of fish and omega-3 fatty acids and risk of coronary heart disease among Japanese: The Japan Public Health Center-Based (JPHC) Study Cohort 1. *Circulation* 2006;113:195.

Lanou AJ, et al. Calcium, dairy products, and bone health in children and young adults: a reevaluation of the evidence. *Pediatrics* 2005;115:736.

Lecarpentier Y. Physiological role of free radicals in skeletal muscles. *J Appl Physiol* 2007;103:1917.

Li WC, et al. Effects of exercise programs on quality of life in osteoporotic and osteopenic postmenopausal women: a systematic review and meta-analysis. *Clin Rehabil* 2009;23(10):888.

Lindsey C, et al. Association of physical performance measures with bone mineral density in postmenopausal women. *Arch Phys Med Rehabil* 2005;86:1102.

Liu JF, et al. Blood lipid peroxides and muscle damage increased following intensive resistance training of female weightlifters. *Ann N Y Acad Sci* 2005; 1042:255.

Lonn E, et al. Effects of long-term vitamin E supplementation on cardiovascular events and cancer: a randomized controlled trial. *JAMA* 2005;293:1338.

Loucks AB. New animal model opens opportunities for research on the female athlete triad. *J Appl Physiol* 2007;103:1467.

Lukaski HC. Vitamin and mineral status: effects on physical performance. *Nutrition* 2004;20:632.

Ma Y, et al. Dietary quality 1 year after diagnosis of coronary heart disease. *J Am Diet Assoc* 2008;108:240.

Maughan RJ, Shirreffs SM. Development of individual hydration strategies for athletes. *Int J Sport Nutr Exerc Metab* 2008;18:457.

Melin A, et al. Energy availability and the female athlete triad in elite endurance athletes. *Scand J Med Sci Sports* 2014; doi: 10.1111/sms.12261.

Melin A, et al. Disordered eating and eating disorders in aquatic sports. *Int J Sport Nutr Exerc Metab* 2014;24:450.

Melin A, et al. The LEAF questionnaire: a screening tool for the identification of female athletes at risk for the female athlete triad. *Br J Sports Med* 2014;48:540.

Mountjoy M, et al. The IOC consensus statement: beyond the Female Athlete Triad—Relative Energy Deficiency in Sport (RED-S). *Br J Sports Med* 2014; 48:491.

Myint PK, et al. Plasma vitamin C concentrations predict risk of incident stroke over 10 y in 20649 participants of the European Prospective Investigation into Cancer Norfolk prospective population study. *Am J Clin Nutr* 2008;87:64.

Nolte HW, et al. Exercise-associated hyponatremic encephalopathy and exertional heatstroke in a soldier: High rates of fluid intake during exercise caused rather than prevented a fatal outcome. *Phys Sportsmed* 2015;43:93.

Noakes TD. Changes in body mass alone explain almost all of the variance in the serum sodium concentrations during prolonged exercise. Has commercial influence impeded scientific endeavour? *Br J Sports Med* 2011;45:475.

Noakes TD. Body cooling as a method for reducing hyperthermia. *S Afr Med J* 1986;70:373.

Noakes TD. *Waterlogged: The Serious Problem of Overhydration in Endurance Sports*. Champaign: Human Kinetics, 2012.

Ormsbee MJ, Bach CW, Baur DA. Pre-exercise nutrition: the role of macronutrients, modified starches and supplements on metabolism and endurance performance. *Nutrients* 2014;6:1782.

Pikosky MA, et al. Increased protein maintains nitrogen balance during exercise-induced energy deficit. *Med Sci Sports Exerc* 2008;40:505.

Popp KL, et al. Bone geometry, strength, and muscle size in runners with a history of stress fracture. *Med Sci Sports Exerc* 2009;41:2145.

Qi L, et al. Whole grain, bran, and cereal fiber intakes and markers of systemic inflammation in diabetic women. *Diabetes Care* 2006;29:207.

Reinking MF, Alexander LE. Prevalence of disordered-eating behaviors in undergraduate female collegiate athletes and nonathletes. *J Athl Train* 2005;40:47.

Rizkalla SW. Glycemic index: is it a predictor of metabolic and vascular disorders? *Curr Opin Clin Nutr Metab Care* 2014;17(4):373.

Rosner MH. Exercise-associated hyponatremia. *Semin Nephrol* 2009;29:271.

Roth EM, Harris WS. Fish oil for primary and secondary prevention of coronary heart disease. *Curr Atheroscler Rep* 2010;12:66.

Siegel AJ, et al. Hyponatremia in marathon runners due to inappropriate arginine vasopressin secretion. *Am J Med* 2007;120:461.e11-7.

Simopoulos AP. Genetic variants in the metabolism of omega-6 and omega-3 fatty acids: their role in the determination of nutritional requirements and chronic disease risk. *Exp Biol Med* 2010;235:785.

Siu PM, et al. Effect of frequency of carbohydrate feedings on recovery and subsequent endurance run. *Med Sci Sports Exerc* 2004;36:315.

Slentz CA, et al. Inactivity, exercise training and detraining, and plasma lipoproteins. STRRIDE: a randomized, controlled study of exercise intensity and amount. *J Appl Physiol* 2007;103:432.

Starnes JW, Taylor RP. Exercise-induced cardioprotection: endogenous mechanisms. *Med Sci Sports Exerc* 2007;39:1537.

Stewart KJ, et al. Exercise effects on bone mineral density relationships to changes in fitness and fatness. *Am J Prev Med* 2005;28:453.

Suh SW, et al. Hypoglycemia, brain energetics, and hypoglycemic neuronal death. *Glia* 2007;55:1280.

Sundgot-Borgen J, et al. How to minimize the health risks to athletes who compete in weight-sensitive sports review and position statement on behalf of the Ad Hoc Research Working Group on Body Composition, Health and Performance, under the auspices of the IOC Medical Commission. *Br J Sports Med* 2013;47:1012.

Thomas-John M, et al. Risk factors for the development of osteoporosis and osteoporotic fractures among older men. *J Rheumatol* 2009;36:1947.

Torstveit MK, Sundgot-Borgen J. Low bone mineral density is two to three times more prevalent in non-athletic premenopausal women than in elite athletes: a comprehensive controlled study. *Br J Sports Med* 2005;39:282.

Torstveit MK, Sundgot-Borgen J. The female athlete triad: are elite athletes at increased risk? *Med Sci Sports Exerc* 2005;37:184.

Venables MC, Jeukendrup AE. Endurance training and obesity: effect on substrate metabolism and insulin sensitivity. *Med Sci Sports Exerc* 2008; 40:495.

Wallis GA, et al. Oxidation of combined ingestion of maltodextrins and fructose during exercise. *Med Sci Sports Exerc* 2005;37:426.

Westerlind KC, Williams NI. Effect of energy deficiency on estrogen metabolism in premenopausal women. *Med Sci Sports Exerc* 2007;39:1090.

Williams PT. Reduced diabetic, hypertensive, and cholesterol medication use with walking. *Med Sci Sports Exerc* 2008;40:433.

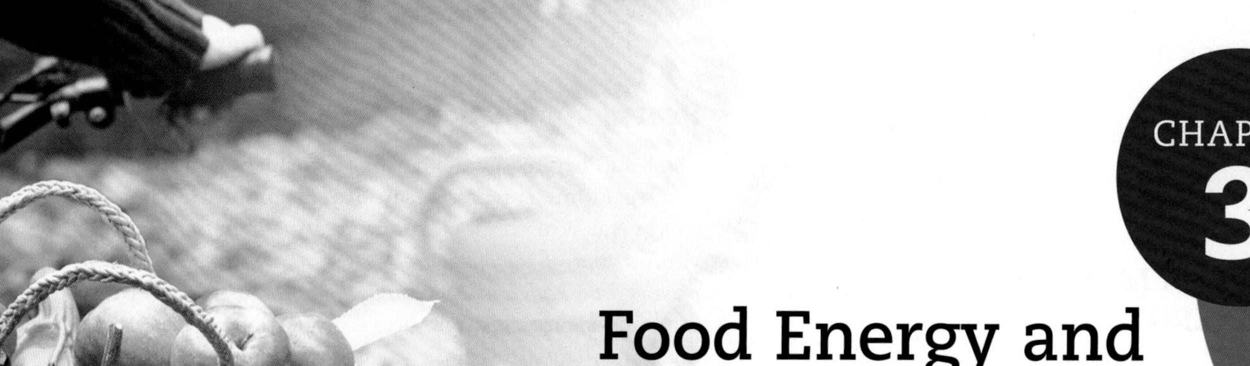

CHAPTER 3

Food Energy and Optimum Nutrition for Physical Activity

CHAPTER OBJECTIVES

- Define *heat of combustion*, *digestive efficiency*, and *Atwater general factors*.
- Compute the energy content of a meal from its macronutrient composition.
- Compare the nutrient and energy intakes of physically active men and women with sedentary counterparts.
- Compare and contrast the MyPlate, Mediterranean Diet Pyramid, and Healthy Eating Plate guides to healthy eating.
- Describe the timing and composition of the pre-event (precompetition) meal, including reasons for limiting lipid and protein intake.
- Summarize effects of low, normal, and high carbohydrate intake on glycogen reserves and subsequent endurance performance.
- For endurance athletes, describe the potential negative effects of consuming a concentrated sugar drink 30 minutes before competition and the ideal composition of a "sports drink."
- Discuss possible reasons why consuming high-glycemic carbohydrates during intense aerobic physical activity enhances endurance performance.
- Define a glucose polymer and give the rationale for adding these compounds to a sports drink.
- Make two general recommendations concerning carbohydrate intake for athletes in intense training.
- Describe the most effective way to replenish glycogen reserves following an intense training regimen or competition.
- Compare and contrast classic carbohydrate loading with modified loading procedures.

ANCILLARIES AT A GLANCE

Visit **http://thePoint.lww.com/MKKESS5e** to access the following resources.

- References: Chapter 3
- Interactive Question Bank
- Appendix A: The Metric System and Conversion Constants in Exercise Physiology
- Appendix B: Dietary Reference Intakes (DRIs): Recommended Vitamin and Mineral Intakes for Individuals
- Appendix SR-3: Nutritive Values for Common Foods, Alcoholic and Nonalcoholic Beverages, and Specialty and Fast-Food Items
- Animation: Digestion of Carbohydrate
- Animation: Glycogen Synthesis

PART 1 Food as Energy

CALORIE—A MEASUREMENT OF FOOD ENERGY

One kilogram–calorie (**kilocalorie [kcal]** or simply calorie) expresses the quantity of heat necessary to raise the temperature of 1 kg (1 L) of water 1°C from 14.5°C to 15.5°C. If a particular food contains 450 kcal, then releasing the potential energy trapped within this food's chemical structure increases the temperature of 450 L of water by 1°C. Different foods contain different amounts of potential energy. For example, one Triple Whopper hamburger with medium French fries and a Coca-Cola from Burger King (**www.bk.com**) contains 1930 kcal (about 60% of kcal from fat in the burger and fries). The equivalent heat energy increases the temperature of 1930 L of water by 1°C.

Gross Energy Value of Foods

Laboratories use **bomb calorimeters (http://chemwiki.ucdavis.edu/Physical_Chemistry/Thermodynamics/Calorimetry/Constant_Volume_Calorimetry)**, similar to the one illustrated in **Figure 3.1**, to measure the total or gross energy value of various food macronutrients. Bomb calorimeters operate on the principle of **direct calorimetry** by measuring the heat liberated as the food burns completely. The bomb calorimeter works as follows:

- A small, insulated chamber filled with oxygen under pressure contains a weighed food portion.
- The food literally explodes and burns when an electric current ignites an electric fuse within the chamber.
- A surrounding water bath absorbs the heat released as the food burns; this heat is termed the *heat of combustion*. An insulating water jacket surrounding the bomb prevents heat loss to the outside environment.
- A sensitive thermometer measures the heat absorbed by the water. For example, the complete combustion of one beef, skinless, 20-oz hot dog and a 1.4-oz bun with mustard and small French fries (2.4 oz) liberates 512 kcal of heat energy. This would raise 5.12 kg (11.3 lb) of water from 32°F (0°C) to it's boiling point, 212°F (100°C).

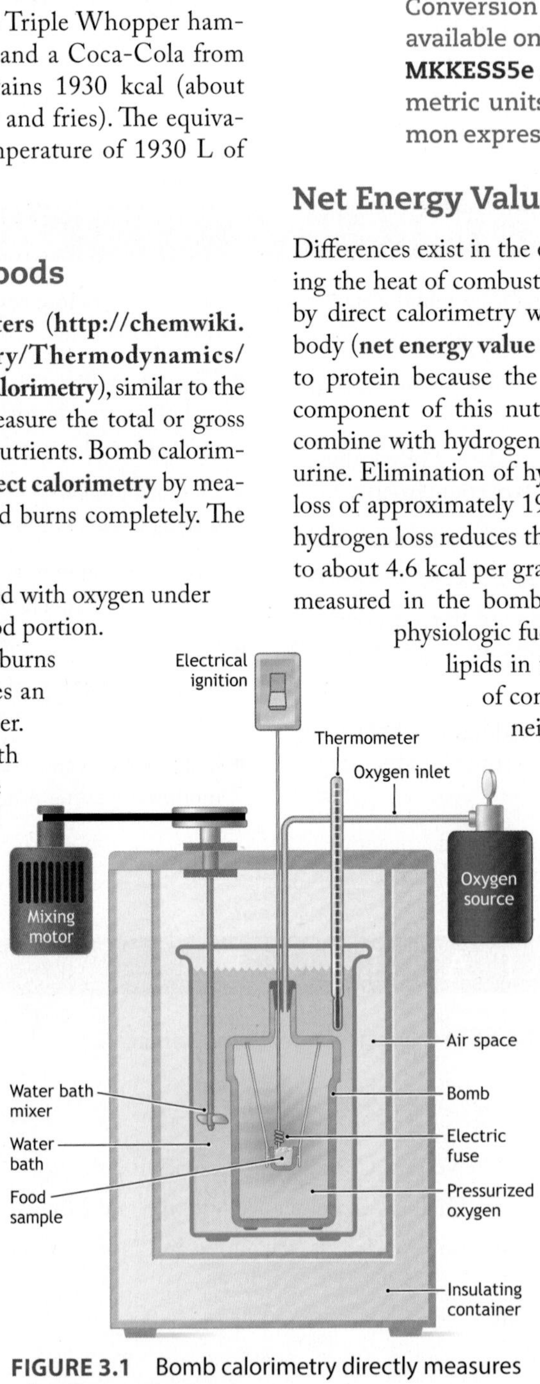

FIGURE 3.1 Bomb calorimetry directly measures a food's energy value.

Heat of Combustion

The heat liberated by the burning or oxidation of food in a bomb calorimeter represents its **heat of combustion** or total energy value of the food. *Burning 1 g of pure carbohydrate yields a heat of combustion of 4.20 kcal, 1 g of pure protein releases 5.65 kcal, and 1 g of pure lipid yields 9.45 kcal.* Most foods in the diet consist of various proportions of these three macronutrients. The caloric value of a given food reflects the *sum* of the heats of combustion for these three macronutrients. Complete lipid oxidation in the bomb calorimeter liberates about 65% more energy per gram than protein oxidation and 120% more energy than carbohydrate oxidation.

thePoint® Appendix A: The Metric System and Conversion Constants in Exercise Physiology available online at **http://thePoint.lww.com/MKKESS5e** shows the relationship between metric units and U.S. units, including common expressions of work, energy, and power.

Net Energy Value of Foods

Differences exist in the energy value of foods when comparing the heat of combustion (gross energy value) determined by direct calorimetry with the *net* energy available to the body (**net energy value of a food**). This pertains particularly to protein because the body cannot oxidize the nitrogen component of this nutrient. In the body, nitrogen atoms combine with hydrogen to form urea, which excretes in the urine. Elimination of hydrogen in this manner represents a loss of approximately 19% of protein's potential energy. The hydrogen loss reduces the body's protein heat of combustion to about 4.6 kcal per gram instead of the 5.65 kcal per gram measured in the bomb calorimeter. In contrast, identical physiologic fuel values exist for carbohydrates and lipids in the body compared with their heats of combustion in the bomb calorimeter as neither contains nitrogen.

Digestive Efficiency

Availability of an ingested macronutrient determines its ultimate caloric yield. *Availability* refers to completeness of digestion and absorption. Normally, about 97% of carbohydrates, 95% of lipids, and 92% of proteins become digested, absorbed, and available for energy conversion. Variation exists in the **digestive efficiency** of protein, ranging from a high of 97% for animal protein to a low of 78% for the protein in dried peas and beans. Furthermore, less energy becomes available from a meal with a high fiber content.

The net kcal value per gram equals 4.0 for carbohydrates, 9.0 for

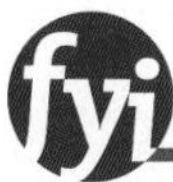

Sports That Promote Marginal Nutrition

Gymnasts, ballet dancers, ice dancers, and weight-class athletes in boxing, wrestling, rowing, and judo engage in arduous training. Owing to the nature of their sport, these athletes continually strive to maintain a lean, light body mass dictated by either esthetic or weight-class considerations. Energy intake often intentionally falls short of energy expenditure, a relative state of malnutrition develops, probably making nutritional supplementation for these athletes beneficial.

Reference: Sousa M, et al. Nutrition and nutritional issues for dancers. *Med Probl Perform Art* 2013;28:119.

lipids, and 4.0 for proteins after considering the average digestive efficiency for each nutrient. These "corrected" heats of combustion, known as the **Atwater general factors**, were named after Wilbur Olin Atwater (1844–1907), an experimental scientist who first described energy release in the calorimeter (**www.sportsci.org/news/history/atwater/atwater.html**).

See the animation "Digestion of Carbohydrate" on **http://thePoint.lww.com/MKKESS5e** for a demonstration of this process.

Energy Value of a Meal

The caloric content of any food can be determined from Atwater values by knowing its composition and weight. For example, based on laboratory analysis of a standard recipe, one can determine the kcal value for 1/2 cup (3.5 oz or about 100 g) of creamed chicken. The macronutrient composition of 1 g of creamed chicken contains 0.2 g of protein, 0.12 g of lipid, and 0.06 g of carbohydrate. Using the Atwater net kcal values, 0.2 g of protein contains 0.8 kcal (0.20 × 4.0), 0.12 g of lipid equals 1.08 kcal (0.12 × 9.0), and 0.06 g of carbohydrate yields 0.24 kcal (0.06 × 4.0). The total caloric value of 1 g of creamed chicken thus equals 2.12 kcal (0.80 + 1.08 + 0.24). A 100-g serving contains 100 times as much or 212 kcal. **Table 3.1** presents the kcal calculations for 3/4 cup (100 g) of vanilla ice cream.

TABLE 3.1 Method of Calculating the Caloric Value of a Food From Its Composition of Macronutrients

Food: Ice cream (vanilla)
Weight: 3/4 cup = 100 g

	Composition		
	Protein	Lipid	Carbohydrate
Percentage	4	13	21
Total grams	4	13	21
In 1 g	0.04	0.13	0.21
Calories per gram	0.16 (0.04 × 4.0 kcal)	1.17 (0.13 × 9.0 kcal)	0.84 (0.21 × 4.0 kcal)

Total calories per gram: 0.16 + 1.17 + 0.84 = 2.17 kcal
Total calories per 100 g: 2.17 × 100 = 217 kcal

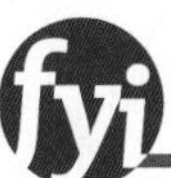

Online Food-Calorie Guides

Computers, smartphones, and tablets make it relatively easy to determine the calorie and nutrient composition of almost any food.

New Rules Go Into Effect

Beginning in late 2016, the U.S. Food and Drug Administration (**www.fda.gov/food/ingredientspackaginglabeling/labelingnutrition/ucm436722.htm**) will require chain restaurants, movie theaters, and pizza parlors, and vending machines, amusement parks, and supermarkets in the United States that sell prepared foods, to include calorie counts on their menus. The new regulations apply to food establishments with 20 or more outlets, including almost every fast-food and sit-down restaurant chain. The rules also will apply to meals or snacks from sit-down restaurants, bakeries, coffee shops, and ice cream stores; foods purchased at drive-through windows; take-out and delivery foods; made-to-order sandwiches; foods ordered from a menu or menu board at a grocery/convenience store or delicatessen; self-serve foods from a salad or hot-food bar at a restaurant or grocery store; and alcoholic drinks, such as cocktails, when the menu lists them.

Government-Sponsored Resources

- **www.nal.usda.gov/fnic/foodcomp/search/**
- **http://ndb.nal.usda.gov/ndb/nutrients/index**
- **www.supertracker.usda.gov/default.aspx**

Other Resources

- **www.calorieking.com/foods/**
- **http://nutritiondata.self.com/**
- **www.thecaloriecounter.com/**
- **http://caloriecount.about.com/**
- **www.fitday.com/**
- **www.myfitnesspal.com**
- **www.fatsecret.com**
- **www.tapandtrack.com/home/index**
- **https://cronometer.com**
- **www.fooducate.com**
- **www.loseit.com**

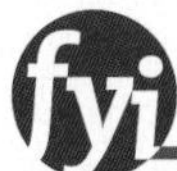

More Lipid Equals More Calories

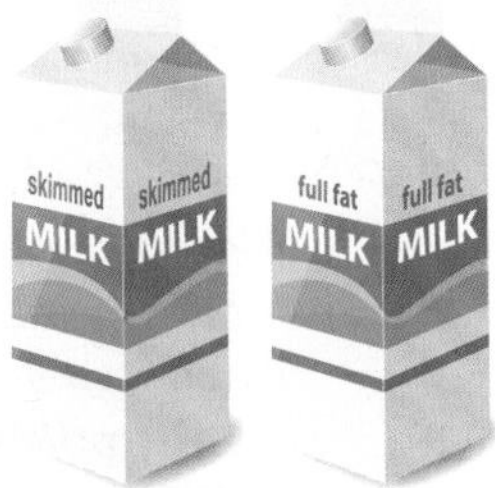

Lipid-rich foods contain a higher energy content than do foods with less fat. For example, one cup of whole milk (4% fat content) contains about 160 kcal, while the same quantity of skimmed milk (0% fat) contains only 90 kcal, and 1 cup of buttermilk (1% fat) contains 110 kcal. If a person who normally consumes 1 quart of whole milk each day switches to skim milk, the total calories ingested each year would be reduced by the equivalent calories in 25 lb of body fat (assuming 3500 kcal per lb of body fat).

Calories Equal Calories

Consider the following five common foods: raw celery, cooked cabbage, cooked asparagus spears, mayonnaise, and salad oil. To consume 100 kcal of each of these foods, you would need to consume 20 stalks of celery, 4 cups of cabbage, or 30 asparagus spears, but only 1 tbsp of mayonnaise or 4/5 ts of salad oil. In other words, a small serving of some foods contains the equivalent energy value as a large quantity of other foods. Viewed from a different perspective, to meet daily energy needs, a sedentary young adult woman would have to consume more than 420 stalks of celery, 84 cups of cabbage, or 630 asparagus spears yet only 1.5 cups of mayonnaise or about 8 oz of salad oil. What is the major difference among these foods? Recall that high-fat foods contain more energy with little water, and foods low in fat or high in water content tend to contain little energy.

A calorie reflects food energy regardless of its source. From an energy standpoint, 100 kcal from mayonnaise equals the same 100 kcal in 20 celery stalks, 100 kcal of Ben and Jerry's Peanut Butter Fudge or Cherry Garcia ice cream, or 30 asparagus spears! The more food consumed, the more kcal consumed. An individual's caloric intake equals the sum of *all* energy consumed from either small or large food quantities. Celery and asparagus spears become "fattening" foods when consumed in excess.

thePoint® Appendix SR-3: Nutritive Values for Common Foods, Alcoholic and Nonalcoholic Beverages, and Specialty and Fast-Food Items, available online at **http://thePoint.lww.com/MKKESS5e**, presents energy and nutritive values for common foods and lists resources for finding values of specialty and fast-food items.

A CLOSER LOOK

The New Nutrition Facts Label

In February, 2014, the US Food and Drug Administration (**www.fda.gov/**) announced changes to the 20-year-old nutrition facts label for packaged foods, for introduction in 2015 (see *upper figure* next page). The last update occurred in 2006 with the addition of *trans* fat to the required list of nutrients. The new NFL reflects the latest dietary recommendations, consensus reports, and national survey data, including the 2010 *Dietary Guidelines for Americans*, nutrient intake recommendations from the Institute of Medicine (IOM), intake data from the National Health and Nutrition Examination Survey (NHANES), and comments from the public. The new label with a refreshed, clean design shown below next to the older version incorporates the latest in nutrition science to make it easier for consumers to make informed food choices and maintain healthy dietary practices. The update focuses on changes in three main areas:

1. **Greater Understanding of Nutrition Science**
   - Requires information about "added sugars." Many experts recommend consuming fewer calories from added sugar because they reduce the intake of nutrient-rich foods while increasing calorie intake.
   - Updates daily values for sodium, dietary fiber, and vitamin D. Daily values, used to calculate the Percent Daily Value listed on the label, help consumers understand the nutrition information in the context of a total daily diet.
   - Requires manufacturers to declare the amount of potassium and vitamin D on the label because these nutrients now have public health significance. Calcium and iron would continue to be required, and vitamins A and C may be included on a voluntary basis.
   - Continues to require "Total Fat," "Saturated Fat," and "*Trans* Fat" on the label, but removes "Calories from Fat" because research shows that the type of fat is more important than the amount of fat.
2. **Updated Serving Size Requirements and New Labeling Requirements for Certain Package Sizes**
   - Changes the serving size requirements to reflect how people eat and drink today, which has changed since serving sizes were first established 20 years ago. By law, the label information on serving sizes must be based on what people actually eat, not on what they should be eating (see *lower figure* next page).
   - Requires that packaged foods, including drinks typically consumed in one sitting, be labeled as a single serving, and that calorie and nutrient information be declared for the entire package. For example, a 20-oz bottle of soda, typically consumed in a single sitting, would be labeled as one serving rather than as more than one serving.
   - For certain packages that are larger and could be consumed in one or multiple sittings, manufacturers have to provide "dual-column" labels to indicate both "per serving" and "per package" calories and nutrient information. Examples would be a 24-oz bottle of soda or a pint of ice cream. This way, people would be able to easily understand how many calories and nutrients they consume if they eat or drink the entire package at one time.
3. **Refreshed Design**
   - Makes calories and serving sizes more prominent to emphasize parts of the label that address current obesity, diabetes, and cardiovascular disease.
   - Shifts the Percent Daily Value to the left of the label so it appears first. This change is important because the Percent Daily Value tells the amount of certain nutrients consumed from a particular food in the context of a total daily diet.
   - Changes the footnote to more clearly explain the meaning of the Percent Daily Value.

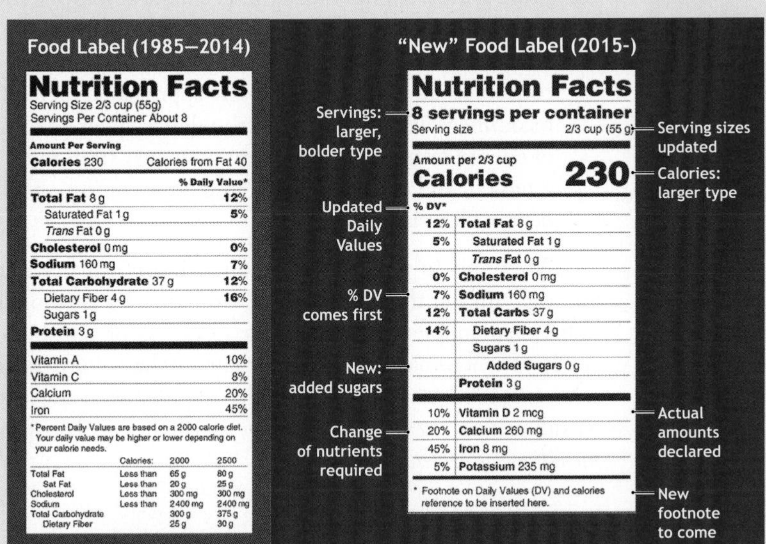

(Adapted from **www.fda.gov/NewsEvents/Newsroom/PressAnnouncements/ucm387418.htm**)

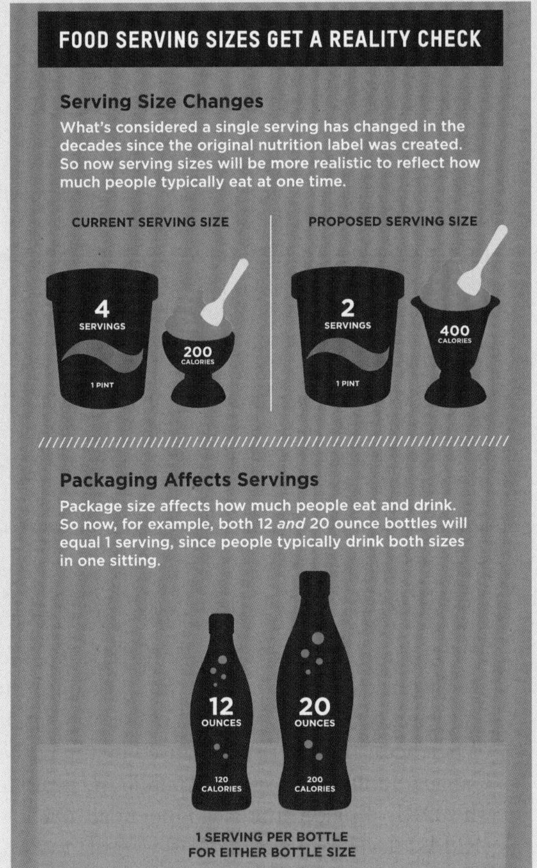

(Adapted from **www.fda.gov/downloads/ForConsumers/ConsumerUpdates/UCM387442.pdf**)

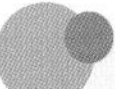

SUMMARY

1. A calorie or kilocalorie (kcal) represents a measure of heat that expresses the energy value of food.
2. Burning food in a bomb calorimeter permits direct quantification of the food's energy content.
3. The heat of combustion represents the amount of heat liberated in a food's complete oxidation.
4. Average gross energy values equal 4.2 kcal per gram for carbohydrates, 9.4 kcal per gram for lipids, and 5.65 kcal per gram for proteins.
5. The coefficient of digestibility represents the proportion of food consumed digested *and* absorbed by the body.
6. Coefficients of digestibility average approximately 97% for carbohydrates, 95% for lipids, and 92% for proteins.
7. The net energy values equal 4 kcal per gram of carbohydrates, 9 kcal per gram of lipids, and 4 kcal per gram of proteins.
8. The net energy values, termed Atwater general factors, provide an estimate of the net energy value of foods in a diet and allow computation of the caloric content of any meal from its carbohydrate, lipid, and protein composition.
9. A calorie represents a unit of heat energy regardless of food source. From an energy standpoint, 500 kcal of chocolate cheesecake topped with homemade whipped cream is no more fattening than 500 kcal of a carrot and lettuce salad, 500 kcal of onion and pepperoni pizza, or 500 kcal of a bagel with Coho salmon, red onions, and sour cream.

THINK IT THROUGH

1. What factors other than the energy value of one's diet should be considered when formulating a healthful approach to weight control?
2. Explain the importance of considering food type in planning a weight loss meal plan.

PART 2 Optimal Nutrition for Physical Activity and Sports

From a nutritional and energy balance perspective, optimal food consumption must supply required nutrients for tissue maintenance, repair, and growth without excessive energy intake. The specific nutrient needs for individuals of different ages and body sizes, with considerations for individual differences, include these four factors:

1. Digestion
2. Storage capacity
3. Nutrient metabolism
4. Daily energy expenditure

Establishing dietary recommendations for physically active men and women remains complicated by specific energy requirements and training demands of particular sports and by individual dietary preferences. Sound nutritional guidelines form the framework for planning and evaluating food intake for individuals who exercise regularly. Part 2 describes nutrient requirements of sedentary and active individuals, including optimal nutrition guidelines for participants in intense physical activity.

NUTRIENT CONSUMPTION OF SEDENTARY AND PHYSICALLY ACTIVE PEOPLE

Many coaches make dietary recommendations based on their "feelings" and past experiences rather than sound research evidence. The fact that athletes often obtain inadequate or incorrect information concerning dietary practices and the role of specific nutrients in exercise exacerbates the problem. Considering the total body of scientific evidence, physically active people and athletes do *not* require additional nutrients beyond those obtained in a balanced diet. *Physically fit individuals, including those involved in increased physical activity, consume foods that more closely approach dietary recommendations than do those foods consumed by less active peers of lower fitness levels.*

Inconsistencies exist among studies that relate diet quality to physical activity level or physical fitness. Relatively crude and imprecise self-reported measures of physical activity, unreliable dietary assessments, or small sample size helps to explain part of the discrepancy. **Table 3.2** contrasts the nutrient and energy intakes with national dietary recommendations of a large population-based cohort of nearly 7959 men and 2453 women classified as low, moderate, and high for cardiorespiratory fitness. The most significant four findings indicate the following:

1. A progressively lower body mass index corresponded with increasing levels of physical fitness for both men and women.
2. Remarkably small differences were seen in energy intake related to physical fitness classification for women (≤94 kcal per day) and men (≤82 kcal per day); the moderate fitness group for both males and females consumed the least calories.
3. Progressively higher dietary fiber intake and lower cholesterol intake occurred in the more fit categories.
4. Men and women with higher fitness levels generally consumed diets that more closely approached dietary recommendations with respect to dietary fiber, percent of energy from total fat, percent of energy from saturated fat, and cholesterol, than did diets consumed by peers of lower fitness levels.

Attention to proper diet does not mean athletes must join the ranks of the more than 87% of Americans who take nutritional supplements, spending in excess of $30 billion yearly to micromanage their nutrient intake (multivitamin sales exceeded $125 million; herbal supplements exceeded $1 billion). *In essence, sound human nutrition represents sound nutrition for athletes.*

fyi Eat More Yet Weigh Less

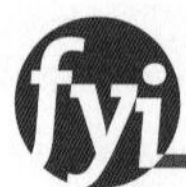

Physically active individuals generally consume more calories per kilogram of body mass than do sedentary counterparts, the extra energy of physical activity accounting for the larger caloric intake. Paradoxically, the most physically active men and women who eat more on a daily basis weigh less than do those who exercise at a lower total caloric expenditure. Regular physical activity allows a person to "eat more yet weigh less" while maintaining a lower percentage of body fat despite the age-related tendency toward weight gain that begins at about age 21 years and continues at about one-half to 1 lb of weight gained yearly for the next 40 years! Physically active persons maintain a lighter and leaner body and a healthier heart disease risk profile despite increased food intake.

DIETARY REFERENCE INTAKES

The **Dietary Reference Intake (DRI) (www.fnic.nal.usda.gov/interactiveDRI/)** represents a system of nutrition recommendations from the IOM of the US National Academy of Sciences. The DRI system, used by the United States and Canada, applies to the general public and health professionals. The DRIs replaced the Recommended Dietary Allowances (RDAs) developed during World War II to investigate issues of nutrition that might impact national defense and used for nutrition recommendations for the armed forces, civilians, and overseas populations who might require food relief. The final RDA guidelines were published in 1941. The RDAs were revised every 5 to 10 years until 1997 when the IOM in cooperation with Canadian scientists developed the DRIs, a more comprehensive individualized approach to nutritional recommendations.

TABLE 3.2 Mean (±SD) Nutrient Intake Based on 3-Day Diet Records by Level of Cardiorespiratory Fitness in 7959 Men and 2453 Women

Variable	Males	Females	Males	Females	Males	Females
	Low Fitness ($N = 786$)	Low Fitness ($N = 233$)	Moderate Fitness ($N = 2457$)	Moderate Fitness ($N = 730$)	High Fitness ($N = 4716$)	High Fitness ($N = 1490$)
Demographic and health data						
Age (y)	47.3 ± 11.1[a,b]	47.5 ± 11.2[b]	47.3 ± 10.3[c]	46.7 ± 11.6	48.1 ± 10.5	46.5 ± 11.0
Apparently healthy (%)	51.5[a,b]	55.4[a,b]	69.1[c]	71.1[c]	77.0	79.3
Current smokers (%)	23.4[a,b]	12.0[a,b]	15.8[c]	9.0[c]	7.8	4.2
BMI ($kg \cdot m^{-2}$)	30.7 ± 5.5[a,b]	27.3 ± 6.7[a,b]	27.4 ± 3.7[c]	24.3 ± 4.9[c]	25.1 ± 2.7	22.1 ± 3.0
Nutrient data						
Energy (kcal)	2378.6 ± 718.6[a]	1887.4 ± 607.5[a]	2296.9 ± 661.9[c]	1793.0 ± 508.2[c]	2348.1 ± 664.3	1859.7 ± 514.7
$kcal \cdot kg^{-1}$	25.0 ± 8.1[a]	27.1 ± 9.4[a]	26.7 ± 8.4[c]	28.1 ± 8.8[c]	29.7 ± 9.2	31.7 ± 9.8
Carbohydrate (% kcal)	43.2 ± 9.4[b]	47.7 ± 9.6[b]	44.6 ± 9.1[c]	48.2 ± 9.0[c]	48.1 ± 9.7	51.1 ± 9.4
Protein (% kcal)	18.6 ± 3.8	17.6 ± 3.7[a]	18.5 ± 3.8	18.1 ± 3.9	18.1 ± 3.8	17.7 ± 3.9
Total fat (% kcal)	36.7 ± 7.2[b]	34.8 ± 7.6[b]	35.4 ± 7.1[c]	33.7 ± 6.8[c]	32.6 ± 7.5	31.3 ± 7.5
SFA (% kcal)	11.8 ± 3.2[b]	11.1 ± 3.3[b]	11.3 ± 3.2[c]	10.6 ± 3.2[c]	10.0 ± 3.2	9.6 ± 3.1
MUFA (% kcal)	14.5 ± 3.2[a,b]	13.4 ± 3.4[a,b]	13.8 ± 3.1[c]	12.8 ± 3.0[c]	12.6 ± 3.3	11.9 ± 3.2
PUFA (% kcal)	7.4 ± 2.2[a,b]	7.5 ± 2.2	7.5 ± 2.2	7.5 ± 2.2	7.4 ± 2.3	7.4 ± 2.4
Cholesterol (mg)	349.5 ± 173.2[b]	244.7 ± 132.8[b]	314.5 ± 147.5[c]	224.6 ± 115.6[c]	277.8 ± 138.5	204.1 ± 103.6
Fiber (g)	21.0 ± 9.5[b]	18.9 ± 8.2[a,b]	22.0 ± 9.7[c]	20.0 ± 8.3[c]	26.2 ± 11.9	23.2 ± 10.7
Calcium (mg)	849.1 ± 371.8[a,b]	765.2 ± 361.8[a,b]	860.2 ± 360.2[c]	774.6 ± 342.8[c]	924.4 ± 386.8	828.3 ± 372.1
Sodium (mg)	4317.4 ± 1365.7	3350.8 ± 980.8	4143.0 ± 1202.3	3256.7 ± 927.7	4133.2 ± 1189.4	3314.4 ± 952.7
Folate (mcg)	336.4 ± 165.2[b]	301.8 ± 157.6[a,b]	359.5 ± 197.0[c]	319.7 ± 196.2	428.0 ± 272.0	356.2 ± 232.5
Vitamin B_6 (mg)	2.4 ± 0.9[b]	2.0 ± 0.8[b]	2.4 ± 0.9[c]	2.0 ± 0.8[c]	2.8 ± 1.1	2.2 ± 0.9
Vitamin B_{12} (mcg)	6.6 ± 5.5[a]	4.7 ± 4.2	6.8 ± 6.0	4.9 ± 4.2	6.6 ± 5.8	5.0 ± 4.2
Vitamin A (RE)	1372.7 ± 1007.3[a,b]	1421.9 ± 1135.3[b]	1530.5 ± 1170.4[c]	1475.1 ± 1132.9[c]	1766.3 ± 1476.0	1699.0 ± 1346.9
Vitamin C (mg)	117.3 ± 80.4[b]	116.7 ± 7.5[b]	129.2 ± 108.9[c]	131.5 ± 140.0	166.0 ± 173.2	153.5 ± 161.1
Vitamin E (AE)	11.5 ± 9.1[b]	10.8 ± 7.5	12.1 ± 8.6[c]	10.3 ± 6.5[c]	13.7 ± 11.4	11.5 ± 8.1

[a]Significant difference between low and moderate fit, $P < 0.05$.

[b]Significant difference between low and high fit, $P < 0.05$.

[c]Significant difference between moderate and high fit, $P < 0.05$.

BMI, body mass index; SFA, saturated fatty acid; PUFA, polyunsaturated fatty acid; MUFA, monounsaturated fatty acid; RE, retinol equivalents; AE, alpha-tocopherol units.

Adapted with permission from Brodney S, et al. Nutrient intake of physically active fit and unfit men and women. *Med Sci Sports Exerc* 2001;33:459.

The current DRI recommendation includes the following:

- **Estimated Average Requirements (EAR)**: expected to satisfy the needs of 50% of the people in an age group based on a scientific literature review.
- **Recommended Dietary Allowances (RDA)**: daily dietary intake level of a nutrient considered sufficient by the Food and Nutrition Board to meet the requirements of 97.5% of healthy individuals in each life stage and sex group. The RDAs, based on the EAR, are approximately 20% higher than the EAR (see Calculating the RDA).
- **Adequate Intake (AI)**: where no RDA has been established, it provides an assumed adequate goal with low risk based on observed or experimentally determined estimates of nutrient intake by a group of apparently healthy persons.
- **Tolerable Upper Intake Levels (UL)**: cautions against excessive intake of nutrients (e.g., vitamin A) that can prove harmful in large amounts. The UL represents the highest level of daily consumption that current data demonstrate cause no side effects in humans when used indefinitely without medical supervision.

The RDA determines the Recommended Daily Value (RDV printed on food labels in the United States and Canada [**Fig. 3.2**]).

The DRIs differ from their predecessor RDAs by focusing more on promoting health maintenance and risk reduction for nutrient-dependent heart disease, diabetes, hypertension, osteoporosis, various cancers, and age-related macular degeneration than preventing the deficiency diseases scurvy (vitamin C

A CLOSER LOOK

Foods and Dietary Patterns That Associate With Reduced Cancer Risk and Improved Survival Following Cancer Diagnosis

Random control scientific studies have clarified many aspects of how foods affect cancer risk, prompting leading organizations to issue recommendations for cancer prevention.[1] In nutritional science, scientific evidence has been insufficient for authorities to issue guidance with confidence. Individuals making daily dietary decisions are impatient for the evolution of scientific consensus. In this situation, it is possible to invoke the *precautionary principle*. This is commonly understood in toxicology and environmental health and may be applicable to nutrition.

The precautionary principle states that if an action or policy has a suspected risk of causing harm to the public (or to the environment), in the absence of scientific consensus that the action or policy is not harmful, the burden of proof that it is *not* harmful falls on those taking an action. For example, the European Union invokes the precautionary principle "when there are reasonable grounds for concern that potential hazards may impact the environment, human, animal or plant health, and when the pertinent data simultaneously preclude a detailed risk evaluation."[2] This approach may play a useful role in cancer prevention due to the limited practicality of randomized controlled trials and the unusually long latency from exposure to cancer diagnoses.[3]

One study developed a set of dietary principles applicable to six areas where evidence exists of a substantial dietary influence, even if inconclusive (see table).[4] The figure presents available evidence of the effects of certain foods on different cancers.

Dietary Areas and Suggestions

Area	Suggested Dietary Guidance
Milk and dairy products	Limiting or avoiding dairy products may reduce the risk of prostate cancer.
Alcohol	Limiting or avoiding alcohol may reduce the risk of cancers of the mouth, pharynx, larynx, esophagus, colon and rectum, and breast.
Red and processed meat	Avoiding red and processed meat may reduce the risk of cancers of the colon and rectum
Meats cooked at high temperature	Avoiding grilled, fried, and broiled meats may reduce the risk of cancers of the colon, rectum, breast, prostate, kidney, and pancreas. In this context, meat refers to red meat, poultry, and fish.
Soy products	Consumption of soy products during adolescence may reduce the risk of breast cancer arising in adulthood. Soy products may also reduce the risk of recurrence and mortality for women previously treated for breast cancer.
Fruits and vegetables	Emphasizing fruits and vegetables in your diet will likely reduce the risk of several common forms of cancer.

Reference: Gonzales RD, et al. Applying the precautionary principle to nutrition and cancer. *J Am Coll Nutr* 2014;28:1.

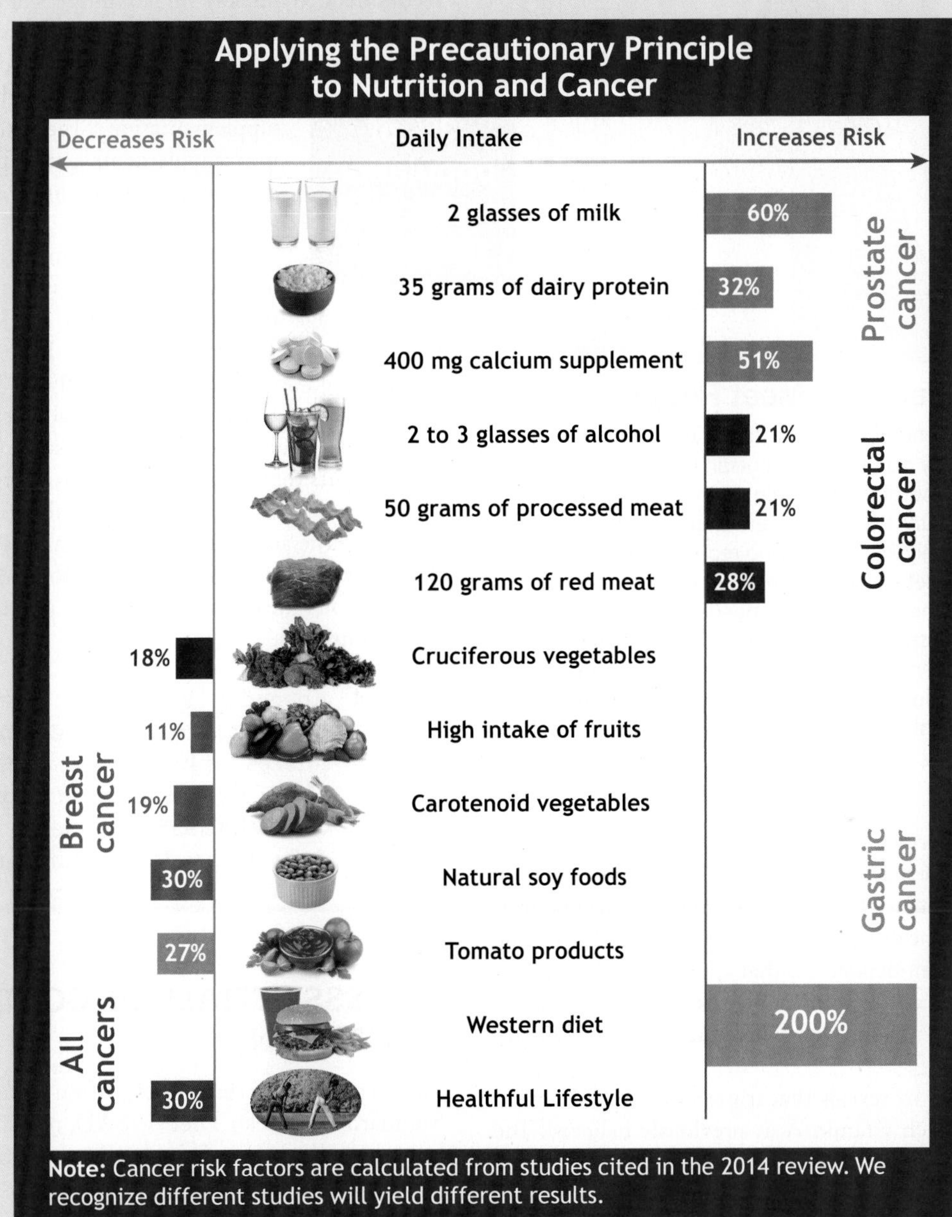

Adapted with permission from Levin S. "Applying the Precautionary Principle to Nutrition and Cancer." Physicians Committee for Responsible Medicine, **www.pcrm.org/health/reports/applying-the-precautionary-principle-to-cancer**; based on Gonzales JF, et al. Applying the precautionary principle to nutrition and cancer. *J Am Coll Nutr* 2014;33:239. doi:10.1080/07315724.2013.866527.

References

1. Kushi LH, et al. American Cancer Society guidelines on nutrition and physical activity for cancer prevention: reducing the risk of cancer with healthy food choices and physical activity. *CA Cancer J Clin* 2012;62:30.
2. Commission of the European Communities: "Communication from the Commission on the Precautionary Principle." Brussels, Belgium: Commission of the European Communities, 2000. Accessed at: **http://eur-lex.europa.eu/legal-content/EN/ALL/?uri= CELEX:52000DC0001**.
3. Blumberg J, et al. Evidence-based criteria in the nutritional context. *Nutr Rev* 2010;68:478.
4. World Cancer Research Fund and the American Institute for Cancer Research: "*Food, Nutrition, Physical Activity, and the Prevention of Cancer: A Global Perspective.*" Washington, DC: American Institute for Cancer Research, 2007.

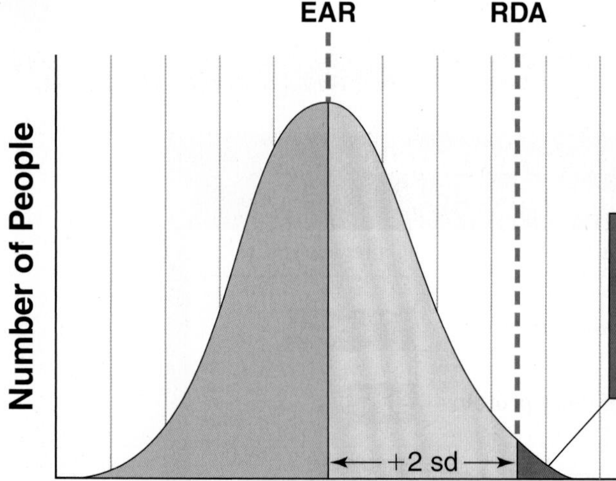

FIGURE 3.2 Theoretical distribution of the number of people adequately nourished by a given nutrient intake. For example, the number of people receiving adequate nutrition with 50 units of the nutrient is greater than that of those receiving only 15 units or who require 75 units. The Recommended Dietary Allowance (RDA) is set at an intake level that would meet the nutrient needs of 97% to 98% of the population (2 standard deviations [SD] above the mean). The Estimated Average Requirement (EAR) represents a nutrient intake value estimated to meet the requirement of 50% of the healthy individuals in a gender and life stage group.

deficiency) or beriberi (vitamin B_1 deficiency). The DRIs provide values for macronutrients and food components of nutritional importance for some phytochemical compounds believed to have health-protecting qualities. The DRI value also includes recommendations that apply to gender and life stages of growth and development based on age including pregnancy and lactation (**www.nap.edu**; search for Dietary Reference Intakes).

The DRI report reveals that fruits and vegetables yield about half as much vitamin A as previously believed. The report also sets a daily maximum intake level for vitamin A in addition to boron, copper, iodine, iron, manganese, molybdenum, nickel, vanadium, and zinc, including specific recommended intakes for vitamins A and K, chromium, copper, iodine, manganese, molybdenum, and zinc. The report concludes that one can meet the daily requirement for the nutrients examined *without* external supplementation. The exception includes iron supplements generally required during pregnancy to meet increased daily requirements.

Well-balanced meals provide an adequate quantity of all vitamins, regardless of a person's age and physical activity level. Similarly, mineral supplements generally confer little benefit because the required minerals occur readily in food and water. Individuals who expend considerable energy in physical activity generally need *not* consume special foods or supplements that increase their micronutrient intake above recommended levels. Also, food intake generally increases to sustain the added energy requirements of high levels of daily physical activity. Additional food through a variety of nutritious meals proportionately increases vitamin and mineral intakes.

Recommended Meal Composition

Suggested composition of a 2500-kcal diet based on recommendations of an expert panel of the Institute of Medicine, National Academies.

	Carbohydrate	Lipid	Protein
Percentage	60	15	25
Kilocalories	150	375	625
Grams	375	94	69
Ounces	13.2	3.3	2.4

Source: www.iom.edu/Reports/2006/Dietary-Reference-Intakes-Essential-Guide-Nutrient-Requirements.aspx

thePoint® Appendix B: Dietary Reference Intakes (DRIs): Recommended Vitamin and Mineral Intakes for Individuals, available at the end of this text and online at **http://thePoint.lww.com/MKKESS5e**, presents recommended daily intakes for vitamins and minerals for different life stage groups.

THE ESSENTIALS OF GOOD NUTRITION

The typical American diet, often referred to as the Standard American Diet or SAD, relies heavily on sugar, fat, salt, and processed foods. This pattern of food intake increases risks for obesity, type 2 diabetes, metabolic syndrome, and other cardiometabolic diseases.

The US government has adopted many different approaches to food consumption for purposes of promoting good health, and in 1980, began issuing ***Dietary Guidelines*** every 5 years (with the most recent issued in January 2015). The guidelines have consistently recommended the basic principles of a healthful diet—*variety*, *balance*, and *moderation*—but have also changed in significant ways to reflect the emerging science.

To their credit, the most recent *Guideline* recommendations emphasize that all Americans including children spend at least *1 hour* (not 30 min as previously recommended) or the equivalent of 400 to 500 kcal expended over the course of each day in moderately intense brisk walking, jogging, swimming, bicycling, or lawn and garden work and housework to maintain overall good health and a

TABLE 3.3 Highlights of the *Dietary Guidelines* for Americans, 2015

Key Recommendation	Overview
Balance calories to manage weight	Calorie balance refers to the relationship between calories consumed from foods and beverages and calories expended in normal body functions (i.e., metabolic processes) and through physical activity. People cannot control the calories expended in metabolic processes, but they can control what they eat and drink, as well as how many calories they use in physical activity.
Foods and food components to reduce	Focus on certain foods and food components that are consumed in excessive amounts and may increase the risk of certain chronic diseases. These include sodium, solid fats (major sources of saturated and *trans* fatty acids), added sugars, and refined grains. Some people also consume too much alcohol.
Foods and nutrients to increase	Increase vegetable and fruit intake; increase intake of fat-free or low-fat milk and milk products (milk, yogurt, cheese, or fortified soy beverages). Choose a variety of protein foods, which include seafood, lean meat and poultry, eggs, beans and peas, soy products, and unsalted nuts and seeds. Replace protein foods that are higher in solid fats with choices that are lower in solid fats and calories and/or are sources of oils. Use oils to replace solid fats where possible.
Building healthy eating patterns	Select an eating pattern that meets nutrient needs over time at an appropriate calorie level. Account for all foods and beverages consumed, and assess how they fit within a total healthy eating pattern. Follow food safety recommendations when preparing and eating foods to reduce risks of foodborne illnesses.
Helping Americans make healthy choices	To reverse trends of increased cardiovascular disease, type 2 diabetes, and some types of cancers, a coordinated system-wide approach is needed that engages all sectors of society, including individuals and families, educators, communities and organizations, health professionals, small and large businesses, and policymakers.

Source: http://www.health.gov/dietaryguidelines/2015.asp#overview

normal body weight. This advice represents a bold increase in activity duration considering that more than 60% of the US population fails to incorporate even a moderate level of physical activity into their lives, and shamefully, 25% do no activity at all.

Table 3.3 highlights the federal *Dietary Guidelines* released in 2015.

MYPLATE: THE HEALTHY EATING GUIDE

MyPlate, which replaced the Food Pyramid in 2011, incorporates the 2015 *Guidelines* to help consumers make better food choices and, to remind Americans to eat healthfully but is not intended to change consumer behavior alone. **Figure 3.3** shows the MyPlate healthy eating icon, which uses a familiar mealtime visual to describe each of the five food groups.

The MyPlate strategy emphasizes more plant-based eating from a variety of vegetables from all five subgroups. Fruits and vegetables occupy half the plate, with vegetables predominating. Grains and proteins make up the other half, with mostly whole grains occupying a majority of that half. The protein category includes meat, poultry, seafood, eggs, and vegetarian beans and peas, nuts, seeds, and tofu. The blue circle indicates dairy products (glass of skim or reduced-fat milk, cheese, or yogurt). MyPlate omits recommendations for daily caloric intake, fat intake, and energy expenditure. Similar to the 2015 *Guidelines*, MyPlate stresses balanced portions among different food categories.

The Web site **www.ChooseMyPlate.gov** provides detailed advice, videos, menus and recipes, food plans, and other educational material about MyPlate and the current Dietary Guidelines for Americans.

Critics of MyPlate Offer Suggestions

Researchers from Harvard's School of Public Health have suggested seven changes to the MyPlate offerings to more closely reflect research in the area. (**www.hsph.harvard.edu/nutritionsource/pyramid-full-story/#References; www.hsph.harvard.edu/nutritionsource/mypyramid-problems/**)

1. Provide information that whole grains are better for health than refined grains.
2. Indicate that some high-protein foods—fish, poultry, beans, nuts—are healthier than red meats and processed meats that often link to various chronic diseases.
3. Be more insistent on including beneficial fats as part of a healthy diet.
4. Differentiate between potatoes and other high-glycemic vegetables that act like sugars in the body.

5. Recommend dairy at every meal, even though little evidence exists that high dairy intake protects against osteoporosis, but evidence exists a high intake can be undesirable.
6. Emphasize the potential negative effect of sugary drinks.
7. Elevate the importance of physical activity.

Alternative Models for Good Nutrition

Healthy Eating Plate

The **Healthy Eating Plate** (**www.hsph.harvard.edu/nutritionsource**) presents a visual guide for eating a healthy meal. This alternative to MyPlate promotes the following:

- **Vegetables**: Eat an abundant variety, but limit potatoes and other high-glycemic starches that have a similar effect on blood sugar as sweets.
- **Fruits**: Choose a rainbow of fruits every day.
- **Whole Grains**: Choose whole grains, such as oatmeal, whole wheat bread, and brown rice, instead of refined grains (white bread and white rice that act like sugar in the body).
- **Healthy Proteins**: Choose fish, poultry, beans, or nuts; limit consumption of red meat and avoid processed meats because these may increase risk of heart disease, type 2 diabetes, colon cancer, and weight gain.
- **Healthy Oils**: Use olive, canola, and other plant oils in cooking, on salads, and at the table because these reduce cholesterol and may prove beneficial to heart function. Limit butter, and avoid *trans* fat.
- **Water**: Drink water, tea, or coffee (with little or no sugar). Limit milk and dairy (1 to 2 servings daily) and juice (1 small glass daily), and avoid sugary drinks.
- **Stay Active**: Increased physical activity should be part of everyone's healthy eating program.

Mediterranean Diet Pyramid

The classic **Mediterranean Diet**, first introduced in 1993 and modified in 2008 (**Fig. 3.4**), created a Mediterranean Diet Pyramid to visually represent a healthy, traditional diet of the Mediterranean region. This diet plan emphasizes the following.

- Replace olive oil for other fats and oils including butter and margarine.
- Make the goal for total fat less than 25% to over 35% of energy (calories); saturated fat not to exceed 7% to 8%.
- Include daily consumption of low to moderate amounts of cheese and yogurt.
- Twice-weekly consumption of low to moderate amounts of fish and poultry.
- Emphasize fresh fruit as the typical daily dessert; minimize high-sugar sweets and saturated fats.
- Reduce red meat consumption to twice monthly (limit to 12 to 16 oz [340 to 450 g]).
- Increase regular physical activity at a level that promotes a healthy weight, fitness, and well-being.
- Emphasize moderate wine consumption (1 to 2 glasses daily for men and 1 glass daily for women).

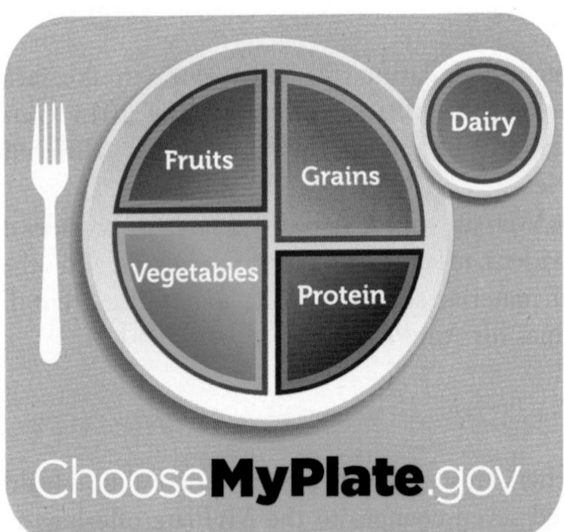

Fruits
- 2 cups a day.
- What counts as a cup?
  One cup of raw or cooked fruit or 100% fruit juice; a half-cup dried fruit.

Vegetables
- 2 1/2 cups a day.
- What counts as a cup?
  One cup of raw or cooked vegetables or vegetable juice; two cups of leafy salad greens.

Dairy
- 3 cups a day.
- What counts as a cup?
  One cup of milk, yogurt, or fortified soy milk; 1 1/2 ounces natural or two ounces processed cheese.

Grains
- 6 ounces a day.
- What counts as an ounce?
  Once slice of bread; a half-cup of cooked rice, cereal, or pasta; one ounce of ready-to-eat cereal.

Protein foods
- 5 1/2 ounces a day.
- What counts as an ounce?
  One ounce of lean meat, poultry or fish; one egg; a tablespoon of peanut butter; a half-ounce of nuts or seeds; a quarter-cup of beans, or peas.

FIGURE 3.3 The MyPlate healthy eating guide. (Adapted from USDA Center for Nutrition Policy and Promotion.)

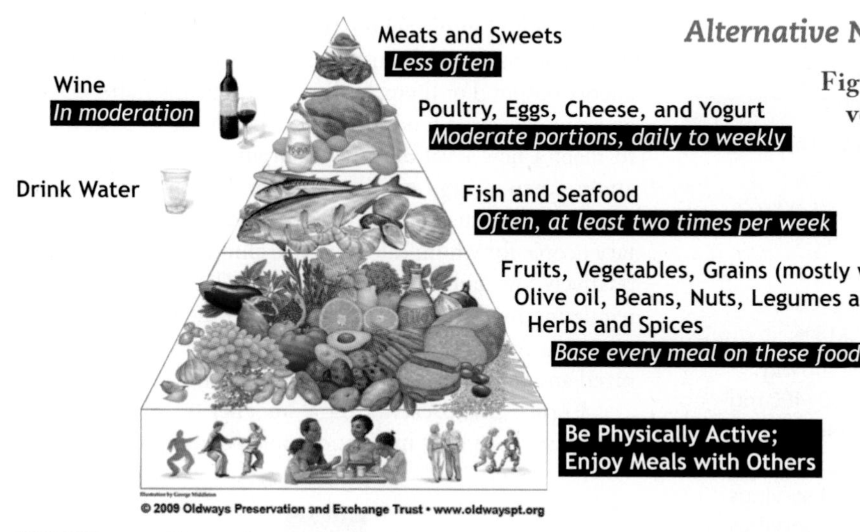

FIGURE 3.4 The Mediterranean Diet Pyramid application to individuals whose diet consists largely of foods from the plant kingdom, or fruits, nuts, vegetables, and all manner of grains, and protein derived from fish, beans, and chicken, with dietary fat composed mostly of monounsaturated fatty acids and with mild alcohol consumption. (Adapted with permission from Oldways Preservation & Exchange Trust, **www.oldwayspt.org**.)

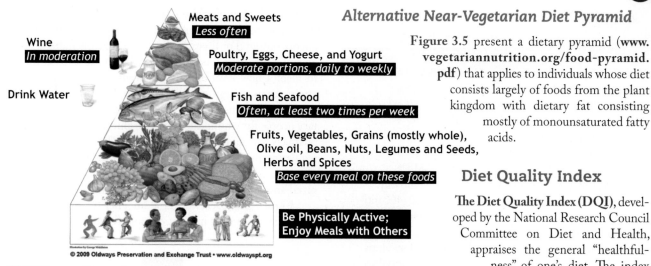

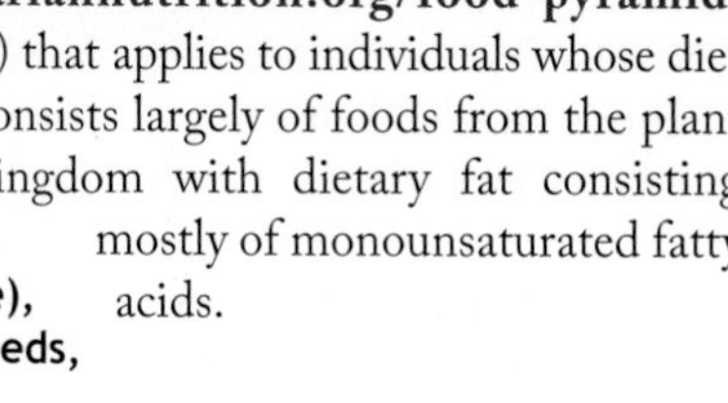

Alternative Near-Vegetarian Diet Pyramid

Figure 3.5 present a dietary pyramid (**www.vegetariannutrition.org/food-pyramid.pdf**) that applies to individuals whose diet consists largely of foods from the plant kingdom with dietary fat consisting mostly of monounsaturated fatty acids.

Diet Quality Index

The Diet Quality Index (DQI), developed by the National Research Council Committee on Diet and Health, appraises the general "healthfulness" of one's diet. The index presented in **Table 3.4** offers a simple scoring schema based on a risk gradient associated with diet and major diet-related chronic diseases. Respondents who meet a given dietary goal receive a score of 0; a score of 1 applies to an intake within 30% of a dietary goal; the score becomes 2 when intake fails to fall within 30% of the goal. The final score equals the total for all eight categories. The index ranges from 0 to 16, with a lower score representing a higher-quality diet. A score of 4 or less reflects a more healthful diet; an index of 10 or higher indicates a less healthful diet that needs improvement.

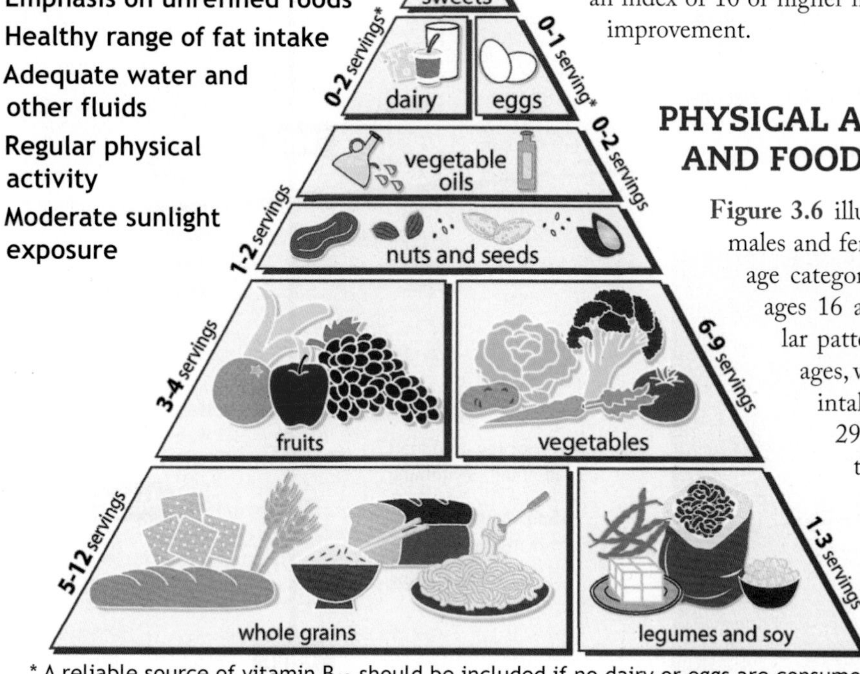

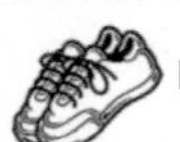

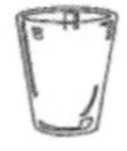

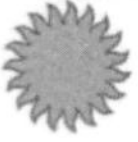

FIGURE 3.5 The Vegetarian Food Pyramid. (Adapted with permission from Loma Linda University, School of Public Health, Department of Nutrition, **www.vegetariannutrition.org/food-pyramid.pdf**.)

PHYSICAL ACTIVITY AND FOOD INTAKE

Figure 3.6 illustrates the average energy intakes for males and females in the US population grouped by age category. Mean energy intakes peak between ages 16 and 29 and decline thereafter. A similar pattern occurs for males and females at all ages, with males reporting higher daily energy intakes than females. Between ages 20 and 29, females consumed 35% fewer kcal than did males on a daily basis (3025 kcal vs. 1957 kcal). With aging, the gender difference in energy intake decreased; at age 70 years, females consumed 25% fewer kcal than did males.

Physical Activity Makes a Difference

Food intake balances easily with daily energy expenditure for individuals who regularly engage in moderate to intense physical activities. Lumber

TABLE 3.4 The Diet Quality Index

Recommendation	Score	Intake
Reduce total lipid intake to 30% or less of total energy	☐ 0 ☐ 1 ☐ 2	<30% >30–40% >40%
Reduce saturated fatty acid intake to less than 10% of total energy	☐ 0 ☐ 1 ☐ 2	<10% 10–13% >13%
Reduce cholesterol intake to less than 300 mg daily	☐ 0 ☐ 1 ☐ 2	<300 mg 300–400 mg >400 mg
Eat 5 or more servings daily of vegetables and fruits	☐ 0 ☐ 1 ☐ 2	≥5 servings 3–4 servings 0–2 servings
Increase intake of starches and other complex carbohydrates by eating 6 or more servings daily of breads, cereals, and legumes	☐ 0 ☐ 1 ☐ 2	≥6 servings 4–5 servings 0–3 servings
Maintain protein intake at moderate levels	☐ 0 ☐ 1 ☐ 2	100% RDA 100–150% RDA >150% RDA
Limit total daily sodium intake to 2400 mg or less	☐ 0 ☐ 1 ☐ 2	≤2400 mg 2400–3400 mg >3400 mg
Maintain adequate calcium intake (approximately the RDA)	☐ 0 ☐ 1 ☐ 2	≥100% RDA 67–99% RDA <67% RDA

Adapted with permission from The Diet Quality Index (DQI), National Research Council Committee on Diet and Health. Patterson RE, Haines PS, Popkin BM. Diet Quality Index (capturing a multidimensional behavior). *J Am Diet Assoc.* 1994;94:57.

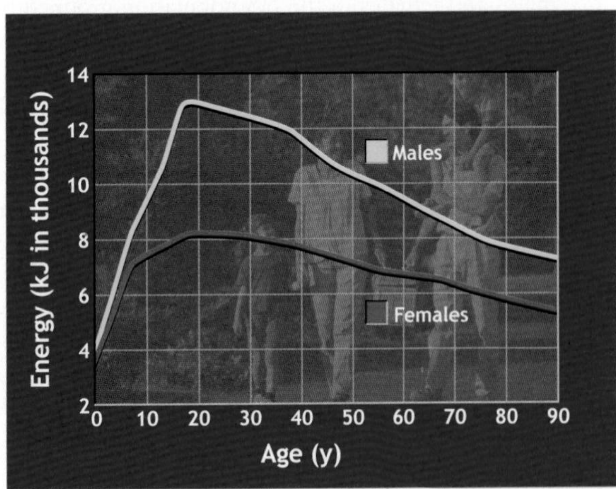

FIGURE 3.6 Average daily energy intake for males and females by age in the US population during the years 1988 to 1990. Multiply by 0.239 to convert kJ to kcal. (Reprinted with permission from McArdle WD, Katch FI, Katch VL. *Exercise Physiology: Nutrition, Energy, and Human Performance.* 8th Ed. Baltimore: Wolters Kluwer Health, 2015, as adapted with permission from Briefel RR, et al. Total energy intake of the U.S. population: the third National Health and Nutrition Examination Survey, 1988–1991. *Am J Clin Nutr* 1995;62(Suppl):1072S.)

workers, for example, who typically expend nearly 4500 kcal daily, unconsciously adjust their energy intake to balance energy output. For them, body weight remains stable despite an extremely large food intake. The balancing of food intake to meet a new level of energy output takes 1 to 2 days to attain a new energy equilibrium. The fine balance between energy expenditure and food intake does not occur in sedentary people for whom caloric intake chronically exceeds their relatively low daily energy expenditure. Lack of precision in regulating food intake at the low end of the physical activity spectrum contributes to "creeping obesity" in highly mechanized and technologically advanced societies.

Figure 3.7 presents data on energy intake from a large sample of elite male and female endurance, strength,

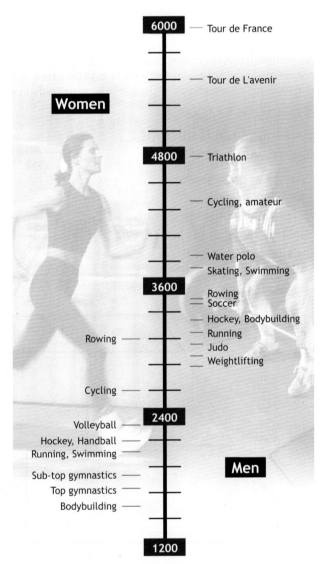

FIGURE 3.7 Daily energy intake (kcal) of elite male and female endurance, strength, and team sport athletes. (Adapted with permission from McArdle WD, Katch FI, Katch VL. *Exercise Physiology: Nutrition, Energy, and Human Performance.* 8th Ed. Baltimore: Wolters Kluwer Health, 2015, as adapted with permission van Erp-Baart AMJ, et al. Nationwide survey on nutritional habits in elite athletes. *Int J Sports Med* 1989;10:53.)

and team sport athletes. For men, daily energy intake ranged between 2900 and 5900 kcal; female competitors consumed 1600 to 3200 kcal. Except for the high-energy intake of athletes at extremes of performance and training, daily energy intake did not exceed 4000 kcal for men or 3000 kcal for women.

Extreme Energy Intake and Expenditure: The Tour de France

During competition or periods of intense training, some sport activities require extreme energy output, sometimes in excess of 1000 kcal • h^{-1} in elite marathoners and professional cyclists, including a correspondingly high-energy intake. For example, the daily energy requirements of elite cross-country skiers during 1 week of training averages 3740 to 4860 kcal for women and 6120 to 8570 kcal for men. **Figure 3.8** shows the variation in daily energy expenditure for a male competitor during the Tour de France professional cycling race. Energy expenditure averaged 6500 kcal daily for nearly 3 weeks during this event. Large daily variation occurred depending on the activity level for a particular day; daily energy expenditure decreased to 3000 kcal on a "rest" day and increased to approximately 9000 kcal when the athlete was cycling over a mountain pass. By combining liquid nutrition with normal meals, the cyclist nearly matched daily energy intake with energy expenditure.

The Precompetition Meal

Athletes often compete in the morning after an overnight fast. Considerable depletion occurs in the body's carbohydrate reserves over 8 to 12 hours without eating (see Chapter 2); thus, precompetition nutrition takes on importance even if the person follows appropriate dietary recommendations. *The precompetition meal provides the athlete with adequate carbohydrate energy and ensures optimal hydration.* Fasting before competition or intense training makes no sense physiologically because it rapidly depletes liver and muscle glycogen and ultimately impairs exercise performance. Consider the following three factors when individualizing an athlete's meal plan:

1. Food preference
2. Psychological set
3. Food digestibility

As a general rule, foods high in lipid and protein should not be consumed on competition days. These foods digest slowly and remain in the digestive tract longer than do carbohydrate foods containing similar calories. The timing of the precompetition meal also deserves consideration. Increased emotional stress and tension depress intestinal absorption because of a decrease in blood flow to the digestive tract. *Generally, 3 hours provides sufficient time to digest and absorb a carbohydrate-rich precompetition meal.*

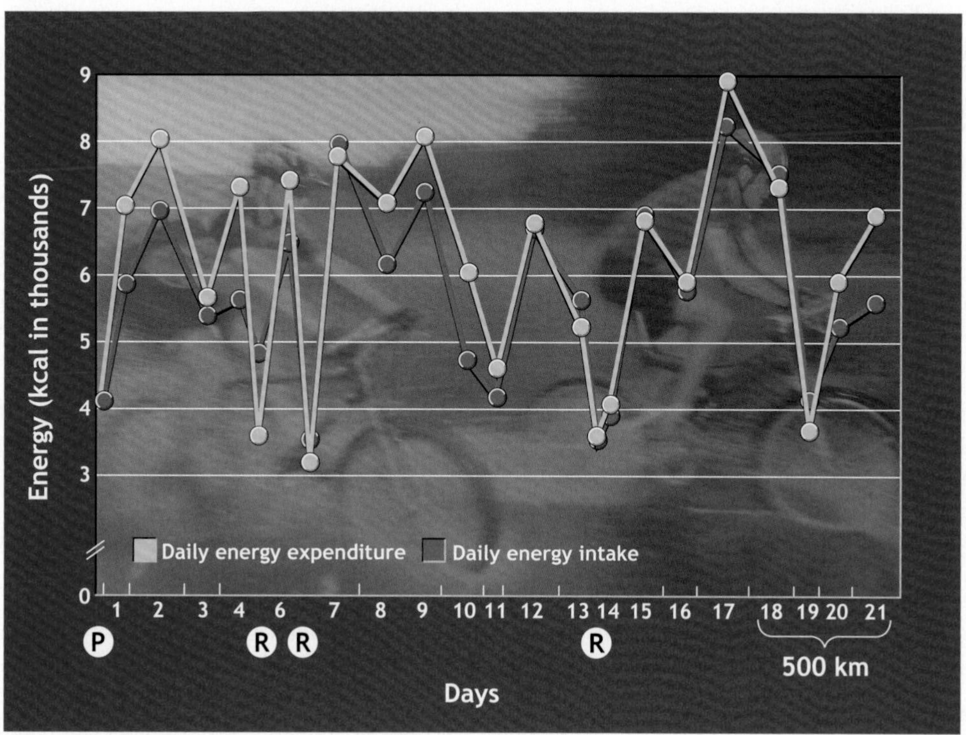

FIGURE 3.8 Daily energy expenditure (*yellow circles*) and energy intake (*red circles*) for a cyclist during the Tour de France competition. For 3 weeks in July, nearly 200 cyclists ride over and around the perimeter of France, covering 2405 miles, more than 100 miles daily (only 1 day of rest), at an average speed of 24.4 mph. Note the extremely high energy expenditure values and ability to achieve energy balance with liquid nutrition plus normal meals. P, stage; R, rest day. (Reprinted with permission from McArdle WD, Katch FI, Katch VL. *Exercise Physiology: Nutrition, Energy, and Human Performance*. 8th Ed. Baltimore: Wolters Kluwer Health, 2015, as adapted with permission from Saris WHM, et al. Adequacy of vitamin supply under maximal sustained workloads; the Tour de France. In: Walter P, et al., eds. *Elevated Dosages of Vitamins*. Toronto: Huber, 1989.)

High Protein: Not the Best Choice

Many athletes become accustomed to and even depend on the classic "steak and eggs" precompetition meal. This meal may satisfy the athlete, coach, and restaurateur, but it can diminish optimal athletic performance.

High-protein precompetition meals should be modified or abolished in favor of those high in carbohydrates for the following five reasons:

1. Dietary carbohydrates, not protein, replenish liver and muscle glycogen previously depleted from an overnight fast.
2. Carbohydrates digest and become absorbed more rapidly than do proteins or lipids; carbohydrates provide energy faster and reduce the feeling of fullness.
3. High-protein meals elevate resting metabolism more than do high-carbohydrate meals because of greater energy requirements for protein's digestion, absorption, and assimilation. Additional metabolic heat, albeit small, places demands on the body's heat-dissipating mechanisms, which impairs exercise performance in hot weather.
4. Protein catabolism for energy facilitates dehydration during exertion because the by-products of amino acid breakdown require water for urinary excretion. Approximately 50 mL of water "accompanies" the excretion of each gram of urea in urine.
5. Carbohydrate provides the main energy nutrient for short-duration anaerobic exercise and prolonged, intense endurance activities.

Ideal Precompetition Meal

The ideal precompetition meal maximizes muscle and liver glycogen storage and provides glucose for intestinal absorption during physical activity. The meal should accomplish these two goals:

1. Contain 150 to 300 g of carbohydrate (3 to 5 g per kg of body mass) in either solid or liquid form
2. Be consumed 3 to 4 hours prior to competition

The benefit of a precompetition meal depends on the athlete maintaining a nutritionally sound meal plan throughout training. Precompetition food cannot correct existing nutritional deficiencies or inadequate nutrient intake during the weeks before competition.

Liquid Meals

Commercially prepared liquid meals offer an alternative to the precompetition meal. They provide the following five benefits:

1. Enhance energy and nutrient intake in training, particularly if daily energy output exceeds energy intake because of the athlete's nutrition mismanagement or lack of interest in food
2. Provide a high-glycemic carbohydrate for glycogen replenishment
3. Contain some lipid and protein to contribute to satiety
4. Supply fluid because these meals exist in liquid form
5. Digest rapidly, thus minimizing intestinal tract residue

Liquid meals prove particularly effective during daylong swimming and track meets or tennis, ice hockey, soccer, field hockey, lacrosse, martial arts, wrestling, volleyball, and basketball tournaments. During tournament competition, the athlete usually has little time for or interest in food. Athletes also can benefit from liquid meals if they experience difficulty maintaining a relatively large body weight required by the sport and/or need a ready source of calories to gain weight.

Carbohydrate Intake Before, During, and After Intense Physical Activity

Intense aerobic activity continued for 1 hour decreases liver glycogen by about 55%, whereas a 2-hour strenuous workout severely depletes glycogen in the liver and the specifically targeted exercised muscle fibers. Even maximal, repetitive, 1- to 5-minute bouts of exertion interspersed with brief rest intervals (e.g., soccer, ice hockey, field hockey, European handball, and tennis) dramatically lower liver and muscle glycogen levels. Carbohydrate supplementation improves prolonged performance capacity and intermittent, high-intensity performance. The "vulnerability" of the body's glycogen stores during intense physical effort has focused research on the potential high-performance benefits of carbohydrate intake just prior to and during exercise. Research also continues to illustrate how to optimize carbohydrate replenishment during the postexercise recovery period.

Before Physical Activity

The potential endurance benefits of consuming simple sugars before more vigorous physical activity remain equivocal. One line of research contends that ingesting rapidly absorbed, high-glycemic carbohydrates within 1 hour before exercising accelerates glycogen depletion and negatively affects endurance performance in three ways as follows:

1. Causes an overshoot in insulin release, thus creating low blood sugar termed **rebound hypoglycemia** that impairs central nervous system function during exercise.
2. Facilitates glucose influx into muscle (through a large insulin release) to increase carbohydrate use as fuel during physical activity.
3. High insulin levels inhibit lipolysis to reduce free fatty acid mobilization from adipose tissue. Greater carbohydrate breakdown and blunted fat mobilization contribute to premature glycogen depletion and early fatigue.

Research has verified that consuming glucose before physical activity increases muscle glucose uptake. It also reduces liver glucose output during physical activity to a degree that *conserves* liver glycogen reserves. From a practical standpoint, one way to eliminate any potential negative effects from pre-exercise simple sugars necessitates ingesting them at least

60 minutes before physical activity. This allows sufficient time to re-establish hormonal balance when physical activity begins.

Pre-exercise Fructose Intake

The small intestine absorbs fructose more slowly than glucose, with only a minimal insulin response without a decline in blood glucose. These observations have stimulated debate about whether fructose might provide a beneficial pre-exercise, exogenous carbohydrate fuel source for prolonged physical activity. The theoretical rationale for fructose appears plausible, but its physical activity benefits remain inconclusive. From a practical standpoint, consuming a high-fructose beverage often produces intestinal cramping, vomiting, and diarrhea, which would negatively impact exercise performance. *After it has been absorbed by the small intestine, fructose also must be converted to glucose in the liver, limiting its rapid availability for energy.*

Glycemic Index and Pre-exercise Food Intake

Use of the glycemic index can help to formulate the composition of the immediate pre-exercise meal. The basic idea is to make glucose available to maintain blood sugar and muscle metabolism without requiring excess insulin release. The objective, to spare glycogen reserves, requires stabilizing blood glucose and optimizing fat mobilization and catabolism. Consuming low-glycemic index foods less than 30 minutes before physical activity allows for a relatively slow rate of glucose absorption into the blood during activity. This eliminates an insulin surge, and also provides a steady supply of "slow-release" glucose from the digestive tract as physical activity progresses. This effect theoretically should benefit long-term, intense activity.

During Physical Activity

Consuming about 60 g (2 oz) of liquid or solid carbohydrates each hour during physical activity benefits long-duration intense activity and repetitive, short bouts of near-maximal effort. Sustained effort below 50% of maximum intensity relies primarily on fat oxidation, with only a relatively small demand on carbohydrate breakdown. Consuming carbohydrate offers little benefit during such activity. In contrast, carbohydrate intake provides supplementary glucose during intense, aerobic activity when glycogen utilization increases greatly. Exogenous carbohydrate accomplishes one or both of the following two goals:

1. Spares muscle glycogen because the ingested glucose provides energy to power the activity.
2. Helps to stabilize blood glucose, which minimizes headaches, light-headedness, nausea, and other symptoms of central nervous system distress.

Maintaining an optimal blood glucose level also supplies muscles with glucose during the later stages of prolonged exercise when glycogen reserves deplete. Consuming carbohydrates while exercising at 60% to 80% $\dot{V}O_{2max}$ **(maximal oxygen uptake)** postpones fatigue by 15 to 30 minutes. This effect offers potential for long-distance endurance runners who often experience muscle fatigue within 90 minutes of running. **Figure 3.9** shows that a single, concentrated carbohydrate intake almost 2 hours into an endurance exercise when blood glucose and glycogen reserves near depletion restores blood glucose levels. This strategy increases carbohydrate availability and delays fatigue because higher blood glucose levels sustain the muscles' energy needs.

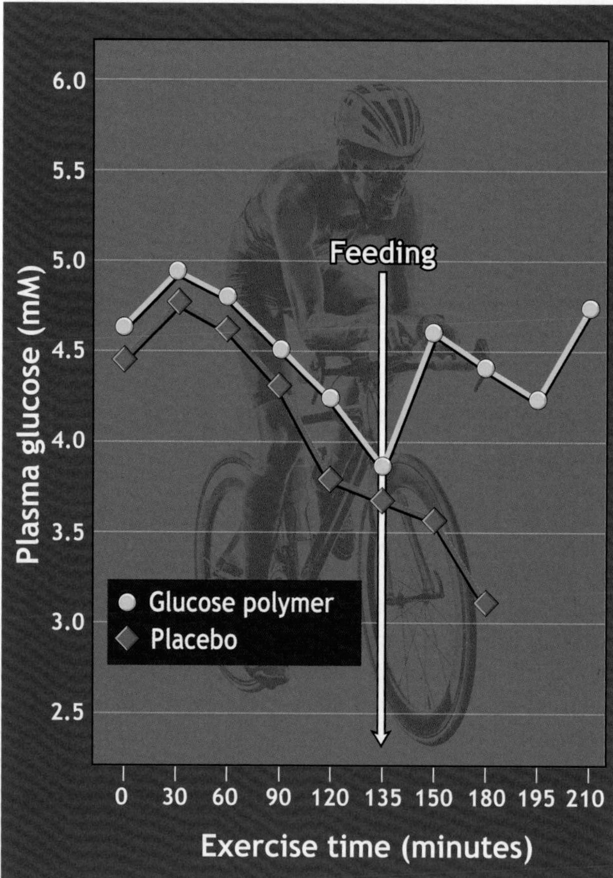

FIGURE 3.9 Average plasma glucose concentration during prolonged intense aerobic exercise when subjects consumed a placebo or glucose polymer (3 g per kg of body mass in a 50% solution). (Reprinted with permission from McArdle WD, Katch FI, Katch VL. *Exercise Physiology: Nutrition, Energy, and Human Performance*. 8th Ed. Baltimore: Wolters Kluwer Health, 2015, as adapted with permission from Coggan AR, Coyle EF. Metabolism and performance following carbohydrate ingestion late in exercise. *Med Sci Sports Exerc* 1989;21:59.)

Postexercise Carbohydrate Intake

To speed glycogen replenishment following a hard bout of training or competition, one should immediately consume carbohydrate-rich, high-glycemic foods, specifically, 50 to 75 g (2 to 3 oz) of moderate- to high-glycemic carbohydrates every 2 hours for a total of 500 g (7 to 10 g per kg body mass) or until consuming a large high-carbohydrate meal. If this strategy is impractical, meals containing 2.5 g of high-glycemic carbohydrates per kg of body mass consumed at 2, 4, 6, 8, and 22 hours after exercise rapidly restores muscle glycogen. For a 70-kg runner, this would amount to a little more than 6 oz of high-glycemic carbohydrate (2.5 g × 70 ÷ 28.4 g per oz = 6 oz).

To rapidly replenish glycogen reserves, avoid legumes, fructose, and dairy products because of their slow rates of intestinal absorption. More rapid glycogen resynthesis occurs by remaining physically inactive during recovery. *Under optimal carbohydrate intake conditions, glycogen replenishes at a rate of about 5% per hour. Even under the best of circumstances, it still would require at least 20 hours to reestablish glycogen stores with glycogen depletion.*

GLUCOSE INTAKE, ELECTROLYTES, AND WATER UPTAKE

Adding carbohydrates to the oral rehydration beverage provides additional glucose energy during prolonged endurance physical activity when the body's glycogen reserves slowly deplete. Determining the optimal fluid/carbohydrate mixture and volume to consume during endurance-type activities takes on importance when the objectives attempt to reduce fatigue and minimize dehydration. Consuming a large, dilute fluid volume may lessen carbohydrate uptake, and concentrated sugar solutions diminish fluid replacement.

The rate of stomach emptying greatly affects the small intestine's fluid and nutrient absorption. Exercise up to an intensity of about 75% $\dot{V}O_{2max}$ minimally (if at all) impacts gastric emptying, and an exercise intensity greater than 75% $\dot{V}O_{2max}$ slows the emptying rate. Gastric volume greatly influences gastric emptying; its rate decreases as stomach volume decreases. *It makes sense to maintain a relatively large stomach fluid volume to speed gastric emptying.*

Consider Fluid Concentration

A key question concerns the possible negative effects of sugar drinks on water absorption from the digestive tract. Gastric emptying slows when ingested fluids contain an excessive concentration of particles in solution (increased osmolality) or possess high caloric content. Any factor that impairs fluid uptake negatively impacts prolonged effort in hot weather, when adequate water intake and absorption play prime roles in the participant's health and safety. Ingesting up to an 8% glucose-sodium oral rehydration beverage causes little negative effect on gastric emptying. This beverage facilitates fluid uptake by the intestinal lumen because active cotransport of glucose and sodium across the intestinal mucosa stimulates water's passive uptake by osmotic action. Water replenishes effectively, and additional glucose uptake contributes to blood glucose maintenance. This glucose can then spare muscle and liver glycogen or provide for blood glucose reserves during the later stage of exercise.

Sodium's Potential Benefit

Two American College of Sports Medicine (ACSM) Position Stands (**http://acsm.org/access-public-information/position-stands**) recommend that sports drinks contain 0.5 to 0.7 g of sodium per liter of fluid consumed during physical activity exceeding 1 hour. They posit this benefits ultraendurance athletes at risk for hyponatremia; we present an opposing point of view to the ACSM recommendations for salt intake supplied by sports drinks (see Chapter 2). In general, exercise-assisted hyponatremia (EAH) results mostly from an unusually large intake of fluid before, during, or following an event, not from salt depletion during activity.

CARBOHYDRATE NEEDS DURING INTENSE TRAINING

Repeated days of strenuous endurance workouts for distance running, swimming, cross-country skiing, and cycling can induce general fatigue that makes training progressively more difficult. Often referred to as "**staleness**," the gradual depletion of glycogen reserves probably triggers this physiologic state. In one experiment in which athletes ran 16.1 km (10 miles) a day for 3 successive days, glycogen in the thigh muscles became nearly depleted, although the athletes' diets contained about 50% carbohydrate. By Day 3, glycogen usage during the run was less than on Day 1, and fat breakdown supplied the predominant fuel to power exercise. No further glycogen depletion occurred when daily dietary carbohydrate increased to 600 g (70% of caloric intake), further supporting the important role of maintaining adequate carbohydrate intake during training.

Diet, Glycogen Stores, and Endurance Capacity

Scientists in the late 1960s observed that endurance performance improved simply by consuming a carbohydrate-rich diet for 3 days before exercising. Conversely, endurance deteriorated when the diet consisted principally of lipids. In one series of classic experiments, subjects consumed one of three diets. The first maintained normal energy intake but supplied the majority of calories from lipids, with only 5% from carbohydrates. The second provided the normal allotment for calories with the typical percentages of the three macronutrients. The third provided 80% of calories as carbohydrates.

The results from this compelling research, illustrated in **Figure 3.10**, show that the glycogen content of leg muscles, expressed as grams of glycogen per 100 g of muscle, averaged 0.6 for subjects who consumed the low-carbohydrate diet, 1.75 for subjects who consumed the typical diet, and 3.75 for subjects who consumed the high-carbohydrate diet. Furthermore, the subjects' endurance capacity varied widely depending on their pre-exercise diet. When subjects consumed the high-carbohydrate diet, endurance more than tripled compared with those consuming the low-carbohydrate diet!

These findings highlight the important role nutrition plays in establishing appropriate energy reserves for physical

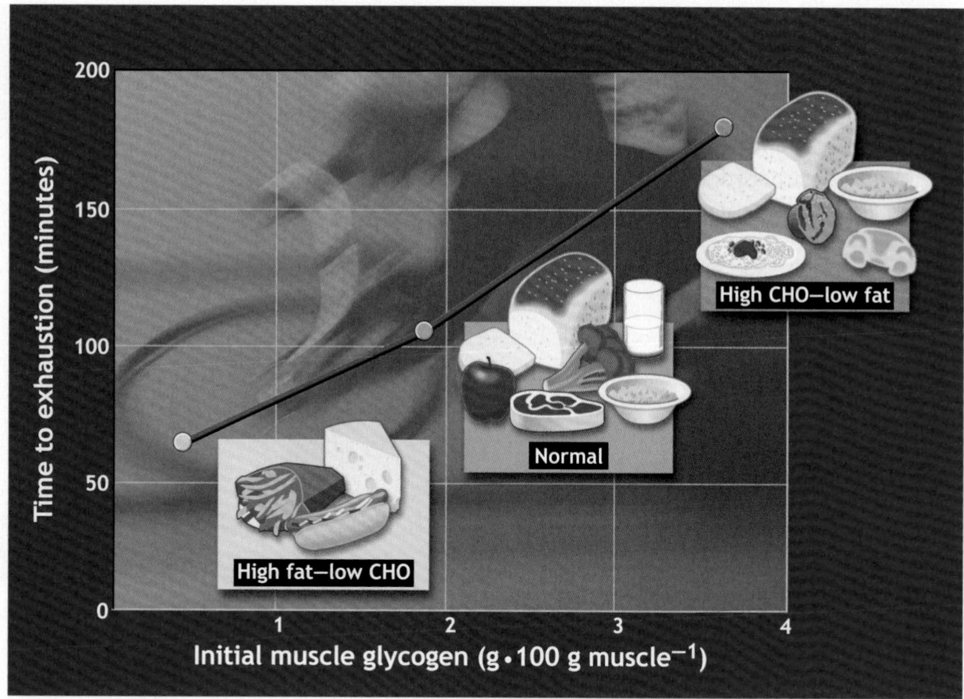

FIGURE 3.10 Classic experiment illustrating the effects of a high-fat–low-carbohydrate (CHO) diet, a normal diet, and a high-carbohydrate–low-fat diet on the quadriceps femoris muscle's glycogen content and duration of endurance exercise on a bicycle ergometer. Endurance time with a high-carbohydrate diet is three times that on a low-carbohydrate diet. (Reprinted with permission from McArdle WD, Katch FI, Katch VL. *Exercise Physiology: Nutrition, Energy, and Human Performance*. 8th Ed. Baltimore: Wolters Kluwer Health, 2015, as adapted with permission from Bergstrom J, et al. Diet, muscle glycogen and physical performance. *Acta Physiol Scand* 1967;71:140.)

activity. A diet deficient in carbohydrates rapidly depletes muscle and liver glycogen. Glycogen depletion subsequently affects performance in maximal, short-term anaerobic effort and prolonged, intense aerobic effort. These observations are germane not only to athletes but also to moderately active people who eat less than the recommended carbohydrate quantity.

fyi Muscle Glycogen Supercompensation Enhanced by Prior Creatine Supplementation

Classic studies suggested a synergy between glycogen storage and creatine supplementation. For example, preceding a glycogen-loading protocol with a creatine-loading protocol (20 g a day for 5 days) produced a 10% greater glycogen packing in the vastus lateralis muscle compared with muscle glycogen levels achieved with only glycogen loading. Increases in creatine and cellular volume with creatine supplementation facilitate subsequent storage of muscle glycogen.

Sources: Hespel P, et al. Creatine supplementation: exploring the role of the creatine kinase/phosphocreatine system in human muscle. *Can J Appl Physiol* 2001;26:S79.

Nelson AG, et al. Muscle glycogen supercompensation is enhanced by prior creatine supplementation. *Med Sci Sports Exerc* 2001;33:1096.

Robinson TM, et al. Role of submaximal exercise in promoting creatine and glycogen accumulation in human skeletal muscle. *J Appl Physiol* 1999 87:598.

Enhanced Glycogen Storage: Carbohydrate Loading

A particular combination of diet plus exercise produces a significant "packing" of muscle glycogen, a procedure termed **carbohydrate loading** or **glycogen supercompensation**. The technique increases muscle glycogen levels more than levels achieved by simply maintaining a high-carbohydrate diet. Glycogen loading packs up to 5 g of glycogen into each 100 g of muscle in contrast to the normal value of 1.7 g. Athletes who follow the classic glycogen-loading procedure (see A Closer Look: *Strategies for Carbohydrate Loading*) maintain enhanced muscle glycogen levels in a resting, non-exercising individual for at least 3 days. This occurs if the diet contains about 60% of total calories as carbohydrate during the maintenance phase.

 See the animation "Glycogen Synthesis" on **http://thePoint.lww.com/MKKESS5e** for a demonstration of this process.

For sports competition and exercise training, a diet containing between 60% and 70% of calories as carbohydrates should adequately maintain muscle and liver glycogen reserves. This diet ensures about twice the level of muscle glycogen compared with that found in sedentary individuals, who typically consume a lower-carbohydrate diet of 50% to 60% carbohydrates. For well-nourished physically active individuals, the supercompensation effect remains relatively small. During intense training, individuals who do not upgrade daily caloric and carbohydrate intakes to meet increased energy demands may experience chronic muscle fatigue and staleness.

Individuals should learn all they can about carbohydrate loading before trying to manipulate their diet and exercise regimens to attain a supercompensation effect. If a person decides to supercompensate after weighing the pros and cons, the new food regimen should be tried in stages during training and not for the first time before competition. For example, a runner should start with a long training run followed by a high-carbohydrate diet. The athlete should maintain a detailed log of how the dietary manipulation affects performance. Subjective feelings should be noted during exercise depletion and replenishment phases. With positive results, the person should then try the complete series of depletion, low-carbohydrate diet, and a high-carbohydrate diet but maintain the low-carbohydrate diet for only 1 day. If no adverse effects appear, the low-carbohydrate diet should be gradually extended to a maximum of 4 days.

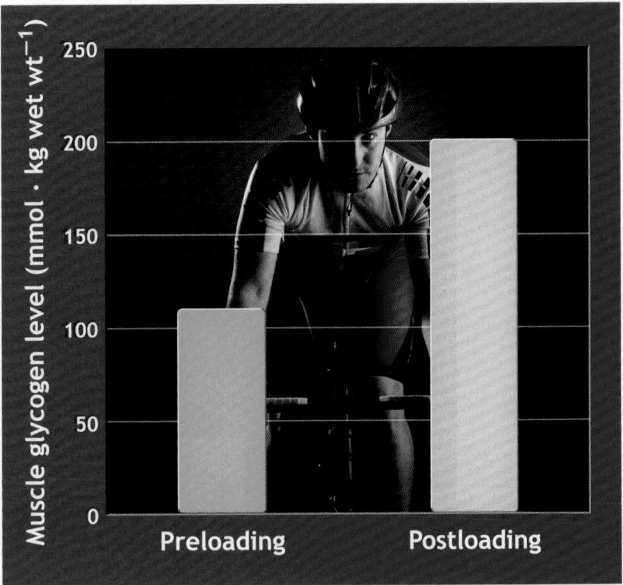

FIGURE 3.11 Muscle glycogen concentration of the vastus lateralis before (preloading) and after 180 seconds of near-maximal intensity cycling and 30 seconds of all-out effort followed by 1 day of high-carbohydrate intake (postloading). (Adapted with permission from McArdle WD, Katch FI, Katch VL. *Sports and Exercise Nutrition*. 4th Ed. Philadelphia: Wolters Kluwer Health, 2013, as reprinted with permission from Fairchild TJ, et al. Rapid carbohydrate loading after short bout of near maximal-intensity exercise. *Med Sci Sports Exerc* 2002;34:980.)

Modified Loading Procedure

The less-stringent, modified dietary protocol removes many of the negative aspects of the classic glycogen-loading sequence. This 6-day protocol does not require prior exercise to deplete glycogen. The athlete trains at about 75% of $\dot{V}O_{2max}$ (85% HR_{max}) for 1.5 hours and then gradually reduces or tapers exercise duration on successive days. Carbohydrates represent approximately 50% of total caloric intake during the first 3 days. Three days before competition, the diet's carbohydrate content then increases to 70% of energy intake, replenishing glycogen reserves to about the same point achieved with the classic loading protocol.

Rapid Loading Procedure: A One-Day Requirement

The 2 to 6 days required to achieve supranormal muscle glycogen levels represents a limitation of typical carbohydrate-loading procedures. Research has evaluated whether a shortened time interval that combines a relatively brief bout of intense exercise with only 1 day of high carbohydrate intake achieves the desired loading effect. Endurance-trained athletes cycled for 150 seconds at 130% of $\dot{V}O_{2max}$, followed by 30 seconds of all-out cycling. In the recovery period, the men consumed 10.3 g · kg-body mass^{-1} of high-glycemic carbohydrate foods. Biopsy data presented in **Figure 3.11** indicated that carbohydrate levels increased 82% in all fiber types of the vastus lateralis muscle after only 24 hours. The increased glycogen storage equaled or exceeded values reported by others using a 2- to 6-day regimen. The short-duration loading procedure benefits individuals who do not wish to disrupt normal training with the time required and potential negative aspects of other loading protocols.

Limited Applicability and Negative Aspects

The potential benefits from carbohydrate loading apply only to intense and prolonged aerobic activities. *Unless the athlete begins competing in a state of depletion, exercising for less than 60 minutes requires only normal carbohydrate intake and glycogen reserves.* Carbohydrate loading and associated high levels of muscle and liver glycogen did not benefit athletes in a 20.9-km (13-mile) run compared with a run after a low-carbohydrate plan. Also, a single, maximal anaerobic exercise for 75 seconds did not improve by increasing muscle glycogen availability above normal through dietary manipulation before the activity.

In most sport competition and exercise training, a daily intake of 60% to 70% of total calories as carbohydrates provides for adequate muscle and liver glycogen reserves. This diet ensures about twice the level of muscle glycogen compared with the 45% to 50% carbohydrate intake of the typical American diet. For well-nourished athletes, any supercompensation effect from carbohydrate loading remains relatively small.

The addition of 2.7 g of water stored with each gram of glycogen makes this a heavy fuel compared with equivalent energy as stored fat. A higher body weight because of water retention often makes the athlete feel heavy, "bloated," and uncomfortable; any extra load also directly adds to the energy cost of weight-bearing running, racewalking, climbing activities, and cross-country skiing. The added energy cost can negate the potential benefits from increased glycogen storage. On the positive side, the water liberated during glycogen breakdown aids somewhat in temperature regulation to benefit physical activity in hot environments.

The classic model for supercompensation is ill advised for individuals with certain health conditions. A dietary carbohydrate overload, interspersed with periods of high lipid or protein intake, may increase blood cholesterol and urea nitrogen levels. This could pose problems to those predisposed to type 2 diabetes and heart disease and those with muscle enzyme deficiencies or renal disease. Failure to eat a balanced diet on a consistent basis may produce mineral and vitamin deficiencies, particularly water-soluble vitamins; these deficiencies may require dietary supplementation. The glycogen-depleted state during the first phase of the glycogen-loading procedure reduces one's capacity to engage in intense training, possibly producing a detraining effect during the loading interval. Dramatically reducing dietary carbohydrate for 3 or 4 days also could set the stage for lean tissue loss because muscle protein serves as gluconeogenic substrate to maintain blood glucose levels with low glycogen reserves.

A CLOSER LOOK

Strategies for Carbohydrate Loading

The importance of muscle glycogen levels to enhance exercise performance remains unequivocal; time to exhaustion during intense aerobic exercise directly relates to the initial glycogen content of the liver and active musculature. Carbohydrate loading provides a strategy to increase initial muscle and liver glycogen levels before prolonged endurance performance.

Classic Carbohydrate-Loading Procedure

Classic carbohydrate loading involves a two-stage procedure.

Stage 1—Depletion

Day 1: Perform exhaustive exercise to deplete muscle glycogen in specific muscles.

Days 2, 3, and 4: Maintain low-carbohydrate food intake with high percentage of protein and lipid in the daily diet.

Stage 2—Carbohydrate Loading

Days 5, 6, and 7: Maintain high-carbohydrate food intake with normal percentage of protein in the daily diet.

Competition Day

Follow high-carbohydrate precompetition meal recommendation.

Specifics of Precompetition Diet-Exercise Plan to Enhance Glycogen Storage

1. Use intense, aerobic physical activity for 90 minutes about 6 days before competition to reduce muscle and liver glycogen stores. Because glycogen loading occurs only in the specific muscles depleted by physical activity, athletes must engage the major muscles involved in their sport.
2. Maintain a low-carbohydrate diet (60 to 100 g per day) for 3 days while training at moderate intensity to further deplete glycogen stores.
3. Switch to a high-carbohydrate diet (400 to 700 g daily) at least 3 days before competition and maintain this intake up to and as part of the precompetition meal.

Sample Meal Plans for Carbohydrate Depletion (Stage 1) and Carbohydrate Loading (Stage 2) Preceding an Endurance Event

Meal	Stage 1	Stage 2
Breakfast	1/2 cup fruit juice 2 eggs 1 slice whole-wheat toast 8 oz whole milk	1 cup fruit juice 1 bowl hot or cold cereal 1 to 2 muffins 1 tbsp butter coffee (cream and sugar)
Lunch	6-oz hamburger 2 slices bread 1 serving salad 1 tbsp mayonnaise and salad dressing 8 oz whole milk	2- to 3-oz hamburger with bun 1 cup juice 1 orange 1 tbsp mayonnaise 1 serving pie or cake
Snack	1 cup yogurt	1 cup yogurt, fruit, or cookies
Dinner	2 to 3 pieces chicken, fried 1 baked potato with sour cream 1/2 cup vegetables 2 tbsp butter iced tea (no sugar)	1–1 1/2 pieces chicken, baked 1 baked potato with sour cream 1 cup vegetables 1/2 cup sweetened pineapple iced tea (sugar) 1 tbsp butter
Snack	1 glass whole milk	1 glass chocolate milk with 4 cookies

Carbohydrate intake averages approximately 100 g or 400 kcal during **stage 1; stage 2** carbohydrate intake increases to 400 to 700 g or about 1600 to 2800 kcal.

SUMMARY

1. Within rather broad limits, a balanced diet from regular food intake provides the nutrient requirements of athletes and others engaged in exercise training and sports competition.
2. MyPlate, formulated by the US government, represents a model for good nutrition for most individuals that emphasizes diverse grains, vegetables, and fruits as major calorie sources, minimizing foods high in animal proteins, lipids, and dairy products.
3. Alternative models for good nutrition include the Healthy Eating Plate, the Mediterranean Diet Pyramid, and the Near-Vegetarian Diet Pyramid.
4. For physically active individuals, consuming 400 to 600 g of low-glycemic polysaccharides should supply 60% to 70% of daily caloric intake.
5. The volume of daily physical activity largely determines energy intake requirements.
6. Daily energy requirements for physically active individuals probably do not exceed 4000 kcal for men and 3000 kcal for women.
7. Under extremes of training and competition, energy intake requirements approach 5000 kcal for women and 9000 kcal for men.
8. The relatively high caloric intakes of physically active men and women usually increase protein, vitamin, and mineral intake above recommended values.
9. The ideal precompetition meal maximizes muscle and liver glycogen storage and enhances glucose for intestinal absorption during exercise.
10. A carbohydrate-rich pre-event meal requires about 3 hours for complete digestion and absorption.
11. Commercially prepared liquid meals offer a practical approach to precompetition nutrition and energy supplementation because they balance nutritive value, contribute to fluid needs, and absorb rapidly in the gut.
12. Consuming low-glycemic index foods immediately before physical activity permits a relatively slow rate of glucose absorption into the blood prior to and during the activity..
13. Stomach fluid volume exerts the greatest effect on gastric emptying rate with the larger volumes producing the greatest rate of emptying.
14. Consuming a 5% to 8% carbohydrate-electrolyte beverage during physical activity in the heat contributes to temperature regulation and fluid balance as effectively as plain water.
15. A person should consume 50 to 75 g of moderate- to high-glycemic carbohydrates every 2 hours for a total of 500 g to speed glycogen replenishment following a bout of intense physical training or competition.
16. It takes at least 20 hours (5% per hour) to fully re-establish pre-exercise glycogen stores.
17. Successive days of intense training gradually deplete glycogen reserves even with the typical carbohydrate intake pattern.
18. A carbohydrate-deficient diet depletes muscle and liver glycogen to profoundly impair performance in maximal, short-term anaerobic physical activity and prolonged, intense aerobic effort.
19. Carbohydrate loading augments prolonged endurance performance but with potentially negative side effects.
20. Modifying the classic carbohydrate-loading procedure enhances glycogen storage without dramatically altering diet and physical activity regimens.

THINK IT THROUGH

1. Under what circumstances would an athlete require nutritional supplementation?
2. An athletic team has three matches scheduled on consecutive days. What should the athletes consume following each day's competition and why?
3. What advice would you give to a sprint runner or swimmer who plans to carbohydrate load for competition?
4. How can physically active men and women who consume the greatest number of calories weigh less than do those who consume fewer calories?
5. In what situations might a protein intake representing twice the RDA still prove inadequate for an individual involved in intense physical training?
6. In what ways can nutritional and energy intake goals for sports training differ from actual competition requirements? Give specific sports examples.
7. From a nutritional perspective, how can a reduced total volume of daily training or taper improve training responsiveness and competitive performance?
8. How would you advise a high school soccer team about sound nutrition with individuals who represent diverse ethnic backgrounds with unique food intake patterns?

KEY TERMS

Adequate intake (AI): Assumed adequate nutritional goal when no RDA has been established; approximates proper nutrient intake of apparently healthy persons.

Atwater general factors: Named after Wilbur Olin Atwater (1844–1907) who first described energy release in the calorimeter as the net kcal value per gram available to the body for each of the macronutrients; 4.0 kcal per gram for carbohydrates, 9.0 kcal per gram for lipids, and 4.0 kcal per gram for proteins.

Bomb calorimeters: Determines total or gross energy value of various food macronutrients by measuring the heat liberated as a food sample burns completely inside the calorimeter.

Carbohydrate loading: Combination diet plus physical activity plan that produces significant "packing" of up to 5 g of glycogen into each 100 g of muscle in contrast to a normal 1.7 g value.

Diet quality index (DQI): Appraises the general "healthfulness" of one's diet based on a scoring schema with a risk gradient associated with diet and major diet-related chronic diseases.

Dietary Guidelines: Provides advice for making food and physical activity choices that promote good health, healthy weight, and disease prevention for Americans aged 2 years and older, including those at increased risk of chronic disease.

Dietary reference intake (DRI): System of nutritional recommendations from the Institute of Medicine (IOM) of the US National Academy of Sciences intended for the general public and health professionals in the United States and Canada.

Digestive efficiency: Amount of ingested chemical energy absorbed by the body relative to the food's total energy content.

Direct calorimetry: Measurement of the amount of heat produced by a subject or food enclosed within an insulated chamber.

Estimated average requirements (EAR): Dietary reference standards based on a review of the scientific literature expected to satisfy the needs of 50% of the people in that life stage and sex group.

Glycogen supercompensation: Application of diet and exercise modification to increase muscle glycogen levels more than levels achieved simply by maintaining a high-carbohydrate diet.

Healthy Eating Plate: Scientific evidence-based visual blueprint for eating a healthful meal.

Heat of combustion: Energy released as heat when a compound undergoes complete combustion with oxygen under standard conditions.

Mediterranean Diet Pyramid: Pyramid icon that lists desirable foods based on the dietary traditions of Crete, Greece, and Southern Italy.

MyPlate: An icon and program designed to remind Americans to eat healthfully for each of five food groups—fruits, vegetables, protein, grains, and dairy (**www.choosemyplate.gov**).

Net Energy Value of a Food: Difference in the energy value of a food determined by direct calorimetry versus the energy available to the body.

One kilogram-calorie (kilocalorie [kcal]): Expresses the quantity of heat necessary to raise the temperature of 1 kg (1 L) of water 1°C (from 14.5°C to 15.5°C).

Rebound hypoglycemia: Ingesting a high insulin index or high glycemic load meal produces a subsequent spike in insulin, which causes blood sugar to decline below pre-ingestion level.

Recommended Dietary Allowances (RDA): Daily dietary intake level of a nutrient considered sufficient by the Food and Nutrition Board to meet the requirements of 97.5% of healthy individuals in each life stage and sex group.

Staleness: Physiological state accompanying overtraining in which the athlete fails to maintain normal training and performance regimens

Tolerable upper intake levels (UL): Highest level of daily consumption without adverse effects when used indefinitely without medical supervision

$\dot{V}O_{2max}$ (maximal oxygen uptake): Maximum rate of oxygen consumption measured during incremental exercise and expressed on an absolute rate as liters of oxygen per minute ($L \cdot min^{-1}$) or a relative rate as milliliters of oxygen per kilogram body mass per minute (e.g., $mL^{-1} \cdot kg^{-1} \cdot min^{-1}$).

SELECTED REFERENCES

Achten J, et al. Higher dietary carbohydrate content during interspersed running training results in a better maintenance of performance and mood state. *J Appl Physiol* 2004;96:1331.

Akabas SR, Dolins KR. Micronutrient requirements of physically active women: what can we learn from iron? *Am J Clin Nutr* 2005;81:1246S.

American College of Sports Medicine, American Dietetic Association, and Dietitians of Canada. Joint Position Statement. Nutrition and athletic performance. *Med Sci Sports Exerc* 2000;32:2130.

American College of Sports Medicine. American College of Sports Medicine position stand. Exercise and fluid replacement. *Med Sci Sports Exerc* 2007;39:377.

Aragon AA, Schoenfeld BJ. Nutrient timing revisited: is there a post-exercise anabolic window? *Nutrients* 2014;6:1782.

Barnett C, et al. Muscle metabolism during sprint exercise in man: influence of sprint training. *J Sci Med Sport* 2004;7:314.

Bartlett JD, et al. Carbohydrate availability and exercise training adaptation: too much of a good thing? *Eur J Sport Sci* 2014;19:1.

Baty JJ, et al. The effect of a carbohydrate and protein supplement on resistance exercise performance, hormonal response, and muscle damage. *J Strength Cond Res* 2007;21:321.

Berardi JM, et al. Postexercise muscle glycogen recovery enhanced with a carbohydrate-protein supplement. *Med Sci Sports Exerc* 2006;38:1106.

Billaut F, Bishop D. Muscle fatigue in males and females during multiple-sprint exercise. *Sports Med* 2009;39:257.

Blacker SD, et al. Carbohydrate vs protein supplementation for recovery of neuromuscular function following prolonged load carriage. *J Int Soc Sports Nutr* 2010;7:2.

Bosch AN, Noakes TD. Carbohydrate ingestion during exercise and endurance performance. *Indian J Med Res* 2005;121:634.

Burgomaster KA, et al. Six sessions of sprint interval training increases muscle oxidative potential and cycle endurance capacity in humans. *J Appl Physiol* 2005;98:1985.

Burke LM. Nutrition for distance events. *J Sports Sci* 2007;25(Suppl 1):S29. Review. Erratum in: *J Sports Sci* 2009;27:667.

Burke LM, et al. Energy and carbohydrate for training and recovery. *J Sports Sci* 2006;24:675.

Burns SF, et al. A single session of resistance exercise does not reduce postprandial lipidemia. *J Sports Sci* 2005;23:251.

Butte NF, et al. Revision of dietary reference intakes for energy in preschool-age children. *Am J Clin Nutr* 2014;100:161.

Cases N, et al. Differential response of plasma and immune cell's vitamin E levels to physical activity and antioxidant vitamin supplementation. *Eur J Clin Nutr* 2005;59:781.

Castell LM, et al. BJSM reviews: A-Z of nutritional supplements: dietary supplements, sports nutrition foods and ergogenic aids for health and performance. Part 8. *Br J Sports Med* 2010;44:468.

Castellani JW, et al. Energy expenditure in men and women during 54h of exercise and caloric deprivation. *Med Sci Sports Exerc* 2006;38:894.

Cochran AJ, et al. Carbohydrate feeding during recovery alters the skeletal muscle metabolic response to repeated sessions of high-intensity interval exercise in humans. *J Appl Physiol* 2010;108:628.

Coggan AR, Coyle EF. Carbohydrate ingestion during prolonged exercise: effects on metabolism and performance. In: Holloszy JO, Ed. *Exercise and Sport Science Reviews*, Vol. 19. Baltimore: Williams & Wilkins, 1991.

Cordain L, et al. Origins and evolutions of the Western diet: health implications for the 21st century. *Am J Clin Nutr* 2005;81:341.

Coyle EF. Fluid and fuel intake during exercise. *J Sports Sci* 2004;22:39.

Currell K, Jeukendrup AE. Superior endurance performance with ingestion of multiple transportable carbohydrates. *Med Sci Sports Exerc* 2008;40:275.

Donaldson CM, et al. Glycemic index and endurance performance. *Int J Sport Nutr Exerc Metab* 2010;20:154. Review.

Erlenbusch M, et al. Effect of high-fat or high-carbohydrate diets on endurance exercise: a meta-analysis. *Int J Sport Nutr Exerc Metab* 2005;15:1.

Fiala KA, et al. Rehydration with a caffeinated beverage during the nonexercise periods of 3 consecutive days of 2-a-day practices. *Int J Sport Nutr Exerc Metab* 2004;14:419.

Food and Nutrition Board, Institute of Medicine. *Dietary Reference Intakes for Energy, Carbohydrates, Fiber, Fat, Protein and Amino Acids*. Washington, DC: National Academy Press, 2002.

Helge JW, et al. Impact of a fat-rich diet on endurance in man: role of the dietary period. *Med Sci Sports Exerc* 1998;30:456.

Heymsfield SB, Gonzalez MC, et al. Weight loss composition is one-fourth fat-free mass: a critical review and critique of this widely cited rule. *Obes Rev* 2014; 15:310.

Hoffman JR, et al. Effect of low-dose, short-duration creatine supplementation on anaerobic exercise performance. *J Strength Cond Res* 2005;19:260, .

Hoffman JR, et al. Effects of beta-hydroxy beta-methylbutyrate on power performance and indices of muscle damage and stress during high-intensity training. *J Strength Cond Res* 2004;18:747.

Horowitz JF, et al. Substrate metabolism when subjects are fed carbohydrates during exercise. *Am J Physiol* 1999;276:E828.

Horowitz JF, et al. Energy deficit without reducing dietary carbohydrate alters resting carbohydrate oxidation and fatty acid availability. *J Appl Physiol* 2005;98:1612.

Horowitz JF. Fatty acid mobilization from adipose tissue during exercise. *Trends Endocrinol Metab* 2003;14:386.

Hulston CJ, Jeukendrup AE. No placebo effect from carbohydrate intake during prolonged exercise. *Int J Sport Nutr Exerc Metab* 2009;19:275.

Iaia FM, et al. Four weeks of speed endurance training reduces energy expenditure during exercise and maintains muscle oxidative capacity despite a reduction in training volume. *J Appl Physiol* 2009;106:73.

Ivy JL, et al. Effect of a carbohydrate-protein supplement on endurance performance during exercise of varying intensity. *Int J Sport Nutr Exerc Metab* 2003; 13:388.

Jeacocke NA, Burke LM. Methods to standardize dietary intake before performance testing. *Int J Sport Nutr Exerc Metab* 2010;20:87. Review.

Jenkins DJ, et al. Glycemic index: an overview of implications in health and disease. *Am J Clin Nutr* 2002;76(Suppl):266S.

Jentjens RL, et al. Oxidation of combined ingestion of glucose and fructose during exercise. *J Appl Physiol* 2004;96:1277.

Jentjens RL, Jeukendrup AE. High rates of exogenous carbohydrate oxidation from a mixture of glucose and fructose ingested during prolonged cycling exercise. *Br J Nutr* 2005;93:485.

Jeukendrup AE, Wallis GA. Measurement of substrate oxidation during exercise by means of gas exchange measurements. *Int J Sports Med* 2005;26:S28.

Kammer L, et al. Cereal and nonfat milk support muscle recovery following exercise. *J Int Soc Sports Nutr* 2009;6:11.

Kerksick C, et al. International Society of Sports Nutrition position stand: nutrient timing. *J Int Soc Sports Nutr* 2008;3;5:17. Erratum in: *J Int Soc Sports Nutr* 2008;5:18.

Khanna GL, Manna I. Supplementary effect of carbohydrate-electrolyte drink on sports performance, lactate removal and cardiovascular response of athletes. *Indian J Med Res* 2005;121:665.

Kirwin JP, et al. A moderate glycemic meal before endurance exercise can enhance performance. *J Appl Physiol* 1998;84:53.

Lambert CP, et al. Macronutrient considerations for the sport of bodybuilding. *Sports Med* 2004;34:317.

Lasheras C, et al. Mediterranean diet and age with respect to overall survival in institutionalized, nonsmoking elderly people. *Am J Clin Nutr* 2000;71:987.

Leiper JB, et al. The effect of intermittent high-intensity running on gastric emptying of fluids in man. *Med Sci Sports Exerc* 2005;37:240.

Liu S, et al. A prospective study of dietary glycemic load, carbohydrate intake, and risk of coronary heart disease in US women. *Am J Clin Nutr* 2000;71:1455.

Margolis LM, et al. Energy requirements of US Army Special Operation Forces during military training. *Nutrients* 2014;12;6(5):1945.

McArdle WD, et al. *Sports and Exercise Nutrition*. 4th Ed. Baltimore: Lippincott Williams & Wilkins, 2013.

Morifuji M, et al. Dietary whey protein increases liver and skeletal muscle glycogen levels in exercise-trained rats. *Br J Nutr* 2005;93:439.

Morrison PJ, et al. Adding protein to a carbohydrate supplement provided after endurance exercise enhances 4E-BP1 and RPS6 signaling in skeletal muscle. *J Appl Physiol* 2008;104:1029.

Noakes TD. Commentary: role of hydration in health and exercise. *BMJ* 2012; 18;345, e4171.

Noakes TD. *Waterlogged: The Serious Problem of Overhydration in Endurance Sports*. Champaign: Human Kinetics, 2012.

Nick JJ, et al. Carbohydrate feedings during team sport exercise preserve physical and CNS function. *Med Sci Sports Exerc* 2005;37:306.

Nutritional Labeling and Education Act (NLEA) Requirements (8/94-2/95): Available at **www.fda.gov/ICECI/InspectionGuides/ucm074948.htm**

Nybo L. CNS fatigue and prolonged exercise: effect of glucose supplementation. *Med Sci Sports Exerc* 2003;35:589.

Pelly F, et al. Catering for the athletes village at the Sydney 2000 Olympic Games: the role of sports dietitians. *Int J Sport Nutr Exerc Metab* 2009; 19:340.

Pi-Sunyer X. Glycemic index and disease. *Am J Clin Nutr* 2002;76(Suppl):290S.

Richmond VL, et al. Energy balance and physical demands during an 8-week arduous military training course. *Mil Med* 2014;179:421.

Riddell MC, et al.. Substrate utilization during exercise with glucose and glucose plus fructose ingestion in boys ages 10–14 yr. *J Appl Physiol* 2001;90:903.

Rodriguez NR, et al. Position of the American Dietetic Association, Dietitians of Canada, and the American College of Sports Medicine: Nutrition and athletic performance. American Dietetic Association; Dietitians of Canada; American College of Sports Medicine. *J Am Diet Assoc* 2009;109:509.

Roy LB, et al. Oxidation of exogenous glucose, sucrose, and maltose during prolonged cycling exercise. *J Appl Physiol* 2004;96:1285.

Saunders MJ, et al. Effects of a carbohydrate-protein beverage on cycling endurance and muscle damage. *Med Sci Sports Exerc* 2004;36:1233.

Sawka MN, et al. Hydration effects on temperature regulation. *Int J Sports Med* 1998;19:S108.

Schoenfeld BJ, et al. The effect of protein timing on muscle strength and hypertrophy: a meta-analysis. *J Int Soc Sports Nutr* 2013;29;10:5.

Shannon KA, et al. Resistance exercise and postprandial lipemia: the dose effect of differing volumes of acute resistance exercise bouts. *Metabolism* 2005; 54:756.

Shirreffs SM, et al. Fluid and electrolyte needs for preparation and recovery from training and competition. *J Sports Sci* 2004;22:57.

Snyder AC. Overtraining and glycogen depletion hypothesis. *Med Sci Sports Exerc* 1998;30:1146.

Sousa M, Carvalho P, et al. Nutrition and nutritional issues for dancers. *Med Probl Perform Art* 2013;28:119.

Sparks MJ, et al. Pre-exercise carbohydrate ingestion: effect of the glycemic index on endurance exercise performance. *Med Sci Sports Exerc* 1998;30:844.

Steinmuller PL, et al. Academy of nutrition and dietetics: revised 2014 standards of practice and standards of professional performance for registered dietitian nutritionists (competent, proficient, and expert) in sports nutrition and dietetics. *J Acad Nutr Diet* 2014;114:631.

Stepto NK, et al. Effect of short-term fat adaptation on high-intensity training. *Med Sci Sports Exerc* 2002;34:449.

Stewart RD, et al. Protection of muscle membrane excitability during prolonged cycle exercise with glucose supplementation. *J Appl Physiol* 2007;103:331.

Tam N, Noakes TD. The quantification of body fluid allostasis during exercise. *Sports Med* 2013;43:1289.

Tharion WJ, et al. Energy requirements of military personnel. *Appetite* 2005;44:47.

Theodorou AS. Effects of acute creatine loading with or without carbohydrate on repeated bouts of maximal swimming in high-performance swimmers. *J Strength Cond Res* 2005;19:265.

Trichopoulou A, et al. Adherence to a Mediterranean diet and survival in a Greek population. *N Engl J Med* 2003;348:2599.

U.S. Food and Drug Administration. Available at: **www.fda.gov/Food/LabelingNutrition/Consumerinformation/ucm078889.htm twoparts panel**

Vogt M, et al. Effects of dietary fat on muscle substrates, metabolism, and performance in athletes. *Med Sci Sports Exerc* 2003;35:952.

Von Duvillard SP, et al. Fluids and hydration in prolonged endurance performance. *Nutrition* 2004;20:651.

Wakshlag JJ, et al. Biochemical and metabolic changes due to exercise in sprint-racing sled dogs: implications for postexercise carbohydrate supplements and hydration management. *Vet Ther* 2004;5:52.

Welsh RS, et al. Carbohydrates and physical/mental performance during intermittent exercise to fatigue. *Med Sci Sports Exerc* 2002;34;723.

Williams MH. *Nutrition for Health, Fitness, and Sport*. 7th Ed. New York: McGraw-Hill, 2009.

Wismann J, Willoughby D. Gender differences in carbohydrate metabolism and carbohydrate loading. *J Int Soc Sports Nutr* 2006;5:3:28.

Yeo WK, et al. Fat adaptation followed by carbohydrate restoration increases AMPK activity in skeletal muscle from trained humans. *J Appl Physiol* 2008; 1051:519.

Zaryski C, Smith DJ. Training principles and issues for ultra-endurance athletes. *Curr Sports Med Rep* 2005;4:165.

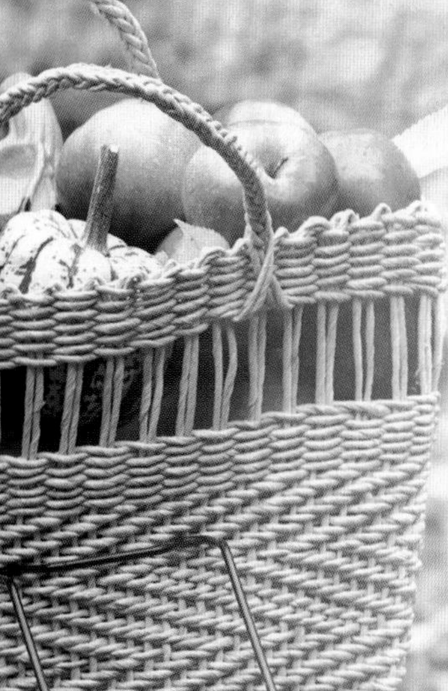

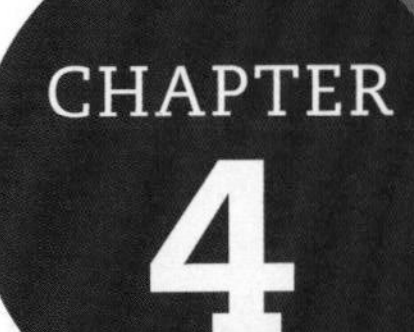

CHAPTER 4

Nutritional and Pharmacologic Aids to Performance

CHAPTER OBJECTIVES

- List four examples of substances alleged to provide ergogenic benefits.
- Summarize research concerning caffeine's potential as an ergogenic aid.
- Explain how glutamine and phosphatidylserine affect exercise performance and training response.
- Describe two positive and two negative ergogenic effects of creatine supplementation.
- Explain how postexercise carbohydrate-protein-creatine supplementation augments resistance-training responses.
- Give the rationale for medium-chain triacylglycerol supplementation as an ergogenic aid.
- Discuss the possible ergogenic benefits and risks of clenbuterol, amphetamines, chromium picolinate, β-hydroxy–β-methylbutyrate, and buffering solutions.
- Discuss the two positive and five negative effects of anabolic steroid use as an ergogenic aid.
- Discuss two positive and two negative effects of using androstenedione as an ergogenic aid.
- Describe medical uses of human growth hormone, including its potential dangers to healthy individuals.
- Describe the rationale for dehydroepiandrosterone (DHEA) as an ergogenic aid.

ANCILLARIES AT A GLANCE

Visit **http://thePoint.lww.com/MKKESS5e** to access the following resources.

- References: Chapter 4
- Interactive Question Bank
- Appendix SR-5: U. S. Olympic Committee (USOC) National Anti-Doping Policy Statement of Prohibited Substances and Methods

Ergogenic aids *include substances and procedures believed to improve exercise capacity, physiologic function, or athletic performance.* From the time of the ancient Olympic Games in 776 BC and probably before, individuals have used many exogenous compounds and concoctions to improve physical performance and augment training responsiveness. This chapter discusses the possible ergogenic role of selected commonly used nutritional and pharmacologic agents. In Chapter 15, we present popular physiologic manipulations and agents used in the sports community to enhance exercise performance.

Considerable literature surrounds different nutritional and pharmacologic ergogenic aids. Product promotional materials often include testimonials and endorsements for untested products from sports professionals and organizations, media publicity, television infomercials, and Web sites. Frequently touted articles quote potential performance benefits from steroids and steroid substitutes, amphetamines, hormones, carbohydrates, amino acids (consumed either singularly or in combination), fatty acids, caffeine, buffering compounds, wheat germ oil, vitamins, minerals, catecholamine agonists, and even marijuana and cocaine. Athletes routinely use many of these substances, believing their use enhances mental and physical functions or training effects for sports performance.

Ergogenic agents exert their influence through six mechanisms:

1. Serve as a central or peripheral nervous system stimulant (e.g., caffeine, choline, amphetamines, alcohol)
2. Increase storage or availability or both of a limiting substrate (e.g., carbohydrate, creatine, carnitine, chromium)
3. Act as a supplemental fuel source (e.g., glucose, medium-chain triacylglycerols [MCTs])

A CLOSER LOOK

A Need to Critically Evaluate Scientific Evidence

Companies expend considerable money and effort to demonstrate a beneficial effect of an "aid." Often, a placebo effect and not the actual "aid" improves performance—the individual performs at a higher level because of the suggestive power of believing that a substance or procedure works. For the exercise professional, the challenge lies in evaluating the scientific merit of articles and advertisements about products and procedures. To separate marketing "hype" from scientific fact, we pose five areas for questioning the validity of research claims concerning the efficacy of chemical, pharmacologic, and nutritional ergogenic aids; these areas include specific questions about the following:

1. Justification/scientific rationale
2. Subjects
3. Research sample and design
4. Conclusions
5. Dissemination of findings

Justification/Scientific Rationale

Does the study represent a "fishing expedition" or is there a sound rationale that the specific treatment should produce an effect? For example, a theoretical basis exists to believe that ingesting creatine elevates intramuscular creatine and phosphocreatine (PCr) to possibly improve short-term power output capacity. In contrast, no rationale exists to hypothesize that hyperhydration, breathing hyperoxic gas, or ingesting MCTs should enhance 100-m dash performance.

Subjects

- **Animals or humans**: Many mammals exhibit similar physiologic and metabolic dynamics, yet significant species differences exist, which often limit generalizations to humans. For example, the models for disease processes, nutrient requirements, hormone dynamics, and growth and development often differ markedly between humans and diverse animal groups.
- **Gender**: Gender-specific responses to the interactions among physical activity, training, and nutrient requirements and supplementation limit generalizability of findings to the gender studied.
- **Age**: Age often interacts to influence the outcome of an experimental treatment. Effective interventions for the elderly may not apply to growing children or young and middle-aged adults.
- **Training status**: Fitness status and training level influence the effectiveness (or ineffectiveness) of a particular diet or supplement intervention. Treatments that benefit the untrained (e.g., chemicals or procedures that enhance neurologic disinhibition) often exert little effect on elite athletes who practice and compete routinely at maximal arousal levels.
- **Baseline nutrition level**: The research should establish the subjects' nutritional status prior to any experimental treatment. Clearly, a nutrient supplement administered to a malnourished group typically improves physical performance and training responsiveness because overall nutrition improves. Nevertheless, such nutritional interventions fail to demonstrate whether the same effects occur if subjects received the supplement with their baseline nutrient intake at recommended levels.

  It should occasion little surprise, for example, that supplemental iron enhances aerobic fitness in a group with iron deficiency anemia. Yet one must not infer that iron supplements provide such benefits to all individuals.
- **Health status**: Nutritional, hormonal, and pharmacologic interventions profoundly impact the diseased and infirm yet offer no benefit to those in "good" health. Research findings from diseased subgroups should not be generalized to healthy populations.

Research Sample and Design

- **Random assignment or self-selection**: The research findings apply only to groups similar to the sample studied. If subject volunteers "self-select" into an experimental group, does the experimental treatment produce the results, or did a change occur from the individual's motivation to take part in the study? For example, desire to enter a weight loss study may elicit behaviors that produce weight loss independent of the experimental treatment *per se*. It is challenging to assign truly random samples of subjects into experimental and control groups. When subjects volunteer to take part in an experiment, they must be randomly assigned to control or experimental conditions, a process termed **randomization**. Under ideal conditions, experiences should be similar for both experimental and control groups, except for the treatment variable.
- **Double-blind, placebo-controlled**: The ideal experiment to evaluate performance-enhancing effects of an exogenous supplement requires that experimental and control subjects remain unaware of or "blinded" to the administered substance. To achieve this goal, subjects receive a similar quantity and/or form of the proposed aid, while control group subjects receive an inert compound or placebo. The placebo treatment evaluates the possibility of subjects performing well or responding better simply because they receive a substance they believe should benefit them (psychological or placebo effect). To further reduce experimental bias from influencing the outcome, those administering the treatment and recording the response must not know which subjects receive the treatment or placebo. In such a **double-blinded experiment**, both investigator and subject remain unaware of the treatment condition. The figure illustrates the design of a double-blind, placebo-controlled study with an accompanying crossover where treatment and placebo conditions reverse.
- **Control of extraneous factors**: Under ideal conditions, experiences should be similar for both experimental and control groups, except for the treatment variable. Random assignment of subjects to control or experimental groups goes a long way to equalize control factors that could influence the study's outcome.
- **Appropriateness of measurements**: Reproducible, objective, and valid measurement tools must evaluate research outcomes. For example, a step test to predict aerobic capacity, or infrared interactance to evaluate body composition components, represents an imprecise tool to answer meaningful questions about the efficacy of a proposed ergogenic aid.

Conclusions

- **Findings should dictate conclusions**: The conclusions of a research study must logically follow from the research findings. Frequently, investigators who study ergogenic aids extrapolate conclusions beyond the scope of their data. The implications and generalizations of research findings must remain within the context of the measurements made, subjects studied, and response magnitude. For example, increases in anabolic hormone levels in response to a dietary supplement reflect just that; they do not necessarily indicate an augmented training responsiveness or improved level of muscular structure or function. Similarly, brief anaerobic power output capacity improvement with creatine supplementation does not justify the conclusion that exogenous creatine improves overall "physical fitness."
- **Appropriate statistical analysis**: Appropriate inferential statistical analysis must quantify the potential that chance caused the research outcome. Other statistics must objectify averages, variability, and degree of association among variables.
- **Statistical versus practical significance**: The finding of statistical significance of a particular experimental treatment only means a high probability exists that the result did *not* occur by chance. One must also evaluate the magnitude of an effect for its real impact on physiology and/or performance. A reduced heart rate of 3 beats a minute during submaximal effort may reach statistical significance, yet have little practical effect on aerobic fitness or cardiovascular function.

Dissemination of Findings

- **Published in peer-reviewed journal**: High-quality research withstands the rigors of critical review and evaluation by colleagues with expertise in the specific area of investigation. **Peer review** provides a measure of quality control over scholarship and interpretation of research findings. Papers or results published in popular magazines or quasi-professional journals do not undergo the same evaluation rigor as those published after peer review. In fact, self-appointed "experts" in sports nutrition and physical fitness pay eager publishers for magazine space to promote their particular viewpoint. In some cases, the expert owns the magazine!
- **Findings reproduced by other investigators**: Findings from one study do not necessarily establish scientific fact. Conclusions become stronger and more generalizable when support emerges from the laboratories of other independent investigators. Consensus reduces the influence of chance, flaws in experimental design, and investigator bias.

(*Continues on next page*)

A CLOSER LOOK (Continued)

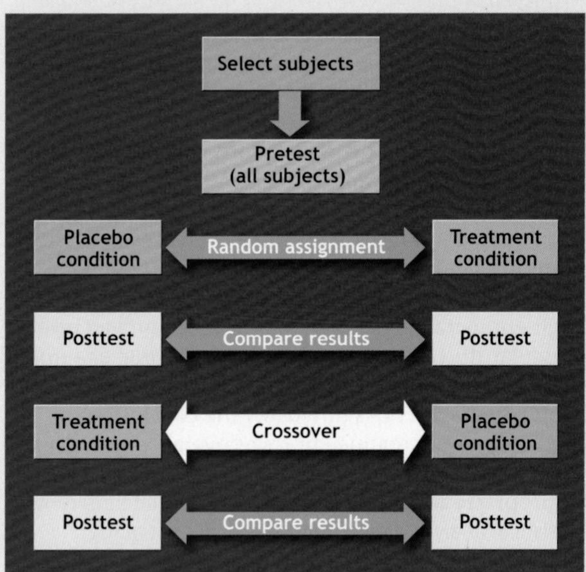

Example of a randomized, double-blind, placebo-controlled, crossover study. Following appropriate subject selection, participants are pretested and then randomly assigned to either the experimental (treatment) or control (placebo) group. Following treatment, a posttest is administered. Participants then cross over into the opposite group for the same time period as in the first condition. A second posttest follows. Comparisons of the posttests determine the extent of a "treatment effect." (Used with permission from McArdle WD, Katch FI, Katch VL. *Exercise Physiology: Nutrition, Energy, and Human Performance*. 8th Ed. Baltimore: Wolters Kluwer Health, 2015.)

4. Reduce or neutralize performance-inhibiting metabolic by-products (e.g., sodium bicarbonate, citrate, pangamic acid, phosphate)
5. Facilitate recovery from strenuous exercise (e.g., high-glycemic carbohydrates)
6. Enhance resistance-training responsiveness (e.g., anabolic steroids, human growth hormone (hGH), or carbohydrate/protein supplements consumed immediately postexercise)

Indiscriminate use of ergogenic substances often increases the likelihood of adverse side effects, which range from benign physical discomfort to life-threatening medical emergencies. Many compounds also fail to conform to labeling requirements and incorrectly identify the product's ingredients and contaminants. For example, supplements available through online sources or in retail establishments often contain steroids and steroidlike substances and stimulants prohibited in sport competition.

For the past 65 years, the use of ergogenic aids, including illegal drugs, to improve competitive achievement in all sports has not abated, nor has the prohibited use of **performance-enhancing drugs (PEDs)**. Neither cycling competitions, track and field, car racing, boxing, mixed martial arts, cricket, weightlifting and bodybuilding, National Basketball Association (NBA), Major League Baseball (MLB), National Football League (NFL), nor Major League Soccer is immune to such practices (**www.ncbi.nlm.nih.gov/pmc/articles/PMC1859606/**).

A Fall From Grace

On June 12, 2012, the U.S. Anti-Doping Agency (USADA), a quasi-governmental agency that polices antidoping in sports in the United States, brought formal doping charges against elite cyclist Lance Armstrong. The accusations alleged that the USADA collected blood samples from Armstrong in 2009 and 2010 that were "fully consistent with blood manipulation including **erythropoietin (EPO)** use and/or blood transfusions." The charges also alleged that "multiple riders with first-hand knowledge" would testify that Armstrong used the blood booster EPO, blood transfusions, testosterone, and masking agents, and that he distributed and administered drugs to other cyclists from 1998 to 2005. In addition to the specific accusations against Armstrong, the charges maintained that his cycling teams engaged in a "doping conspiracy" that involved "team officials, employees, doctors, and elite cyclists of the U.S. Postal Service and Discovery Channel cycling teams."

In June 2012, the USADA formally charged Armstrong with having used PEDs, and in August, they announced disqualification from all his race results since August 1998 (including his seven Tour de France titles) and a lifetime ban from competition. In the words of the USADA's chief executive: "It's a heartbreaking example of win at all costs overtaking the fair and safe option. There is no success in cheating to win." On October 22, 2012, the Union Cycliste Internationale (**www.uci.ch**), the cycling sports governing body, endorsed the USADA's verdict and confirmed both the lifetime ban and the stripping of Armstrong's titles. Armstrong is but one of many examples where tremendously successful athletes have fallen from grace for attempting to "game" the system and have been caught and punished. The most recent admonishment concerning the culture of the Armstrong cheating scandal and total failure of transparency to disclose the extent of the cover-up came from an independent report from the Cycling Independent Reform Commission to the president of the Union Cycliste Internationale (March 8, 2015; **www.uci.ch/mm/Document/News/CleanSport/16/87/99/CIRCReport2015_Neutral.pdf**). One salient conclusion pinpoints the current state of affairs with regard to doping practices:

> In contrast to the findings in previous investigations, which identified systematic doping organised by teams, at the elite level riders who dope now organise their own doping programmes with the help of third parties who are primarily outside the cycling team. At the elite level, doping programmes are generally sophisticated and therefore doctors play a key role in devising programmes that provide performance enhancement whilst minimising the risk of getting caught.

PART 1 Nutritional Ergogenic Aids

BUFFERING SOLUTIONS

Dramatic alterations take place in the chemical balance of intracellular and extracellular fluids during all-out physical activity for durations of 30 to 120 seconds. In activity of these durations, muscle fibers rely predominantly on anaerobic energy transfer, which increases lactate formation with decreased intracellular pH. Increases in acidity inhibit energy transfer and contractile qualities of active muscle fibers. In the blood, increased H^+ and lactate concentrations produce acidosis.

The bicarbonate aspect of the body's **buffering system** defends against increased intracellular H^+ concentration (see Chapter 9). Maintaining high extracellular bicarbonate levels causes rapid H^+ efflux from cells and reduces intracellular acidosis. This process has fueled speculation that increasing the body's bicarbonate or alkaline reserve might enhance subsequent anaerobic performance by delaying decreases in intracellular pH. Research has produced conflicting results based on variations in pre-activity dosages of sodium bicarbonate and type of physical activity to evaluate ergogenic effects.

One study evaluated acute induced metabolic alkalosis effects on short-term fatiguing physical activity that generated considerable lactate accumulation. Six trained middle-distance runners consumed a 300 mg per kg body mass sodium bicarbonate solution or similar amount of calcium carbonate placebo before running an 800-m race or control run without the exogenous substance. Ingesting the alkaline drink increased pH and standard bicarbonate levels before physical activity (**Table 4.1**). Study subjects ran an average 2.9 seconds faster under alkalosis and achieved higher postexercise blood lactate, pH, and extracellular H^+ concentrations compared with placebo or control subjects. Similar ergogenic effects of induced alkalosis also occur on short-term anaerobic performance with sodium citrate.

The ergogenic effect of preexercise alkalosis (not banned by the **World Anti-Doping Agency [WADA]**; **www.wada-ama.org/**) also occurred for physically active women who performed maximal cycling for 60 seconds on separate days under three conditions in a double-blind research design (**Fig. 4.1**): (1) control, no treatment; (2) 300 mg per kg body mass sodium bicarbonate dose in 400 mL of low-calorie flavored water 90 minutes before testing; and (3) placebo of equimolar sodium chloride dose to maintain intravascular fluid status similar to bicarbonate condition administered as the bicarbonate treatment. Cycling capacity represented total work accomplished in the 60-second ride. The inset box in **Figure 4.1** shows that total work (kJ) and peak power output (W) reached higher levels with treatment than under control or placebo conditions. The bicarbonate treatment produced a significantly higher blood lactate level in the immediate and 1-minute postexercise period; the effect explains the greater work capacity attained in the short-term, anaerobic activity trial.

The ergogenic effect of preexercise alkalosis with sodium bicarbonate or sodium citrate before intense, short-term physical activity probably occurs from increased anaerobic energy transfer during physical activity. Increases in extracellular buffering provided by exogenous buffers may facilitate coupled transport of lactate and H^+ across muscle cell membranes into extracellular fluid during fatiguing activity. This would delay decreases in intracellular pH and its subsequent negative effects on muscle function. A 2.9-second faster 800-m race time represents a dramatic and meaningful improvement; it transposes to about 19 m at race pace, bringing a last place finisher to first place in most 800-m races.

TABLE 4.1 Performance Time and Acid-base Profiles for Subjects Under Control, Placebo, and Induced Pre-exercise Alkalosis Conditions Before and Following an 800-m Race

Variable	Condition	Pretreatment	Pre-exercise	Postexercise
pH	Control	7.40	7.39	7.07
	Placebo	7.39	7.40	7.09
	Alkalosis	7.40	7.49[a]	7.18[b]
Lactate ($mmol \cdot L^{-1}$)	Control	1.21	1.15	12.62
	Placebo	1.38	1.23	13.62
	Alkalosis	1.29	1.31	14.29[a]
Standard HCO_3^{-1} ($mEq \cdot L^{-1}$)	Control	25.8	24.5	9.90
	Placebo	25.6	26.2	11.0
	Alkalosis	25.2	33.5[a]	14.30[b]
Performance time (min:s)	Control 2:05.8		Placebo 2:05.1	Alkalosis 2:02.9[c]

[a]Pre-exercise values were significantly higher than pretreatment values.

[b]Alkalosis values were significantly higher than placebo and control values post exercise.

[c]Alkalosis time was significantly faster than control and placebo times.

From Wilkes D, et al. Effects of induced metabolic alkalosis on 800-m racing time. *Med Sci Sports Exerc* 1983;15:277.

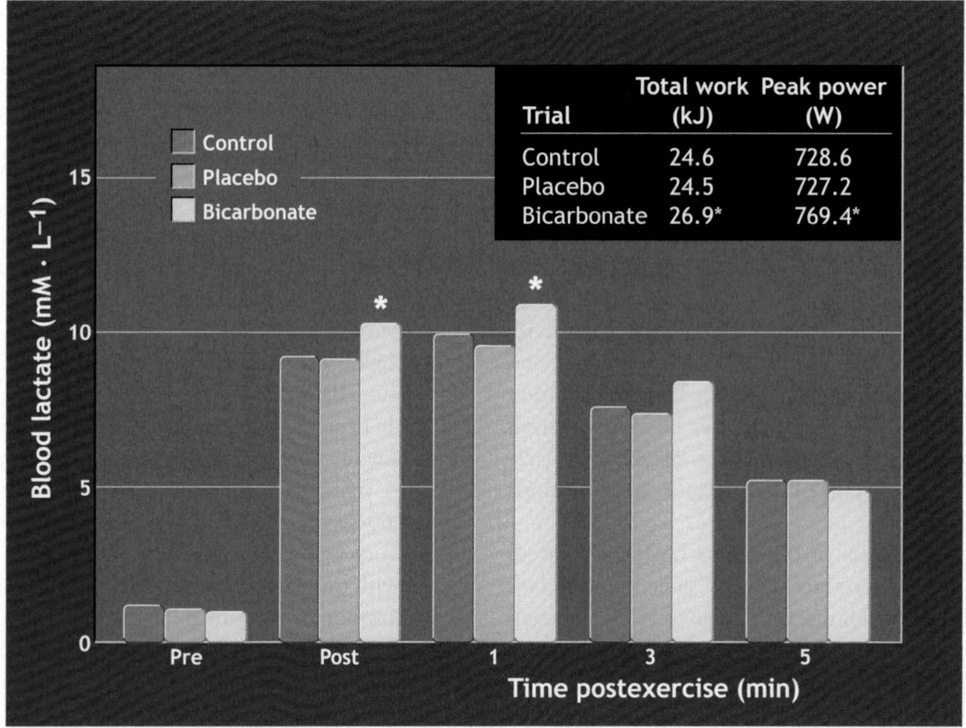

FIGURE 4.1 Effects of bicarbonate loading on total work, peak power output, and postexercise blood lactate levels in moderately trained women. *Significantly higher than either control or placebo. (Used with permission from McArdle WD, Katch FI, Katch VL. *Exercise Physiology: Nutrition, Energy, and Human Performance*. 8th Ed. Baltimore: Wolters Kluwer Health, 2015, as adapted with permission from McNaughton LR, et al. Effect of sodium bicarbonate ingestion on high intensity exercise in moderately trained women. *J Strength Cond Res* 1997;11:98.)

Effects Depend on Dosage and Exercise Anaerobiosis

The interaction between bicarbonate dosage and cumulative anaerobic nature of exercise influences potential ergogenic effects of prephysical activity bicarbonate loading. *For men and women, doses of at least 0.3 g per kg body mass ingested 1 to 2 hours before competition facilitate cellular H^+ efflux.* This enhances a single maximal effort of 1 to 2 minutes or longer-term arm or leg physical activity that produces exhaustion within 6 to 8 minutes. No ergogenic effect occurs for typical resistance training (e.g., squat, bench press, arm curls, leg press). All-out effort lasting less than 1 minute may improve only when performing repetitive physical activity.

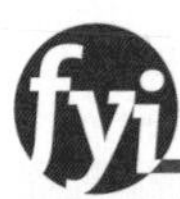

A Huge Disappointment!

World-class female marathoner Rita Jeptoo of Kenya failed an out-of-competition doping test for use of the blood-boosting hormone EPO prior to winning her second consecutive Chicago Marathon on October 12, 2014, in 2:24:35; the win was her fourth straight major marathon victory. Jeptoo won back-to-back titles at the Boston Marathon on April 21, 2014, setting the course record and establishing her personal best of 2:18:57 and made history by becoming the first woman to break the winner's tape in four consecutive races, achieving a perfect 100 points for the 2013–2014 season competition.

What is most disturbing—again—is the relentless pursuit of winning at all costs among highly respected, world-class long-distance runners with a reputation for arduous, difficult training. One only can wonder if other long-distance marathon teammates, both male and female, will become ensnared for participation and complicity in such devious and illegal practices.

Potential Negative Side Effects

Individuals who bicarbonate load often experience abdominal cramps and diarrhea about 1 hour following ingestion. This adverse effect would surely minimize any potential ergogenic effect. Substituting sodium citrate for sodium bicarbonate at a dose of 0.4 to 0.5 g per kg body mass decreases most adverse gastrointestinal effects while still preserving ergogenic benefits.

ANTICORTISOL-PRODUCING COMPOUNDS

The anterior pituitary gland secretes adrenocorticotropic hormone (ACTH), which induces adrenal cortex release of the glucocorticoid hormone **cortisol** or hydrocortisone (see Chapter 12). Cortisol decreases amino acid transport into cells to depress anabolism and stimulate protein breakdown into its amino acid building blocks in all cells except the liver. The liberated amino acids circulate to the liver for gluconeogenesis for energy. Cortisol serves as an insulin antagonist by inhibiting cellular glucose uptake and oxidation.

Prolonged, elevated cortisol serum concentration from exogenous intake ultimately produces three negative effects—excessive protein breakdown, tissue wasting, and negative nitrogen balance. The potential catabolic effect of exogenous cortisol has convinced bodybuilders and others to consume anticortisol supplements hoping they inhibit the body's normal cortisol release. Some believe that depressing cortisol's normal increase following physical activity augments muscular development with resistance training because muscle tissue synthesis progresses unimpeded in recovery. Athletes use glutamine and phosphatidylserine supplements to produce an anticortisol effect.

Glutamine

Glutamine, a nonessential amino acid, exhibits many bodily regulatory functions, one of which provides an anticatabolic effect to enhance protein synthesis. The rationale for glutamine use comes from findings that glutamine supplementation effectively counteracts protein breakdown and muscle wasting from repeated use of exogenous glucocorticoids. In one study with female rats, infusing a glutamine supplement for 7 days countered the normal depressed protein synthesis and skeletal muscle atrophy with chronic glucocorticoid administration. No research addresses the efficacy of excess glutamine altering normal hormonal milieu and training responsiveness in healthy men and women. The potential anticatabolic and glycogen synthesizing effects of exogenous glutamine have promoted speculation that supplementation might benefit resistance-training effects. Daily glutamine supplementation of 0.9 g per kg lean tissue mass in healthy young adults during resistance training for 6 weeks did not affect muscle performance, body composition, or muscle protein degradation compared with a placebo. Research with humans indicates that preexercise glutamine supplementation does not affect immune response following repeated bouts of intense activity. Any objective decision about taking glutamine supplements for ergogenic purposes should await supportive research findings.

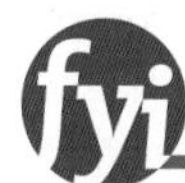

Banned Substances

The World Anti-Doping Agency (WADA; **www.wadaama.org/en/prohibitedlist.ch2**)—an independent foundation created to promote, coordinate, and monitor the war against drugs in sport worldwide—currently bans the following 11 categories of substances:

1. Anabolic-androgenic steroids
2. Hormones and related substances
3. $Beta_2$ agonists
4. Hormone antagonists and modulators
5. Diuretics and other masking agents
6. Stimulants
7. Narcotics
8. Cannabinoids
9. Glucocorticosteroids
10. Alcohol (in particular sports)
11. Beta-blockers (in particular sports)

thePoint® Appendix SR-5, "U.S. Olympic Committee (USOC) National Anti-Doping Policy Statement of Prohibited Substances and Methods" available online at **http://thePoint.lww.com/MKKESS5e**, provides the U.S. Olympic Committee (USOC) National Anti-Doping Policy Statement of Prohibited Substances and Methods. Current 2015 information appears at **www.wada-ama.org/en/Resources/Q-and-A/2013-Prohibited-List/**.

Phosphatidylserine

Phosphatidylserine (PS) represents a glycerophospholipid typical of a class of natural lipids that comprise the structural components of biological membranes, particularly the internal layer of the plasma membrane that surrounds all cells. Speculation exists that PS, through its potential for modulating functional events in cell membranes (e.g., number and affinity of membrane receptor sites), modifies the body's neuroendocrine stress response.

In one study, nine healthy men received 800 mg of PS derived from bovine cerebral cortex in oral form daily for 10 days. Three 6-minute intervals of cycle ergometer activity of increasing intensity induced physical stress. Compared with the placebo condition, the PS treatment diminished ACTH and cortisol release without affecting hGH release. These results confirmed earlier findings by the same researchers that a single intravenous PS injection counteracted hypothalamic-pituitary-adrenal axis activation with physical activity. Soybean lecithin provides the majority of PS supplementation by athletes, yet the research showing physiologic effects used *bovine-derived* PS. Subtle differences in the chemical structure of these two forms of PS may create differences in physiologic action, including the potential for negative effects when using this compound.

β-HYDROXY–β-METHYLBUTYRATE

β-Hydroxy–β-methylbutyrate (HMB), a bioactive metabolite generated in the breakdown of the essential branched-chain amino acid leucine, decreases protein loss during stress by inhibiting protein catabolism. In rats and chicks, less protein breakdown and a slight increase in protein synthesis occurred in muscle tissue *in vitro* exposed to HMB. An HMB-induced increase occurred in fatty acid oxidation in mammalian muscle. Humans synthesize between 0.3 and 1.0 g of HMB daily, depending on HMB in the food ingested, with about 5% from dietary leucine catabolism. Citrus fruit and catfish contain small amounts of HMB. To get a therapeutic dosage, individuals supplement with HMB because of its supposed potential nitrogen-retaining effects to prevent or slow muscle damage, and inhibit muscle proteolysis with intense physical effort.

Research has studied the effects of exogenous HMB on skeletal muscle response to resistance training. In part one of a two-part randomized study (**Fig. 4.2**), 41 young men received 0, 1.5, or 3.0 g of HMB daily at two protein levels, either 117 or 175 g daily for 3 weeks. During this time, the subjects resistance trained for 1.5 hours daily, 3 days a week. In the second study, 28 young men consumed either 0 or 3.0 g of HMB daily and resistance trained for 2 to 3 hours daily, 6 days a week, for 7 weeks.

In the first study, HMB supplementation depressed the activity-induced increase in muscle **proteolysis** reflected by urinary 3-methylhistidine and plasma creatine phosphokinase (CPK) levels during the first 2 training weeks. These biochemical indices of muscle damage were 20% to 60% lower in the HMB-supplemented group. In addition, the supplemented group lifted more total weight (total body strength increase) during each training week (see **Fig. 4.2A**), with the greatest effect in the group receiving the largest HMB supplement. Muscular strength increased 8% in the no-supplement group and more in the HMB-supplemented groups (13% for the 1.5-g group and 18.4% for the 3.0-g group). Added protein (not indicated in the graph) did not affect any of the measurements; one should view this lack of effect in proper context—the "lower" protein quantity (115 $g \cdot d^{-1}$) equaled twice the RDA.

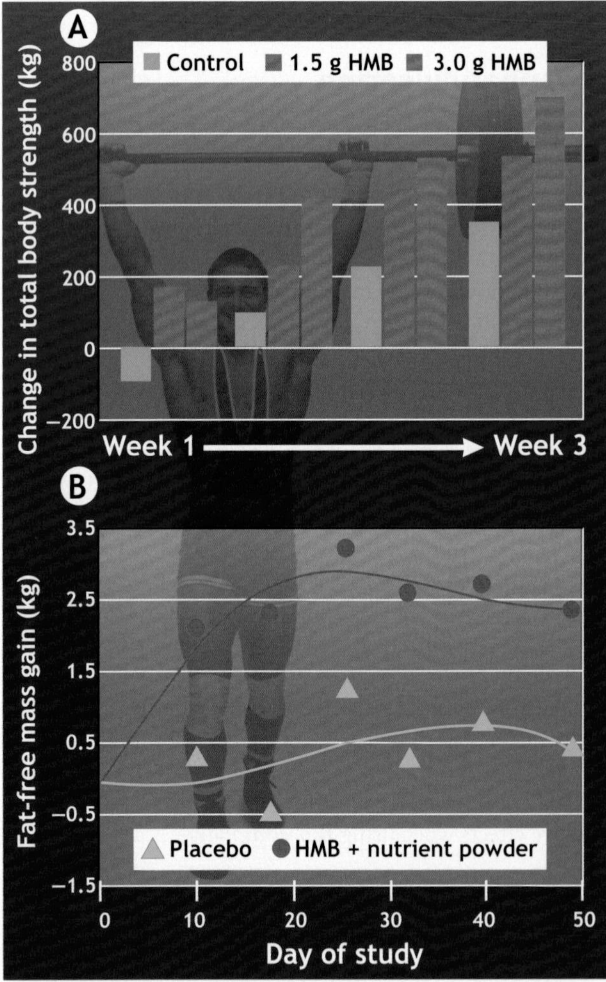

FIGURE 4.2 **A.** Change in muscle strength (total weight lifted in upper-body and lower-body exercises) during study 1 (week 1 to week 3) in subjects who supplemented with HMB. Each group of bars represents one complete set of upper- and lower-body workouts. **B.** Total body electrical conductivity-assessed change in FFM during study 2 for a control group that received a carbohydrate drink (placebo) and a group that received 3 g of Ca-HMB each day mixed in a nutrient powder (HMB + nutrient powder). (Reprinted with permission from Nissen S, et al. Effect of leucine metabolite β-hydroxy–β-methylbutyrate on muscle metabolism during resistance-exercise training. *J Appl Physiol* 1996;81:2095, as adapted with permission from McArdle WD, Katch FI, Katch VL. *Sports and Exercise Nutrition*. 4th Ed. Philadelphia: Wolters Kluwer Health, 2013.)

In the second study, individuals who received HMB supplementation had higher fat-free mass (FFM) than the unsupplemented group at 2 and 4 to 6 weeks of training (see **Fig. 4.2B**).

The mechanism for any HMB effect on muscle metabolism, strength improvement, and body composition remains unknown. Perhaps this metabolite inhibits normal proteolytic processes that accompany intense muscular overload. The results demonstrate an ergogenic effect for HMB supplementation, but it remains unclear just how HMB affects the protein, bone, or water component of FFM. The data in **Figure 4.2B** also indicate potentially transient body composition benefits of supplementation that tend to revert toward the unsupplemented state as training progresses.

Not all research shows beneficial effects of HMB supplementation with resistance training. One study in untrained young men evaluated variations in HMB supplementation of approximately 3 $g \cdot d^{-1}$ versus 6 $g \cdot d^{-1}$ on muscular strength during 8 weeks of whole-body resistance training. The salient finding revealed that HMB supplementation, regardless of dosage, produced *no difference* in most strength results including 1-repetition maximum [1-RM] strength compared with the placebo group. Additional studies must assess the long-term effects of HMB supplements on body composition, training response, and overall health and safety.

CHROMIUM

The trace mineral **chromium** serves as a cofactor to potentiate insulin function, although its precise mechanism of action remains unclear. Chronic chromium deficiency may trigger an increase in blood cholesterol and decrease the body's sensitivity to insulin, thus increasing type 2 diabetes risk. Chromium-rich foods include brewer's yeast, broccoli, wheat germ, nuts, liver, prunes, egg yolks, apples with skins, asparagus, mushrooms, wine, and cheese. Food processing removes chromium from foods in natural form, and strenuous physical activity and associated high carbohydrate intake also promote urinary chromium losses, increasing potential for deficiency.

Chromium's Alleged Benefits

Chromium, touted as a "fat burner" and "muscle builder," is second only to calcium as the largest selling mineral supplement in the United States. Supplement intake of chromium, usually as **chromium picolinate**, often is consumed at levels of 600 μg daily. The combination of chromium with picolinic acid supposedly improves chromium absorption compared with chromium chloride, its inorganic salt.

Most studies that suggest beneficial effects of chromium supplements on body fat and muscle mass incorrectly infer body composition changes from changes in body weight or anthropometric measurements instead of the more appropriate valid assessment methods discussed in Chapter 16. In one study, young men who resistance trained for 6 weeks and supplemented daily with 200 μg (3.85 mmol) of chromium picolinate for 40 days showed a small increase in FFM and decrease in body fat. No data were presented to document increases in muscular strength.

Another study reported increases in body mass without a change in strength or body composition in previously untrained female college students (no change in males) who received daily a 200-μg chromium supplement during a 12-week resistance-training program compared with unsupplemented controls. When collegiate football players received daily supplements of 200 μg of chromium picolinate for 9 weeks, no changes occurred in body composition and muscular strength from intense weightlifting training compared with a control group receiving a placebo.

A double-blind research design involving 36 young men studied the effects of a daily chromium supplement (3.3 to 3.5 mmol either as chromium chloride or chromium picolinate) or a placebo for 8 weeks during resistance training. For each group, dietary intakes of protein, magnesium, zinc, copper, and iron equaled or exceeded recommended levels during training; subjects also had adequate baseline dietary chromium intakes. Chromium supplementation increased serum chromium concentration and urinary chromium excretion equally, regardless of its ingested form. Compared with the placebo treatment, chromium supplementation did *not* affect training-related changes in muscular strength, physique, FFM, or muscle mass.

CREATINE

Meat, poultry, and fish are rich **creatine** sources, containing approximately 4 to 5 g per kg of food weight. The body synthesizes only about 1 to 2 g of this nitrogen-containing organic compound daily, primarily in the kidneys, liver, and pancreas, from the amino acids arginine, glycine, and methionine. Thus, adequate dietary creatine becomes important for obtaining the required amount. The animal kingdom contains the richest creatine-containing foods, making it difficult for vegetarians to obtain ready sources of exogenous creatine.

Creatine supplements, sold as **creatine monohydrate (CrH_2O)**, come as a powder, tablet, capsule, and stabilized liquid. Creatine can be purchased as a nutritional supplement over the counter or via mail order or on the Internet, usually without guarantee of purity. Ingesting a liquid suspension of creatine monohydrate at the relatively high daily dose of 20 to 30 g for up to 2 weeks increases intramuscular concentrations of free creatine and PCr by about 30%. These levels remain high for weeks following only a few days of supplementation. Sports governing bodies have not declared creatine an illegal substance.

Important Component of High-Energy Phosphates

The precise physiologic mechanisms underlying the potential ergogenic effectiveness of supplemental creatine remain poorly understood. The intestinal mucosa serves as a conduit to pass creatine through the digestive tract unaltered for absorption into the bloodstream. Almost all ingested creatine becomes incorporated within skeletal muscle's average concentration of 125 mM per kg dry muscle (range 90 to 160 mM) via insulin-mediated active transport. About 40% of the total exists as free creatine; the remainder combines with phosphate to form PCr. Type II, fast-twitch muscle fibers store about four to six times more PCr than ATP. PCr serves as the cells' "energy reservoir" to provide rapid phosphate-bond energy to resynthesize ATP (refer to Chapter 5), crucial in all-out effort lasting up to 10 seconds. With limited intramuscular PCr, it seems plausible that any increase in PCr availability should potentiate three ergogenic effects:

1. Improve repetitive performance in muscular strength and short-term power activities
2. Augment short bursts of muscular endurance
3. Provide greater muscular overload to enhance resistance-training effectiveness

Consuming Carbohydrate Facilitates Creatine Loading

Consuming creatine with a sugar-containing drink increases creatine uptake and skeletal muscle storage. For 5 days, subjects received either 5 g of creatine four times daily or a 5-g supplement followed 30 minutes later by 93 g of a high-glycemic simple sugar four times daily. For the creatine-only supplement group, muscle PCr increased 7.2%, free creatine 13.5%, and total creatine 20.7%. Larger increases occurred for the creatine plus sugar-supplemented group (14.7% increase in muscle PCr, 18.1% increase in free creatine, and 33.0% increase in total creatine).

Unwanted Side Effects

Anecdotes indicate a possible association between creatine supplementation and cramping in multiple muscle areas during competition or in football players during lengthy practice. This effect may occur for two reasons:

1. Altered intracellular dynamics from increased free creatine and PCr levels
2. Osmotically induced enlarged muscle cell volume (greater cellular hydration) caused by increased creatine content

Consuming creatine can precipitate gastrointestinal tract nausea, indigestion, and difficulty absorbing food. Fortunately, no serious adverse effects requiring medical intervention have been reported from up to 4 years of creatine supplementation.

Desirable Improvements in Performance

Figure 4.3 illustrates positive ergogenic effects of creatine loading on total work accomplished during repetitive sprint cycling performance. Active but untrained men performed sets of maximal 6-second bicycle sprints interspersed with recovery periods of 24, 54, or 84 seconds between sprints to simulate sports conditions. Performance evaluations took place under creatine-loaded (20 g per day for 5 d) or placebo conditions. Supplementation increased muscle creatine levels 49% and PCr levels 13% compared with placebo. Increased intramuscular creatine produced a 6% increase in total work accomplished (251.7 kJ before supplement vs. 266.9 kJ after creatine loaded) compared with the group that consumed the placebo (254.0 kJ before test vs. 252.3 kJ following placebo). Creatine supplements have benefited an on-court "ghosting" routine that involves simulated positional play of competitive squash players. Creatine supplementation also augmented repeated sprint cycle performance following 30 minutes of constant load, submaximal exercise in the heat without disrupting thermoregulatory dynamics. Creatine's benefits to muscular performance also occur in physically active older men.

Figure 4.4 outlines mechanisms of how elevating intramuscular free creatine and PCr with creatine supplementation might enhance exercise performance and training responsiveness. Besides benefiting weightlifting and bodybuilding, improved immediate anaerobic power output capacity benefits sprint running, cycling, swimming, jumping, and all-out, repetitive rapid movements in football and volleyball. Increased intramuscular PCr concentrations also should allow individuals to increase training intensity in strength and power activities.

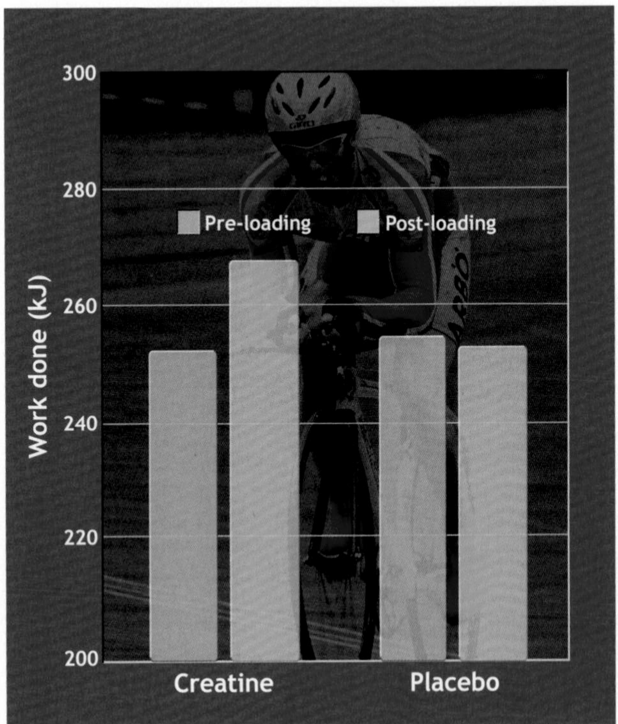

FIGURE 4.3 Effects of creatine loading versus placebo on total work accomplished during long-term (80 min) repetitive sprint cycling performance. (Used with permission from McArdle WD, Katch FI, Katch VL. *Exercise Physiology: Nutrition, Energy, and Human Performance*. 8th Ed. Baltimore: Wolters Kluwer Health, 2015, as adapted with permission from Preen CD, et al. Effect of creatine loading on long-term sprint exercise performance and metabolism. *Med Sci Sports Exerc* 2001;33:814.)

Oral supplements of creatine monohydrate (20 to 25 $g \cdot d^{-1}$) increase muscle creatine and performance in high-intensity exercise, particularly repeated intense muscular effort. The ergogenic effect does not vary between vegetarians and meat eaters. Even daily low 6-g doses for 5 days improve repeated power performance. For Division I football players, creatine supplementation during resistance training increased body mass, lean body mass, cellular hydration, and muscular strength and performance. Similarly, supplementation augmented muscular strength and size during resistance training for 12 weeks.

Taking a high dose of creatine helps to replenish muscle creatine levels following intense exercise. Such metabolic "reloading" facilitates recovery of muscle contractile capacity. This enables athletes to sustain repeated intense exercise efforts. Short-term supplementation in healthy men taking 20 g daily for 5 consecutive days did not detrimentally impact blood pressure, plasma creatine, plasma creatine kinase (CK) activity, or renal responses assessed by glomerular filtration rate or rates of total protein and albumin excretion. For healthy subjects, no differences emerged in plasma content and urine excretion rate for creatinine, urea, and albumin between control subjects and those consuming creatine for between 10 months and 5 years.

Creatine supplementation does *not* significantly improve exercise performance that requires high levels of aerobic energy transfer or cardiovascular and metabolic responses. It also exerts little effect on isometric muscular strength or dynamic muscle force during a single lifting movement.

Effects on Body Mass and Body Composition

Increases in body mass of between 0.5 and 2.4 kg often accompany creatine supplementation independent of short-term changes in testosterone or cortisol concentrations. Research needs to quantify how much of the weight gain occurs from anabolic effects of creatine on muscle tissue synthesis and/or osmotic retention of intracellular water from increased creatine stores.

Creatine Loading

A "loading" phase calls for ingesting 20 to 30 g of creatine daily for 5 to 7 days as a tablet or powder added to liquid. A maintenance phase occurs after the loading phase, during which the person supplements with as little as 2 to 5 g of creatine daily. Individuals who consume vegetarian-type diets have the greatest increase in muscle creatine because of their low creatine content diets. Large increases also characterize "responders," individuals with normally low basal levels of intramuscular creatine who show the greatest response to supplementation.

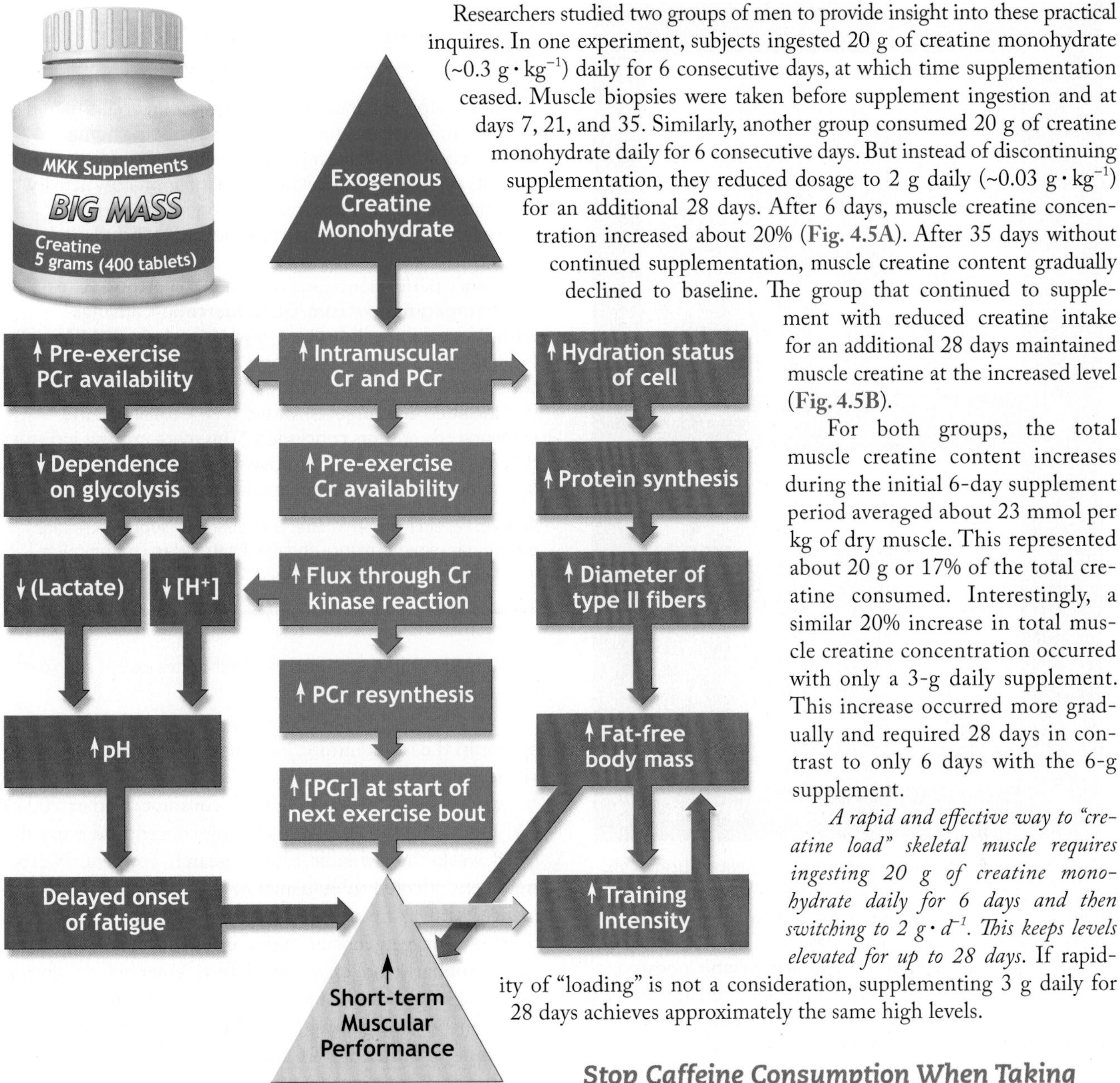

FIGURE 4.4 Mechanisms to explain why increased intracellular creatine (Cr) and phosphocreatine (PCr) might enhance intense, short-term exercise performance and the exercise-training response. (Used with permission from McArdle WD, Katch FI, Katch VL. *Exercise Physiology: Nutrition, Energy, and Human Performance*. 8th Ed. Baltimore: Wolters Kluwer Health, 2015, as adapted with permission from Volek JS, Kraemer WJ. Creatine supplementation: its effect on human muscular performance and body composition. *J Strength Cond Res* 1996;10:200.)

Three practical questions for those desiring to elevate intramuscular creatine with supplementation concern the following:

1. Magnitude and time course of intramuscular creatine increase
2. Dosage required to maintain a creatine increase
3. Rate of creatine loss or "washout" following cessation of supplementation

Researchers studied two groups of men to provide insight into these practical inquires. In one experiment, subjects ingested 20 g of creatine monohydrate (~0.3 $g \cdot kg^{-1}$) daily for 6 consecutive days, at which time supplementation ceased. Muscle biopsies were taken before supplement ingestion and at days 7, 21, and 35. Similarly, another group consumed 20 g of creatine monohydrate daily for 6 consecutive days. But instead of discontinuing supplementation, they reduced dosage to 2 g daily (~0.03 $g \cdot kg^{-1}$) for an additional 28 days. After 6 days, muscle creatine concentration increased about 20% (**Fig. 4.5A**). After 35 days without continued supplementation, muscle creatine content gradually declined to baseline. The group that continued to supplement with reduced creatine intake for an additional 28 days maintained muscle creatine at the increased level (**Fig. 4.5B**).

For both groups, the total muscle creatine content increases during the initial 6-day supplement period averaged about 23 mmol per kg of dry muscle. This represented about 20 g or 17% of the total creatine consumed. Interestingly, a similar 20% increase in total muscle creatine concentration occurred with only a 3-g daily supplement. This increase occurred more gradually and required 28 days in contrast to only 6 days with the 6-g supplement.

A rapid and effective way to "creatine load" skeletal muscle requires ingesting 20 g of creatine monohydrate daily for 6 days and then switching to 2 $g \cdot d^{-1}$. This keeps levels elevated for up to 28 days. If rapidity of "loading" is not a consideration, supplementing 3 g daily for 28 days achieves approximately the same high levels.

Stop Caffeine Consumption When Taking Creatine

Caffeine negates the ergogenic effect of creatine supplementation. To evaluate the effect of pre-exercise caffeine consumption on intramuscular creatine stores and intense exercise performance, subjects consumed either a placebo, a daily creatine supplement (0.5 g per kg body mass), or the same daily creatine supplement plus caffeine of 5 mg per kg body mass for 6 days. Under each condition, subjects performed maximal isokinetic dynamometer intermittent knee extension movements to fatigue. Creatine supplementation with or without caffeine increased intramuscular PCr (evaluated by nuclear magnetic resonance spectroscopy) between 4% and 6%. Dynamic torque production also increased 10% to 23% with creatine compared with placebo.

Consuming caffeine totally negated creatine's ergogenic effect. To optimize benefits, athletes should abstain from caffeine-containing foods and beverages for 2 to 3 days prior to and during creatine loading, training, and competition.

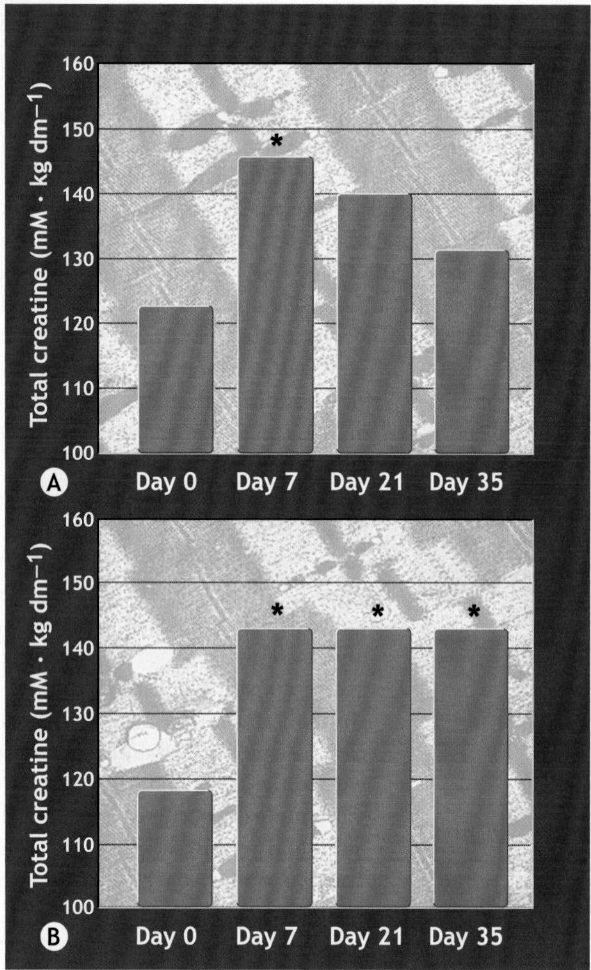

FIGURE 4.5 **A.** Total muscle creatine concentration in six men who consumed 20 g of creatine for 6 consecutive days and then stopped the supplement. Muscle biopsies done before ingestion (day 0) and on days 7, 21, and 35. **B.** Total muscle creatine concentration in nine men who ingested 20 g of creatine for 6 consecutive days and then ingested 2 g of creatine daily for the next 28 days. Muscle biopsies taken before ingestion (day 0) and on days 7, 21, and 35. Values refer to averages per dry mass (dm). *Significantly different from day 0. (Used with permission from McArdle WD, Katch FI, Katch VL. *Exercise Physiology: Nutrition, Energy, and Human Performance*. 8th Ed. Baltimore: Wolters Kluwer Health, 2015, as adapted with permission from Hultman E, et al. Muscle creatine loading in men. *J Appl Physiol* 1996;81:232.)

GINSENG AND EPHEDRINE

The popularity of herbal and botanical remedies has soared as possible ways to improve health, control body weight, and improve exercise performance. Ginseng and ephedrine are marketed as nutritional supplements to "reduce stress," "revitalize," and "optimize mental and physical performance," particularly during times of fatigue and stress.

Ginseng

Used in Asian medicine to prolong life, strengthen and restore sexual function, and invigorate the body, the ginseng root often sold as Panax or Chinese or Korean ginseng, serves no recognized medical use in the United States except as a soothing agent in skin ointments.

Reports of ginseng's ergogenic possibilities often appear in the lay literature, but a review of the research provides little evidence to support its effectiveness for these purposes. For example, volunteers consumed either 200 or 400 mg of the standardized ginseng concentrate every day for 8 weeks in a double-blind research protocol. Neither treatment affected submaximal or maximal exercise performance, ratings of perceived exertion (RPE; see Chapter 13), heart rate, oxygen consumption, or blood lactate concentrations. Similarly, no ergogenic effects emerged on diverse physiologic and performance variables following a 1-week treatment with a ginseng saponin extract administered in two doses of either 8 or 16 mg per kg of body mass. When effectiveness has been demonstrated, the research failed to use adequate controls, placebos, or double-blind testing protocols. *At present, no compelling scientific evidence exists that ginseng supplementation offers any ergogenic benefit for physiologic function or exercise performance.*

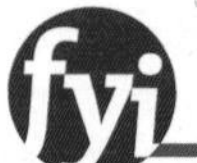

Quercetin Fails the Test

The popular polyphenolic flavinoid quercetin occurs naturally in many fruits, vegetables, and beverages. Some human and animal studies have reported health and performance benefits from its antioxidant and anti-inflammatory activity, including increased mitochondrial biogenesis. Aside from alleged health benefits, marketers have included quercetin in products marketed for ergogenic benefits on endurance performance and maximal oxygen uptake (e.g., **www.stopagingnow.com/QCT/Quercetin-Capsules-with-Bromelain?gclid=Clio7_6ljrUCFcpdpQod9GEAyg**). To evaluate these claims, researchers performed a **meta-analysis** of available research on this topic (seven published studies that included 288 subjects). Based on the totality of the evidence, the authors concluded: "This meta-analysis indicates that quercetin is unlikely to prove ergogenic for aerobic-oriented exercises in trained and untrained individuals."

Source: Pelletier DM, et al. Effects of quercetin supplementation on endurance performance and maximal oxygen consumption: a meta-analysis. *Int J Sport Nutr Exerc Metab* 2013;23:73.

Ephedrine

Unlike ginseng, Western medicine has recognized the potent amphetaminelike compound **ephedrine** with sympathomimetic physiologic effects in several species of the ephedra plant (dried plant stem called ma huang [ma wong, Ephedra sinica]). The medicinal role of this herb has included treating asthma, symptoms of the common cold, hypotension, and urinary incontinence and as a central stimulant to treat depression. Physicians in the United States discontinued ephedrine's use as a decongestant and asthma treatment in the 1930s in favor of safer medications.

Ephedrine exerts both central and peripheral effects, with the latter reflected in increased heart rate, cardiac output, and blood pressure. Ephedrine causes lung bronchodilation because of its β-adrenergic effect. High ephedrine dosages can precipitate hypertension, insomnia, hyperthermia, and cardiac arrhythmias. Other possible side effects include dizziness, restlessness, anxiety, irritability, personality changes, gastrointestinal symptoms, and difficulty concentrating.

The potent physiologic effects of ephedrine have led researchers to investigate its ergogenic potential. No effect of a 40-mg dose of ephedrine occurred on indirect indicators of exercise performance or RPE. The less concentrated pseudoephedrine also produced no effect on $\dot{V}O_{2max}$, RPE, aerobic cycling efficiency, anaerobic power output on the Wingate test, time to exhaustion on a bicycle and 40-km cycling trial, or physiologic and performance measures during 20 minutes of running at 70% of $\dot{V}O_{2max}$ followed by a 5000-m time trial.

FDA Bans Ephedrine

On December 31, 2003, the US federal government announced a ban on the sale of ephedra, the latest chapter in a long story that gained national prominence after the deaths of two football players (a professional NFL all-pro player and a university athlete) were linked to ephedra use in 2001. A little more than 1 month after the death of its player, the NFL became the first sports governing body to ban ephedra. In 2003, the FDA included strong enforcement actions against firms making unsubstantiated claims for their ephedra-containing products. In early 2004, the ban on ephedrine took effect (**www.fda.gov/ola/2003/dietarysupplements1028.html** and **www.cfsan.fda.gov/~dms/ds-ephed.html**). In 2007, the U.S. Supreme Court rejected a lower court's challenge to the FDA's ban of ephedra, which should once and for all curtail sale of the product.

AMINO ACID SUPPLEMENTS AND OTHER DIETARY MODIFICATIONS FOR AN ANABOLIC EFFECT

Many athletes and the lay public regularly consume amino acid supplements, believing they boost testosterone, GH, insulin, and insulinlike growth factor 1 (IGF-1) to improve muscle size and strength and decrease body fat. The rationale for trying such nutritional ergogenic stimulants comes from the clinical use of amino acid infusion or ingestion to regulate anabolic hormones in deficient patients.

Research on healthy subjects does not provide compelling evidence for an ergogenic effect of the generalized use of amino acid supplements on hormone secretion, responsiveness to workouts, or exercise performance. In studies with appropriate design and statistical analysis, supplements of arginine, lysine, ornithine, tyrosine, and other amino acids, either singularly or in combination, produced *no* effect on GH levels or insulin secretion or on diverse measures of anaerobic power and all-out running performance at $\dot{V}O_{2max}$. Elite junior weightlifters who supplemented with all 20 amino acids did not improve physical performance or their resting or exercise-induced responses to testosterone, cortisol, or GH. The indiscriminate use of amino acid supplements at dosages considered pharmacologic rather than nutritional increases risk of direct toxic effects or creation of an amino acid imbalance.

Prudent Means to Possibly Augment an Anabolic Effect

With resistance training, muscle hypertrophy occurs from a shift in the body's normal dynamic state of protein synthesis and degradation to greater tissue synthesis. The normal hormonal milieu for insulin and GH levels in the period following resistance exercise stimulates the muscle fiber's anabolic processes while inhibiting muscle protein degradation. Dietary modifications that increase amino acid transport into muscles, raise energy availability, or increase anabolic hormone levels would theoretically augment a training effect by increasing the rate of anabolism, depressing catabolism, or both. Either effect should create a positive body protein balance to improve muscular growth and strength.

Specific Supplement Timing: A Key to Success

Studies of hormonal dynamics and protein anabolism indicate a transient but potential fourfold increase in protein synthesis with carbohydrate or protein supplements (or both) consumed *immediately following* resistance exercise workouts. This effect of supplementation in the immediate postexercise period also may prove effective for tissue repair and synthesis of muscle proteins following aerobic physical activity.

Drug-free male weightlifters with at least 2 years of resistance-training experience consumed carbohydrate and protein supplements immediately after they completed a standard resistance-training workout. Treatment included one of the following:

1. Pure water placebo
2. Carbohydrate supplement of (1.5 g per kg body mass)
3. Protein supplement (1.38 g per kg body mass)
4. Carbohydrate and protein supplement (1.06-g carbohydrate plus 0.41-g protein per kg body mass) consumed immediately following and then 2 hours after the training session

Compared with the placebo, each nutritive supplement produced a hormonal environment (elevated plasma concentrations of insulin and GH) in recovery conducive to protein synthesis and muscle tissue growth. Such data provide indirect evidence for a possible training benefit of increasing carbohydrate or protein intake (or both) immediately following resistance-training workouts.

A study compared the effects of the strategic consumption of glucose, protein, and creatine before, after, or before and after each resistance-training workout compared with supplementation in the hours not close to the workout (i.e., supplement timing) on muscle fiber hypertrophy, muscular strength, and body composition.

Dietary Supplements: Not What Might Be Expected

In February, 2015, the New York State attorney general's office exposed apparent widespread fraud in the dietary supplement industry. Four major retailers (GNC, Target, Walgreens, and Walmart) were accused of selling contaminated herbal products that either failed to contain the major compounds listed on the label or had them only at trivial levels. Many of those products contained significant quantities of fillers of limited nutritional value.

Unfortunately, the 1994 federal law that applies to supplements—the Dietary Supplement Health and Education Act or DSHEA (**http://ods.od.nih.gov/About/DSHEA_Wording.asp**)—does a better job of protecting the companies that produce the products than protecting the consumers that purchase these products. DSHEA, spearheaded by elected officials with strong financial allegiances to the supplement manufacturing industry, allows companies to attach health claims to their products without providing evidence as to their quality or effectiveness. In essence, the supplement industry is on the "honor system" for self-regulation. Part III - CFR - Code of Federal Regulations Title 21 requires dietary supplement manufacturing facilities to follow strict Good Manufacturing Practices (GMPs). If the FDA identifies violations to FDA GMPs, the FDA has the authority to issue warning letters, seize products, and shut down facilities.

Consumers' Bottom Line: Apply one simple rule before purchasing a supplement—look on the label for one of two seals of approval—either the United States Pharmacopeia (USP) seal shown here, or the NSF seal (shown on their Web site at **www.nsf.org/about-nsf/nsf-mark/**). If one of the seals is not visible on the product label, do *not* buy it!

The following describes the roles of United States Pharmacopeia and of NSF International:

1. United States Pharmacopeia (**www.usp.org**) is an independent, nonprofit organization of scientists that establishes high standards for medicine, food ingredients, and dietary supplements. Supplement companies can volunteer to have their products and facilities tested and reviewed by the USP. Hundreds of products carry the seal.
2. NSF International (**www.nsf.org/services/by-industry/dietary-supplements/**), another nonprofit group, independently tests and certifies products against the only accredited American National Standard for dietary supplements (NSF/ANSI Standard 173) to verify that the ingredients listed on the label are present in the supplement, and there are no harmful levels to humans of specific contaminants. The NSF Certified for Sport program (**www.nsfsport.com/listings/certified_products_results.asp**) screens products for more than 200 banned substances (e.g., steroids, amphetamines, GH).

ConsumerLab (**www.consumerlab.com**) and Labdoor (**https://labdoor.com**) are independent laboratories that test dietary supplements and, for a fee, provide full reports on a variety of protein powders, fish oil, probiotics, vitamin D, and multivitamins.

Resistance-trained men matched for strength were placed in one of two groups: one group consumed a supplement (1 g per kg body weight) of glucose, protein, and creatine immediately before and after resistance training; the other group received the same supplement dose on the workout day in the morning and late evening. Measurements of body composition by dual energy x-ray absorptiometry (DXA; see Chapter 16), strength (1-RM), muscle fiber type, cross-sectional area, contractile protein, creatine, and glycogen content from vastus lateralis muscle biopsies occurred the week prior to and immediately following a 10-week training program. Supplementation in the immediate pre-exercise—postexercise period produced a greater increase in lean body mass and 1-RM strength in two of three measures (**Fig. 4.6**). Greater increases in muscle cross-sectional area of type II muscle fibers and their contractile protein content accompanied body composition changes. These findings demonstrate that supplement timing provides a simple but effective strategy to enhance desirable adaptations from resistance training.

Postexercise Glucose Augments Protein Balance Following Resistance-Training Workouts

Healthy men familiar with resistance training performed eight sets of 10 repetitions of knee extensor exercise at 85% of maximum strength. Immediately following the exercise session and 1 hour later, they received either a glucose supplement of 1.0 g per kg body mass or a placebo of Nutra Sweet. **Figure 4.7A and B** shows that glucose supplementation reduced myofibrillar protein breakdown as reflected by decreased excretion of 3-methylhistidine and urinary nitrogen. Although not statistically significant, glucose supplementation slightly increased the rate of leucine's incorporation into the vastus lateralis over the 10-hour postexercise period (not statistically significant), indicating a more positive postexercise body protein balance. Increased insulin release with glucose intake, which should enhance muscle protein balance in recovery, most likely produced the beneficial effects of postexercise high-glycemic glucose supplementation.

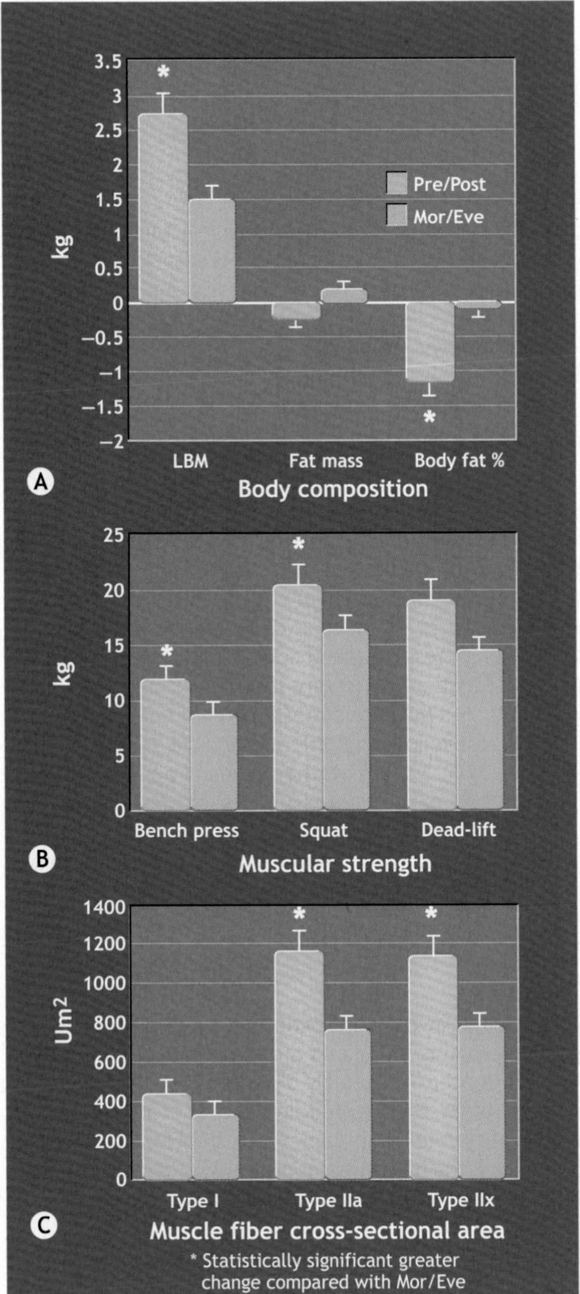

FIGURE 4.6 Effects of consuming a supplement at 1 g per kg of body weight of protein, creatine, and glucose immediately before and following (pre/post) resistance training or in the early morning (Mor) or late evening (Eve) of the training day on changes in body composition **(A)**, 1-RM strength **(B)**, and muscle cross-sectional area **(C)**. (Used with permission from McArdle WD, Katch FI, Katch VL. *Exercise Physiology: Nutrition, Energy, and Human Performance*. 8th Ed. Baltimore: Wolters Kluwer Health, 2015, as adapted with permission from Cribb PJ, Hayes A. Effects of supplement timing and resistance exercise on skeletal muscle hypertrophy. *Med Sci Sports Exerc* 2006;38:1918.)

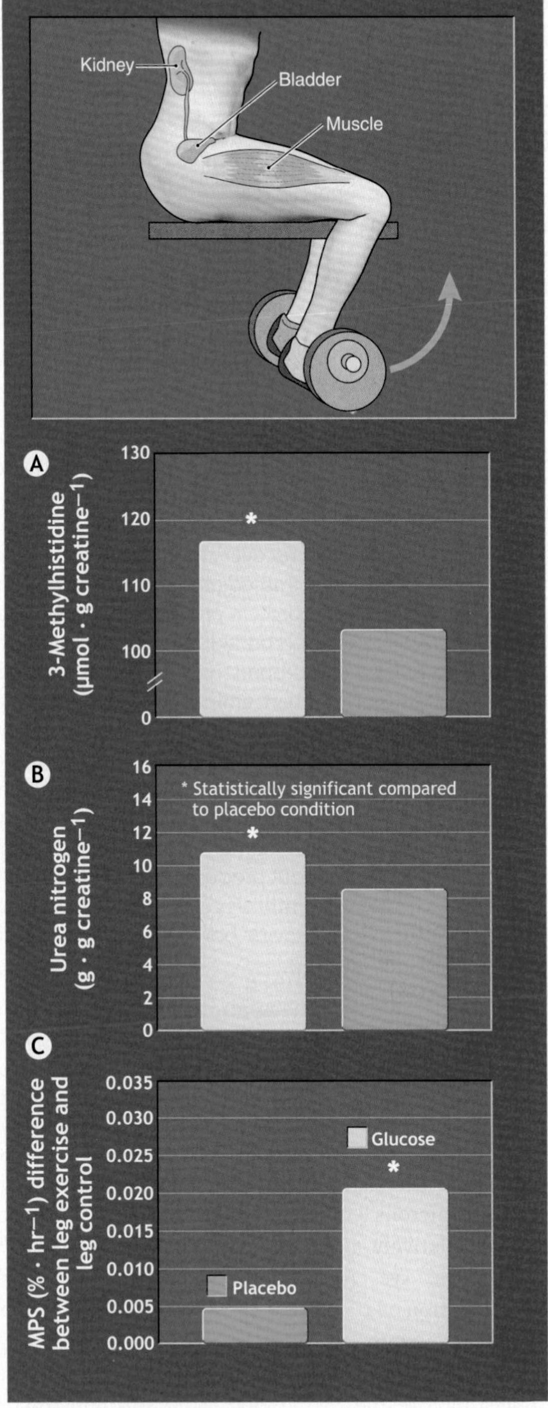

FIGURE 4.7 Effects of glucose (1.0 g per kg body mass) versus NutraSweet placebo, ingested immediately after exercise and 1 hour later, on protein degradation reflected by 24-hour urinary output of **(A)** 3-methylhistidine, **(B)** urinary urea nitrogen, and **(C)** rate of muscle protein synthesis (MPS) measured by vastus lateralis muscle incorporation of leucine (l-[l-13C]). *Bars* for MPS indicate difference between exercise and control leg for glucose and placebo conditions. (Used with permission from McArdle WD, Katch FI, Katch VL. *Exercise Physiology: Nutrition, Energy, and Human Performance*. 8th Ed. Baltimore: Wolters Kluwer Health, 2015, as adapted with permission from Roy BD, et al. Effect of glucose supplement timing on protein metabolism after resistance training. *J Appl Physiol* 1997;82:1882.)

LIPID SUPPLEMENTATION WITH MEDIUM-CHAIN TRIACYLGLYCEROLS

Do high-fat foods or supplements elevate plasma lipid levels to make more energy available during prolonged aerobic physical activity? To answer this question, one must consider two factors. First, consuming triacylglycerols composed of predominantly 12 to 18 carbon long-chain fatty acids *delays* gastric emptying. This negatively affects the rapidity of exogenous fat availability and slows fluid and carbohydrate replenishment, both crucial in intense endurance exercise. Second, after digestion and intestinal absorption (normally a 3- to 4-hr process), long-chain triacylglycerols reassemble with phospholipids, fatty acids, and a cholesterol shell to form fatty droplets called chylomicrons that travel relatively slowly to the systemic circulation via the lymphatic system. In the bloodstream, the tissues remove the triacylglycerols bound to chylomicrons. The relatively slow rate of digestion, absorption, and oxidation of long-chain fatty acids make this energy source undesirable as a supplement to augment energy metabolism in active muscle during exercise.

Medium-chain triacylglycerols (MCTs) provide a more rapid source of fatty acid fuel.

A CLOSER LOOK

Nutrient Timing to Optimize Muscle Response to Resistance Training

An evidence-based nutritional approach can enhance the quality of resistance training and facilitate muscle growth and strength development. This easy-to-follow new dimension to sports nutrition emphasizes not only the specific type and mixture of nutrients but also the timing of nutrient intake. Its goal—to blunt the catabolic state (release of the hormones glucagon, epinephrine, norepinephrine, and cortisol) and activate the natural muscle-building hormones (testosterone, growth hormone, IGF-1, and insulin) to facilitate recovery from physical activity and maximize muscle growth. Optimizing specific nutrient intake occurs in three phases.

Phase 1—Energy Phase

The **energy phase** enhances nutrient intake to spare muscle glycogen and protein, promote muscular endurance, limit immune system suppression, reduce muscle damage, and facilitate recovery in the postexercise period. Consuming a carbohydrate-protein supplement in the immediate pre-exercise period and during exercise extends muscular endurance; the ingested protein promotes protein metabolism, reducing demand for amino acid release from muscle. Carbohydrates consumed during physical activity suppress release of cortisol, which blunts the suppressive effects of exercise on immune system function and lessens the use of branched-chain amino acids (leucine, isoleucine, valine) generated by protein breakdown for energy. The recommended energy phase supplement contains the following nutrients: 20 to 26 g of high-glycemic carbohydrates (glucose, sucrose, maltodextrin), 5 to 6 g of whey protein (rapidly digested, high-quality protein separated from milk in the cheese-making process), 1 g of leucine, 30 to 120 mg of vitamin C, 20 to 60 IU of vitamin E, 100 to 250 mg of sodium, 60 to 100 mg of potassium, and 60 to 220 mg magnesium. Ingestion of the more slowly digested whole protein casein after an activity bout produces similar increases in muscle protein net balance and a short-term net muscle protein synthesis compared with whey protein. Casein and whey protein often combine as supplements to provide both faster-acting and slower-acting protein sources during recovery.

Phase 2—Anabolic Phase

The **anabolic phase** consists of a 45-minute postexercise metabolic window—a period of enhanced insulin sensitivity for muscle glycogen replenishment and muscle tissue repair and synthesis. This shift from catabolic to anabolic state occurs largely by blunting the action of the catabolic hormone cortisol and increasing the anabolic, muscle-building effects of insulin by consuming a standard high-glycemic carbohydrate-protein supplement in liquid form as whey protein or high-glycemic carbohydrates. In essence, the high-glycemic carbohydrate consumed postexercise serves as a nutrient activator to stimulate insulin release, which in the presence of amino acids, increases muscle tissue synthesis and decreases protein degradation. The recommended anabolic phase supplement profile contains the following nutrients: 40 to 50 g of high-glycemic carbohydrates (glucose, sucrose, maltodextrin), 13 to 15 g of whey protein, 1 to 2 g of leucine; 1 to 2 g of glutamine, 60 to 120 mg of vitamin C, and 80 to 400 IU of vitamin E.

Phase 3—Growth Phase

The **growth phase** extends from the end of the anabolic phase to the beginning of the next workout. It represents the time period to maximize insulin sensitivity and maintain an anabolic state to accentuate gains in muscle mass and muscle strength. The first several hours, referred to as the rapid segment, are geared to maintaining increased insulin sensitivity and glucose uptake to maximize glycogen replenishment. The rapid segment also speeds elimination of metabolic wastes via increased blood flow and stimulates tissue repair and muscle growth.

The next 16 to 18 hours, known as the sustained segment, maintain a positive nitrogen balance. This occurs with a relatively high daily protein intake of between 0.91 and 1.2 g of protein per pound of body weight to foster sustained but slower muscle tissue synthesis. An adequate carbohydrate intake emphasizes glycogen replenishment. The recommended growth phase supplement contains the following nutrients: 14 g of whey protein, 2 g of casein, 3 g of leucine, 1 g of glutamine, and 2 to 4 g of high-glycemic carbohydrates.

Sources: Ivy J, Portman R. *Nutrient Timing: The Future of Sports Nutrition*. Laguna Beach: Basic Health Publications, 2004.

Crigg PJ, Hayes A. Effects of supplement timing and resistance exercise on skeletal muscle hypertrophy. *Med Sci Sports Exerc* 2006;38:1918.

MCTs are processed oils, frequently used by patients with intestinal malabsorption and other tissue-wasting diseases. Marketing for the sports enthusiast hypes MCTs as a "fat burner," "energy source," "glycogen sparer," and "muscle builder." Unlike longer-chain triacylglycerols, MCTs contain saturated fatty acids with 8- to 10-carbon atoms along the fatty acid chain. During digestion, they hydrolyze by lipase action in the mouth, stomach, and duodenum to glycerol and medium-chain fatty acids (MCFAs). The water solubility of MCFAs enables them to move rapidly across the intestinal mucosa directly into the bloodstream via the portal vein without necessity of slow chylomicron transport by the lymphatic system as required for long-chain triacylglycerols. In the tissues, MCFAs move through the plasma membrane and diffuse across the inner mitochondrial membrane for oxidation. They pass into the mitochondria largely independent of the carnitine acyl–CoA transferase system; this contrasts with the slower transfer and mitochondrial oxidation rate of long-chain fatty acids. MCTs do not usually store as body fat because of their relative ease of oxidation. Ingesting MCTs rapidly elevates plasma free fatty acids (FFAs). While not definitive, supplementing with these lipids might spare liver and muscle glycogen during intense aerobic exercise.

fyi Beetroot: The New Garden of Ergogenic Eden?

The beetroot, the taproot portion of the beet plant (*Beta vulgaris*), is also known as table beet, garden beet, red or golden beet, or simply beet. In addition to its use as food and food coloring, beetroot has been linked with enhanced exercise endurance, improved blood flow, reduced blood pressure, and favorable effects on postprandial glucose and insulin responses. From a nutritional perspective, beetroot contains potassium; magnesium; iron; vitamins A, B_6, and C; folic acid; carbohydrates; protein; antioxidants; and soluble fiber. Its popularity in the athletic community as a "superfood" is based on claims of recent studies that beets, especially in juices and drinks, act ergogenically via improved muscle oxygenation to enhance exercise tolerance during long-term endurance exercise. Beetroot's rich nitrate content may play a significant modulator role in muscle energetics and oxygen delivery during exercise and subsequent recovery through the body's nitric oxide production cycle. Exercise economy from beetroot supplementation (beetroot shots [70 mL] containing ~4.8 mmol of nitrate) was enhanced in national-level and international-level kayak athletes during laboratory-based tasks predominantly reliant on aerobic energy system pathways. A final recommendation about beetroots' ergogenic benefits awaits further confirming research, but the initial findings are encouraging.

Sources: Jajja A, et al. Beetroot supplementation lowers daily systolic blood pressure in older, overweight subjects. *Nutr Res* 2014;34:868.

Peeling P, et al. Beetroot juice improves on-water 500-m time-trial performance, and laboratory-based paddling economy in national and international-level kayak athletes. *Int J Sport Nutr Exerc Metab* 2014. (In press as of 05.15.15.)

Pinna M, et al. Effect of beetroot juice supplementation on aerobic response during swimming. *Nutrients* 2014;6:605.

Wootton-Beard PC, et al. Effects of a beetroot juice with high neobetanin content on the early-phase insulin response in healthy volunteers. *J Nutr Sci* 2014;3:e9.

Inconclusive Exercise Benefits

Consuming MCTs does not inhibit gastric emptying, but conflicting research concerns their use with physical activity. Ingesting 30 g of MCTs, an estimated maximal amount tolerated in the gastrointestinal tract, before exercising contributed only between 3% and 7% of the total activity energy cost.

Consuming about 3 oz (86 g) of MCT provides interesting results. Endurance-trained cyclists rode for 2 hours at 60% $\dot{V}O_{2max}$; they then immediately performed a simulated 40-km cycling time trial. During each of three rides, they drank 2 L of beverages containing either 10% glucose, a 4.3% MCT emulsion, or 10% glucose plus a 4.3% MCT emulsion. **Figure 4.8** displays the effects of the beverages on average

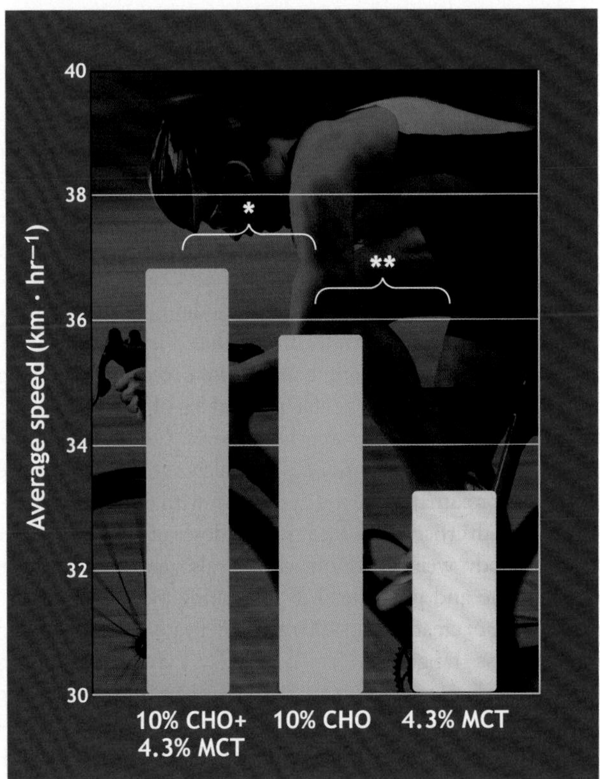

FIGURE 4.8 Effects of carbohydrate (CHO; 10% solution), medium-chain triacylglycerol (MCT; 4.3% emulsion), and carbohydrate 1 MCT (10% CHO 1 4.3% MCT) ingestion during cycling on simulated 40-km time-trial cycling speeds after 2 hours of exercise at 60% of $\dot{V}O_{2max}$. *Significantly faster than10% CHO trials; **Significantly faster than 4.3% MCT trials. (Used with permission from McArdle WD, Katch FI, Katch VL. *Exercise Physiology: Nutrition, Energy, and Human Performance*. 8th Ed. Baltimore: Wolters Kluwer Health, 2015, as adapted with permission from Van Zyl CG, et al. Effects of medium-chain triglyceride ingestion on fuel metabolism and cycling performance. *J Appl Physiol* 1996;80:2217.)

speed in the 40-km trials. Replacing the carbohydrate beverage with only the MCT emulsion impaired exercise performance by approximately 8%. The combined carbohydrate plus MCT solution consumed repeatedly during exercise significantly improved cycling speed by 2.5%. This small but potentially positive ergogenic outcome had the following three effects:

1. Lower total carbohydrate oxidation at a given level of oxygen uptake
2. Higher final circulating FFA and ketone levels
3. Lower final glucose and lactate concentrations

The small endurance performance enhancement with MCT supplementation probably occurred because this exogenous fatty acid source contributed to the total exercise energy expenditure including total fat oxidation in exercise. Consuming MCTs does not stimulate the release of the fat-emulsifying agent bile from the gall bladder. Thus, cramping and diarrhea often accompany an excess intake of this substance. In general, the relatively small alterations in substrate availability and substrate oxidation by increasing FFA availability during moderately intense aerobic exercise have only a small ergogenic effect on exercise capacity.

PYRUVATE

Ergogenic effects have been extolled for **pyruvate**, the 3-carbon end product of the cytoplasmic breakdown of glucose in glycolysis. As a partial replacement for dietary carbohydrate, advocates say that consuming pyruvate enhances endurance performance and promotes fat loss. Pyruvic acid, a relatively unstable chemical, causes intestinal distress. Consequently, various forms of the salt of this acid (e.g., sodium, potassium, calcium, or magnesium pyruvate) are produced in capsule, tablet, or powder form. Supplement manufacturers recommend taking two to four capsules daily, a total of 2 and 5 g of pyruvate spread throughout the day and taken with meals. One capsule usually contains 600 mg of pyruvate. The calcium form of pyruvate contains approximately 80 mg of calcium with 600 mg of pyruvate. Some advertisements recommend doses of one capsule per 20 lb of body weight. Manufacturers also combine creatine monohydrate and pyruvate; 1 g of creatine pyruvate provides about 80 mg of creatine and 400 mg of pyruvate. Recommended pyruvate doses range from 5 to 20 g a day. Pyruvate content in the normal diet ranges between 100 and 2000 mg daily. The largest dietary amounts occur in fruits and vegetables, particularly red apples (500 mg each), with smaller quantities in dark beer (80 mg per 12 oz) and red wine (75 mg per 6 oz).

Effects on Endurance Performance

Two double-blind, crossover studies by the same laboratory showed that 7 days of daily supplementation of a 100-g mixture of pyruvate (25 g) plus dihydroxyacetone (DHA; 75 g, another 3-carbon compound of glycolysis) increased upper-body and lower-body aerobic endurance by 20% compared with exercise with a 100-g supplement of an isocaloric glucose polymer. The pyruvate-DHA mixture increased cycle ergometer time to exhaustion of the legs by 13 minutes (66 min vs. 79 min); upper-body arm-cranking exercise time increased by 27 minutes (133 min vs. 160 min). A reduction also occurred for local muscle and overall body ratings of perceived exertion when subjects exercised with the pyruvate-DHA mixture compared with the placebo. Dosage recommendations range between 2 and 5 g of pyruvate spread throughout the day and consumed with meals.

Proponents of pyruvate supplementation maintain that elevations in extracellular pyruvate augment glucose transport into active muscle. Enhanced "glucose extraction" from blood provides the important carbohydrate energy source to sustain intense aerobic activity while also conserving intramuscular glycogen stores. When the individual's diet contains 55% of total calories as carbohydrate, pyruvate supplementation also increases pre-exercise muscle glycogen levels. Both of these effects—higher pre-exercise glycogen levels and facilitated glucose uptake and oxidation by active muscle—benefit intense endurance exercise similar to how pre-exercise carbohydrate loading and glucose feedings during exercise exert ergogenic effects.

Body Fat Loss

Some research indicates that exogenous pyruvate intake augments body fat loss when accompanied by a low-energy diet. The precise role of pyruvate to facilitate weight loss remains unknown. Consuming pyruvate may stimulate futile metabolic activity—small increases in metabolism not coupled to ATP production, with subsequent wasting of energy. Unfortunately, adverse side effects of a 30- to 100-g daily pyruvate intake include diarrhea and some gastrointestinal

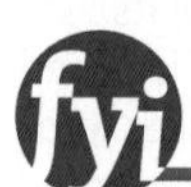

A Way to Enhance Endurance Performance?

Conflicting evidence exists as to the ergogenic efficacy of exogenous nitrate-containing compounds. Supplementing with inorganic nitrate-rich foods (e.g., spinach, lettuce, celery, arugula) or pharmacologic nitrate salts has been advocated as a means to increase the bioavailability of endogenous nitric oxide, a compound involved in regulating numerous bodily functions related to physical activity. Some studies have demonstrated a reduced oxygen cost of submaximal physical activity and enhanced endurance performance in constant load and incremental exercise with nitrate supplementation, perhaps mediated via improvements in muscle contractile efficiency, mitochondrial coupling efficiency, and/or enhanced muscle blood flow brought about by increased levels of nitric oxide in the body. In contrast, other studies have shown no effect of nitrate supplementation on diverse measures of endurance capacity or oxygen cost of submaximal exercise. Dosage, duration of supplementation, fitness level of subjects, and type and duration of physical activity performed may account for the different results.

Sources: Bescòs R, et al. Sodium nitrate supplementation does not enhance performance of endurance athletes. *Med Sci Sports Exerc* 2012;44:2400.

Lansley KE, et al. Acute dietary nitrate supplementation improves cycling time trial performance. *Med Sci Sports Exerc* 2011;43:1125.

Peacock O, et al. Dietary nitrate does not enhance running performance in elite cross-country skiers. *Med Sci Sports Exerc* 2012;44:2213.

gurgling and discomfort. *Until additional studies from independent laboratories reproduce existing findings for exercise performance and body fat loss, one should remain skeptical about the effectiveness of pyruvate supplementation.*

SUMMARY

1. Ergogenic aids consist of substances or procedures that improve physical work capacity, physiologic function, or athletic performance.
2. The strongest research strategies apply a randomized, double-blind, placebo-controlled design.
3. Performance improves by increasing alkaline reserve with sodium bicarbonate or sodium citrate before anaerobic activity.
4. Buffer dosage and the cumulative anaerobic nature of exercise interact to influence the ergogenic effect of bicarbonate or citrate loading.
5. Cortisol decreases amino acid transport into cells, depressing anabolism and stimulating protein catabolism.
6. Blunting cortisol's normal increase following exercise in healthy individuals augments muscular development with resistance training because muscle tissue synthesis progresses unimpeded in recovery.
7. Research fails to show any beneficial effect of chromium supplements on training-related changes in muscular strength, physique, fat-free body mass, or muscle mass.
8. In supplement form, creatine increases intramuscular creatine and PCr, enhances short-term anaerobic power output capacity, and facilitates recovery from repeated bouts of intense effort.
9. Creatine loading occurs by ingesting 20 g of creatine monohydrate for 6 consecutive days. Thereafter, reducing intake to 2 g daily maintains elevated intramuscular levels.
10. No compelling scientific evidence exists to conclude that ginseng supplementation offers positive benefits for physiologic function or performance during physical activity.
11. Significant health risks accompany ephedrine use, prompting the FDA to ban it in 2004 and in 2007; the ban has been upheld by the U.S. Supreme Court.
12. Many resistance-trained athletes supplement with amino acids, either singularly or in combination, to facilitate skeletal muscle protein synthesis.
13. Research generally shows little or no benefits of general amino acid supplementation on levels of anabolic hormones or body composition, muscle size, or exercise performance.
14. Proper timing of carbohydrate-protein-creatine supplementation immediately following resistance training allows for protein synthesis and muscle tissue growth, which are reflected in elevated plasma concentrations of insulin and hGH.
15. MCT may enhance fat metabolism and conserve glycogen during endurance exercise; ingesting about 86 g of MCTs enhances performance by an additional 2.5%.
16. Pyruvate supplementation may augment endurance performance and promote fat loss, the latter attributable to its small effect on metabolic rate increases.

THINK IT THROUGH

1. Respond to the question: "If the government allows some chemicals in food supplements to be sold over the counter, how could they possibly be harmful to an individual?"
2. Advise an Olympic-caliber weightlifter who plans to bicarbonate load because the competitive event requires all-out effort of an anaerobic nature.

PART 2 Pharmacologic Ergogenic Aids

Athletes at all levels of competition often use pharmacologic and chemical agents, believing that a specific drug positively influences technical skills, strength, power, and/or endurance. When winning becomes all-important, cheating to win becomes pervasive, despite scanty "hard" scientific evidence to indicate a performance-enhancing effect of many of these chemicals. Little realistically can be done to prevent athletes using and abusing drugs. This section discusses the most prominent of the pharmacologic chemical agents used by athletes to enhance performance.

CAFFEINE

In January 2004, the International Olympic Committee (IOC) removed **caffeine** from its list of restricted substances. Caffeine belongs to a group of compounds called *methylxanthines* (**www.nlm.nih.gov/medlineplus/caffeine.html**), found naturally in coffee beans, tea leaves, chocolate, cocoa beans, and cola nuts and also added to carbonated beverages and nonprescription medicines listed in **Table 4.2**. Depending on the preparation, 1 cup of brewed coffee contains between 60 and 150 mg of caffeine, instant coffee about 100 mg, brewed tea between 20 and 50 mg, and caffeinated soft drinks approximately 50 mg. As a frame of reference, 2.5 cups of percolated coffee contain 250 to 400 mg, or generally between 3 and 6 mg per kg of body mass. The small intestine's caffeine absorption following ingestion occurs rapidly, reaching peak plasma concentrations between 30 and 120 minutes to exert an influence on the nervous, cardiovascular, and muscular systems. Caffeine's metabolic **half-life** ranges between 3 and 8 hours, which means that it clears from the body fairly rapidly, certainly after a night's sleep.

Caffeine's Ergogenic Effects

A strong base of evidence supports caffeine use to improve exercise performance. Prior research showed that ingesting 330 mg of caffeine in 2.5 cups of regularly percolated coffee 1 hour before exercising extended endurance in intense

TABLE 4.2 Caffeine Content of Common Foods, Beverages, and Over-the-Counter and Prescription Medications

Beverages and Food	Caffeine Content (mg)
Coffee[a]	
Coffee, Starbucks, grande, 16 oz	330
Coffee, Starbucks, tall, 12 oz	260
Coffee, Starbucks, short, 8 oz	180
Coffee, Starbucks, Americano, tall, 12 oz	150
Coffee, Starbucks, latte or cappuccino, grande, 16 oz	150
Brewed, drip method, 8 oz	110–150
Brewed, percolator, 8 oz	64–124
Instant, 8 oz	40–108
Expresso, 1 oz	60-70
Tea, 5-oz cup[a]	
Brewed, 1 min	9–33
Brewed, 3 min	20–46
Brewed, 5 min	20–50
Iced tea, 12 oz; instant tea	12–36
Chocolate	
Baker's semisweet, 1 oz; Baker's chocolate chips, ¼ cup	13
Hot chocolate, 5-oz cup, made from mix	6–10
Milk chocolate, 1 oz	6
Sweet/dark chocolate, 1 oz	20
Baking (unsweetened) chocolate, 1 oz	35
Chocolate bar, 3.5 oz	12–15
Jello chocolate fudge mousse, one serving	12
Ovaltine, one serving	0
Energy drinks	
Red Bull, 8.4 oz	83
Monster, 8 oz	92
AMP, 8 oz	71
5-Hr Energy (regular), 1.9 oz	6
5-Hr Energy (extra strength), 1.9 oz	242
Full Throttle, 8 oz	210
Rockstar, 8 oz	31
NOS, 16 oz	224
Soft drinks, 12 oz can	
Jolt cola (23.5 oz can)	100
Sugar-free Mr. Pibb	59

Beverages and Food (*Continued*)	Caffeine Content (mg)
Mellow Yello, Mountain Dew	53–54
Tab	47
Coca Cola, Diet Coke, 7-Up Gold	46
Shasta Cola, Cherry Cola, Diet Cola	44
Dr. Pepper, Mr. Pibb	40–41
Dr. Pepper, sugar-free	40
Pepsi Cola	38
Diet Pepsi, Pepsi Light, Diet RC, RC Cola, Diet Rite	36

Over-the-Counter Medications	Caffeine Content (mg)
Cold remedies	
Dristan, Coryban-D, Triaminicin, Sinarest	30–31
Excedrin	65
Actifed, Contac, Comtrex, Sudafed	0
Diuretics	
Aqua-Ban	200
Pre-Mens Forte	100
Pain remedies	
Vanquish	33
Anacin, Midol	32
Aspirin, any brand; Bufferin, Tylenol, Excedrin P.M.	0
Stimulants	
Vivarin tablet, NoDoz maximum strength caplet, Caffedrine	200
NoDoz tablet	100
Energets lozenges	75
Weight control aids	
Dexatrim, Dietac	200
Prolamine	140

Prescription Pain Medications	Caffeine Content (mg)
Cafergot	100
Migrol	50
Fiorinal	40
Darvon compound	32

[a]Brewing tea or coffee for longer periods slightly increases the caffeine content.
Data from product labels and manufacturers.

aerobic exercise. Subjects performed on average about 90 minutes of exercise with caffeine, shown as the *orange triangle* in the bottom data line in **Figure 4.9**, and 76 minutes without it (*gold diamond*, bottom data line). Consuming caffeine before exercise increased fat catabolism and reduced carbohydrate oxidation during exercise. Subjects who consumed caffeine exercised for an average of 90.2 minutes compared with 76 minutes in subjects who exercised without caffeine. Even though heart rate and oxygen uptake were similar during the two trials, subjects believed the caffeine made the work seem easier.

Caffeine also provides an ergogenic benefit during maximal swimming performances completed in less than 25 minutes. In a double-blind, crossover experiment, seven male and four female distance swimmers (<25 min for 1500 m) consumed caffeine (6 mg · kg body mass^{-1}) 2.5 hours before swimming 1500 m.

Figure 4.10 illustrates that split times improved with caffeine for each 500-m swim. Total swim time averaged

2% faster with caffeine than without it (20 min, 58.6 s vs. 21 min, 21.8 s). Lower plasma potassium concentration before exercise and higher blood glucose levels following the trial accompanied enhanced performance with caffeine. This suggested that electrolyte balance and glucose availability might be key factors in caffeine's ergogenic effect.

Proposed Mechanisms for Ergogenic Action

A precise explanation remains elusive for the exercise-enhancing boost from caffeine. In all likelihood, the ergogenic effect of caffeine (or other related methylxanthine compounds) in intense endurance exercise occurs from the facilitated use of fat as fuel, thus sparing the body's limited glycogen reserves. In quantities typically administered to humans, caffeine probably acts in one or more of the three following ways:

1. Directly by stimulating adipose tissues to release fatty acids.
2. Indirectly by stimulating epinephrine release from the adrenal medulla; epinephrine then facilitates fatty acid release from adipocytes into plasma. Increased plasma FFA levels, in turn, increase fat oxidation, thus conserving liver and muscle glycogen.
3. Directly produces analgesic effects on the central nervous system and enhances motoneuronal excitability to facilitate motor unit recruitment.

Endurance Effects Often Inconsistent

Prior nutrition may partly account for variation in exercise response after individuals consume caffeine. Group improvements in endurance occur with prior caffeine ingestion, yet individuals who maintain a high carbohydrate intake show reduced FFA mobilization. Individual differences in caffeine sensitivity, tolerance, and hormonal response from short- and long-term patterns of caffeine consumption also affect its ergogenic qualities. Interestingly, caffeine's ergogenic effects are less for caffeine in coffee than an equivalent dose in capsule form. Apparently, components in coffee blunt some of caffeine's actions. Beneficial effects do not occur consistently in habitual caffeine users. This indicates that an athlete should consider "caffeine tolerance" rather than assume caffeine provides a consistent benefit to all people. From a practical standpoint, athletes should omit caffeine-containing foods and beverages 4 to 6 days before competition to optimize caffeine's potential for ergogenic effects.

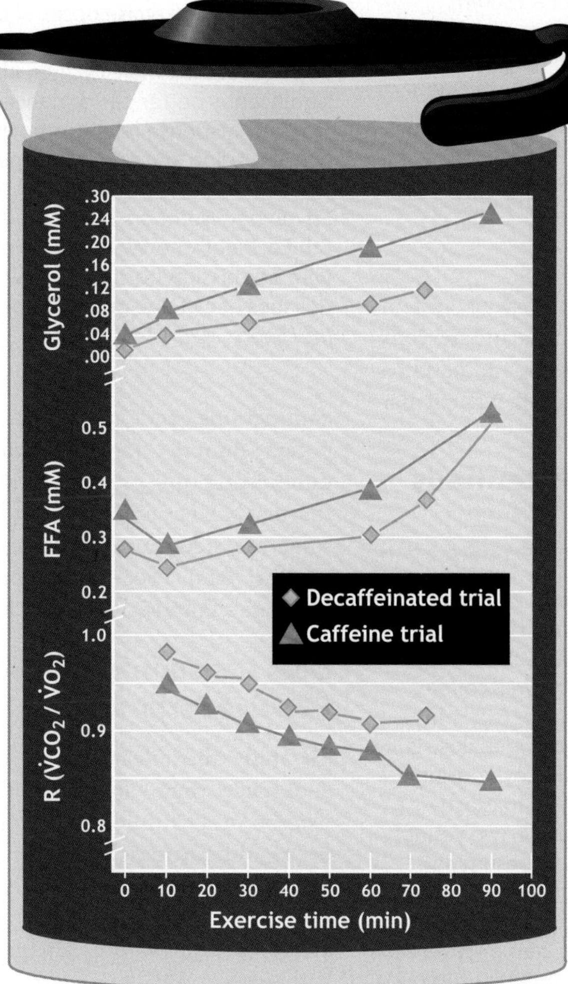

FIGURE 4.9 Average values for plasma glycerol, free fatty acids (FFAs), and the respiratory exchange ratio (R) during endurance exercise trials after ingesting caffeine and decaffeinated liquids. (Used with permission from McArdle WD, Katch FI, Katch VL. *Exercise Physiology: Nutrition, Energy, and Human Performance*. 8th Ed. Baltimore: Wolters Kluwer Health, 2015, as adapted with permission from Costill DL, et al. Effects of caffeine ingestion on metabolism and exercise performance. *Med Sci Sports* 1978;10:155.)

Effects on Muscle

Caffeine can directly act on muscle to enhance exercise capacity. A double-blind research design evaluated voluntary and electrically stimulated muscle actions under "caffeine-free" conditions and following oral administration of 500 mg of caffeine. Electrically stimulating the motor nerve removed central nervous system control and thus quantified caffeine's direct effects on skeletal muscle. Caffeine produced no ergogenic effect on *maximal* muscle force during voluntary or electrically stimulated muscle actions. In contrast, for *submaximal* effort, caffeine increased force output for low-frequency electrical stimulation in both premuscle and postmuscle fatigue. This suggests that caffeine exerts a direct and specific ergogenic effect on skeletal muscle during repetitive low-frequency stimulation. Caffeine may increase sarcoplasmic reticulum's Ca^{2+} permeability, thus enabling this mineral's ready availability for contraction. Caffeine also could influence myofibril Ca^{2+} sensitivity.

Caffeine Warning

Individuals who normally avoid caffeine-containing substances may experience undesirable side effects when they consume it. Caffeine

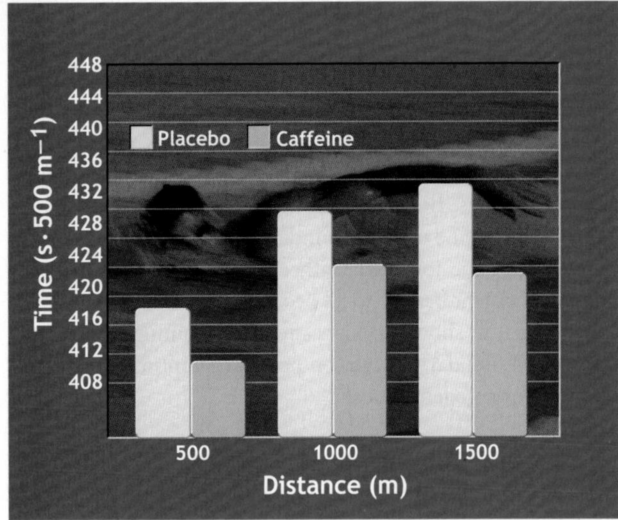

FIGURE 4.10 Split times for each 500 m of a 1500-m time trial with caffeine and placebo. Caffeine produced significantly faster split times. (Used with permission from McArdle WD, Katch FI, Katch VL. *Exercise Physiology: Nutrition, Energy, and Human Performance*. 8th Ed. Baltimore: Wolters Kluwer Health, 2015, as adapted with permission from MacIntosh BR, Wright BM. Caffeine ingestion and performance of a 1500-metre swim. *Can J Appl Physiol* 1995;20:168.)

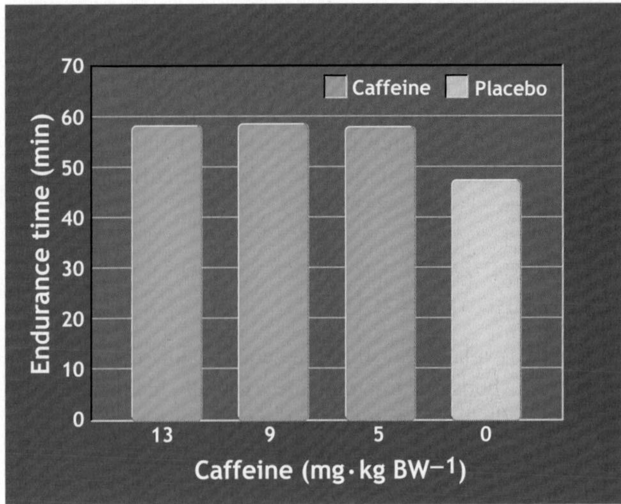

FIGURE 4.11 Endurance performance (time to fatigue) following pre-exercise doses of caffeine in different concentrations. Cycling time (min) represents the average for nine male cyclists. All caffeine trials produced significantly better performance than the placebo condition. No dose-response relationship emerged between caffeine concentration and endurance performance. (Used with permission from McArdle WD, Katch FI, Katch VL. *Exercise Physiology: Nutrition, Energy, and Human Performance*. 8th Ed. Baltimore: Wolters Kluwer Health, 2015, as adapted with permission from Pasman WJ, et al. The effect of different dosages of caffeine on endurance performance time. *Int J Sports Med* 1995;16:225.)

overconsumption stimulates the central nervous system to produce restlessness, headaches, insomnia and nervous irritability, muscle twitching, tremulousness, and psychomotor agitation and trigger premature left-ventricular contractions, and extreme diarrhea. Caffeine acts as a potent diuretic. Excessive consumption may cause an unnecessary pre-exercise fluid loss, negatively affecting thermal balance and performance in a hot environment. In some cases consuming caffeine in concentrated amounts can be fatal (See For Your Information: "Powdered Caffeine's Potentially Lethal Effects.")

fyi Powdered Caffeine's Potentially Lethal Effects

A single teaspoon of powdered (concentrated) caffeine, sold under various names and readily purchased in bulk from online retailers, contains the caffeine equivalent of drinking about 25 consecutive 8-oz cups of brewed coffee, with a total caffeine content of about 6000 mg or 6 g! Sold as an "energy boost" supplement, the recommended dose is 1/16th of a teaspoon, which invites unintended overdosing, as special measuring spoons would be required to exactly measure this amount of the supplement. In 2014, two young men died from a seizure almost instantly after consuming the concentrated powdered caffeine (**www.myhighplains.com/story/d/story/family-looks-to-senate-to-help-ban-powdered-caffei/24870/alph3lxH10q8BQ0-oVfiOA**). Concentrated caffeine use has also been linked in FDA documents to dizziness, delirium, nausea, vomiting, and increased heart rate. Such untoward events have led to initiatives to convince the FDA to ban powdered caffeine.

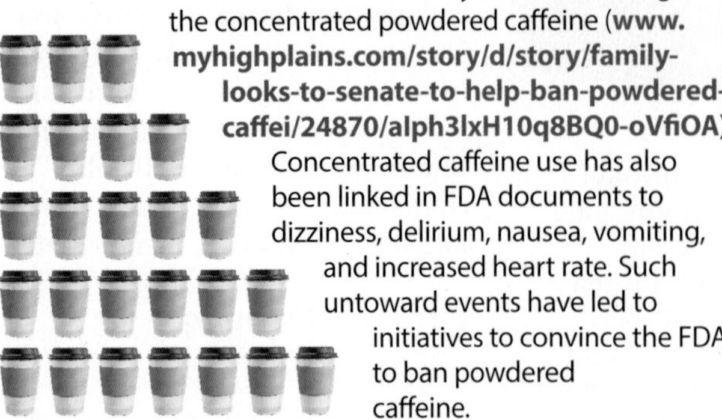

Does Consuming More Caffeine Enhance Exercise Performance?

To study the effects of pre-exercise caffeine intake on endurance time, nine trained, male cyclists received a placebo or a capsule containing 5, 9, or 13 mg of caffeine per kg of body mass 1 hour before cycling at 80% of maximal power output on a $\dot{V}O_{2max}$ test. All caffeine trials showed a 24% improvement in performance *without additional benefit* from caffeine quantities above 5 mg · kg body mass^{-1} (Fig. 4.11).

ANABOLIC STEROIDS

Anabolic steroids available for therapeutic use in oral, injectable, and transdermal forms became prominent in the early 1950s to treat patients deficient in natural androgens or with muscle-wasting diseases. Other legitimate steroid uses include treatment for osteoporosis and severe breast cancer and to counter the excessive decline in lean body mass and increase in body fat observed among elderly men, people with HIV, and individuals undergoing kidney dialysis.

Anabolic steroids (popular names include Dianabol, Anadrol, Deca Durabolin, Parabolin, and Winstrol) became an integral part of the high-technology scene of competitive American sports beginning in the 1950s. Widespread steroid use is believed to have started with the 1955 US weightlifting team's use of Dianabol, the modified, synthetic testosterone molecule methandrostenolone. A new era of competitive athletes "drugging" to presumably gain a competitive advantage created a plethora of newly created anabolic steroid forms.

Steroid Structure and Action

Anabolic steroids function similarly to the male hormone testosterone. By binding with special receptor sites mainly on muscle, testosterone contributes to male secondary sex characteristics that include gender differences in muscle mass and strength that develop at puberty onset. The hormone's androgenic or masculinizing effects are attenuated by synthetically manipulating the steroid's chemical structure to increase muscle growth from anabolic tissue building and nitrogen retention. Nevertheless, the masculinizing effect of synthetically derived steroids still occurs despite chemical alteration, particularly in women.

Athletes who take steroids do so typically during the active years of their athletic careers. They combine multiple steroid preparations in oral and injectable form because they believe various androgens differ in their physiologic action. This practice, called **stacking**, progressively increases the drug dosage, called **pyramiding**, usually during 6- to 12-week cycles. The drug quantity often far exceeds the recommended medical dose. The athlete then alters the drug dosage or combines it with other prescription-only drugs before competition to minimize chances of detection during random drug testing.

The difference between dosages used in research studies and the excess typically used by athletes has contributed to a credibility gap between scientific findings (often, no effect of steroids) and what most in the athletic community know to be true. One often pictures steroid abusers as extremely muscular bodybuilders, but abuse also occurs among competitive athletes in road cycling, tennis, track and field, American collegiate and professional football, canoeing, auto racing, swimming, and other highly competitive sport activities. A 2000 survey of United States Powerlifting Team members indicated that up to two-thirds used androgenic-anabolic steroids, with many athletes obtaining black market drugs. Misinformed individuals usually take massive and prolonged dosages without medical monitoring and consequently suffer harmful alterations in physiologic function. Steroid abuse among adolescents and its accompanying risks, including extreme virilization and premature cessation of bone growth, are particularly worrisome: survey research has confirmed that boys and girls as young as 11 years of age use anabolic-androgenic steroids. Teenagers cite improved athletic performance as the most common reason for taking steroids, yet many acknowledge enhanced appearance as a main reason. Boys of short stature believe that taking steroids stimulates gains in muscular development to make them more "manly," and possibly trigger a growth spurt! In this regard, a body image dysphoria may contribute to anabolic steroid abuse among teenagers and adults.

The relatively small residual androgenic effect of steroids can precipitate aggressiveness or so-called **roid rage**, extreme competitiveness, and hoped for resistance to fatigue. Such disinhibitory central nervous system effects allow the athlete to train harder for a longer duration or believe that augmented training effects have actually occurred. Abnormal alterations in mood, including psychiatric dysfunction, also have been attributed to androgen use.

Research with animals suggests that anabolic steroid treatment, when combined with exercise and adequate protein intake, stimulates protein synthesis and increases muscle protein content. In contrast, research also shows no benefit from steroid treatment on the leg muscle weight of rats subjected to functional overload by surgically removing the synergistic muscle. The researchers concluded that anabolic steroid treatment did not complement functional overload to augment muscle development. Effects of steroids on humans remain difficult to interpret. Some studies with steroids show augmented body mass gains and reduced body fat in men who train, but other studies show no effects on strength and power or body composition, even with sufficient energy and protein intake to support an anabolic effect. When steroid use produced body weight gains, the compositional nature of these gains in water, muscle, and fat remained unclear. The fact that steroid use remains widespread among top-level athletes worldwide suggests it serves as a potent substance with considerable credibility.

Dosage as a Key Factor

Much of the confusion regarding ergogenic effectiveness of anabolic steroids results from variations in experimental design, poor controls, differences in specific drugs and dosages (50 to >200 mg per day vs. the usual medical dosage of 5 to 20 mg), treatment duration, training intensity, measurement techniques, previous experience as subjects, individual variation in response, and nutritional supplementation.

Researchers studied 43 healthy men with some resistance training experience. Diet (energy and protein intake) and physical activity (standard weightlifting thrice weekly) were controlled, with steroid dosage exceeding previous human studies (600 mg of testosterone enanthate injected weekly or placebo).

Changes from baseline average values were evaluated for FFM assessed by hydrostatic weighing (refer to Chapter 16), triceps and quadriceps cross-sectional muscle areas assessed by magnetic resonance imaging, and muscle strength repetition maximum (1-RM) following 10 weeks of testosterone treatment. The men who received the hormone and continued to train gained about 0.5 kg (1 lb) of lean tissue weekly, with no increase in body fat over the relatively brief treatment period. Even the group that received the drug but did not train increased their muscle mass and strength compared with the group receiving the placebo, yet the increases in this group were lower than the group that trained while taking testosterone.

Urine Testing for Steroids (and Other Banned Substances)

Urine testing has remained the primary "gold standard" method to detect illicit drug use in athletes. Testing consists of two steps:

1. The first step is a screening test. Screening tests are usually done by immunoassay methods.
2. If the first screen turns out positive for traces of banned PEDs, a second step known as the confirmation test is then applied to samples that test positive during the screening test. The confirmation test in most laboratories relies on mass spectrometry (testing labs are certified by the Substance Abuse and Mental Health Services Administration [SAMHSA], a branch of the U.S. Department of Health and Human Services; **www.samhsa.gov**). This precise analytical methodology assesses the mass-to-charge ratio of charged particles in a particular chemical substance. The sample, after vaporization, creates charged particles following electron beam bombardment, which are further analyzed to determine the precise amount of the chemical present. The distinct pattern or "signature" made by the molecules in the chemical deflected by the field is compared with known patterns of chemicals. Besides the detection of steroids, testing may detect other banned substances, including alcohol, amphetamines, methamphetamine, MDMA (ecstasy), barbiturates, phenobarbital, benzodiazepines, cannabis, cocaine, cotinine (breakdown product of nicotine), morphine, tricyclic antidepressants (TCAs), lysergic acid diethylamide (LSD), methadone, and phencyclidine (PCP, angel dust, supergrass). Testing time to obtain confirmation results can range from 1 day for barbiturates to 3 to 30 days for steroids (**www.deadiversion.usdoj.gov/drugs_concern/pcp.htm**).

Risks of Anabolic Steroid Abuse

Table 4.3 lists some known harmful side effects from anabolic steroid abuse. Prolonged high dosages of steroids, often

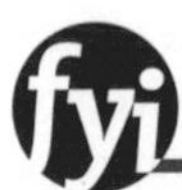

Diuretics Can Mask Drug Use

Diuretics facilitate the kidney's urine production. In clinical use, they control hypertension and reduce water retention or edema via reduced blood volume and total body water. For the athlete wishing to escape detection for illicit drug use, increased urine production with a diuretic reduces the urine's banned drug concentration, decreasing the likelihood of its discovery (**www.ncbi.nlm.nih.gov/pmc/articles/PMC2962812/**).

TABLE 4.3 Side Effects and Medical Risks of Anabolic Steroid Use

System	Adverse Effect	Reversibility
Cardiovascular (male and female)	Increased LDL cholesterol	Yes
	Decreased HDL cholesterol	Yes
	Hypertension	Yes
	Elevated triglycerides	Yes
	Arteriosclerotic heart disease	No
	High blood pressure	Possible
Reproductive (male)	Testicular atrophy	Possible
	Gynecomastia (breast enlargement)	Possible
	Impaired spermatogenesis	Yes
	Altered libido (impotence)	Yes
	Male pattern baldness	No
	Enlarged prostate gland	Possible
	Pain in urinating	Yes
Reproductive (female)	Menstrual dysfunction	Yes
	Altered libido	Yes
	Clitoral enlargement	No
	Deepening voice	No
	Male pattern baldness	No
	Breast reduction	No
Hepatic (male and female)	Elevated liver enzymes	Yes
	Jaundice	Yes
	Hepatic tumors	No
	Peliosis	No
Endocrine (male and female)	Altered glucose tolerance	Yes
	Decreased FSH, LH	Yes
	Acne	Yes
Musculoskeletal (male and female)	Premature epiphyseal closure (stunted growth)	No
	Tendon degeneration, ruptures	No
	Swelling of feet or ankles	Yes
Central nervous (male and female)	Mood swings	Yes
	Violent behavior	Yes
	Depression	Yes
	Psychoses/delusions	Yes
Other	Hepatoma (liver cancer)	Yes
	Bad breath	Yes
	Nausea and vomiting	Yes
	Sleep problems	Yes
	Impaired judgment	Yes
	Paranoid jealousy	Yes
	Increased risk of blood poisoning and infections	No

at levels 10 to 200 times the therapeutic recommendation, can impair normal testosterone endocrine function. A study of five male power athletes showed that 26 weeks of steroid administration reduced serum testosterone to less than half the level measured when the study began, with the effect lasting throughout a 12- to 16-week follow-up period. Infertility, reduced sperm concentrations (azoospermia), and decreased testicular volume pose additional problems for male steroid users.

Other accompanying male hormonal alterations during steroid use in men include a sevenfold increase in estradiol concentration, the major female hormone. The higher estradiol level represents an average value for normal women and possibly explains the anabolic steroid-induced **gynecomastia** (breast enlargement). Furthermore, steroids have been shown to cause the following four responses:

1. Chronic prostate gland stimulation and increased size
2. Injury and functional alterations in cardiovascular function and myocardial cell cultures
3. Possible pathologic ventricular growth and dysfunction when combined with resistance training
4. Increased blood platelet aggregation, which can compromise cardiovascular health and function and possibly increase the risk of stroke and acute myocardial infarction from blood clots

Steroid Abuse and Life-Threatening Disease

Concern regarding the risk of chronic steroid use centers on evidence about possible links between androgen abuse and abnormal liver function. Androgen metabolism occurs almost exclusively in the liver, thus making the liver susceptible to damage from long-term steroid use and toxic excess. One of the serious effects of androgens on the liver and sometimes splenic tissue occurs when the liver develops randomly distributed localized blood-filled lesions or cysts, a condition called **peliosis hepatis**. In extreme cases, the liver eventually fails or intra-abdominal hemorrhage develops, ending in death. These potentially serious side effects may occur even when a physician prescribes the drug in the recommended dosage.

Some athletes take steroids on and off for years, with dosages exceeding typical therapeutic levels. Reports of other negative effects in user include significantly increased chromosome damage, apoptosis, and necrosis in exfoliated cells from the oral mucosa compared to control nonusers, perhaps triggering incubators of the carcinogenic process leading to destructive disease states.

Steroid Use and Plasma Lipoproteins

Anabolic steroid use, particularly of the orally active 17-alkylated androgens in healthy men and women, can negatively impact plasma lipoproteins by lowering high-density lipoprotein cholesterol (HDL-C), elevating both low-density lipoprotein cholesterol (LDL-C) and total cholesterol, and lowering the HDL-C:LDL-C ratio. Weightlifters who took anabolic steroids averaged 26 $mg \cdot dL^{-1}$ for HDL-C compared with 50 $mg \cdot dL^{-1}$ for weightlifters not taking these drugs. Reduced HDL-C to this level considerably increases coronary artery disease risk.

Specific Female Concerns

Females have additional concerns about dangers from anabolic steroids. These include virilization (more apparent than in men), disruption of normal growth pattern by premature closure of bone growth plates, altered menstrual function, dramatic increase in sebaceous gland size, acne, hirsutism (excessive body and facial hair), generally irreversible voice deepening, decreased breast size, enlarged clitoris (clitoromegaly), and hair loss (alopecia areata). Declines also occur in serum levels of luteinizing hormone, follicle-stimulating hormone, progesterone, and estrogens. These may negatively affect follicle formation, ovulation, and menstrual function.

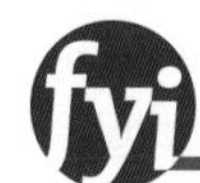

American College of Sports Medicine (ACSM; www.acsm.org) Position Statement on the Use of Anabolic-Androgenic Steroids in Sports

The American College of Sports Medicine (ACSM) issued the following position statement based on a comprehensive survey of the world literature and analysis of claims made for and about anabolic-androgenic steroid efficacy to improve human physical performance (**www.acsm.org/access-public-information/position-stands**):

1. Anabolic-androgenic steroids in the presence of an adequate diet and training can contribute to increases in body weight, often in the lean mass compartment.
2. The gains in muscular strength achieved through high-intensity exercise and proper diet can occur by the increased use of anabolic-androgenic steroids in some individuals.
3. Anabolic-androgenic steroids do not increase aerobic power or capacity for muscular exercise.
4. Anabolic-androgenic steroids have been associated with adverse effects on the liver, cardiovascular, reproductive system, and psychological status in therapeutic trials and in limited research on athletes. Until further research is completed, the potential hazards of the use of anabolic-androgenic steroids in athletes must include those found in therapeutic trials.
5. The use of anabolic-androgenic steroids by athletes is contrary to the rules and ethical principles of athletic competition as set forth by many of the sports governing bodies. The ACSM supports these ethical principles and deplores the use of anabolic-androgenic steroids by athletes.

ANDROSTENEDIONE: A STEROID ALTERNATIVE?

Androstenedione, an intermediate or precursor hormone between DHEA and testosterone, helps the liver to synthesize other biologically active steroid hormones. Normally produced by the adrenal glands and gonads, androstenedione (also marketed as Andromax, Finaflex 1-ANDRO, and Androstat 100) converts to testosterone through enzymatic action in various body tissues. Some androstenedione also converts into estrogens. Many physically active individuals have taken this over-the-counter nutritional supplement, believing it produces endogenous testosterone to enable them to train harder, build more muscle mass, and repair and recover from injury more rapidly. Initially marketed as a dietary supplement and antiaging drug, androstenedione occurs naturally in meat and extracts of some plants and is touted on the Internet as "a metabolite that is only one step away from the biosynthesis of testosterone." The NFL (**www.nfl.com**), National Collegiate Athletic Association (NCAA; **www.ncaa.com**), Men's Professional Tennis Association (**www.atpworldtour.com**), WADA, and IOC ban its use because these organizations believe it provides an unfair competitive advantage and may endanger health, similar to anabolic steroids. The IOC banned for life the 1996 Olympic shot-put gold medalist because he used androstenedione; androstenedione remains a banned substance by the IOC and U.S. Olympic Committee. In 2004, the FDA banned androstenedione because of its potent anabolic and androgenic effects and accompanying health risks.

Alcohol Drinks for Fluid Replacement: Not a Good Idea!

Alcohol exaggerates the dehydrating effect of exercise in a warm environment. It acts as a potent diuretic in two ways by:

1. Depressing antidiuretic hormone release from the posterior pituitary
2. Diminishing the arginine vasopressin response

These two effects impair thermoregulation during heat stress, placing the athlete at increased risk for heat distress.

Many athletes consume alcohol-containing beverages *after* exercising or sports competition; thus, the question arises as to whether alcohol impairs rehydration in recovery. Alcohol's effect on rehydration has been studied after exercise-induced dehydration equal to approximately 2% of body mass. Subjects consumed a rehydration fluid volume equivalent to 150% of fluid lost and containing 0%, 1%, 2%, 3%, or 4% alcohol. Urine volume produced during the 6-hour study period directly related to the beverages' alcohol concentration; greater alcohol consumed produced more urine. The increase in recovery plasma volume compared with the dehydrated state averaged 8.1% when the rehydration fluid contained no alcohol but only 5.3% for the beverage with 4% alcohol content. *The bottom line is that alcohol-containing beverages impede rehydration.*

Alcohol acts as a peripheral vasodilator, so it should never be consumed during extreme cold exposure or to facilitate recovery from hypothermia. A good "stiff drink" does not warm you up. Currently, debate exists as to whether moderate alcohol intake exacerbates body cooling during mild cold exposure.

Sources: Shirreffs SM, Maughan RJ. The effect of alcohol consumption on fluid retention following exercise-induced dehydration in man. *J Physiol* 1995;489:33P.

Shirreffs SM, Maughan RJ. The effect of alcohol consumption on the restoration of blood and plasma volume following exercise-induced dehydration in man. *J Physiol* 1996;491:64P.

Summary of Eight Research Findings Concerning Androstenedione

1. No favorable effect on muscle mass
2. No favorable effect on muscular performance
3. No favorable alteration in body composition
4. No favorable effects on muscle protein synthesis or tissue anabolism
5. Elevates plasma testosterone concentrations
6. Elevates a variety of estrogen subfractions
7. Impairs the blood lipid profile in apparently healthy men
8. Increases the likelihood of testing positive for steroid use

TETRAHYDROGESTRINONE: THE HIDDEN STEROID

Tetrahydrogestrinone (THG or "The Clear") represents an anabolic steroid specifically designed to escape detection by normal drug testing. Developed by an American nutritional supplement company, THG is closely related to the banned anabolic steroids gestrinone and trenbolone. It has affinity to the androgen and progesterone receptors, but not the estrogen receptor. At the cell's nucleus, THG binds to the androgen receptor. Here, it changes the expression of a variety of genes, turning on several anabolic and androgenic functions. This "designer drug" was made public in 2003 when the USADA (**www.usantidoping.org**), which oversees drug testing for all sports federations under the US Olympic umbrella, was contacted by an anonymous track and field coach claiming several top athletes used the drug. The same coach subsequently provided the USADA with a syringe containing THG that the USADA then used to develop a new test for its detection. The USADA then reanalyzed 350 urine samples from participants at the June 2003 US track and field championships and 100 samples from random out-of-competition tests. Six athletes tested positive.

The source of the THG was traced to a company that analyzed blood and urine from athletes and then prescribed a series of supplements to compensate for vitamin and mineral deficiencies. Among its clients were high-profile athletes in many professional and amateur sports. The ability to develop an undetectable steroid points to the disturbing ready market for such drugs among athletes who are prepared to try almost any substance to achieve success. THG served as the drug of choice for several high-profile Olympic gold medal winners, including sprinter Marion Jones, who resigned from her athletic career in 2007 after admitting to using THG prior to the 2000 Sydney Olympics, and New York Yankees' first baseman Jason Giambi. Although it is difficult to document illegal drug abuses among specific high-profile athletes in different sports worldwide, the IOC disqualified 30 athletes, mainly in biathlon and cross-country skiing, from participating in the 2010 winter Olympics after they tested positive for a variety of banned substances, including hGH. In the 2014 Sochi Winter Olympics, two Russian biathlon athletes tested positive for prohibited substances prior to competition and were banned from competition.

Prior to the 2012 summer London Olympics, Italian 50-km walk 2008 Beijing Olympics champion Alex Schwazer was banned from further competition until 2016 after testing positive for EPO. Doping is a criminal offense in Italy. His companion, Olympic bronze medalist figure skater Carolina Kostner, received a 16-month ban from competition for assisting Schwazer in covering up his doping, In the February 2014 Sochi Winter Olympics, three biathalon athletes (two Russian and one Lithuanian) tested positive for recombinant EPO prior to competition and were banned from competition. At one point, 300 international competitors had either received or were awaiting sanctions for illegal drug use, including some double violators who were banned in 1 year, served their suspension, and then were banned again following additional competition violations. Confirmed examples of doping violations and disqualification through December, 2014 include Turkish hammer thrower Elif Akbas (2013), Australian swimmer Anthony Alozie (2013), female Russian shot-putter Anna Avdeyeva (2013), female sprinter Anna Yagupova (2014), French marathoner Abraham Kiprotich (2013), and Finnish cross-country skier Juha Lallukka, whose ban was upheld after the Court of Arbitration for Sport in Lausanne, Switzerland (CAS; **www.tas-cas.org/news**), validated WADA's testing protocol for the hGH banned substance infraction.

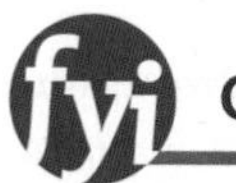

Competitive Athletes Beware

Elite athletes who take androstenedione can fail a urine test for the banned anabolic steroid nandrolone because the supplement often contains contaminates with trace amounts as low as 10 mg of 19-norandrosterone, the standard marker for nandrolone use. Many androstenedione preparations are grossly mislabeled. Analysis of nine different brands of 100-mg doses indicates wide fluctuations in overall content of androstenedione ranging from 0 to 103 mg, with one brand contaminated with testosterone.

Sources: Abbate V, et al. Anabolic steroids detected in bodybuilding dietary supplements—a significant risk to public health. *Drug Test Anal* 2014. (Doi 10.1002/dta.1728.)

Judkins C, Prock P. Supplements and inadvertent doping—how big is the risk to athletes. *Med Sport Sci* 2013;59:143.

Kamber M, et al. Nutritional supplements as a source for positive doping cases? *Int J Sport Nutr Exerc Metab* 2001;11:258.

Vaclavik L, et al. Mass spectrometric analysis of pharmaceutical adulterants in products labeled as botanical dietary supplements or herbal remedies: a review. *Anal Bioanal Chem* 2014;406:6767.

CLENBUTEROL: ANABOLIC STEROID SUBSTITUTE

Extensive random testing of competitive athletes for anabolic steroid use has produced a number of steroid substitutes obtainable on the illicit health food, mail order, and "black market" drug network. One such drug, the sympathomimetic amine **clenbuterol** (trade names Clenasma, Monores, Novegan, Prontovent, and Spiropent), remains popular among athletes because of its purported tissue-building and fat-reducing benefits. Typically, when bodybuilders discontinue steroid use before competition to avoid detection and possible disqualification, they substitute clenbuterol to maintain a steroid effect.

Clenbuterol, one of a group of chemical compounds classified as a β-adrenergic agonist (e.g., albuterol, clenbuterol, salbutamol, salmeterol, and terbutaline), is not approved for human use in the United States, but is commonly prescribed abroad as an inhaled bronchodilator to treat obstructive pulmonary disorders. Clenbuterol facilitates responsiveness of adrenergic receptors to circulating epinephrine, norepinephrine, and other adrenergic amines (**http://livertox.nlm.nih.gov/Beta2AdrenergicAgonists.htm**). A review of animal studies (no human studies exist) indicates that when sedentary, growing livestock receive clenbuterol in dosages in excess of those prescribed in Europe for human use for bronchial asthma, clenbuterol increases skeletal and cardiac muscle protein deposition and slows fat gain by enhancing lipolysis. Clenbuterol also has been experimentally used in animals with some success to counter the muscle-wasting effects of aging, immobilization, malnutrition, and zero-gravity exposure. The enlarged muscle size from clenbuterol treatment came from decreases in protein breakdown and increases in protein synthesis. Clenbuterol treatment induced muscular hypertrophy in young male rats but also inhibited longitudinal bone growth. Negative effects of clenbuterol and salbutamol affected mechanical properties and microarchitecture of animals' trabecular bone. An increase of muscle mass with enhanced bone fragility increases fracture risk when β_2-agonists are included as part of a doping regimen.

Reported short-term side effects in humans accidentally "overdosing" from eating animals that were treated with clenbuterol include muscle tremor, agitation, palpitations, muscle cramps, rapid heart rate, and headache. Despite such negative side effects, supervised use of clenbuterol may prove beneficial for humans with muscle wasting from disease, forced immobilization, and aging. Unfortunately, no data exist for its potential toxicity level in humans or its efficacy and safety in long-term use. Clearly, clenbuterol use cannot be justified and should not be used as an ergogenic aid.

HUMAN GROWTH HORMONE: THE STEROID COMPETITOR

Human growth hormone (hGH or GH), also known as somatotropic hormone, competes with anabolic steroids in the illicit market of alleged tissue-building PEDs. This hormone, produced by the pituitary gland's adenohypophysis, facilitates tissue-building processes and normal human growth. Specifically, hGH stimulates bone and cartilage growth, enhances fatty acid oxidation, and slows glucose and amino acid breakdown. Reduced hGH secretion (about 50% less at age 60 than at age 30) accounts for some of the decrease in FFM and increase in fat mass that accompany aging; reversal occurs with exogenous hGH supplements produced by genetically engineered bacteria.

Children with kidney failure or those hGH-deficient take hGH to help stimulate long bone growth. hGH use appeals to strength and power athletes because, at physiologic levels, it stimulates amino acid uptake and protein synthesis by muscle while enhancing fat breakdown and conserving glycogen reserves.

Research produced equivocal results concerning true benefits of hGH supplementation to counter the loss of muscle mass, thinning bones, increased body fat (particularly abdominal fat), and depressed energy levels. For example, 16 previously sedentary young men who participated in a 12-week resistance-training program received daily recombinant hGH ($40\ g \cdot kg^{-1}$) or a placebo. FFM, total body water, and whole-body protein synthesis (attributed to increased nitrogen retention in lean tissue other than skeletal muscle) increased more in the hGH recipients, with no differences between groups in fractional rate of protein synthesis in skeletal muscle, torso and limb circumferences, or muscle function in dynamic and static strength measures.

One of the largest studies to date determined the effects of hGH on changes in the body composition and functional capacity of healthy men and women who ranged in age from the mid-1960s to the late 1980s. Men who took hGH gained 7 lb of lean body mass and lost a similar amount of fat mass compared to a group taking a placebo. Women gained about 3 lb of lean body mass and lost 5 lb of body fat while comparable values remained unchanged for the placebo group. The subjects remained sedentary and did not change their diet over the 6-month study duration. Unfortunately, serious side effects affected between 24% and 46% of the subjects. These included swollen feet and ankles, joint pain, carpal tunnel syndrome (swelling of tendon sheath over a nerve in the wrist), and development of a diabetic or prediabetic condition. As in previous research, no effects occurred for hGH treatment on measures of muscular strength or endurance capacity despite increases in lean body mass.

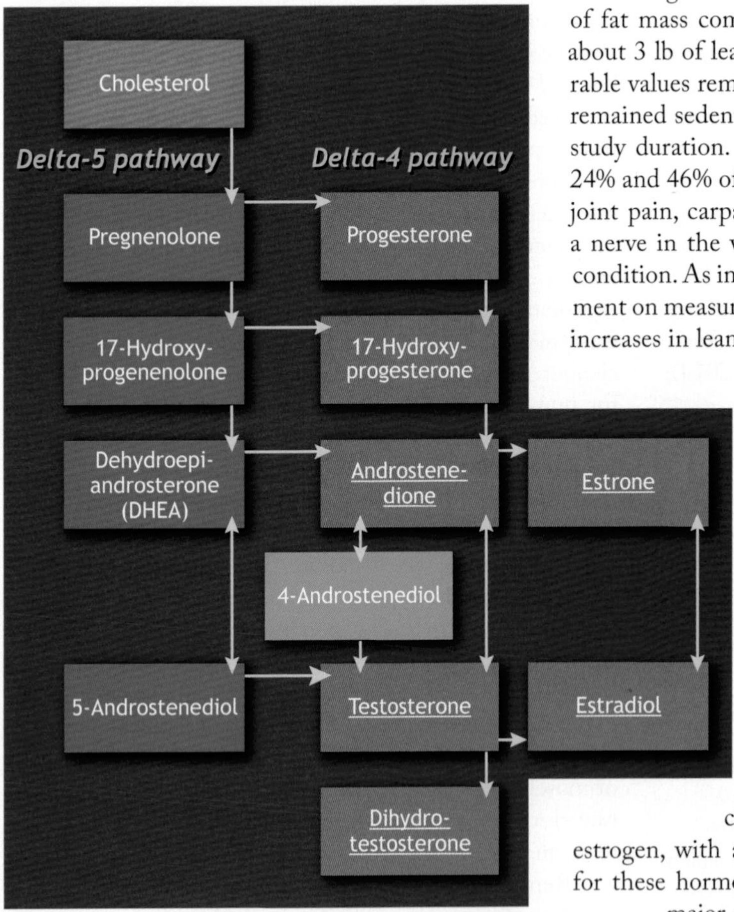

FIGURE 4.12 Outline of metabolic pathways for dehydroepiandrosterone (DHEA), androstenedione, and related compounds. *Directional arrows* signify one-way and two-way conversions. Compounds underlined are DHEA-precursor products currently available on the market. (Used with permission from McArdle WD, Katch FI, Katch VL. *Exercise Physiology: Nutrition, Energy, and Human Performance*. 8th Ed. Baltimore: Wolters Kluwer Health, 2015.)

DHEA: "WONDER DRUG?"

Use of synthetic **dehydroepiandrosterone (DHEA)** (marketed under the names *Prastera*, *Fidelin*, and *Fluasterone*) among athletes and the general population raises concerns from safety and effectiveness issues. DHEA and its sulfated ester, DHEAS, are relatively weak steroid hormones synthesized from cholesterol in the adrenal cortex. The quantity of DHEA (commonly referred to as "*mother hormone*") produced by the body surpasses all other known steroids; its chemical structure closely resembles the sex hormones testosterone and estrogen, with a minute amount of DHEA serving as a precursor for these hormones for men and women. **Figure 4.12** outlines the major pathways for synthesizing DHEA, androstenedione, and related compounds. The *yellow* directional arrows signify one-way and two-way conversions, including intermediate compounds. Those underlined serve as DHEA-precursor products currently available on the market. For example, androstenedione, the popular 19-carbon steroid hormone produced in gonads and adrenal glands, serves as an intermediary step that eventually forms testosterone, estrone, and estradiol. These conversions require specialized enzymes (e.g., 17β-hydroxysteroid dehydrogenase for testosterone and aromatase for estrone and estradiol). Many of these **prohormone** compounds can only be purchased with a medical prescription and, in the case of androstenedione, may produce undesirable estrogenic side effects including breast enlargement or tenderness, ankle and leg swelling, appetite loss, water retention, vomiting, abdominal cramping, and bloating.

DHEA occurs naturally in the body, so the FDA exerts no control over its distribution or claims for its action and effectiveness. The lay press, Internet sites, mail order catalogs, and the health food industry describe DHEA as a "superhormone" to increase testosterone production; preserve youth; protect against heart disease, cancer, diabetes, and osteoporosis; invigorate sex drive; facilitate lean tissue gain and body fat loss; enhance mood and memory; extend life; and boost immunity to a variety of infectious diseases (including AIDS). The WADA and USOC include DHEA on their banned substance lists at zero-tolerance levels.

Figure 4.13 illustrates the generalized trend for plasma DHEA levels during a lifetime plus six common claims made by manufacturers for DHEA supplements. For boys and girls, DHEA levels are substantial at birth and then decline sharply. A steady increase in DHEA production occurs from age 6 to 10, an occurrence that some researchers believe contributes to the beginning of puberty and sexuality. This is followed by a rapid increase, with peak production, higher in young men than young women, reached between ages 18 and 25.

In contrast to the glucocorticoid and mineralocorticoid adrenal steroids whose plasma levels remain relatively high with aging, a long, steady decline in DHEA occurs after age 30. By age 75, plasma levels decrease to only about 20% of the value in young adulthood. This trend has fueled speculation that DHEA plasma levels might serve as a biochemical marker of biologic aging and disease susceptibility. Popular reasoning concludes that supplementing with DHEA diminishes the negative effects of aging by increasing plasma levels to more youthful concentrations. Many people supplement with this hormone "just in case" it proves beneficial, without concern for its long-term safety.

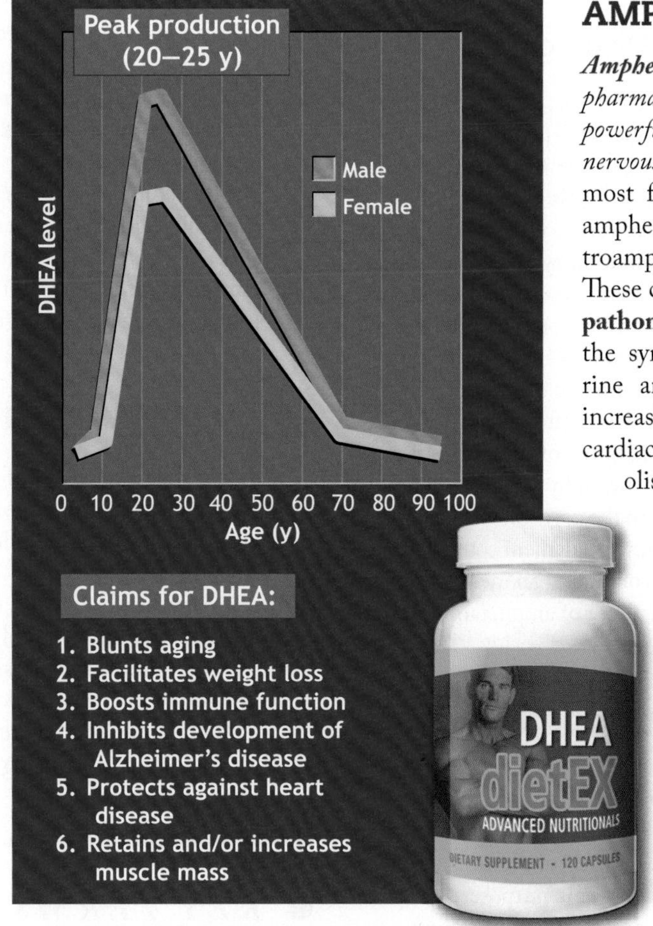

FIGURE 4.13 Generalized trend for plasma levels of DHEA for men and women over a lifetime. (Adapted with permission from McArdle WD, Katch FI, Katch VL. *Sports and Exercise Nutrition*. 4th Ed. Philadelphia: Wolters Kluwer Health, 2013.)

DHEA Safety

In 1994, the FDA reclassified DHEA from the category of unapproved new drug with a prescription required for use to a dietary supplement for sale over-the-counter without a prescription. Despite its quantitative significance as a hormone, researchers know little about DHEA's relationship to health and aging, cellular or molecular mechanisms of action, and possible receptor sites and the potential for negative side effects from exogenous dosage, particularly among young adults with normal DHEA levels. *The appropriate DHEA dosage for humans has not been determined.* Concern exists about possible harmful effects on blood lipids, glucose tolerance, and prostate gland health, particularly because medical problems associated with hormone supplementation often do not appear until years after their first use. *Despite its popularity among exercise enthusiasts, no data support an ergogenic effect of exogenous DHEA among young adult men and women.*

AMPHETAMINES

Amphetamines *or "pep pills" consist of pharmacologic compounds that exert a powerful stimulating effect on central nervous system function.* Athletes most frequently use the compounds amphetamine (Benzedrine) and dextroamphetamine sulfate (Dexedrine). These compounds, referred to as **sympathomimetics**, mimic the actions of the sympathetic hormones epinephrine and norepinephrine to trigger increases in blood pressure, heart rate, cardiac output, breathing rate, metabolism, and blood glucose. Taking 5 to 20 mg of amphetamine usually produces an effect that lasts for 30 to 90 minutes. Amphetamines supposedly increase alertness, wakefulness, and augment work capacity by depressing sensations of muscle fatigue. The deaths of two famed cyclists in the 1960s during competitive road racing were attributed to amphetamine use for just such purposes. Soldiers in World War II commonly "popped" amphetamines to increase their alertness and reduce fatigue, and athletes use amphetamines for the same purpose.

Serious Amphetamine Dangers

Amphetamine dangers include the following:

- Continual use can lead to physiologic or emotional drug dependency. This often causes cyclical dependency on "uppers" (amphetamines) or "downers" (barbiturates). Barbiturates blunt or tranquilize the "hyper" state brought on by amphetamines.
- General side effects include headache, tremulousness, agitation, insomnia, nausea, dizziness, and confusion, all of which negatively impact sports performance.
- Prolonged use eventually requires more of the drug to achieve the same effect because drug tolerance increases; this may aggravate and even precipitate cardiovascular and serious psychologic disorders. Medical risks include hypertension, stroke, sudden death, and glucose intolerance.
- Ongoing use may inhibit or suppress the body's normal mechanisms to perceive and respond to pain, fatigue, and heat stress, severely jeopardizing health and safety.
- Prolonged high doses produce weight loss, paranoia, psychosis, repetitive compulsive behavior, and nerve damage.

Amphetamines and Athletic Performance

Athletes take amphetamines to get "up" psychologically for competition. On the day or evening before a contest, competitors often feel nervous or irritable and have difficulty relaxing. Under these circumstances, a barbiturate induces sleep. The athlete then regains the "hyper" condition by taking an "upper." This undesirable cycle of depressant-to-stimulant becomes dangerous because the stimulant acts abnormally after barbiturate intake. Knowledgeable and prudent sports professionals urge banning amphetamines from athletic competition. Most athletic governing groups have rules regarding athletes who use amphetamines. Ironically, the majority of research indicates that amphetamines do not enhance physical performance. Perhaps their greatest influence is in the psychological realm, as naive athletes believe that taking any supplement contributes to superior performance. A placebo containing an inert substance often produces results identical to those of amphetamines.

SUMMARY

1. Caffeine exerts an ergogenic effect in extending aerobic exercise duration by increasing fat utilization for energy, thus conserving glycogen reserves.
2. Anabolic steroids comprise a group of pharmacologic agents frequently used for ergogenic purposes.
3. Anabolic steroids function similar to the hormone testosterone; with resistance training, they may increase muscle size, strength, and power.
4. Undesirable side effects accompany anabolic steroid use including infertility; reduced sperm concentrations; decreased testicular volume; gynecomastia; connective tissue damage that decreases tendon tensile strength and elastic compliance; chromosome damage, apoptosis, and necrosis in exfoliated cells; and increased risk of stroke and acute myocardial infarction.
5. Androstenedione supplementation does not impact basal serum concentrations of testosterone or training response for muscle size, strength, and body composition.
6. Androstenedione supplementation includes the potentially negative effects of lowered HDL-C on heart disease risk and elevated serum estrogen level on gynecomastia risk and possibly pancreatic and other cancers.
7. THG often escapes detection using normal drug testing, which caused the initiation of retesting urine samples from competitors in diverse sports.
8. The β_2-adrenergic agonist clenbuterol increases skeletal muscle mass and slows fat gain in animals to counter the effects of aging, immobilization, malnutrition, and tissue-wasting pathology.
9. Debate exists about whether healthy people who take hGH augment muscular hypertrophy when combined with resistance training.
10. DHEA is a relatively weak steroid hormone synthesized from cholesterol by the adrenal cortex.
11. DHEA levels steadily decrease throughout adulthood, but research does not indicate a DHEA ergogenic effect.
12. Little credible evidence exists that amphetamines or "pep pills" aid exercise performance or psychomotor skills any better than inert placebos.
13. Amphetamine side effects include drug dependency, headache, dizziness, confusion, and stomach upset.

THINK IT THROUGH

1. Discuss the importance of the psychologic or "placebo" effect to evaluate claims for the effectiveness of particular nutrients, chemicals, or procedures as ergogenic aids.
2. If testosterone, hGH, and DHEA occur naturally in the body, what harm could exist in supplementing with these "natural" compounds?
3. Outline the main points you would make in a talk to a high school football team concerning whether they should consider using performance-enhancing chemicals and hormones.

KEY TERMS

Amphetamines: Group of pharmacologic compounds that exert powerful stimulating effects on central nervous system function.

Anabolic steroids: Chemical compounds that function similarly to the male hormone testosterone.

Androstenedione: Intermediate precursor hormone between DHEA and testosterone used by the body to synthesize testosterone and estrogen; aids the liver in synthesizing other biologically active steroid hormones.

ß-Hydroxy–ß-methylbutyrate (HMB): Bioactive metabolite generated in the breakdown of the essential branched-chain amino acid leucine; decreases protein loss during stress by inhibiting protein catabolism.

Buffering system: Defends against increased intracellular H^+ concentration.

Caffeine: Group of lipid-soluble purines (proper chemical name 1,3,7-trimethylxanthine) occurring naturally in coffee beans, tea leaves, chocolate, cocoa beans, and cola nuts and often added to carbonated beverages and nonprescription medicines. Also serves as a central nervous system stimulant that temporarily attenuates drowsiness and restores alertness.

Chromium: Trace mineral that serves as a cofactor for a low–molecular-weight protein that potentiates insulin functions.

Chromium picolinate: Popular chelated picolinic acid combination that purportedly yields better chromium absorption than does chromium chloride.

Clenbuterol: Compound classified as β_2-adrenergic agonist (e.g., albuterol [salbutamol], bitolterol, salmeterol, metaproterenol, pirbuterol, terbutaline, and formoterol), which facilitates adrenergic receptor responsiveness to circulating epinephrine, norepinephrine, and other adrenergic amines.

Cortisol: Releasing factor that stimulates the anterior pituitary gland to release adrenocorticotropic hormone (ACTH), which induces the adrenal cortex to discharge the glucocorticoid hormone cortisol (hydrocortisone); decreases amino acid transport into the cell, which depresses anabolism and stimulates protein breakdown to its building block amino acids in all cells except the liver.

Creatine: Nitrogen-containing organic acid synthesized from the nonessential amino acids arginine, glycine, and methionine and as part of PCr ("the energy reservoir") that supplies immediate phosphate-bond energy to resynthesize ATP.

Creatine monohydrate (CrH_2O): Popular form of creatine sold in supplemental form as a powder, tablet, capsule, and stabilized liquid.

Dehydroepiandrosterone (DHEA): The body's most produced known steroid with a chemical structure closely resembling testosterone and estrogen; serves as a weak steroid hormone that the adrenal cortex synthesizes primarily from cholesterol.

Diuretics: Facilitate the kidney's urine production and in steroid-using athletes may reduce the urine's concentration of a banned or illegal substance, potentially decreasing the probability of its discovery.

Double-blinded experiment: Both investigator and subjects remain unaware of the treatment condition.

Ephedrine: Potent amphetaminelike alkaloid compound with sympathomimetic physiologic effects; present in several species of the ephedra plant.

Ergogenic aids: Substances and procedures believed to improve exercise capacity, physiologic function, and/or athletic performance.

Erythropoietin (EPO): Glycoprotein hormone produced by the kidney and liver, which controls red blood cell production via its effect on bone marrow red blood cell precursors.

Glutamine: Plasma and skeletal muscle amino acid accounting for more than half of the muscles' free amino acid pool; augments protein synthesis via its anticatabolic effects.

Gynecomastia: Anabolic steroid side effect that results in excessive male mammary gland development.

Half-life: Time required for the concentration of a biological substance to reach half of its original value.

Human growth hormone (hGH or GH): Hormone produced by the pituitary gland's adenohypophysis; potent anabolic and lipolytic agent in tissue-building processes and growth. Also stimulates bone and cartilage growth, enhances fatty acid oxidation, and reduces breakdown of glucose and amino acid.

Medium chain triacylglycerols (MCTs): Processed oils containing saturated fatty acids with 8- to 10-carbon atoms along the fatty acid chain frequently produced for patients with intestinal malabsorption and other tissue-wasting diseases; provide a more rapid source of fatty acid fuel than their longer chain counterparts.

Meta-analysis: application of quantitative statistical methods to analyze results of separate but similar experiments or studies to identify patterns among study results.

Peer review: Colleagues with expertise in a targeted area of scientific investigation and research provide critical assessment and evaluation of research by others, usually for manuscript submission to scientific journals and grant application process.

Peliosis hepatis: Development of localized blood-filled lesions; serious medical condition with potentially fatal consequences, often from longer-term anabolic steroid abuse.

Performance-enhancing drugs (PEDs): Substances used to improve performance; usually in reference to anabolic steroids or their precursors; stimulants; cognition enhancers; painkillers; sedatives and blood boosters (EPO) used by athletes

Phosphatidylserine (PS): Glycerophospholipid typical of a natural lipid class that constitutes the structural components of the internal layer of the plasma membrane that surrounds all cells; modifies the neuroendocrine stress response.

Prohormone: Inactive precursor compound that converts to its functioning hormone.

Proteolysis: Protein breakdown during digestion into simpler, soluble substances including peptides and amino acids.

Pyramiding: Progressively altering drug dosage, usually in multiple day, weekly, and monthly cycles.

Pyruvate: Three-carbon end product of cytoplasmic glucose breakdown in glycolysis. Ergogenic effects of exogenous pyruvate may act as a partial dietary carbohydrate replacement to augment endurance performance and promote fat loss.

Randomization: Volunteer participants in an experiment must be assigned at random (no definite plan, pattern, or sequence so the assignment has an equal probability of occurrence) to a control or experimental condition.

Roid rage: Outbursts of physical or verbal anger, frustration, extreme mood swings, combativeness, and agressiveness in anabolic steroid users.

Stacking: Doping process combining multiple steroid preparations in oral and injectable form.

Sympathomimetics: Stimulant compounds that mimic the effects of neurotransmitter substances of the sympathetic nervous system including catecholamines and dopamine.

Tetrahydrogestrinone (THG or "The Clear"): Anabolic steroid specifically designed to escape detection by normal drug testing that has affinity to androgen and progesterone receptors, but not the estrogen receptor; closely related to the banned anabolic steroids gestrinone and trenbolone.

World Anti-Doping Agency (WADA): Independent foundation to promote, coordinate, and monitor the war against drugs in sport worldwide (**www.wada-ama.org**).

SELECTED REFERENCES

Ali A, et al. The effect of caffeine ingestion during evening exercise on subsequent sleep quality in females. *Int J Sports Med* 2015. (In Press as of 05.15.15.)

An SM, et al. Effect of energy drink dose on exercise capacity, heart rate recovery and heart rate variability after high-intensity exercise. *J Exerc Nutrition Biochem* 2014;18:31.

Angell PJ, et al. Anabolic steroid use and longitudinal, radial, and circumferential cardiac motion. *Med Sci Sports Exerc* 2012;44;583.

Armstrong LE, et al. Caffeine, fluid-electrolyte balance, temperature regulation, and exercise-heat tolerance. *Exerc Sport Sci Rev* 2007;35:135.

Bassit RA, et al. Effect of short-term creatine supplementation on markers of skeletal muscle damage after strenuous contractile activity. *Eur J Appl Physiol* 2010;108:945.

Baty JJ, et al. The effect of a carbohydrate and protein supplement on resistance exercise performance, hormonal response, and muscle damage. *J Strength Cond Res* 2007;21:321.

Bellinger PM, et al. Effect of combined ß-alanine and sodium bicarbonate supplementation on cycling performance. *Med Sci Sports Exerc* 2012;44:1545.

Betts JA, Stevenson E. Should protein be included in CHO-based sports supplements? *Med Sci Sports Exerc* 2011;43:1244.

Bhasin S, et al. The effects of supraphysiological doses of testosterone on muscle size and strength in normal men. *N Engl J Med* 1996;335:1.

Bishop D, et al. Induced metabolic alkalosis affects muscle metabolism and repeated-sprint activity. *Med Sci Sports Exerc* 2004;36:807.

Blackman MR, et al. Growth hormone and sex steroid administration in healthy aged women and men: a randomized controlled trial. *JAMA* 2002;288:2282.

Bortolotti H, et al. Performance during a 20-km cycling time-trial after caffeine ingestion. *J Int Soc Sports Nutr* 2014;11:45.

Buck CL, et al. Sodium phosphate as an ergogenic aid. *Sports Med* 2013;43:425.

Bunsawat K, et al. Caffeine delays autonomic recovery following acute exercise [Epub ahead of print]. *Eur J Prev Cardiol* October 8, 2014. pii: 2047487314554867.

Burke LM, Maughan RJ. The Governor has a sweet tooth—mouth sensing of nutrients to enhance sports performance. *Eur J Sport Sci* 2014;27:1.

Cellini M, et al. Dietary supplements: physician knowledge and adverse event reporting. *Med Sci Sports Exerc* 2013;45:23.

Coggan AR, et al. Effect of acute dietary nitrate intake on maximal knee extensor speed and power in healthy men and women. *Nitric Oxide* 2014. (In press as of 05.15.15.)

Collier SR, et al. Oral arginine attenuates the growth hormone response to resistance exercise. *J Appl Physiol* 2006;101:848.

Darvishi L, et al. The use of nutritional supplements among male collegiate athletes. *Int J Prev Med* 2013;4:S68.

Decorte NS, et al. Effects of acute salbutamol inhalation on quadriceps force and fatigability. *Med Sci Sports Exerc* 2008;40:1220.

DeLorey DS, et al. Prior exercise speeds pulmonary O_2 uptake kinetics by increases in both local muscle O_2 availability and O_2 utilization. *J Appl Physiol* 2007;103:771.

Deuster PA, et al. A-Z of nutritional supplements: dietary supplements, sports nutrition foods and ergogenic aids for health and performance: part 46. *Br J Sports Med* 2013;47:809.

Do Carmo EC, et al. Anabolic steroid associated to physical training induces deleterious cardiac effects. *Med Sci Sports Exerc* 2011;43:1836.

Douroudos I, et al. Dose-related effects of prolonged $NaHCO_3$ ingestion during high-intensity exercise. *Med Sci Sports Exerc* 2006;38:1746.

Eibye, K, et al. Formoterol concentrations in blood and Urine: the World Anti-Doping Agency 2012 Regulations. *Med Sci Sports Exerc* 2013;45:16.

Eichner ER. Fatal caffeine overdose and other risks from dietary supplements. *Curr Sports Med Rep* 2014;13:353.

Erskine RM, et al. Whey protein does not enhance the adaptations to elbow flexor resistance training. *Med Sci Sports Exerc* 2012;44:1791.

Faulkner SH, et al. Reducing muscle temperature drop after warm-up improves sprint cycling performance. *Med Sci Sports Exerc* 2013;45:359.

Fleck SJ, et al. Anaerobic power effects of an amino acid supplement containing no branched amino acids in elite competitive athletes. *J Strength Cond Res* 1995;9:132.

Godfrey RJ, et al. A-Z of nutritional supplements: dietary supplements, sports nutrition foods and ergogenic aids for health and performance: part 45. *Br J Sports Med* 2013;47:659.

Gordon SE, et al. The influence of age and exercise modality on growth hormone bioactivity in women. *Growth Horm IGF Res* 2014;24:95.

Hackett DA, et al. Training practices and ergogenic aids used by male bodybuilders. *J Strength Cond Res* 2013;27:1609.

Hogervorst E, et al. Caffeine improves physical and cognitive performance during exhaustive exercise. *Med Sci Sports Exerc* 2008;40:1841.

Ihalainen J, et al. Acute leukocyte, cytokine and adipocytokine responses to maximal and hypertrophic resistance exercise bouts. *Eur J Appl Physiol* 2014;114:2607.

Judkins C, Prock P. Supplements and inadvertent doping—how big is the risk to athletes. *Med Sport Sci* 2013;59:143.

Kraemer WJ, et al. Effects of amino acids supplement on physiological adaptations to resistance training. *Med Sci Sports Exerc* 2009;41:1111.

Kraemer WJ, et al. Growth hormone, exercise, and athletic performance: a continued evolution of complexity. *Curr Sports Med Rep* 2010;9:242.

Kraemer WJ, et al. The order effect of combined endurance and strength loadings on force and hormone responses: effects of prolonged training. *Eur J Appl Physiol* 2014;114:867

Kraemer WJ, et al. The effects of exercise training programs on plasma concentrations of proenkephalin Peptide F and catecholamines. *Peptides* 2015; 64:74.

Kraemer WJ, et al. Influence of HMB supplementation and resistance training on cytokine responses to resistance exercise. *J Am Coll Nutr* 2014;33:247.

Leenders M, et al. Protein supplementation during resistance-type exercise training in the elderly. *Med Sci Sports Exerc* 2013;45:543.

Lönnberg M, Lundby C. Detection of EPO injections using a rapid lateral flow isoform test. *Anal Bioanal Chem* 2013;405:9685.

Lukaski HC, et al. Chromium supplementation and resistance training: effects on body composition, strength, and trace element status of men. *Am J Clin Nutr* 1996;63:954.

Maughan RJ. Quality assurance issues in the use of dietary supplements, with special reference to protein supplements. *J Nutr* 2013;143:1843S.

McNaughton LR, et al. Ergogenic effects of sodium bicarbonate. *Curr Sports Med Rep* 2008;7:230.

Meinhardt U, et al. The effects of growth hormone on body composition and physical performance in recreational athletes: a randomized trial. *Ann Intern Med* 2010;152:568.

Mohr M, et al. Caffeine intake improves intense intermittent exercise performance and reduces muscle interstitial potassium accumulation. *J Appl Physiol* 2011;111:1373.

Morrison PJ, et al. Adding protein to a carbohydrate supplement provided after endurance exercise enhances 4E-BP1 and RPS6 signaling in skeletal muscle. *J Appl Physiol* 2008;104:1029.

Müller W, Maughan RJ. The need for a novel approach to measure body composition: is ultrasound an answer? *Br J Sports Med* 2013;47:1001.

Neves M Jr, et al. Beneficial effect of creatine supplementation in knee osteoarthritis. *Med Sci Sports Exerc* 2011;43:1538.

Northgraves MJ, et al. Effect of lactate supplementation and sodium bicarbonate on 40 km cycling time trial performance. *J Strength Cond Res* 2014;28:273.

O'Connor DM, Crowe MJ. Effects of six weeks of beta-hydroxy-beta-methylbutyrate (HMB) and HMB/creatine supplementation on strength, power, and anthropometry of highly trained athletes. *J Strength Cond Res* 2007;21:419.

Outlaw JJ, et al. Acute effects of a commercially-available pre-workout supplement on markers of training: a double-blind study. *J Int Soc Sports Nutr* 2014;11:40.

Palisin T, Stacy JJ. Beta-hydroxy-methylbutyrate and its use in athletics. *Curr Sports Med Reports* 2005;4:220.
Parkinson AB, Evans NA. Anabolic androgenic steroids: a survey of 500 users. *Med Sci Sports Exerc* 2006;38:644.
Peeling P, et al. Beetroot juice improves on-water 500 m time-trial performance, and laboratory-based paddling economy in national and international-level Kayak athletes. *Int J Sport Nutr Exerc Metab* 2014. (In press as of 05.15.15.)
Saremi A, et al. Effects of oral creatine and resistance training on serum mostatin and GASP-1. *Mol Cell Endocrinol* 2010;317:25.
Schubert MM, Astorino TA. A systematic review of the efficacy of ergogenic aids for improving running performance. *J Strength Cond Res* 2013;27:1699.
Scott AT, et al. Caffeinated carbohydrate gel ingestion improves 2000 metre rowing performance. *Int J Sports Physiol Perform* 2015;10:464.
Shearer J, Graham TE. Performance effects and metabolic consequences of caffeine and caffeinated energy drink consumption on glucose disposal. *Nutr Rev* 2014;72:121.
Sökmen B, et al. Caffeine use in sports: considerations for the athlete. *J Strength Cond Res* 2008;22:978.
Spriet LL, et al. Legal pre-event nutritional supplements to assist energy metabolism. *Essays Biochem* 2008;22:978.
Spriet LL. Exercise and sport performance with low doses of caffeine. *Sports Med* 2014;44:175.
Souza JP, et al. Chromosome damage, apoptosis, and necrosis in exfoliated cells of oral mucosa from androgenic anabolic steroids users. *J Toxicol Environ Health A* 2015;78:67.
Sterczala AJ, et al. Similar hormonal stress and tissue damage in response to national collegiate athletic association division I football games played in two consecutive seasons. *J Strength Cond Res* 2014;28:3234.
Tipton KD, et al. Acute response of net muscle protein balance reflects 24-h balance after exercise and amino acid ingestion. *Am J Physiol* 2003;284:E76.
Tipton KD, et al. Ingestion of casein and whey proteins result in muscle anabolism after resistance exercise. *Med Sci Sports Exerc* 2004;36:2073.
Vierck JL, et al. The effects of ergogenic compounds on myogenic satellite cells. *Med Sci Sports Exerc* 2003;35:769.
Vistisen B, et al. Minor amounts of plasma medium-chain fatty acids and no improved time trial performance after consuming lipids. *J Appl Physiol* 2003;95:2434.
Whittaker JP, et al. Effect of aerobic interval training and caffeine on blood platelet function. *Med Sci Sports Exerc* 2013;45:342.
Wilson GJ, et al. Effects of beta-hydroxy-beta-methylbutyrate (HMB) on exercise performance and body composition across varying levels of age, sex, and training experience: a review. *Nutr Metab (Lond)* 2008;3:5.
Wolfe RR. Regulation of muscle protein by amino acids. *J Nutr* 2002; 132:3219S.
Xu ZR, et al. Clinical effectiveness of protein and amino acid supplementation on building muscle mass in elderly people: a meta-analysis. *PLoS One* 2014;9:e109141.
Yang Y, et al. Resistance exercise enhances myofibrillar protein synthesis with graded intakes of whey protein in older men. *Br J Nutr* 2012;108:1.
Yau AM, et al. Short-term dietary supplementation with fructose accelerates gastric emptying of a fructose but not a glucose solution. *Nutrition* 2014;30:1344.

SECTION III

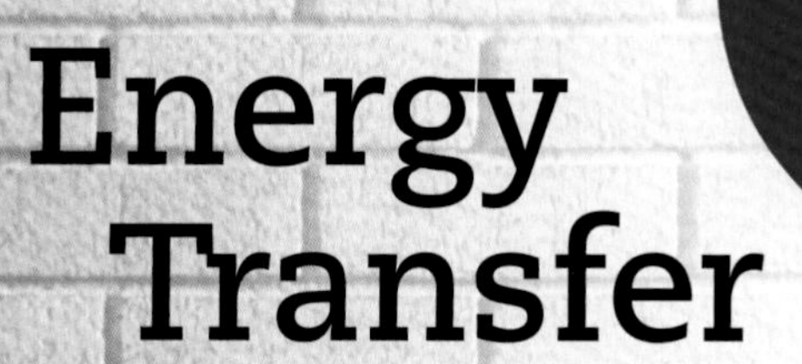

Energy Transfer

Biochemical reactions that do not use oxygen generate considerable energy for short durations. This rapid energy generation becomes crucial in maintaining a high performance standard in sprint activities and other bursts of all-out physical activity. In contrast, longer-duration aerobic activity extracts energy more slowly from food catabolism through chemical reactions that require oxygen's continual use. Three factors impact how to plan effective training to enhance performance:

1. Understand basic information about how muscle tissue generates energy to sustain physical activity
2. Recognize the sources that provide that energy
3. Determine energy requirements of diverse physical activities

This section presents a broad overview of human energy transfer during rest and physical activity. We emphasize how the body's cells extract chemical energy bound within food molecules and transfer it to a common compound that powers every form of human biologic work. We focus on food nutrients and processes of energy transfer that play pivotal roles in sustaining physiologic function during light, moderate, and strenuous physical activity, including laboratory techniques to assess diverse human energy transfer capacities.

I often say that when you can measure what you are speaking about, and express it in numbers, you know something about it; but when you cannot measure it, when you cannot express it in numbers, your knowledge is of a meagre and unsatisfactory kind.

— *Lord Kelvin (William Thomson, 1st Baron) (1824–1907), English physicist and mathematician*

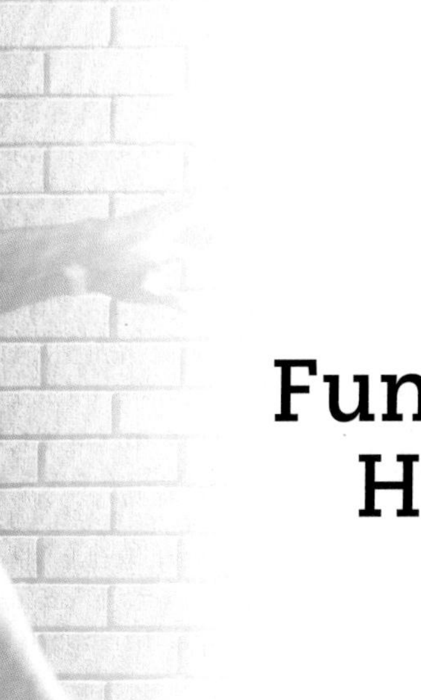

CHAPTER 5

Fundamentals of Human Energy Transfer

CHAPTER OBJECTIVES

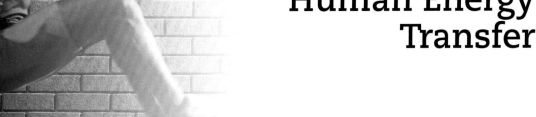

- Describe the first law of thermodynamics related to energy balance and biologic work.
- Define *potential energy* and *kinetic energy* and give two examples of each.
- Give two examples of exergonic and endergonic chemical processes within the body, and indicate their importance.
- State the second law of thermodynamics, and give two practical applications.
- Identify and give examples of three forms of biologic work.
- Discuss the major roles of enzymes and coenzymes in bioenergetics.
- Identify the high-energy phosphates, and discuss their contributions in powering biologic work.
- Outline the process of electron transport–oxidative phosphorylation.
- Explain oxygen's main role in human energy metabolism.
- Describe how anaerobic energy release occurs in cells.
- Describe lactate formation during progressively increasing intensity of physical effort.
- Outline the general pathways of the citric acid cycle during macronutrient catabolism.
- Contrast the adenosine triphosphate yield from carbohydrate, fat, and protein catabolism.
- Explain the statement, "Fats burn in a carbohydrate flame."

ANCILLARIES AT A GLANCE

Visit **http://thePoint.lww.com/MKKESS5e** to access the following resources.

- References: Chapter 5
- Interactive Question Bank
- Animation: Alanine-Glucose Cycle
- Animation: Biochemical Reactions of Cori Cycle
- Animation: Catabolism
- Animation: Chemical Reactions of Mitochondrion
- Animation: Citric Acid Cycle
- Animation: Electron Transport
- Animation: Energy Transfer Chain
- Animation: Exercise and Blood Flow
- Animation: Glycolysis
- Animation: Hydrolysis
- Animation: Muscle Contraction
- Animation: Oxygen Consumption
- Animation: Triacylglycerol Breakdown

The body's capacity to extract energy from food nutrients and transfer it to skeletal muscle's contractile elements determines the capacity for physical movement. Energy transfer occurs through thousands of complex chemical reactions that require the proper mixture of macronutrients and micronutrients continually fueled by oxygen. The term **aerobic** describes such oxygen-requiring energy reactions. In contrast, **anaerobic** energy reactions generate energy rapidly from chemical reactions without oxygen. *The anaerobic and aerobic breakdown of ingested food nutrients provides the energy source to synthesize the chemical fuel that powers all forms of biologic work.*

This chapter presents an overview of the different energy forms and factors that impact energy generation. The chapter also discusses how the body obtains energy to power its diverse functions. A basic understanding of carbohydrate, fat, and protein catabolism and concurrent anaerobic and aerobic energy transfer provides the basis for much of the subject matter content of exercise physiology. Knowledge about human bioenergetics guides the practical basis to formulate sport-specific training regimens, recommending activities for physical fitness and weight control, and advocating prudent dietary modifications for specific sport requirements.

PART 1 Energy—The Capacity for Work

Unlike the physical properties of matter, one cannot define **energy** in concrete terms of size, shape, or mass. Rather, the term *energy* suggests a dynamic state related to change; thus, the presence of energy emerges only when change occurs. Within this context, energy relates to the performance of work and the occurrence of change. Stated somewhat differently, as work increases, so does energy transfer.

The **first law of thermodynamics**, one of the most important principles related to biologic work, states that energy cannot be created or destroyed; rather it is transformed from one form to another without being depleted. In essence, this law describes the immutable principle of the **conservation of energy**. *In the body, chemical energy stored within the macronutrient's bonds does not immediately dissipate as heat during energy metabolism. Instead, a large portion remains as chemical energy, which the musculoskeletal system then changes into mechanical energy and then ultimately to heat energy.*

POTENTIAL AND KINETIC ENERGY

***Potential energy** and **kinetic energy** constitute the system's total energy.* **Figure 5.1** shows potential energy as energy of position, similar to water at the top of a mountain or dam before it flows downstream. In the example of flowing water, the energy change is proportional to the water's vertical drop; the greater the vertical drop, the greater water's potential energy at the top. A waterwheel inserted into the flow of the falling water, as practiced for many centuries in countries around the world, could harness some of the energy to produce useful work.

Other examples of potential energy include bound energy within the internal structure of a battery, a stick of dynamite, or a macronutrient before release of its stored energy in human metabolism. *Releasing potential energy transforms the basic ingredient into kinetic energy of motion.* In some cases, bound energy in one substance directly transfers to other substances to increase their potential energy. Energy transfers of this type provide the required energy for the body's chemical work of **biosynthesis**. In this process, specific building-block atoms of carbon, hydrogen, oxygen, and nitrogen become activated and join other atoms and molecules to synthesize important biologic compounds and tissues. Some newly created compounds provide structure as in bone or each cell's outer lipid-containing plasma membrane. The synthesized compounds adenosine triphosphate (ATP) and phosphocreatine (PCr) provide the main source of the cell's energy requirements.

ENERGY-RELEASING AND ENERGY-CONSERVING PROCESSES

The term **exergonic** describes any physical or chemical process that releases or frees up energy to its surroundings. Such reactions represent "downhill" processes; they produce a decline in free energy—"useful" energy for biologic work that encompasses all of the cell's energy-requiring, life-sustaining processes. In contrast, **endergonic** chemical processes store or absorb energy; these reactions represent "uphill" processes

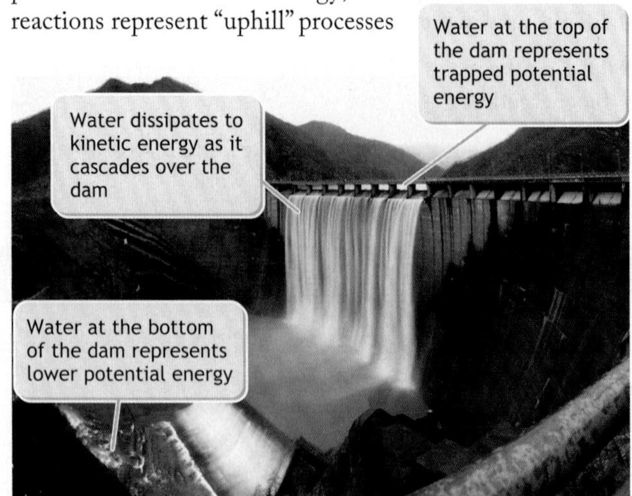
Water at the top of the dam represents trapped potential energy
Water dissipates to kinetic energy as it cascades over the dam
Water at the bottom of the dam represents lower potential energy

FIGURE 5.1 High-grade potential energy capable of performing work degrades to a useless form of kinetic energy. In the example of falling water over a dam, the water at the crest, before it cascades to the next level, represents potential energy. All of this potential energy dissipates to kinetic energy (heat) as the water crashes to the surface below. (Reprinted with permission from McArdle WD, Katch FI, Katch VL. *Exercise Physiology: Nutrition, Energy, and Human Performance.* 8th Ed. Baltimore: Wolters Kluwer Health, 2015.)

and proceed with an increase in free energy for biologic work. Sometimes, exergonic processes link or couple with endergonic reactions to transfer a portion of the energy to the endergonic process.

Changes in free energy occur when the bonds in the reactant molecules form new product molecules but with different bonding. The equation that expresses these changes, under conditions of constant temperature, pressure, and volume, takes the following form:

$$\Delta G = \Delta H - T\Delta S$$

The symbol Δ designates change. The change in free energy represents a keystone of chemical reactions. In exergonic reactions, ΔG is negative (−ΔG); the products contain *less* free energy than do the reactants, with the energy differential released as heat. For example, when hydrogen unites with oxygen to form water, 68 kcal per mole (substance molecular weight in gram) of free energy are released in the following reaction:

$$H_2 + O \rightarrow H_2O$$
$$-\Delta G\ 68\ kcal \cdot mol^{-1}$$

In the reverse endergonic reaction, ΔG remains positive (+ΔG) because the product contains *more* free energy than do the reactants. The infusion of 68 kcal of energy per mole of water causes the water molecule's chemical bonds to split apart, freeing the original hydrogen and oxygen atoms. This "uphill" process of energy transfer provides the hydrogen and oxygen atoms with their original energy content to satisfy the principle of the first law of thermodynamics—energy conservation.

$$H_2 + O \leftarrow H_2O + \Delta G\ 68\ kcal \cdot mol^{-1}$$

Energy transfer in cells follows the same principles in the waterfall-waterwheel example. Carbohydrate, lipid, and protein macronutrients possess considerable potential energy. The formation of product substances progressively reduces the nutrients' original potential energy

A CLOSER LOOK

The Discovery of Adenosine Triphosphate

The history of the discovery of ATP reads like a mystery dating back to the 1860s in France and the work of Nobel Laureate Louis Pasteur (1822–1895). During one of his experiments with yeast, Pasteur proposed that this micro-organism's ability to degrade sugar to carbon dioxide and alcohol (ethanol) was strictly a living or, as Pasteur called it, "vitalistic" function of the yeast cell. He hypothesized that if the yeast cell died, the fermentation process would cease.

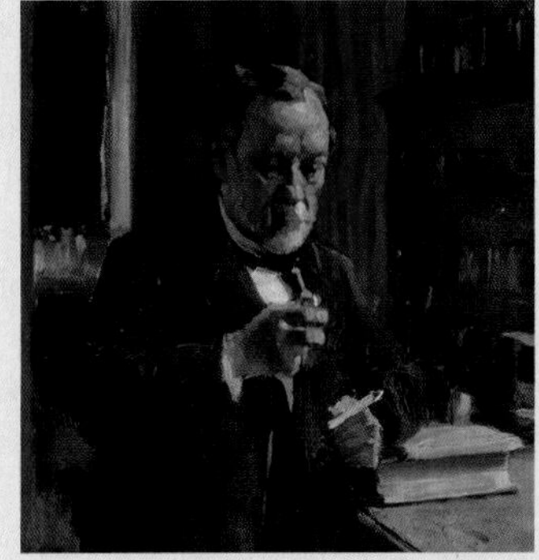

French Nobel Laureate Chemist Louis Pasteur (1822–1895)

In 1897, German chemist and eventual 1907 Chemistry Nobel Prize winner Eduard Buchner (1860–1917) made a chance observation that proved Pasteur wrong. His discovery revolutionized the study of physiologic systems and represented the beginning of the modern science of biochemistry. Searching for therapeutic uses for protein, he concocted a thick paste of freshly grown yeast and sand in a large mortar and pressed out the yeast cell juice. The gummy liquid proved unstable and could not be preserved by techniques available at that time. One of his laboratory assistants suggested adding a large amount of sugar to the mixture, a technique used by the assistant's wife to preserve fruit.

To everyone's surprise, what seemed like a silly solution worked: the nonliving juice from the yeast cells converted the sugar to carbon dioxide and alcohol and directly contradicting Pasteur's prevailing theory.

In 1905, British biochemist Arthur Harden (1865–1940; 1929 Nobel Prize in Chemistry) and Australian biochemist William Young (1878–1942) observed, as had their German predecessors, that the fermenting ability of yeast juice decreased gradually with time and could be restored only by adding fresh boiled yeast juice or blood serum. Crude yeast juice pressed through a gelatin film yielded a filtrate free of protein. The filtrate and protein were completely inert. Vigorous fermentation began when the filtrate and protein recombined. They called this combination "zymase"; it consisted of the filtrate "cozymase" and the protein residue "apozymase." Many years passed before the two components were accurately analyzed and identified as containing "coenzyme" compounds. In addition, the apozymase consisted of many proteins, each a specific catalyst in sugar breakdown.

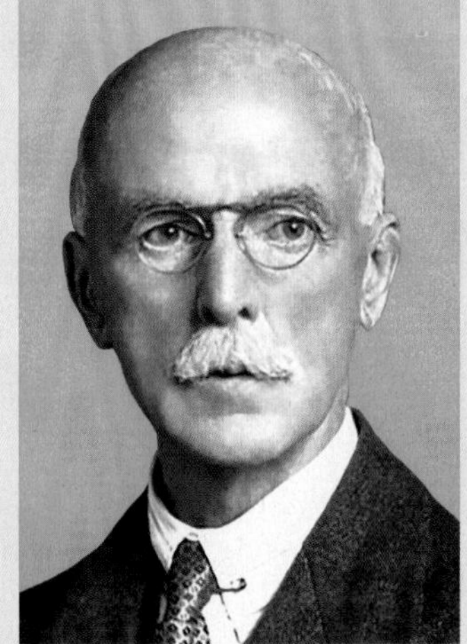

English Nobel Laureate Biochemist Sir Arthur Harden (1865–1940)

In 1929, young German scientist Karl Lohmann (1898–1978) working in the laboratory of eventual Nobel Prize recipient Otto Meyerhoff (1884–1950; **www.nobelprize.org/nobel_prizes/medicine/laureates/1922/meyerhof-bio.html**) studied the "energy" source responsible for cellular reactions involving yeast and sugar. Working with yeast juice, Lohmann discovered that an unstable substance in the cozymase filtrate degraded the sugar. This energizing substance contained the nitrogen-containing compound adenine linked to the sugar ribose and three phosphate groups, a substance we now know as ATP. The potential energy stored in the "high-energy bonds" link the ATP molecule's phosphate groups. The splitting of these phosphate bonds releases the energy for *all* biologic work.

with corresponding increases in kinetic energy. Enzyme-regulated transfer systems harness or conserve some of this chemical energy in new compounds for biologic work. In essence, living cells serve as transducers with the capacity to extract and harness chemical energy stored within a compound's atomic structure. Conversely, and equally important, they also bond atoms and molecules together, raising them to a higher potential energy level.

The transfer of potential energy in any spontaneous process always proceeds in a direction that *decreases* capacity to perform work. **Entropy** refers to the degree of unpredictability or disorder in a closed thermodynamic system and, when related to the system's total energy availability, means little energy availability from the system to produce work. It also applies to the tendency of potential energy to convert to kinetic energy of motion with a lower capacity for work and reflects the **second law of thermodynamics**. This important principle applies to and is nicely illustrated by the common flashlight battery—the electrochemical energy stored within its cells slowly dissipates, even when the battery remains unused. The energy from sunlight also continually degrades to heat energy when light strikes and becomes absorbed by a surface. Food and other chemicals represent excellent potential energy storage depots, yet this energy continually declines as the compounds decompose through normal oxidative processes. Energy, similar to water, always runs downhill to decrease the potential energy. *Ultimately, all the potential energy in a system degrades to the unusable form of kinetic or heat energy.*

ENERGY INTERCONVERSIONS

Figure 5.2 shows energy categorized into one of six forms: chemical, mechanical, heat, light, electric, and nuclear. During energy conversions, a loss of potential energy from

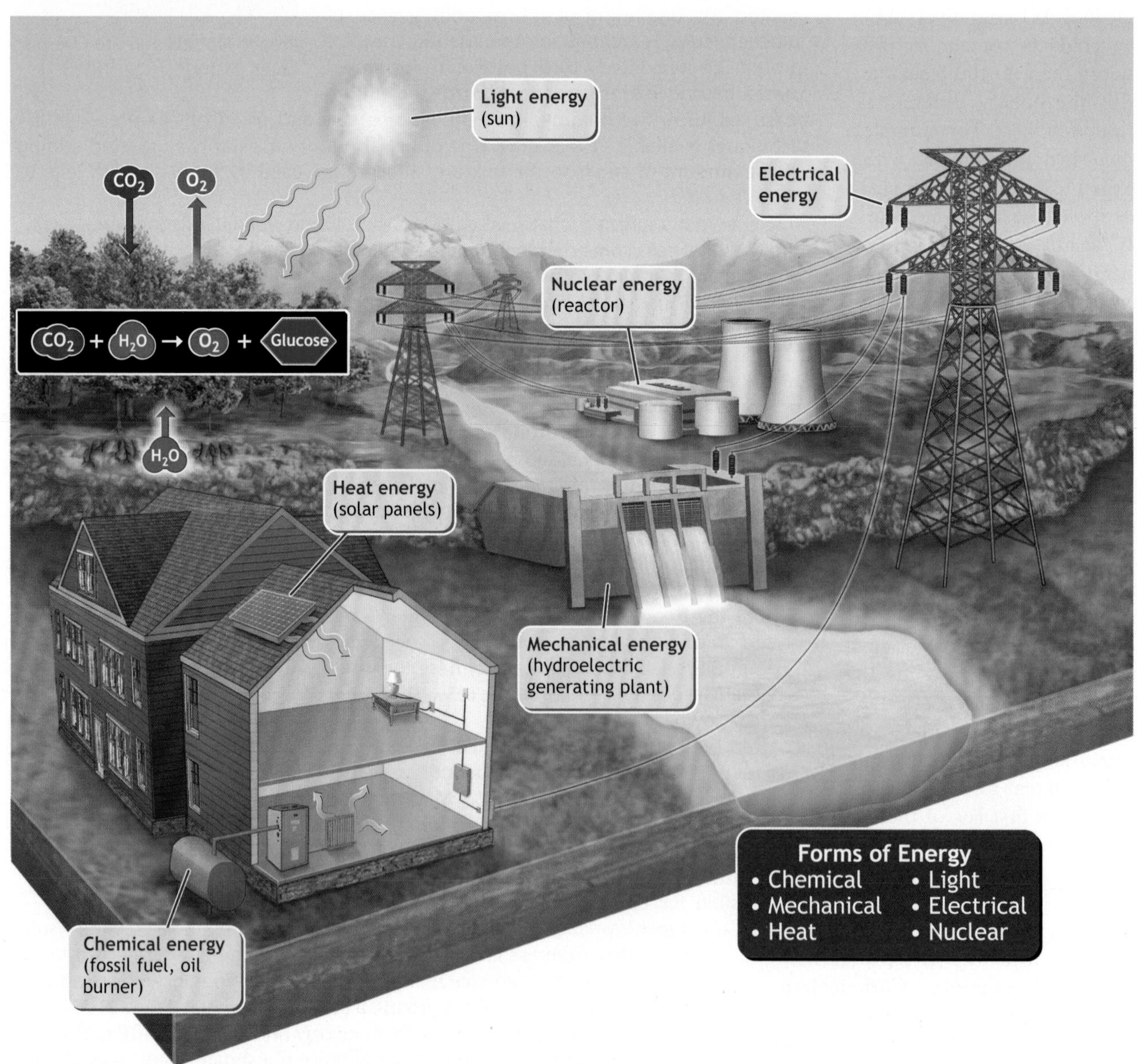

FIGURE 5.2 Interconversions among six forms of energy. (Reprinted with permission from McArdle WD, Katch FI, Katch VL. *Exercise Physiology: Nutrition, Energy, and Human Performance*. 8th Ed. Baltimore: Wolters Kluwer Health, 2015.)

one source often produces a temporary increase in the potential energy of another source. In this way, nature harnesses vast quantities of potential energy for useful purposes. Even under such favorable conditions, the net flow of energy in the biologic world still moves toward entropy, ultimately producing a loss of a system's total potential energy.

Examples of Energy Conversions

In living cells, **photosynthesis** and **respiration** represent the most fundamental examples of energy conversion.

Photosynthesis

Figure 5.3 depicts the dynamics of photosynthesis, an endergonic process powered by the sun's energy. The pigment chlorophyll located within the leaf cell's large organelles, the chloroplasts, absorbs radiant or solar energy to synthesize glucose from carbon dioxide and water, with oxygen flowing freely to the environment. The plant also converts carbohydrates to lipids and proteins for storage as a future reserve for energy and growth. Animals then ingest plant nutrients to serve their own energy needs. *In essence, solar energy coupled with photosynthesis powers the animal world with food and oxygen.*

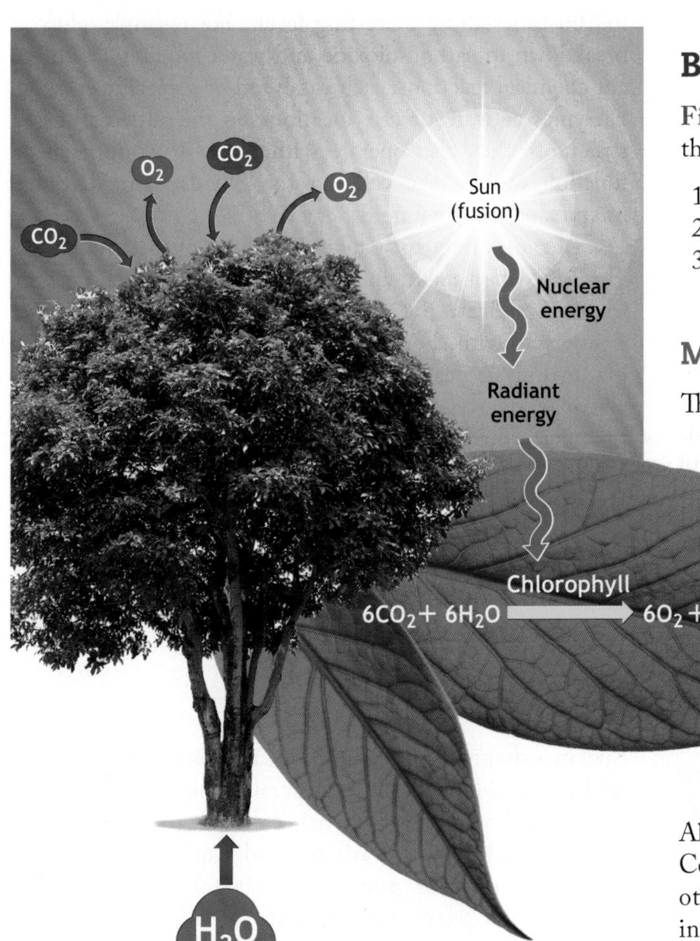

FIGURE 5.3 The endergonic process of photosynthesis in plants, algae, and some bacteria serves as the mechanism to synthesize carbohydrates, lipids, and proteins. In this example, a glucose molecule forms when carbon dioxide binds with water with a positive free energy (useful energy) change ($+\Delta G$). (Reprinted with permission from McArdle WD, Katch FI, Katch VL. *Exercise Physiology: Nutrition, Energy, and Human Performance*. 8th Ed. Baltimore: Wolters Kluwer Health, 2015.)

Cellular Respiration

Figure 5.4 illustrates the exergonic reactions of respiration, the reverse of photosynthesis, as the plant's stored energy is recovered for biologic work shown in the bottom three panels. In these exergonic reactions in the presence of oxygen, the cells extract the chemical energy stored in the carbohydrate, lipid, and protein molecules. For glucose displayed in the top box, this set of reactions releases 689 kcal per mole (180 g) oxidized. *A portion of energy released during cellular respiration becomes conserved in other chemical compounds in energy-requiring processes; the remaining energy flows to the environment as heat.*

BIOLOGIC WORK IN HUMANS

Figure 5.4 also illustrates that biologic work takes one of three forms:

1. **Mechanical work** of muscle contraction
2. **Chemical work** that synthesizes cellular molecules
3. **Transport work** that concentrates various substances in the intracellular and extracellular fluids

Mechanical Work

The most obvious example of energy transformation occurs from **mechanical work** generated by muscle action and subsequent movement. The molecular motors in a muscle fiber's protein filaments directly convert chemical energy into the mechanical energy of movement. The cell's nucleus represents another example of the body's mechanical work, where contractile elements literally tug at the chromosomes to produce cell division.

Chemical Work

All cells perform **chemical work** for maintenance and growth. Continuous synthesis of cellular components takes place as other components degrade. An example of chemical work includes muscle tissue synthesis in response to chronic resistance-training overload.

Transport Work

Cellular materials normally flow "downhill" from an area of higher to lower concentration. This passive **diffusion** process does not require energy. To maintain proper physiologic functioning, certain chemicals require transport "uphill" against their normal concentration gradients from an area of lower to higher concentration. **Active transport** describes

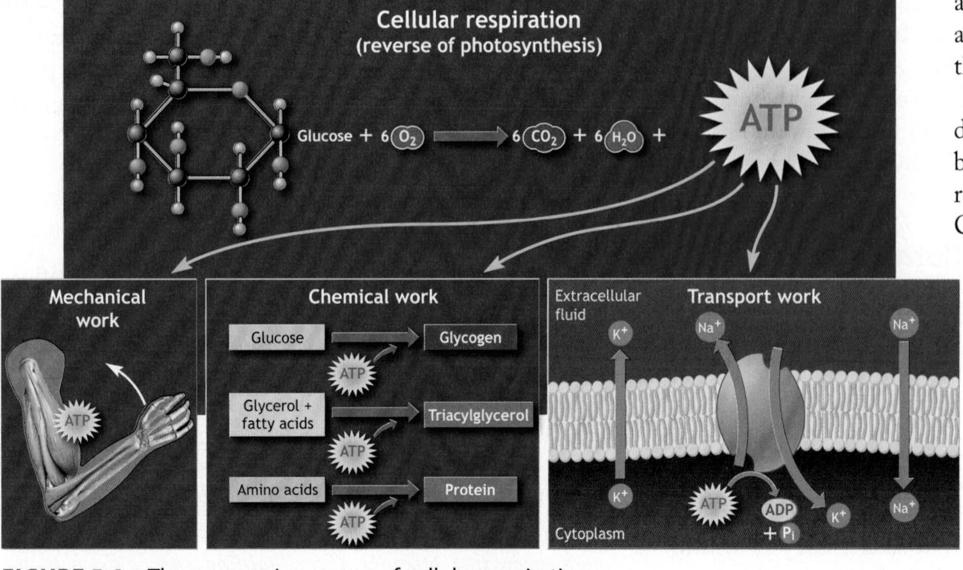

FIGURE 5.4 The exergonic process of cellular respiration. Exergonic reactions, such as the burning of gasoline or the oxidation of glucose, release potential energy. This produces a negative standard free energy change (i.e., reduction in total energy available for work, or $-\Delta G$). In this illustration, cellular respiration harvests the potential energy in food to form ATP. Subsequently, the energy in ATP powers all forms of biologic work. (Adapted with permission from McArdle WD, Katch FI, Katch VL. *Exercise Physiology: Nutrition, Energy, and Human Performance*. 8th Ed. Baltimore: Wolters Kluwer Health, 2015.)

this energy-requiring process. Secretion and resorption in the kidney tubules use active transport mechanisms, as does neural tissue to establish the proper electrochemical gradients surrounding its plasma membranes. These more "quiet" forms of biologic work require a continual expenditure of stored chemical energy.

FACTORS AFFECTING BIOENERGETICS

The limits of exercise intensity ultimately depend on the rate that cells extract, conserve, and transfer chemical energy in the food nutrients to skeletal muscle's contractile filaments. *The sustained pace of the world-class marathon runner at close to 90% of maximum aerobic capacity or the speed achieved by the sprinter in all-out activity directly reflects the body's capacity to transfer chemical energy into mechanical work.* Enzymes and coenzymes control the rate of energy release during chemical reactions.

Enzymes as Biological Catalysts

*An **enzyme**, a highly specific and large protein catalyst, tremendously accelerates the forward and reverse rates of chemical reactions without being consumed or changed in the reaction.* Enzymes only govern reactions that normally take place but at a reduced rate. Enzyme action takes place without altering equilibrium constants and the total energy released or the change in free energy.

Enzymes possess the distinctive property of not being readily altered by the reactions they interact with. Consequently, enzyme turnover remains relatively low, and specific enzymes are continually reused. A typical mitochondrion can contain up to 10 billion enzyme molecules, each responsible for millions of cellular operations. During strenuous physical activity, the rate of enzyme activity increases exponentially as energy demands increase up to 100 times those of resting levels. For example, glucose breakdown to carbon dioxide and water requires 19 different chemical reactions, each catalyzed by a specific enzyme. Enzymes activate precise locations on the surfaces of cell structures; they also operate within the structure itself or function outside the cell—in the bloodstream, digestive mixture, or intestinal fluids.

Enzymes frequently take the names of their functions. The suffix-*ase* usually appends to the enzyme whose prefix often indicates its mode of operation or the substance it interacts with. For example, hydrol*ase* adds water during hydrolysis reactions, prote*ase* interacts with protein, oxid*ase* adds oxygen to a substance, and ribonucle*ase* splits ribonucleic acid (RNA). **Table 5.1** lists six classifications of enzymes, and their typical actions, and provides examples of each.

 See the animation "Hydrolysis" on **http://thePoint.lww.com/MKKESS5e** for a demonstration of this process.

Reaction Rates

Enzymes do not all operate at the same rate—some operate relatively slowly while others operate rapidly. Consider the enzyme carbonic anhydrase that catalyzes the hydration of carbon dioxide to form carbonic acid. Carbonic anhydrase's maximum **turnover number** of 800,000 represents the number of moles of substrate that react to form a product per mole of enzyme per unit time. In contrast, the turnover number for tryptophan synthetase is only two to catalyze the final step in tryptophan synthesis. Enzymes often work cooperatively. While one substance "turns on" at a particular site, its neighbor "turns off" until the process ends. The operation can then reverse, with one enzyme becoming inactive and the other active. Cellular pH and temperature dramatically impact enzyme activity. For some enzymes, peak activity

TABLE 5.1 Six Classifications of Enzymes

Name (Example)	Action
Oxidoreductases (lactate dehydrogenase)	Catalyze oxidation-reduction reactions where the substrate oxidized is regarded as hydrogen or electron donor; includes dehydrogenases, oxidates, oxygenases, reductases, peroxidases, and hydroxylases.
Transferases (hexokinase)	Catalyze the transfer of a group (e.g., the methyl group or a glycosyl group) from one compound regarded as donor to another compound regarded as acceptor; include kinases, transcarboxylases, and transaminases.
Hydrolases (lipase)	Catalyze reactions that add water; includes esterases, phosphatases, and peptidases.
Lyases (carbonic anhydrase)	Catalyze reactions that cleave C–C, C–O, C–N, and other bonds by different means than by hydrolysis or oxidation. Includes synthases, deaminases, and decarboxylases.
Isomerases (phosphoglycerate mutase)	Catalyze reactions that rearrange molecular structure; include isomerases and epimerases. These enzymes catalyze changes within one molecule.
Ligases (pyruvate carboxylase)	Catalyze bond formation between two substrate molecules with concomitant hydrolysis of the diphosphate bond in ATP or a similar triphosphate.

requires relatively high acidity, but others function optimally on the alkaline side of neutrality. The pH optimum for lipase in the stomach, for example, ranges from 4.0 to 5.0, but in the pancreas, the optimum lipase pH increases to 8.0.

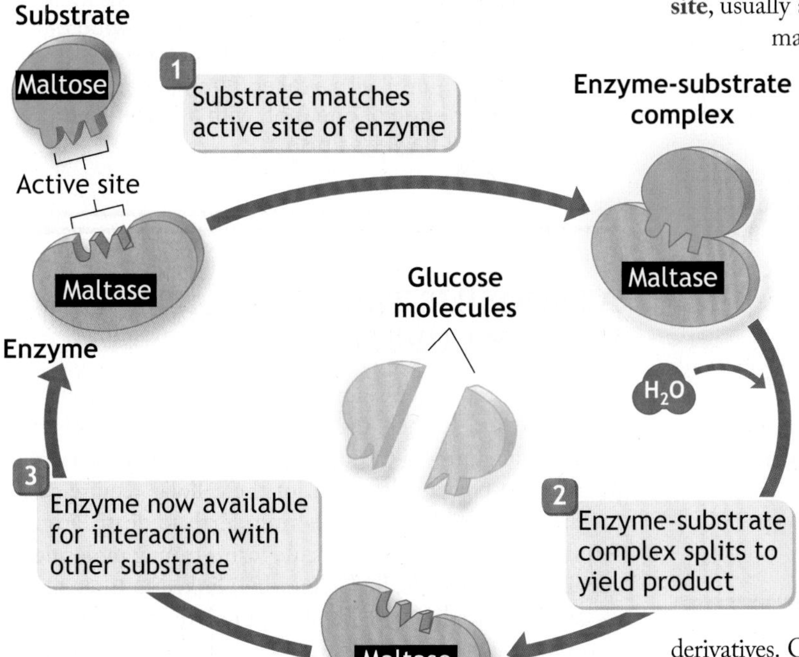

FIGURE 5.5 Sequence of steps in the "lock-and-key mechanism" of an enzyme with its substrate. The example shows how two monosaccharide glucose molecules form when maltase interacts with its disaccharide substrate maltose. (Adapted with permission from McArdle WD, Katch FI, Katch VL. *Exercise Physiology: Nutrition, Energy, and Human Performance*. 8th Ed. Baltimore: Wolters Kluwer Health, 2015.)

Mode of Enzyme Action

How an enzyme interacts with its specific substrate represents a unique characteristic of an enzyme's three-dimensional globular protein structure. Interaction works similarly to a key fitting a lock. The enzyme "turns on" when its **active site**, usually a groove, cleft, or cavity on the protein's surface, matches in a "perfect fit" with the substrate's active site (see **Fig. 5.5**, step 1). Upon forming an enzyme-substrate complex, the splitting of chemical bonds forms a new product with new bonds (see **Fig. 5.5**, step 2), freeing the enzyme to interact on additional substrate (see **Fig. 5.5**, step 3). This lock-and-key mechanism serves a protective function so only the correct, specific enzyme activates a specific substrate.

Coenzymes

Some enzymes remain totally dormant unless activated by additional substances termed **coenzymes**. These complex nonprotein substances facilitate enzyme action by binding the substrate with its specific enzyme. Coenzymes then regenerate to assist in further but similar reactions. The metallic ions iron and zinc play coenzyme roles as do the B vitamins and their derivatives. Oxidation-reduction reactions use the B vitamins riboflavin and niacin, while other vitamins serve as transfer agents for groups of compounds in other metabolic processes. A coenzyme requires less specificity in its action than does an enzyme because the coenzyme impacts additional but different reactions. Coenzymes either act as a "cobinder" or serve as a temporary carrier of intermediary products in the reaction. For example, the coenzyme **nicotinamide adenine dinucleotide (NAD^+)** forms NADH to transport hydrogen atoms and electrons that split from food fragments during energy metabolism.

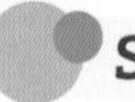

SUMMARY

1. The first law of thermodynamics states that the body does not produce, consume, or use up energy; rather, it transforms it from one form into another as physiologic systems undergo continual change.
2. Potential energy and kinetic energy constitute a system's total energy.
3. Potential energy is the energy of position and form; kinetic energy is the energy of motion.
4. The release of potential energy transforms this energy into kinetic energy of motion.
5. The term *exergonic* describes any physical or chemical process resulting in the release or freeing of energy to its surroundings.
6. *Endergonic* chemical processes store or absorb energy.
7. The second law of thermodynamics describes the tendency for potential energy to degrade to kinetic energy with a lower capacity to perform work.
8. Total energy in an isolated system remains constant; a decrease in one form of energy matches an equivalent increase in another form.
9. Biologic work takes one of three forms: mechanical work (work of muscle contraction), chemical work (synthesizing cellular molecules), and transport work (concentrating various substances in the intracellular and extracellular fluids).
10. An enzyme, a highly specific and large protein catalyst, tremendously accelerates the forward and reverse rates of chemical reactions within the body without being consumed or changed in the reaction.
11. All enzymes do not operate at the same rate; some operate relatively slowly, while others work more rapidly; pH and temperature dramatically affect enzyme activity.
12. Coenzymes are nonprotein substances that facilitate enzyme action and bind substrate to its specific enzyme.

THINK IT THROUGH

1. From a metabolic perspective, why is destruction of the rain forests throughout the world counterproductive for humans?
2. In terms of metabolism, why is body temperature maintained within a relatively narrow range?

PART 2 Phosphate-Bond Energy

The human body receives a continual chemical energy supply to perform its many complex and interrelated functions. Energy derived from food oxidation does not release suddenly at some kindling temperature because the body, unlike a mechanical engine, cannot directly harness heat energy. Rather, intricate enzymatically controlled reactions within the cell's relatively cool, watery medium extract chemical energy trapped within carbohydrate, fat, and protein's molecular bonds. This extraction process reduces energy loss and substantially enhances energy transformation efficiency. Fortunately, the body can directly use chemical energy for many forms of biologic work ranging from ciliary movement in the GI tract, nerve impulse transmission to propagate electrical signaling in the heart's four chambers, to the finely coordinated finger, hand, and arm and shoulder muscle actions required to master a Beethoven piano concerto. **Adenosine triphosphate (ATP)**, the special carrier for free energy, provides energy for all cellular functions.

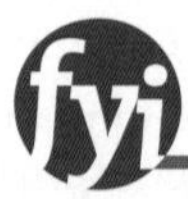

fyi High-Energy Phosphates

To appreciate the importance of the intramuscular high-energy phosphates during physical activity, consider activities in which success requires brief but intense bursts of maximal effort for only up to 8 seconds; these include aspects of American football, tennis, track and field, golf, volleyball, field hockey, baseball, weightlifting, and chopping wood or performing the Salchow figure skating jump with a takeoff from a back inside edge of one foot, with a graceful and flawless finish.

ADENOSINE TRIPHOSPHATE: THE ENERGY CURRENCY

Energy in food does not transfer directly to cells for biologic work. Rather, the stored "macronutrient energy" releases and funnels through ATP, the energy-rich compound, that powers almost all of the cellular requirements for the body's trillions of cells from birth to death. **Figure 5.6** shows how an **ATP** molecule forms from a molecule of adenine and ribose (called adenosine) linked to three phosphate molecules. The two bonds that link the two outermost phosphates, termed **high-energy bonds**, represent a huge stored chemical energy depot.

A tight coupling exists between the breakdown of the macronutrient energy molecules and ATP synthesis, the latter "capturing" a significant portion of the released energy. **Coupled reactions** occur in pairs; the breakdown of one compound provides energy for synthesizing another compound. To meet cellular energy needs, water binds ATP in the process of **hydrolysis**. This operation splits the outermost phosphate bond from the ATP molecule.

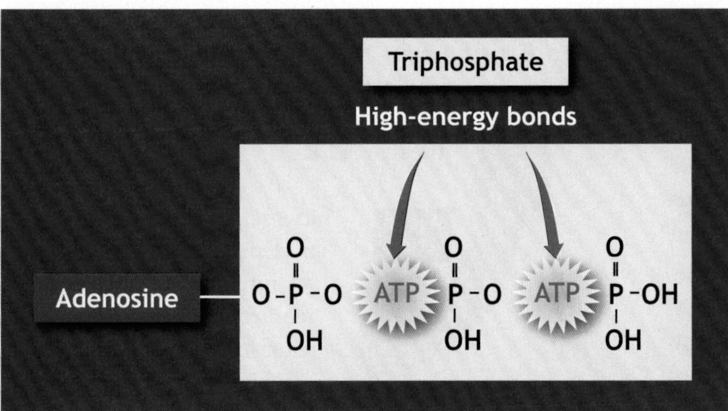

FIGURE 5.6 Adenosine triphosphate (ATP), the energy currency of the cell. The starbursts represents the high-energy bonds.

Anabolism uses energy to synthesize new compounds. For example, many glucose molecules join together to form the larger, complex glycogen molecule; similarly, glycerol and fatty acids combine to synthesize **triacylglycerols (triglyceride)**, and amino acids bind together to create larger protein molecules. Each reaction starts with simple compounds and groups them as building blocks to form larger, more intricate compounds.

Catabolic reactions release energy to form ADP. During this hydrolytic process, adenosine triphosphatase catalyzes the reaction when ATP joins with water. For each mole of ATP degraded to ADP, the outermost phosphate bond divides and liberates approximately 7.3 kcal of **free energy**, making it available for further biological functions.

$$ATP + H_2O \xrightarrow{ATPase} ADP + Pi - \Delta G\ 7.3\ kcal \cdot mol^{-1}$$

The enzyme accelerates hydrolysis to form a new compound, **adenosine diphosphate (ADP)**. In turn, these reactions couple to other reactions that incorporate the "freed" phosphate-bond chemical energy. The ATP molecules transfer the energy produced during catabolic reactions to power chemical reactions to further synthesize other new compounds. In essence, this energy receiver–energy donor cycle represents the cells' two major energy-transforming activities:

1. Form and conserve ATP from food's potential energy
2. Use extracted energy from ATP to power biologic work

Figure 5.7 illustrates examples of anabolic and catabolic reactions involving coupled chemical energy transfer. All of the energy released from catabolizing one compound does not dissipate as heat; rather, a portion remains conserved within the chemical structure of the newly formed compound. A new highly "energized" ATP molecule represents the common energy transfer "vehicle" in most coupled biologic reactions.

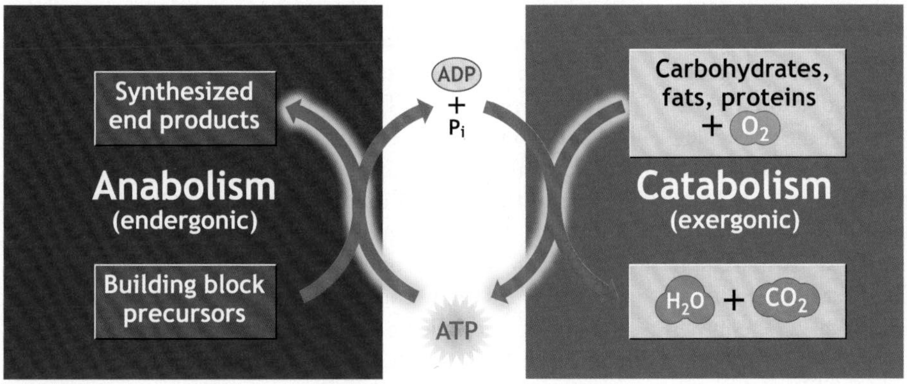

The symbol ΔG refers to the standard free energy change measured under laboratory conditions, which seldom occur in the body (25°C; 1 atmosphere pressure; concentrations maintained at 1 molal at pH = 7.0). In the intracellular environment, the value may approach 10 kcal · mol^{-1}. The free energy liberated in ATP hydrolysis reflects the energy *difference* between reactant and end products. This reaction generates considerable useful energy.

The splitting of ATP and liberation of energy allows for direct energy transfer to other energy-requiring molecules. In muscle, for example, this energy activates specific sites on the muscle's contractile elements causing them to shorten. *Energy from ATP powers all forms of biologic work; thus, ATP is considered the cell's "energy currency."* **Figure 5.8** illustrates ATP's general role as energy currency, depicting it as a starburst that power all forms of biologic work: glandular secretion, nerve transmission, muscle work, circulation, tissue synthesis, and digestion.

FIGURE 5.7 Catabolism-anabolism interactions. Continual recycling of ATP for biologic work of macronutrient synthesis (anabolic or endergonic processes) and its subsequent reconstruction from ADP and a phosphate ion (Pi) via oxidation of the stored macronutrients (catabolic or exergonic processes). (Adapted with permission from McArdle WD, Katch FI, Katch VL. *Exercise Physiology: Nutrition, Energy, and Human Performance*. 8th Ed. Baltimore: Wolters Kluwer Health, 2015.)

The splitting of ATP takes place immediately without oxygen. The cell's capability for ATP breakdown generates energy for rapid use for all biologic activities including muscle action. Think of anaerobic energy release as a backup power source relied on to deliver energy in *excess* of aerobic energy production. There are literally hundreds of examples in your own daily routines of this type of energy production. Lifting your hand to turn the page of this book or lifting a fork occurs *without* the need for oxygen in the energy-requiring process. Other sport-related

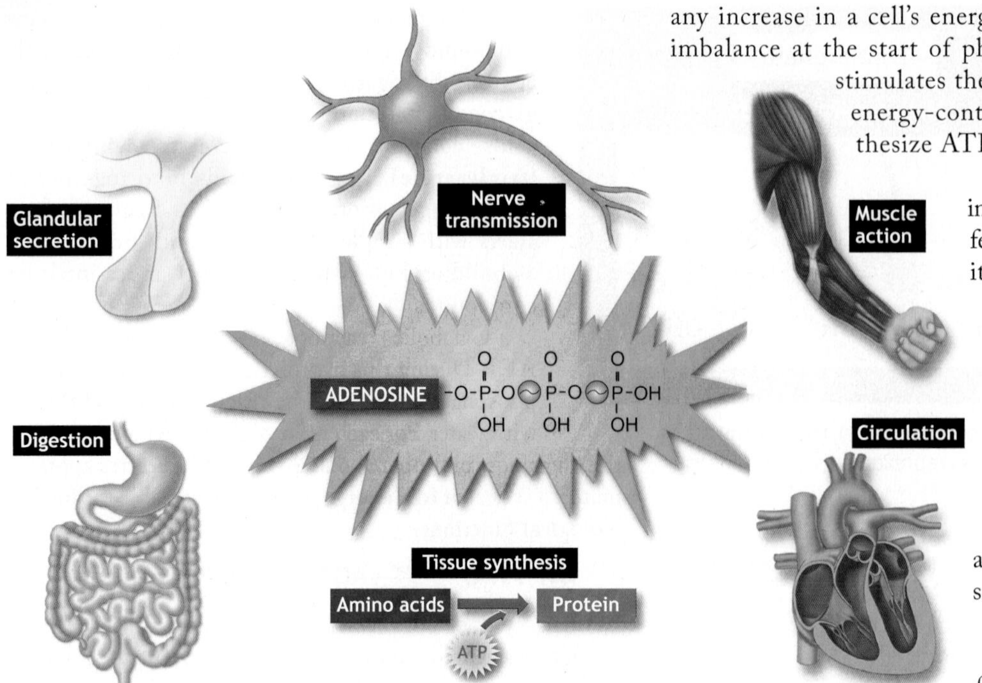

FIGURE 5.8 Structure of ATP, the energy currency that powers all forms of biologic work. The symbol ⊖ represents high-energy bonds. (Adapted with permission from McArdle WD, Katch FI, Katch VL. *Exercise Physiology: Nutrition, Energy, and Human Performance.* 8th Ed. Baltimore: Wolters Kluwer Health, 2015.)

examples of immediate anaerobic energy release include smashing a golfball, spiking a volleyball, doing a pushup, or jumping up in the air. Each of these movements requires an immediate burst of energy to complete the muscle action.

Adenosine Triphosphate: A Limited Currency

A limited quantity of ATP serves as the energy currency for all cells. In fact, at any one time, the body stores about 80 to 100 g or in the range of 2.5 to 3.5 oz of ATP. This provides enough intramuscular stored energy for several seconds of explosive, all-out activity. A limited quantity of "stored" ATP represents an additional advantage because of the molecule's heaviness. Biochemists estimate that a sedentary person each day uses an amount of ATP equal to about 75% of body mass. For a female who weighs 140 lb or 63.5 kg, the ATP equivalent would equal about 105 lb or 47 kg. A marathon run that generates about 20 times resting energy expenditure over a 3-hour time period would require a total ATP equivalent of about 80 kg!

Cells store only a small quantity of ATP, so it must be resynthesized continually at its rate of use. This provides a tremendously useful biologic mechanism to regulate cellular energy metabolism. By maintaining only a small amount of ATP, its relative concentration and corresponding ADP concentration change rapidly with any increase in a cell's energy demands. An ATP:ADP imbalance at the start of physical activity immediately stimulates the breakdown of other stored energy-containing compounds to resynthesize ATP.

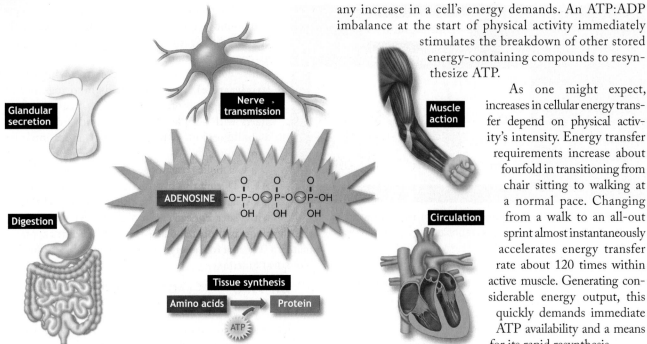

As one might expect, increases in cellular energy transfer depend on physical activity's intensity. Energy transfer requirements increase about fourfold in transitioning from chair sitting to walking at a normal pace. Changing from a walk to an all-out sprint almost instantaneously accelerates energy transfer rate about 120 times within active muscle. Generating considerable energy output, this quickly demands immediate ATP availability and a means for its rapid resynthesis.

Diverse Processes for Generating ATP

The body maintains a continuous ATP supply through different metabolic pathways. Some are located in the cell's cytosol and involve anaerobic processes (rapid glycolysis—see Part 3 of this chapter), whereas others operate within mitochondria relying on reactions that generate ATP aerobically via the citric acid cycle (CAC) and respiratory chain reactions. **Figure 5.9** illustrates these two diverse ATP generating processes to power biologic work.

PHOSPHOCREATINE: THE ENERGY RESERVOIR

The hydrolysis of a phosphate from another intracellular high-energy phosphate compound—**phosphocreatine** (PCr, also known as creatine phosphate [CP])—provides some energy for ATP resynthesis. PCr, similar to ATP, releases considerable energy when the bond splits between the creatine and phosphate molecules. PCr hydrolysis begins at the onset of intense physical activity as in all-out sprinting, does not require oxygen, and reaches a maximum in about 8 to 12 seconds. Thus, PCr can be considered a "reservoir" of high-energy phosphate bonds. **Figure 5.10** illustrates the release and creation of phosphate-bond energy in ATP and PCr. The term high-energy phosphates or **phosphagens** describes these two stored intramuscular compounds.

In each reaction, the white arrows point in both directions to indicate reversible reactions. In other words, creatine (Cr) and inorganic phosphate from ATP can join again to reform PCr. This also holds true for ATP, where joining

FIGURE 5.9 Diverse ways to produce ATP. The body maintains a continuous ATP supply through different metabolic pathways: Some are located in the cell's cytosol, whereas others operate within the mitochondria. Reactions that harness cellular energy to generate ATP aerobically—the citric acid cycle and respiratory chain (including β-oxidation)—reside within the mitochondria. (Adapted with permission from McArdle WD, Katch FI, Katch VL. *Sports and Exercise Nutrition*. 4th Ed. Philadelphia: Wolters Kluwer Health, 2013.)

ADP with Pi re-forms ATP (**Fig. 5.10**, top). ATP resynthesis occurs if sufficient energy exists to rejoin an ADP molecule with one Pi molecule. The hydrolysis of PCr "fuels" this energy.

Cells store PCr in considerably larger quantities than ATP. PCr mobilization for energy takes place almost instantaneously and does not require oxygen. Interestingly, ADP concentration in the cell stimulates the activity level of **creatine kinase (CK)**, the enzyme that facilitates PCr breakdown to Cr and ATP. This provides a crucial feedback mechanism known as the **creatine kinase reaction** that forms ATP from the high-energy phosphates.

The **adenylate kinase reaction** represents another single-enzyme–mediated reaction for ATP regeneration. The reaction uses two ADP molecules to produce one molecule of ATP and AMP as follows:

$$2\ ADP \xleftrightarrow{\text{Adenylate kinase}} ATP + AMP$$

The creatine kinase and adenylate kinase reactions not only augment how well the muscles almost instantaneously increase energy output (i.e., increase ATP availability) but also produce the molecular by-products AMP, Pi, ADP that activate the initial stages of glycogen and glucose breakdown in cell fluids and the mitochondrion's aerobic pathways.

INTRAMUSCULAR HIGH-ENERGY PHOSPHATES

The energy released from ATP and PCr breakdown within muscle sustains all-out running, cycling, or swimming for 5 to 8 seconds. In the 100-m sprint, for example, the body cannot maintain maximum speed for longer than this duration. During the last few seconds, runners actually slow down, with the winner slowing the least. From an energy perspective, the winner most effectively supplies and uses the limited quantity of phosphate-bond energy.

In almost all sports, the energy transfer capacity of the ATP-PCr high-energy phosphates, termed the "**immediate energy system**," plays a crucial role in success or failure of some phase of performance. If all-out effort continues beyond about 8 seconds or if moderate activity continues for much longer periods, ATP resynthesis requires an additional energy source other than PCr. Without additional ATP resynthesis, the "fuel" supply diminishes and intense movement ceases. The foods we consume and store provide the energy to continually recharge cellular ATP and PCr supplies.

Identifying Important Energy Sources

Identifying predominant energy sources required for a particular sport or activities of daily living forms the basis for an effective physical training program. Football and baseball, for example, require a high-energy output for only brief time periods. These performances rely almost exclusively on energy transfer from the intramuscular high-energy phosphates. Developing this immediate energy system becomes important when training to improve performance in these activities. Chapter 13 discusses specific training to optimize different energy systems' power-output capacity.

Phosphorylation: Chemical Bonds Transfer Energy

Biologic work occurs in the body when compounds relatively low in potential energy "juice up" from energy transfer via high-energy phosphate bonds. ATP serves as the ideal energy-transfer agent. In one respect, ATP's phosphate bonds "trap" a large portion of the original food molecules' potential energy. ATP then transfers this energy to other compounds to raise them to a higher activation level. **Phosphorylation** refers to energy transfer through phosphate bonds.

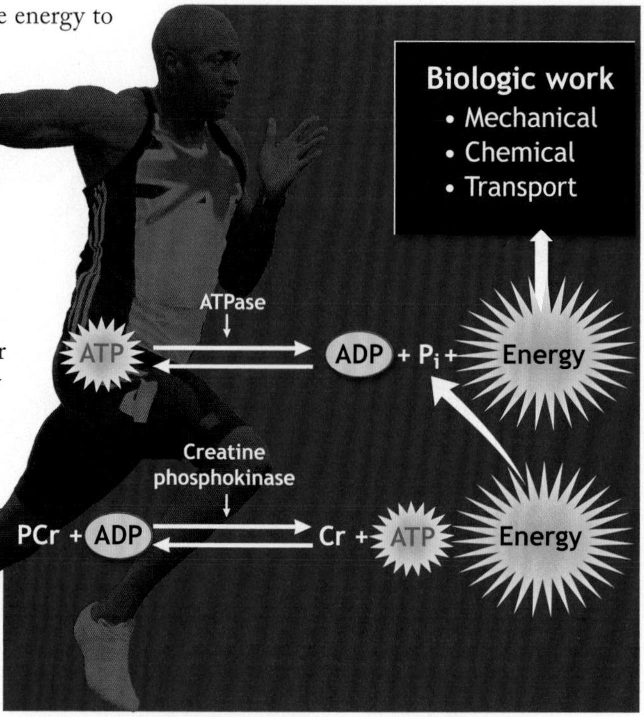

FIGURE 5.10 ATP and PCr provide anaerobic sources of phosphate-bond energy. The energy liberated from the hydrolysis (splitting) of PCr rebonds ADP and Pi to form ATP. (Adapted with permission from McArdle WD, Katch FI, Katch VL. *Sports and Exercise Nutrition*. 4th Ed. Philadelphia: Wolters Kluwer Health, 2013.)

CELLULAR OXIDATION

The energy for phosphorylation comes from **oxidation** or "biologic burning" of carbohydrate, lipid, and protein macronutrients. A molecule becomes **reduced** when it accepts electrons from an electron donor. In turn, the molecule that gives up the electron becomes **oxidized**.

Oxidation reactions (those donating electrons) and **reduction reactions** (those accepting electrons) remain tightly coupled because every oxidation reaction coincides with a reduction reaction. *In essence, cellular oxidation–reduction constitutes the mechanism for energy metabolism.* The stored carbohydrate, fat, and protein molecules continually provide hydrogen atoms for this process. The complex but highly efficient **mitochondria (micro.magnet.fsu.edu/cells)**, the cell's "energy factories," have carrier molecules that remove electrons from hydrogen (oxidation) and eventually pass them to oxygen (reduction). Oxidation-reduction reactions synthesize the high-energy phosphate ATP.

Electron Transport

Figure 5.11 illustrates hydrogen oxidation and accompanying electron transport to oxygen. During cellular oxidation, hydrogen atoms are not merely turned loose in cell fluids. Rather, highly specific **dehydrogenase enzymes** catalyze hydrogen's release from nutrient substrates. The coenzyme part of the dehydrogenase (usually the niacin-containing coenzyme, NAD^+) accepts pairs of electrons or in essence energy from hydrogen. While the substrate oxidizes and loses hydrogen's electrons, NAD^+ gains one hydrogen and two electrons and reduces to NADH; the other hydrogen appears as H^+ in cell fluid.

The riboflavin-containing coenzyme **flavin adenine dinucleotide (FAD)** represents the other important electron acceptor that oxidizes food fragments. FAD also catalyzes dehydrogenations and accepts electron pairs. Unlike NAD^+, FAD transforms into $FADH_2$ with the addition of both hydrogens. This distinct difference between NAD^+ and FAD produces a different total number of ATP in the respiratory chain (see next page).

The NADH and $FADH_2$ formed in macronutrient breakdown represent energy-rich molecules as they carry the electrons with a high-energy transfer potential. Cytochromes, a series of iron-protein electron carriers, then pass pairs of electrons carried by NADH and $FADH_2$ in "bucket brigade" fashion on the mitochondria's inner membranes. The iron portion of each cytochrome exists in either its oxidized (ferric or Fe^{3+}) or reduced (ferrous or Fe^{2+}) ionic state. By accepting an electron, the ferric portion of a specific cytochrome reduces to its ferrous form. In turn, ferrous iron donates electrons to the next cytochrome, and so on down the "bucket brigade." By shuttling between these two iron forms, the cytochromes transfer electrons to their ultimate destination, where they reduce oxygen to form water. The NAD^+ and FAD then recycle for subsequent reuse in energy metabolism.

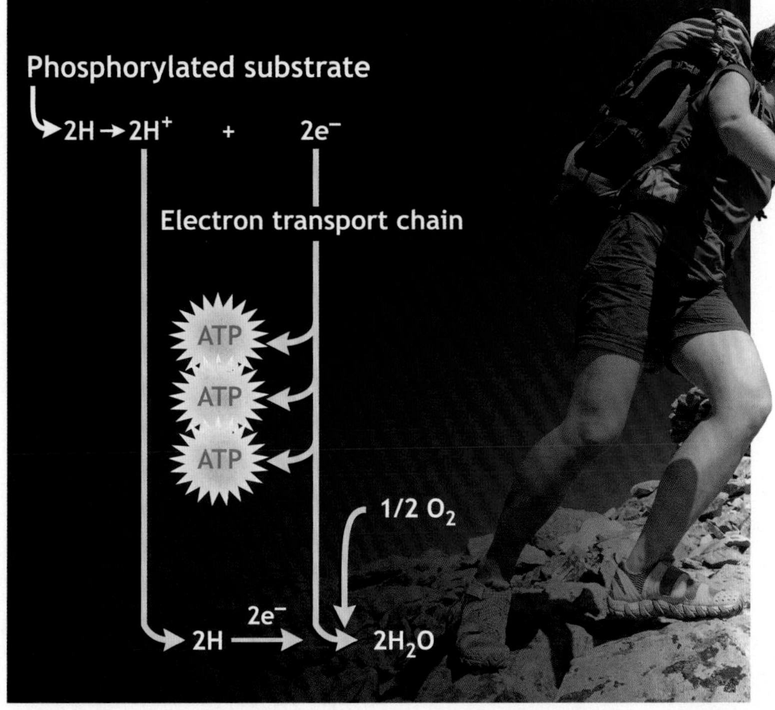

FIGURE 5.11 General scheme for oxidizing hydrogen (removing electrons) and the accompanying electron transport. In this process, oxygen is reduced (gain of electrons) and water forms. The liberated energy powers the synthesis of ATP from ADP. (Adapted with permission from McArdle WD, Katch FI, Katch VL. *Exercise Physiology: Nutrition, Energy, and Human Performance*. 8th Ed. Baltimore: Wolters Kluwer Health, 2015.)

Electron transport by specific carrier molecules constitutes the **respiratory chain (electron transport chain)**, the final common pathway where electrons extracted from hydrogen pass to oxygen. *For each pair of hydrogen atoms, two electrons flow down the chain and reduce one oxygen atom to form water.* Of the five specific cytochromes, only the last one, **cytochrome oxidase** (cytochrome aa_3 with a strong oxygen affinity), discharges its electron directly to oxygen. **Figure 5.12A and B** shows the harnessing of potential energy to kinetic energy in industry using a turbine waterwheel, and in the body, via the respiratory chain route for hydrogen oxidation, electron transport, and energy transfer. In both examples, note the transition at the left in going from higher potential energy at the top to lower potential energy at the bottom. The respiratory chain releases free energy in relatively small amounts. In several of the electron transfers, energy conservation occurs by forming high-energy phosphate bonds.

See the animation "Electron Transport" on **http://thePoint.lww.com/MKKESS5e** for a demonstration of this process.

Oxidative Phosphorylation

Oxidative phosphorylation refers to how ATP forms during electron transfer from NADH and $FADH_2$ with the eventual involvement of molecular oxygen. This crucial cellular metabolic process represents the cells' primary means to extract and trap chemical energy in the high-energy phosphates. *More than 90% of ATP synthesis takes place in the respiratory chain by oxidative reactions coupled with phosphorylation.*

Think of oxidative phosphorylation as a waterfall divided into several separate cascades by the waterwheels located at different heights. **Figure 5.12A** depicts the waterwheels harnessing the energy of the falling water; similarly, electrochemical energy generated via electron transport in the respiratory chain becomes harnessed and transferred (or coupled) to ADP. The energy in NADH transfers to ADP to reform ATP at three distinct coupling sites during electron transport, displayed in **Figure 5.12B**. Oxidation of hydrogen and subsequent phosphorylation occurs as follows:

$$\mathbf{NADH + H^+ + 3ADP + 3P_i + \tfrac{1}{2}O_2 \rightarrow NAD^+ + H_2O + 3ATP}$$

In this reaction, three ATP form for each NADH and H^+ oxidized. If $FADH_2$ originally donates hydrogen, only two ATP molecules form for each hydrogen pair oxidized. This occurs because $FADH_2$ enters the respiratory chain at a lower energy level at a point beyond the first ATP synthesis site.

Biochemists have recently adjusted their accounting transpositions regarding energy conservation in the aerobic pathway resynthesis of an ATP molecule. Energy provided by NADH and $FADH_2$ oxidation resynthesizes ADP to ATP. Additional energy (H^+) also is required to shuttle the NADH from the cell's cytoplasm across the mitochondrial membrane to deliver H^+ to electron transport. This added energy exchange of NADH shuttling across the mitochondrial membrane reduces the net ATP yield for glucose metabolism and changes ATP's overall production efficiency (see Part 3 of this chapter). The oxidation of one NADH molecule produces on average only 2.5 ATP molecules. This decimal value for ATP does not indicate formation of half of an ATP molecule but instead indicates the average ATP number produced per NADH oxidation with the energy for mitochondrial transport subtracted. When $FADH_2$ donates hydrogen, then on average only 1.5 molecules of ATP form for each hydrogen pair oxidized.

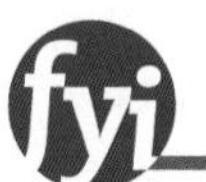

"OIL RIG"

To remember that oxidation involves the *loss* of electrons and reduction involves their *gain*, use OIL RIG:

OIL = **O**xidation **I**nvolves **L**oss
RIG = **R**eduction **I**nvolves **G**ain

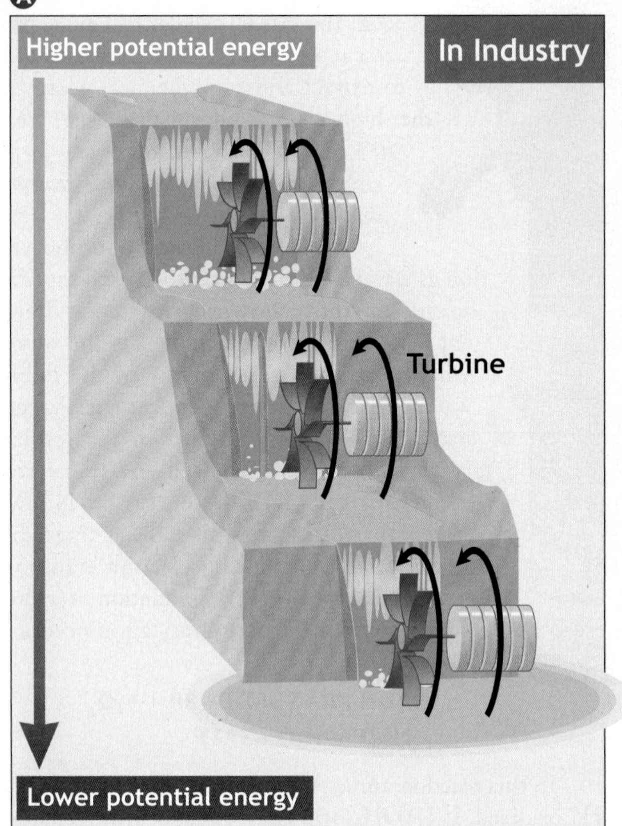

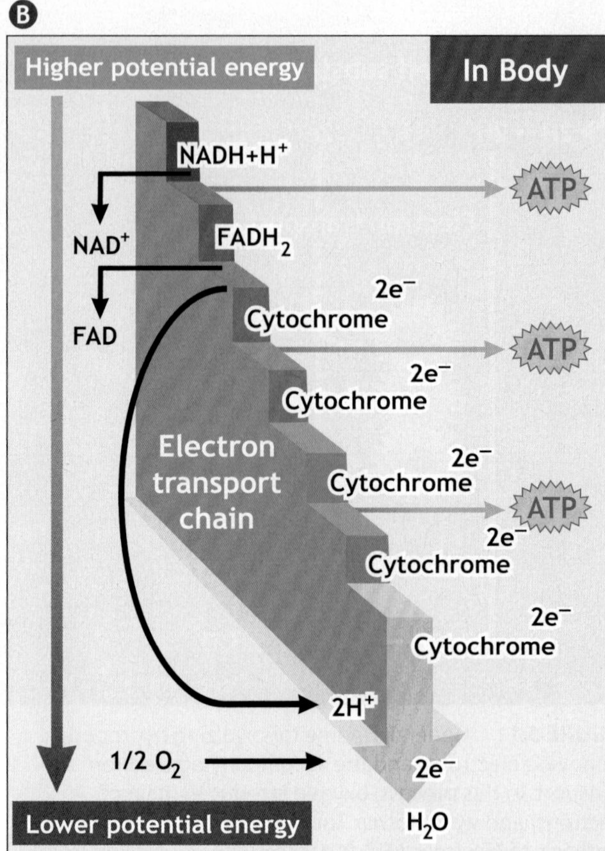

FIGURE 5.12 Examples of harnessing potential energy. **A.** In industry, energy from falling water becomes harnessed to turn the waterwheel, which in turn performs mechanical work. **B.** In the body, the electron transport chain removes electrons from hydrogens for ultimate delivery to oxygen. In oxidation-reduction, much of the chemical energy stored within the hydrogen atom does not dissipate to kinetic energy but instead is conserved within ATP. (Adapted with permission from McArdle WD, Katch FI, Katch VL. *Sports and Exercise Nutrition*. 4th Ed. Philadelphia: Wolters Kluwer Health, 2013.)

Efficiency of Electron Transport and Oxidative Phosphorylation

Each mole of ATP formed from ADP conserves approximately 7 kcal of energy. Because 2.5 moles of ATP regenerate from the total of 52 kcal of energy released to oxidize 1 mole of NADH, about 18 kcal (7 kcal · mol^{-1} × 2.5) conserves as chemical energy. This represents a relative efficiency of 34% to harness chemical energy via electron transport–oxidative phosphorylation (18 kcal ÷ 52 kcal × 100). The remaining 66% of the energy dissipates as heat. If the intracellular energy change for ATP synthesis approaches 10 kcal · mol^{-1}, then energy conservation efficiency approximates 50%. Considering that a steam engine transforms its fuel into useful energy at only about 30% efficiency, the value of 34% or above for the human body represents a relatively high-efficiency rate.

Oxygen's Role in Energy Metabolism

Continual ATP resynthesis during coupled oxidative phosphorylation of macronutrients has three prerequisites:

1. Availability of the reducing agents NADH or $FADH_2$
2. Presence of oxygen as a terminal oxidizing agent
3. Sufficient quantity of enzymes and metabolic machinery in the tissues to make the energy transfer reactions "go" at an appropriate sequence and rate

Satisfying these three conditions causes hydrogen and electrons to continually shuttle down the respiratory chain. The hydrogens combine with oxygen to form water, and the electrons pass on to form the high-energy ATP molecule. During strenuous activity, inadequacy in oxygen delivery (prerequisite 2) or its rate of utilization (prerequisite 3) creates a relative imbalance between hydrogen release and oxygen's final acceptance of them. If either condition occurs, electrons flowing down the respiratory chain "back up" and hydrogens accumulate bound to NAD^+ and FAD. Without oxygen, the temporarily "free" hydrogens require another molecule to bind with. In a subsequent section, we explain how lactate forms when the compound pyruvate temporarily binds these excess hydrogens or electrons; lactate formation allows electron transport–oxidative phosphorylation to proceed relatively unimpeded at a given intensity.

Aerobic energy metabolism refers to the energy-generating catabolic reactions during which oxygen serves as the final electron acceptor in the respiratory chain to form water when it combines with hydrogen. Some might posit that the term **aerobic metabolism (cellular respiration)** is misleading because oxygen does not participate directly in ATP synthesis. Nevertheless, oxygen's presence at the "end of the respiratory chain sequence" largely determines an individual's capacity for ATP production.

SUMMARY

1. Energy release occurs in miniscule amounts during complex, enzymatically controlled reactions to enable more efficient energy transfer and conservation.
2. Approximately 40% of the potential energy in food nutrients transfers to the high-energy compound ATP.
3. Splitting of ATP's terminal phosphate bond liberates free energy to power all forms of biologic work.
4. ATP represents the cell's energy currency, although its limited quantity amounts to only about 3.5 oz.
5. PCr interacts with ADP to form ATP; this nonaerobic, high-energy reservoir replenishes ATP rapidly. ATP and PCr are collectively referred to as "high-energy phosphates."
6. Phosphorylation represents energy transfer as energy-rich phosphate bonds. In this process, ADP and Cr continually recycle into ATP and PCr.
7. Cellular oxidation occurs on the inner lining of mitochondrial membranes; it involves transferring electrons from NADH and $FADH_2$ to molecular oxygen, thus releasing and transferring chemical energy to combine ATP from ADP plus a phosphate ion.
8. During aerobic ATP resynthesis, molecular hydrogen combines with oxygen to form water, making oxygen the final electron acceptor in the respiratory chain.

THINK IT THROUGH

1. Explain why it is imprecise to refer to the body's energy *"production."*
2. Discuss implications of the second law of thermodynamics to measure energy expenditure.

PART 3 Energy Release From Food

The energy release from macronutrient breakdown serves one crucial purpose: to phosphorylate ADP to reform ATP, known as the most important energy-rich compound. Macronutrient catabolism favors generating phosphate-bond energy, yet the specific pathways of degradation differ depending on the nutrients metabolized.

Figure 5.13 outlines the six macronutrient fuel sources that supply substrate for oxidation and subsequent ATP regeneration:

1. Muscle cells' storage of triacylglycerol and glycogen molecules
2. Blood glucose derived from liver glycogen
3. Free fatty acids derived from triacylglycerols in the liver and adipocytes
4. Intramuscular- and liver-derived amino acid carbon skeletons
5. Anaerobic reactions in the cytosol in the initial phase of glucose or glycogen breakdown, which generate a relatively small amount of ATP
6. Phosphorylation of ADP by PCr under enzymatic control by creatine kinase and adenylate kinase

fyi Glucose is Not Retrievable From Fatty Acids

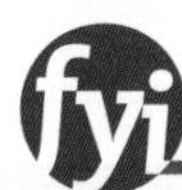

Cells synthesize glucose from pyruvate and other 3-carbon compounds. Glucose, however, cannot form from the 2-carbon acetyl fragments from β-oxidation of fatty acids. Consequently, fatty acids *cannot* readily provide energy for such tissues as the brain and nerve cells rely on glucose almost exclusively as a fuel source. A large portion of dietary lipid occurs in triacylglycerol form. Triacylglycerol's glycerol component can yield glucose, but the glycerol molecule contains only 3% or 6% of the 57 carbon atoms in the molecule. Thus, fat from dietary sources or stored in adipocytes does not provide an adequate potential glucose source; about 95% of the fat molecule cannot be converted to glucose.

CARBOHYDRATE ENERGY RELEASE

Carbohydrates' primary function supplies energy for cellular work. Our discussion of nutrient energy metabolism begins with carbohydrate for five reasons:

1. Carbohydrate represents the *only* macronutrient whose potential energy generates ATP both with oxygen (aerobically) and without oxygen (anaerobically). The anaerobic breakdown of carbohydrate becomes important in vigorous physical activity that requires rapid energy release above levels supplied only by aerobic metabolic reactions.
2. Carbohydrate supplies about half the body's energy requirements during light and moderate aerobic activity.
3. Processing fat for energy through the metabolic mill requires some carbohydrate catabolism.
4. Aerobic breakdown of carbohydrate for energy occurs at about *twice* the rate as energy generated from lipid breakdown. Thus, depleting glycogen reserves

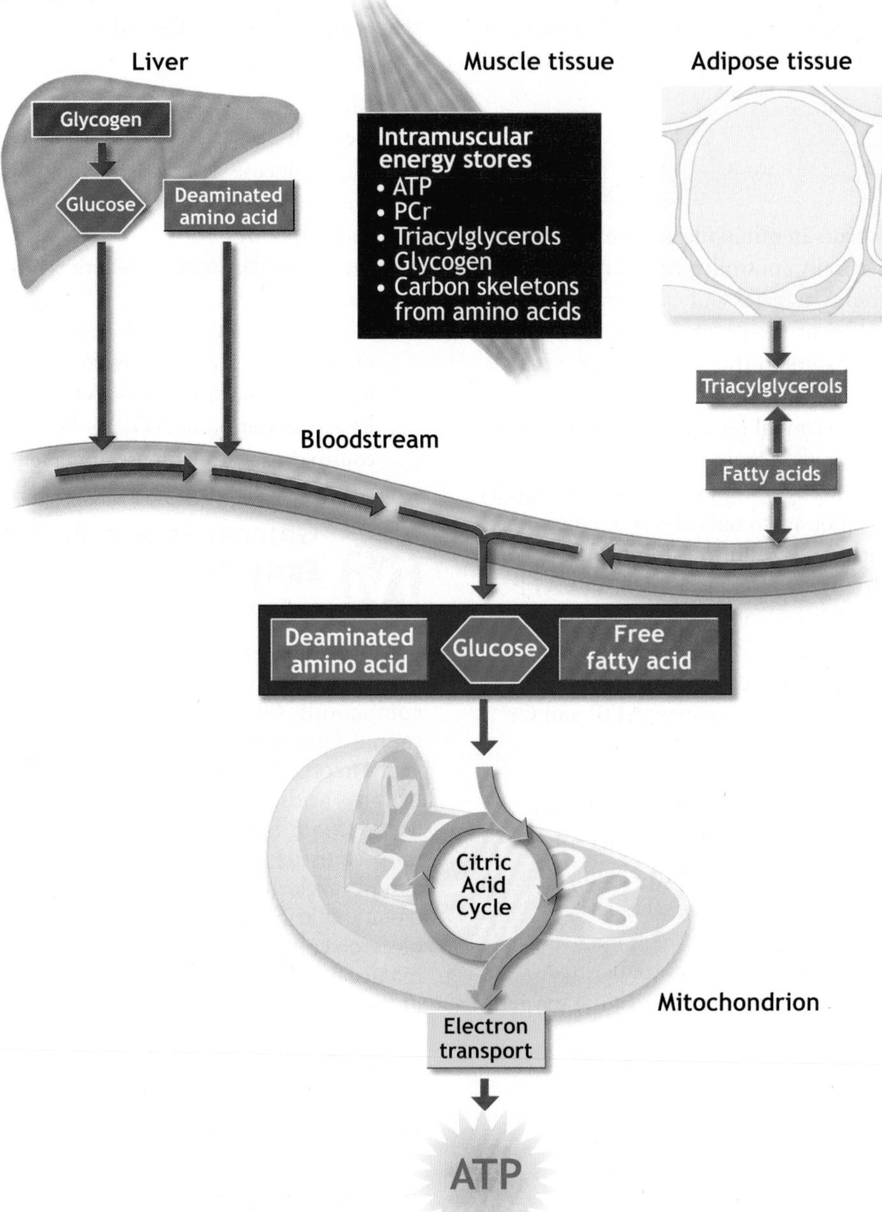

FIGURE 5.13 Fuel sources that supply substrate to regenerate ATP. The liver provides a rich source of amino acids and glucose, while adipocytes generate large quantities of energy-rich fatty acid molecules. After their release, the bloodstream delivers these compounds to the muscle cell. Most of the cells' energy production takes place within the mitochondria. Mitochondrial proteins carry out their roles in oxidative phosphorylation on the inner membranous walls of this architecturally elegant complex. The intramuscular energy sources consist of the high-energy phosphates ATP and PCr and triacylglycerols, glycogen, and amino acids. (Adapted with permission from McArdle WD, Katch FI, Katch VL. *Exercise Physiology: Nutrition, Energy, and Human Performance*. 8th Ed. Baltimore: Wolters Kluwer Health, 2015.)

reduces power output. In intense aerobic activity as in marathon running, athletes can experience nutrient-related fatigue, a state associated with muscle and liver glycogen depletion.

5. To function optimally, the central nervous system requires an uninterrupted carbohydrate supply.

The complete breakdown of 1 mole or 180 g of glucose to carbon dioxide and water yields a maximum of 686 kcal of free energy available for work.

$$C_6H_{12}O_2 + 6O_2 \rightarrow 6CO_2 + 6H_2O - \Delta G\ 686\ \text{kcal} \cdot \text{mol}^{-1}$$

Recall that the synthesis of 1 mole of ATP from ADP plus a phosphate ion requires 7.3 kcal of energy. Coupling all of the energy from glucose oxidation to phosphorylation could theoretically form 94 moles of ATP per mole of glucose (686 kcal ÷ 7.3 kcal · mole^{-1} = 94 moles). In muscle, phosphate bond formation conserves only 34% or 233 kcal of energy, with the remainder dissipated as heat. As such, glucose breakdown regenerates 32 moles of ATP (233 kcal ÷ 7.3 kcal · mole^{-1} = 32 moles) with an accompanying free energy gain of 233 kcal. One additional ATP forms if carbohydrate breakdown begins with glycogen.

Anaerobic Versus Aerobic Glycolysis

Two forms of carbohydrate breakdown occur in a series of fermentation reactions collectively termed **glycolysis** ("the dissolution of sugar") or the Embden-Meyerhof pathway, named for its two German chemist discoverers (Otto Meyerhof  [1884–1951], 1922 Nobel Prize in Chemistry [**www.nobelprize.org/nobel_prizes/medicine/laureates/1922/meyerhof-bio.html**], and Gustav Embden [1874–1933], first to explain all the steps involved in converting **glycogen** to **lactic acid**). In one form, lactate formed from pyruvate becomes the end product. In the other form, pyruvate remains the end product. With pyruvate as the end substrate, carbohydrate catabolism proceeds and couples to further break down in the CAC with ATP from subsequent electron transport production. This form of carbohydrate breakdown, sometimes termed *aerobic* (with oxygen) *glycolysis*, is a relatively *slower* process resulting in substantial ATP formation. In contrast, glycolysis that results in lactate formation, referred to as *anaerobic* (without oxygen) *glycolysis*, represents more rapid but limited ATP production. The net formation of either lactate or pyruvate depends more on the relative glycolytic and mitochondrial activities than molecular oxygen's presence. The relative demand for rapid or slow ATP production determines either the rapid or slow form of glycolysis. The glycolytic process itself, from beginning substrate to ending lactate or pyruvate substrate, does not involve oxygen. Two terms describe glycolysis—*rapid* anaerobic glycolysis and *slower* aerobic glycolysis.

See the animations "Glycolysis" and "Catabolism" on **http://thePoint.lww.com/MKKESS5e** for a demonstration of these processes.

Lactic Acid Versus Lactate

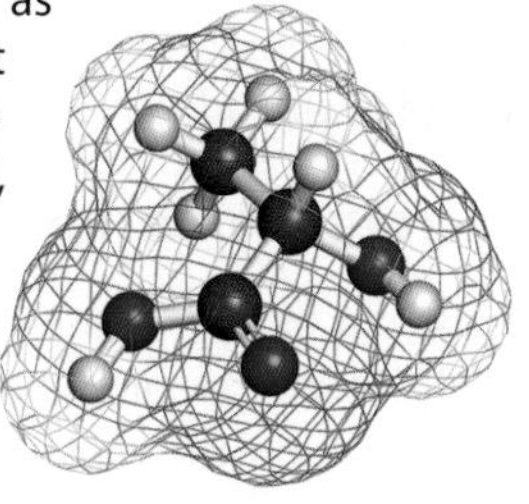

Lactic acid ($C_3H_6O_3$), also known as "milk acid," and *lactate* should not be used interchangeably as they are not the same substance. Lactic acid, an acid formed during anaerobic glycolysis, quickly dissociates to release a hydrogen ion (H^+). In the molecular model, the white spheres represent hydrogen atoms attached to the 3 black carbon atoms, and the three red atoms are oxygen. Following the dissociation, the remaining compound binds with a positively charged sodium or potassium ion to form the acid salt called lactate. Under physiological conditions, the majority of lactic acid dissociates and presents as lactate.

Glucose to Glycogen and Glycogen to Glucose

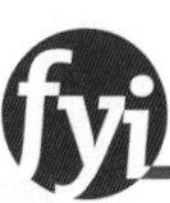

The cytoplasm of liver and muscle cells contains glycogen granules and enzymes for glycogen synthesis (glycogenesis) and breakdown (glycogenolysis). Normally following a meal, the glucose molecule shown schematically does not accumulate in blood; rather, surplus glucose follows one of three strategies: (1) it enters the pathways of energy metabolism, (2) it stores as the complex molecule glycogen, or (3) it converts to fat for storage in subcutaneous tissues, internal organs, or accumulates in the viscera, most notably the abdominal region. During high cellular activity, blood glucose oxidizes via the glycolytic pathway, CAC, or respiratory chain to form ATP (glycogenolysis). In contrast, low cellular activity (and/or depleted glycogen reserves) inactivates key glycolytic enzymes, which results in surplus glucose forming glycogen (**glycogenesis**).

Energy Release From Glucose: Rapid Anaerobic Glycolysis

Rapid anaerobic glycolysis occurs in the cytoplasm, the watery medium of the cell outside the mitochondrion (**Fig. 5.14**). The term **glycogenolysis** describes these reactions when they initiate from stored glycogen. In a way, glycolytic reactions represent a more primitive form of energy transfer, well developed in amphibians, reptiles, fish, and marine mammals. In humans, the cells' limited capacity for rapid glycolysis plays a crucial role during physical activities that require maximal effort for up to 90-second duration. Note the six ATPs produced during glycolysis reactions.

In reaction 1, ATP acts as a phosphate donor to phosphorylate glucose to glucose 6-phosphate. In most tissues, this "traps" the glucose molecule in the cell. In the presence of the enzyme *glycogen synthase*, glucose links or polymerizes with other glucose molecules to form a large glycogen molecule. Liver and kidney cells contain the enzyme **phosphatase** that splits the phosphate from glucose 6-phosphate. This frees glucose from the cell for transport throughout the body. During energy metabolism, glucose 6-phosphate changes to fructose 6-phosphate. At this stage, no energy extraction occurs, yet some energy incorporates into the original glucose molecule at the expense of one ATP molecule. In a sense, phosphorylation "primes the pump" to continue energy metabolism. The fructose 6-phosphate molecule gains an additional phosphate and changes to fructose 1,6-diphosphate under control of **phosphofructokinase (PFK)**. The activity level of this enzyme probably limits the rate of glycolysis during maximum-effort activity. Fructose 1,6-diphosphate then splits into two phosphorylated molecules with three-carbon chains (*3-phosphoglyceraldehyde*), which further decompose to *pyruvate* in five successive reactions. Fast-twitch (type II) muscle fibers described in Chapter 14 contain relatively large quantities of PFK, making them ideally suited to generate anaerobic energy via glycolysis.

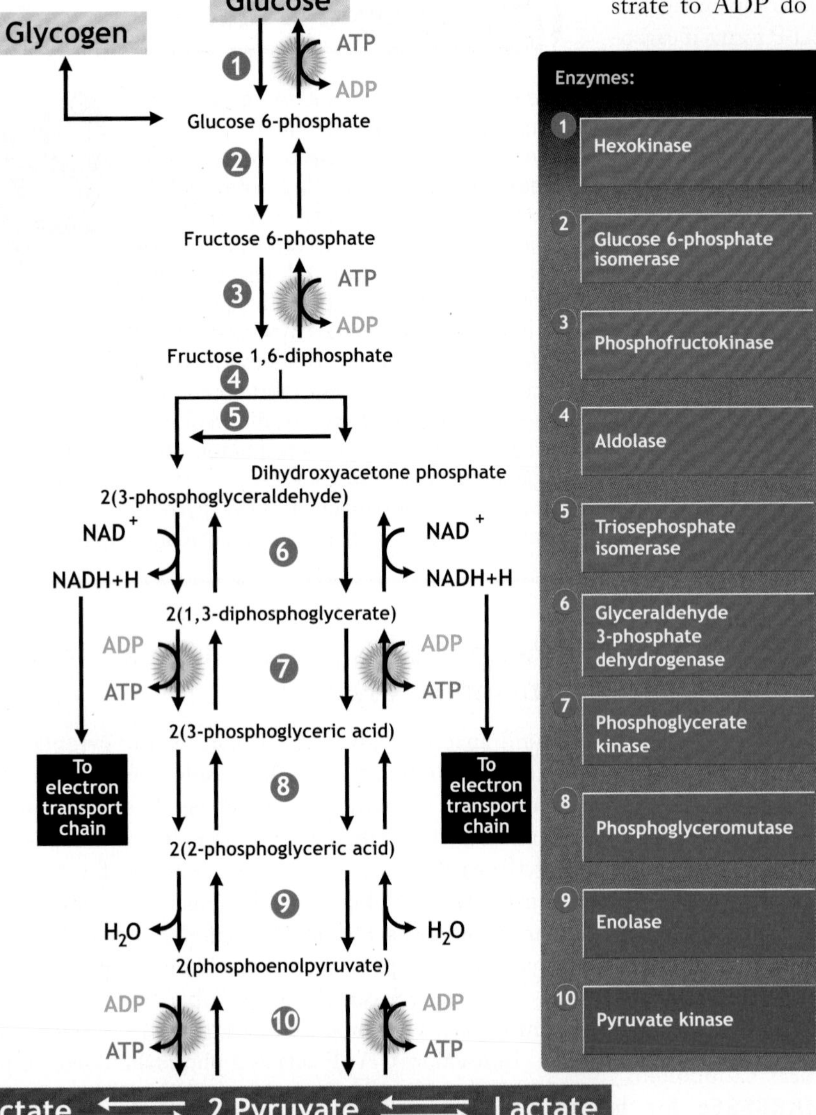

FIGURE 5.14 Glycolysis: a series of 10 enzymatically controlled chemical reactions creates two molecules of pyruvate from the anaerobic breakdown of glucose. Lactate forms when NADH oxidation does not keep pace with its formation in glycolysis. Enzymes *(numbers in the red circles)* play a key regulatory role in these metabolic reactions. (Adapted with permission from McArdle WD, Katch FI, Katch VL. *Sports and Exercise Nutrition*. 4th Ed. Philadelphia: Wolters Kluwer Health, 2013.)

Substrate-Level Phosphorylation in Rapid Anaerobic Glycolysis

Most energy generated in glycolysis does not resynthesize ATP but instead dissipates as heat. In reactions 7 and 10 in **Figure 5.14**, the energy released from the glucose intermediates stimulates the direct transfer of phosphate groups to ADP, generating four ATP molecules. Two molecules of ATP were used in the initial phosphorylation of the glucose molecule, allowing glycolysis to generate a *net gain* of 2 ATPs. Note that these specific energy transfers from substrate to ADP do not require molecular oxygen. Rather, energy directly transfers via phosphate bonds in the anaerobic reactions called **substrate-level phosphorylation**. Energy conservation during rapid glycolysis operates at an efficiency of about 30%.

Rapid glycolysis generates only about 5% of the total ATP during the glucose molecule's complete degradation. Examples of activities that rely heavily on ATP generated by rapid glycolysis include sprinting at the end of a mile run, swimming all-out from start to finish in a 50- and 100-m swim, routines on gymnastics apparatus, and sprint running up to 200 m.

Hydrogen Release During Rapid Anaerobic Glycolysis

During rapid glycolysis, two pairs of hydrogen atoms strip away from the glucose substrate, and their electrons are passed to NAD^+ to form NADH (see **Fig. 5.14**). Normally, if the respiratory chain processed these electrons directly, 2.5 molecules of ATP would generate for each NADH molecule oxidized. Skeletal muscle mitochondria remain impermeable to NADH formed in the cytoplasm during glycolysis. Consequently, the electrons from NADH outside the mitochondrial shuttle indirectly into the mitochondria. In skeletal muscle, this route ends with electrons passing to FAD to form $FADH_2$ at a point below the first ATP formation (see **Fig. 5.12B**). Thus, 1.5 rather than 2.5 ATP molecules form when the respiratory chain oxidizes cytoplasmic NADH. Two molecules of NADH form in glycolysis, allowing subsequent coupled electron transport–oxidative phosphorylation to aerobically generate four ATP molecules.

Lactate Formation

Sufficient oxygen bathes the cells during light-to-moderate levels of energy metabolism. The hydrogens (electrons) stripped from the substrate and carried by NADH oxidase within mitochondria to form water when oxygen joins with them. In a biochemical sense, a "steady rate" exists because hydrogen oxidizes at about the same rate it becomes available. This condition of aerobic glycolysis forms pyruvate as the end product.

In strenuous physical activity, when energy demands exceed either oxygen supply or utilization rate, the respiratory chain cannot process all of the hydrogen joined to NADH. Continued release of anaerobic energy in glycolysis depends on NAD^+ availability for oxidizing 3-phosphoglyceraldehyde (see reaction 6 in **Fig. 5.14**); otherwise, the rapid rate of glycolysis "grinds to a halt." During rapid or anaerobic glycolysis, NAD^+ "frees up" as pairs of "excess" nonoxidized hydrogens combine temporarily with pyruvate to form lactate, catalyzed by the enzyme lactate dehydrogenase in the reversible reaction displayed in **Figure 5.15**.

During rest and moderate activity, some lactate continually forms and readily oxidizes for energy in neighboring muscle fibers with high oxidative capacity or in more distant tissues such as the heart and ventilatory muscles. Lactate also provides an indirect precursor of liver glycogen. Consequently, lactate does not accumulate because its removal rate equals its production rate. One of the benefits of physical training is that increased endurance capacity enhances lactate clearance or turnover during higher-intensity physical activities.

A direct chemical pathway exists for liver glycogen synthesis from dietary carbohydrate. Liver glycogen synthesis also occurs indirectly from conversion of the 3-carbon precursor lactate to glucose. Erythrocytes and adipocytes contain glycolytic enzymes, and skeletal muscle possesses the largest quantity, making any lactate-to-glucose conversion likely to occur in muscle.

The temporary storage of hydrogen with pyruvate represents a distinctive aspect of energy metabolism because it provides a ready "collector" for temporary storage of the rapid glycolysis end product. After lactate forms in muscle, it takes one of two routes:

1. Diffuses into the interstitial space and blood for buffering and removal from the site of energy metabolism
2. Provides a gluconeogenic substrate for glycogen synthesis

Through each of these routes, glycolysis continues to supply anaerobic energy for ATP resynthesis. This avenue for extra energy remains temporary if blood and muscle lactate levels increase and ATP formation fails to keep pace with its rate of use. Fatigue soon sets in and performance deteriorates. Increased intracellular acidity under anaerobic conditions likely modulates fatigue by inactivating some energy transfer enzymes, which likely impair muscle's contractile properties.

fyi The Discoverers of the Cori Cycle

The Cori cycle was named in honor of husband and wife biochemists Gerty Theresa Cori (Radnitz; 1897–1957; first American woman to win a Nobel Prize in science, and first woman to be awarded the Nobel Prize in Physiology or Medicine, 1947) and Carl Ferdinand Cori (1896–1984; 1947 Nobel Prize in Physiology or Medicine), who discovered the course of the catalytic conversion of glycogen. They shared the Nobel Prize for their work with Argentine physiologist Bernardo Alberto Houssay (1896–1984) for his discovery of the part contributed by the hormone of the anterior pituitary lobe in sugar metabolism. Besides the role of intermediates in carbohydrate metabolism, Gerty Cori also investigated diseases related to glycogen storage that led to discovering the cause of four different disease complications of glycogen storage.

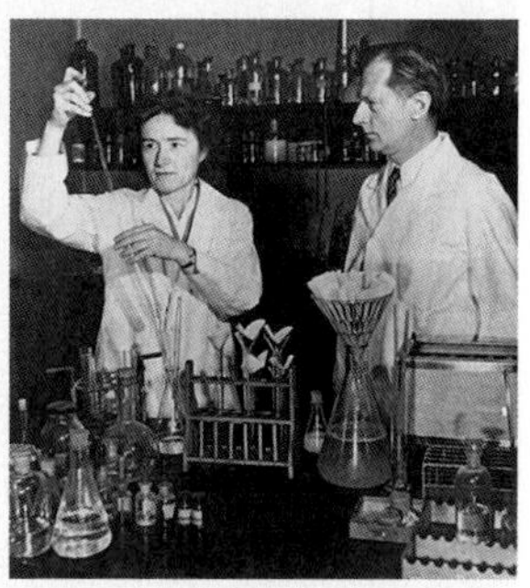

Gerty and Carl Ferdinand Cori. (Image courtesy Smithsonian Institution Archives.)

The animation "Biochemical Reactions of Cori Cycle," available on **http://thePoint.lww.com/MKKESS5e**, demonstrates this process.

FIGURE 5.15 Under physiologic conditions within muscle, lactate forms when hydrogens from NADH combine temporarily with pyruvate. This frees up NAD to accept additional hydrogens generated in glycolysis. (Adapted with permission from McArdle WD, Katch FI, Katch VL. *Exercise Physiology: Nutrition, Energy, and Human Performance*. 8th Ed. Baltimore: Wolters Kluwer Health, 2015.)

Lactate: A Valuable "Waste Product"

Lactate should not be viewed as a metabolic waste product. To the contrary, it accumulates with intense activity as a valuable chemical energy source. When sufficient oxygen becomes available during recovery or when activity pace slows, NAD^+ scavenges hydrogens attached to lactate, subsequently oxidizing them to form ATP. Recall that one pyruvate molecule + 2 hydrogens form one lactate molecule. This means that the pyruvate molecules' carbon skeletons reformed from lactate during physical activity become either oxidized for energy or synthesized to glucose during gluconeogenesis in muscle itself or in the liver via the **Cori cycle** (**Fig. 5.16**). The Cori cycle removes lactate and uses it to replenish glycogen reserves depleted from intense movement.

Lactate Shuttle: Blood Lactate as an Energy Source

Isotope tracer studies show that lactate produced in fast-twitch muscle fibers and other tissues circulates to other fast- or slow-twitch fibers for conversion to pyruvate. Pyruvate, in turn, converts to acetyl-CoA for entry into the CAC for aerobic energy metabolism. This process of **lactate shuttling** among cells enables glycogenolysis in one cell to

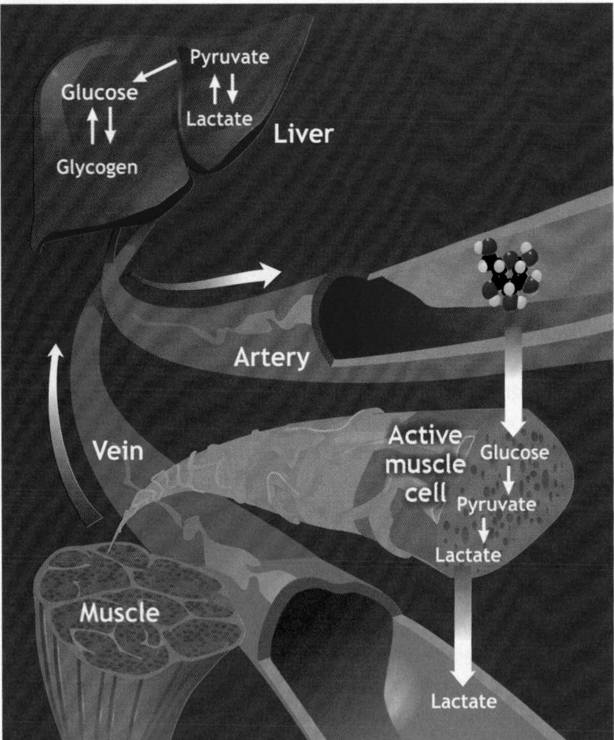

FIGURE 5.16 The biochemical reactions of the Cori cycle in the liver synthesize glucose from the lactate released from active muscles. This gluconeogenic process helps to maintain carbohydrate reserves. (Adapted with permission from McArdle WD, Katch FI, Katch VL. *Sports and Exercise Nutrition*. 4th Ed. Philadelphia: Wolters Kluwer Health, 2013.)

supply other cells with fuel for oxidation. *This makes muscle not only a major site of lactate production but also a primary tissue for lactate removal via oxidation.*

fyi Free Radicals Formed During Increased Aerobic Metabolism

The passage of electrons along the electron transport chain can form reactive oxygen species (ROS), free radical molecules with unpaired electrons or an open electron shell making them highly reactive. These reactive free radicals bind quickly to other molecules that promote potential damage to the combining molecule. Free radical formation in muscle, for example, may contribute to muscle fatigue or soreness, or a potential reduction in metabolic potential in some athletes. There is increased interest in monitoring the oxidative stress status of athletes followed by appropriate antioxidant supplement use.

Source: Hadžović-Džuvo A. Oxidative stress status in elite athletes engaged in different sport disciplines. *Bosn J Basic Med Sci* 2014;14:56.

Slow Aerobic Glycolysis Energy Release: The Citric Acid Cycle

The rapid anaerobic glycolysis reactions release only about 5% of the potential energy within the original glucose molecule. This means that extracting the remaining energy must occur by an additional metabolic pathway, which in this case occurs when pyruvate irreversibly converts to acetyl-CoA, a form of acetic acid. Acetyl-CoA enters the second stage of carbohydrate breakdown known as slow aerobic glycolysis (also termed the **citric acid cycle [CAC], Krebs cycle, or tricarboxylic acid cycle**).

Figure 5.17 shows the metabolic reactions of pyruvate to acetyl-CoA. Each 3-carbon pyruvate molecule loses a carbon when it joins with a CoA molecule to form acetyl-CoA and carbon dioxide. The reaction from pyruvate proceeds in one direction only.

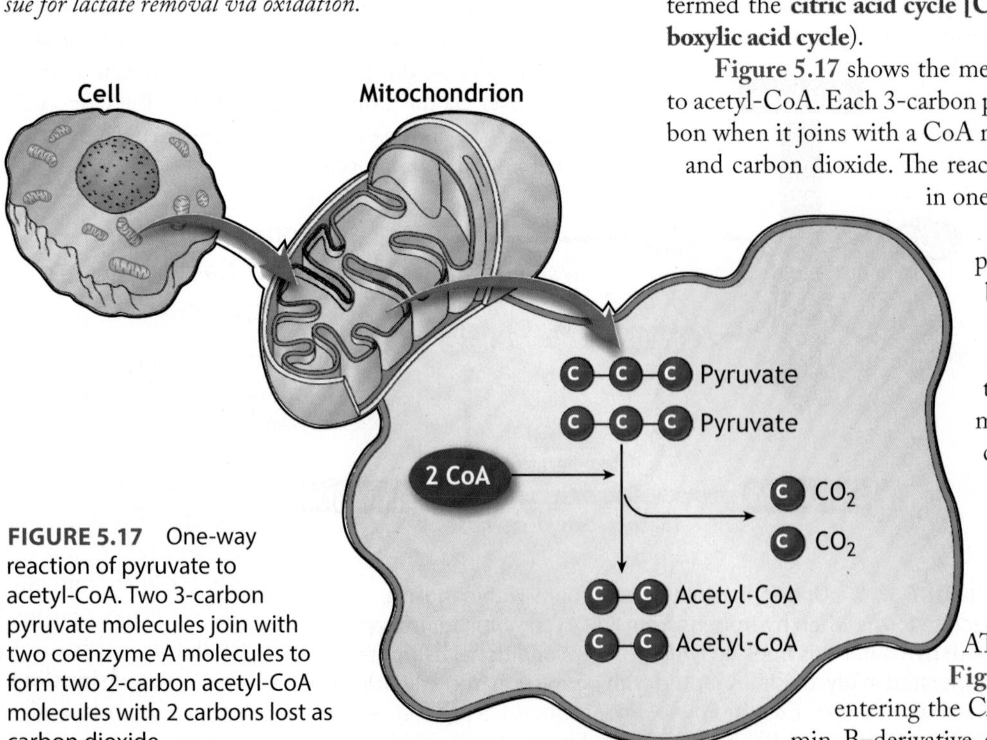

FIGURE 5.17 One-way reaction of pyruvate to acetyl-CoA. Two 3-carbon pyruvate molecules join with two coenzyme A molecules to form two 2-carbon acetyl-CoA molecules with 2 carbons lost as carbon dioxide.

Figure 5.18 illustrates two phases of complete pyruvate breakdown starting with the glycolytic production of acetyl-CoA. This molecule then enters the CAC within mitochondria and degrades to carbon dioxide and hydrogen atoms (phase 1). In phase 2, hydrogen atom oxidation occurs during electron transport–oxidative phosphorylation to regenerate ATP.

Figure 5.19 shows pyruvate entering the CAC by joining with the vitamin B–derivative coenzyme A ("A" stands for

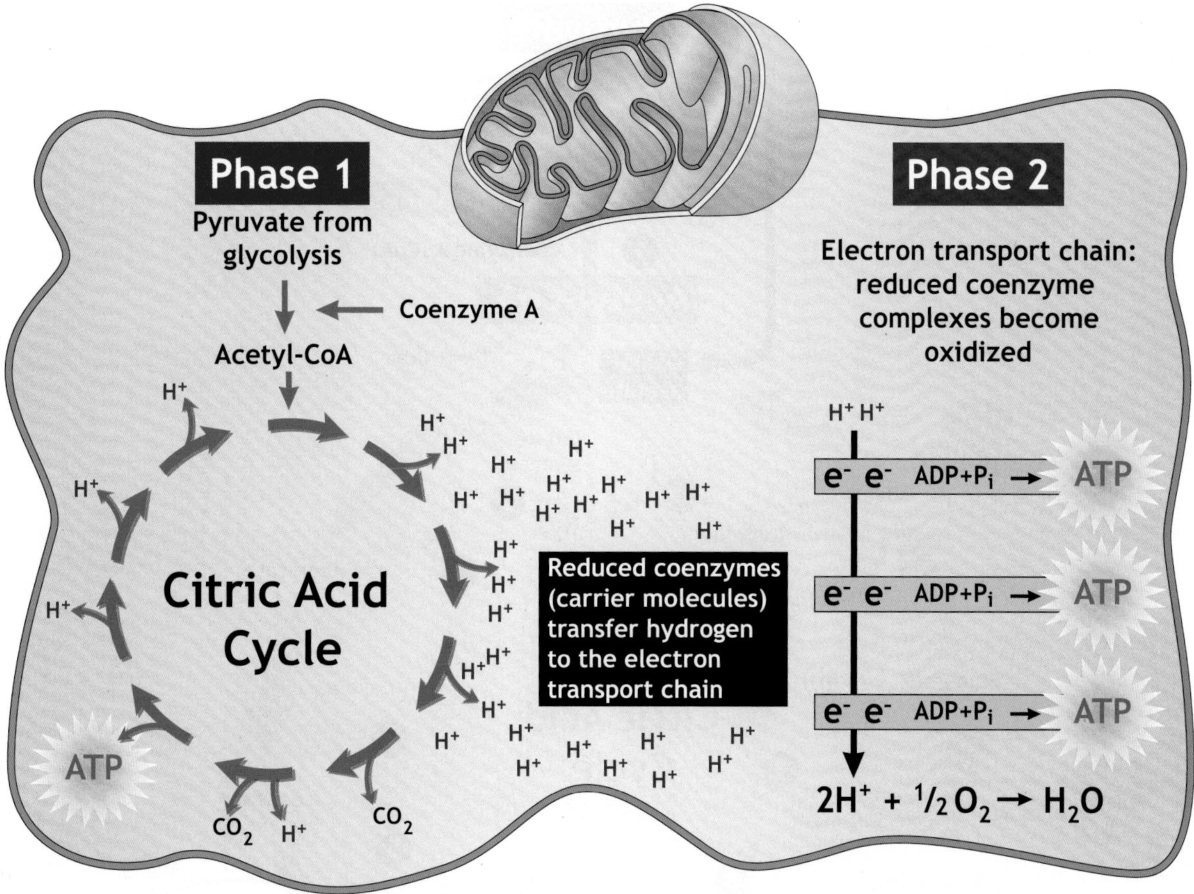

FIGURE 5.18 Aerobic energy metabolism. Phase 1. In the mitochondria, the citric acid cycle generates hydrogen atoms during acetyl-CoA breakdown. Phase 2. Significant quantities of ATP regenerate when these hydrogens oxidize via the aerobic process of electron transport–oxidative phosphorylation (electron transport chain). (Adapted with permission from McArdle WD, Katch FI, Katch VL. *Sports and Exercise Nutrition*. 4th Ed. Philadelphia: Wolters Kluwer Health, 2013.)

acetic acid) to form the 2-carbon compound acetyl-CoA. This process releases two hydrogens, which transfers their electrons to NAD^+, forming one molecule of carbon dioxide as follows:

$$\textbf{Pyruvate} + \textbf{NAD}^+ + \textbf{CoA} \rightarrow \textbf{Acetyl} - \textbf{CoA} + \textbf{CO}_2 + \textbf{NADH} + \textbf{H}^+$$

The acetyl portion of acetyl-CoA joins with oxaloacetate to form citrate (the same 6-carbon citric acid compound found in citrus fruits), which then proceeds through the CAC. This cycle continues to operate because it retains the original oxaloacetate molecule to join with a new acetyl fragment.

Each acetyl-CoA molecule entering the CAC releases two carbon dioxide molecules and four pairs of hydrogen atoms. One molecule of ATP also regenerates directly by substrate-level phosphorylation from CAC reactions (reactions 7 and 8; **Fig. 5.19**). As summarized at the bottom of **Figure 5.19**, four hydrogens release when acetyl-CoA forms from the two pyruvate molecules created in glycolysis, with an additional 16 hydrogens released in the CAC (acetyl-CoA hydrolysis) for a total of 20 hydrogens. *The primary function of the CAC generates electrons (H^+) for passage in the respiratory chain to NAD^+ and FAD.*

Oxygen does not directly participate in CAC reactions. The chemical energy within pyruvate transfers to ADP through electron transport–oxidative phosphorylation. With adequate oxygen, enzymes, and substrate, NAD^+ and FAD regenerate, allowing CAC metabolism to proceed unimpeded. The three components of aerobic metabolism are the CAC, electron transport, and oxidative phosphorylation.

 See the animation "Citric Acid Cycle" on **http://thePoint.lww.com/MKKESS5e** for a demonstration of this process.

Net Energy Transfer From Glucose Catabolism

Figure 5.20 summarizes the skeletal muscle pathways for energy transfer during glucose breakdown. A net gain of two ATP molecules form from substrate-level phosphorylation in glycolysis; similarly, 2 ATP molecules come from acetyl-CoA degradation in the CAC. The 24 released hydrogen atoms and their subsequent oxidation are accounted for as follows:

1. Four extramitochondrial hydrogens (2 NADH) generated in rapid glycolysis yield 5 ATPs during oxidative phosphorylation.

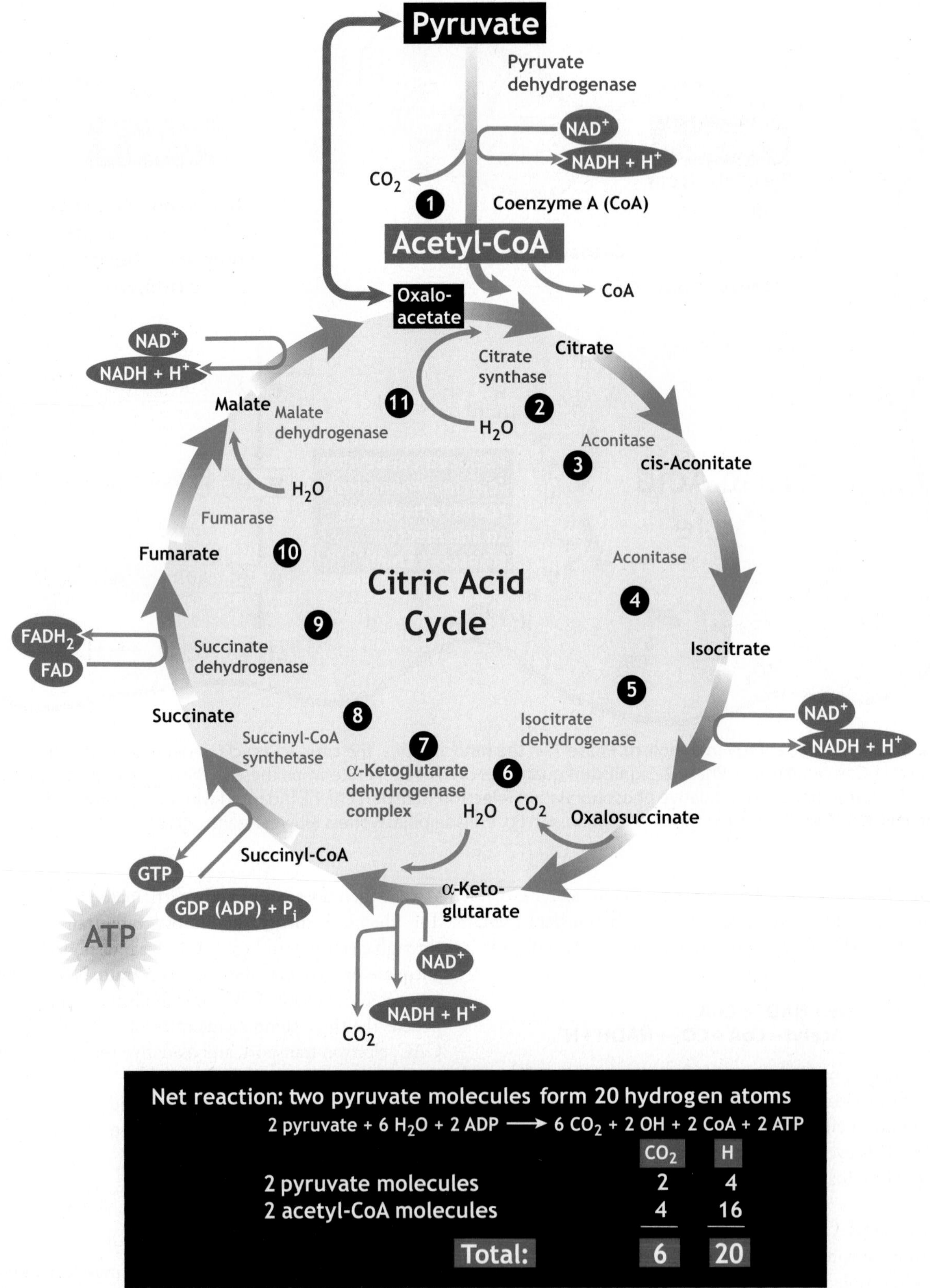

FIGURE 5.19 Flow sheet for the release of hydrogen and carbon dioxide in the mitochondrion during the breakdown of one pyruvate molecule. All values are doubled when computing the net gain of hydrogen and carbon dioxide because two molecules of pyruvate form from one glucose molecule in glycolysis. The three enzymes denoted in purple play key roles in this regulatory process. (See also **http://thePoint.lww.com/MKKESS5e** for the animation "Chemical Reactions of Mitochondrion.") (Adapted with permission from McArdle WD, Katch FI, Katch VL. *Sports and Exercise Nutrition*. 4th Ed. Philadelphia: Wolters Kluwer Health, 2013.)

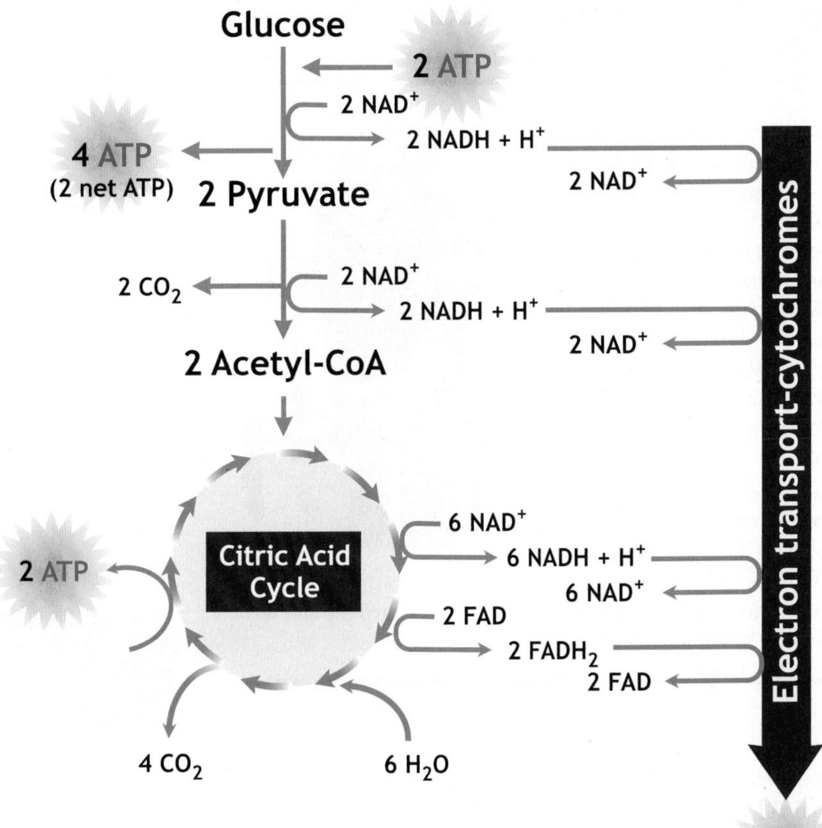

Net ATP from glucose metabolism

Source	Reaction	Net ATP
Substrate phosphorylation	Glycolysis	2
2 H_2 (4 H^+)	Glycolysis	5
2 H_2 (4 H^+)	Pyruvate → Acetyl-CoA	5
Substrate phosphorylation	Citric acid cycle	2
6 H_2 (12 H^+)	Citric acid cycle	15
2 H_2 (4 H^+)	Citric acid cycle	3
	Total:	32 ATP

FIGURE 5.20 A net yield of 32 ATPs from energy transfer during the complete oxidation of one glucose molecule in glycolysis, citric acid cycle, and electron transport. (Adapted with permission from McArdle WD, Katch FI, Katch VL. *Sports and Exercise Nutrition*. 4th Ed. Philadelphia: Wolters Kluwer Health, 2013.)

2. Four hydrogens (2 NADH) released in the mitochondrion when pyruvate degrades to acetyl-CoA yield 5 ATPs.
3. The CAC via substrate-level phosphorylation produces two guanosine triphosphates (GTPs; a molecule similar to ATP).
4. Twelve of the 16 hydrogens (6 NADH) released in the CAC yield 15 ATPs (6 NADH × 2.5 ATPs per NADH = 15 ATPs).
5. Four hydrogens joined to FAD (2 $FADH_2$) in the CAC yield 3 ATPs.

The glucose molecule's complete breakdown yields 34 ATPs. Two ATPs initially phosphorylate glucose, making 32 ATP molecules equal the net ATP yield from glucose catabolism in skeletal muscle. Whereas 4 ATP molecules form directly from substrate-level phosphorylation (glycolysis and CAC), 28 ATP molecules regenerate during oxidative phosphorylation.

Some biochemistry and exercise physiology textbooks quote a net yield of 36 to 38 ATP molecules from glucose catabolism. This depends on which shuttle system, the glycerol-phosphate or malate-aspartate pathway, transports NADH with H^+ into the mitochondrion and the ATP yield per NADH oxidation used in the computations. One must temper the *theoretical* values for ATP yield in energy metabolism in light of recent biochemical experiments that suggests an overestimate because only 30 to 32 ATP actually enter the cell's cytoplasm. The added energy cost to transport ATP out of the mitochondria may

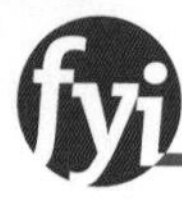

The Fat Burning Activity Zone to Optimize Fat Use

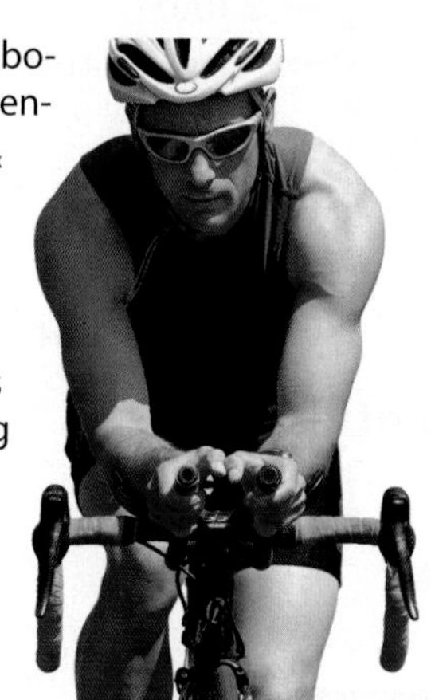

Research suggests that lipid metabolism maximizes at an average intensity of about 55% to 72% $\dot{V}O_{2max}$ and 68% to 79% of HR_{max} in conditioned cyclists. Above these zones, lipid metabolism decreases and switches to a predominance of carbohydrate metabolism. This suggests the necessity of exercising within these zones for sufficient duration to realize maximum fat burn.

Sources: Achten J, et al. Determination of the exercise intensity that elicits maximal fat oxidation. *Med Sci Sports Exerc* 2002;34:92.

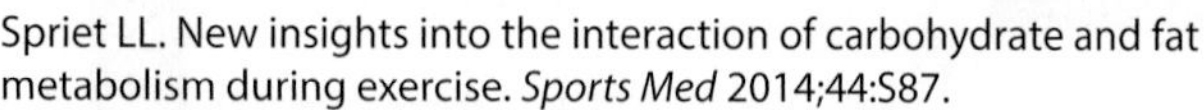

Spriet LL. New insights into the interaction of carbohydrate and fat metabolism during exercise. *Sports Med* 2014;44:S87.

help to explain the differences between theoretical versus actual ATP yield.

ENERGY RELEASE FROM LIPID

Stored fat represents the body's most plentiful potential energy source. Relative to carbohydrate and protein, stored fat provides almost unlimited energy. The fuel reserves in an average college-aged man represent between 60,000 and 100,000 kcal of energy from triacylglycerol in fat cells (adipocytes) and about 3000 kcal from intramuscular triacylglycerol stored in close proximity to muscle mitochondria. In contrast, the carbohydrate energy reserve only contributes about 2000 kcal to the total available energy pool.

Three specific energy sources for fat catabolism are as follows:

1. Triacylglycerols stored directly within the muscle fiber in close proximity to the mitochondria, with more in slow-twitch than in fast-twitch muscle fibers
2. Circulating triacylglycerols in lipoprotein complexes that hydrolyze on a tissue's capillary endothelial surface
3. Adipose tissue that provides circulating **free fatty acids (FFAs)** mobilized from triacylglycerols in adipose tissue

Figure 5.21 presents an overview of fatty acid mobilization and fat use. Triacylglycerol breaks down into its glycerol and fatty acid components. Blood transports FFAs released from adipocytes and bound to plasma albumin. Energy releases when triacylglycerols stored within the muscle fiber also degrade to glycerol and fatty acids. Triacylglycerol breakdown proceeds as follows:

$$\textbf{Triacylglycerol} + 3H_2O \xrightarrow{\text{lipase}} \textbf{Glycerol} + 3\textbf{Fatty acids}$$

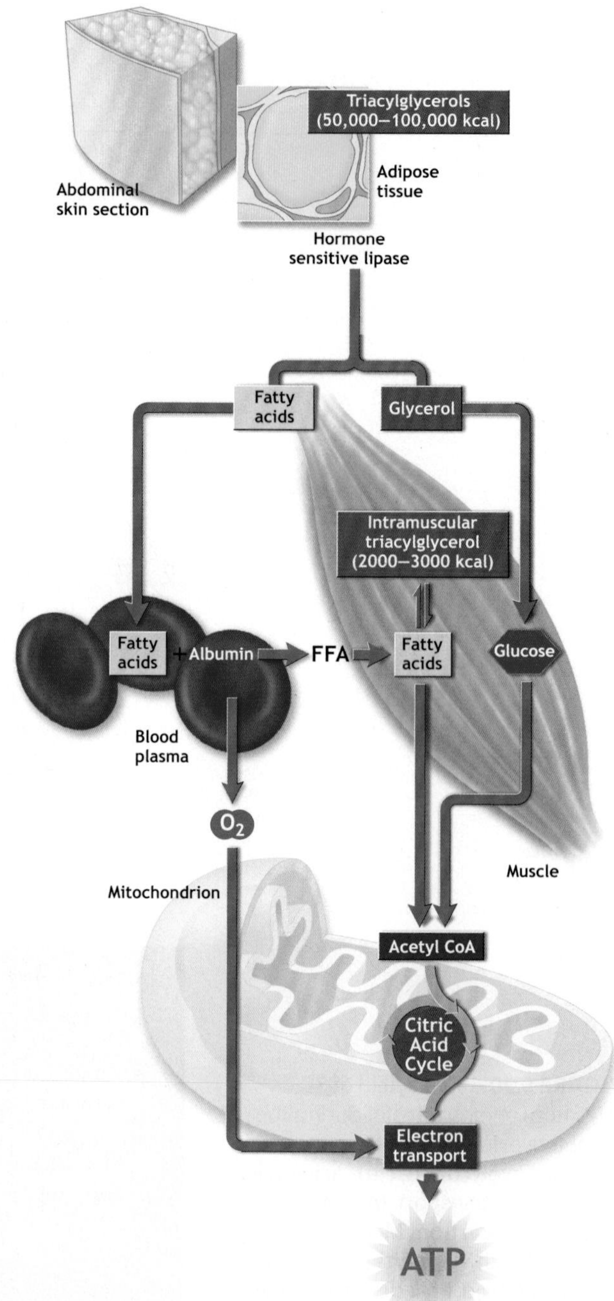

FIGURE 5.21 Dynamics of fat mobilization and fat use. Hormone-sensitive lipase stimulates triacylglycerol breakdown into its glycerol and fatty acid components. The blood transports free fatty acids (FFAs) released from adipocytes and bound to plasma albumin. Energy is released when triacylglycerols stored within the muscle fiber also degrade to glycerol and fatty acids. (Adapted with permission from McArdle WD, Katch FI, Katch VL. *Exercise Physiology: Nutrition, Energy, and Human Performance*. 8th Ed. Baltimore: Wolters Kluwer Health, 2015.)

Adipocytes: Site of Fat Storage and Mobilization

All cells store some fat, but adipose tissue represents an active and major supplier of fatty acid molecules. Adipocytes synthesize and store triacylglycerol, with these fat droplets occupying up to 95% of the cell's volume. When fatty acids diffuse from the adipocyte and enter the circulation, nearly all of them bind to plasma albumin for transport to the body's tissues as FFAs. Fat utilization as an energy substrate varies in synchrony with blood flow in active tissue. As blood flow increases with physical movement, adipose tissue releases more FFA to active muscle for energy metabolism. The activity level of **lipoprotein lipase (LPL)** facilitates the local cells' uptake of fatty acids for energy use or re-esterification (resynthesis) of stored triacylglycerol in muscle and adipose tissue.

FFAs do not exist as truly "free" entities. At the muscle site, FFAs release from the albumin-FFA complex to move across the plasma membrane. Inside the muscle cell, FFAs either esterify to form intracellular triacylglycerol or bind with intramuscular proteins to enter the mitochondria for energy metabolism. Medium- and short-chain fatty acids do not depend on this carrier-mediated means of transport, as most diffuse freely into the mitochondria.

Glycerol and Fatty Acid Breakdown

Figure 5.22 summarizes the pathways for the breakdown of the triacylglycerol molecule's glycerol through the CCA and fatty acid components via **β-oxidation** and electron transport chain.

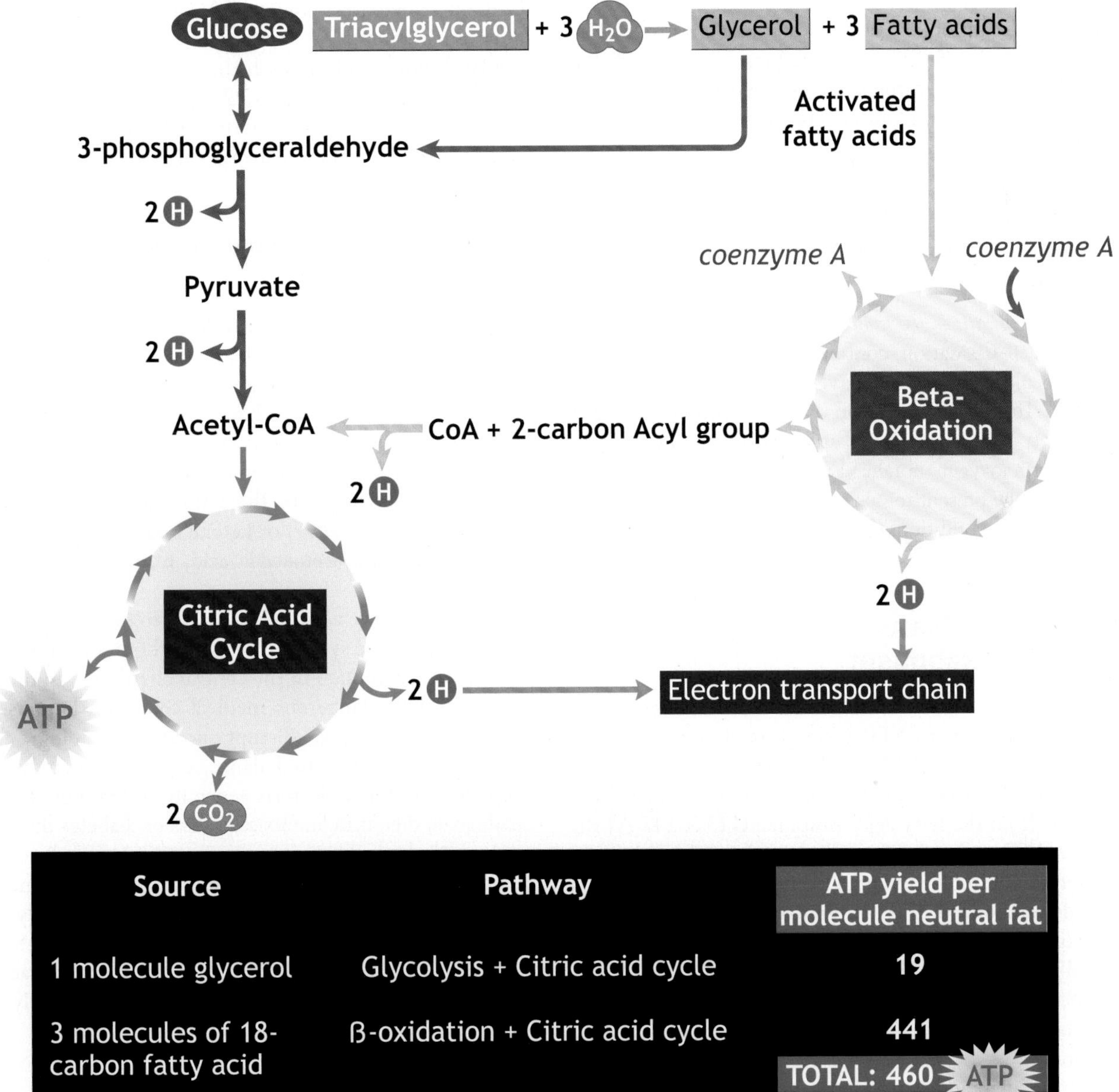

Source	Pathway	ATP yield per molecule neutral fat
1 molecule glycerol	Glycolysis + Citric acid cycle	19
3 molecules of 18-carbon fatty acid	β-oxidation + Citric acid cycle	441
		TOTAL: 460 ATP

FIGURE 5.22 General schema for the breakdown of a triacylglycerol molecule's glycerol and fatty acid components. Glycerol enters the energy pathways during glycolysis. Fatty acids prepare to enter the citric acid cycle through β-oxidation. The electron transport chain accepts hydrogens released during glycolysis, β-oxidation, and citric acid cycle metabolism. (See also **http://thePoint.lww.com/MKKESS5e** and the animation "Triacylglycerol Breakdown.") (Adapted with permission from McArdle WD, Katch FI, Katch VL. *Exercise Physiology: Nutrition, Energy, and Human Performance*. 8th Ed. Baltimore: Wolters Kluwer Health, 2015.)

Glycerol

The anaerobic reactions of glycolysis accept glycerol as 3-phosphoglyceraldehyde, which then degrades to pyruvate to form ATP by substrate-level phosphorylation. Hydrogen atoms pass to NAD^+ and the CAC oxidizes pyruvate. The complete degradation of the single glycerol molecule in a triacylglycerol synthesizes 19 ATP molecules. Glycerol also provides carbon skeletons for glucose synthesis. *Glycerol's gluconeogenic role becomes prominent when glycogen reserves deplete from carbohydrate dietary restriction, extended-duration physical activity, or high-intensity training.*

Fatty Acids

In the mitochondrion, the fatty acid molecule transforms to acetyl-CoA during β-oxidation reactions. This involves the successive release of 2-carbon acetyl fragments split from the fatty acid's long chain, a four-step process:

1. ATP phosphorylates the reactions.
2. Water is added.
3. Hydrogens pass to NAD^+ and FAD.
4. Acetyl-CoA forms when coenzyme A joins the acetyl fragment.

This acetyl unit is the same as that generated from glucose breakdown. β-Oxidation continues until the entire fatty acid molecule degrades to acetyl-CoAs that directly enter the CAC. The respiratory chain oxidizes hydrogen released during fatty acid catabolism. Fatty acid breakdown relates directly with oxygen uptake. For β-oxidation to proceed, oxygen must be present to join with hydrogen. Without oxygen (anaerobic conditions), hydrogen remains joined with NAD^+ and FAD and fat catabolism ceases.

Total Energy Transfer From Fat Catabolism

For each 18-carbon fatty acid molecule, 147 molecules of ADP phosphorylate to ATP during β-oxidation and CAC metabolism (see **Fig. 5.22**). Each triacylglycerol molecule contains three fatty acid molecules to form 441 ATP molecules from the fatty acid components (3 × 147 ATP). Also, 19 ATP molecules form during glycerol breakdown to generate 460 molecules of ATP for each triacylglycerol molecule catabolized. This represents a considerable energy yield compared to the net 32 net ATPs formed when a skeletal muscle catabolizes one glucose molecule. The efficiency of energy conservation for fatty acid oxidation amounts to about 40%, a value slightly higher than glucose oxidation.

Intracellular and extracellular lipid molecules usually supply between 30% and 80% of the energy for biologic work, depending on three factors in each individual:

1. Nutritional status
2. Current level of training
3. Intensity and duration of physical activity

Fat serves as the primary energy fuel for physical activity and recovery when intense, long-duration activity depletes glycogen. Furthermore, enzymatic adaptations occur with prolonged exposure to a high-fat, low-carbohydrate diet because this dietary regimen enhances fat oxidation capacity during physical activity.

Fats Burn in a Carbohydrate Flame

Interestingly, fatty acid breakdown depends in part on a continual background level of carbohydrate breakdown. Recall that acetyl-CoA enters the CAC by combining with oxaloacetate to form citrate (see **Fig. 5.19**). Depletion of carbohydrate decreases pyruvate production during glycolysis. Diminished pyruvate further reduces CAC intermediates, slowing CAC activity. Fatty acid degradation in the CAC depends on sufficient oxaloacetate availability to combine with the acetyl-CoA formed during β-oxidation (see **Fig. 5.22**). With diminished carbohydrate stores, the oxaloacetate level becomes inadequate and reduces fat catabolism. In this sense, *fats burn in a carbohydrate flame.*

Metabolism Under Low-Carbohydrate Conditions

Oxaloacetate converts to pyruvate (see **Fig. 5.19**; note the *two-way arrow* between oxaloacetate and pyruvate), which then can be synthesized to glucose. This occurs with inadequate carbohydrates (perhaps from fasting, prolonged physical activity, or diabetes) that are unavailable to combine with acetyl-CoA to form citrate. The liver converts the acetyl-CoA derived from the fatty acids into strong acid metabolites called *ketones* or ketone bodies. The three major ketone bodies are acetoacetic acid, β-hydroxybutyric acid, and acetone.

Ketones serve as a fuel primarily to muscles and minimally to nervous system tissues. Without ketone catabolism, they accumulate in the central circulation to produce the potentially dangerous medical condition **ketosis**. The high acidity of ketosis disrupts normal physiologic function, especially acid-base balance, and can ultimately prove dangerous to health. Ketosis generally occurs more from an inadequate diet as in anorexia nervosa or diabetes than from prolonged physical activity, as active muscle uses ketones as a fuel. One telltale sign of the ketotic state is chronic bad breath. Resuming normal carbohydrate intake usually helps curb the condition (minimum daily carbohydrate intake of 3 to 4 oz or about 100 g). During physical activity, aerobically trained individuals use ketones more effectively than untrained individuals.

Slower Energy Release From Fat

A rate limit exists for how active muscles use fatty acids. Aerobic training enhances this limit, but the rate of energy generated solely by fat breakdown still represents only about half of the value achieved with carbohydrate as the chief aerobic energy source. This explains why muscle glycogen

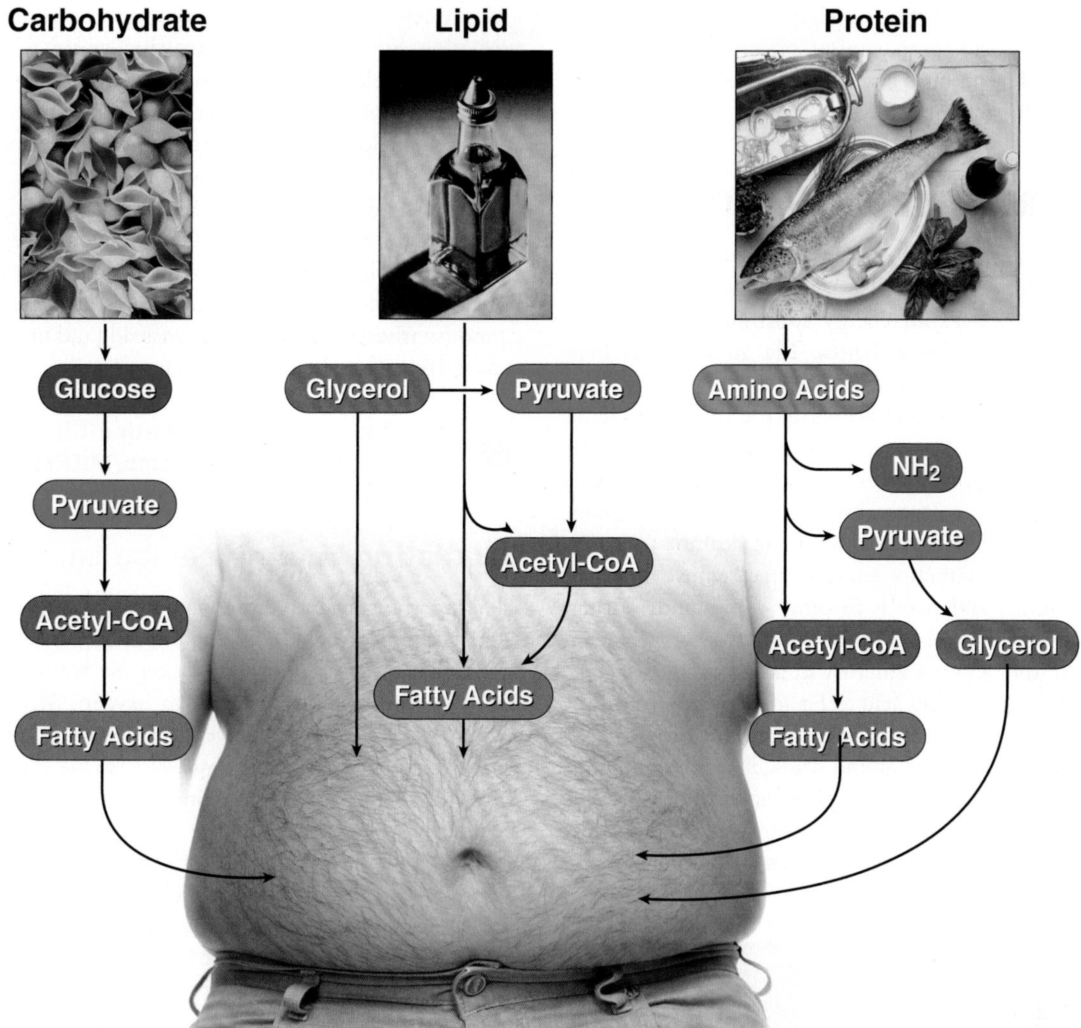

FIGURE 5.23 Metabolic fate of macronutrient energy surplus.

depletion decreases the intensity a muscle can sustain a desired level of aerobic power output. Just as the hypoglycemic condition coincides with a "central" or neural fatigue, exercising with depleted muscle glycogen causes "peripheral" or local muscle fatigue.

Excess Macronutrients Convert to Fat

Excess energy intake from any fuel source can prove counterproductive. **Figure 5.23** shows how too much of any macronutrient converts to fatty acids, which then accumulate as excess body fat, typically in the abdominal area. Surplus dietary carbohydrate first fills the glycogen reserves. When these reserves fill, excess carbohydrate converts to triacylglycerols for storage in adipose tissue. Excess dietary fat calories move quickly into the body's fat deposits. After they have been deaminated, the carbon residues of excess amino acids from protein readily convert to fat.

Hormones Affect Fat Metabolism

Four hormones—epinephrine, norepinephrine, glucagon, and growth hormone—augment lipase activation and subsequent lipolysis and FFA mobilization from adipose tissue. Plasma concentrations of these lipogenic hormones increase during physical activity to continually supply active muscles with energy-rich substrate. An intracellular mediator, **adenosine 3′,5′-cyclic monophosphate (cyclic AMP)**, activates hormone-sensitive lipase and thus regulates fat breakdown. Various lipid-mobilizing hormones that themselves do not enter the cell activate cyclic AMP. Circulating lactate, ketones, and especially insulin inhibit cyclic AMP activation. Physical training–induced increases in the activity level of skeletal muscle and adipose tissue lipases enhance fat use for energy during moderate physical activity. This includes biochemical and vascular adaptations in muscles themselves. Paradoxically, excess body fat decreases fatty acid availability during physical activity. Chapter 12 presents a more detailed evaluation of hormone regulation during physical activity and training.

Availability of fatty acid molecules regulates fat catabolism or synthesis. Following a meal, when energy metabolism remains relatively low, digestive processes increase FFA and triacylglycerol delivery to cells; this in turn stimulates triacylglycerol synthesis. In contrast, moderate physical activity increases fatty acid use for energy, which reduces FFA and triacylglycerol cellular concentration. The decrease in intracellular FFAs stimulates triacylglycerol breakdown into glycerol and fatty acid components. Concurrently, hormonal release triggered by physical activity stimulates adipose tissue lipolysis to further augment FFA delivery to active muscle.

ENERGY RELEASE FROM PROTEIN

Figure 5.24 illustrates how protein supplies intermediates at three different levels that have energy-producing capabilities. Protein acts as an energy substrate during long-duration, endurance-type activities. The amino acids first convert to a molecular form that readily enters pathways for energy release. These include primarily the branched-chain amino acids leucine, isoleucine, valine, glutamine, and aspartic acid. This conversion requires removing nitrogen from the amino acid molecule, a process known as deamination (refer to Chapter 2). The liver serves as the main deamination site. Skeletal muscle also contains enzymes that remove nitrogen from amino acids and pass it to other compounds during transamination. Removal of nitrogen usually occurs when an amine group from a donor amino acid transfers to an acceptor acid from a new amino acid (refer to Chapter 2). In this way, the muscle directly taps the energy from the carbon skeleton by-products of donor amino acids. Enzyme levels for transamination favorably adapt to physical training; this may further facilitate protein's use as an energy substrate. Only when an amino acid loses its nitrogen-containing amine group does the remaining compound contribute to ATP formation. Some amino acids are **glucogenic**; when deaminated, they yield intermediate products for glucose synthesis via gluconeogenesis. In the liver, for example, pyruvate forms when alanine loses its amino group and gains a double-bond oxygen, allowing glucose synthesis from pyruvate. This gluconeogenic method serves as an important adjunct to the Cori cycle to provide glucose when glycogen reserves diminish during prolonged physical activity. Similar to fat and carbohydrate molecules, some amino acids are **ketogenic** and cannot synthesize to glucose but instead (and unfortunately) synthesize to fat when consumed in excess!

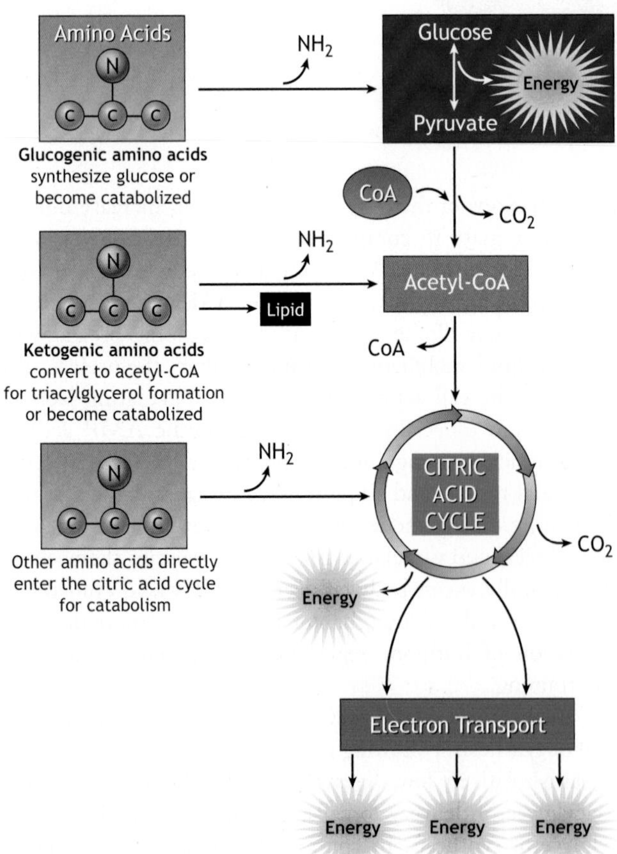

FIGURE 5.24 Protein-to-energy pathways.

See the animation "Alanine-Glucose Cycle" on **http://thePoint.lww.com/MKKESS5e** for a demonstration of this process.

Regulating Energy Metabolism

Electron transfer and subsequent energy release normally tightly couple to ADP phosphorylation. Without ADP availability for ATP phosphorylation, electrons do not shuttle down the respiratory chain to oxygen. *Metabolites that either inhibit or activate enzymes at key control points in the oxidative pathways modulate regulatory control of glycolysis and the CAC.* Each pathway contains at least one enzyme considered *rate limiting* because the enzyme controls the overall speed of that pathway's reactions. *Cellular ADP concentration exerts the greatest effect on the rate-limiting enzymes that control macronutrient energy metabolism.* This mechanism for respiratory control makes sense because any increase in ADP signals a need to supply energy to restore diminished ATP levels. Conversely, high cellular ATP levels indicate a relatively low-energy requirement. From a broader perspective, ADP concentrations function as a cellular *feedback mechanism* to maintain a relative constancy or homeostasis in the level of energy currency required for biologic work. Other rate-limiting modulators include cellular levels of phosphate, cyclic AMP, AMP-activated protein kinase (AMPK), calcium, NAD^+, citrate, and pH. More specifically, ATP and NADH serve as enzyme inhibitors, and intracellular calcium, ADP, and NAD^+ function as activators. This form of chemical feedback allows rapid metabolic adjustment to the cells' energy needs. Within a resting cell, the ATP concentration considerably exceeds ADP's concentration by about 500:1. A decrease in the ATP:ADP ratio and intramitochondrial NADH:NAD^+ ratio, as occurs when physical activity begins, signals a need to increase the metabolism of stored nutrients. In contrast, relatively low levels of energy demand maintain high ratios of ATP to ADP and NADH to NAD^+, both depressing the rate of metabolic energy metabolism.

Independent Effects

No single chemical regulator dominates mitochondrial ATP production. Experiments ***in vitro*** (outside the living organism) and ***in vivo*** (within the living organism) show that changes in each of these compounds independently alter oxidative phosphorylation rate. All compounds exert regulatory effects, each contributing differentially depending on three factors:

1. Energy demands
2. Intracellular conditions
3. Specific tissues involved

THE METABOLIC MILL

The "metabolic mill" illustrated in **Figure 5.25** depicts the CAC as the essential "connector" between macronutrient energy and ATP's chemical energy. The CAC plays a much more important role than simply degrading pyruvate produced during glucose catabolism. Fragments from other organic compounds formed from fat and protein breakdown provide energy during CAC metabolism. Deaminated residues of excess amino acids enter the CAC at various intermediate stages. In contrast, the glycerol fragment of triacylglycerol catabolism gains entrance via the glycolytic pathway. Fatty acids oxidize via β-oxidation to acetyl-CoA, which then directly enters the CAC.

The CAC also serves as a metabolic hub to provide intermediates to synthesize nutrients for tissue maintenance and growth. For example, excess carbohydrates provide glycerol and acetyl fragments to synthesize triacylglycerol. Acetyl-CoA also functions as the starting point for synthesizing cholesterol and many hormones. In contrast, fatty acids do not contribute to glucose synthesis because pyruvate's conversion to acetyl-CoA does not reverse (notice the red *one-way downward arrow* in **Fig. 5.25**). Many carbon compounds generated in CAC reactions provide the organic starting points to synthesize nonessential amino acids. Amino acids with carbon skeletons resembling CAC intermediates after deamination synthesize to glucose.

A CLOSER LOOK

Estimating Individual Protein Requirements

Total body protein remains constant when nitrogen intake from protein in food balances its excretion in the feces, urine, and sweat. An imbalance in the body's nitrogen content provides (1) an accurate estimate of either protein's depletion or accumulation and (2) the adequacy of dietary protein intake. Nitrogen balance evaluation can estimate human protein requirements under various conditions including intense physical training.

The magnitude and direction of nitrogen balance in individuals engaged in physical training depends on five interrelated factors:

1. Training status
2. Quality and quantity of consumed protein
3. Total energy intake
4. Current glycogen levels
5. Intensity, duration, and mode of physical activity performed

Measuring Nitrogen Balance

- **Nitrogen Intake.** Estimate protein intake (in grams) by carefully measuring total food consumed over a 24-hour period. Determine nitrogen quantity (in grams) by assuming protein contains 16% of nitrogen. Then:
- Total nitrogen intake (g) = Total protein intake (g) × 0.16
- **Nitrogen Output.** Researchers determine nitrogen output by collecting all of the nitrogen excreted over the same period that assessed nitrogen intake. This involves collecting nitrogen loss from urine, lungs, sweat, and feces. A simplified method estimates nitrogen output by measuring urinary urea nitrogen (UUN; plus 4 g to account for other sources of nitrogen loss):

Total nitrogen output = UUN + 4 g

Example

Male, age 22; total body mass 75 kg; total energy intake (food diary) 2100 kcal; protein intake (food diary) 63 g; UUN (collection and analysis of urine output) 8 g

$$\begin{aligned}\textbf{Nitrogen balance} &= \textbf{nitrogen intake (g)} - \textbf{nitrogen output (g)}\\ &= \mathbf{(6.3\,g \times 0.16) - (8\,g + 4\,g)}\\ &= \mathbf{-1.92\,g}\end{aligned}$$

This example shows that a daily negative nitrogen balance of −1.92 g occurred because estimated protein catabolized in metabolism exceeded its replacement through dietary protein. To correct this deficiency and achieve nitrogen or protein balance, the person would need to increase his daily protein intake.

Estimated Daily Protein Needs

Condition	Protein Needs g · kg BW
Normal, healthy	0.8–1.0
Fever, fracture, infection	1.5–12.0
Protein depleted	1.5–2.0
Extensive burns	1.5–3.0
Intensive training	1.0–2.0

Estimating Individual Protein Requirements

The table estimates average protein needs of adults under different conditions. For a healthy person who weighs 70 kg, the protein requirement equals 56 g.

$$\mathbf{0.8\,g \cdot kg^{-1} \times 70\,kg = 56\,g}$$

The same person with a chronic infection or in a protein-depleted state would require an upper-range estimate of 140 g of protein daily.

$$\mathbf{2.0\,g \cdot kg^{-1} \times 70\,kg = 140\,g}$$

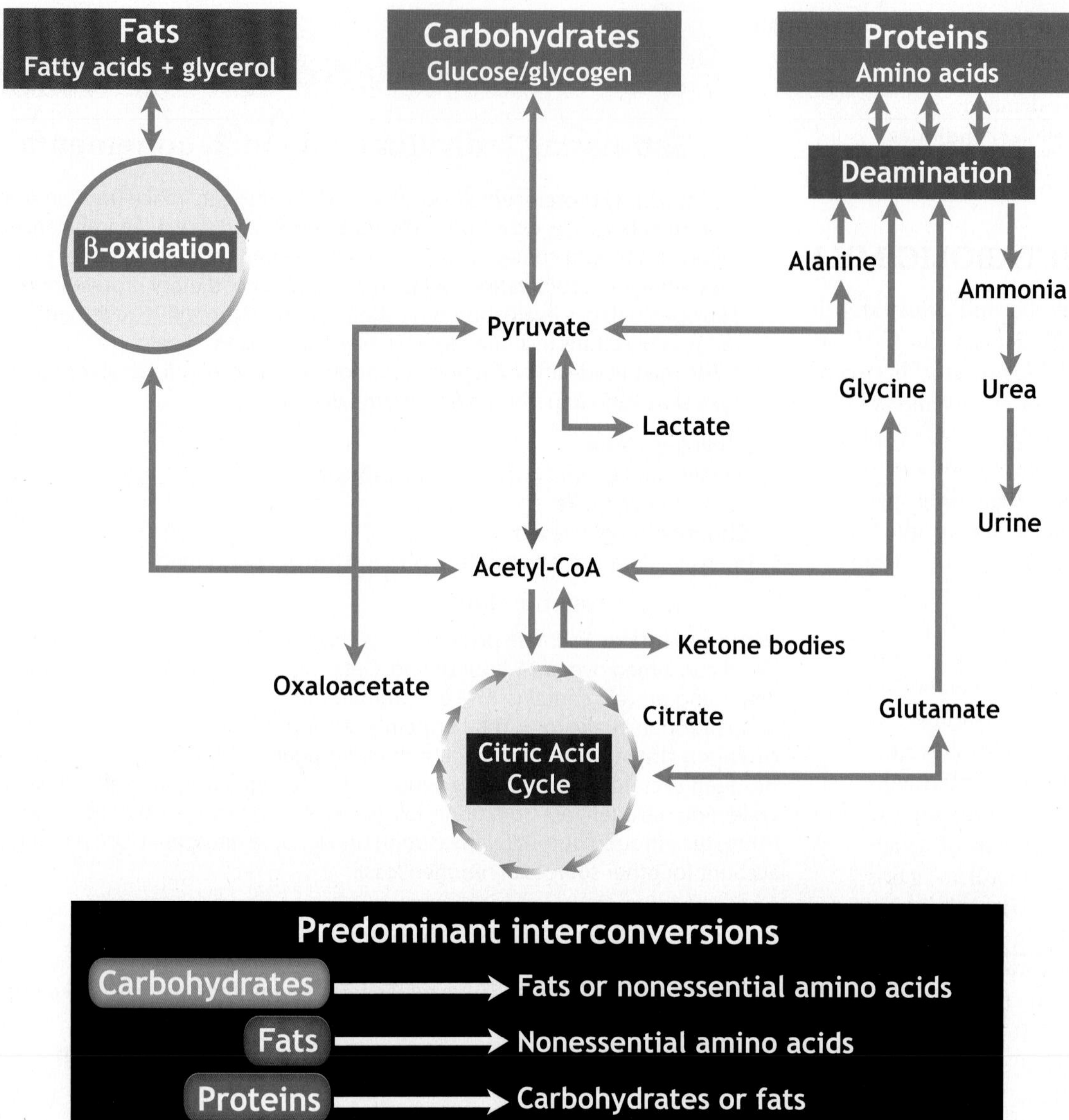

FIGURE 5.25 The "metabolic mill" allows important interconversions for catabolism and anabolism among carbohydrates, fats, and proteins. (Adapted with permission from McArdle WD, Katch FI, Katch VL. *Sports and Exercise Nutrition*. 4th Ed. Philadelphia: Wolters Kluwer Health, 2013.)

SUMMARY

1. Complete breakdown of 1 mole of glucose liberates 689 kcal of energy. Of this total, ATP's bonds conserve about 233 kcal (34%), with the remainder dissipated as heat.
2. During glycolytic reactions in the cell's cytosol, a net of 2 ATP molecules form during anaerobic substrate-level phosphorylation.
3. In intense physical activity when hydrogen oxidation does not keep pace with its production, pyruvate temporarily binds hydrogen to form lactate.
4. In mitochondria, the second stage of carbohydrate breakdown converts pyruvate to acetyl-CoA, which then progresses through the CAC.
5. Hydrogen atoms released during glucose breakdown oxidize via the respiratory chain, with the energy generated coupling to ADP phosphorylation.
6. Oxidation of one glucose molecule in skeletal muscle yields a net gain of 32 ATP molecules.
7. Adipose tissue serves as an active and major supplier of fatty acid molecules.
8. Breakdown of a triacylglycerol molecule yields approximately 460 ATP molecules.
9. Fatty acid catabolism requires oxygen.
10. Protein can serve as an energy substrate.
11. When deamination removes nitrogen from an amino acid molecule, the remaining carbon skeleton can enter metabolic pathways to produce ATP aerobically.
12. Numerous interconversions take place among the food nutrients; fatty acids are an exception because they cannot synthesize to glucose.
13. Fatty acids require a minimum level of carbohydrate breakdown for their continual catabolism for energy in the metabolic mill.

14. Cellular ADP concentration exerts the greatest effect on the rate-limiting enzymes that control energy metabolism.

THINK IT THROUGH

1. How does aerobic and anaerobic energy metabolism affect optimal energy transfer capacity for a 100-m sprinter, 400-m hurdler, and marathon runner?
2. Explain how elite marathoners can run 26.2 miles at a pace of 5 minutes per mile, yet very few can run just 1 mile in 4 minutes?
3. In prolonged aerobic marathon running, explain why physical activity capacity diminishes when glycogen reserves deplete even though stored fat contains more than adequate energy reserves.
4. Explain if it makes sense for weightlifters and sprint athletes to have a high capacity to consume oxygen.

KEY TERMS

Active site: Groove, cleft, or cavity on an enzyme's protein surface that joins in a "perfect fit" with a specific substrate's active site.

Active transport: Molecular movement of a substance through a cell membrane in a direction against its concentration gradient; requires an input of ATP energy.

Adenosine 3′,5′-cyclic monophosphate (cyclic AMP): A second messenger important in many biological processes; used in the metabolic process of intracellular signal transduction.

Adenosine diphosphate (ADP): End product of energy transfer composed of three structural components: a sugar backbone attached to a molecule of adenine and two phosphate groups bonded to a ribose carbon molecule.

Adenosine triphosphate (ATP): The energy currency of life present in the cytoplasm and nucleoplasm of every cell; stores energy that powers physiological mechanisms for all bodily function. Composed of a sugar backbone attached to an adenine molecule and three phosphate groups bonded to a ribose carbon molecule.

Adenylate kinase reaction: Single-enzyme–mediated reaction for ATP regeneration that catalyzes the interconversion of adenine nucleotides and plays an important role in cellular energy balance: ATP + AMP = ADP + ADP.

Aerobic: ATP generated from oxygen requiring chemical reactions.

Aerobic metabolism (cellular respiration): Mitochondrial (aerobic) metabolic reactions and processes to convert biochemical energy from macronutrients into ATP.

Anaerobic: ATP generated from chemical reactions not requiring oxygen.

β-Oxidation: Fatty acid molecules break down in mitochondria to generate acetyl-CoA, which then enters the citric acid cycle; the electron transport chain then oxidizes NADH and $FADH_2$ to generate ATP.

Biosynthesis: A multistep, enzyme-catalyzed process by living organisms that results in the formation of complex compounds from simple substances.

Chemical work: Work accomplished by cells for synthesizing new molecules (anabolism) or cellular breakdown of existing molecules (catabolism).

Citric acid cycle (CAC), Krebs cycle, or tricarboxylic acid cycle: Series of chemical reactions by all aerobic organisms to generate energy through oxidation of carbohydrate, lipid, and protein into carbon dioxide and ATP.

Coenzymes: Nonprotein chemical compounds that bind with enzymes for participation in biochemical transformations.

Conservation of energy: Energy of an isolated system remains constant or conserved over time; energy can be neither created nor be destroyed, but can change in form.

Cori cycle: Lactate produced by anaerobic glycolysis in muscle moves to the liver for conversion to glucose, which then returns to muscle and metabolizes back to lactate.

Coupled reactions: Reactions that occur in pairs, such that breakdown of one compound provides energy for building another compound.

Creatine kinase (CK): Also known as creatine phosphokinase (CPK) or phosphocreatine kinase. An enzyme expressed by various tissues and cell types; catalyzes the conversion of creatine and consumes ATP to create phosphocreatine (PCr) and ADP.

Creatine kinase reaction: Reaction in which creatine kinase catalyzes the conversion of creatine + ATP to create PCr, ADP, and free energy release.

Cytochrome oxidase: Last enzyme in the respiratory electron transport chain; receives an electron from each of four cytochrome c molecules and transfers them to one oxygen molecule, converting molecular oxygen to two molecules of water.

Dehydrogenase enzymes: Specific enzymes including FAD and NAD^+ that catalyze hydrogen's release from nutrient substrates.

Diffusion: Passive net movement of atoms, ions, or molecules from a region of higher concentration to lower concentration.

Endergonic: "Uphill" energy processes that store or absorb energy, which proceed with an increase in free energy for biologic work.

Energy: Dynamic state related to change; the presence of energy emerges only when change occurs, and energy relates to the performance of work and occurrence of change.

Entropy: Degree of unpredictability or disorder in a closed thermodynamic system; when related to the system's total energy availability; it indicates little energy availability from the system to produce work.

Enzymes: Protein molecules that act as selective catalysts, which greatly accelerate the rate and specificity of metabolic reactions.

Exergonic: "Downhill" metabolic processes that produce a decline in free or "useful" energy for biologic work.

First law of thermodynamics: The total energy of an isolated system remains constant, so that energy can be transformed from one form to another but cannot be created or destroyed.

Flavin adenine dinucleotide (FAD): Important redox cofactor involved in energy metabolism; accepts two electrons and two protons to become $FADH_2$, which then oxidizes to produce ATP.

Free energy: Portion of energy available to perform thermodynamic work; for each mole of ATP degraded to ADP the outermost phosphate bond splits and liberates approximately 7.3 kcal of free energy.

Free fatty acids (FFAs): Naturally occurring fatty acids with a chain of an even number of carbon atoms ranging from 4 to 28; derived either from triacylglycerols or phospholipids and called "free" fatty acids when unattached to other molecules.

Glucogenic: Deaminated amino acids yield intermediate products for glucose synthesis via gluconeogenesis.

Glycogenesis: Process of glycogen synthesis, where glucose molecules add to chains of glycogen for storage from action of the enzyme hexokinase or glucokinase.

Glycogenolysis: Breakdown of glycogen to glucose from action of the enzyme glycogen phosphorylase.

Glycolysis: Series of 10 metabolic reactions in the cell's cytoplasm that convert glucose into pyruvate and release free forms of ATP and NADH + H.

High-energy bonds: Phosphate-phosphate bonds formed in high-energy compounds such as adenosine diphosphate and triphosphate; the splitting of the bonds transfers the released energy to other cellular substances.

Hydrolysis: Cleavage of chemical bonds by addition of water to a molecule, thus altering the molecule's molecular structure; for example, sucrose separation in hydrolysis yields glucose and fructose.

Immediate energy system: Single–enzyme mediated energy transfer of the ATP-PCr high-energy phosphates with "fast" but limited energy.

***In vitro*:** *Outside* a living organism.

***In vivo*:** *Inside* a living organism.

Ketogenic: Deaminated amino acids yield intermediate products for fat synthesis.

Ketosis: Elevated levels of ketone bodies (acetone, acetoacetic acid, beta-hydroxybutyric acid) during prolonged fasting, starvation, or following a ketogenic diet where most of the body's energy supply comes from ketone bodies in the blood, with potentially fatal consequences from dehydration and depressed pH.

Kinetic energy: Energy that associates with a system in motion; refers to the work needed to accelerate an object of a given mass, expressed as kcal or SI unit joule (J).

Lactate: Carboxylic acid produced from pyruvate via the enzyme lactate dehydrogenase (LDH) in fermentation during both anaerobic and aerobic metabolism.

Lactate shuttling: Intracellular and intercellular lactate movement; lactate produced at sites with high rates of glycolysis and glycogenolysis shuttles to adjacent or remote sites including heart or other skeletal muscles for use as a gluconeogenic precursor or substrate for oxidation.

Lipoprotein lipase (LPL): Water-soluble enzyme that hydrolyzes triacylglycerols in lipoproteins into two free fatty acids.

Mechanical work: Force acting on an object that results in the object's displacement in the direction of the force such that Work = Force × Distance traveled + Energy.

Mitochondria: Cell's "power plants" that generate most of its ATP supply; also involved in cell signaling, cellular differentiation, cell death, and cell cycle and cell growth control.

Nicotinamide adenine dinucleotide (NAD^+): Coenzyme found in all living cells involved in redox reactions that carry electrons from one reaction to another; also found in cells as an oxidizing agent.

Oxidation: Refers to electron loss or increase in oxidation state by a molecule, atom, or ion; usually coupled with reduction.

Oxidation reactions: Reactions that donate electrons.

Oxidative phosphorylation: Mitochondrial metabolic pathway to reform ATP.

Oxidized: When a molecule releases electrons.

Phosphagens: Alternate name for high-energy phosphates.

Phosphatase: Dedicated enzyme that removes a phosphate group from its substrate.

Phosphocreatine: Phosphorylated creatine molecule that donates a phosphate group to ADP to form ATP during or immediately following intense muscular or neuronal effort.

Phosphofructokinase (PFK): Rate-limiting enzyme in glycolytic pathway that phosphorylates fructose 6-phosphate in glycolysis.

Phosphorylation: Process of adding a high-energy phosphate bond to other compounds to raise their activation level; occurs at the substrate level during glycolysis (anaerobic) or coupled oxidative phosphorylation (aerobic) metabolism.

Photosynthesis: Process used by plants and other organisms to convert light energy from the sun to drive carbohydrate synthesis.

Potential energy: Energy stored in a system that associates with position in space; when released, potential energy transfers to kinetic energy and is expressed as kcal or SI unit joule (J).

Reduced: Gain of electrons or a decrease in oxidation state of a molecule, atom, or ion; usually coupled with oxidation and electron loss.

Reduction reactions: Chemical reactions that accept electrons.

Respiration: Cellular process in which the nutrients' molecular structures transform into a useful form of energy.

Respiratory chain (electron transport chain): Series of chemical reactions that involve compounds that transfer electrons from electron donors to electron acceptors via redox reactions that couple electron transfer with proton transfer (H^+ ions) to drive ATP synthesis.

Second law of thermodynamics: Dissipation of potential energy to the unusable form of kinetic or heat energy.

Substrate-level phosphorylation: Anaerobic metabolic reactions form ATP by direct transfer and donation of a phosphate group to ADP; usually refers to ATP production during glycolysis.

Triacylglycerols (triglycerides): Lipid molecules formed by combining glycerol molecule with three fatty acid molecules; function as either saturated or unsaturated molecules with respect to their H^+ ion number.

Turnover number: Number of substrate moles that react to form a product per mole of enzyme per unit time.

SELECTED REFERENCES

Achten J, Jeukendrup AE. Optimizing fat oxidation through exercise and diet. *Nutrition* 2004;20:716.

Alberts B, et al. *Essential Cell Biology*. 4th Ed. New York: Garland Publishers, 2013.

Åstrand PO, et al. *Textbook of Work Physiology. Physiological Bases of Exercise*. 4th Ed. Champaign: Human Kinetics, 2003.

Aveseh M, et al. Endurance training increases brain lactate uptake during hypoglycemia by up regulation of brain lactate transporters. *Mol Cell Endocrinol* 2014;394:29.

Barnes BR, et al. 5'-AMP-activated protein kinase regulates skeletal muscle glycogen content and ergogenics. *FASEB J* 2005;19:773.

Berg JM, et al. *Biochemistry*. 7th Ed. San Francisco: W.H. Freeman, 2010.

Binzoni T. Saturation of the lactate clearance mechanisms different from the "lactate shuttle" determines the anaerobic threshold: prediction from the bioenergetic model. *J Physiol Anthropol Appl Human Sci* 2005;24:175.

Brooks GA, et al. *Exercise Physiology: Human Bioenergetics and Its Applications*. 4th Ed. New York: McGraw-Hill, 2004.

Brooks GA. Cell-cell and intracellular lactate shuttles. *J Physiol* 2009; 587:5591.

Brooks GA. Bioenergetics of exercising humans. *Compr Physiol* 2012;2:537.

Brooks GA. What does glycolysis make and why is it important. *J Appl Physiol* 2010;108:1450.

Campbell MK, Farrel SO. *Biochemistry*. 8th Ed. Belmont: Brooks/Cole, 2014.

Carr DB, et al. A reduced-fat diet and aerobic exercise in Japanese Americans with impaired glucose tolerance decreases intra-abdominal fat and improves insulin sensitivity but not beta-cell function. *Diabetes* 2005;54:340.

DiNuzzo M, et al. Changes in glucose uptake rather than lactate shuttle take center stage in subserving neuroenergetics: evidence from mathematical modeling. *J Cereb Blood Flow Metab* 2010;30:586.

Emhoff CA, et al. Direct and indirect lactate oxidation in trained and untrained men. *J Appl Physiol* 2013;115:829.

Emhoff CA, et al. Gluconeogenesis and hepatic glycogenolysis during exercise at the lactate threshold. *J Appl Physiol* 2013;114:297.

Enqvist JK, et al. Energy turnover during 24 hours and 6 days of adventure racing. *J Sports Sci* 2010;28:947.

Fatouros IG, et al. Oxidative stress responses in older men during endurance training and detraining. *Med Sci Sports Exerc* 2004;36:2065.

Ferrier DR. *Biochemistry (Lippincott Illustrated Reviews Series)*. Philadelphia: Lippincott Williams & Wilkins/Wolters Kluwers, 2013.

Fox SI. *Human Physiology*. 12th Ed. New York: McGraw-Hill, 2010.

Gimenez P, et al. Changes in the energy cost of running during a 24-h treadmill exercise. *Med Sci Sports Exerc* 2013;45:1807.

Hashimoto T, Brooks GA. Mitochondrial lactate oxidation complex and an adaptive role for lactate production. *Med Sci Sports Exerc* 2008;40:486.

Hauser T, et al. Comparison of calculated and experimental power in maximal lactate-steady state during cycling. *Theor Biol Med Model* 2014;11:25.

Henderson GC, et al. Plasma triglyceride concentrations are rapidly reduced following individual bouts of endurance exercise in women. *Eur J Appl Physiol* 2010;109:721.

Henderson GC, et al. Pyruvate shuttling during rest and exercise before and after endurance training in men. *J Appl Physiol* 2004;97:317.

Horton R. *Principles of Biochemistry*. 4th Ed. Englewood Cliffs: Prentice-Hall, 2005.

Jeukendrup AE, Wallis GA. Measurement of substrate oxidation during exercise by means of gas exchange measurements. *Int J Sports Med* 2005;26:S28.

Jones DE, et al. Abnormalities in pH handling by peripheral muscle and potential regulation by the autonomic nervous system in chronic fatigue syndrome. *J Intern Med* 2010;267:394.

Jorgensen SB, et al. Role of AMPK in skeletal muscle metabolic regulation and adaptation in relation to exercise. *J Physiol* 2006;574:17.

Kiens B. Skeletal muscle lipid metabolism in exercise and insulin resistance. *Physiol Rev* 2006;86:205.

Li J, et al. Interstitial ATP and norepinephrine concentrations in active muscle. *Circulation* 2005;111:2748.

Marieb EN, Hoehn K. *Human Anatomy and Physiology*. 9th Ed. Redwood City: Pearson Education/Benjamin Cummings, 2012.

Messonnier LA, et al. Lactate kinetics at the lactate threshold in trained and untrained men. *J Appl Physiol* 2013;114:1593.

Monleon D, et al. Metabolomic analysis of long term spontaneous exercise in mice suggests increased lipolysis and altered glucose metabolism when animals are at rest. *J Appl Physiol* 2014;117:1110.

Moore DR, et al. Post-exercise protein ingestion increases whole body net protein balance in healthy children. *J Appl Physiol* 2014;117:1493.

Moran L, et al. *Principles of Biochemistry*. 5th Ed. Redwood City: Pearson Education, 2011.

Nelson DL, Cox MM. *Lehninger Principles of Biochemistry*. 6th Ed. New York: WH Freeman, 2012.

Ormsbee MJ, et al. Pre-exercise nutrition: the role of macronutrients, modified starches and supplements on metabolism and endurance performance. *Nutrients* 2014;6:1782.

Peres SB, et al. Endurance exercise training increases insulin responsiveness in isolated adipocytes through IRS/PI3-kinase/Akt pathway. *J Appl Physiol* 2005; 98:1037.

Petibois C, Deleris G. FT-IR spectrometry analysis of plasma fatty acyl moieties selective mobilization during endurance exercise. *Biopolymers* 2005;77:345.

Revan S, et al. Short duration exhaustive running exercise does not modify lipid hydroperoxide, glutathione peroxidase and catalase. *J Sports Med Phys Fitness* 2010;50:235.

Ricquier D. Respiration uncoupling and metabolism in the control of energy expenditure. *Proc Nutr Soc* 2005;64:47.

Roepstorff C, et al. Regulation of oxidative enzyme activity and eukaryotic elongation factor 2 in human skeletal muscle: influence of gender and exercise. *Acta Physiol Scand* 2005;184:215.

Rose AJ, Richter EA. Skeletal muscle glucose uptake during exercise: how is it regulated? *Physiology* 2005;20:260.

Rouis M, et al. Relationship between vertical jump and maximal power output of legs and arms: effects of ethnicity and sport. *Scand J Med Sci Sports* 2014; In Press as of 03.16.15.

Schamroth C. Adverse effects of the 'Noakes' diet on dyslipidaemia. *Cardiovasc J Afr* 2014;25:192.

Tarnopolsky M. Protein requirements for endurance athletes. *Nutrition* 2004;20:662.

Tauler P, et al. Pre-exercise antioxidant enzyme activities determine the antioxidant enzyme erythrocyte response to exercise. *J Sports Sci* 2005;23:5.

van Loon LJ. Use of intramuscular triacylglycerol as a substrate source during exercise in humans. *J Appl Physiol* 2004;97:1170.

Veldhorst MA, et al. Presence or absence of carbohydrates and the proportion of fat in a high-protein diet affect appetite suppression but not energy expenditure in normal-weight human subjects fed in energy balance. *B J Nutr* 2010;22:1.

Venables MC, et al. Determinants of fat oxidation during exercise in healthy men and women: a cross-sectional study. *J Appl Physiol* 2005;98:160.

Watson JD, Berry A. *DNA: The Secret of Life*. New York: Knopf, 2003.

Widmaier EP, et al. *Vander's Human Physiology: The Mechanism of Body Function*. 13th Ed. New York: McGraw-Hill, 2013.

Wu JW, et al. Inborn errors of cytoplasmic triglyceride metabolism. *J Inherit Metab Dis* 2015;38:85.

Human Energy Transfer During Physical Activity

CHAPTER OBJECTIVES

- Identify the body's three energy systems, and explain their relative contributions to exercise intensity and duration.
- Describe differences in blood lactate threshold between sedentary and aerobically trained individuals.
- Outline the time course for oxygen uptake during 10 minutes of moderately intense physical activity.
- Draw a figure showing the relationship between oxygen uptake and exercise intensity during progressively increasing increments of exercise to maximum.
- Describe the oxygen deficit and debt and how these factors might help to explain individual differences in exercise performance.
- Differentiate between the body's two types of muscle fibers and their influence in energy transfer.
- Explain two differences in the pattern of recovery oxygen uptake from steady-rate moderate and non–steady-rate exhaustive physical activity, and discuss two factors that account for the excess postexercise oxygen consumption (EPOC) from each activity mode.
- Outline two optimal recovery procedures from steady-rate and non–steady-rate physical activity.
- Discuss the rationale for intermittent exercise applied to interval training.

ANCILLARIES AT A GLANCE

Visit **http://thePoint.lww.com/MKKESS5e** to access the following resources.

- References: Chapter 6
- Interactive Question Bank

Physical activity provides the greatest stimulus to increase energy metabolism. In sprint running and cycling, whole-body energy output in world-class competitors exceeds 40 to 50 times their resting energy expenditure. During less intense but sustained marathon running, energy requirements still exceed resting level by 20 to 25 times. This chapter explains how the body's different energy systems interact to transfer energy during rest and various physical activity intensities.

IMMEDIATE ENERGY: THE ADENOSINE TRIPHOSPHATE–PHOSPHOCREATINE SYSTEM

Performances of short duration and high intensity, including the 100-m sprint, 25-m swim, smashing a tennis ball during the serve, or thrusting a heavy weight upward, require an immediate and rapid energy supply. The two high-energy phosphates **adenosine triphosphate (ATP)** and **phosphocreatine (PCr)** stored within muscles almost exclusively provide this energy. ATP and PCr collectively are termed **phosphagens.**

Each kilogram (kg) of skeletal muscle stores approximately 5 millimoles (mmol) of ATP and 15 mmol of PCr. For a person with 30 kg of muscle mass, this amounts to between 570 and 690 mmol of phosphagens. If physical activity activates 20 kg of muscle, then stored phosphagen energy could power a brisk walk for 1 minute, a slow run for 20 to 30 seconds, or all-out sprint running and swimming for about 6 to 8 seconds. In the 100-m dash, for example, the body cannot maintain maximum speed for longer than 8 seconds, and the runner actually slows down toward the end of the race. *Thus, the quantity of intramuscular phosphagens substantially influences "all-out" performance for brief durations.* The enzyme creatine kinase triggers PCr hydrolysis to resynthesize ATP to regulate phosphagen breakdown rate.

SHORT-TERM GLYCOLYTIC (LACTATE-FORMING) ENERGY SYSTEM

The intramuscular phosphagens must continually and rapidly resynthesize for strenuous activity to continue beyond a brief period. During intense effort, intramuscular stored glycogen provides the energy source to phosphorylate ADP during anaerobic **glycogenolysis**, forming lactate (see Chapter 5, Figs. 5.14 and 5.15).

With inadequate oxygen supply and utilization, all of the hydrogens formed in rapid glycolysis fail to oxidize; in this case, pyruvate converts to lactate in the chemical reaction, Pyruvate + 2H → Lactate. This conversion enables continuation of rapid ATP formation by anaerobic substrate-level phosphorylation. Anaerobic energy for ATP resynthesis from glycolysis can be viewed as "reserve fuel" activated when the oxygen demand:oxygen utilization ratio exceeds 1:1. This occurs during the last phase "sprint" of a 1-mile race. Relatively fast ATP production from rapid glycolysis also remains crucial during a 440-m run or 100-m swim and in multiple-sprint activities such as ice hockey, field hockey, rugby, and soccer. These activity examples require rapid energy transfer that exceeds that supplied by stored phosphagens. When the intensity of "all-out" effort decreases to extend its duration, lactate buildup correspondingly decreases.

Lactate Accumulation

Chapter 5 pointed out that some lactate still forms even during rest. Lactate removal by the heart muscle and nonactive skeletal muscle balances this lactate production without "net" lactate buildup. Blood lactate accumulates in tissue and blood only when its removal fails to match its production. *Aerobic activities induce metabolic and tissue adaptations to increase lactate removal rates so lactate only accumulates at higher exercise intensities.* **Figure 6.1** illustrates the general relationship in endurance athletes and untrained individuals between oxygen uptake expressed as a percentage of maximum and blood lactate level during light, moderate, and strenuous physical activity. In both groups during light and moderate activity, aerobic metabolism adequately meets energy demands. Nonactive tissues rapidly oxidize any lactate that forms, permitting blood lactate to remain fairly stable without net blood lactate accumulation, even though oxygen uptake increases.

For healthy, untrained persons, blood lactate begins to accumulate and rise in an exponential manner at about 50% to 55% of the maximal capacity for aerobic metabolism. The traditional explanation for blood lactate accumulation in physical activity assumed a relative tissue hypoxia. When glycolytic metabolism predominates, nicotinamide adenine dinucleotide (NADH) production exceeds the cell's capacity to shuttle its hydrogen electrons through the respiratory chain. This occurs from insufficient oxygen supply or

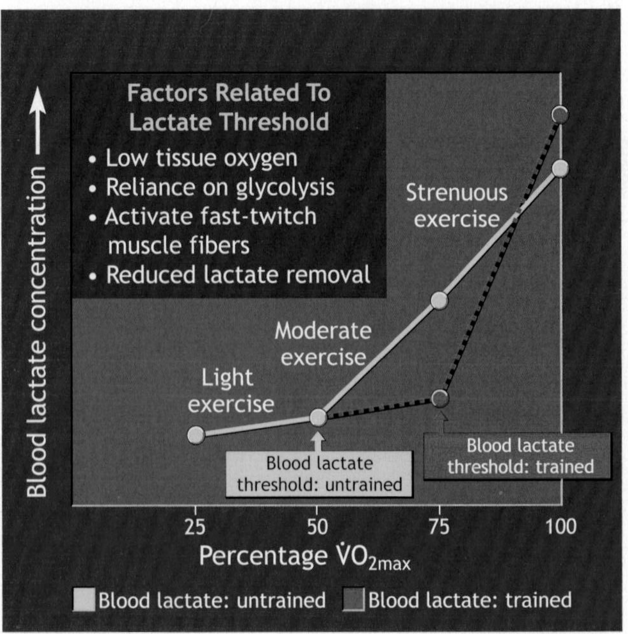

FIGURE 6.1 Blood lactate concentration for trained and untrained subjects at different levels of exercise expressed as a percentage of maximal oxygen uptake ($\dot{V}O_{2max}$).

tissue level use, or even by epinephrine and norepinephrine stimulation independent of tissue hypoxia. The imbalance in hydrogen release and subsequent oxidation causes two hydrogens to attach to a pyruvate molecule. The original pyruvate with two additional hydrogens forms a new molecule—lactic acid, which changes to lactate in the body and begins to accumulate.

Radioactive tracer studies that label carbon in the glucose molecule spawned an alternate hypothesis to explain lactate buildup in muscle and its subsequent appearance in blood. Lactate continuously forms in muscle during rest and moderate physical activity. About 70% of the lactate oxidizes, 20% converts to glucose in muscle and liver, and 10% synthesizes to amino acids. Thus, no *net* lactate accumulates because blood lactate concentration remains stable. *Blood lactate accumulates only when its disappearance by oxidation or substrate conversion does not match its production rate.*

Adaptations from aerobic training allow high rates of lactate turnover at a given movement intensity; lactate begins to accumulate at higher intensity levels following training than in the untrained state. Another adaptation includes the tendency for **lactate dehydrogenase (LDH)** in fast-twitch muscle fibers to favor the conversion of pyruvate to lactate. In contrast, the LDH level in slow-twitch fibers favors lactate-to-pyruvate conversion. Recruitment of fast-twitch fibers with increasing intensity of effort therefore favors lactate formation, independent of tissue oxygenation.

Lactate production and accumulation accelerate as exercise intensity increases. In such cases, the muscle cells can neither meet the additional energy demands aerobically nor oxidize lactate at its formation rate. A similar pattern exists for untrained subjects and endurance athletes, except the threshold for lactate buildup, termed the **blood lactate threshold (LT)**, occurs at a *higher percentage* of the trained persons' aerobic capacity. Trained endurance individuals perform steady-rate aerobic activity at intensities between 80% and 90% of maximum capacity for aerobic metabolism. In Chapter 13, we discuss the concept of the blood lactate threshold related to endurance performance.

fyi Lactic Acid and pH

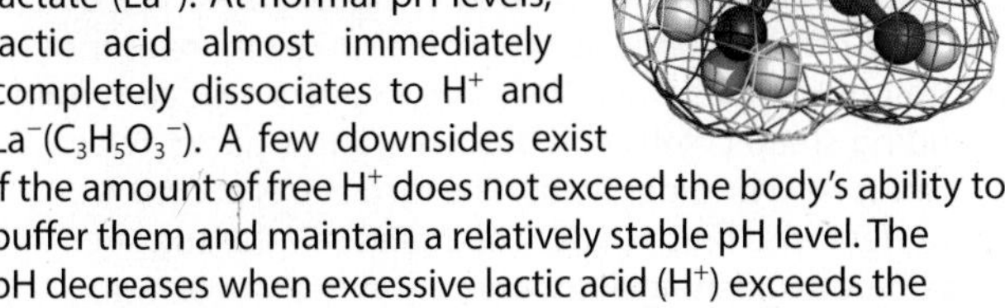

The body's primary challenge regards hydrogen ions (H^+) dissociating from lactic acid, rather than dissociated lactate (La^-). At normal pH levels, lactic acid almost immediately completely dissociates to H^+ and $La^-(C_3H_5O_3^-)$. A few downsides exist if the amount of free H^+ does not exceed the body's ability to buffer them and maintain a relatively stable pH level. The pH decreases when excessive lactic acid (H^+) exceeds the body's immediate buffering capacity. Discomfort occurs and performance subsequently decreases as the blood becomes more acidic.

Lactate-Producing Capacity

Specific sprint-power anaerobic training produces high blood lactate levels during maximal physical activity. Sprint-power athletes often achieve 20% to 30% higher blood lactate levels than those of untrained counterparts during maximal short-duration activity. One or more of the following three mechanisms helps to explain this training response:

1. Improved motivation with training
2. Increased intramuscular glycogen stores with training allow a greater contribution of energy via anaerobic glycolysis
3. Increased training-induced glycolytic-related enzymes, particularly phosphofructokinase; the 20% increase in glycolytic enzymes does not achieve the two- to threefold increase in aerobic enzymes with endurance training

Blood Lactate as an Energy Source

In Chapter 5 we emphasized how blood lactate serves as substrate for gluconeogenesis and a direct fuel source for active muscle. Isotope tracer studies of muscle and other tissues reveal that lactate produced in fast-twitch muscle fibers circulates to other fast- or slow-twitch fibers for conversion to pyruvate. Pyruvate, in turn, converts to acetyl-CoA for entry to the citric acid cycle for aerobic energy metabolism. Such **lactate shuttling** between cells enables glycogenolysis in one cell to supply other cells with fuel for oxidation. *This makes muscle not only a major site of lactate production but also a primary tissue for lactate removal via oxidation.*

A muscle oxidizes much of its produced lactate without releasing lactate into the blood. The liver also accepts muscle-generated lactate from the bloodstream and synthesizes it to glucose through the Cori cycle's gluconeogenic reactions (outlined in Chapter 5). Glucose derived from lactate takes one of two routes:

1. It returns in the blood to skeletal muscle for energy metabolism.
2. It synthesizes to glycogen for storage.

These two uses of lactate make this anaerobic byproduct of intense physical activity a valuable metabolic substrate and certainly not an unwanted "waste" product.

LONG-TERM ENERGY: THE AEROBIC SYSTEM

Glycolysis releases anaerobic energy rapidly, with only a relatively small total ATP yield. In contrast, aerobic metabolic reactions provide for the greatest portion of energy transfer, particularly when activity duration exceeds 2 to 3 minutes.

Oxygen Uptake During Physical Activity

The upward-bending yellow curve in **Figure 6.2** illustrates oxygen uptake during each minute of a 20-minute slow jog continued at a steady pace. The vertical *y* axis indicates the uptake of oxygen (referred to as **oxygen uptake or oxygen consumption**); the horizontal *x* axis displays time. The abbreviation $\dot{V}O_2$ indicates oxygen uptake, where the V denotes the volume consumed; the dot placed above the $\dot{V}$ expresses oxygen uptake as a per minute value. Oxygen uptake during any minute can be determined easily by locating time on the *x* axis and its corresponding point for oxygen uptake on the *y* axis. For example, after running 4 minutes, oxygen uptake equals approximately 17 $mL \cdot kg^{-1} \cdot min^{-1}$.

Oxygen uptake increases rapidly during the first minutes of activity and reaches a relative plateau between minutes 4 and 6. It then remains relatively stable thereafter. The flat portion or plateau of the best-fitting curve

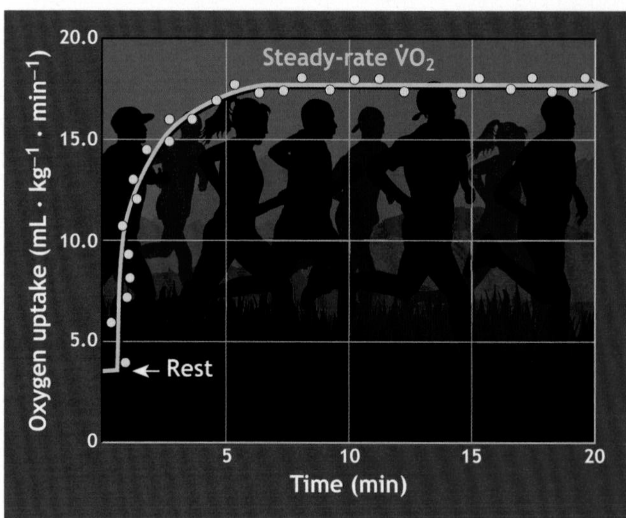

FIGURE 6.2 Time course of oxygen uptake during continuous jogging at a slow pace. The *dots* along the curve represent measured values of oxygen uptake determined by open-circuit spirometry.

Ultimate Aerobic Challenge

By combining extreme distances with rugged terrain, heat, cold, elevation, and route-finding difficulties, three competitions surely represent the ultimate aerobic and physiologic challenge for those who finish.

Marathon des Sables Marathon des Sables (www.darbaroud.com/en)

Founded in 1986 with 23 competitors, this race in the south Moroccan desert is characterized as the "toughest footrace on Earth." Participants complete the equivalent of five and a half marathons over 5 to 6 days, covering a total of 156 miles and traversing the desert over dunes, mountains, wind-formed waves of sand, dry riverbed valleys, and desert storms. The longest single stage covers 57 miles. Outdoor temperatures typically exceed 100°F (37.8°C). Competitors carry their own supplies, including food, clothing, sleeping bag, and other survival-type items (a small ration of water is provided daily). Female champion ultra endurance athlete Nikki Kimball, the woman's winner of the 2014 race, prepared daily reports of her trials and tribulations of the run (**www.irunfar.com/2014/04/nikki-kimballs-2014-marathon-des-sables-race-report.html**).

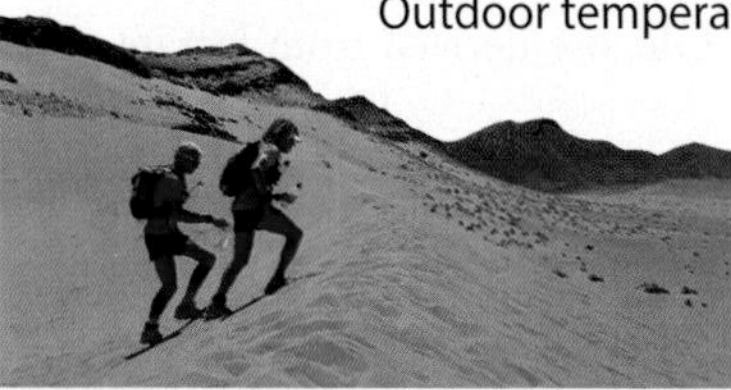

In the 29th Marathon des Sables in 2014, 917 competitors out of 1029 were able to finish. (Reprinted from **www.marathondessables.com/archives/29mds/en/medias-gb/photos/category/3-07-04-etape-stage-n-2-erg-znaigui-oued-moungarf-41-km.html**.)

Badwater 135 Ultramarathon (www.badwater.com/index.html)

The Badwater 135 Ultramarathon starts in Lone Pine, CA, and climbs to the finish at Mt. Whitney Portal at 10,000 feet (3048 m). Runners trek across the Owens Valley to a 5500-foot dirt road ascent to the ghost town of Cerro Gordo, followed by a run to the entrance to Darwin, and then a final dramatic ascent to the highest paved point on Mt. Whitney. The last part of the race goes 13 miles continuously uphill with a 5000-foot (1524 m) elevation gain. The 135 mile nonstop footrace in mid-July features approximately 100 runners, triathletes, adventure racers, and mountaineers who endure extreme heat—120°F (48.9°C), high winds, and over 17,000 feet (5200 m) of cumulative vertical ascent and 12,700 feet (3900 m) of cumulative descent.

Hardrock 100-Mile Run (www.hardrock100.com/)

Located in the San Juan Range in Southern Colorado, this race begins and ends in Silverton, CO, with the loop course covering 100.5 miles at an average elevation of 11,186 feet (3410 m). Participants traverse more than 33,992 vertical feet of climb during the competition (67,984 feet total elevation change). Finishers trek 13 times above 13,000 feet (3962 m) and once at 14,048 feet (4282 m) over the summit of Handies Peak. The course covers rugged terrain including steep climbs and descents, snow packs, river crossings, and boulder fields. The race starts at 6:00 AM, so runners who finish in over 40 hours see the sun set twice before finishing. Runners continue at night using flashlights or headlamps. The cutoff time for finishing the race is 48 hours.

to represent the data points indicates the **steady rate of aerobic metabolism**—a balance between energy required by the body and rate of aerobic ATP production. Oxygen-consuming reactions supply the energy for steady-rate physical activity; any lactate produced either oxidizes or reconverts to glucose in the liver, kidneys, and skeletal muscles. *No net accumulation of blood lactate occurs under steady-rate metabolic conditions.*

Many Steady Rate Levels

For some individuals, lying in bed, working around the house, and playing an occasional round of golf represent the activity spectrum for steady-rate energy metabolism. In contrast, a champion marathon runner covers 26.2 miles in slightly more than 2 hours yet still can maintain a steady rate of aerobic metabolism. This sub–5-minute-per-mile pace represents a truly magnificent physiologic-metabolic accomplishment. Maintenance of the required level of aerobic metabolism necessitates well-developed functional capacities of many physiologic systems that deliver adequate oxygen to active muscles and process oxygen within muscle cells for aerobic ATP production.

Oxygen Deficit

Note that the oxygen uptake curve in **Figure 6.2** does not increase instantaneously to a steady rate at the start of physical activity. In other words, it does not rise up vertically to the steady rate level. Instead, in the first minute of activity, oxygen uptake remains considerably below the steady-rate level even if the energy requirement remains essentially unchanged throughout the activity period. The temporary "lag" in oxygen uptake occurs because ATP and PCr provide the muscles' immediate energy requirements without the

A CLOSER LOOK

Overtraining: Too Much of a Good Thing

Intense and prolonged training can produce overtraining, staleness, or burnout. The overtrained condition reflects more than just a short-term inability to train hard or a slight dip in competition-level performance; rather, it involves a more chronic fatigue experienced during physical activity and subsequent recovery periods. Overtraining associates with sustained poor exercise performance, frequent infections particularly of the upper respiratory tract, general malaise and loss of interest in high-level training, and injuries. The specific symptoms of overtraining are highly individualized, with those outlined below most common. Little is known about the cause of this syndrome, although researchers suspect neuroendocrine alterations that affect the sympathetic nervous system, including alterations in immune function. These symptoms persist unless the athlete rests, with complete recovery requiring weeks or even months.

Carbohydrates' Possible Role in Overtraining

A gradual depletion of the body's carbohydrate reserves with repeated strenuous training exacerbates the overtraining syndrome. A pioneering study showed that after 3 successive days of running 16.1 km (10 miles), glycogen in the thigh muscle became nearly depleted. This occurred even though the runners' diets contained 40% to 60% of total calories as carbohydrates. In addition, glycogen use on the third day of the run averaged about 72% less than on day 1. The mechanism by which repeated occurrences of glycogen depletion may contribute to overtraining remains unclear.

Tapering Often Helps

Overtraining symptoms may range from mild to severe. They more often occur in highly motivated individuals when a large increase in training occurs abruptly and when the overall training program does not include sufficient rest and recovery.

Overtraining symptoms often occur before season-ending competition. To achieve peak performance, athletes should reduce their training volume and increase their carbohydrate intake for at least several days before competition—a practice called *tapering*. The goal attempts to provide time for muscles to resynthesize glycogen to maximal levels and allow them to heal from training-induced damage.

Overtraining Signs and Symptoms

1. **Performance-Related Symptoms**
   - Consistent performance decline
   - Persistent fatigue and sluggishness
   - Excessive recovery required after competitive events
   - Inconsistent performance
2. **Physiologic Symptoms**
   - Decrease in maximum work capacity
   - Frequent headaches or stomachaches
   - Insomnia
   - Persistent low-grade stiffness and muscle or joint soreness
   - Frequent constipation or diarrhea
   - Unexplained loss of appetite and body mass
   - Amenorrhea
   - Elevated resting heart rate on waking
3. **Psychologic Symptoms**
   - Depression
   - General apathy
   - Decreased self-esteem
   - Mood changes
   - Difficulty concentrating
   - Loss of competitive drive

need for oxygen. Even with experimentally increased oxygen availability and increased oxygen diffusion gradients at the tissue level, the initial increase in exercise oxygen uptake *always* calculates lower than the steady-rate oxygen uptake. Owing to the interaction of intrinsic inertia in cellular metabolic signals and enzyme activation and the relative sluggishness of oxygen delivery to mitochondria, the hydrogens produced in energy metabolism do not immediately oxidize and combine with oxygen. Instead a deficiency always exists in the oxygen uptake response to a new, higher steady-rate, regardless of activity mode or activity intensity.

The ***oxygen deficit*** *quantitatively represents the difference between the total oxygen consumed during physical activity and an additional amount that would have been consumed if a steady-rate aerobic metabolism occurred immediately at the initiation of activity.* Energy provided during the deficit phase represents, at least conceptually, a predominance of anaerobic energy transfer. Stated in metabolic terms, the oxygen deficit represents the quantity of energy produced from stored intramuscular phosphagens plus energy contributed from rapid glycolytic reactions. This yields enough phosphate-bond energy until oxygen uptake and energy demands reach steady rate.

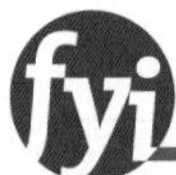

Oxygen Uptake and Body Size

To adjust for the effects of variations in body size on oxygen uptake (i.e., bigger people usually consume more oxygen), researchers frequently express oxygen uptake in terms of body mass (relative oxygen uptake) as milliliters of oxygen per kilogram of body mass per minute ($mL \cdot kg^{-1} \cdot min^{-1}$). At rest for a 70-kg person, this averages about 3.5 $mL \cdot kg^{-1} \cdot min^{-1}$ or 1 metabolic equivalent (MET) or 245 $mL \cdot min^{-1}$ (absolute oxygen uptake). Other means of relating oxygen uptake to aspects of body size and body composition include milliliters of oxygen per kilogram of fat-free body mass per minute ($mL \cdot kg\ FFM^{-1} \cdot min^{-1}$) and sometimes milliliters of oxygen per square centimeter of muscle cross-sectional area per minute ($mL \cdot cm\ MCSA^{-2} \cdot min^{-1}$).

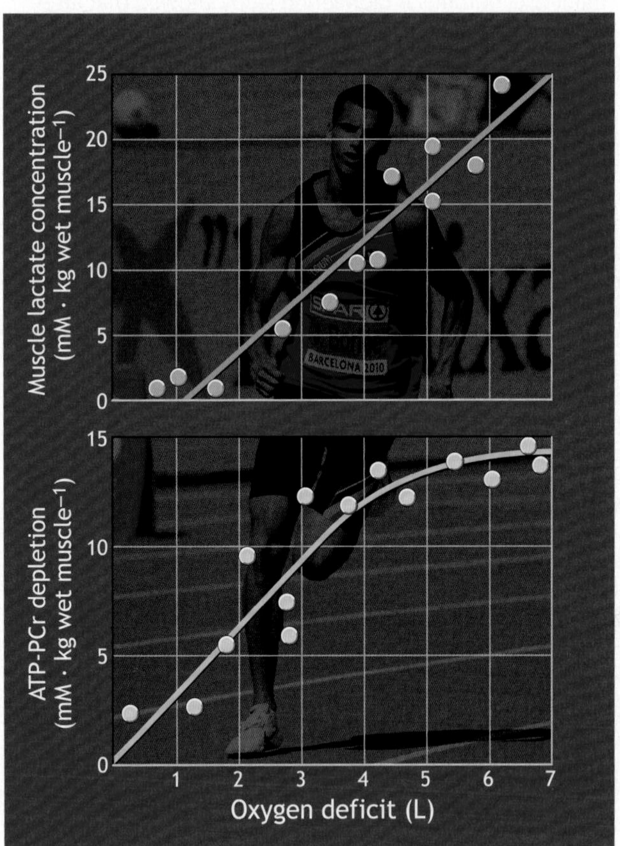

FIGURE 6.3 Muscle ATP and PCr depletion and muscle lactate concentration plotted versus oxygen deficit. (Reprinted with permission from McArdle WD, Katch FI, Katch VL. *Exercise Physiology: Nutrition, Energy, and Human Performance*. 8th Ed. Baltimore: Wolters Kluwer Health, 2015; as adapted with permission from Karlsson J. Muscle ATP, PCr and lactate in submaximal and maximal exercise. In: Pernow B, Saltin B, eds. *Muscle Metabolism During Exercise*. New York: Plenum Press, 1971.)

Figure 6.3 depicts the relationship between the size of the oxygen deficit and the energy contribution from the ATP-PCr and lactic acid energy systems. Physical activity that generates about a 3- to 4-L oxygen deficit substantially depletes the intramuscular high-energy phosphates. Consequently, this intensity continues only on a "pay-as-you-go" basis; ATP must be replenished continually through either glycolysis or aerobic breakdown of carbohydrate, fat, and protein. Interestingly, lactate begins to increase in active muscle before the phosphagens attain their lowest levels. This means that glycolysis contributes anaerobic energy early in vigorous activity before full utilization of the high-energy phosphates. *Energy for physical activity does not merely result from a series of energy systems that "switch on" and "switch off" like a light switch. Rather, a muscle's energy supply represents a smooth transition between anaerobic and aerobic sources, with considerable overlap from one source of energy transfer to another.*

Oxygen Deficit in Trained and Untrained Individuals

Figure 6.4 shows the oxygen uptake response to submaximal cycle ergometer or treadmill activity for a trained and an untrained person. Trained and untrained individuals show similar values for steady-rate $\dot{V}O_2$ during light and moderate physical activity. A trained person achieves the steady-rate quicker; comparatively, this person has a smaller oxygen deficit for the same exercise duration. This indicates that the trained person consumes more total oxygen during physical activity with a proportionately smaller anaerobic energy transfer component. The following three aerobic training

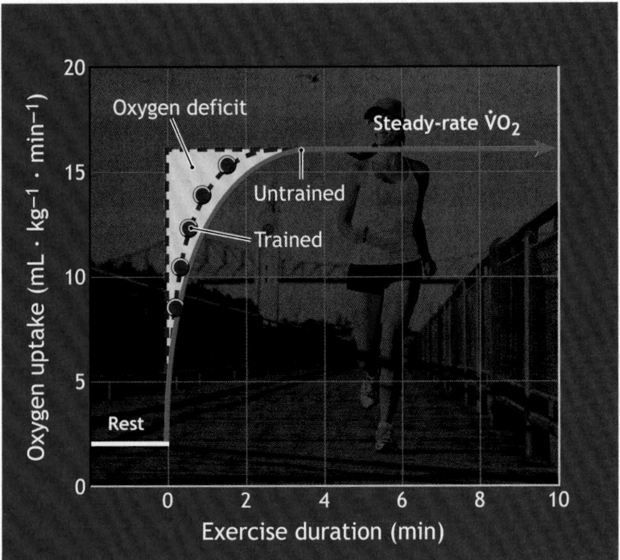

FIGURE 6.4 Oxygen uptake and oxygen deficit for trained and untrained individuals during submaximum cycle ergometer exercise. Both individuals reach the same steady-rate $\dot{V}O_2$, but the trained person reaches it at a faster rate, reducing the oxygen deficit. (Adapted with permission from McArdle WD, Katch FI, Katch VL. *Exercise Physiology: Nutrition, Energy, and Human Performance*. 8th Ed. Baltimore: Wolters Kluwer Health, 2015.)

adaptations facilitate increased capacity to generate ATP aerobically when activity begins:

1. More rapid increase in muscle bioenergetics
2. Increase in overall cardiac output
3. Disproportionately large regional blood flow to active muscle complemented by cellular aerobic adaptations

MAXIMAL OXYGEN UPTAKE ($\dot{V}O_{2MAX}$)

Figure 6.5 depicts oxygen uptake during a series of constant-speed runs up six progressively steeper "hills." simulated in the laboratory. This occurs by increasing treadmill elevation, step bench height, and/or stepping rate; increasing resistance to pedaling at a constant rate on a bicycle ergometer; and increasing rate of water flow toward the swimmer in a swim flume. Each successive "hill" requires a greater energy output that places additional demand on capacity for aerobic ATP resynthesis. During the first several hills, $\dot{V}O_2$ increases rapidly, with each new steady-rate value in direct proportion to exercise intensity. The runner maintains speed up the two last hills, but $\dot{V}O_2$ fails to increase as rapidly or to the same extent as in the previous hills. No increase in $\dot{V}O_2$ occurs during the run up the last hill. The region in yellow at the top right of the figure where oxygen uptake plateaus or increases only slightly with additional increases in exercise intensity represents the greatest amount of oxygen the individual can consume—also called **maximal oxygen uptake, maximal aerobic power, aerobic capacity,** or simply **$\dot{V}O_{2max}$**. Energy transfer via anaerobic glycolysis allows performance of more intense physical activity with resulting lactate accumulation. Under these conditions, the runner soon becomes exhausted and stops running.

The $\dot{V}O_{2max}$ provides a quantitative measure of a person's capacity for aerobic ATP resynthesis. This makes $\dot{V}O_{2max}$ an important indicator of how well a person can maintain intense activity for longer than 4 or 5 minutes. Attainment of a high $\dot{V}O_{2max}$ has important physiologic meanings in addition to its role in sustaining energy metabolism during

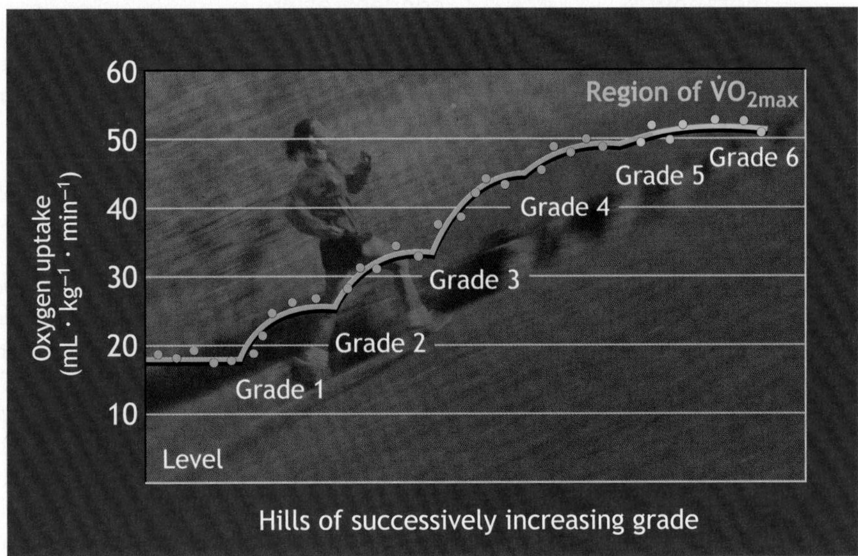

FIGURE 6.5 Attainment of maximal oxygen uptake ($\dot{V}O_{2max}$) while running up hills of progressively increasing slope. $\dot{V}O_{2max}$ occurs in the region (designated by *yellow data points* along the *yellow part* of the curve and not a single point) where further increases in exercise intensity produce a less-than-expected increase (or no increase) in oxygen uptake. *Dots* represent measured values of oxygen uptake while traversing the hills. (Reprinted with permission from McArdle WD, Katch FI, Katch VL. *Exercise Physiology: Nutrition, Energy, and Human Performance*. 8th Ed. Baltimore: Wolters Kluwer Health, 2015.)

physical activity. A high $\dot{V}O_{2max}$ requires the integrated and high-level response of diverse physiologic support systems. **Figure 6.6** illustrates pulmonary ventilation, hemoglobin concentration, blood volume and cardiac output, peripheral blood flow, and cellular metabolic capacity. In subsequent chapters, we discuss various aspects of $\dot{V}O_{2max}$, including its physiologic significance, measurement, and role in determining physical performance and cardiovascular well-being.

ENERGY TRANSFER IN FAST- AND SLOW-TWITCH MUSCLE FIBERS

Two distinct muscle fibers types exist in humans, each generating ATP differently. **Fast-twitch (FT) or type II muscle fibers** have two primary subdivisions, type IIa and type IIx. Each fiber type possesses rapid contraction speed and high capacity for anaerobic ATP production via glycolysis. The subdivision type IIa fiber also possesses relatively high aerobic capacity. Type II fibers engage during change-of-pace and stop-and-go sports like basketball, field hockey, lacrosse, soccer, and ice hockey. They also increase force output when running or cycling up hills while maintaining a constant speed or during all-out effort that requires rapid, powerful movements that depend almost exclusively on energy-derived from anaerobic metabolism.

The second fiber type, the **slow-twitch (ST) or type I muscle fiber**, generates energy primarily through aerobic pathways. This fiber possesses a slower contraction speed compared with fast-twitch fibers. Capacity to generate ATP aerobically relates to the type I fiber's numerous large mitochondria including high levels of enzymes required for aerobic metabolism to sustain fatty acid catabolism. Slow-twitch muscle fibers primarily support continuous activities requiring a steady rate of aerobic energy transfer. Fatigue in prolonged running associates with glycogen depletion in the leg muscles' type I and type IIa fibers. More than likely, the predominance of slow-twitch muscle fibers contributes to high blood lactate thresholds among elite endurance athletes.

Athletes who excel in different sporting high-power versus endurance activities typically have a large percentage of the specific muscle fiber type that supports the sport's energy demands. For example, **Figure 6.7** illustrates muscle-fiber composition of two athletes in sports that rely on distinctly different energy transfer systems favored by specific muscle fiber type predominance. For the 50-m sprint swim champion (left panel), type II fibers represent nearly 80% of the total muscle fibers, whereas the endurance cyclist (right panel) possesses 80% type I fibers. From a practical perspective, most sports require relatively slow, sustained muscle actions interspersed with short bursts of powerful effort (e.g., basketball, soccer, lacrosse, field hockey). Not surprisingly, these activities require an approximate equal percentage and activation of both fiber types.

The preceding discussion suggests that a muscle's predominant fiber type contributes to success in certain sports or physical activities. Chapter 14 explores this idea more fully. This includes consideration of metabolic, contractile, and fatigue characteristics of each fiber type, their various subdivisions and proposed classification system, and exercise training effects.

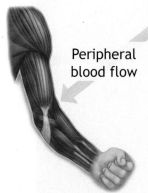

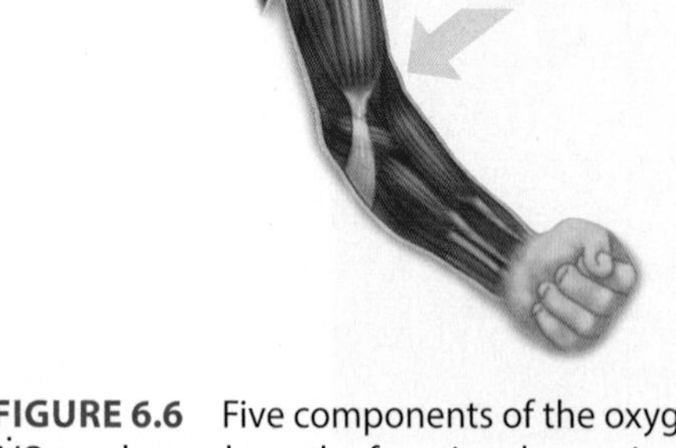

FIGURE 6.6 Five components of the oxygen transport system. The physiologic significance of $\dot{V}O_{2max}$ depends on the functional capacity and integration of systems required for oxygen supply, transport, delivery, and use. (Adapted with permission from McArdle WD, Katch FI, Katch VL. *Exercise Physiology: Nutrition, Energy, and Human Performance*. 8th Ed. Baltimore: Wolters Kluwer Health, 2015; Lung and heart images adapted with permission from Moore KL, Dalley AF, Agur AMR. *Clinically Oriented Anatomy*. 7th Ed, as used with permission from Agur AMR, Dalley AF. *Grant's Atlas of Anatomy*. 13th Ed. Baltimore: Wolters Kluwer Health, 2013.)

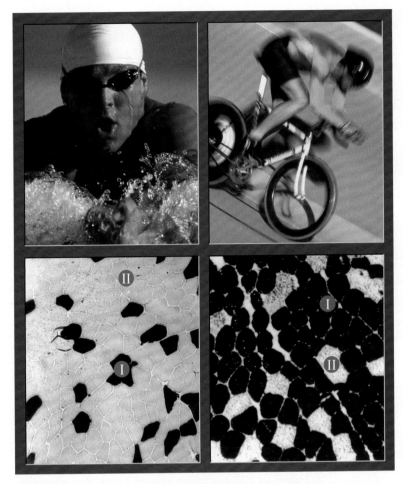

FIGURE 6.7 Differences in muscle-fiber type composition between a sprint swimmer and endurance cyclist. The type I and type II muscle fibers were sampled from the vastus lateralis muscle and stained for myofibrillar ATPase after incubation at pH 4.3. Type I fibers stain dark, while type II fibers remain unstained. (Reprinted with permission from McArdle WD, Katch FI, Katch VL. *Exercise Physiology: Nutrition, Energy, and Human Performance*. 8th Ed. Baltimore: Wolters Kluwer Health, 2015; photos and photomicrographs courtesy of Dr. R. Billeter, School of Life Sciences, University of Nottingham, Great Britain.)

ENERGY SPECTRUM OF PHYSICAL ACTIVITY

Figure 6.8 depicts the relative contributions of anaerobic and aerobic energy sources for various durations of maximal physical activity. The data represent estimates from all-out treadmill running and stationary bicycling laboratory experiments. The data also relate to other activities by juxtaposing the appropriate time relationships. For example, a 100-m sprint run equates to any all-out 10-second activity, but an 800-m run lasts approximately 2 minutes. All-out effort for 1 minute includes the 400-m sprint in track, a 100-m swim, and repeated full-court presses during a basketball game.

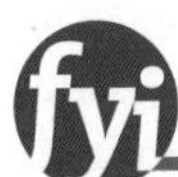

Difficult to Excel in All Sports

An understanding of the energy requirements of various physical activities partly explains why a world record holder in the 1-mile run does not achieve similar success in long-distance running events. Conversely, premier marathoners usually cannot run 1 mile in less than 4 minutes, yet they complete a 26-mile race averaging just under a 5-minute-per-mile pace.

Intensity and Duration Determine the Blend of Energy Use

The body's energy transfer systems can be viewed along a continuum of exercise bioenergetics. Anaerobic sources supply most of the energy for fast movements and during increased resistance to movement at a given speed. Also, when movement begins at either fast or slow speed, as in performing a front handspring to starting a marathon run, the intramuscular phosphagens provide immediate anaerobic energy for the required initial burst of muscle actions.

At the short-duration extreme of maximum effort, the intramuscular phosphagens supply the major energy for physical activity. The ATP-PCr and lactic acid systems contribute about half of the energy required for "best-effort exercise" lasting 2 minutes, with aerobic reactions contributing the remainder. Top performance in all-out, 2-minute bouts requires well-developed capacities for aerobic *and* anaerobic metabolism. Five to 10 minutes of intense middle-distance running and swimming or stop-and-go basketball and soccer demand greater aerobic energy transfer. Longer duration marathon running, distance swimming and cycling, recreational jogging, cross-country skiing, and hiking and backpacking require continual energy from aerobic resources without reliance on lactate's contribution.

Intensity and duration determine the energy system and metabolic mixture use during physical activity. The aerobic system predominates in low-intensity effort, with fat serving as the primary fuel source. The liver markedly increases its glucose release to active muscle as activity progresses from lower to higher intensity. Simultaneously, glycogen stored within active muscle serves as the predominant carbohydrate energy source during the early stages of physical activity and with increasing intensity of effort. *The advantage of selective dependence on carbohydrate metabolism during near-maximum aerobic activity lies in its two times more rapid energy transfer capacity compared with fat and protein fuels.* Compared with fat, carbohydrate also generates close to 6% greater energy per unit of oxygen consumed. As activity continues with accompanying muscle glycogen depletion, progressively

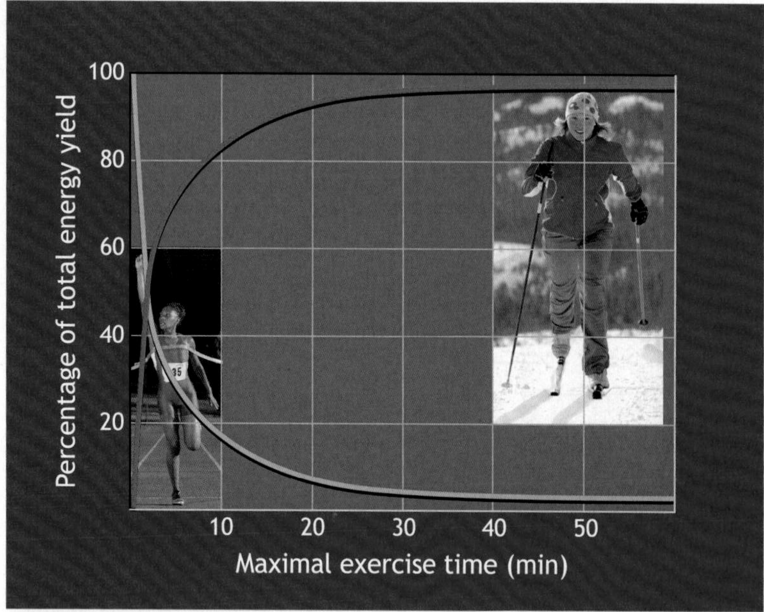

Duration of maximal exercise

	Seconds			Minutes					
	10	30	60	2	4	10	30	60	120
Percentage anaerobic	90	80	70	50	35	15	5	2	1
Percentage aerobic	10	20	30	50	65	85	95	98	99

FIGURE 6.8 Relative contribution of aerobic and anaerobic energy metabolism during maximal physical effort of various durations. Note that 2 minutes of maximal effort requires about 50% of the energy from combined aerobic and anaerobic processes. A world-class 4-minute-mile pace derives approximately 65% of its energy from aerobic metabolism, with the remainder generated from anaerobic processes. A 2.5-hour marathon, in contrast, generates almost all of its energy from aerobic processes. (Adapted with permission from Åstrand PO, Rodahl K. *Textbook of Work Physiology*. New York: McGraw-Hill, 1977.)

more intramuscular triacylglycerols and circulating free fatty acids (FFAs) supply substrate for ATP production. In maximal anaerobic effort, carbohydrate serves as the sole contributor to ATP production in mainstream glycolytic reactions.

A sound approach to training to ensure optimal physiologic and metabolic adaptations first analyzes an activity for its specific energy components and then establishes a task-specific training regimen. Improved capacity for energy transfer should translate to improved performance.

Nutrient-Related Fatigue

Severe liver and muscle glycogen depletion during intense prolonged aerobic effort induces fatigue despite sufficient oxygen availability to muscle and an almost unlimited energy supply from stored fat. Endurance athletes commonly refer to this extreme sensation of fatigue as **"bonking" or hitting the wall**. The image of hitting the wall suggests an inability to continue exercising, which in reality does not occur, although pain occurs in the active muscles and effort intensity drops off markedly. Skeletal muscle does not contain the phosphatase enzyme present in the liver that helps to free glucose from liver cells; this means that relatively inactive muscle retains all of its stored glycogen. Controversy exists as to why liver and muscle glycogen depletion during longer duration activity reduces exercise capacity. Three factors are involved:

1. The central nervous system's use of blood glucose for energy
2. Muscle glycogen's role as a "primer" in fat catabolism
3. The slower rate of energy release from fat compared with carbohydrate oxidation

OXYGEN UPTAKE DURING RECOVERY: THE SO-CALLED OXYGEN DEBT

Bodily processes do not immediately return to resting levels following most physical activities. In light activity (e.g., golf, archery, bowling, walking), return to a prior resting condition takes place rapidly and often progresses unnoticed. Intense physical activity such as running full speed for 800 m or trying to swim 200 m "all-out" requires considerable time for body processes to return to resting levels. The difference in recovery from light and strenuous activity relates largely to the specific metabolic and physiologic processes during each activity mode.

British Nobel physiologist Archibal Vivian Hill (1886–1977; **http://www.nobelprize.org/nobel_prizes/medicine/laureates/1922/hill-bio.html**), referred to oxygen uptake during recovery as **oxygen debt**. Contemporary researchers no longer use this term. Instead, **recovery oxygen uptake or excess postexercise oxygen consumption (EPOC)** now defines the excess oxygen uptake above the resting level in recovery. This specifically refers to the total oxygen consumed following physical activity in excess of a pre-exercise baseline level.

Figure 6.9 illustrates oxygen uptake during physical activity and recovery from different movement intensities. Light aerobic activity (**A**), with rapid attainment of steady-rate $\dot{V}O_2$, produces a small oxygen deficit. The magnitude of recovery $\dot{V}O_2$, approximates the size of the oxygen deficit when activity begins. Recovery proceeds rapidly. Oxygen uptake follows a logarithmic curve, decreasing by about 50% over each subsequent 30-second period until attaining the preactivity level.

Oxygen uptake, usually expressed as $mL \cdot min^{-1}$, $L \cdot min^{-1}$, or $mL \cdot kg^{-1} \cdot min^{-1}$ during steady-rate and non–steady-rate activity and recovery, plots as a logarithmic function related to time. The function increases in activity or decreases in recovery by a constant fraction for each unit of time as oxygen uptake approaches an asymptote or level value. Consider the example of recovery from 10 minutes of steady-rate physical activity at an oxygen uptake of 2000 mL • min^{-1}. If recovery $\dot{V}O_2$ decreased by half over 30 seconds, then $\dot{V}O_2$ would equal 1000 mL • min^{-1} at 30-second recovery and 500 mL • min^{-1} at 60 seconds, with the resting value of 250 mL • min^{-1} achieved in about 90 seconds.

Moderate-to-intense aerobic activity (**Fig. 6.9B**) requires a longer time to achieve steady-rate $\dot{V}O_2$ and creates a larger oxygen deficit than does less intense effort. Consequently, it takes longer for the recovery oxygen uptake to return to preactivity levels. The $\dot{V}O_2$ recovery curve demonstrates an initial rapid decline, similar to recovery from light activity, followed by a more gradual decline to baseline resting levels. In **Figure 6.9A and B**, computing the oxygen deficit and recovery $\dot{V}O_2$ relies on steady-rate $\dot{V}O_2$ to represent physical activity's oxygen or energy requirement. **Figure 6.9C** shows that all-out, exhaustive physical effort does not produce a steady-rate $\dot{V}O_2$. Such effort demands a larger energy requirement than aerobic processes can supply. Consequently, anaerobic energy transfer increases and blood lactate accumulates, with considerable time required to achieve complete recovery to approximately resting values. Failure to achieve steady-rate $\dot{V}O_2$ makes it unfeasible to accurately quantify the true oxygen deficit.

Each of the curves in **Figure 6.9** shows that $\dot{V}O_2$ in recovery always exceeds resting $\dot{V}O_2$, independent of intensity. The excess $\dot{V}O_2$ has classically been termed *oxygen debt* or *recovery oxygen uptake*, with the newer preferred term the excess postexercise oxygen consumption or EPOC (indicated by the *darker purple* shaded area under each recovery curve in A, B, and C. EPOC computes as the total $\dot{V}O_2$ in recovery minus the total $\dot{V}O_2$ theoretically consumed at rest during the recovery period. For example, if a total of 5.5 L of oxygen were consumed in recovery until attaining the resting value of 0.310 L • min^{-1}, and recovery required 10 minutes, the recovery $\dot{V}O_2$ would equal 5.5 L – 3.1 L (0.310 L × 10 minutes) or 2.4 L. In this example, the preceding period caused physiologic alterations during activity *and* during recovery that required an additional 2.4-L $\dot{V}O_2$ before returning to pre-exercise rest. These calculations assume that resting $\dot{V}O_2$ remains unaltered during activity and recovery. As we discuss later in the section on Contemporary Concepts, this assumption may not be entirely correct, particularly following strenuous physical activity.

The three curves in **Figure 6.9** illustrate two important characteristics of recovery $\dot{V}O_2$:

1. With mild aerobic activity of relatively short duration and little disruption in body temperature and hormonal milieu, about half of the total recovery oxygen uptake occurs within 30 seconds, and complete recovery within 2 to 4 minutes. The decline in $\dot{V}O_2$ in **Figure 6.9A** follows a single-component exponential curve termed the **fast component of recovery oxygen uptake**.
2. Recovery from strenuous activity presents a different picture, presumably because three factors—blood lactate, body temperature, and thermogenic hormone levels—increase substantially. A second phase of recovery exists in addition to the fast component of the recovery phase called the **slow component of recovery oxygen uptake**. Depending on the intensity and duration of the prior physical activity, the slow component can

A CLOSER LOOK

Establishing Cardiovascular Fitness Categories

Cardiovascular fitness reflects the maximal amount of oxygen consumed during each minute of near-maximal exercise. Values for maximal oxygen uptake, or $\dot{V}O_{2max}$, generally are expressed in milliliters of oxygen per kilogram of body mass per minute (mL • kg^{-1} • min^{-1}). Individual values can range from about 10 mL • kg^{-1} • min^{-1} in cardiac patients to 80 or 90 mL • kg^{-1} • min^{-1} in world-class runners and cross-country skiers. Men and women distance runners, swimmers, cyclists, and cross-country skiers generally attain $\dot{V}O_{2max}$ values nearly double those of sedentary persons.

Researchers have measured the $\dot{V}O_{2max}$ of thousands of individuals of different ages. The average values and respective ranges for men and women of different ages establish category values to classify individuals for cardiovascular fitness. The table presents a five-part classification based on data from the literature for nonathletes.

Cardiovascular Fitness Classifications ($\dot{V}O_{2max}$ Values are in mL • kg^{-1} • min^{-1})

		Fitness Classification				
Gender	Age	Poor	Fair	Average	Good	Excellent
Male	≤29	≤24.9	25–33.9	34–43.9	44–52.9	≥53
	30–39	≤22.9	23–30.9	31–41.9	42–49.9	≥50
	40–49	≤19.9	20–26.9	27–38.9	39–44.9	≥45
	50–59	≤17.9	18–24.9	25–37.9	38–42.9	≥43
	60–69	≤15.9	16–22.9	23–35.9	36–40.9	≥41
Female	≤29	≤23.9	24–30.9	31–38.9	39–48.9	≥49
	30–39	≤19.9	20–27.9	28–36.9	37–44.9	≥45
	40–49	≤16.9	17–24.9	25–34.9	35–41.9	≥42
	50–59	≤14.9	15–21.9	22–33.9	34–39.9	≥40
	60–69	≤12.9	13–20.9	21–32.9	33–36.9	≥37

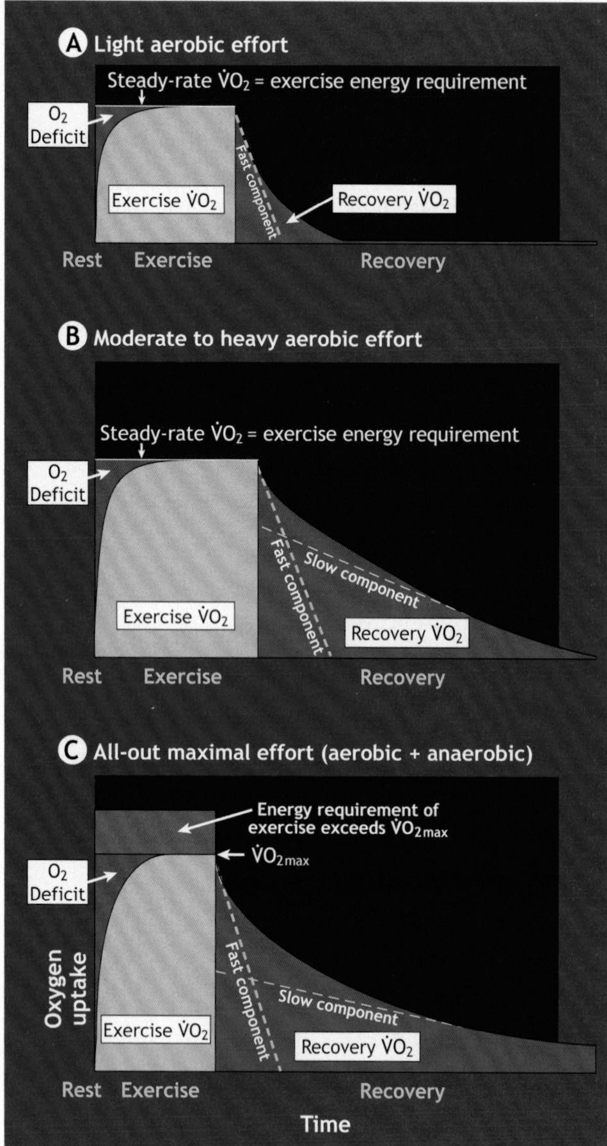

FIGURE 6.9 Oxygen uptake during physical activity and in recovery from **(A)** light steady-rate effort, **(B)** moderate-to-intense steady-rate effort, and **(C)** all-out exhaustive effort that does not produce a steady rate of aerobic metabolism. Note that the exercise oxygen requirement depicted by the purple rectangle above the exercise $\dot{V}O_2$ curve at $\dot{V}O_{2max}$ exceeds the actual exercise oxygen uptake.

take up to 24 hours to return to the pre-exercise $\dot{V}O_2$. Even with shorter, intermittent bouts of "supermaximal" effort (e.g., three 2-minute bouts at 108% $\dot{V}O_{2max}$ interspersed with 3-minute rest intervals), recovery $\dot{V}O_2$ depictd in **Figure 6.9C** can remain elevated for 1 hour or longer.

Trained subjects have a faster rate of recovery $\dot{V}O_2$ when exercising at either the same absolute or relative intensities compared to untrained counterparts. More than likely, training adaptations that facilitate a rapid achievement of steady-rate oxygen uptake also facilitate a rapid recovery process.

Metabolic Dynamics of Recovery Oxygen Uptake

Traditional View: A.V. Hill's 1922 Oxygen Debt Theory

In 1922, Nobel laureate A.V. Hill and colleagues first coined the term *oxygen debt*. These pioneer scientists discussed energy metabolism during physical activity and recovery in financial-accounting terms. The body's carbohydrate stores were likened to energy "credits." Expending stored credits during physical activity incurred an energy "debt." The greater the energy "deficit" or use of available stored energy credits, the larger the energy debt. Hill believed that the recovery $\dot{V}O_2$ represented the cost of repaying this debt—hence the term *oxygen debt*.

Lactate accumulation from the anaerobic component of physical activity represented the use of glycogen, the stored energy credit. The ensuing oxygen debt served two purposes:

1. Reestablish the original glycogen stores or credits by synthesizing approximately 80% of the lactate back to glycogen in the liver via the Cori cycle
2. Catabolize the remaining lactate through the pyruvate–citric acid cycle pathway, with the new ATP presumably powering glycogen resynthesis from lactate

The early explanation of the dynamics of recovery oxygen uptake was subsequently termed the "*lactic acid theory of oxygen debt*."

In 1933 following the work of Hill, researchers at the Harvard Fatigue Laboratory (**http://hper.usu.edu/files/uploads/Courses/Fall%202010/PEP/PEP-2000-Harvard-Fatigue-Lab.pdf**) deduced that the initial phase of recovery $\dot{V}O_2$ terminated before blood lactate could decline. They showed that a physically active individual could incur an oxygen debt of almost 3 L without appreciable blood lactate accumulation. To resolve these findings, they proposed two phases of oxygen debt:

1. **Alactic or alactacid oxygen debt** (meaning without lactate buildup)
2. **Lactic acid or lactacid oxygen debt** (associated with elevated blood lactate levels)

These two explanations persisted because the early chemical methodology did not allow them to measure ATP and PCr replenishment or the relationship between blood lactate and glucose and glycogen levels.

Testing Hill's Oxygen Debt Theory

Acceptance of Hill's explanation for the lactic acid phase of the oxygen debt requires evidence that in recovery, the major portion of lactate produced during physical activity resynthesizes to glycogen. The evidence indicates otherwise. When researchers infused radioactive-labeled lactate into rat muscle, more than 75% of it appeared as radioactive carbon dioxide, with the remaining 25% synthesized to glycogen. In experiments with humans, no substantial replenishment of glycogen occurred 10 minutes following strenuous activity even though blood lactate levels decreased significantly. Contrary to Hill's theory, the heart, liver, kidneys, and skeletal muscle incorporate a major portion of the blood lactate produced during physical activity as an energy substrate during the activity and in recovery.

An Updated Explanation for EPOC

Research during the last two decades provides a contemporary explanation for the appearance of the postexercise elevated $\dot{V}O_2$. Current thinking centers on an elevated aerobic metabolism during recovery to restore the body's processes to pre-exercise conditions, in contrast to repayment of borrowed "energy credits."

In short-duration, light-to-moderate activity, recovery $\dot{V}O_2$ generally replenishes the high-energy phosphates depleted by the activity. Recovery typically proceeds within several minutes. In longer duration intense aerobic activity of 60 minutes or more, recovery $\dot{V}O_2$ remains elevated for longer durations and can take hours to return to baseline values. The increase in recovery $\dot{V}O_2$ does not fully relate to lactate accumulation. Rather, disequilibriums in other physiologic functions elevate the recovery metabolism.

In exhaustive physical effort with its large anaerobic component and lactate accumulation, a small portion of EPOC resynthesizes lactate to glycogen. This gluconeogenic mechanism would probably progress during activity mainly in trained individuals. A significant component of EPOC relates to physiologic processes that occur during recovery. Such factors likely account for the considerably larger EPOC than oxygen deficit in prolonged aerobic activity and exhaustive anaerobic activity. Body temperature, for example, rises about 5.4°F (3°C) during extended, intense aerobic activity and remains elevated for several hours in recovery. Elevated body temperature directly stimulates metabolism to increase recovery $\dot{V}O_2$.

fyi Seven Possible Causes of Excess Postexercise Oxygen Consumption

1. Resynthesis of ATP and PCr
2. Resynthesis of blood lactate to glycogen (Cori cycle)
3. Oxidation of blood lactate in energy metabolism
4. Restoration of oxygen to blood, tissue fluids, and myoglobin
5. Thermogenic effects of elevated core temperature
6. Thermogenic effects of epinephrine and norepinephrine
7. Increased recovery pulmonary and circulatory dynamics and other elevated levels of physiologic function

Implications of EPOC for Physical Activity and Recovery

Understanding EPOC dynamics provides a basis for structuring activity intervals to optimize recovery. No appreciable lactate accumulates either with steady-rate aerobic activity or with 5- to 10-second bouts of all-out effort powered by the intramuscular high-energy phosphates. Recovery progresses rapidly, and activity can begin again with only a short rest period, with passive recovery the most desirable. In contrast, prolonged durations of anaerobic effort lasting longer than 2 minutes produce considerable lactate buildup in active muscles and blood, with disruption in most physiologic-support systems. As such, recovery $\dot{V}O_2$ often requires additional time to return to preactivity baseline levels. Prolonged recovery between activity intervals would impair performance in basketball, hockey, soccer, tennis, and badminton. In a practical sense, an athlete pushed to a high level of anaerobic metabolism may not fully recover during brief time-out periods or intermittent intervals of less intense physical activity.

Procedures for speeding recovery from physical activity generally are classified as active or passive. In **active recovery**, often termed "cooling down" or "tapering off," the individual performs submaximal effort with large muscle groups, believing that continued physical activity prevents muscle cramps and stiffness and facilitates lactate removal and overall recovery. In **passive recovery**, the person usually lies down, presuming that total inactivity reduces the resting energy requirements and thus "frees" oxygen to fuel recovery. Modifications of passive recovery have included massage, cold showers, maintenance of specific body positions, and consuming cold liquids.

Optimal Recovery From Steady-Rate Physical Activity

Most people easily can perform physical activity below 55% to 60% of $\dot{V}O_{2max}$ in steady rate with essentially no blood lactate accumulation. Passive procedures produce the most rapid recovery at this intensity level because physical activity elevates total metabolism and delays recovery.

Optimal Recovery From Non–Steady-Rate Physical Activity

Blood lactate accumulates when physical activity intensity exceeds the maximum steady-rate level and lactate formation in muscle exceeds its removal rate. With increasing intensity, blood lactate levels rise sharply and the exerciser soon becomes exhausted. Although the precise mechanisms for exhaustion during anaerobic activity remain unclear, blood lactate levels provide an objective indication of the *relative* strenuousness of physical activity; it also may reflect the adequacy of recovery. Lactate anions induce a fatiguing effect on skeletal muscle independent of associated reductions in pH, so any procedure that accelerates lactate removal probably augments subsequent physical performance.

Performing aerobic physical activity in recovery accelerates blood lactate removal. The optimal level of recovery activity ranges between 30% and 45% $\dot{V}O_{2max}$ for cycling and 55% to 60% $\dot{V}O_{2max}$ when the recovery involves running. This difference between activity modes reflects a more localized muscle involvement in bicycling, which lowers the threshold for blood lactate accumulation. In a practical application following a moderately strenuous workout, one should not just lie down to rest following the workout. Instead, remain active by walking or engaging in other "light" recovery activity.

Figure 6.10 illustrates the proposed relationship between blood lactate removal rate and percent $\dot{V}O_{2max}$ during recovery. The graph illustrates that optimal recovery intensity probably ranges between 30% and 40% $\dot{V}O_{2max}$. Facilitated lactate removal with active recovery likely results from increased blood perfusion through the "lactate-using" liver, heart, and inspiratory muscles. Increased blood flow through muscle in active recovery also enhances lactate removal because this tissue readily oxidizes lactate via citric acid cycle metabolism.

Intermittent Activity and Recovery: The Interval Training Approach

One approach to performing physical activity that normally produces exhaustion within several minutes if performed continuously requires exercising *intermittently* with preestablished spacing of activity and rest intervals. The physical conditioning strategy of **interval training** characterizes this approach. This training regimen applies different work-to-rest intervals with supermaximal effort to overload the energy transfer systems. For example, with all-out movement of up to 8 seconds' duration, intramuscular high-energy phosphates provide most of the

A CLOSER LOOK

How to Measure Work on a Treadmill, Cycle Ergometer, and Step Bench

The most common ergometers to quantify work include treadmills, cycle and arm-crank ergometers, stair steppers, and rowers.

Work and Power

Work (*W*) represents application of force (*F*) through a distance (*D*):

$$W \times F \times D$$

Power (*P*) represents work (*W*) performed per unit time (*T*):

$$P = F \times D \div T$$

Units of measurement to express work include kg-m, foot-pounds (ft-lb), joules (J), Newton-meters (Nm), and kilocalories (kcal); units of measurement for power are kg-m · min^{-1}, Watts (1 W = 6.12 kg-m · min^{-1}), and kcal · min^{-1}.

For example, for a body mass of 70 kg and vertical jump score of 0.5 m, the work accomplished would equal 35 kilogram-meters (kg-m) (70 kg × 0.5 m). If the person were to accomplish work in the vertical jump of 35 kg-m in 500 milliseconds (0.500 seconds; 0.008 minutes), the power attained would equal 4375 kg-m · min^{-1}.

Calculation of Treadmill Work

The treadmill is a moving conveyor belt with variable angle of incline and speed. Work performed equals the product of the weight (mass) of the person (*F*) and the vertical distance (*D*) achieved walking or running up the incline. Vertical distance equals the sine of the treadmill angle (theta or θ) multiplied by the distance traveled along the incline (treadmill speed × time).

$$W = \text{Body mass}\ (F) \times \text{Vertical distance}\ (D)$$

Example

For an angle θ of 8 degrees (measured with an inclinometer or determined by knowing the percent grade of the treadmill), the sine of angle θ equals 0.1392 (see table). The vertical distance represents treadmill speed multiplied by exercise duration multiplied by sine θ. For example, vertical distance on the incline while walking at 5000 m · h^{-1} for 1 hour equals 696 m (5000 × 0.1392). If a 50-kg person walked at an incline of 8 degrees (percent grade ~14%) for 60 minutes at 5000 m · h^{-1}, work accomplished computes as:

$$\begin{aligned} W &= F \times \text{Vertical distance}\ (\text{sine}\ \theta \times D) \\ &= 50\ \text{kg} \times (0.1392 \times 5000\ \text{m}) \\ &= 34{,}800\ \text{kg-m} \end{aligned}$$

The value for power equals 34,800 kg-m ÷ 60 minutes or 580 kg-m · min^{-1}.

Degree θ	Sine θ	Tangent θ	Percent Grade (%)
1	0.0175	0.0175	1.75
2	0.0349	0.0349	3.49
3	0.0523	0.0523	5.23
4	0.0698	0.0698	6.98
5	0.0872	0.0872	8.72
6	0.1045	0.1051	10.51
7	0.1219	0.1228	12.28
8	0.1392	0.1405	14.05
9	0.1564	0.1584	15.84
10	0.1736	0.1763	17.63
15	0.2588	0.2680	26.80
20	0.3420	0.3640	36.40

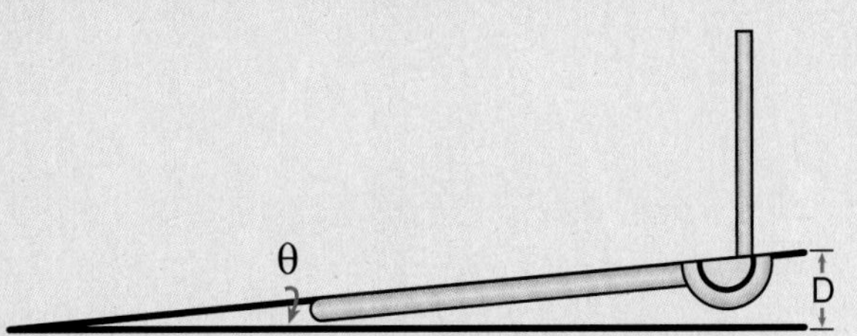

Calculation of Cycle Ergometer Work

The typical mechanically braked cycle ergometer contains a flywheel with a belt around it connected by a small spring at one end and an adjustable tension lever at the other end. A pendulum balance indicates the resistance against the flywheel as it turns. Increasing belt tension increases flywheel friction, which increases pedaling resistance. The force (flywheel friction) represents braking load in kg or kiloponds (kp = force acting on 1-kg mass at the normal acceleration of gravity). The distance traveled equals number of pedal revolutions times flywheel circumference.

Example

A person pedaling a bicycle ergometer with a 6-m flywheel circumference at 60 rpm for 1 minute covers a distance (D) of 360 m each minute (6 m × 60). If the frictional resistance on the flywheel equals 2.5 kg, total work computes as:

$$\begin{aligned} W &= F \times D \\ &= \textbf{Frictional resistance} \times \textbf{Distance traveled} \\ &= \textbf{2.5 kg} \times \textbf{360 m} \\ &= \textbf{900 kg-m} \end{aligned}$$

Power generated by the effort equals 900 kg-m in 1 minute or 900 kg-m · min^{-1} (900 kg-m ÷ 1 minute).

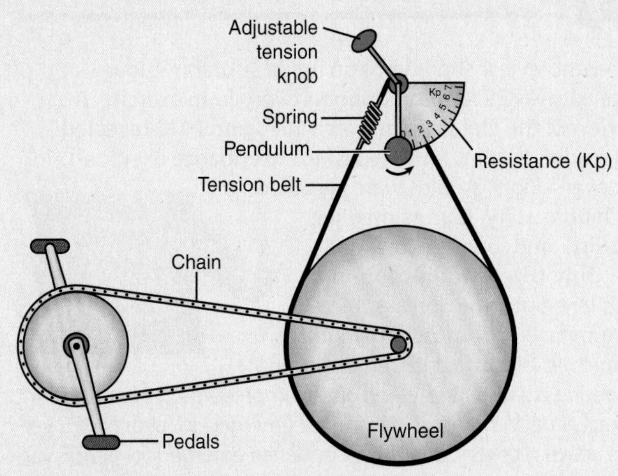

Calculation of Bench Stepping Work

Only the vertical (positive) work can be calculated in bench stepping. Distance (*D*) computes as bench height multiplied by the number of steps by the person; force (*F*) equals the person's body mass (kg).

Example

If a 70-kg person steps on a bench 0.375 m high (14.8 inch) at a rate of 30 steps per minute for 10 minutes, total work computes as:

$$\begin{aligned} W &= F \times D \\ &= \textbf{Body mass, kg} \times (\textbf{Vertical distance, m} \\ &\quad \times \textbf{Steps per min} \times \textbf{10 minute}) \\ &= \textbf{70 kg} \times (\textbf{0.375 m} \times \textbf{30} \times \textbf{10}) \\ &= \textbf{7875 kg-m} \end{aligned}$$

Power generated during stepping equals 787 kg-m · min^{-1} (7875 kg-m ÷ 10 minutes).

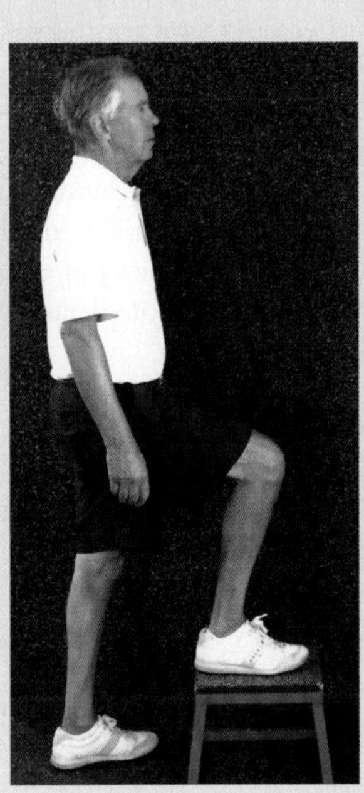

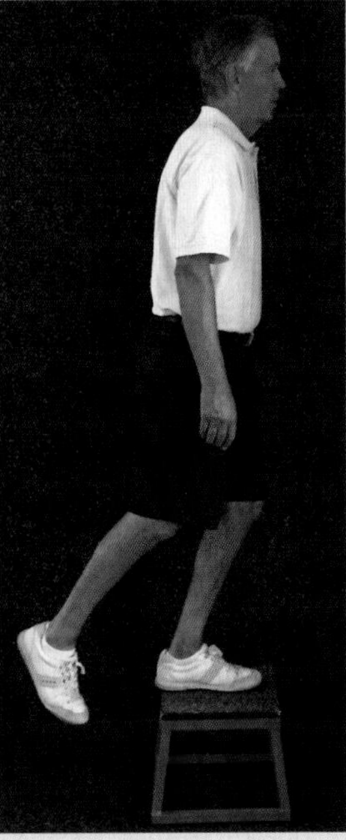

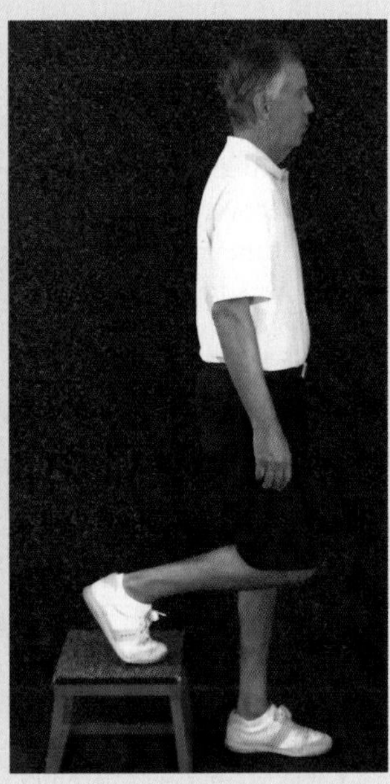

Does Neuromuscular Electrical Stimulation (NMES) During Recovery Work?

A recent review sheds light on use of subtetanic low-intensity NMES for promoting recovery from exercise. A review of the literature between 1970 and 2012 revealed 13 studies that investigated NMES to enhance exercise recovery. Eight studies were classified as high quality, four as medium quality, and one as low quality. Only three studies found a positive outcome for a subjective measure of muscle pain, three for improved blood lactate removal, one for lowering creatine kinase, and one for improvement in subsequent exercise performance. No evidence emerged to favor NMES versus active recovery, and mixed evidence emerged for NMES versus passive recovery for the rate of blood lactate removal. The authors concluded that while some subjective benefits exist for NMES during postexercise recovery, the overwhelming evidence fails to support NMES for enhancing subsequent exercise performance, including maximal exercise.

Sources: Malone JK, et al. Neuromuscular electrical stimulation (NMES) during recovery from exercise: A systematic review. *J Strength Cond Res* 2014;28:2478.

Malone JK, et al. Neuromuscular electrical stimulation; no enhancement of recovery from maximal exercise. *Int J Sports Physiol Perform* 2014;9:791.

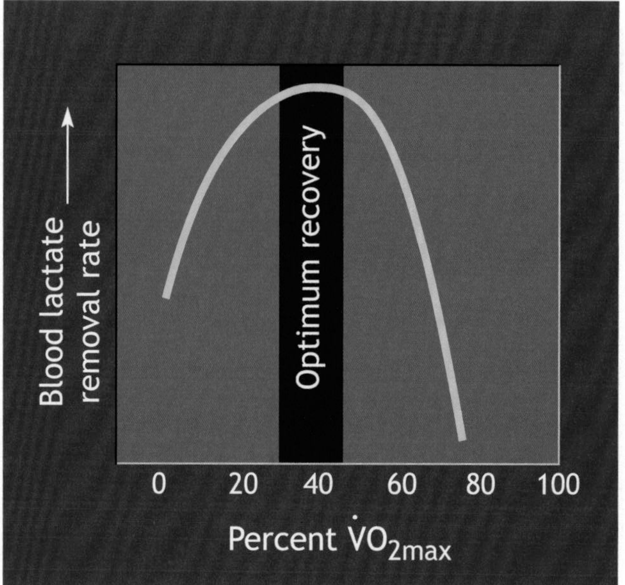

FIGURE 6.10 The yellow inverted curve depicts the generalized relationship between exercise intensity expressed as percent $\dot{V}O_{2max}$ and blood lactate removal rate. (Adapted with permission from McArdle WD, Katch FI, Katch VL. *Exercise Physiology: Nutrition, Energy, and Human Performance*, 8th Ed. Baltimore: Wolters Kluwer Health, 2015, as adapted with permission from Dodd S, et al. Blood lactate disappearance at various intensities of recovery exercise. *J Appl Physiol: Respir Environ Exerc Physiol* 1984;57:1462.)

energy with only minimal reliance on the glycolytic pathway. Rapid recovery occurs from such short duration activity that enables resuming a subsequent bout of intense activity within a few minutes.

Table 6.1 summarizes the results of a classic series of experiments that combined physical activity and rest intervals. On one day, the subject ran at a speed that would normally exhaust him within 5 minutes. The continuous run covered about 0.8 mile, and the runner attained a $\dot{V}O_{2max}$ of 5.6 $L \cdot min^{-1}$. A high blood lactate level owing to substantial anaerobic metabolism verified a relative state of exhaustion (last column in the table). On another day, he ran at the same fast speed but intermittently, with periods of 10 seconds of running and 5 seconds of recovery. During 30 minutes of intermittent running, the time running amounted to 20 minutes and the distance covered equaled 4 miles, compared with less than 5 minutes and 0.8 miles with a continuous run! The effectiveness of the intermittent activity protocol becomes more impressive considering that blood lactate remained low, even though $\dot{V}O_2$ averaged 5.1 $L \cdot min^{-1}$ (91% $\dot{V}O_{2max}$) during the 30-minute period. The stability in blood lactate indicated that a relative balance existed between the energy requirements of physical activity and aerobic energy transfer within the muscles throughout activity and rest intervals.

Manipulating the duration of physical activity and rest intervals can effectively overload a specific energy-transfer system. When the rest interval increased from 5 to 10 seconds, $\dot{V}O_2$ averaged 4.4 $L \cdot min^{-1}$; 15-second work and 30-second recovery intervals produced only a 3.6 L $\dot{V}O_2$. For each 30-minute bout of intermittent running, the runner achieved a longer distance and substantially lower blood lactate level than when running continuously at the same intensity. We discuss interval training in more detail in Chapter 13.

TABLE 6.1 Classic Study Results With Intermittent Physical Activity

Exercise-Rest Periods	Total Distance Run (Yards)	Average Oxygen Uptake ($L \cdot min^{-1}$)	Blood Lactate Level ($mg \cdot dL\ Blood^{-1}$)
4-min continuous	1422	5.6	150
10-s exercise 5-s rest	7294	5.1	44
10-s exercise 10-s rest	5468	4.4	20
15-s exercise 30-s rest	3642	3.6	16

From data of Christenson EH, et al. Intermittent and continuous running. *Acta Physiol Scand* 1960;60:269.

SUMMARY

1. The major energy pathway for ATP production differs depending on intensity and duration of physical effort.
2. Intense, short duration physical activity (100-m dash, weightlifting) derives energy primarily from the intramuscular phosphagens ATP and PCr (immediate energy system).
3. Relatively intense activity of 1 to 2 minutes requires energy mainly from the reactions of anaerobic glycolysis (short-term energy system).
4. The long-term aerobic system predominates as activity progresses beyond several minutes duration.
5. The steady-rate oxygen uptake represents a balance between an activity's energy requirements and aerobic ATP resynthesis.
6. The oxygen deficit represents the difference between the exercise oxygen requirement and the actual oxygen consumed.
7. The maximum oxygen uptake or $\dot{V}O_{2max}$ quantitatively represents the maximum capacity for aerobic ATP resynthesis.
8. Human muscle fibers have unique metabolic and contractile properties. The two major fiber types include low glycolytic, high oxidative, slow-twitch fibers and low oxidative, high glycolytic, fast-twitch fibers.
9. Forming a sound basis for creating optimal training regimens relies on understanding the energy spectrum of physical activity.
10. Bodily processes do not immediately return to resting levels following cessation of physical activity. The difference in recovery from light and strenuous activity relates largely to the specific metabolic and physiologic processes in each activity.
11. Moderate activity performed during recovery (active recovery) from strenuous physical activity facilitates recovery compared with passive procedures (inactive recovery).
12. Active recovery performed below the point of blood lactate accumulation speeds lactate removal.
13. Proper spacing of activity and rest intervals optimizes workouts geared toward training a specific energy transfer system.

THINK IT THROUGH

1. If the maximal oxygen uptake represents such an important measure of a person's capacity to resynthesize ATP aerobically, why does the person with the highest $\dot{V}O_2$ not always achieve the best marathon run performance?
2. How does an understanding of the energy spectrum of exercise help to formulate optimal training for improving specific exercise performance?
3. Why is it atypical for athletes to excel at both short- and long-distance running?
4. How would you answer the question: At what level of physical activity does the body switch to anaerobic energy metabolism?
5. If athletes generally perform marathon running under intense but steady-rate aerobic conditions, explain why some competitors have diminished capacity to sprint to the finish.

KEY TERMS

Active recovery: Low- to moderate-level physical activity during recovery from previous physical activity.

Adenosine triphosphate (ATP): High-energy phosphate stored within cells; considered the energy currency of life that provides the energy for all forms of biologic work.

Alactic or alactacid oxygen debt: Quantitative amount of oxygen consumed during the fast component of the postexercise oxygen uptake curve.

Blood lactate threshold (LT): Lactate inflection point or anaerobic threshold (AT), representing the exercise intensity where lactate begins to accumulate in the blood; sometimes designates exercise intensity point between anaerobic and aerobic metabolism.

"Bonking" or hitting the wall: Terms used in endurance activities that describe a condition related to depletion of liver and muscle glycogen stores manifested by sudden-onset muscular fatigue and depressed energy transfer.

Fast component of recovery oxygen uptake: Mathematical expression of the rapid portion of the decline in the oxygen uptake curve during the postexercise recovery.

Fast-twitch (FT) or type II muscle fibers: Type of muscle fiber identified by myosin ATPase activity staining, subdivided into type IIA and type IIX based on their unique metabolic and biochemical characteristics.

Glycogenolysis: Conversion of glycogen in muscle and liver to glucose-1-phosphate and glycogen by glycogen phosphorylase.

Interval training: Discontinuous or intermittent physical activity involving multiple bouts of high-intensity exercise intervals interspersed with recovery periods.

Lactate dehydrogenase (LDH): Enzyme catalyzing the conversion and reconversion of pyruvate to lactate, and conversion and reconversion of NADH to NAD^+.

Lactate shuttling: Hypothesis describing movement of lactate intracellularly and intercellularly based on observations that anaerobic and aerobic conditions continuously form and utilize lactate.

Lactic acid or lactacid oxygen debt: Quantitative amount of oxygen consumed during the slow component of the postexercise oxygen uptake curve.

Maximal oxygen uptake, maximal aerobic power, aerobic capacity, $\dot{V}O_{2max}$: Highest rate of oxygen uptake measured during incremental exercise; considered a fundamental measure of physiologic functional capacity for physical activity.

Oxygen debt: Term coined by British Nobel laureate A.V. Hill to describe energy metabolism during recovery from physical activity in financial-accounting terms, where the body's carbohydrate stores were likened to energy "credits."

Oxygen deficit: Quantitative difference between total oxygen consumed during an activity and additional oxygen that would have been consumed if a steady-rate aerobic metabolism occurred immediately at physical activity initiation.

Oxygen uptake or oxygen consumption or $\dot{V}O_2$: Quantity of oxygen consumed expressed as a rate per unit time as liters of oxygen per minute ($L \cdot min^{-1}$) or in milliliters of oxygen per kilogram body mass per minute ($mL \cdot kg^{-1} \cdot min^{-1}$).

Passive recovery: Inactivity during recovery following physical activity.

Phosphagens: High-energy storage compounds (chiefly ATP and PCr), also known as high-energy phosphates, chiefly found in muscular tissue in animals; act as reservoirs of phosphate bond energy, donating phosphoryl groups for ATP synthesis when supplies are low.

Phosphocreatine (PCr): Phosphorylated creatine molecule that provides a rapid reserve of high-energy phosphates in skeletal muscle and the brain.

Recovery oxygen uptake or excess postexercise oxygen consumption (EPOC): Oxygen uptake during recovery following cessation of physical activity, above a resting level, to restore the body to a resting state.

Slow component of recovery oxygen uptake: Mathematical expression of the slower portion of the decline in the oxygen uptake curve during the postexercise recovery continuing to the pre-exercise resting oxygen uptake level.

Slow-twitch (ST) or type I muscle fiber: Type of muscle fiber identified by myosin ATPase activity staining, and referred to as type I.

Steady rate of aerobic metabolism: Oxygen uptake in submaximal effort that represents a rate of physical activity or energy exchange where aerobic metabolism predominately fulfills the energy requirement.

SELECTED REFERENCES

Abboud GJ, et al. Effects of load-volume on EPOC after acute bouts of resistance training in resistance-trained men. *J Strength Cond Res* 2013;27:1936.

Aisbett B, Le Rossignol P. Estimating the total energy demand for supra-maximal exercise using the VO_2-power regression from an incremental exercise test. *J Sci Med Sport* 2003;6:343.

Arend M, et al. The effect of inspiratory muscle warm-up on submaximal rowing performance. *J Strength Cond Res* 2014;1:213.

Baltan S. Can lactate serve as an energy substrate for axons in good times and in bad, in sickness and in health? *Metab Brain Dis* 2015;30:25.

Beneke R. Methodological aspects of maximal lactate steady state-implications for performance testing. *Eur J Appl Physiol* 2003;89:95.

Berg K, et al. Oxygen cost of sprint training. *J Sports Med Phys Fitness* 2010;50:25.

Berger NJ, et al. Influence of continuous and interval training on oxygen uptake on-kinetics. *Med Sci Sports Exerc* 2006;38:504.

Borsheim E, Bahr R. Effect of exercise intensity, duration and mode on post-exercise oxygen consumption. *Sports Med* 2003;33:1037.

Bourdin M, et al. Laboratory blood lactate profile is suited to on water training monitoring in highly trained rowers. *J Sports Med Phys Fitness* 2004;44:337.

Breen L, et al. No effect of carbohydrate-protein on cycling performance and indices of recovery. *Med Sci Sports Exerc* 2010;42:1140.

Brooks GA. Bioenergetics of exercising humans. *Compr Physiol* 2012;2:537.

Burt DG, et al. Effects of exercise-induced muscle damage on resting metabolic rate, sub-maximal running and post-exercise oxygen consumption. *Eur J Sport Sci* 2014;14:337.

Callison ER, Berg KE, Slivka DR. Grunting in tennis increases ball velocity but not oxygen cost. *J Strength Cond Res* 2014;28:1915.

Campos EZ, et al. The effects of physical fitness and body composition on oxygen consumption and heart rate recovery after high-intensity exercise. *Int J Sports Med* 2012;33:621.

Carter H, et al. Effect of prior exercise above and below critical power on exercise to exhaustion. *Med Sci Sports Exerc* 2005;37:775.

Chan HH, Burns SF. Oxygen consumption, substrate oxidation, and blood pressure following sprint interval exercise. *Appl Physiol Nutr Metab* 2013;38:182.

Chiappa GR, et al. Blood lactate during recovery from intense exercise: impact of inspiratory loading. *Med Sci Sports Exerc* 2008;40:111.

Christensen PM, et al. Leg oxygen uptake in the initial phase of intense exercise is slowed by a marked reduction in oxygen delivery. *Am J Physiol Regul Integr Comp Physiol* 2013;305:R313.

Cleuziou C, et al. Dynamic responses of O2 uptake at the onset and end of exercise in trained subjects. *Can J Appl Physiol* 2003;28:630.

Crommett AD, Kinzey SJ. Excess postexercise oxygen consumption following acute aerobic and resistance exercise in women who are lean or obese. *J Strength Cond Res* 2004;18:410.

Da Silva RL, Brentano MA, et al. Effects of different strength training methods on postexercise energetic expenditure. *J Strength Cond Res* 2010;24:2255.

Dupont G, et al. Effect of short recovery intensities on the performance during two Wingate tests. *Med Sci Sports Exerc* 2007;39:1170.

Emhoff CA, et al. Direct and indirect lactate oxidation in trained and untrained men. *J Appl Physiol* 2013;115:829.

Emhoff CA, et al. Gluconeogenesis and hepatic glycogenolysis during exercise at the lactate threshold. *J Appl Physiol* 2013;114:297.

Ferguson RA, et al. Effect of muscle temperature on rate of oxygen uptake during exercise in humans at different contraction frequencies. *J Exp Biol* 2002;205:981.

Ferreira LF, et al. Dynamics of skeletal muscle oxygenation during sequential bouts of moderate exercise. *Exp Physiol* 2005;90:393.

Gardner A, et al. A comparison of two methods for the calculation of accumulated oxygen deficit. *J Sports Sci* 2003;21:155.

Gordon D, et al. Influence of blood donation on oxygen uptake kinetics during moderate and heavy intensity cycle exercise. *Int J Sports Med* 2010;31:298.

Greer BK, et al. EPOC comparison between isocaloric bouts of steady-state aerobic, intermittent aerobic, and resistance training. *Res Q Exerc Sport* 2015;12:1.

Grey TM, et al. Effects of age and long-term endurance training on VO_2 kinetics. *Med Sci Sports Exerc* 2015;47:289.

Gunnarsson TP, et al. Effect of intensified training on muscle ion kinetics, fatigue development and repeated short term performance in endurance trained cyclists. *Am J Physiol Regul Integr Comp Physiol* 2013;305:R8.

Hill DW, et al. Effect of plasma donation and blood donation on aerobic and anaerobic responses in exhaustive, severe-intensity exercise. *Appl Physiol Nutr Metab* 2013;38:551.

Hughson RL. Oxygen uptake kinetics: historical perspective and future directions. *Appl Physiol Nutr Metab* 2009;34:840.

Ingham SA, et al. Comparison of the oxygen uptake kinetics of club and Olympic champion rowers. *Med Sci Sports Exerc* 2007;39:865.

Isaacs K, et al. Modeling energy expenditure and oxygen consumption in human exposure models: accounting for fatigue and EPOC. *Expo Sci Environ Epidemiol* 2008;18:289.

Iwayama K, et al. Transient energy deficit induced by exercise increases 24-h fat oxidation in young trained men. *J Appl Physiol* 2015;118:80.

Jeppesen TD, et al. Lactate metabolism during exercise in patients with mitochondrial myopathy. *Neuromuscul Disord* 2013;23:629.

Kaikkonen P, et al. Heart rate variability is related to training load variables in interval running exercises. *Eur J Appl Physiol* 2012;112:829.

Kang J, et al. Evaluation of physiological responses during recovery following three resistance exercise programs. *J Strength Cond Res* 2005;19:305.

Koppo K, Bouckaert J. Prior arm exercise speeds the VO_2 kinetics during arm exercise above the heart level. *Med Sci Sports Exerc* 2005;37:613.

LeCheminant JD, et al. Effects of long-term aerobic exercise on EPOC. *Int J Sports Med* 2008;29:53.

Lira VA, et al. Autophagy is required for exercise training-induced skeletal muscle adaptation and improvement of physical performance. *FASEB J* 2013; 27:4184.

Lyons S, et al. Excess post-exercise oxygen consumption in untrained men following exercise of equal energy expenditure: comparisons of upper and lower body exercise. *Diabetes Obes Metab* 2007;9:889.

Mann TN, et al. Effect of exercise intensity on post-exercise oxygen consumption and heart rate recovery. *Eur J Appl Physiol* 2014;114:1809.

Markovitz GH, et al. On issues of confidence in determining the time constant for oxygen uptake kinetics. *Br J Sports Med* 2004;38:553.
Matsuo T, et al. Cardiorespiratory fitness level correlates inversely with excess post-exercise oxygen consumption after aerobic-type interval training. *BMC Res Notes* 2012;5:646.
McLaughlin JE, et al. A test of the classic model for predicting endurance running performance. *Med Sci Sports Exerc* 2010;42:991.
Mendonca GV, et al. Effects of walking with blood flow restriction on excess post-exercise oxygen consumption. *Int J Sports Med* 2015. (In Press as of 05.18.15.)
Menzies P, et al. Blood lactate clearance during active recovery after an intense running bout depends on the intensity of the active recovery. *J Sport Sci* 2010;28:975.
Messonnier LA, et al. Lactate kinetics at the lactate threshold in trained and untrained men. *J Appl Physiol* 2013;114:1593.
Messonnier LA, et al. Lactate kinetics at the lactate threshold in trained and untrained men. *J Appl Physiol* 2013;114:1593.
Nanas S, et al. Heart rate recovery and oxygen kinetics after exercise in obstructive sleep apnea syndrome. *Clin Cardiol* 2010;33:46.
Naimo MA, et al. High-intensity interval training has positive effects on performance in ice hockey players. *Int J Sports Med* 2015;36:61.
Peinado AB. Responses to increasing exercise upon reaching the anaerobic threshold, and their control by the central nervous system. *BMC Sports Sci Med Rehabil* 2014;6:17.
Pringle JS, et al. Effect of pedal rate on primary and slow-component oxygen uptake responses during heavy-cycle exercise. *J Appl Physiol* 2003;94:1501.
Robergs R, et al. Influence of pre-exercise acidosis and alkalosis on the kinetics of acid-base recovery following intense exercise. *Int J Sport Nutr Exerc Metab* 2005;15:59.
Sahlin K, et al. Prior heavy exercise eliminates VO_2 slow component and reduces efficiency during submaximal exercise in humans. *J Physiol* 2005;564:765.
Schaal K, et al. Effect of recovery mode on postexercise vagal reactivation in elite synchronized swimmers. *Appl Physiol Nutr Metab* 2013;38:126.
Scott CB, Kemp RB. Direct and indirect calorimetry of lactate oxidation: implications for whole-body energy expenditure. *J Sports Sci* 2005;23:15.
Sloth M, et al. Effects of sprint interval training on and aerobic exercise performance: a systematic review and meta-analysis. *Scand J Med Sci Sports* 2013;23:e341.
Soultanakis HN, et al. Impact of cool and warm water immersion on 50-m sprint performance and lactate recovery in swimmers. *J Sports Med Phys Fitness* 2015;55:267.
Stupnicki R, et al. Fitting a single-phase model to the post-exercise changes in heart rate and oxygen uptake. *Physiol Res* 2010;59:357.
Tahara Y, et al. Fat-free mass and excess post-exercise oxygen consumption in the 40 minutes after short-duration exhaustive exercise in young male Japanese athletes. *J Physiol Anthropol* 2008;27:139.
Takken T, et al. Cardiopulmonary exercise testing in congenital heart disease: equipment and test protocols. *Neth Heart J* 2009;17:339.
Van Hall G. Lactate kinetics in human tissues at rest and during exercise. *Acta Physiol* 2010;199:499.
Van Hall G, et al. Leg and arm lactate and substrate kinetics during exercise. *Am J Physiol Endocrinol Metab* 2003;284:E193.
Whipp BJ. The slow component of O2 uptake kinetics during heavy exercise. *Med Sci Sports Exerc* 1994;26:1319.
Wilkerson DP, et al. Effect of prior multiple-sprint exercise on pulmonary O2 uptake kinetics following the onset of perimaximal exercise. *J Appl Physiol* 2004;97:1227.
Williams AM, et al. High-intensity interval training speeds the adjustment of pulmonary O_2 uptake, but not muscle deoxygenation, during moderate-intensity exercise transitions initiated from low and elevated baseline metabolic rates. *J Appl Physiol* 2013;114:1550.
Wiltshire EV, et al. Massage impairs post exercise muscle blood flow and "lactic acid" removal. *Med Sci Sports Exerc* 2010;42:1062.
Winlove MA, et al. Influence of training status and exercise modality on pulmonary O2 uptake kinetics in pre-pubertal girls. *Eur J Appl Physiol* 2010; 108:1169.
Zarzeczny R, et al. Anaerobic capacity of amateur mountain bikers during the first half of the competition season. *Biol Sport* 2013;30:189.
Zhang Z, et al. Comparisons of muscle oxygenation changes between arm and leg muscles during incremental rowing exercise with near-infrared spectroscopy. *J Biomed Opt* 2010;15:017007.

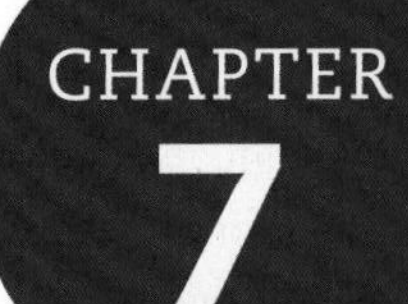

Measuring and Evaluating Energy-Generating Capacities During Physical Activity

CHAPTER OBJECTIVES

- Compare and contrast concepts of measurement, evaluation, and prediction.
- Explain specificity and generality applied to performance and physiologic function.
- Describe two procedures to administer two practical "field tests" to evaluate the power output capacity of ATP-PCr catabolism (immediate energy system).
- Describe a commonly used test to evaluate the power output capacity of glycolysis (short-term energy system).
- Compare the differences between direct and indirect calorimetry.
- Compare the differences between open- and closed-circuit spirometry.
- Describe two different open-circuit spirometry measurement systems.
- Define the term respiratory quotient (RQ), including its use and importance.
- Explain three factors that influence the respiratory exchange ratio (RER).
- Define maximal oxygen uptake ($\dot{V}O_{2max}$), including its physiological significance.
- Define graded exercise test.
- List three criteria that indicate when a person reaches "true" $\dot{V}O_{2max}$ and $\dot{V}O_{2peak}$ during a graded exercise test.
- Outline three commonly used treadmill protocols to assess $\dot{V}O_{2max}$.
- Explain how physical activity mode, heredity, training state, gender, body composition, and age affect $\dot{V}O_{2max}$.
- Describe two procedures to predict $\dot{V}O_{2max}$ from a submaximal walking "field test."
- Outline a typical protocol to administer a step test to predict $\dot{V}O_{2max}$.
- List three assumptions using submaximal physical activity heart rate to predict $\dot{V}O_{2max}$.

ANCILLARIES AT A GLANCE

Visit **http://thePoint.lww.com/MKKESS5e** to access the following resources.

- References: Chapter 7
- Interactive Question Bank
- Appendix C: Metabolic Computations in Open-Circuit Spirometry

All individuals possess the *capability* for anaerobic and aerobic energy metabolism, although the *capacity* for each energy transfer form varies considerably among individuals. These differences illustrate the **individual differences** concept in metabolic capacity for physical activity. A person's capacity for energy transfer, and for many other physiologic functions, does not exist as a general factor for all activities. Rather, it depends largely on activity mode and training status. A high maximal oxygen uptake ($\dot{V}O_{2max}$) assessed during running, for example, does not necessarily ensure a similar $\dot{V}O_{2max}$ assessed in swimming or rowing. The differences in $\dot{V}O_{2max}$ within an individual for different activities that activate different muscle groups emphasize the **specificity of metabolic capacity**. In contrast, some individuals with high $\dot{V}O_{2max}$ in one physical activity mode can also possess an above-average aerobic power in other diverse activities—illustrating the **generality of metabolic capacity**. *For the most part, more specificity exists than generality in metabolic and physiologic functions.* In this chapter, we discuss the rationale for measurement of energy expenditure at rest and during physical activity. We also discuss different performance and physiologic tests to evaluate the capacity of the three energy transfer systems discussed in Chapter 6.

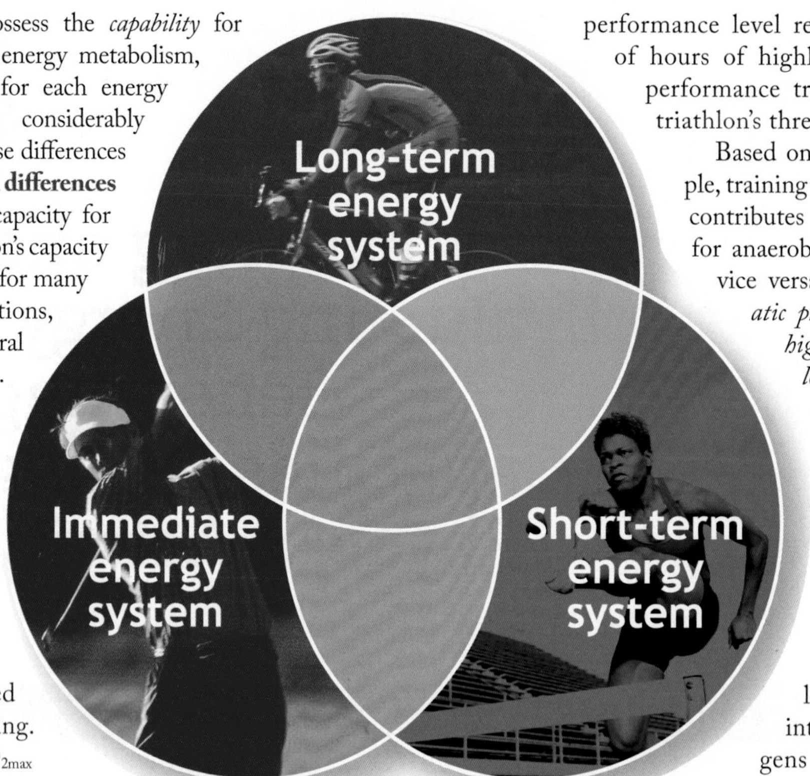

FIGURE 7.1 Specificity-generality of the three systems of energy transfer. When considering only two systems, their overlap represents generality and the remainder specificity. (Reprinted with permission from McArdle WD, Katch FI, Katch VL. *Exercise Physiology: Nutrition, Energy, and Human Performance*. 8th Ed. Baltimore: Wolters Kluwer Health, 2015.)

OVERVIEW OF ENERGY TRANSFER CAPACITY DURING PHYSICAL ACTIVITY

Figure 7.1 illustrates the specificity-generality concept of energy capacities. The nonoverlapped or single color areas (red, blue, green) represent *specificity* of physiologic and performance functions, while the overlapped areas with a blend of four adjacent colors represent *generality* of functions. For each energy system, specificity exceeds generality; rarely do individuals excel in markedly different activities, as for example sprint running and distance running. Both activities involve running, but their physiologic and energy system requirements differ markedly. Many world-class triathletes seem to possess "generalized" capacities for the diverse aerobic activities, yet their high performance level results from thousands of hours of highly specific sports and performance training in *each* of the triathlon's three demanding events.

Based on the specificity principle, training for high aerobic power contributes little to one's capacity for anaerobic energy transfer and vice versa. *The effects of systematic physical training remain highly specific for neurologic, physiologic, and metabolic responses.*

Figure 7.2 illustrates the anaerobic and aerobic energy transfer system's involvement for different all-out effort durations. At initiation of either high- or low-speed movements, intramuscular phosphagens provide immediate nonaerobic energy for muscle action. Following the first few seconds of movement, rapid-glycolytic energy provides an increasingly greater proportion of the total energy requirements. Continuation of activity, although at a lower intensity, places a progressively greater demand on aerobic metabolic pathways for ATP resynthesis.

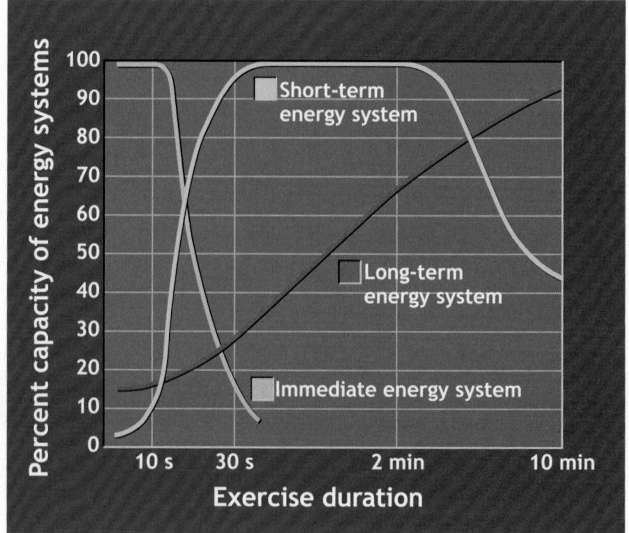

FIGURE 7.2 Three systems of energy transfer and percentage use of their total capacity during all-out physical activity of different durations. (Adapted with permission from McArdle WD, Katch FI, Katch VL. *Exercise Physiology: Nutrition, Energy, and Human Performance*. 8th Ed. Baltimore: Wolters Kluwer Health, 2015.)

PART 1

Measuring and Evaluating the Immediate and Short-Term Energy Systems

PHYSIOLOGIC AND PERFORMANCE TESTS

Two general approaches assess anaerobic power and capacity for both immediate and short-term physical activity responses:

1. **Physiologic tests** measure changes in ATP and PCr levels *metabolized* or lactate *produced* from anaerobic metabolism.
2. **Performance tests** quantify *external work performed* or *power generated* during brief- and short-duration, intense activity that demands a high level of anaerobic energy transfer.

Both approaches assumes that short-duration, intense activity could not occur without a high level of anaerobic energy transfer; measuring such work or power indirectly can gauge or predict anaerobic energy utilization.

Physiologic Tests to Assess the Immediate Energy System

American football, weightlifting, and other short-duration, maximal-effort activities that require rapid energy release rely nearly exclusively on energy from intramuscular high-energy phosphates. Performance tests that maximally activate the ATP-PCr energy system serve as practical field tests to evaluate the capacity for "immediate" energy transfer. Two assumptions underlie the use of performance test scores to infer the power-generating capacity of the high-energy phosphates:

1. ATP-PCr hydrolysis regenerates all ATP at maximal power output.
2. Adequate ATP and PCr exist to support maximal effort for about a 6-second duration.

Physiologic and biochemical measures to evaluate energy-generating capacity of the immediate energy system include the following:

1. Size of intramuscular ATP-PCr pool
2. ATP and PCr depletion rates in all-out, brief-duration activity

ATP and PCr depletion rates provide the most direct estimate and correlate highly with physical performance assessments of the immediate energy system. For example, one experiment using the muscle biopsy technique determined muscle PCr depletion at different intervals of a 100-m sprint. Compared with resting values (22 mmol · kg wet weight^{-1}), PCr decreased by 60% during the first 40 m (<6 s) and only another 20% for the remainder of the sprint. It remains nearly impossible with current technology to readily obtain precise biochemical data during brief duration all-out effort. Researchers must rely on the "face validity" of the various specific performance measures as satisfactory markers to evaluate capacity for ATP-PCr energy transfer in physical activity.

IMMEDIATE ENERGY SYSTEM PERFORMANCE TESTS

Anaerobic power and capacity performance tests serve as practical "field tests" to evaluate the **immediate energy system**. These maximal effort power tests rely on maximal activation of intramuscular ATP-PCr energy reserves. They often evaluate the **time-rate of doing work** (i.e., work accomplished per unit of time). The following formula computes power output (*P*):

$$P = (F \times D) \div T$$

where F equals force generated, D equals distance through which the force moves, and T equals effort duration. **Watts** represent a common expression of power; 1 watt equals 0.73756 ft-lb · s^{-1} or 6.12 kg-m · min^{-1}.

Maximal effort short-term performance tests for 1 to 10 seconds reflect energy transfer of the immediate ATP-PCr energy system. Maximal tests of 10 to 60 seconds reflect utilization of the slower glycolytic energy system.

Jumping Power Test

Common physical fitness test batteries have included jump-and-reach and standing broad jump tests (see *A Closer Look: Predicting Power of the Immediate Energy System Using a Vertical Jump Test*) to evaluate the ATP-PCr system. The jump-and-reach test score equals the difference between a person's maximum standing reach and maximum jump-and-touch height. For the broad jump, the score represents the horizontal distance covered in a maximal-effort leap from a semicrouched position. Both tests purport to measure leg power, but they probably do not achieve the goal of evaluating a person's true ATP and PCr power output capacity owing to their brief application of muscular effort.

Other Immediate Energy Performance-Power Tests

Examples of other tests to evaluate individual differences in immediate power from the intramuscular high-energy phosphates include brief sprint running or cycling, shuttle runs, and localized arm cranking, or simulated stair climbing, rowing, or skiing. In the Québec 10-second test of leg cycling power using a stationary cycle ergometer, subjects perform two all-out, 10-second rides at a frictional resistance equal to 0.09 kg per kg of body mass with 10 minutes of rest between repeat bouts. Cycling begins by pedaling as fast as possible after applying the friction load and continues all-out for 10 seconds. Performance represents the average of the two tests reported in peak joules (or kcal) per kg of body mass and total joules (or kcal) per kg body mass.

The 40-yard sprint test is routinely administered to test for anaerobic performance of professional American football players. Unfortunately, this relates poorly to "football speed" *per se*, yet continues to be used. Several researchers have suggested replacing this test with a more sport-specific repeat, short-duration sprint test from the "down" position that includes multiple directional changes. Large interindividual and intraindividual differences exist in brief-duration performance and its physiologic correlates, so it becomes problematic to develop reliable and valid tests for specific sport performances.

First, low interrelationships exist among different power output capacity test scores. Low interrelationships suggest a high degree of task specificity. This means the best sprint runner may not necessarily be the best sprint swimmer, sprint cyclist, stair sprinter, repetitive volleyball leaper, or sprint-arm cranker. The same metabolic reactions generate energy to power each performance, yet energy transfer occurs predominantly within specific muscles activated by the activity. Furthermore, each specific test requires different neurologic skill components. The predominance of neuromuscular task specificity predicts that the outcome from any one test will likely differ from results on another test.

Specific sports training can change an athlete's performance on anaerobic power tests. *Such tests also serve as excellent self-testing and motivational tools and provide the actual movement-specific activity for training the immediate energy system.*

A CLOSER LOOK

Predicting Power of the Immediate Energy System Using a Vertical Jump Test

Peak anaerobic power output for brief duration underlies success in many sport activities. The vertical jump test has become a widely used measure of "explosive" peak anaerobic power.

Vertical Jump Test

The vertical jump measures the highest distance jumped from a semicrouched position. The specific protocol follows.

1. Establish standing reach height. The individual stands with the shoulder adjacent to a wall with the feet flat on the floor before reaching up as high as possible to touch the wall with the longest finger. Measure the distance (in cm) from the wall mark to the floor.
2. Bend the knees to roughly a 90-degree angle, and place both arms back in a winged position.
3. Thrust forward and upward, touching as high as possible on the wall; no foot or leg movement is permitted before jumping.
4. Perform three trials of the jump test, and use the highest score to represent the individual's "best" vertical jump height.
5. Compute the vertical jump height as the difference between the standing reach height and the vertical jump height in centimeters.

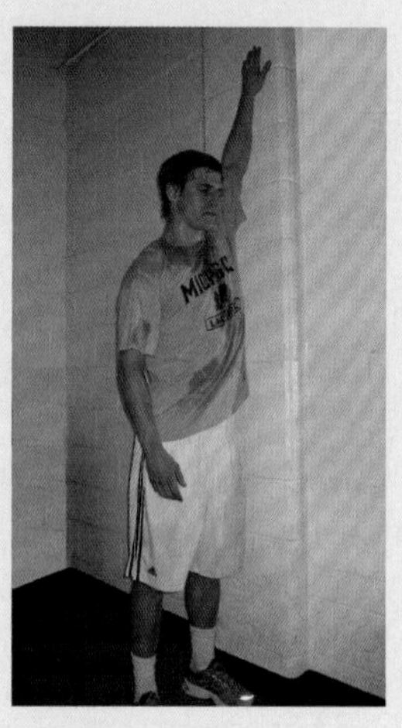

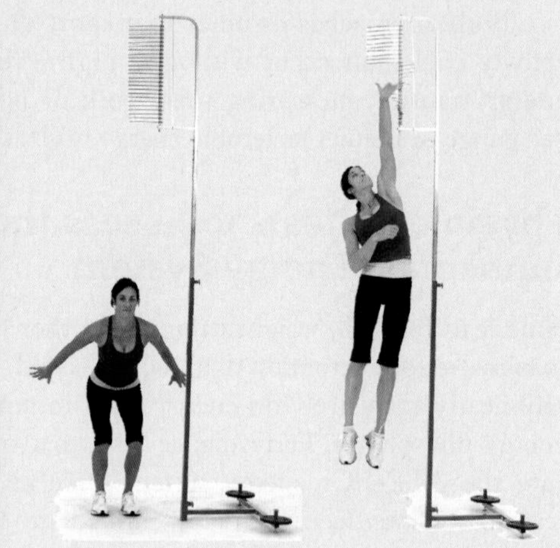

Interchangeable Expressions for Energy and Work

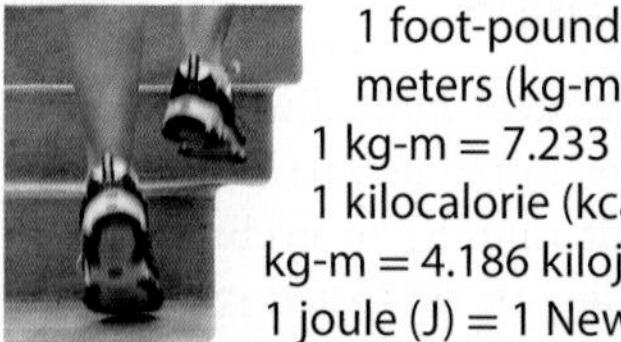

1 foot-pound (ft-lb) = 0.13825 kilogram-meters (kg-m)
1 kg-m = 7.233 ft-lb = 9.8066 joules
1 kilocalorie (kcal) = 3.0874 ft-lb = 426.85 kg-m = 4.186 kilojoules (kJ)
1 joule (J) = 1 Newton-meter (Nm)
1 kilojoule (kJ) = 1000 J = 0.23889 kcal

THE SHORT-TERM, SLOWER GLYCOLYTIC ENERGY SYSTEM

The anaerobic reactions of the **short-term energy system (rapid glycolysis)** do not imply that aerobic metabolism remains unimportant at this stage of physical effort or that oxygen-consuming reactions have failed to "switch on." To the contrary, the aerobic energy contribution begins early in activity. The energy requirement in brief, intense effort significantly exceeds energy generated by hydrogen's oxidation

Anaerobic Power Output Equation

The following equation predicts peak anaerobic power output from the immediate energy system in watts (PAP_W) from vertical jump height in centimeters (VJ_{cm}) and body weight in kilograms (BW_{kg}). The equation applies to males and females:

$$PAP_W = (60.7 \times VJ_{cm}) + (45.3 \times BW_{kg}) - 2055$$

Example

A 21-year-old man weighing 78 kg records a vertical jump height of 43 cm (standing reach height = 185 cm; vertical jump height = 228 cm); predict peak anaerobic power output in watts.

$$\begin{aligned} PAP_W &= (60.7 \times VJ_{cm}) + (45.3 \times BW_{kg}) - 2055 \\ &= (60.7 \times 43\ cm) + (45.3 \times 78\ kg) - 2055 \\ &= 4088.5\ W \end{aligned}$$

Applicability to Males and Females

For comparison purposes, average peak power output measured with this protocol averages 4620.2 W (SD = ±822.5 W) for males and 2993.7 W (SD = ±542.9 W) for females.

References

Clark MA, Lucett SC, eds. *NASM Essentials of Personal Fitness Training*. Baltimore: Lippincott Williams & Wilkins, 2010:103.

Sayers S, et al. Cross-validation of three jump power equations. *Med Sci Sports Exerc* 1999;31:572.

Pinto MD, et al. Differential effects of 30-s vs. 60-s static muscle stretching on vertical jump performance. Effects of volume stretching on jump performance. *J Strength Cond Res* 2014;28:3440.

fyi High-Intensity Interval Training Reduces Fat in Overweight Young Males

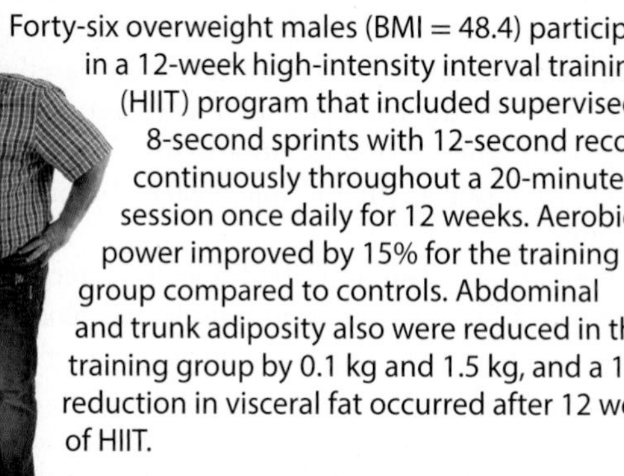

Forty-six overweight males (BMI = 48.4) participated in a 12-week high-intensity interval training (HIIT) program that included supervised 8-second sprints with 12-second recovery continuously throughout a 20-minute session once daily for 12 weeks. Aerobic power improved by 15% for the training group compared to controls. Abdominal and trunk adiposity also were reduced in the training group by 0.1 kg and 1.5 kg, and a 17% reduction in visceral fat occurred after 12 weeks of HIIT.

Sources: Heydari M, et al. The effect of high-intensity intermittent exercise on body composition of overweight young males. *J Obes* 2012;2012:480467.

Giannaki CD, et al. Eight weeks of a combination of high intensity interval training and conventional training reduce visceral adiposity and improve physical fitness: a group-based intervention. *J Sports Med Phys Fitness* 2015. (In Press as of 06.04.15.)

in the respiratory chain. This means anaerobic reactions of glycolysis predominate, presumably with large quantities of lactate accumulating within the active muscle and ultimately appearing in the blood.

No specific criteria exist to indicate when a person reaches a maximal anaerobic effort. In fact, one's level of self-motivation, including external factors in the test environment, likely influence test scores. *Researchers often use the blood lactate level to reveal the short-term energy system's degree of activation.*

Activation of the Short-Term Glycolytic Energy System

Blood Lactate Levels

Considerable blood lactate accumulates from glycolytic energy pathway activation during maximal short-duration activity. Thus, blood lactate levels often reflect this energy system's capacity.

Figure 7.3 presents data from 10 college men who performed 10 all-out bicycle ergometer rides of different durations on different days on the Katch test (see "Performance Tests of Short-Term Glycolytic Power" later in this chapter). Subjects included men involved

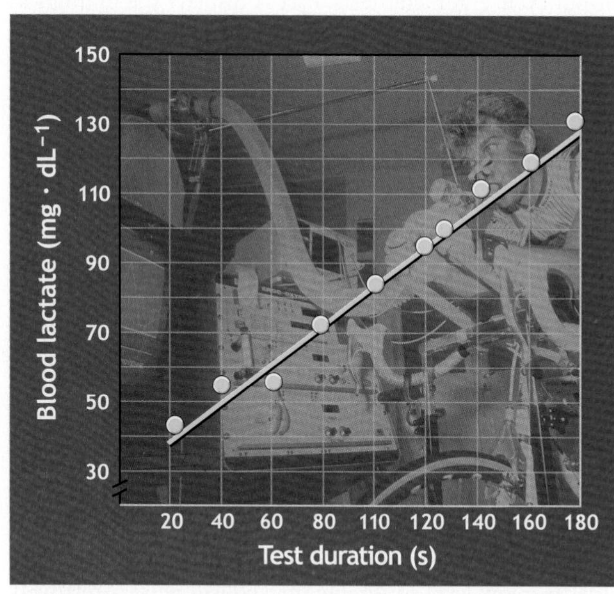

FIGURE 7.3 Pedaling a stationary bicycle ergometer at each subject's highest possible power output increases blood lactate in direct proportion up to 3 minutes. Each value represents the average of 10 subjects. (Data from the Applied Physiology Laboratory, University of Michigan.)

in physical conditioning programs and varsity athletics. Unaware of test duration, the men were urged to turn as many revolutions as possible. The researchers measured venous blood lactate before and immediately following each test and throughout recovery. The plotted points represent the average peak blood lactate values at the end of cycling for each test. Blood lactate levels increased proportionally with test duration and total work output of all-out cycling. The highest blood lactates occurred at the end of 3 minutes, averaging about 130 mg in each 100 mL of blood (~16 mmol).

Physiologists also have traditionally interpreted the appearance of "excess" lactate in muscle and blood following physical activity to indicate contributions of anaerobic metabolism to the activity's energy requirement. Muscle or venous blood lactate was routinely used to verify steady-rate physical activity or magnitude of glycolytic activity consequent to non–steady-rate effort. This view now appears overly simplistic in light of research showing lactate's role as a metabolic intermediate rather than a metabolic "dead end" whose only fate involves pyruvate reconversion (see Chapter 6). Lactate in different tissues serves as an important substrate in energy-storing *and* energy-generating pathways. Lactate measured during or following physical activity does not necessarily reflect absolute anaerobic energy transfer levels via glycolysis. With increasing intensity, including near-maximal and **supermaximal effort levels**, greater lactate production reflects increasing ATP resynthesis from anaerobic pathways. Anaerobic glycolysis and PCr degradation provide about 70% of the total energy yield for 30 seconds of all-out physical effort, with aerobic pathways generating the remaining energy.

Figure 7.4 shows estimates of the relative contribution of each metabolic pathway during three different duration all-out cycle ergometer tests. Part A displays the findings as a percentage of total work output, and part B reports estimated kilojoules (kJ) and kcal of energy (1 kJ = 4.2 kcal). Note the progressive change in the percentage contribution of each of the energy systems to the total work output with increasing duration of effort.

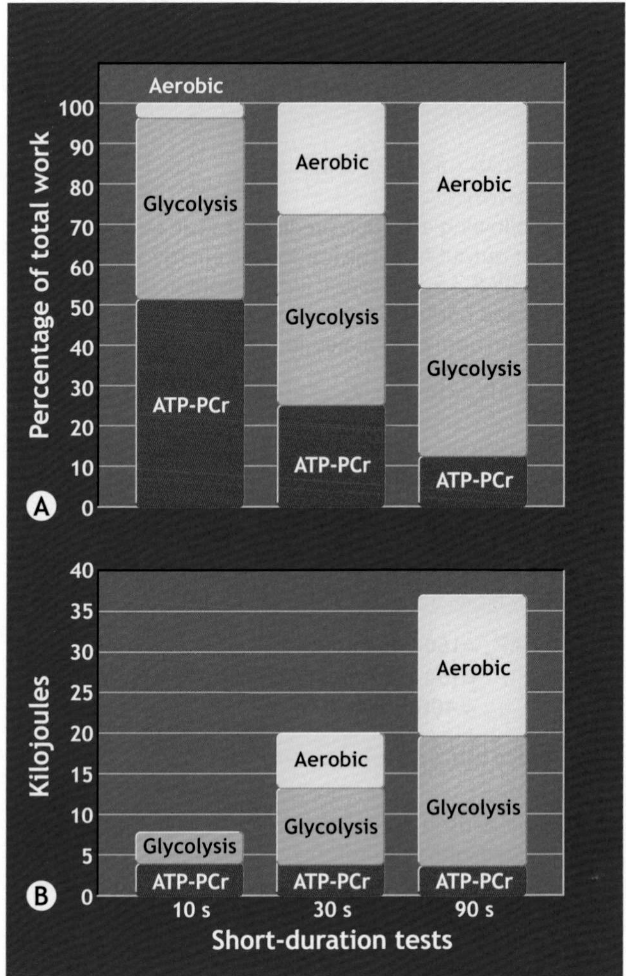

FIGURE 7.4 Relative contribution of each energy system to total work accomplished in three short-duration exercise tests. **A.** Percentage of total work output. **B.** Total kilojoules of energy. Test results based on Katch test protocol (see section "Performance Test Evaluation of the Short-Term Energy System"). (Adapted with permission from McArdle WD, Katch FI, Katch VL. *Exercise Physiology: Nutrition, Energy, and Human Performance*. 8th Ed. Baltimore: Wolters Kluwer Health, 2015; data from Applied Physiology Laboratory, University of Michigan.)

Glycogen Depletion

Energy derived from the short-term energy system depends on the glycogen quantity stored within specific muscles activated by physical activity. The pattern of glycogen depletion in these muscles indicates the glycolytic contribution.

Figure 7.5 shows that glycogen depletion rate in the quadriceps femoris muscle during bicycle activity closely parallels physical activity intensity. With steady-rate physical activity at about 30% of $\dot{V}O_{2max}$, a substantial muscle glycogen reserve remains even after cycling for 180 minutes because a low level of aerobic metabolism powers relatively light physical activity. This means large quantities of fatty acids provide energy with only moderate stored glycogen use. The most rapid and pronounced glycogen depletion occurs at the two most intense workloads. This makes sense from a metabolic standpoint because glycogen provides the only stored nutrient for anaerobic ATP resynthesis. Thus, glycogen assumes high priority in "metabolic mill" chemical reactions during such strenuous effort.

Performance Tests of Short-Term Glycolytic Power

Cycle Ergometer Tests

Short-term energy system activation occurs in maximal work for up to 3 minutes duration. Testing this energy transfer capacity usually involves all-out runs or cycling, including resistance training using repetitive lifting of a certain percentage of

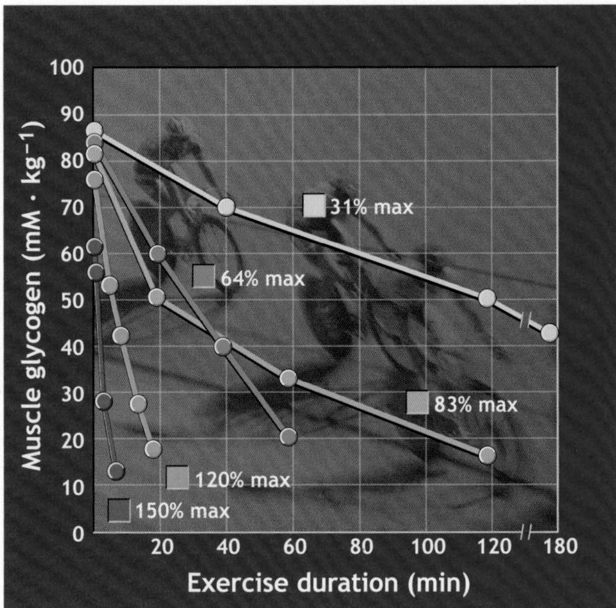

FIGURE 7.5 Glycogen depletion from the vastus lateralis of the quadriceps femoris muscles during bicycle exercise of different intensities and durations. Exercise at 31% of $\dot{V}O_{2max}$ (the lightest workload) caused some depletion of muscle glycogen, but the most rapid depletion occurred during exercise between 83% and 150% of $\dot{V}O_{2max}$. (Adapted with permission from McArdle WD, Katch FI, Katch VL. *Exercise Physiology: Nutrition, Energy, and Human Performance*. 8th Ed. Baltimore: Wolters Kluwer Health, 2015; as adapted with permission from Gollnick PD. Selective glycogen depletion pattern in human muscle fibers after exercise of varying intensity and at varying pedaling rates. *J Physiol* 1974;241:45.)

maximum, and shuttle and agility runs. Five factors impact physical performance on such tests:

1. Age
2. Gender
3. Skill
4. Motivation
5. Body size

These confounding factors inhibit researchers from selecting a suitable single criterion test to develop normative standards for glycolytic energy capacity. A test that maximally engages only leg muscles cannot adequately assess short-term anaerobic capacity for upper-body activity such as rowing, arm cranking, or swimming. *Considered within the framework of specificity, the performance test must closely replicate the activity or sport for which energy capacity is evaluated. In most cases, the actual activity serves as the "best" test.*

In 1973, the **Katch test** of all-out stationary cycling of short duration estimated the power of the anaerobic energy systems. Subsequent extension of this work created a stationary bicycle test with frictional resistance against the flywheel preset at a high load (6 kg for men; 5 kg for women). Subjects turned as many revolutions as possible in 40 seconds, with pedal rate continuously recorded with a microswitch assembly. Peak cycling power reported in watts during any portion of the test represented the subject's anaerobic power, whereas total work accomplished indicated anaerobic capacity expressed in joules. A later modification of this test, the popular **Wingate test** of anaerobic power, involves 30 seconds of supermaximal effort on either an arm-crank or leg-cycle ergometer. Body mass determines resistance to pedaling (originally set to 0.075 kg per kg body mass but may exceed 0.12 kg in well-trained athletes) with resistance applied within 3 seconds after overcoming the initial inertia and unloaded frictional resistance. **Peak power** represents the highest mechanical power generated during any 3- to 5-second period of the test; **relative power** represents peak power divided by body mass. **Anaerobic fatigue** represents the percentage decline in power output during the test, while **anaerobic capacity** denotes total work accomplished over the 30 seconds. **Rate of fatigue** corresponds to the decline in power relative to the peak value. The Katch and Wingate tests assume peak power output reflects the energy-generating capacity of the high-energy phosphates, while average power reflects glycolytic capacity.

With these tests, what is the contrast between the terms *power* and *capacity?* The original intention was to create measures of anaerobic performance, similar to aerobic performance as a measure of power. Unfortunately, some authors incorrectly use *capacity* to infer total work (joules) but use power scores (joules $\cdot$ s^{-1} = watts) to represent this entity. To represent anaerobic power in this context, the term *capacity* must be a power score (much like $\dot{V}O_{2max}$) and not a work score; thus, the term watts denotes the correct expression. The joule is used to compute total anaerobic work.

A Closer Look: Predicting Anaerobic Power and Capacity using the Wingate Cycle Ergometer Test in this chapter outlines procedures on the Wingate cycle ergometer test to determine anaerobic power and capacity. **Table 7.1** presents normative standards for average and peak power outputs in young, physically active men and women during the Wingate cycling test. Performance scores, blood lactate concentrations, and peak heart rates show high test–retest reproducibility and moderate validity compared with other anaerobic capacity criteria. Elite volleyball and ice hockey players have achieved the highest Wingate power scores.

Other Anaerobic Performance Tests

Anaerobic power run tests include all-out runs from 200 to 800 m and sport-specific run tests. For example, soccer player evaluation typically relies on repeat, 20-m all-out shuttle run-tests of varying distances and durations. Sport-specific, ultra-short tests exist for tennis, basketball, ice skating, and swimming. These tests attempt to specifically mimic and evaluate actual performance and to assess training success.

TABLE 7.1 Wingate Percentile Norms for Average Power and Peak Power for Physically Active Young Adult Men and Women

% Rank	Male		Female		Male		Female	
	Average Power Watts	Average Power Watts · kg BM[-1a]	Average Power Watts	Average Power Watts · kg BM[-1a]	Peak Power Watts	Peak Power Watts · kg BM[-1a]	Peak Power Watts	Peak Power Watts · kg BM[-1a]
90	662	8.24	470	7.31	822	10.89	560	9.02
80	618	8.01	419	6.95	777	10.39	527	8.83
70	600	7.91	410	6.77	757	10.20	505	8.53
60	577	7.59	391	6.59	721	9.80	480	8.14
50	565	7.44	381	6.39	689	9.22	449	7.65
40	548	7.14	367	6.15	671	8.92	432	6.96
30	530	7.00	353	6.03	656	8.53	399	6.86
20	496	6.59	336	5.71	618	8.24	376	6.57
10	471	5.98	306	5.25	570	7.06	353	5.98

[a]W • kg BM^{-1}, watts per kilogram of body mass.

Adapted with permission from Maud PJ, Schultz BB. Norms for the Wingate anaerobic test with comparisons in another similar test. *Res Q Exerc Sport* 1989;60:144.

Children's Reduced Anaerobic Power

Children perform poorer on tests of short-term anaerobic power compared with adolescents and young adults. Children's lower muscle glycogen concentrations and rates of glycogen utilization may partly account for this difference. Children have less lower leg muscle strength related to body mass compared with adults, further diminishing their anaerobic exercise performance.

Gender Differences in Anaerobic Performance

Differences in body composition, physique, muscular strength, or neuromuscular factors do not fully explain the considerable difference in anaerobic power capacity between women and men. Supermaximal cycling exercise, for example, elicited a higher peak oxygen deficit in men than in women per unit of fat-free leg volume. This difference persisted even after considering gender differences in active muscle mass. Similar observations occur for gender differences in anaerobic capacity in children and adolescents.

A CLOSER LOOK

Predicting Anaerobic Power and Capacity Using the Wingate Cycle Ergometer Test

The Wingate cycle ergometer test represents the most popular test to assess anaerobic capacity. Developed at the Wingate Institute in Israel in the 1970s, its scores reliably determine peak anaerobic power and anaerobic fatigue.

The Test

A mechanically braked bicycle ergometer serves as the testing device. After warming up for 3 to 5 minutes, the subject begins pedaling as fast as possible without resistance. Within 3-seconds, a fixed resistance is applied to the flywheel; the subject continues to pedal "all out" for 30 seconds. An electrical, mechanical, or computer interface counter continuously records flywheel revolutions in 5-second intervals. Total work during the 30 seconds computes in joules, and power computes as joules • s^{-1}, or watts.

Resistance

Flywheel resistance equals 0.075 kg per kg body mass. For a 70-kg person, the flywheel resistance would equal 5.25 kg (70 kg × 0.075). Resistance often increases to 0.10 kg per kg body mass or higher (up to 0.12 kg) when testing power- and sprint-type athletes. The Wingate test was originally designed using the Swedish Monarch cycle ergometer (**http://monarkexercise.se/?lang=en**). The unit of resistance was the former standard Swedish unit of force called the *kilopond (kp)*. Its measurement represented a cleverly engineered system composed of a basket containing a weight representing the braking force applied to the flywheel, equal to the weight of the basket and its contents. The criterion standard corresponded to the weight of a 1 kg mass; hence, 1 kp has come to represent 1 kg. The proper unit of force when using the Monarch bike should be kp-m • min^{-1}, not kg-m • min^{-1}. When Sweden joined the European Union, it switched to the Newton (N), the SI unit of force, Note that 1 kp corresponds to the force exerted by Earth's gravity (9.80665 m • s^{-2}) on 1 kilogram of mass; thus, 1 kg force equals 9.80665 Newtons (N).

Test Scores

1. **Peak power (PP) output**—The highest power output, observed during the first 5-second exercise interval, indicates the energy-generating capacity of the immediate energy system, which

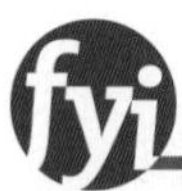

Benefits of Enhanced Alkaline Reserve

Altering pre-exercise acid-base balance in the direction of alkalosis can temporarily but significantly enhance short-term, intense performance (see Chapter 4). Run times improve by consuming a buffering solution of sodium bicarbonate before an anaerobic effort. This effect is accompanied by higher blood lactate and extracellular H^+ concentrations, which indicate increased anaerobic energy contribution.

These findings suggest the possibility of gender-related biologic differences in anaerobic capacity. If this possibility proves correct, then physical testing that focuses on anaerobic performance would further highlight performance differences between men and women to a greater degree than typically expected. For physical testing in the occupational setting, all-out anaerobic testing may exacerbate existing gender differences in performance scores. This would further adversely impact female performance scores.

Factors Affecting Anaerobic Performance

Three factors impact individual differences in anaerobic performance.

1. **Specific training:** Training for brief all-out exercise can positively enhance the glycolytic system's capacity to generate energy. Short-term supermaximal training produces higher blood and muscle lactate levels and greater muscle glycogen depletion compared with untrained counterparts; better performances usually correlate with higher blood lactate levels.

represents the intramuscular high-energy phosphates ATP and PCr. PP, expressed in watts ($1\ W = 6.12\ kp\text{-}m \cdot min^{-1}$), computes as Force in Newtons (kp resistance × acceleration due to gravity) × Distance (number of revolutions × distance per revolution) ÷ Time in minutes (5 s = 0.0833 min).

2. **Relative peak power (RPP) output**—Peak power output (W) relative to body mass: PP ÷ Body mass (kg).
3. **Anaerobic fatigue (AF)**—Percentage decline in power output during the test; AF is thought to represent the total capacity to produce ATP via the immediate and short-term energy systems. AF computes as (Highest 5-s PP – Lowest 5-s PP) ÷ Highest 5-s PP × 100.
4. **Anaerobic work (AW)**—Total work accomplished in watts for the 30-second test duration.

Example

A male weighing 73.3 kg performs the Wingate test on a Monark cycle ergometer (6.0 m traveled per pedal revolution) with an applied resistance or force of 5.5 kp (73.3 kg body mass × 0.075 = 5.497, rounded to 5.5 kg); pedal revolutions for each 5 seconds interval equal 12, 10, 8, 7, 6, and 5 (48 total revolutions in 30 s).

Calculations

1. **Peak power output**

$$\begin{aligned} PP &= Force \times Distance \div Time \\ &= (5.5\ kp \times 9.8\ m \cdot s^{-2}) \times (12\ rev \times 6\ m/rev) \div 5 \\ &= 776.8\ kg \cdot m^{-2} \cdot s^{-3} \\ &= 776.8\ N \cdot m \cdot s^{-2} \\ &= 776.8\ W \end{aligned}$$

2. **Relative peak power output**

$$\begin{aligned} RPP &= PP \div Body\ mass, kg \\ &= 776.8\ W \div 73.3\ kg \\ &= 10.6\ W \cdot kg^{-1} \end{aligned}$$

3. **Anaerobic fatigue**

$$AF = (Highest\ PP - Lowest\ PP) \div Highest\ PP \times 100$$
$$[Highest\ PP = Force \times Distance \div Time = 55\ kp \times 9.8\ m \cdot s^{-2} \times (12\ rev \times 6\ m) \div 0.0833\ min = 4753.9\ kp\text{-}m \cdot min^{-1}, or\ 776.8\ W]$$

4. **Anaerobic work**

$$\begin{aligned} AW &= Force \times Total\ Distance\ (in\ 30\ s) \\ &= (5.5\ kg \times 9.8\ m \cdot s^{-2}) \times [(12\ rev + 10\ rev + 8\ rev + 7\ rev + 6\ rev + 5\ rev) \times 6\ m] \\ &= 15{,}523\ joules, or\ 15.5\ kJ \end{aligned}$$

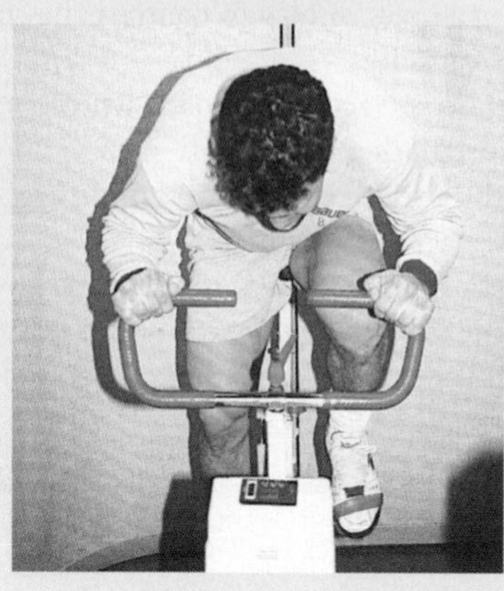

2. **Buffering of acid metabolites:** Anaerobic training might enhance short-term energy transfer by increasing the body's buffering capacity or alkaline reserve to enhance greater lactate production; unfortunately, no data confirm that trained individuals have a superior buffering capacity.
3. **Motivation:** Individuals with greater "pain tolerance," "toughness," or ability to "push" beyond the discomforts of fatiguing physical activity accomplish more anaerobic work and generate greater blood lactate levels and glycogen depletion. Such "toughness" usually increases with intense training.

SUMMARY

1. The contribution of anaerobic and aerobic energy transfer depends largely on physical activity intensity and duration.
2. For sprint and strength-power activities, primary energy transfer involves immediate and short-term anaerobic energy systems.
3. The long-term aerobic energy system becomes progressively more important in activities lasting longer than 2 minutes.
4. Appropriate physiologic measurements and performance tests provide estimates of each energy system's capacity at a particular time or reveal changes consequent to specific training programs.
5. The 30-second, all-out Wingate test evaluates peak power and average power capacity from the glycolytic pathway.
6. Training status, motivation, and acid-base regulation contribute to differences among individuals in the capacities of the immediate and short-term energy system.

THINK IT THROUGH

1. How can one reconcile observations that certain individuals perform exceptionally well in multiple physical activity modes and thus appear to be "natural" athletes?
2. Give two examples of how to contrast the concepts of power and capacity.
3. How would you react to the coach who says, "You can't train for speed; it's a genetic gift"?
4. Explain why a triathlete should train in each of the sport's three aerobic events.
5. Considering training specificity, describe how to test immediate energy system power output capacity of volleyball players, swimmers, and soccer players.

PART 2 Measurement and Evaluation of the Aerobic Energy System at Rest and During Submaximal and Maximal Physical Activity

All metabolic processes within the body ultimately result in heat production. The heat production rate from cells, tissues, or even the whole body operationally defines the energy metabolism rate. The **calorie** represents the basic unit of heat measurement, and *calorimetry* refers to measurement of heat transfer. **Direct calorimetry** and **indirect calorimetry**, two different measurement approaches illustrated in **Figure 7.6**, accurately quantify human energy transfer.

DIRECT CALORIMETRY

Direct calorimetry assesses human energy metabolism by measuring heat production similar to the method that deter-

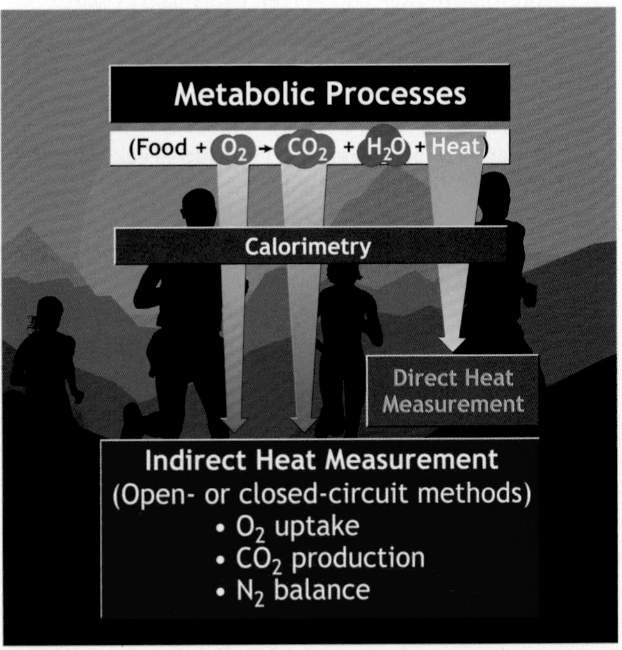

FIGURE 7.6 Measurement of the body's rate of heat production directly assesses metabolic rate. Heat production (metabolic rate) can also be estimated indirectly by measuring the exchange of carbon dioxide and oxygen during the breakdown of food macronutrients and nitrogen excretion. (Adapted with permission from McArdle WD, Katch FI, Katch VL. *Exercise Physiology: Nutrition, Energy, and Human Performance*. 8th Ed. Baltimore: Wolters Kluwer Health, 2015.)

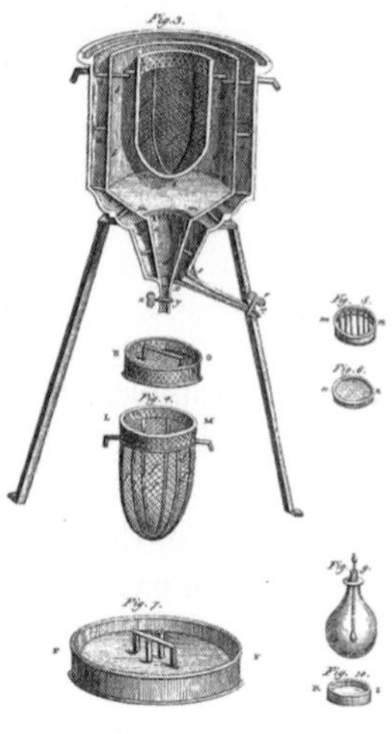

mines a food's energy value in the bomb calorimeter (see Chapter 3). The early experiments of French chemist Antoine Lavoisier (1743–1794) and his contemporaries (**http://scienceworld.wolfram.com/biography/Lavoisier.html**; **www.encyclopedia.com/topic/Antoine-Laurent_Lavoisier.aspx**) in the 1770–1780s provided the impetus to directly measure energy expenditure during rest and physical activity in animals and humans. In his classic experiment, Lavoisier collaborated with French mathematician Pierre Simon de Laplace (1749–1827; **www-history.mcs.st-and.ac.uk/Biographies/Laplace.html**) on problems in respiration chemistry. Their experiments with guinea pigs in 1780 were first to quantify oxygen consumed and carbon dioxide produced by metabolism using the first ice calorimeter they built as shown above.

Over a 10-hour period, approximately 3 g of carbonic acid were collected from an animal breathing pure oxygen. In a second experiment, they placed a guinea pig into a wire cage, which in turn was placed into a double-walled container. Ice packed into the double walls of the outer container maintained a constant temperature; ice between the cage and the inner container's walls melted from of the animal's body heat. During 24 hours, 13 oz (370 g) of ice melted. Lavoisier and Laplace concluded that total heat produced by the animal equaled the amount of heat required to melt the ice. Lavoisier and his colleagues paved the way for future studies of energy balance by initially recognizing that the elements carbon, hydrogen, nitrogen, and oxygen involved in metabolism appeared neither suddenly nor disappeared mysteriously. Rather, these elements reconfigured in a predictable sequence during combustion. Lavoisier supplied basic truths: only oxygen participates in animal respiration, and the "caloric" liberated during respiration is itself the result of the combustion.

The **human calorimeter** illustrated in **Figure 7.7** consists of an airtight chamber where a person lives and works for extended durations. A known volume of water at a specified temperature circulates through a series of coils at the top of the chamber. Circulating water absorbs the heat produced and radiated by the individual. Insulation protects the entire chamber, so any change in water temperature relates directly to the individual's energy metabolism. Chemicals continually remove moisture and absorb carbon dioxide from the person's exhaled air. Oxygen added to the air recirculates through the chamber.

Professors Wilber Olin Atwater (1844–1907, a chemist; **www.sportsci.org/news/history/atwater/atwater.html**) and Edward Bennet Rosa (1861–1921, a physicist; **www.nasonline.org/publications/biographical-memoirs/memoir-pdfs/rosa-e-b.pdf**) in the 1890s built and perfected the first human calorimeter of major scientific significance. Their elegant calorimetric experiments relating energy input to energy expenditure successfully verified the ***law of the conservation of energy*** and validated the relationship between direct and indirect calorimetry.

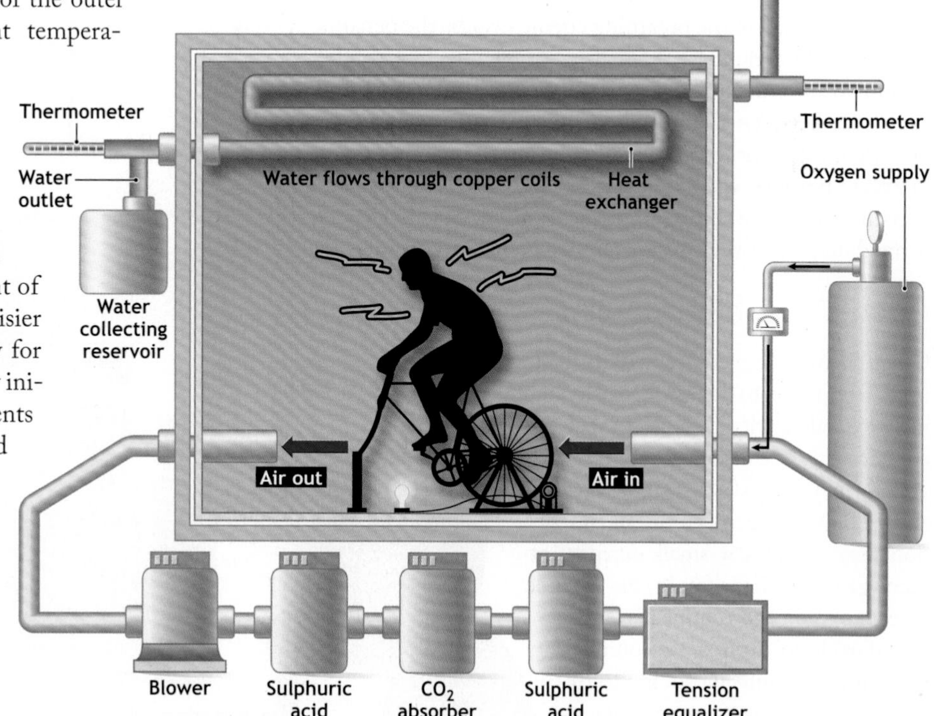

FIGURE 7.7 A human calorimeter directly measures the body's rate of energy metabolism (heat production). In the Atwater-Rosa calorimeter, a thin sheet of copper lines the interior wall to which heat exchangers attach overhead and through which cold water passes. Water cooled to 35.6°F (2°C) moves at a high flow rate, absorbing the heat radiated from the subject during exercise. As the subject rests, warmer water flows at a slower rate. In the original bicycle ergometer shown in the schematic, the rear wheel contacts the shaft of a generator that powers a light bulb. In later versions of ergometers, copper composed part of the rear wheel. The wheel rotated through the field of an electromagnet to produce an electric current for determining power output. (Reprinted with permission from McArdle WD, Katch FI, Katch VL. *Exercise Physiology: Nutrition, Energy, and Human Performance*. 8th Ed. Baltimore: Wolters Kluwer Health, 2015.)

The **Atwater-Rosa Calorimeter** consisted of a small chamber where the subject lived, ate, slept, and exercised on a first-generation bicycle ergometer devised by their colleague and chemist Francis Gano Benedict (1870–1957; **www.sportsci.org/news/history/benedict/benedict.html**). Experiments lasted from several hours to 13 days; during some experiments, subjects cycled continuously for up to 16 hours, expending more than 10,000 kcal. The calorimeter's operation required 16 people working in teams of eight for 12-hour shifts.

INDIRECT CALORIMETRY

All energy-releasing reactions in the body ultimately depend on the use of oxygen. By measuring a person's oxygen uptake, researchers obtain an *indirect* yet accurate estimate of energy expenditure. **Closed-circuit spirometry** and **open-circuit spirometry** represent the two indirect calorimetric methods.

Closed-Circuit Spirometry

Figure 7.8 illustrates closed-circuit spirometry developed in the late 1800s for use in hospitals and research laboratories to estimate resting energy expenditure. The subject breathes 100% oxygen from a prefilled spirometer. The spirometer in this application represents a "closed system" because the person rebreathes only the gas in the chamber without outside air entering the system. A soda lime canister of potassium hydroxide placed in the breathing circuit absorbs the person's exhaled carbon dioxide. A rotating drum attached to the calibrated spirometer turns at a known speed and records the difference between the initial and final oxygen volumes to provide a value for oxygen uptake during the measurement interval. Because of its bulkiness and size, this system remains unsuitable during any type of physical activity performed outside of the spirometer's immediate footprint.

Open-Circuit Spirometry

Open-circuit spirometry represents the most widely used technique to measure oxygen uptake during physical activity. A subject inhales ambient air with a constant composition of 20.93% oxygen, 0.03% carbon dioxide, and 79.04% nitrogen. The nitrogen fraction also includes a small quantity of inert gases. Differences in the volume percent oxygen and volume percent carbon dioxide in expired air compared with inspired ambient air indirectly reflect the ongoing energy metabolism process. The analysis of two factors—volume of inspired and expired air breathed during a specified time period and composition of expired air—allows computation of oxygen uptake.

Three common open-circuit, indirect calorimetric procedures—bag technique, portable spirometry, and computerized instrumentation—assess oxygen uptake during physical activity.

Bag Technique

Figure 7.9 depicts the bag technique. In this example, a subject rides a stationary bicycle ergometer wearing headgear containing a two-way, high-velocity, low-resistance breathing valve. Ambient air passes through one side of the valve and exits out the other side. The expired air then passes into either large canvas or plastic bags or rubber meteorological balloons or directly through a meter that measures gas flow to quantify air volume. An aliquot of expired air is analyzed for its oxygen and carbon dioxide composition, with subsequent calculation of $\dot{V}O_2$ and calorie expenditure.

thePoint® **Appendix C: Metabolic Computations in Open-Circuit Spirometry, available online at http://thePoint.lww.com/MKKESS5e, provides the step-by-step procedure for calculating oxygen uptake, carbon dioxide production, and the respiratory quotient using open-circuit spirometry.**

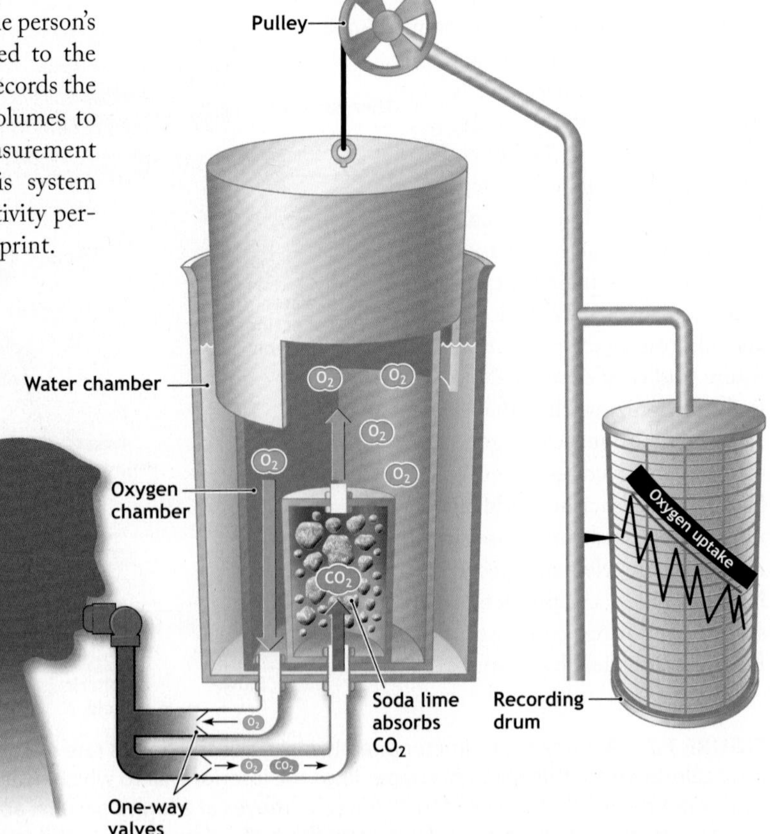

FIGURE 7.8 The closed-circuit method uses a spirometer prefilled with 100% oxygen. As the subject rebreathes from the spirometer, soda lime removes the expired air's carbon dioxide. The difference between the initial and final volumes of oxygen in the calibrated spirometer indicates oxygen uptake during the measurement interval. (Reprinted with permission from McArdle WD, Katch FI, Katch VL. *Exercise Physiology: Nutrition, Energy, and Human Performance*. 8th Ed. Baltimore: Wolters Kluwer Health, 2015.)

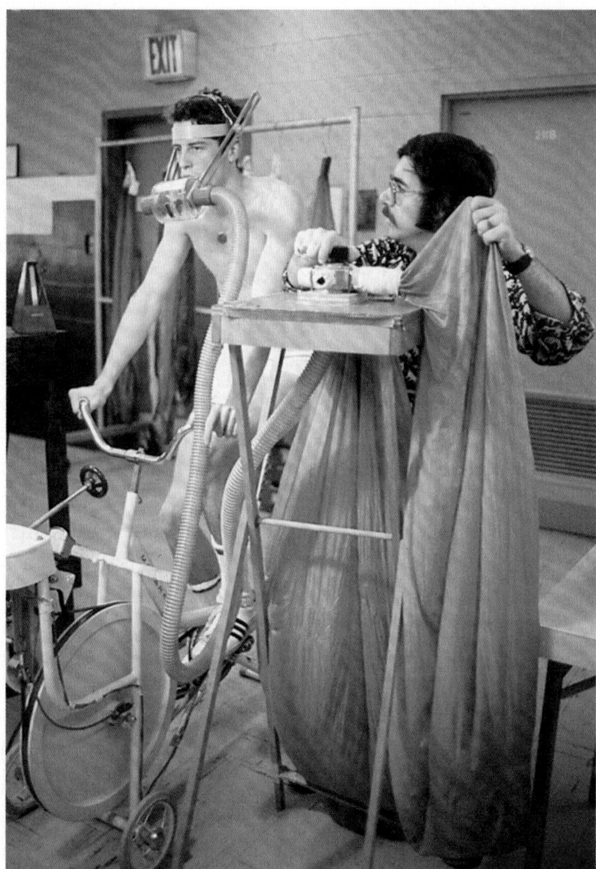

FIGURE 7.9 Oxygen uptake measurement by open-circuit spirometry (bag technique) during stationary cycle ergometer exercise. (Reprinted with permission from McArdle WD, Katch FI, Katch VL. *Exercise Physiology: Nutrition, Energy, and Human Performance*. 8th Ed. Baltimore: Wolters Kluwer Health, 2015.)

Portable Spirometry

German scientists in the early 1940s perfected a lightweight, portable system to indirectly determine the energy expended during physical activity. The original apparatus was devised by German physiologist Nathan Zuntz (1847–1920) and featured in several of his 430 published studies of animals and humans relating to respiratory gas exchange at different altitudes.

As shown at the top of the next column, the device made it possible for the first time to measure O_2 consumed and CO_2 produced during ambulation. Later iterations of the device included assessment of the energy expenditure during war-related combat-type activities while traveling over different terrain with full battle gear, operating transportation vehicles including tanks and aircraft, and simulating tasks that soldiers would encounter during combat. The 3 kg box-shaped device, worn like a backpack, allowed the soldier freedom of movement while collecting the expired air in a small, orange-colored aliquot rubber bag (similar to a balloon that fills with air into a sphere) for later analysis of oxygen and carbon dioxide concentrations, while a sensitive meter within the device monitored gas flow or ventilation volume for each minute of the activity. This device (worn by the golfer in the illustration below) was the same as that worn to measure $\dot{V}O_2$ and estimate energy expenditure during military field operations, including hundreds of common household and recreational activities.

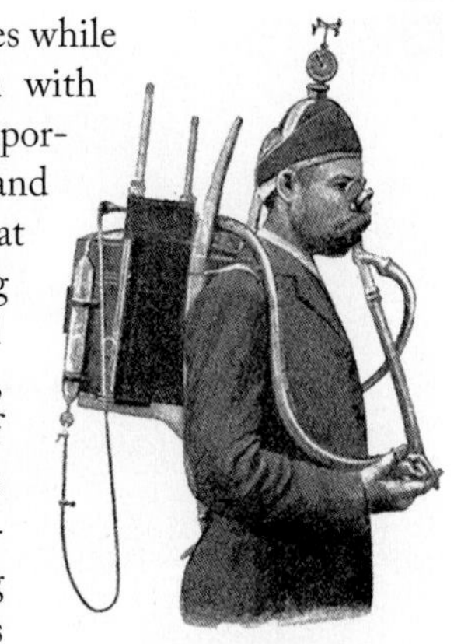

Courtesy Max Planck Institute for the History of Science, Berlin/ Virtual Lab; **http://mpiwg-berlin.mpg/technology/data?id=tec1715**

Following those early studies with portable spirometry, many different portable systems have been designed, tested, and used in numerous commercial applications. For the most part, these portable systems use the latest advances in computer technology to produce acceptable results when compared with more fixed, dedicated desktop systems or the traditional bag system. **Figure 7.10** shows applications of a commercially available portable metabolic collection system. Newer systems on the horizon include a smart "systems" watch paired with a smartphone that incorporates microelectromechanical system (MEMS) actuators and optical sensors (visual and infrared) to record physiological data. Older systems, for example, rely on electrical conductivity to monitor heart rate, while the new pulse measuring devices rely on next-generation optical sensors. Such sensors interface with the watch electronics to allow for detailed record keeping, with arrays of microphones for auditory feedback (and multiple cameras to detect changes in skin color) to assess physiological parameters during training, competition, and general fitness activities. In these applications, an onboard computer performs the metabolic calculations based on electronic signals it receives from micro-designed sensors that measure oxygen and carbon dioxide concentrations in expired air, including ventilatory flow dynamics and volumes. Data are stored on microchips for later analyses. Such advanced systems also include automated blood pressure, heart rate, water vapor, and temperature monitors and preset instructions to regulate speed, duration, and workload of a treadmill, bicycle ergometer, stepper, rower, swim flume, resistance device, or other exercise apparatus.

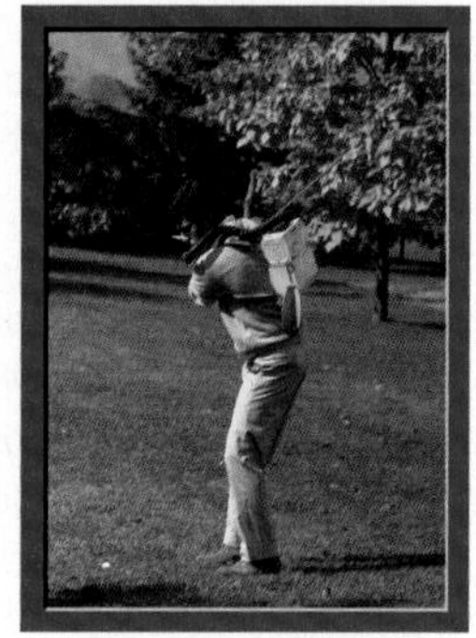

Kilocalorie Equivalent for 1 Liter Oxygen

Assuming the combustion of a mixed diet, a rounded value of 5.0 kcal per L of oxygen consumed designates the appropriate conversion factor for estimating energy expenditure from oxygen uptake under steady-rate conditions of aerobic metabolism.

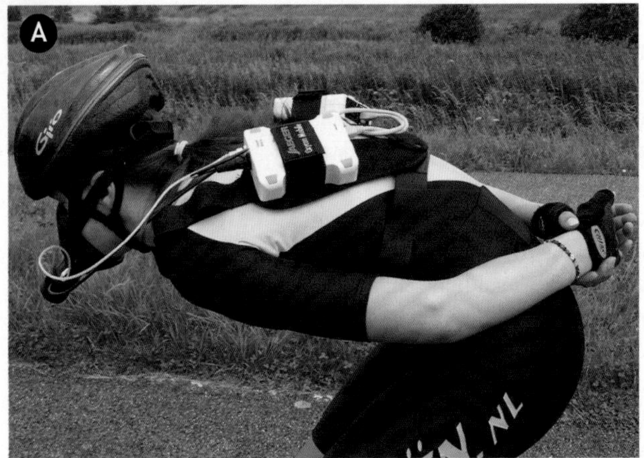

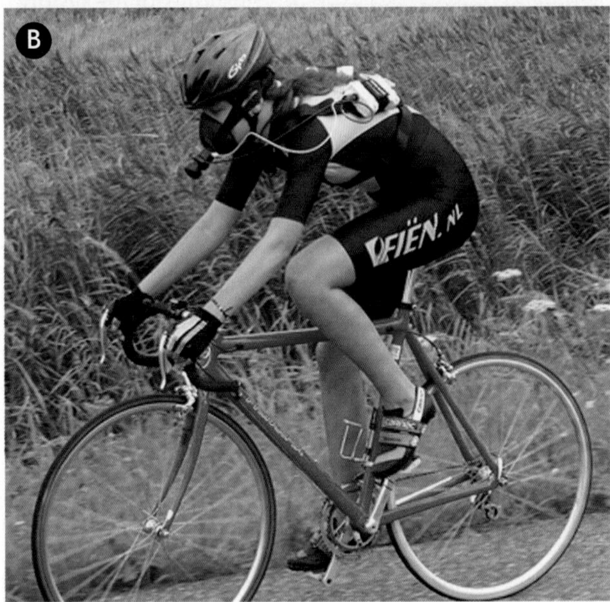

FIGURE 7.10 Portable metabolic collection systems use the latest in miniature computer technology. Built-in oxygen and carbon dioxide analyzer cells coupled with a highly sensitive micro-flow meter measure oxygen uptake by the open-circuit method during different activities such as **(A)** in-line skating and **(B)** cycling. (Adapted with permission from McArdle WD, Katch FI, Katch VL. *Sports and Exercise Nutrition*. 4th Ed. Philadelphia: Wolters Kluwer Health, 2013.)

Calibration Required

Regardless of the apparent sophistication of a particular automated system, the output data can only reflect accuracy of the measuring device. Accuracy and validity of measurement devices require careful and frequent ***calibration*** *using established reference standards.* This calibration process includes purchasing gases of known composition (e.g., 18.5% and 16.82% O_2) verified by a precise analysis system, then analyzing these gases with the laboratory's analysis method to determine the "closeness" of agreement. This procedure also verifies the oxygen concentration in ambient air (20.93% O_2), thus providing three data points within the typical physiological range for comparison between laboratory analysis and criterion gas composition. By knowing how well laboratory assessment compares to the known samples (in this case 16.82%, 18.5%, and 20.93% O_2), any discrepancy can serve as a "correction factor" applied to gas samples collected during an actual experiment that measures oxygen uptake. This validation process remains a crucial part of metabolic gas collection procedures. Prudent laboratory techniques also require regular calibration of the analyzer that measures carbon dioxide percentage and the meter that measures the air volume breathed during an experiment.

DIRECT VERSUS INDIRECT CALORIMETRY

Energy metabolism studied simultaneously using direct and indirect calorimetry provides convincing evidence for validity of the indirect method. Atwater and Rosa, the two scientists who devised the human calorimeter described previously, compared the two calorimetric methods in the early 1900s for 40 days with three men who lived in calorimeters similar to the one shown in **Figure 7.7**. Their daily energy outputs averaged 2723 kcal when measured directly by heat production and 2717 kcal when computed indirectly using closed-circuit measures of oxygen uptake. Other experiments with animals and humans based on moderate physical activity also demonstrated close agreement between direct and indirect methods; in most instances, the difference averaged less than ±1%. In the classic Atwater and Rosa calorimetry experiments, the ±0.2% method error represents a remarkable achievement in equipment design and construction, given that these experiments used handmade instruments.

DOUBLY LABELED WATER TECHNIQUE

The **doubly labeled water technique** developed in the early 1950s estimated the energy output of small animals (**www.fao.org/docrep/005/y3800m/y3800m02.htm**). Since then, cost reductions and refinements in this isotope-based method allow for its use to safely estimate total and average daily energy expenditure of groups of children and adults in free-living conditions without the normal constraints imposed by laboratory procedures. Few studies routinely use this method because of the expense in using doubly labeled water and the need for sophisticated measurement equipment. Nevertheless, its measurement does serve as a criterion or standard to validate other methods that estimate habitual total daily energy expenditure patterns over prolonged periods.

The subject consumes a quantity of water with a known concentration of the heavy, nonradioactive forms of the stable isotopes of heavy hydrogen (^2H– deuterium) and oxygen (^{18}O or oxygen-18)—hence the term *doubly labeled water*. The isotopes distribute throughout all bodily fluids. Labeled hydrogen leaves the body as water in sweat, urine, and pulmonary water vapor (^2H_2O), and labeled oxygen exits as both water ($H_2{}^{18}O$) and carbon dioxide ($C^{18}O_2$)

produced during macronutrient oxidation during energy metabolism. Differences between the two isotope elimination rates determined by an isotope ratio mass spectrometer relative to the body's normal background levels estimate total CO_2 production during the measurement period. Oxygen uptake is estimated based on CO_2 production and an assumed (or measured) respiratory quotient or RQ value of 0.85 (see the section "Respiratory Quotient").

Under normal circumstances, urine or saliva analysis before consuming the doubly labeled water serves as control baseline values for ^{18}O and ^{2}H. Ingested isotopes require about 5 hours to distribute throughout body water. Researchers measure enriched urine or saliva sample initially and then every day (or week) thereafter for the study's duration, usually up to 3 weeks. The progressive decrease in the two isotope sample concentrations permits computation of CO_2 production rate and hence $\dot{V}O_2$. The doubly labeled water technique provides an ideal way to assess total energy expenditure of individuals over extended durations, including bed rest and extreme activities such as climbing the Himalayan mountains (**http://ngm.nationalgeographic.com/2013/06/125-everest-maxed-out/jenkins-text**), cycling the Tour de France (**www.letour.com/us/**), trekking across Antarctica, and participating in the Iditarod (**http://iditarod.com**), military activities, extravehicular activities in space (**http://spaceflight.nasa.gov/shuttle/reference/faq/eva.html**), and extreme endurance swims (**www.channelswimmingassociation.com**).

Computerized Instrumentation

With advances in computer and microprocessor technology, exercise scientists can rapidly measure metabolic and physiologic responses to physical activity. Computers interface with at least three instruments: a system to continuously sample the subject's expired air volume, and oxygen and carbon dioxide analyzers to measure the expired air mixture's composition. The computer performs metabolic calculations in real time based on electronic signals it receives from the instruments. A data printout or graphic display of the data appears throughout the measurement period, including transmission of the electronic signals directly to a smart watch for personal or medical use. Sharing of such data with physicians and healthcare providers opens up new vistas in patient health services, without the constraints of office visits. For example, interval training workouts on a beach in South Africa can be instantly reviewed tens of thousands of miles away, whether by a physician in Boston, MA monitoring a post-cardiac transplant patient or a coach assessing heart rate response during a promising athlete's high intensity interval training (HIIT) workouts. **Figure 7.11** depicts a typical computerized system to assess and monitor metabolic and physiologic responses during physical activity. The flowchart in the figure illustrates the sequence of events, usually breath by breath, to compute ventilation volume and amount of oxygen consumed and carbon dioxide produced during the measurement period.

Caloric Transformation for Oxygen

Bomb calorimeter studies show that approximately 4.82 kcal release when a blend of carbohydrate, lipid, and protein burns in 1 L of oxygen. Even with large variations in the metabolic mixture, this **caloric value for oxygen** varies within ±2% to 4%.

An energy-oxygen equivalent of 5.0 kcal per liter provides a convenient yardstick to transpose any aerobic physical activity to a caloric or energy frame of reference. Indirect calorimetry through oxygen uptake measurement provides the basis to quantify the caloric cost of physical activity.

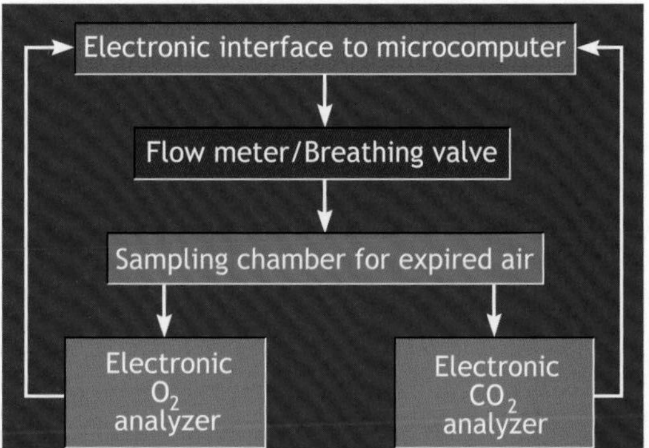

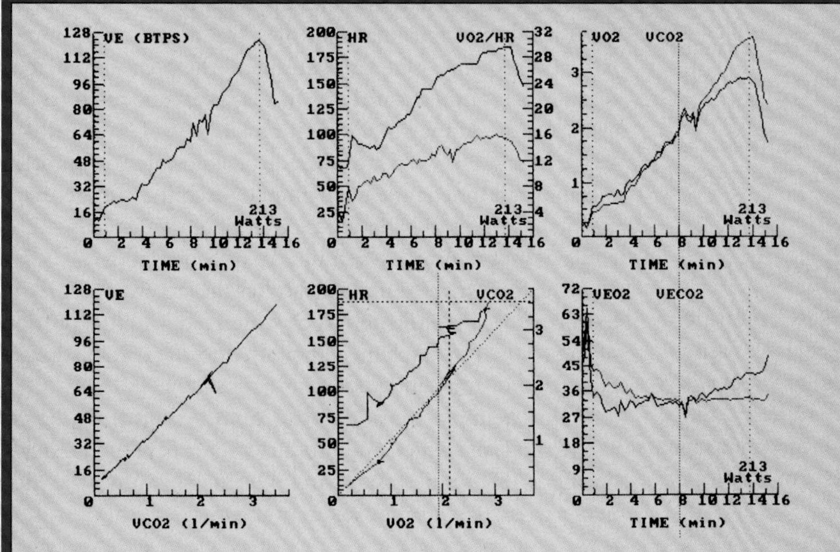

FIGURE 7.11 Computer systems approach to collect, analyze, and monitor physiologic and metabolic data. (Adapted with permission from McArdle WD, Katch FI, Katch VL. *Exercise Physiology: Nutrition, Energy, and Human Performance*. 8th Ed. Baltimore: Wolters Kluwer Health, 2015.)

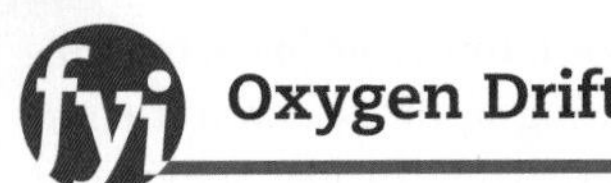

Oxygen Drift

Exercise $\dot{V}O_2$ increases when performing under three conditions:

1. An intensity level greater than about 70% $\dot{V}O_{2max}$
2. An intensity level at a lower percentage of $\dot{V}O_{2max}$ but for prolonged durations (>30 min)
3. Physical activity in hot, humid environments for prolonged periods

$\dot{V}O_2$ increases occur, but the energy requirement of effort does not change. This increase in oxygen uptake, independent of the "real" cost of the activity, spuriously increases the "true" activity energy cost as estimated by indirect calorimetry. The *upward drift* in $\dot{V}O_2$ results from increasing blood levels of catecholamines, lactate accumulation (with intense activity), shifting substrate utilization (to greater carbohydrate use), increased energy cost of higher pulmonary ventilation, and increased body temperature.

RESPIRATORY QUOTIENT

Complete oxidation of a molecule's carbon and hydrogen atoms to carbon dioxide and water end products requires different amounts of oxygen because of inherent chemical differences in carbohydrate, lipid, and protein composition. Consequently, the substrate metabolized determines the quantity of carbon dioxide produced relative to oxygen consumed. The **respiratory quotient (RQ)** refers to the following ratio of metabolic gas exchange:

$$RQ = CO_2 \text{ produced} \div O_2 \text{ consumed}$$

The RQ helps approximate the nutrient mixture catabolized for energy during rest and aerobic physical activity. Also, the caloric equivalent for oxygen differs depending on the nutrients oxidized, so precisely determining the body's heat or kcal production requires information about both oxygen uptake and RQ.

Respiratory Quotient for Carbohydrate

All of the oxygen consumed in carbohydrate combustion oxidizes carbon in the carbohydrate molecule to carbon dioxide. This occurs because the ratio of hydrogen to oxygen atoms in carbohydrates always exists in the same 2:1 ratio as in water. The complete oxidation of one glucose molecule requires six oxygen molecules and produces six molecules of carbon dioxide and water as follows:

$$C_6H_{12}O_6 + 6O_2 \rightarrow 6CO_2 + 6H_2O$$

Gas exchange during glucose oxidation produces an equal number of CO_2 molecules to O_2 molecules consumed; therefore, RQ for carbohydrate equals 1.00:

$$RQ = 6CO_2 \div 6O_2 = 1.00$$

Respiratory Quotient for Lipid

The chemical composition of lipids differs from carbohydrates because lipids contain considerably fewer oxygen atoms in proportion to hydrogen and carbon atoms. Consequently, lipid catabolism for energy requires considerably more oxygen relative to carbon dioxide production. Palmitic acid, a typical fatty acid, oxidizes to carbon dioxide and water to produce 16 carbon dioxide molecules for every 23 oxygen molecules consumed. The following equation summarizes this exchange to compute RQ:

$$C_{16}H_{32}O_2 + 23O_2 \rightarrow 16CO_2 + 16H_2O$$
$$RQ = 16CO_2 \div 23O_2 = 0.696$$

Generally, a value of 0.70 represents the RQ for lipid, ranging between 0.69 and 0.73 depending on the oxidized fatty acid's carbon chain length.

Respiratory Quotient for Protein

Proteins do not oxidize to carbon dioxide and water during energy metabolism. Rather, the liver first deaminates or removes nitrogen from the amino acid molecule; then the body excretes the nitrogen and sulfur fragments in the urine, sweat, and feces. The remaining "keto acid" fragment oxidizes to carbon dioxide and water to provide energy for biologic work. To achieve complete combustion, short-chain keto acids require more oxygen than carbon dioxide produced. For example, the protein albumin oxidizes as follows:

$$C_{72}H_{112}N_2O_{22}S + 77O_2 \rightarrow 63CO_2 + 38H_2O + SO_3 + 9CO(NH_2)_2$$
$$RQ = 63CO_2 \div 77O_2 = 0.818$$

The general value 0.82 characterizes the RQ for protein.

Nonprotein RQ

The RQ computed from compositional analysis of expired air usually reflects catabolism of a blend of carbohydrates, fats, and proteins. One can determine the precise contribution of each of these nutrients to the metabolic mixture. For example, the kidneys excrete approximately 1 g of urinary nitrogen for every 5.57 to 6.25 g (classic value) of protein metabolized for energy. Each gram of excreted nitrogen represents a carbon dioxide production of approximately 4.8 L and a corresponding oxygen uptake of about 6.0 L.

The following example illustrates the stepwise procedure to calculate the **nonprotein RQ**, which refers to that portion of the respiratory exchange attributed to the combustion of only carbohydrate and fat, excluding protein.

This example considers data from a subject who consumes 4.0 L of oxygen and produces 3.4 L of carbon dioxide during a 15-minute rest period. During this time, the kidneys excrete 0.13 g of nitrogen in the urine.

- *Step 1.* 4.8 L CO_2 per g protein metabolized × 0.13 g = 0.62 L CO_2 produced in protein catabolism
- *Step 2.* 6.0 L O_2 per g protein metabolized × 0.13 g = 0.78 L O_2 consumed in protein catabolism
- *Step 3.* Nonprotein CO_2 produced = 3.4 L CO_2 − 0.62 L CO_2 = 2.78 L CO_2

TABLE 7.2 Thermal Equivalents of Oxygen for the Nonprotein Respiratory Quotient, Including Percentage kcal and Grams Derived From Carbohydrate and Fat

Nonprotein RQ	kcal per Liter O_2 Uptake	Percentage kcal Derived From		Grams per Liter O_2 Uptake	
		Carbohydrate	Fat	Carbohydrate	Fat
0.707	4.686	0.0	100.0	0.000	.496
0.71	4.690	1.1	98.9	.012	.491
0.72	4.702	4.8	95.2	.051	.476
0.73	4.714	8.4	91.6	.900	.460
0.74	4.727	12.0	88.0	.130	.444
0.75	4.739	15.6	84.4	.170	.428
0.76	4.750	19.2	80.8	.211	.412
0.77	4.764	22.8	77.2	.250	.396
0.78	4.776	26.3	73.7	.290	.380
0.79	4.788	29.9	70.1	.330	.363
0.80	4.801	33.4	66.6	.371	.347
0.81	4.813	36.9	63.1	.413	.330
0.82	4.825	40.3	59.7	.454	.313
0.83	4.838	43.8	56.2	.496	.297
0.84	4.850	47.2	52.8	.537	.280
0.85	4.862	50.7	49.3	.579	.263
0.86	4.875	54.1	45.9	.621	.247
0.87	4.887	57.5	42.5	.663	.230
0.88	4.887	60.8	39.2	.705	.213
0.89	4.911	64.2	35.8	.749	.195
0.90	4.924	67.5	32.5	.791	.178
0.91	4.936	70.8	29.2	.834	.160
0.92	4.948	74.1	25.9	.877	.143
0.93	4.961	77.4	22.6	.921	.125
0.94	4.973	80.7	19.3	.964	.108
0.95	4.985	84.0	16.0	1.008	.090
0.96	4.998	87.2	12.8	1.052	.072
0.97	5.010	90.4	9.6	1.097	.054
0.98	5.022	93.6	6.4	1.142	.036
0.99	5.035	96.8	3.2	1.186	.018
1.00	5.047	100.0	0	1.231	.000

From Zuntz N. Ueber die Bedeutung der verschiedenen Nährstoffe als Erzeuger der Muskelkraft. [*Arch Gesamta Physiol* Bonn, Germany: LXXXIII, 557–571, 1901], *Pflügers Arch Physiol* 1901;83:557.

- *Step 4.* Nonprotein O_2 consumed = 4.0 L O_2 – 0.78 L O_2 =3.22 L O_2
- *Step 5.* Nonprotein RQ = 2.78 ÷ 3.22 = 0.86

Table 7.2 presents thermal energy equivalents for oxygen uptake for different nonprotein RQ values, and percentage of fat and carbohydrate catabolized for energy. For the 0.86 nonprotein RQ computed in the previous example, each liter of oxygen consumed liberates 4.875 kcal. For this RQ, 54.1% of the nonprotein calories derive from carbohydrate and 45.9% come from fat. The total 15-minute heat production at rest attributable to fat and carbohydrate catabolism equals 15.70 kcal (4.875 kcal · L^{-1} × 3.22 L O_2); the energy from protein breakdown equals 3.51 kcal (4.5 kcal · L^{-1} × 0.78 L O_2). The total energy from protein and nonprotein macronutrient combustion during the 15-minute period equals 19.21 kcal (15.70 kcal nonprotein + 3.51 kcal protein).

Mixed Diet Respiratory Quotient

During activities that range from complete bed rest to mild aerobic walking or slow jogging, the RQ seldom reflects oxidation of pure carbohydrate or pure fat. Instead, metabolizing

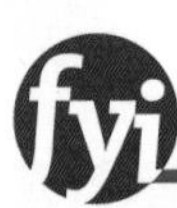

Respiratory Quotient versus Respiratory Exchange Ratio

The respiratory exchange ratio (RER) or R, the ratio of the amount of CO_2 produced to amount of O_2 consumed, represents physiologic occurrences on a total body level. In contrast, the RQ, the ratio of the amount of CO_2 produced to the amount of O_2 consumed and the same as R, represents the gas exchange ratio on the cellular level from substrate metabolism.

a mixture of nutrients occurs with an RQ intermediate between 0.70 and 1.00. *For most purposes, we assume an RQ of 0.82 from the metabolism of a mixture of 40% carbohydrate and 60% fat by applying the caloric equivalent of 4.825 kcal per liter of oxygen for the energy transformation.* Using 4.825 kcal, the maximum error possible in estimating energy metabolism from steady-rate oxygen uptake equals about ±4%.

RESPIRATORY EXCHANGE RATIO

Application of the RQ requires the assumption that the O_2 and CO_2 exchange measured at the lungs reflects cellular level gas exchange from nutrient metabolism. This assumption remains reasonably valid for rest and during steady-rate light to moderate aerobic physical activity conditions with minimal lactate accumulation. Various factors can alter the exchange of oxygen and carbon dioxide in the lungs so the gas exchange ratio no longer reflects *only* the substrate mixture in cellular energy metabolism. For example, carbon dioxide elimination increases during hyperventilation because breathing increases to disproportionately high levels compared with intrinsic metabolic demands. By overbreathing, the normal level of CO_2 in the blood decreases because the gas "blows off" in expired air. A corresponding increase in oxygen uptake does not accompany this additional CO_2 elimination. Consequently, the exchange ratio often exceeds 1.00. *Respiratory physiologists refer to the ratio of carbon dioxide produced to oxygen consumed under such conditions as the* **respiratory exchange ratio, R, or RER.** This ratio computes in exactly the same manner as RQ. An increase in the respiratory exchange ratio above 1.00 cannot be attributed to foodstuff oxidation.

Exhaustive physical activity presents another situation where R usually exceeds 1.00. To maintain proper acid-base balance, sodium bicarbonate in the blood "neutralizes" or buffers the lactate generated during anaerobic metabolism in the following reaction:

$$HLa + NaHCO_3 \rightarrow NaLa + H_2CO_3 \rightarrow H_2O + CO_2 \rightarrow \text{Lungs}$$

Lactate buffering produces the weaker carbonic acid. In the pulmonary capillaries, carbonic acid catabolizes to its carbon dioxide and water components to allow carbon dioxide to readily exit the lungs. The R increases above 1.00 because buffering adds "extra" CO_2 to expired air above the quantity normally released during cellular energy metabolism.

Lower R values also occur following exhaustive activity when carbon dioxide remains in body fluids to replenish bicarbonate that buffered the accumulating lactate. This action reduces expired carbon dioxide without affecting oxygen uptake; this decreases R to below 0.70.

MAXIMAL OXYGEN UPTAKE ($\dot{V}O_{2max}$)

$\dot{V}O_{2max}$ (also called aerobic power) represents the greatest amount of oxygen a person can use to produce ATP aerobically on a per-minute basis, usually during intense, endurance-type activities. The data in **Figure 7.12** illustrate that persons who engage in sports that require sustained,

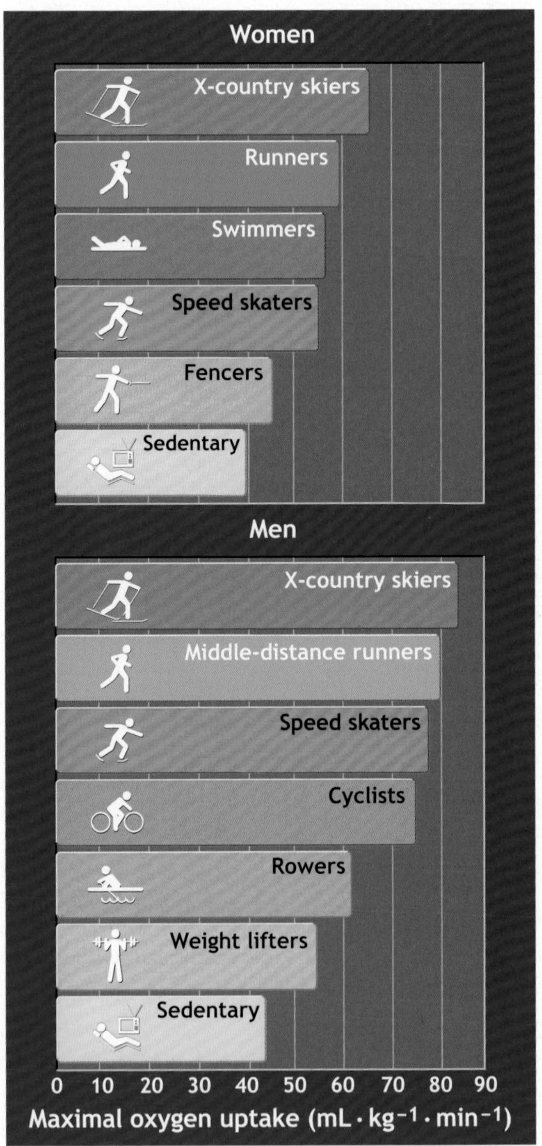

FIGURE 7.12 Maximal oxygen uptake of male and female Olympic-caliber athletes in different sport categories compared with healthy sedentary subjects. (Adapted with permission from McArdle WD, Katch FI, Katch VL. *Exercise Physiology: Nutrition, Energy, and Human Performance*. 8th Ed. Baltimore: Wolters Kluwer Health, 2015; as adapted with permission from Saltin B, Åstrand PO. Maximal oxygen consumption in athletes. *J Appl Physiol* 1967;23:353.)

intense exertion possess large capacities for aerobic energy transfer.

Male and female competitors in distance running, swimming, bicycling, rowing, and cross-country skiing have nearly twice the aerobic capacity as sedentary individuals. This does not mean that only $\dot{V}O_{2max}$ determines endurance capacity. Other factors at the muscle level such as capillary density, enzymes, and muscle fiber type, strongly influence capacity to sustain physical activity at a high $\dot{V}O_{2max}$ percentage (i.e., achieve a high blood lactate threshold). $\dot{V}O_{2max}$, however, does provide useful information about the capacity of the long-term energy system. Attaining one's $\dot{V}O_{2max}$ requires integration of the ventilatory, cardiovascular, and neuromuscular systems; this gives significant physiologic "meaning" to this metabolic measure. *In essence, $\dot{V}O_{2max}$ represents a fundamental measure in exercise physiology and serves as a standard to compare performance estimates of aerobic capacity and endurance fitness.*

Tests for $\dot{V}O_{2max}$ rely on activities with sufficient intensity and duration to activate large muscle groups to properly engage maximal aerobic energy transfer. Typical tasks include treadmill walking or running, bench stepping, or cycling; tethered and flume swimming and swim-bench ergometry; and simulated rowing, skiing, in-line roller skating, stair-climbing, ice skating, and arm-crank ergometry. Considerable research effort has been directed toward development and standardization of $\dot{V}O_{2max}$ tests and norms that consider age, gender, state of training, and body composition. This Internet site summarizes twenty-one $\dot{V}O_{2max}$ assessment tests utilizing track running, swimming, cycling, step-climbing, non-exercise data and step-test data (see **A Closer Look: Using a Step Test To Predict $\dot{V}O_{2max}$** in this chapter) to predict $\dot{V}O_{2max}$ (**www.brianmac.co.uk/vo2max.htm**).

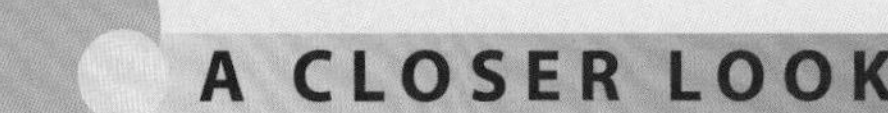

A CLOSER LOOK

The Weir Method to Calculate Energy Expenditure

In 1949, a Scottish physician and physiologist from Glasgow University, J.B. Weir, presented a simple method to estimate caloric expenditure ($kcal \cdot min^{-1}$) from measures of pulmonary ventilation and expired oxygen percentage, accurate to within ±1% of the traditional RQ method.

Basic Equation

Weir demonstrated the following formula could calculate energy expenditure if total energy production from protein breakdown equaled 12.5%, a reasonable percentage for most people:

$$kcal \cdot min^{-1} = \dot{V}_{E(STPD)} \times (1.044 - 0.0499 \times \%O_{2E})$$

where $\dot{V}_{E(STPD)}$ represents expired minute ventilation ($L \cdot min^{-1}$) corrected to STPD conditions and $\%O_{2E}$ represents expired oxygen percentage. The value in parentheses ($1.044 - 0.0499 \times \%O_{2E}$) represents the "Weir factor." The table displays Weir factors for different $\%O_{2E}$ values. To use the table, locate the $\%O_{2E}$ and corresponding Weir factor. Compute energy expenditure in $kcal \cdot min^{-1}$ by multiplying the Weir factor by $\dot{V}_{E(STPD)}$

Example

A person runs on a treadmill and $\dot{V}_{E(STPD)} = 50\ L \cdot min^{-1}$ and $\%O_{2E} = 16.0\%$. Compute energy expenditure by the Weir method as follows:

$$\begin{aligned} kcal \cdot min^{-1} &= \dot{V}_{E(STPD)} \times (1.044 - [0.0499 \times \%O_{2E}]) \\ &= 50 \times (1.044 - [0.0499 \times 16.0]) \\ &= 50 \times 0.2456 \\ &= 12.3 \end{aligned}$$

Weir also derived the following equation to calculate $kcal \cdot min^{-1}$ from RQ and $\dot{V}O_2$ in $L \cdot min^{-1}$:

$$kcal \cdot min^{-1} = ([1.1 \times RQ] + 3.9) \times \dot{V}O_2$$

Weir Factors

Weir	$\%O_{2E}$ Factor	Weir	$\%O_{2E}$ Factor	Weir	$\%O_{2E}$ Factor
14.50	0.3205	16.20	0.2366	17.90	0.1508
14.60	0.3155	16.30	0.2306	18.00	0.1468
14.70	0.3105	16.40	0.2256	18.10	0.1408
14.80	0.3055	16.50	0.2206	18.20	0.1368
14.90	0.3005	16.60	0.2157	18.30	0.1308
15.00	0.2955	16.70	0.2107	18.40	0.1268
15.10	0.2905	16.80	0.2057	18.50	0.1208
15.20	0.2855	16.90	0.2007	18.60	0.1168
15.30	0.2805	17.00	0.1957	18.70	0.1109
15.40	0.2755	17.10	0.1907	18.80	0.1068
15.50	0.2705	17.20	0.1857	18.90	0.1009
15.60	0.2656	17.30	0.1807	19.00	0.0969
15.70	0.2606	17.40	0.1757	19.10	0.0909
15.80	0.2556	17.50	0.1707	19.20	0.0868
15.90	0.2506	17.60	0.1658	19.30	0.0809
16.00	0.2456	17.70	0.1608	19.40	0.0769
16.10	0.2406	17.80	0.1558		

If $\%O_{2E}$ (expired oxygen percentage) does not appear in the table, compute individual Weir factors as $1.044 - 0.0499 \times \%O_{2E}$.

From Weir JB. New methods for calculating metabolic rates with special reference to protein metabolism. *J Physiol* 1949;109:1.

$\dot{V}O_{2max}$ Criteria

A leveling-off or peaking-over in oxygen uptake during increasing exercise intensity, displayed in **Figure 7.13**, *signifies attainment of maximum capacity for aerobic metabolism (i.e., a "true" $\dot{V}O_{2max}$).* When this accepted criterion is not met or local muscle fatigue in the arms or legs rather than central circulatory dynamics limits test performance, the term **peak oxygen uptake ($\dot{V}O_{2peak}$)** usually describes the highest oxygen uptake value during the test.

The data in **Figure 7.13** reflect oxygen uptake with progressive increases in treadmill intensity; the test terminates when the subject decides to stop even when prodded to continue. For the average oxygen uptake values of 18 subjects plotted in this figure, the highest $\dot{V}O_2$ occurred before subjects attained their maximum performance. The peaking-over criterion substantiates attainment of a true $\dot{V}O_{2max}$.

Peaking-over or slight decreases in $\dot{V}O_2$ do not always occur with increases in effort intensity. The highest $\dot{V}O_2$ usually occurs during the last minute of physical activity without the $\dot{V}O_{2max}$ plateau criterion. Additional criteria for establishing $\dot{V}O_{2max}$ (and $\dot{V}O_{2peak}$) include three metabolic and physiologic responses:

1. Failure for $\dot{V}O_2$ versus exercise intensity to increase by some value usually expected from previous observations with the particular test ($\dot{V}O_{2max}$ criterion)
2. Blood lactate levels that attain at least 70 or 80 mg per 100 mL of blood, or about 8 to 10 mmol to ensure the subject significantly exceeded the lactate threshold with near-maximal effort ($\dot{V}O_{2peak}$ criterion)
3. Attainment of near age-predicted maximum heart rate, or an R value in excess of 1.00, which indicates that the subject exercised at close to the maximum intensity ($\dot{V}O_{2peak}$ criterion)

Aerobic Power Tests

Many different standardized tests assess $\dot{V}O_{2max}$. Such tests remain independent of muscle strength, speed, body size, and skill, with the exception of specialized swimming, rowing, and ice skating tests.

The $\dot{V}O_{2max}$ test may require a continuous 3- to 5-minute "supermaximal" effort, but it usually consists of pre-established increments in effort intensity referred to as a **graded exercise test (GXT)** until the subject stops. Some researchers have imprecisely termed the end point "exhaustion," but the subject can terminate the test for many reasons, with exhaustion only one possibility. A variety of psychologic or motivational factors can influence this decision instead of true physiologic exhaustion. It can take considerable urging and encouragement to convince subjects to attain their "real" $\dot{V}O_{2max}$. Children and adults encounter particular difficulty if they have little prior experience performing to maximum with its associated central

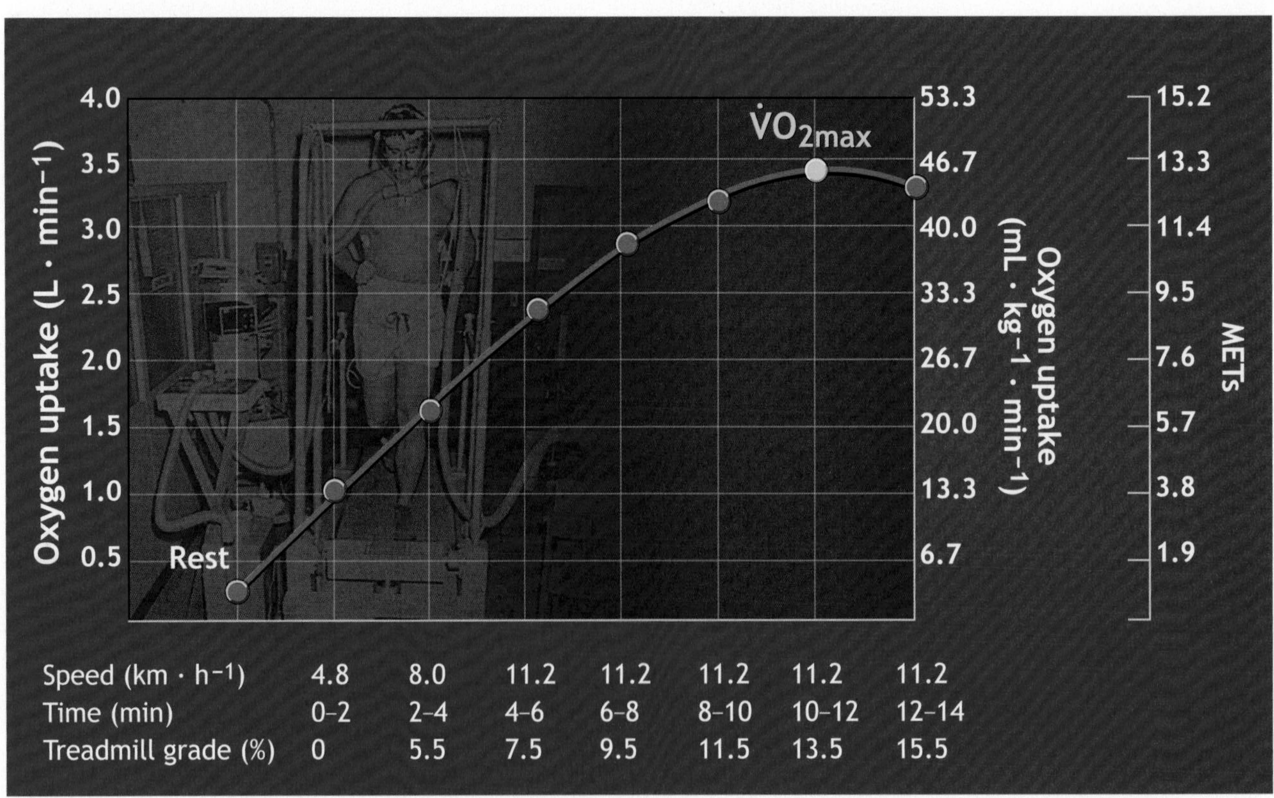

FIGURE 7.13 Peaking-over in oxygen uptake with increasing treadmill exercise intensity. Each point represents the average oxygen uptake of 18 sedentary males. The region where oxygen uptake fails to increase the expected amount or even decreases slightly with increasing intensity represents the $\dot{V}O_{2max}$. (Adapted with permission from McArdle WD, Katch FI, Katch VL. *Exercise Physiology: Nutrition, Energy, and Human Performance*. 8th Ed. Baltimore: Wolters Kluwer Health, 2015; data from the Applied Physiology Laboratory, University of Michigan.)

(cardiorespiratory) and peripheral (local muscular) discomforts. *Attaining a plateau in oxygen uptake during the* $\dot{V}O_{2max}$ *test requires high motivation and a large anaerobic component because of the maximal exercise requirement.*

Comparisons Among $\dot{V}O_{2max}$ Tests

Two types of $\dot{V}O_{2max}$ tests are typically used:

1. **Continuous GXT test:** No rest between exercise increments
2. **Discontinuous GXT test:** Several minutes of rest between exercise increments

The data in **Table 7.3** compare $\dot{V}O_{2max}$ scores measured by six common continuous and discontinuous treadmill and bicycle procedures.

Only a small 8-mL difference occurred in $\dot{V}O_{2max}$ between continuous and discontinuous bicycle tests, with $\dot{V}O_{2max}$ averaging 6.4% to 11.2% below treadmill values. The largest difference among any of the three treadmill running tests equaled only 1.2%. The walking-only test, in contrast, elicited $\dot{V}O_{2max}$ scores about 7% above values achieved on the bicycle but 5% less than the average for the three run tests.

Subjects reported local discomfort in their thigh muscles during intense effort on both bicycle tests. In walking, subjects reported discomfort in the lower back and calf muscles, particularly at higher treadmill elevations. The running tests produced little local discomfort, but subjects experienced general fatigue categorized as feeling "winded." In healthy subjects, a continuous treadmill run remains the method of choice for administrative ease. Total time to administer the test averaged slightly more than 12 minutes, whereas the discontinuous running test averaged about 65 minutes. One also can achieve $\dot{V}O_{2max}$ with

A CLOSER LOOK

Using a Step Test to Predict $\dot{V}O_{2max}$

Recovery heart rate from a standardized stepping activity can classify individuals with reasonable accuracy on cardiovascular fitness and $\dot{V}O_{2max}$.

The Test

Individuals step to a four-step cadence ("up-up-down-down") on a bench 16¼ inches high, the height of standard gymnasium bleachers. Women perform 22 complete step-ups per minute to a metronome set at 88 beats per minute; men use 24 step-ups per minute at a metronome setting of 96 beats per minute. Stepping begins after a brief demonstration and practice period. Following stepping, the person remains standing while another person measures the pulse rate at the carotid or radial artery for a 15-second period 5 to 20 seconds into recovery. Fifteen-second recovery heart rate converts to beats per minute (15 s HR × 4), which converts to a percentile ranking for predicted $\dot{V}O_{2max}$ (see table).

Equations

The following equations predict $\dot{V}O_{2max}$ ($mL \cdot kg^{-1} \cdot min^{-1}$) from step-test heart rate recovery for men and women ages 18 to 24:

$$\textbf{Men: } \dot{V}O_{2max} = 111.33 - (0.42 \times \text{step-test pulse rate, } b \cdot min^{-1})$$

$$\textbf{Women: } \dot{V}O_{2max} = 65.81 - (0.1847 \times \text{step-test pulse rate, } b \cdot min^{-1})$$

The *Predicted* $\dot{V}O_{2max}$ columns of the table present the $\dot{V}O_{2max}$ values for men and women from different recovery heart rate scores.

Percentile Ranking for Recovery Heart Rate and Predicted $\dot{V}O_{2max}$ ($mL \cdot kg^{-1} \cdot min^{-1}$) for Male and Female College Students

Percentile	Recovery HR Females	Predicted $\dot{V}O_{2max}$	Recovery HR Males	Predicted $\dot{V}O_{2max}$
100	128	42.2	120	60.9
95	140	40.0	124	59.3
90	148	38.5	128	57.6
85	152	37.7	136	54.2
80	156	37.0	140	52.5
75	158	36.6	144	50.9
70	160	36.3	148	49.2
65	162	35.9	149	48.8
60	163	35.7	152	47.5
55	164	35.5	154	46.7
50	166	35.1	156	45.8
45	168	34.8	160	44.1
40	170	34.4	162	43.3
35	171	34.2	164	42.5
30	172	34.0	166	41.6
25	176	33.3	168	40.8
20	180	32.6	172	39.1
15	182	32.2	176	37.4
10	184	31.8	178	36.6
5	196	29.6	184	34.1

Sources: McArdle WD, et al. Percentile norms for a valid step test in college women. *Res Q* 1973;44:498.

McArdle WD, et al. Reliability and interrelationships between maximal oxygen uptake, physical work capacity, and step test scores in college women. *Med Sci Sports* 1972;4:182.

TABLE 7.3 Average Maximal Oxygen Uptakes for 15 College Students During Continuous (Cont.) and Discontinuous (Discont.) Tests on the Bicycle and Treadmill

Variable	Bicycle		Treadmill			
	Discont.	Cont.	Discont. Walk-Run	Cont. Walk	Discont. Run	Cont. Run
$\dot{V}O_{2max}$, $mL \cdot min^{-1}$	3691 ± 453	3683 ± 448	4145 ± 401	3944 ± 395	4157 ± 445	4109 ± 424
$\dot{V}O_{2max}$, $mL \cdot kg^{-1} \cdot min^{-1}$	50.0 ± 6.9	49.9 ± 7.0	56.6 ± 7.3	56.6 ± 7.6	55.5 ± 7.6	55.5 ± 6.8

Values are means ± standard deviation.

$\dot{V}O_{2max}$, maximal oxygen uptake.

Adapted from McArdle WD, et al. Comparison of continuous and discontinuous treadmill and bicycle tests for max $\dot{V}O_2$. *Med Sci Sport* 1973;5:156.

a continuous exercise protocol during which intensity increases progressively in 15-second intervals. With such an approach, total test time averages only about 5 minutes for bicycle or treadmill modes.

Commonly Used Treadmill Protocols

Figure 7.14 summarizes six commonly used treadmill protocols to assess $\dot{V}O_{2max}$ in healthy individuals and individuals with cardiovascular disease. Common features include manipulation of test duration and treadmill speed and grade. The Harbor treadmill test (example F), referred to as a ramp test, is unique because treadmill grade increases every minute up to 10 minutes by a constant amount that ranges from 1% to 4% depending on the subject's fitness. This quick procedure linearly increases oxygen uptake to the maximum level. Healthy individuals and monitored cardiac patients tolerate the protocol without problems.

Manipulating Test Protocol to Increase $\dot{V}O_{2max}$

On completion of a $\dot{V}O_{2max}$ test, one assumes the tester has made every attempt to "push" the subject to near limits of performance. This effort includes verbal encouragement from laboratory staff and peers or a monetary incentive. If the test meets the usual physiologic criteria, one assumes the test score represents the subject's "true" $\dot{V}O_{2max}$.

In one study, 44 sedentary and trained men and women performed a continuous treadmill $\dot{V}O_{2max}$ test to the point of so-called "exhaustion" in which they refused to continue exercising. They then recovered for 2 minutes before performing a second $\dot{V}O_{2max}$ test. During active recovery from test 1, the researchers lowered the treadmill grade at least 2.5% below the final grade of the previous test and reduced running speed from 11.0 to 9.0 $km \cdot h^{-1}$ for the trained subjects and from 9.0 to 6.0 $km \cdot h^{-1}$ for the sedentary subjects. After 2 minutes, treadmill speed increased to the test 1 speed for 30 seconds and percent grade increased to the final grade achieved in test 1. Treadmill grade increased every 2 minutes thereafter until the subjects again terminated the test. Subjects received strong verbal encouragement during both tests, particularly during the last minutes of activity.

The $\dot{V}O_{2max}$ scores averaged a statistically significant 1.4% higher value on test 2. This small difference was almost double the difference typically measured between two final oxygen uptake readings on continuous or discontinuous tests. A "booster" test following a normally administered aerobic capacity test can increase the final oxygen uptake, illustrating the need to pay careful attention to $\dot{V}O_{2max}$ administrative techniques.

Factors Affecting $\dot{V}O_{2max}$

The most important factors that influence $\dot{V}O_{2max}$ include exercise test mode and the person's heredity, training state, gender, body composition, and age.

Exercise Testing Mode

Variations in $\dot{V}O_{2max}$ during different test modes reflect the quantity of activated muscle mass. Experiments that measured $\dot{V}O_{2max}$ on the same subjects during treadmill exercise produced the highest values. Bench stepping generates $\dot{V}O_{2max}$ scores nearly identical to treadmill values and higher than bicycle ergometer values. With arm-crank exercise, a person's aerobic capacity reaches only about 70% of treadmill $\dot{V}O_{2max}$.

For skilled but untrained swimmers, $\dot{V}O_{2max}$ during swimming records about 20% below treadmill values. Definite test specificity exists in this form of activity mode because trained collegiate swimmers achieved $\dot{V}O_{2max}$ values swimming only 11% below treadmill values; some elite competitive swimmers equal or even exceed their treadmill $\dot{V}O_{2max}$ scores during an aerobic capacity swimming test. Similarly, a distinct exercise and training specificity occurs among competitive racewalkers who achieve oxygen uptakes during walking that equal $\dot{V}O_{2max}$ values during treadmill running. If competitive cyclists pedal at their fastest competition rate, they also achieve $\dot{V}O_{2max}$ values equivalent to their treadmill scores.

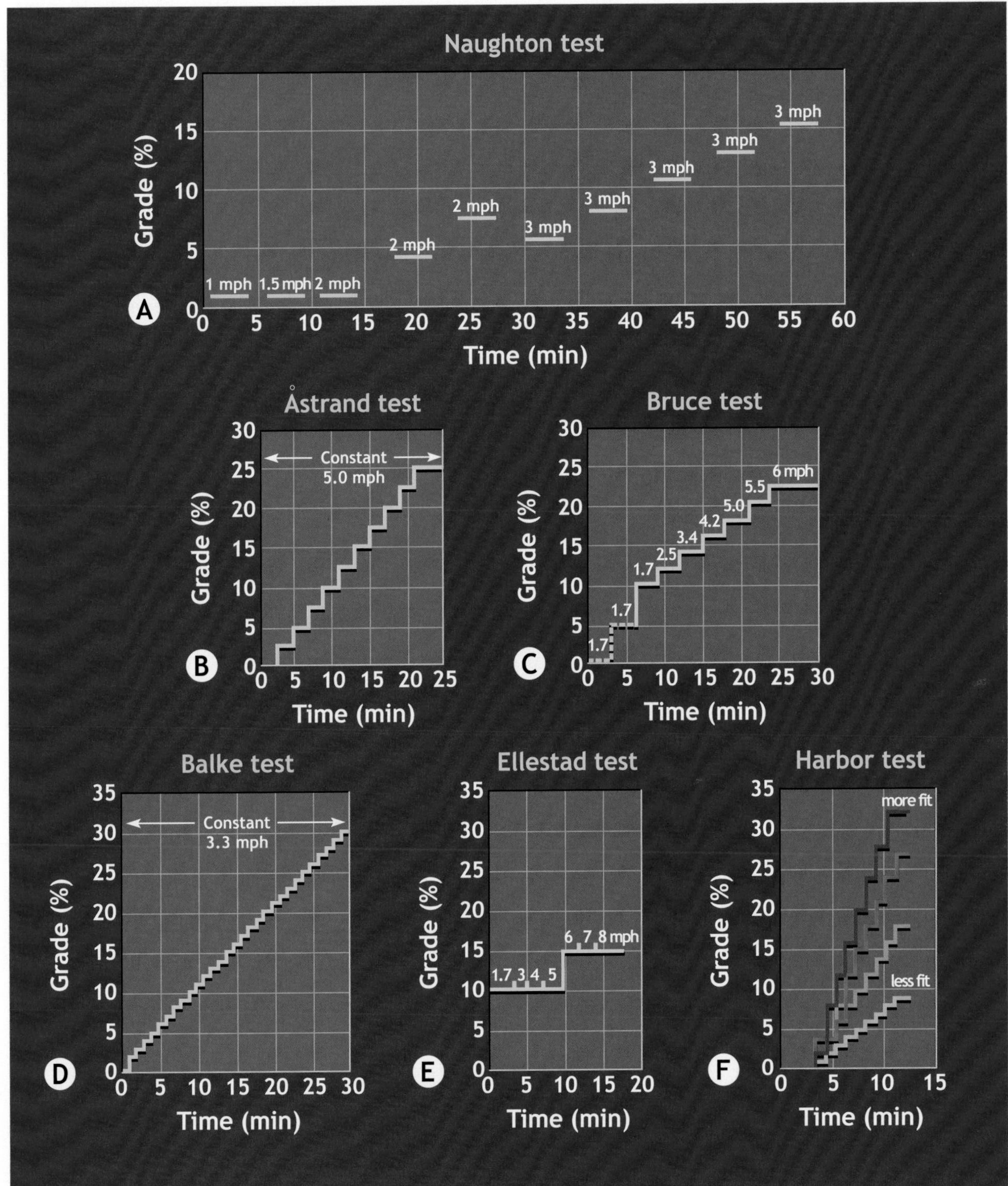

FIGURE 7.14 Six commonly used treadmill protocols to assess $\dot{V}O_{2max}$. **A.** Naughton protocol. Three-minute exercise periods of increasing intensity alternate with 3 minutes of rest. Exercise periods vary in % grade and speed. **B.** Åstrand protocol. Constant speed at 5 mph. After 3 minutes at 0% grade, the grade increases 2½% every 2 minutes. **C.** Bruce protocol. Grade and/or speed change every 3 minutes Omit the 0% and 5% grades for healthy subjects. **D.** Balke protocol. After 1 minute at 0% grade and 1 minute at 2% grade, the grade increases 1% per minute; speed is maintained at 3.3 mph. **E.** Ellestad protocol. Initial grade of 10% and later grade of 15%, while speed increases every 2 or 3 minutes. **F.** Harbor protocol. After 3 minutes of walking at a comfortable speed, the grade increases at a constant preselected amount each minute: 1%, 2%, 3%, or 4%, so that the subject achieves $\dot{V}O_{2max}$ in approximately 10 minutes. (Adapted with permission from McArdle WD, Katch FI, Katch VL. *Exercise Physiology: Nutrition, Energy, and Human Performance*. 8th Ed. Baltimore: Wolters Kluwer Health, 2015; as adapted with permission from Wasserman K, et al. *Principles of Exercise Testing and Interpretation*. 2nd Ed. Philadelphia: Lea & Febiger, 1994.)

In healthy subjects, the treadmill represents the laboratory apparatus of choice to determine $\dot{V}O_{2max}$. The treadmill easily quantifies and regulates effort intensity. Compared with other modes, subjects achieve one or more of the criteria more easily on the treadmill to establish $\dot{V}O_{2max}$ or $\dot{V}O_{2peak}$. Bench stepping or bicycle exercise serves as suitable alternatives under nonlaboratory "field" conditions.

Heredity

A frequent question concerns the relative contribution of heredity to physiologic function and exercise performance. For example, to what extent does heredity determine the extremely high aerobic capacities of endurance athletes? Some researchers have focused on the question of how genetic variability accounts for differences among individuals in physiologic and metabolic capacity.

Early studies were conducted on 15 pairs of identical twins (same heredity because they came from the same fertilized egg) and 15 pairs of fraternal twins (did not differ from ordinary siblings because they result from separate fertilization of two eggs) raised in the same city by parents with similar socioeconomic backgrounds. The researchers concluded that heredity alone accounted for up to 93% of the observed differences in $\dot{V}O_{2max}$. Subsequent investigations of larger groups of brothers, fraternal twins, and identical twins indicate a much smaller but still important influence of inherited factors on aerobic capacity and endurance performance.

Current estimates of the genetic effect ascribe about 20% to 30% for $\dot{V}O_{2max}$*, 50% for maximum heart rate, and 70% for physical working capacity.* Future research will ultimately determine the exact upper limit of genetic determination, but present data show that inherited factors contribute *considerably* to physiologic functional capacity and performance. A large genotype dependency also exists for the potential to improve aerobic and anaerobic power and adaptations of most muscle enzymes to training. In other words, members of the same twin pair show almost identical responses to physical training.

A CLOSER LOOK

Predicting $\dot{V}O_{2max}$ Using Age for Sedentary, Physically Active, and Endurance-Trained Individuals

For most individuals, $\dot{V}O_{2max}$ declines approximately 0.4 mL · kg^{-1} · min^{-1} each year or 4.0 mL · kg^{-1} · min^{-1} each decade. With aging, sedentary individuals may have twofold faster $\dot{V}O_{2max}$ rates of decline. Heredity undoubtedly plays an important role, as does the well-documented decrement in muscle mass. Thus, for both active and sedentary persons, it is possible to predict $\dot{V}O_{2max}$ for classification purposes from age alone.

Equations

The accompanying table presents different equations to predict $\dot{V}O_{2max}$ using only age as the predictor variable.

Example 1: Endurance-Trained Man, Age 55 y (Equation 3)

$$\begin{aligned}\text{Predicted } \dot{V}O_{2max} &= 77.2 - 0.46\ (\text{age, y})\\ &= 77.2 - 0.46\ (55)\\ &= 51.7\ \text{mL} \cdot \text{kg}^{-1} \cdot \text{min}^{-1}\end{aligned}$$

Example 2: Active Woman, Age 21 y (Equation 2)

$$\begin{aligned}\text{Predicted } \dot{V}O_{2max} &= 61.4 - 0.39\ (\text{age, y})\\ &= 61.4 - 0.39\ (21)\\ &= 53.2\ \text{mL} \cdot \text{kg}^{-1} \cdot \text{min}^{-1}\end{aligned}$$

Example 3: 23-Year-Old Woman of Unknown Fitness Status (Equation 4)

$$\begin{aligned}\text{Predicted } \dot{V}O_{2max} &= 53.7 - 0.537\ (\text{age, y})\\ &= 53.7 - 0.537\ (23)\\ &= 41.4\ \text{mL} \cdot \text{kg}^{-1} \cdot \text{min}^{-1}\end{aligned}$$

Equations to Predict $\dot{V}O_{2max}$ (mL · kg^{-1} · min^{-1}) from Age

Group	Equation	Correlation
1. Sedentary[a]	Predicted $\dot{V}O_{2max}$ = 54.2 – 0.40 (age, y)	$r = 0.88$
2. Moderately active[b]	Predicted $\dot{V}O_{2max}$ = 61.4 – 0.39 (age, y)	$r = 0.80$
3. Endurance trained[c]	Predicted $\dot{V}O_{2max}$ = 77.2 – 0.46 (age, y)	$r = 0.89$
4. Alternate equations (independent of relative fitness status) *Males:* Predicted $\dot{V}O_{2max}$ = 59.48 – 0.46 (age, y) *Females:* Predicted $\dot{V}O_{2max}$ = 53.7 – 0.537 (age, y)		

[a] No physical activity.
[b] Occasional physical activity, about 2 d · wk^{-1}.
[c] Physical activity = 3 d · wk^{-1} for at least 1 full year.

Sources: Wilson TM, Seals DR. Meta-analysis of the age-associated decline in maximal aerobic capacity in men: relation to habitual aerobic status. *Med Sci Sports Exerc* 1995;31:S385.

Jackson AS, et al. Changes in aerobic power of women age 20–64 y. *Med Sci Sports Exerc* 1996;28:884.

Training State

Maximal oxygen uptake must be evaluated relative to the person's training status at the time of measurement. Aerobic capacity with training improves between 6% and 20%, although increases have attained 50% more than pretraining levels. As would be expected, the largest $\dot{V}O_{2max}$ improvements occur among the most sedentary individuals.

Gender

$\dot{V}O_{2max}$ expressed in mL · kg^{-1} · min^{-1} for women typically averages 15% to 30% below values for men. Even among trained athletes, the disparity ranges between 10% and 20%. Such differences increase considerably when expressing $\dot{V}O_{2max}$ as an absolute value in L · min^{-1} rather than relative to body mass as mL · kg^{-1} · min^{-1} or fat-free body mass as mL · kg FFM^{-1} · min^{-1}. Among world-class male and female cross-country skiers, a 43% lower $\dot{V}O_{2max}$ for women (6.54 vs. 3.75 L · min^{-1}) decreased to 15% (83.8 vs. 71.2 mL · kg^{-1} · min^{-1}) when using the athletes' body mass in the $\dot{V}O_{2max}$ ratio expression.

Apparent gender difference in $\dot{V}O_{2max}$ has been attributed to differences in body composition and blood's hemoglobin concentration. Untrained young adult women possess about 26% body fat, while the corresponding value for men averages approximately 15%. Trained athletes have a lower body fat percentage, yet trained women possess significantly more body fat than male counterparts. Consequently, males generate more total aerobic energy simply because of their larger muscle mass and lower total fat than females.

Men also show a 10% to 14% greater concentration of hemoglobin than women. This difference in the blood's oxygen-carrying capacity enables males to circulate more oxygen during physical activity and gives them an edge in aerobic capacity.

Differences in normal physical activity level between an "average" or "typical" male and female also provide a possible explanation for the $\dot{V}O_{2max}$ gender difference. Even among prepubertal children, boys exhibit a higher physical activity level in daily life.

Despite these possible limitations, the aerobic capacity of physically active women exceeds that of sedentary men. In this regard, female cross-country skiers have $\dot{V}O_{2max}$ scores 40% higher than untrained men of the same age.

Body Composition

Differences in body mass among individuals explain roughly 70% of the differences in $\dot{V}O_{2max}$ expressed in L · min^{-1}. Thus, meaningful comparisons of $\dot{V}O_{2max}$ when expressed in L · min^{-1} become difficult among individuals who differ in body size or body composition. This has led to the common practice of expressing oxygen uptake by body surface area (BSA), body mass (BM), fat-free body mass (FFM), or even limb volume (i.e., dividing the $\dot{V}O_{2max}$ scores by BSA, FFM, or BM) in the belief that $\dot{V}O_{2max}$ remains independent of the respective divisor.

TABLE 7.4 Different Ways to Express Oxygen Uptake

Variable	Female	Male	%Difference[a]
$\dot{V}O_{2max}$, L · min^{-1}	2.00	3.50	−43
$\dot{V}O_{2max}$, mL · min^{-1}	40.0	50.0	−20
$\dot{V}O_{2max}$, mL · kg FFM^{-1} · min^{-1}	53.3	58.8	-9.0
Body mass, kg	50	70	−29
Percent body fat	25	15	+67
FFM, kg	37.5	59.5	−37

[a]Female minus male.

FFM, fat-free mass; $\dot{V}O_{2max}$, maximal oxygen uptake.

Table 7.4 present typical oxygen uptake values for an untrained man and woman who differ considerably in body mass. The percentage difference in $\dot{V}O_{2max}$ between these individuals, when expressed in L · min^{-1} amounts to 43%. The woman still exhibited about a 20% lower value when expressing $\dot{V}O_{2max}$ related to body mass (mL · kg^{-1} · min^{-1}); the difference shrank to 9% when divided by FFM.

Similar findings occur for $\dot{V}O_{2peak}$ for men and women during arm-cranking exercise. Adjusting arm-crank $\dot{V}O_{2peak}$ for variations in arm and shoulder size equalizes values between men and women. This suggests gender differences in aerobic capacity largely reflect the size of the active muscle mass. Such observations foster arguments that no "true" gender difference exist in active muscle mass capacity to generate ATP aerobically.

Age

Changes in $\dot{V}O_{2max}$ relate to chronological age, yet limitations exist in drawing inferences from cross-sectional studies of different aged people. The available data provide insight into the possible effects of aging on physiologic function.

Absolute Values

Maximal oxygen uptake expressed in L · min^{-1} increases dramatically during the growth years. A longitudinal study that measured children's $\dot{V}O_{2max}$ in the same individuals over a prolonged time period showed that absolute values increase from about 1.0 L · min^{-1} at age 6 to 3.2 L · min^{-1} at age 16. $\dot{V}O_{2max}$ in girls peaks at about age 14 and declines thereafter. At age 14, the difference in $\dot{V}O_{2max}$ (L · min^{-1}) between boys and girls approximated 25%, with the spread reaching 50% 2 years later.

Relative Values

When expressed relative to body mass, $\dot{V}O_{2max}$ remains constant at about 53 mL · kg^{-1} · min^{-1} between ages 6 and 16 for boys. In contrast, relative $\dot{V}O_{2max}$ in girls gradually decreases from 52.0 mL · kg^{-1} · min^{-1} at age 6 to 40.5 mL · kg^{-1} · min^{-1}

at age 16. Greater accumulation of body fat in young women helps to explain this discrepancy.

A longitudinal study of a cohort of more than 3000 women and 16,000 men aged 20 to 96 from the Aerobics Center Longitudinal Study who completed serial health examinations including maximal treadmill testing during 1974 to 2006 illustrates the effects of age on aerobic capacity (**www.cooperinstitute.org/research/study/acls.cfm**). *Beyond age 35, $\dot{V}O_{2max}$ declines at a nonlinear rate that accelerates after age 45 so that by age 60, it averages 11% below values for 35-year-old men and 15% below values for 35-year-old women.* Active adults retain a relatively high $\dot{V}O_{2max}$ at all ages, but their aerobic power still declines with advancing years. Research continues to show that one's habitual level of physical activity through middle age determines changes in $\dot{V}O_{2max}$ to a greater extent than does chronological age.

$\dot{V}O_{2max}$ PREDICTIONS FROM WALKING AND RUNNING PERFORMANCE AND ACTIVITY HEART RATE

Directly measuring $\dot{V}O_{2max}$ requires an extensive laboratory and equipment, not to mention considerable motivation on the subject's part to perform "all out." In addition, maximal effort can be hazardous to nonconditioned adults due to undiagnosed medical conditions, lack of proper medical clearance, and lack of established guidelines for appropriate safeguards and supervision.

In view of these requirements, alternative tests can predict $\dot{V}O_{2max}$ from submaximal performance tests. The most popular $\dot{V}O_{2max}$ predictions use walking and running performance. These tests are easily administered and performed by large groups without need for a formal laboratory setting. Running tests assume $\dot{V}O_{2max}$ largely determines distance run in a specified time (>5 or 6 min). The first of the running tests to predict $\dot{V}O_{2max}$ required subjects to run-walk for 15 minutes covering as much distance as possible; a 1968 revision of the test shortened duration to 12 minutes or 1.5 miles.

Research findings suggest that aerobic capacity prediction should be approached with caution when using walking and running performance. Establishing a consistent level of motivation and effective pacing becomes critical for inexperienced subjects. Some individuals may run too fast early in the run and slow down or even stop as the test and fatigue progresses. Other individuals may begin too slowly and continue this way, so their final run score reflects inappropriate pacing or motivation rather than physiologic and metabolic capacity.

Factors other than $\dot{V}O_{2max}$ determine walking-running performance. Five factors contribute to the final $\dot{V}O_{2max}$ predicted score:

1. Body mass
2. Body fatness
3. Economy of effort
4. Percentage of aerobic capacity sustainable without blood lactate buildup
5. Psychological factors

$\dot{V}O_{2max}$ Predictions From Heart Rate

Common tests to predict $\dot{V}O_{2max}$ from physical activity or postactivity heart rates use a standardized submaximal exercise regimen on a bicycle ergometer, motorized treadmill, or step bench. Such tests make use of the essentially linear or straight-line relationship between heart rate and oxygen uptake for various intensities of light to moderately intense activity. The slope of this relationship (i.e., rate of HR increase per unit of $\dot{V}O_2$ increase) reflects the individual's $\dot{V}O_{2max}$. It is estimated by drawing a best-fit straight line through several submaximum points that relate heart rate and oxygen uptake or exercise intensity, and then extending the line to an assumed maximum heart rate (HR_{max}) for the person's age.

Figure 7.15 applies this extrapolation procedure for a trained and untrained subject. Four submaximal measures during bicycle exercise provided the data points to draw the heart rate–oxygen uptake or HR-$\dot{V}O_2$ line. Each person's HR-$\dot{V}O_2$ line tends to be linear, but the slope of the individual lines can differ considerably largely from variations in

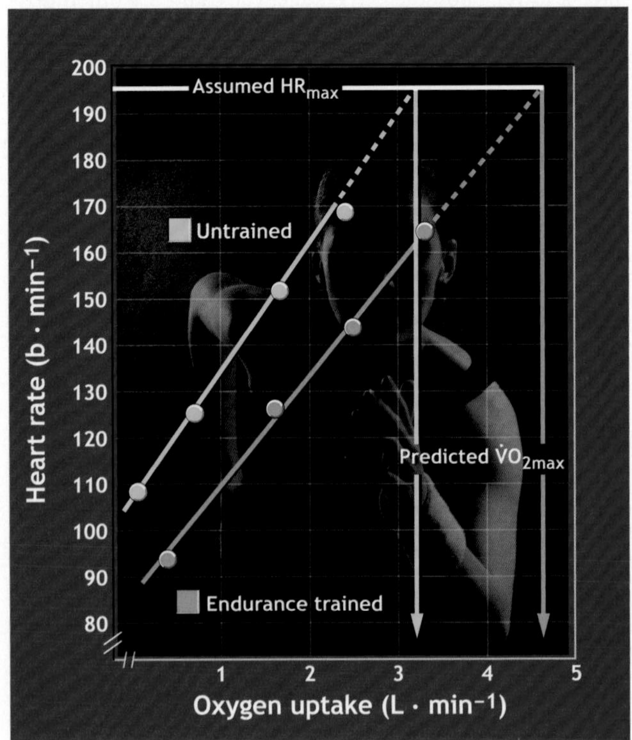

FIGURE 7.15 Extrapolating the linear relationship between submaximal heart rate and oxygen uptake up to an assumed maximum heart rate during graded exercise by an untrained subject and an endurance-trained subject. (Adapted with permission from McArdle WD, Katch FI, Katch VL. *Exercise Physiology: Nutrition, Energy, and Human Performance.* 8th Ed. Baltimore: Wolters Kluwer Health, 2015.)

how much blood the heart pumps with each beat or stroke volume. A person with a relatively high aerobic power can accomplish more activity and achieves a higher oxygen uptake before attaining their HR_{max} than a less "fit" person. The person with the lowest heart rate increase tends to have the highest capacity and largest $\dot{V}O_{2max}$. The data in **Figure 7.15** predict $\dot{V}O_{2max}$ by extrapolating the HR-$\dot{V}O_2$ line to a heart rate of 195 b • min^{-1}, the assumed maximum heart rate for these college-age subjects.

The following four assumptions limit the accuracy of predicting $\dot{V}O_{2max}$ from submaximal exercise heart rate:

1. **Linearity of the HR-$\dot{V}O_2$ (effort, intensity) relationship.** Various intensities of light to moderately intense physical activity meet this assumption. For some subjects, the HR-$\dot{V}O_2$ line curves or asymptotes at intense effort levels in a direction that predicts a larger than expected increase in oxygen uptake per unit increase in heart rate. Oxygen uptake increases more than predicted through linear extrapolation of the HR-$\dot{V}O_2$ line, thus *underestimating* $\dot{V}O_{2max}$.
2. **All subjects have similar maximum heart rates.** The standard deviation for the average maximum heart rate for individuals of the same age averages about ±10 b • min^{-1}. The $\dot{V}O_{2max}$ of a 25-year-old person with a maximum heart rate of 185 b • min^{-1} would be *overestimated* if the HR-$\dot{V}O_2$ line extrapolated to an assumed maximum heart rate for this age group of 195 b • min^{-1}. The opposite would occur if this subject's maximum heart rate equaled 210 b • min^{-1}. HR_{max} also decreases with age. Without considering this age effect, older subjects would consistently be *overestimated* by assuming a maximum heart rate of 195 b • min^{-1}, which represents the appropriate estimation for 25 year olds.
3. **Assumed constant exercise economy.** The predicted $\dot{V}O_{2max}$ varies from variability in exercise economy when estimating submaximal $\dot{V}O_2$ from a particular exercise level. For a subject with low economy (i.e., $\dot{V}O_2$ higher than assumed), the $\dot{V}O_{2max}$ would be *underestimated* because heart rate increases from the additional oxygen cost of uneconomical physical activity. The opposite occurs for a person with high exercise economy. The variation among individuals in $\dot{V}O_2$ during walking, stepping, or cycling does not usually exceed ±6%. Also, seemingly small modifications in

A CLOSER LOOK

A Walking Test to Predict $\dot{V}O_{2max}$

A walking test devised in the 1980s for use on large groups predicts $\dot{V}O_{2max}$ (L • min^{-1}) from the following variables (see Equation 1): body weight (W) in pounds; age (A) in years; gender (G): 0 = female, 1 = male; time (T1) for the 1-mile track walk expressed as minutes and hundredths of a minute; and peak heart rate (HR_{peak}) in beats • min^{-1} at the end of the last quarter mile (measured as a 15-s pulse immediately after the walk × 4 to convert to b • min^{-1}). The test consisted of having individuals walk 1 mile as fast as possible without jogging or running.

For most individuals, $\dot{V}O_{2max}$ ranged within ±0.335 L • min^{-1} (±4.4 mL • kg^{-1} • min^{-1}) of actual $\dot{V}O_{2max}$. This prediction method applies to a broad segment of the general population ages 30 to 69).

Equations

Equation 1

Predicts $\dot{V}O_{2max}$ in L • min^{-1}:

$$\begin{aligned}\dot{V}O_{2max} = {} & 6.9652 + (0.0091 \times W) \\ & - (0.0257 \times A) \\ & + (0.5955 \times G) - (0.224 \times T1) \\ & - (0.0115 \times HR_{peak})\end{aligned}$$

Equation 2

Predicts $\dot{V}O_{2max}$ in mL • kg^{-1} • min^{-1}:

$$\begin{aligned}\dot{V}O_{2max} = {} & 132.853 - (0.0769 \times W) \\ & - (0.3877 \times A) + (6.315 \times G) \\ & - (3.2649 \times T1) \\ & - (0.1565 \times HR_{peak})\end{aligned}$$

Example

Predict $\dot{V}O_{2max}$ (mL • kg^{-1} • min^{-1}) from the following data: gender, female; age, 30 years; body weight, 155.5 lb; T1, 13.56 minute; HR_{peak}, 145 b • min^{-1}.

Substituting the above values in Equation 2:

$$\begin{aligned}\dot{V}O_{2max} = {} & 132.853 - (0.0769 \times 155.5) \\ & - (0.3877 \times 30.0) + (6.315 \times 0) \\ & - (3.2649 \times 13.56) \\ & - (0.1565 \times 145) \\ = {} & 132.853 - (11.96) - (11.63) \\ & + (0) - (44.27) - (22.69) \\ = {} & 42.3\ mL \cdot kg^{-1} \cdot min^{-1}\end{aligned}$$

Reference

Kline G, et al. Estimation of $\dot{V}O_{2max}$ from a one-mile track walk, gender, age, and body weight. *Med Sci Sports Exerc* 1987;19:253.

test procedures profoundly affect the metabolic cost of physical activity. Allowing individuals to support themselves with treadmill handrails reduces the oxygen cost by up to 30%. Also, failure to maintain a preset cadence on a bicycle, elliptical trainer, rowing machine, or step bench will dramatically alter the oxygen requirement.

4. **Day-to-day variation in activity heart rate.** Even under highly standardized conditions, an individual's submaximal heart rate varies by about ±5 beats per minute with day-to-day testing at the same intensity. This variation in activity heart rate represents an additional error source.

Considering these four limitations, $\dot{V}O_{2max}$ predicted from submaximal heart rate generally falls within 10% to 20% of the person's measured $\dot{V}O_{2max}$. *Clearly, this represents an unacceptably large error for research purposes.* These tests are better suited in the health club environment for general fitness screening and classification.

A Word of Caution About Predictions

All predictions involve some type of error. The total error, referred to as the **standard error of estimate (SEE)**, computes from the original equation that generated the prediction. Errors of estimate are expressed in units of the predicted variable or as a percentage. For example, suppose the $\dot{V}O_{2max}$ in $mL \cdot kg^{-1} \cdot min^{-1}$ prediction from a walking test equals 55 $mL \cdot kg^{-1}$ min^{-1} and the SEE of the predicted score equals ±10 $mL \cdot kg^{-1} \cdot min^{-1}$. In reality, this means the actual $\dot{V}O_{2max}$ probably ranges within ±10 $mL \cdot kg^{-1} \cdot min^{-1}$ of the predicted value or between 45 and 65 $mL \cdot kg^{-1} \cdot min^{-1}$. This amount of error is referred to as the 68% likelihood range. In this case, it represents a relatively large error, equivalent to ±18.2% of the actual value, resulting in a less than useful predicted score because the true score falls within such a broad range of possible values. *The take home message seems clear—one cannot judge the usefulness of predicted scores without knowing the magnitude of the error.* Whenever making predictions, the predicted score should be interpreted relative to the magnitude of prediction error. Fortunately, $\dot{V}O_{2max}$ prediction proves useful in appropriate situations when one cannot directly measure the $\dot{V}O_{2max}$ and when the SEE remains small.

SUMMARY

1. Direct and indirect calorimetry determine the body's rate of energy expenditure.
2. Direct calorimetry measures actual heat production in an insulated calorimeter.
3. Indirect calorimetry infers energy expenditure from oxygen uptake and carbon dioxide production using closed- or open-circuit spirometry.
4. All energy-releasing reactions ultimately depend on oxygen use.
5. Measuring oxygen uptake during steady-rate physical activity provides an indirect yet accurate estimate of energy expenditure.
6. Three common open-circuit, indirect calorimetric procedures to measure oxygen uptake during physical activity are portable spirometry, bag technique, and computerized instrumentation.
7. Complete oxidation of each nutrient requires a different quantity of oxygen uptake compared with carbon dioxide production.
8. The ratio of carbon dioxide produced to oxygen consumed or RQ provides important information about the nutrient mixture catabolized for energy.
9. The RQ averages 1.00 for carbohydrate, 0.70 for fat, and 0.82 for protein.
10. For each RQ value, a corresponding caloric value exists for 1 L of oxygen consumed.
11. The RQ-kcal relationship determines energy expenditure during steady-rate physical activity with a high degree of accuracy.
12. During strenuous physical activity, the respiratory exchange ratio (R or RER) does not represent specific substrate use because of nonmetabolic production of carbon dioxide in lactate buffering or from activity hyperventilation or processes related to recovery.
13. $\dot{V}O_{2max}$ provides reliable and important information about power of the long-term aerobic energy system, including functional capacity of various physiologic support systems.
14. A leveling-off or peaking-over in oxygen uptake during increasing exercise intensity signifies attainment of maximum capacity for aerobic metabolism (i.e., a "true" $\dot{V}O_{2max}$).
15. The term *peak oxygen uptake* ($\dot{V}O_{2peak}$) describes the highest oxygen uptake when the accepted criteria for $\dot{V}O_{2max}$ is not met or local muscle fatigue in the arms or legs rather than central circulatory dynamics limits test performance.
16. Different standardized test protocols measure $\dot{V}O_{2max}$; they remain independent of muscle strength, speed, body size, and skill, with the exception of specialized swimming, rowing, and ice skating tests.
17. The $\dot{V}O_{2max}$ test may require a continuous 3- to 5-minute "supermaximal" effort but usually consists of progressive increments in exercise intensity referred to as a graded exercise test or GXT.
18. Two types of $\dot{V}O_{2max}$ tests involve either a continuous test without rest between exercise increments or a discontinuous test with several minutes of rest between exercise increments.
19. Important factors that influence $\dot{V}O_{2max}$ include activity mode, training state, heredity, gender, body composition, and age.
20. Differences in body mass explain roughly 70% of the differences among individuals in absolute $\dot{V}O_{2max}$ expressed in $L \cdot min^{-1}$.
21. Changes in $\dot{V}O_{2max}$ generally relate inversely to chronological age.

22. Tests to predict $\dot{V}O_{2max}$ from submaximal physiologic and performance data prove useful to classify individuals into discrete fitness categories.
23. The validity of heart rate prediction equations relies on the following assumptions: linearity of the HR-$\dot{V}O_2$ line, similar maximal heart rate for individuals of the same age, a constant exercise economy, and relatively small day-to-day variation in physical activity heart rate.
24. Field methods to predict $\dot{V}O_{2max}$ are better suited in the health club environment for general fitness screening and classification.

THINK IT THROUGH

1. How have exercise physiologists determined between 70% and 80% of the energy during the last phases of a marathon run comes from fat combustion?
2. What rationale underlies early experiments that quantified energy metabolism of small animals by measuring the rate that ice melted in an insulated container that surrounded the animal?
3. Discuss pros and cons of predicting $\dot{V}O_{2max}$ from submaximal variables.
4. Explain how oxygen uptake translates to heat production during all modes of physical activity.
5. Justify measuring only CO_2 to measure energy expenditure during steady-rate physical activity.
6. Discuss four variables that influence an individual's $\dot{V}O_{2max}$.
7. Explain why $\dot{V}O_{2max}$ values do not always agree when measured directly in the laboratory and predicted with a 12-minute run-walk test.

KEY TERMS

Anaerobic capacity: Total mechanical work in a given time period during short-duration maximal effort.

Anaerobic fatigue: Percentage decline in power output during short-duration maximal effort.

Anaerobic work (AW): Total work accomplished in watts for the 30-second test duration.

Atwater-Rosa calorimeter: First human calorimeter to measure energy metabolism. Designed by research scientists W.O. Atwater and E.B. Rosa in the 1890s, it consisted of a small chamber where the subject lived, ate, slept, and performed daily cycle ergometer exercise.

Calibration: Method to assess accuracy (validity) and consistency (reliability) of a measurement instrument.

Caloric value for oxygen: Energy release in kcal measured by bomb calorimetry for a given nutrient when burned in 1 L oxygen.

Calorie: Quantity of heat necessary to raise the temperature of 1 kg (1 L) of water 1°C from 14.5°C to 15.5°C.

Closed-circuit spirometry: Uses principles of indirect calorimetry to estimate energy expenditure. The subject rebreathes 100% oxygen from a prefilled spirometer with a canister of soda lime placed in the breathing circuit to absorb the exhaled carbon dioxide. The difference between initial and final oxygen volumes indicates the oxygen uptake during the measurement interval.

Continuous GXT test: Graded exercise test where increments of intensity and duration continue without rest periods until the subject will not successfully complete a full exercise increment.

Direct calorimetry: Directly measuring heat as kcal transferred directly from combustion of food in a bomb calorimeter or heat produced by a person in a human calorimeter.

Discontinuous GXT test: Graded exercise test where increments of intensity and duration continue for a preset time interspersed with rest periods until the subject will not successfully complete a full exercise increment.

Doubly labeled water technique: Isotope-based method using ^2H or deuterium and oxygen ^{18}O or oxygen-18 to safely estimate total and average daily energy expenditure of groups of children and adults in free-living conditions without the normal constraints imposed by laboratory procedures.

Generality of metabolic capacity: Individuals with a high $\dot{V}O_{2max}$ in one mode of physical activity also possess above-average aerobic capacity in other diverse forms of activity.

Graded exercise test (GXT): Laboratory exercise test that involves progressive increases in intensity (speed, resistance) or duration until the subject voluntarily stops exercising.

Human calorimeter: Special human chamber for purposes of directly measuring heat production.

Immediate energy system: Energy system that derives from the catabolism of ATP-PCr energy reserves.

Indirect calorimetry: Method of calculating heat production of living organisms by measuring either carbon dioxide production or oxygen uptake or both over a given duration.

Individual differences: True differences *among* individuals on test variables such as $\dot{V}O_{2max}$; distinguished from trial-to-trial differences *within* an individual.

Katch test: "All-out" stationary cycling test of short duration to estimate power of the anaerobic energy systems. Frictional resistance is 6 kg for men and 5 kg for women, and test duration 40 seconds.

Lactate buffering: Lactate generated during anaerobic metabolism undergoes buffering to reduce its acidic effect as, for example, sodium bicarbonate (in blood) buffers excess lactic acid.

Law of the conservation of energy: The total energy of an isolated system that can neither be created nor destroyed but changes from one form to another.

Nonprotein RQ: Portion of the respiratory exchange attributed to only carbohydrate and fat combustion excluding protein.

Open-circuit spirometry: Subject inhales ambient air (20.93% O_2, 0.03% CO_2, and 79.04% N_2), such that differences between inspired and expired gas concentrations reflect the ongoing process of oxygen uptake and thus energy metabolism.

Peak oxygen uptake ($\dot{V}O_{2peak}$): The highest measured oxygen uptake value during a test when the accepted $\dot{V}O_{2max}$ criteria are not met, or local arm or leg muscle fatigue rather than central circulatory dynamics limit test performance.

Peak power: Highest mechanical power output measured in watts generated during a short-duration maximal physical effort.

Rate of fatigue: Rate of decline in power output relative to peak power output.

Relative peak power (RPP) output: Peak power output (W) relative to body mass: PP ÷ body mass (kg).

Relative power: Peak power output divided by body weight as $W \cdot kg^{-1} \cdot min^{-1}$.

Respiratory exchange ratio (R or RER): Computes the same as RQ, and reflects the ratio of carbon dioxide produced to oxygen consumed under conditions of nonsteady-rate physical activity.

Respiratory quotient (RQ): Ratio of carbon dioxide produced to oxygen consumed with complete oxidation of a nutrient measured during steady-rate metabolic conditions; calculated as RQ = CO_2 produced ÷ O_2 consumed.

Short-term energy system (rapid glycolysis): Energy system that derives from glucose breakdown in glycolysis; refers to rapid glycolytic production of ATP resulting in lactate formation.

Specificity of metabolic capacity: Individuals with a high $\dot{V}O_{2max}$ in one form of exercise do not possess above-average aerobic capacity in other diverse activities.

Standard error of estimate (SEE): Error component calculated as the standard deviation of scores on a repeated test variable, as, for example, multiple resting heart rate scores taken in succession over 5 minutes; the standard deviation of the prediction errors.

Supermaximal effort levels: Work output that is considerably above effort that produces an individual's $\dot{V}O_{2max}$.

Time-rate of doing work: Work accomplished per unit of time; usually referred to as "power" ($P = (F \times D) \div T$ where F equals force generated, D equals distance through which the force moves, T equals time).

Watts: Expression of power; 1 W = 0.73756 ft-lb $\cdot$ s^{-1} or 6.12 kg-m $\cdot$ min^{-1}.

Wingate test: Test to assess the anaerobic energy system power output using all-out stationary cycling for 30-second of supermaximal effort with resistance of 0.075 kg per kg body weight.

SELECTED REFERENCES

Aisbett B, et al. The influence of pacing during 6-minute supra-maximal cycle ergometer performance. *J Sci Med Sport* 2003;6:187.

Álvarez C, et al. Eight weeks of combined high intensity intermittent exercise normalized altered metabolic parameters in women. *Rev Med Chil* 2014;142:458.

Amann M, et al. An evaluation of the predictive validity and reliability of ventilatory threshold. *Med Sci Sports Exerc* 2004;36:1716.

Anderson O. *Running Science*. Champaign: Human Kinetics Press, 2013.

Angius L, et al. Measurement of pulmonary gas exchange variables and lactic anaerobic capacity during field testing in elite indoor football players. *J Sports Med Phys Fitness* 2013;53:46.

Armstrong N, Welsman JR. Assessment and interpretation of aerobic fitness in children and adolescents. *Exerc Sport Sci Rev* 1994;22:435.

Atwater WO, Rosa EB. *Description of a New Respiration Calorimeter and Experiments on the Conservation of Energy in the Human Body*. Bulletin No. 63, U.S. Department of Agriculture, Office of Experiment Stations. Washington, DC: Government Printing Office, 1899.

Baker J, et al. Anaerobic performance in obese populations: underestimation of power profiles. *Asian J Sports Med* 2013;4:82.

Balke B, Ware RW. An experimental study of fitness of Air Force personnel. *U S Armed Forces Med J* 1959;10:675.

Balmer J, et al. Mechanically braked Wingate powers: agreement between SRM, corrected and conventional methods of measurement. *J Sports Sci* 2004; 22:661.

Bar-Or O. The Wingate anaerobic test: an update on methodology, reliability, and validity. *Sports Med* 1987;4:381.

Bentley DJ, McNaughton LR. Comparison of W(peak), $\dot{V}O_2$(peak) and the ventilation threshold from two different incremental exercise tests: relationship to endurance performance. *J Sci Med Sport* 2003;6:422.

Bergstrom HC, et al. Physiologic responses to a thermogenic nutritional supplement at rest, during low-intensity exercise, and during recovery from exercise in college-aged women. *Appl Physiol Nutr Metab* 2013;38:988.

Binzoni T. Saturation of the lactate clearance mechanisms different from the "lactate shuttle" determines the anaerobic threshold: prediction from the bioenergetic model. *J Physiol Anthropol Appl Human Sci* 2005;24:175.

Blain G, et al. Assessment of ventilatory thresholds during graded and maximal exercise test using time varying analysis of respiratory sinus arrhythmia. *Br J Sports Med* 2005;39:448.

Bosquet L, et al. Methods to determine aerobic endurance. *Sports Med* 2002;32:675.

Bouchard C, et al. Familial resemblance for in the sedentary state: the HERITAGE Family Study. *Med Sci Sports Exerc* 1998;30:252.

Bouchard C, et al. Genetics of aerobic and anaerobic performance. *Exerc Sport Sci Rev* 1992;20:27.

Bouchard C, et al. Genomic predictors of the maximal O_2 uptake response to standardized exercise training programs. *J Appl Physiol* 2011;110:1160.

Bouchard C, Pérusse L. Heredity, activity level, fitness, and health. In: Bouchard C, et al., eds. *Physical Activity, Fitness, and Health*. Champaign: Human Kinetics, 1994.

Bouchard C, et al. Testing anaerobic power and capacity. In: MacKougall J, et al., eds. *Physiological Testing of the High Performance Athlete*. Champaign: Human Kinetics Press, 1991:175222.

Bouchard C, et al. Familial resemblance for $\dot{V}O_{2max}$ in the sedentary state: the Heritage family study. *Med Sci Sports Exerc* 1998;30:252.

Bouhlel H, et al. Effect of Ramadan observance on maximal muscular performance of trained men. *Clin J Sport Med* 2013;23:222.

Brooks GA. Intra- and extra-cellular lactate shuttles. *Med Sci Sports Exerc* 2000;32:790.

Buchfuhrer MJ, et al. Optimizing the exercise protocol for cardiopulmonary assessment. *J Appl Physiol* 1983;55:1558.

Buchheit M, et al. Predicting changes in high-intensity intermittent running performance with acute responses to short jump rope workouts in children. *J Sports Sci Med* 2014;13:476.

Buresh R, Berg K. Scaling oxygen uptake to body size and several practical applications. *J Strength Cond Res* 2002;16:46.

Buskirk ER, Hodgson JL. Age and aerobic power: the rate of change in men and women. *Fed Proc* 1997;46:1824.

Busso T, et al. A comparison of modelling procedures used to estimate the power-exhaustion time relationship. *Eur J Appl Physiol* 2010;108:257.

Cain SM. Mechanisms which control $\dot{V}O_2$ near $\dot{V}O_{2max}$: an overview. *Med Sci Sports Exerc* 1995;27:60.

Canavan PK, Vescovi JD. Evaluation of power prediction equations: peak vertical jumping power in women. *Med Sci Sports Exerc* 2004;36:1589.

Carey P, et al. Comparison of oxygen uptake during maximal work on the rowing ergometer. *Med Sci Sports* 1974;6:101.

Castellani JW, et al. Energy expenditure in men and women during 54 h of exercise and caloric deprivation. *Med Sci Sports Exerc* 2006;38:894.

Conway JM, et al. Comparison of energy expenditure estimates from doubly labeled water, a physical activity questionnaire, and physical activity records. *Am J Clin Nutr* 2002;75:519.

Cooper K. Correlation between field and treadmill testing as a means for assessing maximal oxygen intake. *JAMA* 1968;203:201.
Cooper SM, et al. A simple multistage field test for the prediction of anaerobic capacity in female games players. *Br J Sports Med* 2004;38:784.
Coquart JB, et al. Prediction of peak oxygen uptake from sub-maximal ratings of perceived exertion elicited during a graded exercise test in obese women. *Psychophysiology* 2009;46:1150.
Crandall CG, et al. Evaluation of the Cosmed K2 portable telemetric oxygen uptake analyzer. *Med Sci Sports Exerc* 1994;26:108.
Dallmeijer AJ, et al. Test-retest reliability of the 20-sec Wingate Test to assess anaerobic power in children with cerebral palsy. *Am J Phys Med Rehabil* 2013;92:762.
de Sousa MV, et al. Carbohydrate beverages attenuate bone resorption markers in elite runners. *Metabolism* 2014;63:1536.
Doolittle TL, Bigbee R. The twelve-minute run-walk: a test of cardiorespiratory fitness of adolescent boys. *Res Q* 1968;39:41.
Duncan GE, et al. Applicability of $\dot{V}O_{2max}$ criteria: discontinuous versus continuous protocols. *Med Sci Sports Exerc* 1997;29:273.
Dunn SL, et al. The effect of a lifestyle intervention on metabolic health in young women. *Diabetes Metab Syndr Obes* 2014;7:437.
Ekelund U, et al. Energy expenditure assessed by heart rate and doubly labeled water in young athletes. *Med Sci Sports Exerc* 2002;34:1360.
Eston R, et al. Prediction of maximal oxygen uptake in sedentary males from a perceptually regulated, sub-maximal graded exercise test. *J Sports Sci* 2008;26:131.
Fairshter RD, et al. A comparison of incremental exercise tests during cycle and treadmill ergometry. *Med Sci Sports Exerc* 1983;15:549.
Ferguson RJ, et al. A maximal oxygen uptake test during ice skating. *Med Sci Sports* 1969;1:207.
Fleg JL, et al. Accelerated longitudinal decline of aerobic capacity in healthy older adults. *Circulation* 2005;112:674.
Flinn S, et al. Differential effect of metabolic alkalosis and hypoxia on high-intensity cycling performance. *J Strength Cond Res* 2014;28:2852.
Flouris AD, et al. Prediction of $\dot{V}O_{2max}$ from a new field test based on portable indirect calorimetry. *J Sci Med Sport* 2010;13:70.
George JD, et al. Non-exercise estimation for physically active college students. *Med Sci Sports Exerc* 1997;29:415.
Gergley T, et al. Specificity of arm training on aerobic power during swimming and running. *Med Sci Sports Exerc* 1984;16:349.
Gladden LB. Muscle as a consumer of lactate. *Med Sci Sports Exerc* 2000;32:764.
Gladden LB. The role of skeletal muscle in lactate exchange during exercise: introduction. *Med Sci Sports Exerc* 2000;32:753.
Gonnissen HK, et al. Overnight energy expenditure determined by whole-body indirect calorimetry does not differ during different sleep stages. *Am J Clin Nutr* 2013;98:867.
Gore JC, et al. CPX/D underestimates O_2 in athletes compared with an automated Douglas bag system. *Med Sci Sports Exerc* 2003;35:1341.
Hagberg JM, et al. Specific genetic markers of endurance performance and $\dot{V}O_{2max}$. *Exerc Sport Sci Rev* 2001;29:15.
Haldane JS, Priestley JG. *Respiration*. New York: Oxford University Press, 1935.
Hetzler RK, et al. Development of a modified Margaria-Kalamen anaerobic power test for American football athletes. *Strength Cond Res* 2010;24:978.
Hirvonen J, et al. Breakdown of high-energy phosphate compounds and lactate accumulation during short supramaximal exercise. *Eur J Appl Physiol* 1987;56:253.
Howley ET, et al. Criteria for maximal oxygen uptake: review and commentary. *Med Sci Sports Exerc* 1995;27:1292.
Iacono AD, et al. Improving fitness of elite handball players: small-sided games vs. high-intensity intermittent training. *J Strength Cond Res* 2015;29:835.
Jackson A, et al. Role of lifestyle and aging on the longitudinal change in cardiorespiratory fitness. *Arch Intern Med* 2009;169:1781.
Jéquier E, Schutz Y. Long-term measurements of energy expenditure in humans using a respiration chamber. *Am J Clin Nutr* 1983;38:989.
Jo E. Influence of recovery duration after a potentiating stimulus on muscular power in recreationally trained individuals. *J Strength Cond Res* 2010;24:343.
Joao P, et al. Physical and physiological demands of beach volleyball game: an analysis based on GPS. World Congress of Performance Analysis of Sport X. Opatija, Croatia, September 3–6, 2014. Abstract.
Jones AM. Influence of dietary nitrate on the physiological determinants of exercise performance: a critical review. *Appl Physiol Nutr Metab* 2014;39:1019.
Jurca R, et al. Assessing cardiorespiratory fitness without performing exercise testing. *Am J Prev Med* 2005;29:185.
Kannan U, et al. Effect of exercise intensity on lipid profile in sedentary obese adults. *J Clin Diagn Res* 2014;8:BC08.
Kasch FW, et al. A comparison of maximal oxygen uptake by treadmill and step test procedures. *J Appl Physiol* 1966;21:1387.
Katch FI, et al. Maximal oxygen intake, endurance running performance, and body composition in college women. *Res Q* 1973;44:301.
Katch V, et al. A steady-paced versus all-out cycling strategy for maximal work output of short duration. *Res Q* 1976;47:164.
Katch V. Body weight, leg volume, leg weight and leg density as determiners of short duration work performance on the bicycle ergometer. *Med Sci Sports* 1974;6:267.
Katch V. Kinetics of oxygen uptake and recovery for supramaximal work of short duration. *Eur J Appl Physiol* 1973;31:197.
Katch VL, et al. Optimal test characteristics for maximal anaerobic work on the bicycle ergometer. *Res Q* 1977;48:319.
Kiely C, et al. Hemodynamic responses during graded and constant-load plantar flexion exercise in middle-aged men and women with type 2 diabetes. *J Appl Physiol* 2014;117:755.
Kline G, et al. Estimation of from a one-mile track walk, gender, age, and body weight. *Med Sci Sports Exerc* 1987;19:253.
Klissouras V, et al. Adaptation to maximal effort: genetics and age. *J Appl Physiol* 1973;35:288.
Koffranyi E, Michaelis HF. Ein tragbarer apparat zur bestimmung des gasstoffwechsels. *Arbeitsphysiologie* 1940;11:148.
Kohler RM, et al. Peak power during repeated Wingate trials: implications for testing. *J Strength Cond Res* 2010;24:370.
Krogh A, Lindhard J. The relative value of fat and carbohydrate as sources of muscular energy. *Biochem J* 1920;14:290.
Kyröläinen H. Comparison between direct and predicted maximal oxygen uptake measurement during cycling. *Mil Med* 2013;178:234.
Lamberts RP, Davidowitz KJ. Allometric scaling and predicting cycling performance in (well-) trained female cyclists. *Int J Sports Med* 2014;35:217.
Lau PW, et al. Effects of high-intensity intermittent running exercise in overweight children. *Eur J Sport Sci* 2014;11:1.
Little JP, et al. A practical model of low-volume high-intensity interval training induces mitochondrial biogenesis in human skeletal muscle: potential mechanisms. *J Physiol* 2010;588.
Loe H, et al. Aerobic capacity reference data in 3816 healthy men and women 20–90 years. *PLoS One* 2013;8:e64319.
Maes HH, et al. Inheritance of physical fitness in 10-yr-old twins and their parents. *Med Sci Sports Exerc* 1996;28:1479.
Magel JR, Faulkner JA. Maximum oxygen uptake of college swimmers. *J Appl Physiol* 1967;22:929.
Maksud MG, Coutts KD. Application of the Cooper twelve-minute run-walk to young males. *Res Q* 1971;42:54.
Margaria R, et al. Measurement of muscular power (anaerobic) in man. *J Appl Physiol* 1966;21:1662.
Mayhew JL, Salm PC. Gender differences in anaerobic power tests. *Eur J Appl Physiol* 1990;60:133.
McArdle WD, et al. Metabolic and cardiorespiratory response during free swimming and treadmill walking. *J Appl Physiol* 1971;30:733.
McArdle WD, et al. Reliability and inter-relationships between maximal oxygen intake, physical work capacity, and step-test scores in college women. *Med Sci Sports* 1972;4:182.
McArdle WD, et al. Specificity of run training on VO_{2max} and heart rate changes during running and swimming. *Med Sci Sports* 1978;10:16.
McLester JR, et al. Effects of standing vs. seated posture on repeated Wingate performance. *J Strength Cond Res* 2004;18:816.
McMurray RG, et al. Predicted maximal aerobic power in youth is related to age, gender, and ethnicity. *Med Sci Sports Exerc* 2002;34:145.
Medbo JL, et al. Relative importance of aerobic and anaerobic energy release during short-lasting exhausting exercise. *J Appl Physiol* 1989;67:1881.
Meredith CN, et al. Body composition and aerobic capacity in young and middle-aged endurance-trained men. *Med Sci Sports Exerc* 1987;19:557.
Missitzi J, et al. Heritability in neuromuscular coordination: implications for motor control strategies. *Med Sci Sports Exerc* 2004;36:233.
Montgomery HE, et al. Human gene for physical performance. *Nature* 1998;393:221.
Montoye HJ, et al. *Measuring Physical Activity and Energy Expenditure*. Boca Raton: Human Kinetics, 1996.
Moore A, Murphy A. Development of an anaerobic capacity test for field sport athletes. *J Sci Med Sport* 2003;6:275.
Murgatroyd RR, James WPT. Energy measurement in man by direct calorimetry. In: Björntorp P, et al., eds. *Recent Advances in Obesity Research*. London: John-Libby, 1982.
Mustelin L, et al. Genetic influences on physical activity in young adults: a twin study. *Med Sci Sports Exerc* 2012;44:1293.
Nascimento PC, et al. The effect of prior exercise intensity on oxygen uptake kinetics during high-intensity running exercise in trained subjects. *Eur J Appl Physiol* 2015;115:147.
Newton RL, et al. The energy expenditure of sedentary behavior: a whole room calorimeter study. *PLoS One* 2013;8:e63171.
Nieman DC, et al. Validity of COSMED's quark CPET mixing chamber system in evaluating energy metabolism during aerobic exercise in healthy male adults. *Res Sports Med* 2013;21:136.
Nikooie R, et al. Noninvasive determination of anaerobic threshold by monitoring the %SpO2 changes and respiratory gas exchange. *J Strength Cond Res* 2009;23:2107.
Okada Triana R, et al. Can information on remaining time modulate psycho-physiological parameters during an intermittent exercise? *J Sports Med Phys Fitness* 2014. (InPress as of 06.05.15.)
Ouergui I, et al. Anaerobic upper and lower body power measurements and perception of fatigue during a kick boxing match. *J Sports Med Phys Fitness* 2013;53:455.

Padulo J, et al. A paradigm of uphill running. *PLoS One* 2013;8:e69006.
Panissa VL, et al. Acute effect of high-intensity aerobic exercise performed on treadmill and cycle ergometer on strength performance. *J Strength Cond Res* September 25, 2014.
Porszasz J, et al. A treadmill ramp protocol using simultaneous changes in speed and grade. *Med Sci Sports Exerc* 2003;35:1596.
Potteiger JA, et al. Relationship between body composition, leg strength, anaerobic power, and on-ice skating performance in division I men's hockey athletes. *J Strength Cond Res* 2010;24:1755.
Rampinini E, et al. Accuracy of GPS devices for measuring high-intensity running in field-based team sports. *Int J Sports Med* 2015;36:49.
Ravussin E, et al. Determinants of 24-hour energy expenditure in man: methods and results using a respiratory chamber. *J Clin Invest* 1986;78:1568.
Rico-Sanz J, et al. Familial resemblance for muscle phenotypes in the HERITAGE Family Study. *Med Sci Sports Exerc* 2003;35:1360.
Robertson HT. Imaging tools for the investigation of human gas exchange. *J Appl Physiol* 2013;115:309.
Rowland TW. Does peak reflect in children? *Med Sci Sports Exerc* 1993; 25:689.
Rumpler W, et al. Repeatability of 24-hour energy expenditure measurements in humans by indirect calorimetry. *Am J Clin Nutr* 1990;51:147.
Sartor F, et al. Estimation of maximal oxygen uptake via submaximal exercise testing in sports, clinical, and home settings. *Sports Med* 2013;43:865.
Schafer MA, et al. Intensity selection and regulation using the OMNI scale of perceived exertion during intermittent exercise. *Appl Physiol Nutr Metab* 2013;38:960.
Scholander PF. Analyzer for accurate estimation of respiratory gases in one-half cubic centimeter samples. *J Biol Chem* 1947;167:235.
Schutz Y, Deurenberg P. Energy metabolism: overview of recent methods used in human studies. *Ann Nutr Metab* 1996;40:183.
Scott B, et al. The maximally accumulated oxygen deficit as an indicator of anaerobic capacity. *Med Sci Sports Exerc* 1991;23:618.
Scribbans TD, et al. Heart rate during basketball game play and volleyball drills accurately predicts oxygen uptake and energy expenditure. *J Sports Med Phys Fitness* 2014 October 17.
Seiler S, et al. The fall and rise of the gender difference in elite anaerobic performance 1952–2006. *Med Sci Sports Exerc* 2007;39:534.
Sentija D, et al. The effects of strength training on some parameters of aerobic and anaerobic endurance. *Coll Antropol* 2009;33:111.
Slinde F, et al. Minnesota leisure time activity questionnaire and doubly labeled water in adolescents. *Med Sci Sports Exerc* 2003;35:1923.
Snell PG, et al. Maximal oxygen uptake as a parametric measure of cardiorespiratory capacity. *Med Sci Sports Exerc* 2007;39:103.
Souissi N, et al. Diurnal variation in Wingate test performances: influence of active warm-up. *Chronobiol Int* 2010;27:640.
Sparks SA, et al. The effect of carrying a portable respiratory gas analysis system on energy expenditure during incremental running. *Appl Ergon* 2013;44:55.
Sparks SA, et al. The energy demands of portable gas analysis system carriage during walking and running. *Ergonomics* 2013;56:1901.
Speakman JR. The history and theory of the doubly labeled water technique. *Am J Clin Nutr* 1998;68:932S.
Spencer MR, Gastin PB. Energy system contribution during 200-m to 1500-m running in highly trained athletes. *Med Sci Sports Exerc* 2001;33:157.
Stanula A, et al. The role of aerobic capacity in high-intensity intermittent efforts in ice-hockey. *Biol Sport* 2014;31:193.
Strømme SB, et al. Assessment of maximal aerobic power in specially trained athletes. *J Appl Physiol* 1977;42:833.
Stroud MA, et al. Energy expenditure using isotope-labeled water (2H18O), exercise performance, skeletal muscle enzyme activities and plasma biochemical parameters in humans during 95 days of endurance exercise with inadequate energy intake. *Eur J Appl Physiol* 1997;76:243.
Suminski RR, et al. The effect of habitual smoking on measured and predicted $\dot{V}O_2$(max). *J Phys Act Health* 2009;6:667.
Taylor HL, et al. Maximal oxygen intake as an objective measure of cardiorespiratory performance. *J Appl Physiol* 1955;8:73.
Tiainen K, et al. Heritability of maximal isometric muscle strength in older female twins. *J Appl Physiol* 2004;96:173.
Uth N, et al. Estimation of VO_{2max} from the ratio between HR_{max} and HR_{rest}—the heart rate ratio method. *Eur J Appl Physiol* 2004;91:111.
Vandenberghe K, et al. No effect of glycogen level on glycogen metabolism during high intensity exercise. *Med Sci Sports Exerc* 1995;27:1278.
Vandewalle H, et al. Standard anaerobic exercise test. *Sports Med* 1987;4:268.
Vogel JA, et al. An analysis of aerobic capacity in a large United States population. *J Appl Physiol* 1986;60:494.
Waldron M, Highton J. Fatigue and pacing in high-intensity intermittent team sport: an update. *Sports Med* 2014;44:1645.
Wang L, et al. Time constant of heart rate recovery after low level exercise as a useful measure of cardiovascular fitness. *Conf Proc IEEE Eng Med Biol Soc* 2006;1:1799.
Wasserman K, et al. *Principles of Exercise Testing and Interpretation.* 3rd Ed. Baltimore: Lippincott Williams & Wilkins, 1999.
Wedin JO, Henriksson AE. Postgame elevation of cardiac markers among elite floorball players. *Scand J Med Sci Sports* 2014. doi: 10.1111/sms.12304.
Weltman A, et al. Exercise recovery, lactate removal, and subsequent high intensity exercise performance. *Res Q* 1977;48:786.
Weltman A, et al. The lactate threshold and endurance performance. *Adv Sports Med Fitness* 1989;2:91.
Westerterp KR, et al. Comparison of doubly labeled water with respirometry at low- and high-activity levels. *J Appl Physiol* 1988;65:53.
Westerterp KR. Physical activity and physical activity induced energy expenditure in humans: measurement, determinants, and effects. *Front Physiol* 2013;4:90.
Weyand PG, et al. Peak oxygen deficit during one- and two-legged cycling in men and women. *Med Sci Sports Exerc* 1993;25:584.
White GE, et al. The effect of various cold-water immersion protocols on exercise-induced inflammatory response and functional recovery from high-intensity sprint exercise. *Eur J Appl Physiol* 2014;114:2353.
Wideman L, et al. Assessment of the Aerosport TEEM 100 portable metabolic measurement system. *Med Sci Sports Exerc* 1996;28:509.
Wiedemann MS, Bosquet L. Anaerobic Work Capacity derived from isokinetic and isoinertial cycling. *Int J Sports Med* 2010;31:89.
Wilmore JH. Influence of motivation on physical work capacity and performance. *J Appl Physiol* 1968;24:459.
Yamashita N, et al. Two percent hypohydration does not impair self-selected high intensity intermittent exercise performance. *J Strength Cond Res* 2015; 29:116.
Yoon BL, et al. $\dot{V}O_{2max}$, protocol duration, and the $\dot{V}O_2$ plateau. *Med Sci Sports Exerc* 2007;39:1186.
Zagatto AM, et al. Validity of the running anaerobic sprint test for assessing anaerobic power and predicting short-distance performance. *J Strength Cond Res* 2009;23:1820.
Zajac A, et al. The diagnostic value of the 10- and 30-second Wingate test for competitive athletes. *J Strength Cond Res* 1999;13:16.
Zeimetz GA, et al. Quantifiable changes in oxygen uptake, heart rate, and time to target heart rate when hand support is allowed during treadmill exercise. *J Cardiac Rehabil* 1985;11:525.

CHAPTER

8

Energy Expenditure During Rest and Physical Activity

CHAPTER OBJECTIVES

- Define basal metabolic rate and indicate three factors that affect it.
- Explain the effect of body weight on the energy cost of different forms of physical activity.
- Identify three factors that contribute to the total daily energy expenditure.
- Outline two different classification systems to rate physical activity intensity.
- Describe two ways to predict resting daily energy expenditure.
- Explain concepts of exercise efficiency and exercise economy.
- List three factors that affect energy cost of walking and running.
- Identify three factors that contribute to lower exercise economy of swimming compared with running.

ANCILLARIES AT A GLANCE

Visit **http://thePoint.lww.com/MKKESS5e** to access the following resources.

- References: Chapter 8
- Interactive Question Bank

PART 1 Energy Expenditure During Rest

Three factors shown in **Figure 8.1** determine the **total daily energy expenditure (TDEE)**:

1. Resting metabolic rate (includes basal and sleeping conditions plus the added energy cost of arousal)
2. Thermogenic influence of consumed food
3. Energy expended during physical activity and recovery

BASAL (RESTING) METABOLIC RATE

The **basal metabolic rate (BMR)** represents the minimum energy required for an individual to sustain the body's functions in the waking state. Measuring oxygen uptake under the following three standardized conditions quantifies this requirement:

1. No food consumed for a minimum of 12 hours before measurement; the **postabsorptive state** describes this condition
2. No undue muscular exertion for at least 12 hours before assessment
3. Measured after the person has been lying quietly for 30 to 60 minutes in a dimly lit, temperature-controlled, thermoneutral room

Maintaining controlled conditions provides a way to study relationships among energy expenditure and body size, gender, and age. The BMR also establishes a baseline for implementing a prudent program of weight control by food restraint, physical activity, or both. In most instances, basal values measured in the laboratory remain only marginally lower than values for **resting metabolic rate (RMR)** measured under less strict conditions (e.g., 3 to 4 h following a light meal without physical activity.) The discussions that follow use the terms *basal metabolism* and *resting metabolism* interchangeably.

INFLUENCE OF BODY SIZE ON RESTING METABOLISM

Body surface area (BSA) frequently provides a common denominator to express basal metabolism. The standard expression unit for the BMR is kilocalories per square meter of BSA per hour or $kcal \cdot m^{-2} \cdot h^{-1}$. **Figure 8.2**

fyi: Regular Physical Activity Slows Decreases in Basal Metabolism With Age

Increases in body fat and decreases in fat-free mass (FFM) largely explain the 2% decline in BMR per decade through adulthood. Endurance and resistance activities offset the decrease in resting metabolism with aging. For example, an accompanying 8% increase in resting metabolism occurs when 50- to 65-year-old men increase their FFM with intense resistance training.

illustrates that at all ages, BMR averages 5% to 10% lower in females compared with males. A female's larger percentage body fat and smaller muscle mass in relation to body size helps explain her lower metabolic rate per unit surface area. From ages 20 to 40, average values for BMR equal 38 $kcal \cdot m^{-2} \cdot h^{-1}$ for men and 36 $kcal \cdot m^{-2} \cdot h^{-1}$ for women. For a more precise BMR estimate, the actual average value for a specific age should be read directly from the curves. A person's RMR in $kcal \cdot min^{-1}$ can be estimated and converted to a total daily resting requirement with the value for heat production (BMR) in **Figure 8.2** combined with the appropriate surface area value.

ESTIMATING RESTING DAILY ENERGY EXPENDITURE

The curves in **Figure 8.2** estimate a person's **resting daily energy expenditure (RDEE)**. To estimate the total metabolic rate per hour, multiply the BMR value by the person's calculated BSA expressed in meters squared. This hourly total provides important information to estimate the daily energy baseline requirement for caloric intake.

Accurate assessment of BSA poses a considerable challenge. Experiments in the early 1900s provided the data to determine BSA via a simple prediction using only body mass (kg) and stature (m). The studies clothed eight men and two women in tight, whole-body underwear and applied melted paraffin and paper strips to prevent modification of their body surface measure. After removing the treated cloth, it was cut into flat pieces to

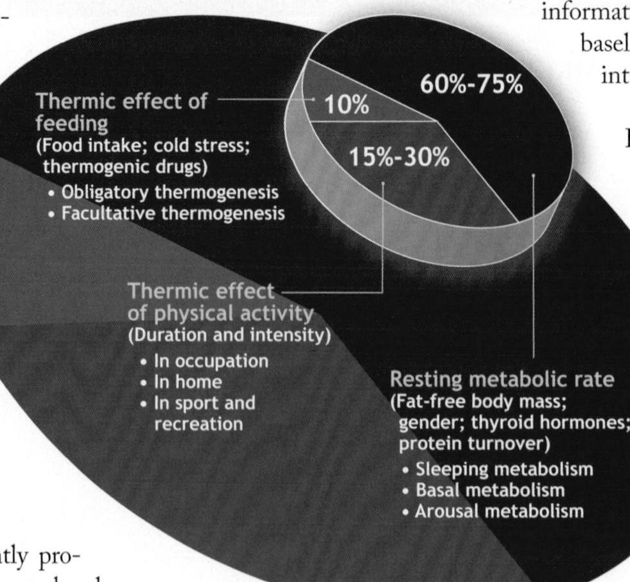

FIGURE 8.1 Components of total daily energy expenditure (TDEE).

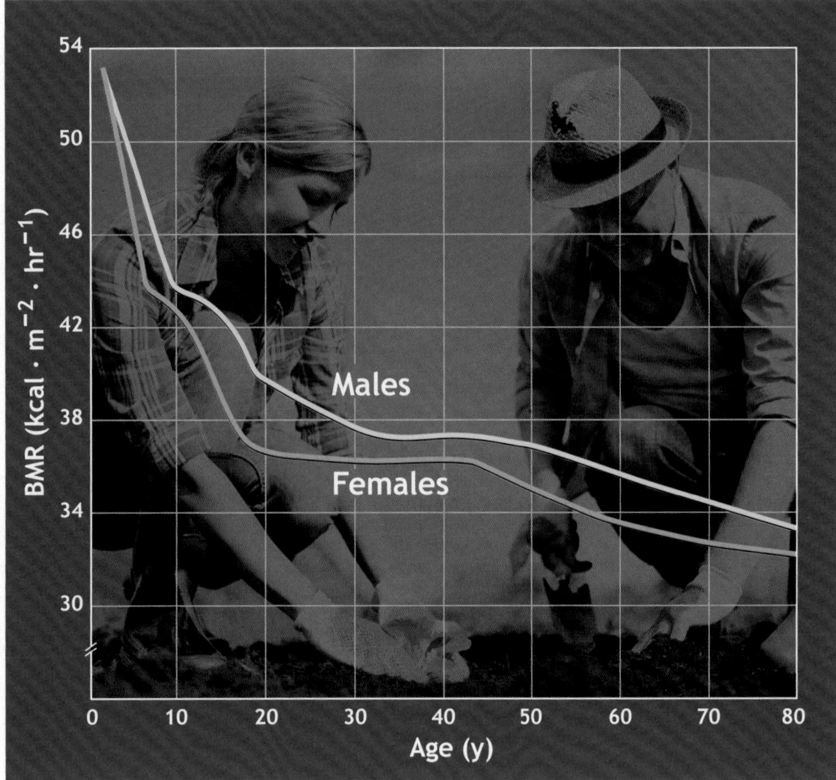

FIGURE 8.2 Basal metabolic rate (BMR) as a function of age and gender. (Adapted with permission from McArdle WD, Katch FI, Katch VL. *Exercise Physiology: Nutrition, Energy, and Human Performance*. 8th Ed. Baltimore: Wolters Kluwer Health, 2015; data from Altman PL, Dittmer D. *Metabolism*. Bethesda: Federation of American Societies for Experimental Biology, 1968.) (Adapted with permission from Ravussin E, et al. Determination of 24-hour energy expenditure in man: Methods and results using a respiratory chamber. *J Clin Invest* 1986;78:1568.)

precisely measure BSA (length × width). The close relationship between stature and body mass and BSA culminated in the following empirical formula to quantify BSA:

$$\textbf{BSA, m}^2 = 0.20247 \times \text{Stature}^{0.725} \times \text{Body mass}^{0.425}$$

Stature is height in meters (multiply inches by 0.254 to convert to meters), and body mass is weight in kilograms (divide pounds by 2.205 to convert to kilograms). For example, BSA computations for a man 70 inches tall (1.778 m) who weighs 165.3 lb (75 kg) are as follows:

$$\begin{aligned} \text{BSA} &= 0.20247 \times 1.778^{0.725} \times 75^{0.425} \\ &= 0.20247 \times 1.51775 \times 6.2647 \\ &= 1.925 \text{ m}^2 \end{aligned}$$

For a 20-year-old man, the estimated BMR equals 36.5 kcal · m^{-2} · h^{-1}. If his surface area were 1.925 m^2 as in the calculation above, the hourly energy expenditure would equal 70.3 kcal (36.5 × 1.925 m^2). On a 24-hour basis, this amounts to an RDEE of 1686 kcal (70.3 kcal × 24 h).

PREDICTING RESTING ENERGY EXPENDITURE

Body mass (BM in kilograms), stature (*S* in centimeters), and age (*A* in years) can successfully predict RDEE with sufficient accuracy using the following equations for women and men:

$$\textbf{Women: } \text{RDEE} = 655 + (9.6 \times \text{BM}) + (1.85 \times S) - (4.7 \times A)$$

$$\textbf{Men: } \text{RDEE} = 66.0 + (13.7 \times \text{BM}) + (5.0 \times S) - (6.8 \times A)$$

Examples

Woman

$$\text{BM} = 62.7 \text{ kg}; S = 172.5 \text{ cm}; A = 22.4 \text{ y}.$$

$$\begin{aligned} \text{RDEE} &= 655 + (9.6 \times 62.7) + (1.85 \times 172.5) - (4.7 \times 22.4) \\ &= 655 + 601.92 + 319.13 - 105.28 \\ &= 1471 \text{ kcal} \end{aligned}$$

Man

$$\text{BM} = 80 \text{ kg}; S = 189.0 \text{ cm}; A = 30 \text{ y}.$$

$$\begin{aligned} \text{RDEE} &= 66.0 + (13.7 \times 80) + (5.0 \times 189.0) - (6.8 \times 30.0) \\ &= 66.0 + 1096 + 945 - 204 \\ &= 1903 \text{ kcal} \end{aligned}$$

CONTRIBUTION OF DIVERSE TISSUES TO RESTING METABOLIC RATE

Table 8.1 presents estimates of absolute and relative energy needs, expressed as oxygen uptake in mL · min^{-1} and as a percentage of the resting metabolism of different organs and tissues of adults. The brain and skeletal muscles consume about the same total quantity of oxygen even though the brain weighs only 1.6 kg (2.3% of body mass) while muscle constitutes almost 50% of body mass. For children, brain metabolism represents nearly 50% of total resting energy expenditure. This similarity in metabolism does not transfer to maximal physical activity because energy generated by active muscle increases nearly 100 times; the total energy expended by the brain increases only marginally.

THREE FACTORS AFFECT TOTAL DAILY ENERGY EXPENDITURE

The three most important factors that affect TDEE are physical activity, dietary-induced thermogenesis, and climate. Pregnancy also affects TDEE through its impact on the energy cost of diverse modes of physical activity from the progressive increase in body weight.

Physical Activity

Physical activity profoundly impacts human energy expenditure. World-class athletes can nearly double their daily caloric outputs during 3 or 4 hours of physical training. Most people can sustain metabolic rates that average 10 times their resting value during "big muscle" fast walking, running, cycling, and swimming. *Physical activity generally accounts for 15% and 30% of TDEE.*

Dietary-Induced Thermogenesis

Consuming food increases energy metabolism from the energy-requiring processes of digesting, absorbing, and assimilating nutrients. **Dietary-induced thermogenesis** or **DIT**, also termed **thermic effect of food (TEF)**, typically achieves maximum 1 hour following feeding. This effect depends on food quantity and food types consumed. The magnitude of DIT ranges between 10% and 35% of the ingested food energy. A meal of pure protein, for example, produces a

A CLOSER LOOK

Estimate Resting Daily Energy Expenditure From Fat-Free Body Mass

The following equation predicts RDEE from fat-free body mass (see Chapter 16):

$$\text{RDEE}\ (\text{kcal} \cdot 24\ \text{h}^{-1}) = 370 + 21.6\ (\text{FFM, kg})$$

The data in the table were computed from the equation above; the equation applies to males and females over a wide range of body weights:

Example

A male who weighs 90.9 kg at 21% body fat has an estimated FFM of 71.7 kg. Rounding to 72 kg translates to an RDEE of 1925 kcal per 24 hours or 8047 kJ per 24 hours (8.08 MJ).

Estimation of Resting Daily Energy Expenditure (RDEE) Based on Fat-Free Body Mass (FFM)

FFM (kg)	RDEE[a] (kcal)[b]	FFM (kg)	RDEE (kcal)	FFM (kg)	RDEE (kcal)
30	1018	58	1623	86	2228
31	1040	59	1644	87	2249
32	1061	60	1666	88	2271
33	1083	61	1688	89	2292
34	1104	62	1709	90	2314
35	1126	63	1731	91	2336
36	1148	64	1752	92	2357
37	1169	65	1774	93	2379
38	1191	66	1796	94	2400
39	1212	67	1817	95	2422
40	1234	68	1839	96	2444
41	1256	69	1860	97	2465
42	1277	70	1882	98	2487
43	1299	71	1904	99	2508
44	1320	72	1925	100	2530
45	1342	73	1947	101	2552
46	1364	74	1968	102	2573
47	1385	75	1990	103	2595
48	1407	76	2012	104	2616
49	1428	77	2033	105	2638
50	1450	78	2055	106	2660
51	1472	79	2076	107	2681
52	1493	80	2098	108	2703
53	1515	81	2120	109	2724
54	1536	82	2141	110	2746
55	1558	83	2163	111	2768
56	1580	84	2184	112	2789
57	1601	85	2206	113	2811

[a] Prediction equation for RDEE derived as the weighted mean constants from studies of large samples of males and females.

[b] To convert kcal to kJ, multiply by 4.18; to convert kcal to MJ, multiply by 0.0042.

Data from Katch V. *Exercise Physiology Laboratory*. Ann Arbor: University of Michigan, 1985.

TABLE 8.1 Oxygen Uptake of Various Body Tissues at Rest for a 65-kg Man

Organ	Oxygen Uptake ($mL \cdot min^{-1}$)	Percentage of Resting Metabolism
Liver	67	27
Brain	47	19
Heart	17	7
Kidneys	26	10
Skeletal muscle	45	18
Remainder	48	19
Total	250	100

Adapted with permission from McArdle WD, Katch FI, Katch VL. *Exercise Physiology: Nutrition, Energy, and Human Performance*. 8th Ed. Baltimore: Wolters Kluwer Health, 2015.

thermic effect often equaling 25% of the meal's total energy content.

Advertisements routinely tout the high thermic effect of protein consumption to promote a high-protein diet for weight loss. Advocates maintain that fewer calories ultimately become available to the body compared with a lipid- or carbohydrate-rich meal of similar caloric value. This point has some validity, but other factors must be considered in formulating a prudent weight loss program. These include potentially harmful strain on kidney and liver function induced by excessive protein, and cholesterol-synthesizing effects of saturated fatty acids contained in higher protein content foods from the animal kingdom. Well-balanced meal plans require a blend of macronutrients with adequate vitamins and minerals. When combining physical activity with food restriction for weight loss, carbohydrate, not protein intake, provides energy for physical activity and conserves lean tissue invariably lost through food-restricted dietary plans.

Individuals with poor body weight control often display a depressed thermic response to eating, an effect likely related to genetic predisposition. Over many years, this connection can contribute to considerable body fat accumulation. If a person's lifestyle includes regular moderate physical activity, then the thermogenic effect represents only a small percentage of TDEE. Also, exercising following a meal further stimulates the normal thermic response to food consumption. This supports the wisdom of "going for a brisk walk" within a few minutes after eating.

Climate

Environmental factors influence RMR. The resting metabolism of people living in tropical climates, for example, averages 5% to 20% higher than counterparts in more temperate regions. Physical activity performed in hot weather also imposes a small 5% elevation in metabolic load that translates to correspondingly higher oxygen uptake compared with the same work performed in a thermoneutral environment. Three factors directly produce an increased environmentally induced thermogenic effect:

1. Elevated core temperature
2. Additional energy required for sweat gland activity
3. Altered circulatory dynamics

Cold environments increase energy metabolism depending on the body's fat content and thermal quality of clothing. During extreme cold stress, resting metabolism can triple because shivering generates heat to maintain a stable core temperature referred to as **shivering thermogenesis**. The effects of cold stress during physical activity become most evident in cold water from the extreme difficulty of maintaining a stable core temperature in this hostile environment.

Pregnancy

Maternal cardiovascular dynamics follow normal response patterns. Moderate physical activity presents no greater physiologic stress to the mother than that imposed by the additional weight gain and possible encumbrance of fetal tissue. Pregnancy does not compromise the absolute value for aerobic capacity expressed in $L \cdot min^{-1}$. As pregnancy progresses, increases in maternal body weight add to the physical activity effort during weight-bearing walking, jogging, and stair climbing and may reduce the economy of movement. Pregnancy, particularly the last trimester, increases pulmonary ventilation at a given submaximal effort intensity. Progesterone elevation during pregnancy increases respiratory center sensitivity to carbon dioxide, which directly stimulates maternal hyperventilation.

SUMMARY

1. BMR reflects the minimum energy required for vital functions in the waking state.
2. BMR relates inversely to age and gender, averaging 5% to 10% lower in women than in men.
3. FFM and percentage of body fat largely account for age and gender differences in BMR.
4. TDEE represents the sum of energy required in resting metabolism, the thermic effect of food, and energy generated in physical activity.
5. Body mass, stature, age, and FFM provide for accurate estimates of RDEE.
6. Physical activity, dietary-induced thermogenesis, environmental factors, and pregnancy significantly impact the TDEE.
7. *Dietary-induced thermogenesis* (*DIT*) refers to the increase in energy metabolism attributable to digestion, absorption, and food nutrient assimilation.
8. Exposure to hot and cold environments increases the TDEE up to 5%.

THINK IT THROUGH

1. Discuss three factors contributing to TDEE. Explain which factor contributes the most.
2. Discuss the notion that for some individuals, a calorie ingested really is not a calorie in its potential for energy storage.
3. What would be the ideal prescription to optimize increases in TDEE?
4. Discuss why middle-aged men and women should maintain or increase muscle mass for purposes of weight control.

PART 2 Energy Expenditure During Physical Activity

An understanding of resting energy metabolism provides an important frame of reference to appreciate the human potential to substantially increase daily energy output. According to numerous surveys, *physical inactivity* accounts for about one-third to one-half of a person's waking hours (e.g., watching television, lounging around the home, playing video games, and other sedentary-type activities). Consider this example:

> Over a 10-year period, say from ages 20 to 30, an individual sleeps 8 hours nightly with 16 hours available for daily activity participation. However, the person remains sedentary for 5 hours each day. Over the 10 years, this amount of "sedentariness" equates with about 18,250 hours of idle time, 640 days of inactivity, or 2.1 years spent at essentially resting metabolism!

In our view, this presents a huge opportunity for individuals of all ages to engage in meaningful physical activity, thereby considerably boosting TDEE. Actualizing this potential depends on the intensity, duration, and mode of physical activity performed (not necessarily standard exercise forms).

Researchers have measured energy expended during hundreds of everyday activities such as brushing teeth, chewing gum, fidgeting, house cleaning, grocery shopping, supervising children's playtime, watching TV, working on a computer, mowing the lawn, walking the dog, driving a car, playing ping-pong, bowling, dancing, swimming, and rock climbing. Even physical activity during space flight and equipment repair and rendezvous missions outside the space craft has been quantified.

Consider an activity such as rowing continuously at 30 strokes per minute for 30 minutes. How can we determine the number of calories "burned" during the 30 minutes? If the amount of oxygen consumed averages $2.0\ L \cdot min^{-1}$ during each minute of rowing, then in 30 minutes the rower would consume 60 L of oxygen. A reasonably accurate estimate of the energy expended in rowing can be made because 1 L of oxygen generates about 5 kcal of energy. In this example, the rower expends 300 kcal (60 L × 5 kcal) during the activity. This value represents the **gross energy expenditure** for the activity duration.

The 300 kcal of energy cannot all be attributed solely to rowing because this value also includes the resting requirement during the 30-minute row. The rower's BSA of $2.04\ m^2$, estimated from the formula BSA, $m^2 = 0.20247 \times Stature^{0.725} \times Body\ mass^{0.425}$ (body mass = 81.8 kg; stature = 1.83 m), multiplied by the average BMR for gender ($38\ kcal \cdot m^{-2} \cdot h^{-1} \times 2.04\ m^2$) gives the resting metabolism per hour. This value would equate to 78 kcal in 1 hour or 39 kcal "burned" over 30 minutes.

Based on these computations, the **net energy expenditure** attributable solely to rowing equals gross energy expenditure (300 kcal) minus the requirement for rest (39 kcal for the same time period) or approximately 261 kcal expended. One estimates TDEE by determining the time spent in daily activities (using a paper diary or electronic smart watch sensor device or other body metric recorder) and quantifying the activities' corresponding energy requirements.

CLASSIFICATION OF PHYSICAL ACTIVITIES BY ENERGY EXPENDITURE

All of us at one time or another have performed some type of physical work we would classify as exceedingly "difficult." This includes walking up a long flight of subway or train station stairs, shoveling a snow-filled driveway, sprinting to catch a bus, loading and unloading furniture from a truck, digging trenches, skiing or snowshoeing through a snowstorm, or running at a faster than normal pace for 10 minutes in soft beach sand. Two factors affect how researchers rate the difficulty of a particular task:

1. *Duration of effort*
2. *Intensity of effort*

Both factors can vary considerably. Running a 26-mile marathon at various speeds illustrates this point. One world-class runner maintains maximum pace and completes the race in a little more than 2 hours. Another runner selects a slower, more "leisurely" pace and completes the run in 3 hours (or even 4 to 5 h). In these examples, the intensity of physical activity differentiates the performance. In another situation, two people run at the same speed, but one runs twice as long as the other. Here, activity duration differentiates performance.

RATING "STRENUOUSNESS" OF PHYSICAL ACTIVITY

Several classification systems rate sustained physical activity for "strenuousness." One system recommends classification of work by the ratio of energy required for the task to the resting energy requirement. This system employs the **physical activity ratio (PAR)**. For example, light work for men elicits an oxygen uptake or energy expenditure up to three times the resting requirement. Heavy work encompasses physical activity requiring six to eight times resting metabolism, whereas maximal work includes any task that requires metabolism to increase nine times or more above rest. As a frame of reference, most industrial jobs and household tasks require less than three times resting energy expenditure. These work classifications rated in multiples of resting metabolism average slightly lower for women because of their generally lower aerobic capacity. Work classification based on the PAR model rates the strenuousness of occupational tasks at a somewhat lower level than typical classifications for general physical activity. This occurs because occupational and industrial work usually extends for much longer durations than does physical activity training and often requires the use of a smaller muscle mass performed under varying and stressful environmental conditions and physical constraints.

Using Metabolic Equivalents

Oxygen uptake and kilocalories commonly express differences in physical activity intensity. As an alternative, a convenient way to express intensity classifies physical effort as multiples of resting energy expenditure with a unitless measure. To this end, scientists have developed the concept of **metabolic equivalents (METs)**. One MET represents an adult's average seated resting oxygen uptake or energy expenditure—about 250 mL $O_2 \cdot min^{-1}$, 3.5 mL $O_2 \cdot kg^{-1} \cdot min^{-1}$, 1 $kcal \cdot kg^{-1} \cdot h^{-1}$, or 0.017 $kcal \cdot kg^{-1} \cdot min^{-1}$ (1 $kcal \cdot kg^{-1} \cdot h^{-1} \div 60\ min \cdot h^{-1} = 0.017$). Using these data as a frame of reference, a 2-MET activity requires twice as much energy expended at rest and so on.

The MET provides a convenient way to rate intensity from a resting baseline. Conversion from METs to $kcal \cdot min^{-1}$ requires knowledge of body mass and the following conversion: 1.0 $kcal \cdot kg^{-1} \cdot h^{-1}$ = 1 MET. For example, if a person who weighs 70 kg bicycles at 10 mph, which is listed as a 10-MET activity, the corresponding kilocalorie expenditure calculates as follows:

$$\begin{aligned} 10.0\ \text{METs} &= 10.0\ kcal \cdot kg^{-1} \cdot h^{-1} \times 70\ kg \div 60\ min \\ &= 700\ kcal \div 60\ min \\ &= 11.7\ kcal \cdot min^{-1} \end{aligned}$$

Table 8.2 presents a five-level classification scheme of physical activity based on energy expenditure and corresponding MET levels for untrained men and women.

Heart Rate to Estimate Energy Expenditure

For each person, heart rate (HR) and oxygen uptake ($\dot{V}O_2$) relate linearly throughout a broad range of aerobic physical activity intensities. By knowing this precise relationship, activity HR provides an estimate of $\dot{V}O_2$, and thus energy expenditure, during physical activity. This approach has served as a surrogate when $\dot{V}O_2$ cannot easily be measured as for example during a sport, recreational, or household activity. In soccer, for example, it would be extremely difficult to monitor $\dot{V}O_2$ for a midfielder (or almost any position for that matter) during a game. In addition, player safety would be severely compromised if players had to compete wearing a portable oxygen update apparatus that covered the nose and mouth (see Fig. 8.7 later in this chapter). In contrast, attaching a portable HR monitor to the skin surface, or a smartphone watch or other compact, miniaturized device that continuously records the HR during the activity, would be relatively simple, unobtrusive, and without safety concerns. Once the HR-$\dot{V}O_2$ relationship had been determined in the laboratory independently from the activity (e.g., the midfielder position), only HR during a representative portion of the activity would serve as the surrogate to infer the corresponding $\dot{V}O_2$, and hence energy expenditure.

TABLE 8.2 Five-Level Classification of Physical Activity Based on Physical Activity Intensity

	Energy Expenditure[a]			
		MEN		
LEVEL	$kcal \cdot min^{-1}$	$L \cdot min^{-1}$	$mL \cdot kg^{-1} \cdot min^{-1}$	METs
Light	2.0–4.9	0.40–0.99	6.1–15.2	1.6–3.9
Moderate	5.0–7.4	1.00–1.49	15.3–22.9	4.0–5.9
Heavy	7.5–9.9	1.50–1.99	23.0–30.6	6.0–7.9
Very heavy	10.0–12.4	2.00–2.49	30.7–38.3	8.0 -9.9
Unduly heavy	12.5–	2.50–	38.4–	10.0–
		WOMEN		
LEVEL	$kcal \cdot min^{-1}$	$L \cdot min^{-1}$	$mL \cdot kg^{-1} \cdot min^{-1}$	METs
Light	1.5–3.4	0.30–0.69	5.4–12.5	1.2–2.7
Moderate	3.5–5.4	0.70–1.09	12.6–19.8	2.8–4.3
Heavy	5.5–7.4	1.10–1.49	19.9–27.1	4.4–5.9
Very heavy	7.5–9.4	1.50–1.89	27.2–34.4	6.0–7.5
Unduly heavy	9.5–	1.90–	34.5–	7.6–

[a] $L \cdot min^{-1}$ based on 5 kcal per liter of oxygen; $mL \cdot kg^{-1} \cdot min^{-1}$ based on 65-kg man and 55-kg woman; 1 MET equals average resting oxygen uptake of 3.5 $mL \cdot kg^{-1} \cdot min^{-1}$.

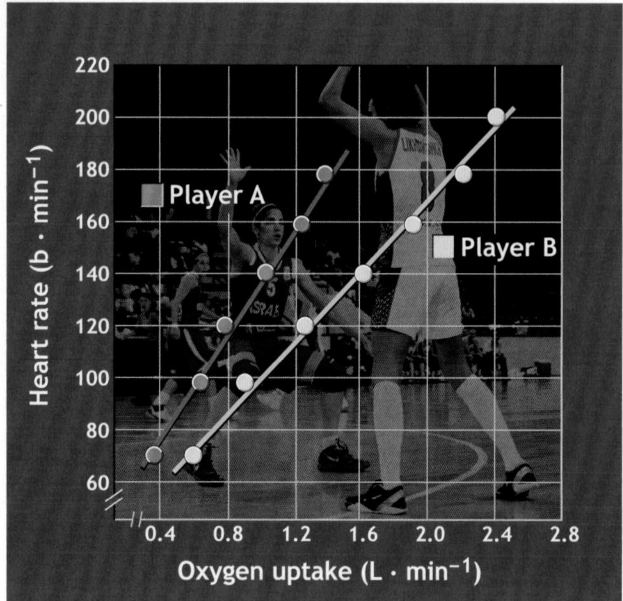

FIGURE 8.3 Linear relationship between heart rate and oxygen uptake for two women collegiate basketball players of different aerobic fitness levels. Measurements made during a graded exercise test on a motor-driven treadmill. (Adapted with permission from Laboratory of Applied Physiology, Queens College, NY.)

Figure 8.3 presents data for two members of a nationally ranked women's basketball team during a laboratory treadmill running test. The HR for each woman increased linearly with intensity—a proportionate increase in HR accompanied each increase in oxygen uptake. However, a similar HR for each athlete did not correspond to the same level of oxygen uptake because the slope or rate of change of the HR-$\dot{V}O_2$ line differed considerably between the women. For a given increase in oxygen uptake, the HR of subject B increased less than did that for subject A. For player A, a HR of 140 b · min^{-1} corresponds to an oxygen uptake of 1.08 L · min^{-1}. The same HR for player B corresponds to an oxygen uptake of 1.60 L · min^{-1}.

A major consideration when using HR to estimate oxygen uptake lies in the similarity between the laboratory assessment of the HR-$\dot{V}O_2$ line and the specific *in vivo* field activity applied to this relationship. Not unexpectedly, factors other than oxygen uptake influence HR response to physical activity. These include environmental temperature, emotional state, previous food intake, body position, muscle groups exercised, continuous or discontinuous nature of the activity, and whether the muscles act statically or more dynamically. During aerobic dance, for example, higher HRs occur while dancing at a specific oxygen uptake than at the same oxygen uptake while walking or running on a treadmill. Natural arm position movement during an activity, or when muscles act statically in a straining-type activity, produces consistently higher HRs than dynamic leg activity at any submaximal oxygen uptake. Consequently, applying HRs during upper-body or static activity to a HR-$\dot{V}O_2$ line established during running or cycling *overpredicts* the criterion oxygen uptake.

ENERGY COST OF RECREATIONAL AND SPORT ACTIVITIES

Table 8.3 illustrates the energy cost among diverse recreational and sport activities. Notice, for example, that volleyball requires about 3.6 kcal per minute (216 kcal per h) for a person who weighs 71 kg (157 lb). The same person expends more than twice this energy, or 546 kcal per hour, swimming the front crawl. Viewed somewhat differently, 25 minutes spent swimming expends about the same number of calories as playing 1 hour of recreational volleyball. If the pace of the swim increases or the volleyball game becomes more intense, energy expenditure increases proportionately.

TABLE 8.3 Gross Energy Cost (kcal · min^{-1}) for Selected Recreational and Sports Activities in Relation to Body Mass[a]

Activity	kg lb	50 110	53 117	56 123	59 130	62 137	65 143	68 150	71 157	74 163	77 170	80 176	83 183
Volleyball		2.5	2.7	2.8	3.0	3.1	3.3	3.4	3.6	3.7	3.9	4.0	4.2
Aerobic dancing		6.7	7.1	7.5	7.9	8.3	8.7	9.2	9.6	10.0	10.4	10.8	11.2
Cycling, leisure		5.0	5.3	5.6	5.9	6.2	6.5	6.8	7.1	7.4	7.7	8.0	8.3
Tennis		5.5	5.8	6.1	6.4	6.8	7.1	7.4	7.7	8.1	8.4	8.7	9.0
Swimming, slow crawl		6.4	6.8	7.2	7.6	7.9	8.3	8.7	9.1	9.5	9.9	10.2	10.6
Touch football		6.6	7.0	7.4	7.8	8.2	8.6	9.0	9.4	9.8	10.2	10.6	11.0
Running, 8 min/mile		10.8	11.3	11.9	12.5	13.11	3.6	14.2	14.8	15.4	16.0	16.5	17.1
Skiing, uphill racing		13.7	14.5	15.3	16.2	17.0	17.8	18.6	19.5	20.3	21.1	21.9	22.7

Note: Energy expenditure computes as the number of minutes of participation multiplied by the kilocalorie value in the appropriate body weight column. For example, the kilocalorie cost of 1 hour of tennis for a person weighing 150 lb equals 444 kcal (7.4 kcal × 60 min).

[a]Data from Katch F, et al. *Calorie Expenditure Charts*. Ann Arbor: Fitness Technologies Press, 1996. © Fitness Technologies Press. Used with permission of Fitness Technologies Press.

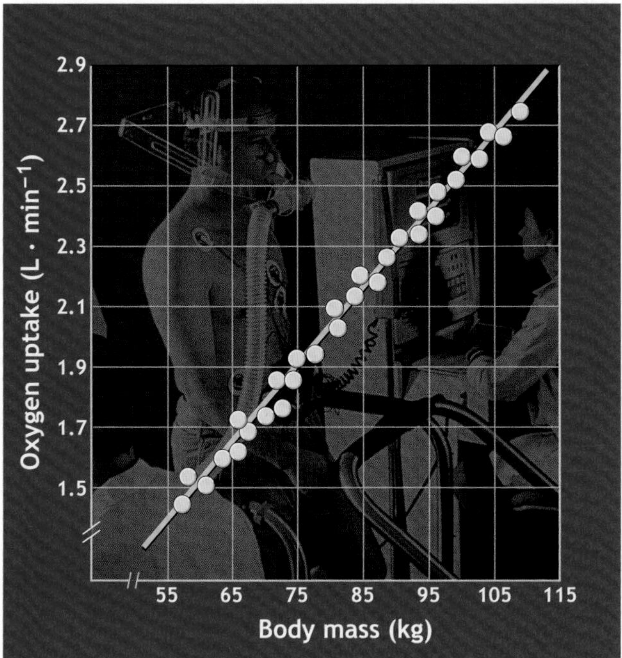

FIGURE 8.4 Relationship between body mass and oxygen uptake measured during submaximal, brisk treadmill walking. (Adapted with permission from Laboratory of Applied Physiology, Queens College, NY.)

Effect of Body Mass

Body size plays an important contributing role in energy requirements. **Figure 8.4** illustrates that heavier people expend more energy to perform the same activity than people weighing less. This occurs because energy expended during **weight-bearing activity** increases directly with the body mass transported. *Such a strong relationship means that one can predict energy expenditure during walking or running from body weight with almost as much accuracy as measuring oxygen uptake under controlled laboratory conditions.* In **non–weight-bearing (weight-supported activity)**, such as stationary cycling, little relationship exists between body weight and energy cost.

From a practical standpoint, walking and other weight-bearing activities require a substantial calorie burn for heavier people. Notice in **Table 8.3** that playing tennis or volleyball requires considerably greater energy expenditure for a person who weighs 83 kg than for someone who weighs 62 kg. Expressing caloric cost of weight-bearing activity relative to body mass, as kilocalories per kilogram of body mass per minute ($kcal \cdot kg^{-1} \cdot min^{-1}$), greatly reduces the difference in energy expenditure among individuals of different body weights. Nonetheless, the absolute energy cost of the activity ($kcal \cdot min^{-1}$) remains greater for the heavier person simply because of the extra body weight.

AVERAGE DAILY RATES OF ENERGY EXPENDITURE

A committee of the US Food and Nutrition Board (**www.iom.edu/en**) proposed various norms to represent average rates of energy expenditure for men and women in the United States. These values apply to people with occupation energy expenditures between sedentary and active and who participate in some recreational activities such as weekend swimming, golf, hiking, and tennis. **Table 8.4** reveals that the average daily energy expenditure ranges between 2900 and 3000 kcal for men and 2200 kcal for women between the ages of 15 and 50 years.

TABLE 8.4 Average Rates of Energy Expenditure for Men and Women Living in the United States[a]

	Age (y)	Body Mass		Stature		Energy Expenditure
		(kg)	(lb)	(cm)	(in)	(kcal)
Males	15–18	66	145	176	69	3000
	19–24	72	160	177	70	2900
	25–50	79	174	176	70	2900
	51+	77	170	173	68	2300
Females	15–18	55	120	163	64	2200
	19–24	58	128	164	65	2200
	25–50	63	138	163	64	2200
	50+	65	143	160	63	1900

Activity	Average Time Spent During the Day Time (h)
Sleeping and lying down	8
Sitting	6
Standing	6
Walking	2
Recreational activity	2

[a]The information in this table was designed for the maintenance of practically all healthy people in the United States.

Data from Food and Nutrition Board, National Research Council. *Recommended Dietary Allowances, Revised.* Washington: National Academy of Sciences, 1989.

The lower part of the table confirms that a typical person spends about 75% of their day in sedentary activities. This predominance of physical *inactivity* has prompted some sociologists to refer to the modern-day American as *homosedentarius*.

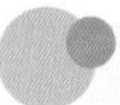

SUMMARY

1. Energy expenditure can be expressed in gross or net terms. Gross or total values include the resting energy requirement during the activity phase; net energy expenditure reflects the energy cost of the activity that excludes resting metabolism over an equivalent time period.
2. Daily rates of energy expenditure classify different occupations and sports professions. Within any classification, variability exists from energy expended in recreational or on-the-job pursuits.
3. Different classification systems rate the strenuousness of physical activities. These include ratings based on energy cost expressed in kcal • min^{-1}, oxygen requirement in L • min^{-1}, or multiples of the RMR (METs).
4. HR during physical activity estimates energy expenditure from a laboratory-determined individual's HR-$\dot{V}O_2$ line.
5. Researchers apply the HRs during recreational, sport, or occupational activity to the HR-$\dot{V}O_2$ line to estimate oxygen uptake.
6. Diverse factors that influence HR act independently of the oxygen uptake so estimates of energy cost using HR response are limited to only select types of physical activities.
7. Average TDEE ranges between 2900 and 3000 kcal for men and 2200 kcal for women aged 15 to 50 years.

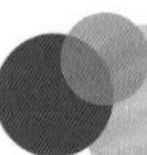

THINK IT THROUGH

1. What circumstances would cause a particular physical task to be rated "strenuous" in intensity by one person but only "moderate" by another?
2. Discuss the limitations of using physical activity HR to estimate the energy cost of vigorous resistance training based on an HR-$\dot{V}O_2$ line determined from treadmill walking.

PART 3 Energy Expenditure During Walking, Running, and Swimming

TDEE depends largely on the type, intensity, and duration of physical activity. The following sections explore energy expenditure for walking, running, and swimming. These activities play an important role in weight control, physical conditioning, and cardiac rehabilitation.

EFFICIENCY AND ECONOMY OF HUMAN MOVEMENT

Three factors largely determine success in aerobic endurance performance:

1. Aerobic capacity ($\dot{V}O_{2max}$)
2. Ability to sustain effort at a large percentage of $\dot{V}O_{2max}$
3. Efficiency of energy use or movement economy

Exercise physiologists consider a high $\dot{V}O_{2max}$ a prerequisite for success in endurance activities. Among long-distance runners with nearly identical aerobic powers who compete in elite levels of competition, however, other factors often explain success in competition. For example, a performance edge would clearly exist for an athlete able to run at a higher percentage of $\dot{V}O_{2max}$ (i.e., higher blood lactate threshold [LT]) than competitors. Similarly, the runner who maintains a given pace with relatively low energy expenditure or greater movement economy maintains a competitive advantage.

Efficiency of Human Movement

The energy expenditure related to external work represents a fraction of the total energy utilized when an individual engages in physical activity—the remainder appears as heat. **Mechanical efficiency (ME)** indicates the percentage of the total chemical energy expended (denominator) that contributes to the external work output (numerator). Within this context:

$$\text{ME (\%)} = \frac{\text{Work Output}}{\text{Energy Expended}} \times 100$$

Force, acting through a vertical distance (F × D) and usually recorded as foot-pounds (ft-lb) or kilogram-meters (kg-m), represents external work accomplished or work output. External work output is determined routinely during cycle ergometry, or stair climbing and bench stepping that require lifting the body mass vertically. In horizontal walking or running, work output cannot be computed because technically, external work does not occur. Reciprocal leg and arm movements negate each other, and the body achieves no net gain in vertical distance. If a person walks or runs up a grade, the work component depends on body mass and vertical distance or lift achieved during the activity interval (see Chapter 6, "A Closer Look: *How to Measure Work on a Treadmill, Cycle Ergometer, and Step Bench*"). Work output converts to kilocalories using these standard conversions:

$$1\ \text{kcal} = 426.8\ \text{kg-m}$$
$$1\ \text{kcal} = 3087.4\ \text{ft-lb}$$
$$1\ \text{kcal} = 1.5593\ 10^{-3}\ \text{hp} \cdot \text{h}^{-1}$$
$$1\ \text{watt} = 0.01433\ \text{kcal} \cdot \text{min}^{-1}$$
$$1\ \text{watt} = 6.12\ \text{kg-m} \cdot \text{min}^{-1}$$

Steady-rate oxygen uptake during physical activity represents the energy input portion of the efficiency equation (denominator). To obtain common units, the oxygen uptake converts to energy units (1.0 L O_2 = 5.0 kcal; see

fyi Changes in Mechanical Efficiency During a Competitive Season Related to Training Volume and Intensity

Cyclists who spend time training at or above their LT increase gross efficiency cycling compared to preseason and postseason. The increase in gross efficiency averages a modest 1%, yet this can make a difference in winning or losing, and posting a rider's best times.

Source: Hopker J, et al. Changes in cycling efficiency during a competitive season. *Med Sci Sports Exer* 2009;41:912.

Table 7.2 for precise calorific transformations based on the nonprotein RQ).

Three terms express efficiency—gross, net, and delta. Each expression, calculated differently, exhibits a particular advantage. Each calculation method assumes a submaximal steady-rate condition and requires expression of work output and energy expenditure be expressed in the same units—typically kilocalories. Applying the different calculation methods to the same activity modality yields varying results for ME that range from 8% to 25% using gross calculations, 10% to 30% using net calculations, and 24% to 35% using delta calculations.

Gross Mechanical Efficiency

Gross mechanical efficiency, the most frequently calculated measure of efficiency, applies when one requires specific rates of work and speed, or in nutritional studies that expresses energy expenditure over extended durations. Gross efficiency computations use the total oxygen uptake during the activity.

For example, suppose a 15-minute ride on a stationary bicycle generated 13,300 kg-m of work or 31.2 kcal (13,300 kg-m ÷ 426.8 kcal per kg-m). The oxygen consumed to perform the work totaled 25 L with an RQ of 0.88, which indicates that each liter of oxygen uptake generated an energy equivalent of 4.9 kcal (see Table 7.2). Thus, the activity required 122.5 kcal (25 L × 4.9 kcal). ME (%) computes as follows:

$$\text{Gross ME (\%)} = \frac{\text{Work Output}}{\text{Energy Expended}} \times 100$$

$$= \frac{31.2\text{ kcal}}{122.5\text{ kcal}} \times 100$$

$$= 25.5\%$$

As with all machines, the human body's efficiency to produce mechanical work falls considerably below 100%. The energy required to overcome internal and external friction becomes the biggest factor affecting ME. Overcoming friction represents essentially wasted energy because it accomplishes no external work; consequently, work input *always* exceeds work output. The ME of human locomotion in most walking, running, and cycling activities ranges between 20% and 30%.

Net Mechanical Efficiency

Net mechanical efficiency involves subtracting the resting energy expenditure from the total energy expended during activity. This calculation indicates the efficiency of the work *per se*, unaffected by the energy expended to sustain the body at rest. Net ME calculates as follows:

$$\text{Net ME (\%)} = \frac{\text{Work Output}}{\text{Energy Expended Above Rest}} \times 100$$

Resting energy output is determined for the same time duration as the work output.

In the previous example for gross ME, if the resting oxygen uptake equaled 250 mL · min^{-1} (0.25 L · min^{-1}) and RQ equaled 0.91 (4.936 kcal · L O_2^{-1}; 0.250 L · min^{-1} × 4.936 = 1.234 kcal · min^{-1}), the net ME computes as:

$$\text{Net ME (\%)} = \frac{31.2\text{ kcal}}{122.5\text{ kcal} - (1.234\text{ kcal}\cdot\text{min}^{-1} \times 15\text{ min})} \times 100$$

$$= 30\%$$

Delta Efficiency

Delta efficiency calculates as the *relative* energy cost of performing an additional increment of work; that is, the ratio of the difference between work output at two work output levels to the *difference* in energy expenditure determined for the two exercise levels.

$$\text{Delta }(\Delta)\text{ Efficiency} = \frac{\text{Differences in Work Output Between Two Exercise Levels}}{\text{Difference in Energy Expended Between Two Exercise Levels}} \times 100$$

For example, suppose an individual cycles at 100 watts for 5 minutes (100 W = 1.433 kcal · min^{-1}) at a steady-rate oxygen uptake of 1.70 L · min^{-1} with an RQ of 0.83 (4.838 kcal · L O_2^{-1}). This corresponds to an energy expenditure of 8.23 kcal · min^{-1}. The person then completes another 5 minutes at 200 watts (200 W = 2.866 kcal · min^{-1}) at a steady-rate oxygen uptake of 2.80 L · min^{-1} with an RQ of 0.90 (4.924 kcal · L O_2^{-1}). This results in an energy expenditure of 13.8 kcal · min^{-1}. Delta efficiency computes as:

$$\text{Delta }(\Delta)\text{ Efficiency} = \frac{\text{Differences in Work Output Between Two Exercise Levels}}{\text{Differences in Energy Expended Between Two Exercise Levels}} \times 100$$

$$= \frac{2866\text{ kcal}\cdot\text{min}^{-1} - 1.433\text{ kcal}\cdot\text{min}^{-1}}{13.79\text{ kcal}\cdot\text{min}^{-1} - 8.23\text{ kcal}\cdot\text{min}^{-1}} \times 100$$

$$= \frac{1.433\text{ kcal}\cdot\text{min}^{-1}}{5.56\text{ kcal}\cdot\text{min}^{-1}} \times 100$$

$$= 25.8\%$$

Delta efficiency remains the calculation of choice when assessing efficiency of treadmill activity because it is impossible to determine work output accurately during horizontal movement.

Factors Influencing Physical Activity Efficiency

Seven factors influence exercise efficiency:

1. **Work rate**: Efficiency generally decreases as work rate increases because of the curvilinear, rather than linear, relation between energy expenditure and work. As work rate increases, total energy expenditure increases disproportionately to work output, resulting in a lowered ME.
2. **Movement speed**: Every individual has an optimum speed of movement for any given work rate. Generally, the optimum movement speed increases as power output increases (i.e., higher power outputs require greater movement speed to create optimum efficiency). Any deviation from the optimal movement speed decreases efficiency. Low efficiencies at slow speeds most likely result from inertia (i.e., increased energy expended to overcome internal starting and stopping). Declines in efficiency at high speeds can result from increases in muscular friction, with resulting increases in internal work and energy expenditure.
3. **Extrinsic factors**: Improvements in equipment design have increased efficiency in many physical activities. For example, lighter and softer running shoes with different insole cushioning properties permit running at a given speed with a lower energy expenditure, thus increasing movement efficiency; changes in clothing have produced a similar effect (e.g., lighter, more absorbent fabrics and more hydrodynamic full-body swim suits).
4. **Muscle fiber composition**: Activation of slow-twitch muscle fibers produces greater efficiency than the same work accomplished by fast-twitch fibers. Slow-twitch fibers require less ATP per unit work than do fast-twitch fibers. Thus, individuals with a higher percentage of slow-twitch muscle fibers exhibit increased ME.
5. **Fitness level**: More fit individuals perform a given task at a higher efficiency from decreased energy expenditure for the non–exercise-related functions of temperature regulation, increased circulation, and waste product removal.
6. **Body composition**: Overweight individuals perform a given activity, particularly weight-bearing walking and running, at a lower efficiency from the increased energy cost of transporting extra poundage.
7. **Technique**: Improved technique produces fewer extraneous body movements, resulting in a lower energy expenditure and hence higher efficiency. The golf swing serves as a prime example. Millions of men and women expend considerable "energy" trying to direct the ball where they want it to go—most of the time with less than perfect execution. In contrast, tour golfers seemingly waste little "energy" in coordinating the feet, legs, hips, shoulders, and arms as they strike the ball on a preplanned trajectory in a precise, coordinated manner that looks "effortless."

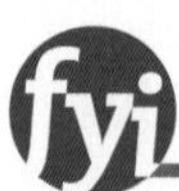

Elite Runners Run More Economically

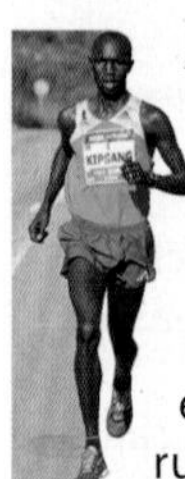

At a particular speed, elite endurance runners run at a lower oxygen uptake than less trained or less successful counterparts of similar age. This holds for 8- to 11-year-old cross-country runners and adult marathoners. Elite distance athletes, as a group, run with 5% to 10% greater economy than well-trained middle-distance runners.

ECONOMY OF HUMAN MOVEMENT

The concept of exercise economy also encompasses the relation between energy input and energy output. For **economy of human movement**, the quantity of energy to perform a particular task relative to performance quality represents an important concern. In a sense, many of us assess economy by visually comparing the ease of movement among highly trained athletes. It does not require a trained eye to discriminate the ease of effort in comparisons of elite swimmers, skiers, golfers, dancers, gymnasts, and platform divers with less proficient counterparts who seem to expend considerable "wasted energy" to perform the same tasks. Anyone who has learned a new sport recalls the difficulties encountered performing basic movements that with proper practice became automatic and indeed "effortless."

Physical Activity Oxygen Uptake Reflects Movement Economy

A common method to assess differences in movement economy between individuals evaluates the steady-rate oxygen uptake during a specific activity at a set power output or speed. This approach only applies to steady-rate physical activity that mirrors oxygen uptake with energy expenditure. *At a given submaximal running, cycling, or swimming speed, an individual with greater movement economy consumes less oxygen.* Economy takes on importance during longer duration activities in which aerobic capacity and the task's oxygen requirements largely determine success. *All else being equal, a training adjustment that improves economy of effort directly translates to improved performance.*

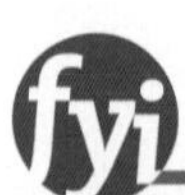

Running Economy Improves With Age

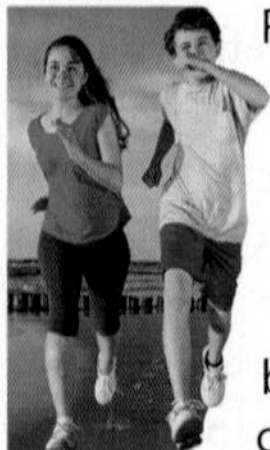

Running economy improves steadily from ages 10 to 18 years. This partly explains the relatively poor performance of young children in distance running and their progressive improvement throughout adolescence. Improved endurance occurs even though aerobic capacity relative to body mass (mL $O_2 \cdot kg^{-1} \cdot min^{-1}$) remains relatively constant during this time.

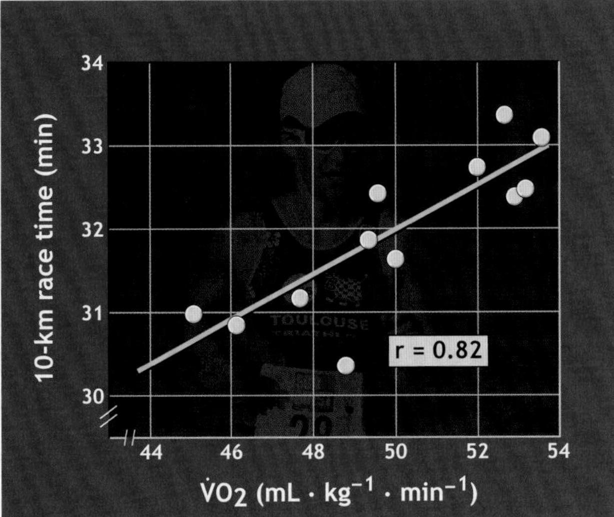

FIGURE 8.5 Relationship between submaximal oxygen uptake running at 268 m · min^{-1} and 10-km race time in elite male runners of comparable aerobic capacity. (Adapted with permission from Morgan DW, Craib M. Physiological aspects of running economy. *Med Sci Sports Exerc* 1992;24:456.)

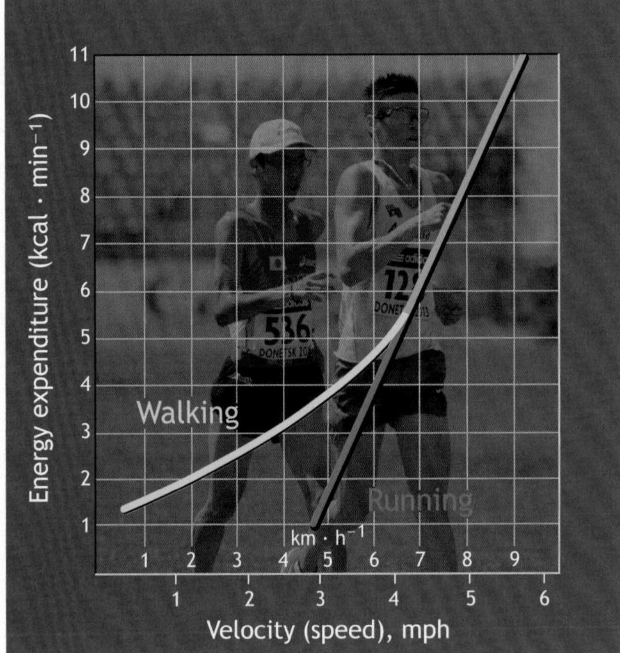

FIGURE 8.6 Energy expenditures while walking on a level surface at different speeds. The *line* represents a compilation of values reported in the literature.

Figure 8.5 relates running economy to endurance performance in elite athletes of comparable aerobic fitness. Clearly, athletes with greater running economies (i.e., lower oxygen uptake at the same running pace) achieve better performance.

No single biomechanical factor accounts for individual differences in running economy. Significant variation in economy at a particular running speed occurs even among trained runners. In general, improved running economy results from years of arduous run training with particular attention to training specific *movement* patterns in running. Short-term training that emphasizes only "proper techniques" of running (e.g., arm movements and body alignment) probably does not improve running economy. Distance runners who lack an economical stride-length pattern benefit from a short-term program of audiovisual feedback that focuses on optimizing stride length.

ENERGY EXPENDITURE AND ECONOMY DURING WALKING

Walking, the most common form of activity for most individuals, represents the major type of physical activity that falls outside the realm of sedentary living. **Figure 8.6** displays the combined research from five countries on energy expenditure of men walking at speeds from 1.5 to 9.5 km · h^{-1} (0.9 to 5.9 mph). The relationship between walking speed and oxygen uptake remains approximately linear between 3.0 and 5.0 km · h^{-1} (1.9 and 3.1 mph); as walking economy decreases at faster speeds, the relationship curves upward with a disproportionate increase in energy expenditure with increasing speed. This explains why, per unit distance traveled, faster but less-efficient walking speeds require more total calories expended per unit distance traveled. In **Figure 8.6**, note the intersection of the two straight lines referred to as the **crossover velocity**, which occurs at about 6.5 km · h^{-1} (4.0 mph). At this juncture, running becomes more economical than walking.

Competition Walking

The energy expended by Olympic-caliber walkers has been assessed at various speeds walking and running on a treadmill. Their competitive walking speeds average a remarkable 13.0 km · h^{-1} (11.5 to 14.8 km · h^{-1} or 7.1 to 9.2 mph) over distances ranging from 1.6 to 50 km. At world record speed that equals about 15.6 km · h^{-1} (9.7 mph) for men and 14.2 km · h^{-1} (8.8 mph) for women, the crossover velocity occurs at about 8.0 km · h^{-1} (4.97 mph) when running becomes more economical than walking. The oxygen uptake of race walkers during treadmill walking at competition speeds averages only slightly lower than the highest oxygen uptake measured for these athletes during treadmill running. Also, a linear relationship exists between oxygen uptake and walking at speeds above 8 km · h^{-1}, but the slope of the line was *twice* as steep compared with running at the same speeds. The athletes could walk at velocities up to 16 km · h^{-1} (9.9 mph) and attain oxygen uptakes as high as those while running; the economy of walking faster than 8 km · h^{-1} averaged half of running at similar speeds.

Effects of Body Mass

Body mass predicts energy expenditure with reasonable accuracy at horizontal walking speeds ranging from 3.2 to 6.4 km · h^{-1} (~2.0 to 4.0 mph) for people of diverse body size and composition. The predicted values for energy expenditure during walking listed in **Table 8.5** fall within ±15% of the actual energy expenditure for men and women of different body weights up to 91 kg (200 lb). On a daily basis, the estimated energy expended while walking would only be in error by about 50 to 100 kcal, assuming the person walks intermittently for 2 hours throughout the day. Extrapolations are appropriate for heavier individuals but with some loss in accuracy.

Effects of Terrain and Walking Surface

Table 8.6 summarizes the influence of terrain and walking surface type on energy cost of walking. Similar economies exist for level walking on a grass track or paved surface. Not surprisingly, energy cost almost doubles walking in sand compared with walking on a hard surface; in soft snow, metabolic cost increases threefold compared with treadmill walking. A brisk walk along a sandy beach or in freshly fallen snow provides excellent activity for programs designed to "burn" calories or improve physiologic fitness. For people who tend to gain weight during winter months, walking in the snow provides an excellent way to expend additional calories while still reaping the benefits of an intense, aerobic workout.

Footwear Effects

It requires considerably more energy to carry added weight on the feet or ankles than to carry similar weight attached to the torso. For a weight equal to 1.4% of body mass placed on the ankles, the energy cost of walking increases an average 8% or nearly six times more than with the same weight carried on the torso. In a practical sense, energy cost of locomotion during walking and running increases when wearing boots than wearing running shoes. Adding an additional 100 g or about 3 oz to each shoe increases oxygen uptake by 1% during moderate-speed running. The implication of these

A CLOSER LOOK

Predicting Energy Expenditure During Treadmill Walking and Running

An almost linear relationship exists between energy expenditure (oxygen uptake) and walking speeds between 3.0 and 5.0 km · h^{-1} (1.9 and 3.1 mph), and running at speeds faster than 8.0 km · h^{-1} (5 to 10 mph; see **Fig. 8.6**). Adding the resting oxygen uptake to the oxygen requirements of the horizontal and vertical components of the walk or run makes it possible to estimate total (gross) exercise oxygen uptake ($\dot{V}O_2$) and energy expenditure.

Basic Equation

$\dot{V}O_{2max}$ (mL · kg^{-1} · min^{-1}) = Resting component (1 MET [3.5 mL O_2 · kg^{-1} · min^{-1}]) + Horizontal component (speed [m · min^{-1}] × oxygen uptake of horizontal movement) + Vertical component (percentage grade × speed [m · min^{-1}] × oxygen uptake of vertical movement)

To convert mph to m · min^{-1}, multiply by 26.82; to convert m · min^{-1} to mph, multiply by 0.03728.

Walking

Oxygen uptake of the horizontal component of movement equals 0.1 mL · kg^{-1} · min^{-1} and 1.8 mL · kg^{-1} · min^{-1} for the vertical component.

Running

Oxygen uptake of the horizontal component of movement equals 0.2 mL · kg^{-1} · min^{-1} and 0.9 mL · kg^{-1} · min^{-1} for the vertical component.

Predicting Energy Expenditure of Treadmill Walking

Problem

A 55-kg person walks on a treadmill at 2.8 mph (2.8 × 26.82 = 75 m · min^{-1}) up a 4% grade. Calculate (1) $\dot{V}O_2$ (mL · kg^{-1} · min^{-1}), (2) METs, and (3) energy expenditure (kcal · min^{-1}).

Note: Express % grade as a decimal value (i.e., 4% grade = 0.04)

Solution

1. $\dot{V}O_2$ (mL · kg^{-1} · min^{-1}) = Resting component + Horizontal component + Vertical component

$$\dot{V}O_2 = \text{Resting } \dot{V}O_2 (\text{mL} \cdot \text{kg}^{-1} \cdot \text{min}^{-1}) + [\text{speed} (\text{m} \cdot \text{min}^{-1}) \times 0.1\ \text{mL} \cdot \text{kg}^{-1} \cdot \text{min}^{-1}] + [\%\ \text{grade} \times \text{speed} (\text{m} \cdot \text{min}^{-1}) \times 1.8\ \text{mL} \cdot \text{kg}^{-1} \cdot \text{min}^{-1}]$$

$$= 3.5 + (75 \times 0.1) + (0.04 \times 75 \times 1.8)$$

$$= 3.5 + 7.5 + 5.4$$

$$= 16.4\ \text{mL} \cdot \text{kg}^{-1} \cdot \text{min}^{-1}$$

2. $$\text{METs} = \dot{V}O_2 (\text{mL} \cdot \text{kg}^{-1} \cdot \text{min}^{-1}) \div 3.5\ \text{mL} \cdot \text{kg}^{-1} \cdot \text{min}^{-1}$$

$$= 16.44 \div 3.5$$

$$= 4.7$$

$$3.\ \text{kcal}\cdot\text{min}^{-1} = \dot{V}O_2(\text{mL}\cdot\text{kg}^{-1}\cdot\text{min}^{-1}) \times \text{Body mass (kg)} \times 5.05\ \text{kcal}\cdot\text{LO}_2^{-1}$$
$$= 16.4\ \text{mL}\cdot\text{kg}^{-1}\cdot\text{min}^{-1} \times 55\ \text{kg} \times 5.05\ \text{kcal}\cdot\text{L}^{-1}$$
$$= 0.902\ \text{L}\cdot\text{min}^{-1} \times 5.05\ \text{kcal}\cdot\text{L}^{-1}$$
$$= 4.6$$

Predicting Energy Expenditure of Treadmill Running

Problem

A 55-kg person runs on a treadmill at 5.4 mph ($5.4 \times 26.82 = 145\ \text{m}\cdot\text{min}^{-1}$) up a 6% grade. Calculate (1) in $\text{mL}\cdot\text{kg}^{-1}\cdot\text{min}^{-1}$, (2) METs, and (3) energy expenditure ($\text{kcal}\cdot\text{min}^{-1}$).

Solution

$$1.\ \dot{V}O_2(\text{mL}\cdot\text{kg}^{-1}\cdot\text{min}^{-1}) = \text{Resting component} + \text{Horizontal component} + \text{Vertical component}$$

$$\dot{V}O_2 = \text{Resting } \dot{V}O_2(\text{mL}\cdot\text{kg}^{-1}\cdot\text{min}^{-1}) + [\text{speed}(\text{m}\cdot\text{min}^{-1}) \times 0.2\ \text{mL}\cdot\text{kg}^{-1}\cdot\text{min}^{-1}] + [\%\ \text{grade} \times \text{speed}(\text{m}\cdot\text{min}^{-1}) \times 0.9\ \text{mL}\cdot\text{kg}^{-1}\cdot\text{min}^{-1}]$$
$$= 3.5 + (145 \times 0.2) + (0.06 \times 145 \times 0.9)$$
$$= 3.5 + 29.0 + 7.83$$
$$= 40.33\ \text{mL}\cdot\text{kg}^{-1}\cdot\text{min}^{-1}$$

$$2.\ \text{METs} = \dot{V}O_2(\text{mL}\cdot\text{kg}^{-1}\cdot\text{min}^{-1}) \div 3.5\ \text{mL}\cdot\text{kg}^{-1}\cdot\text{min}^{-1}$$
$$= 40.33 \div 3.5$$
$$= 11.5$$

$$3.\ \text{kcal}\cdot\text{min}^{-1} = \dot{V}O_2(\text{mL}\cdot\text{kg}^{-1}\cdot\text{min}^{-1}) \times \text{Body mass (kg)} \times 5.05\ \text{kcal}\cdot\text{LO}_2^{-1}$$
$$= 40.33\ \text{mL}\cdot\text{kg}^{-1}\cdot\text{min}^{-1} \times 55\ \text{kg} \times 5.05\ \text{kcal}\cdot\text{L}^{-1}$$
$$= 2.22\ \text{L}\cdot\text{min}^{-1} \times 5.05\ \text{kcal}\cdot\text{L}^{-1}$$
$$= 11.2$$

Adapted with permission from *ACSM Guidelines for Exercise Testing and Prescription*. 9th Ed. Baltimore: Lippincott Williams & Wilkins, 2014.

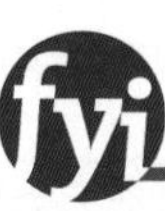

Edward Payson Weston: Walker Extraordinaire

Born in 1839, when life span averaged 40 years, Edward Payson Weston (1839–1929) in his prime would walk 50 to 100 miles a day. In 1861, he walked 453 miles from Boston to Washington, DC, in 10 days and 10 hours to attend Lincoln's inauguration on March 4. The new 16th president, Abraham Lincoln, gave Weston a congratulatory handshake, which inspired Weston to compete in many professional "pedestrian" competitions. These included 6-day ultramarathon races before huge crowds in New York City's Madison Square Garden and in London's Agricultural Hall. At age 71, Weston was the first to walk across America from Los Angeles to New York City, covering approximately 3600 miles in 88 days, averaging 41 miles daily. In his mid-80s, Weston still walked 25 miles a day. Other notable achievements included walking from Philadelphia to New York, a distance of over 100 miles, in less than 24 hours; at age 68, he repeated his Maine-to-Chicago walk of 1867, beating his prior time by over 24 hours. In 1909, Weston walked for 100 days, covering a distance of nearly 4000 miles from New York City to San Francisco following many routes not on the standard trail of that time.

Weston, a professional race walker and early American advocate of vigorous physical activity, died in 1929 at age 90, 2 years after being struck by a New York City taxicab that ironically caused him to lose the use of his legs!

findings seems clear for the design of running shoes, hiking and climbing boots, and work boots traditionally required in mining, forestry, firefighting, and the military. Small changes in shoe weight produce large changes in economy of locomotion because heavier shoes increase energy expenditure thus lowering economy. The cushioning properties of shoes also impact energy expenditure. A softer-soled running shoe reduces oxygen cost of running at moderate speed by about 2.4% compared with a similar shoe with a firmer cushioning system, although softer-soled shoes weighed only an additional 31 g or 1.1 oz. The preceding observations about terrain, footwear, and economy of locomotion indicate that, at the extreme, one could dramatically elevate energy cost by walking in soft sand at rapid speed wearing heavy work

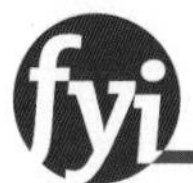

A Considerable Energy Output

During a marathon, elite athletes generate a steady-rate energy expenditure of about 25 kcal per minute for the run duration. Among elite rowers, a 5- to 7-minute competition generates about 36 kcal a minute!

TABLE 8.5 Prediction of Energy Expenditure (kcal · min^{-1}) From Speed of Level Walking and Body Mass

Speed		Body Mass							
		kg	36	45	54	64	73	82	91
mph	km · h^{-1}	lb	80	100	120	140	160	180	200
2.0	3.22		1.9	2.2	2.6	2.9	3.2	3.5	3.8
2.5	4.02		2.3	2.7	3.1	3.5	3.8	4.2	4.5
3.0	4.83		2.7	3.1	3.6	4.0	4.4	4.8	5.3
3.5	5.63		3.1	3.6	4.2	4.6	5.0	5.4	6.1
4.0	6.44		3.5	4.1	4.7	5.2	5.8	6.4	7.0

How to use the chart: A 54-kg (120-lb) person who walks at 3.0 mph (4.83 km · h^{-1}) expends 3.6 kcal · min^{-1}.
This person would expend 216 kcal during a 60-min walk (3.6 × 60).

boots and ankle weights. A more prudent and less cumbersome approach would advocate unweighted race walking or running on a firmer surface.

Use of Handheld and Ankle Weights

The impact force on the legs during running equals about three times body mass, while the amount of leg shock with walking reaches only about 30% of this value.

Ankle weights increase energy cost of walking to values usually observed for running. This benefits people who want to use only walking as a relatively low-impact training modality yet require intensities of effort higher than normal walking speeds provide. Handheld weights also increase walking energy cost, particularly when arm movements accentuate a pumping action. Despite this apparent benefit, this procedure may disproportionately elevate systolic blood pressure from increased intramuscular tension while gripping the weight. For individuals with clinical hypertension or coronary heart disease, an unnecessarily "induced" elevated blood pressure would contraindicate using handheld weights. For these individuals, increasing running speed or distance offers a better alternative than handheld or ankle weights.

TABLE 8.6 Effect of Different Terrain on the Energy Expenditure of Walking Between 5.2 and 5.6 km · h^{-1}

Terrain[a]	Correction Factor[b]
Paved road (similar to a grass track)	0.0
Plowed field	1.5
Hard snow	1.6
Sand dune	1.8

[a]First entry from Passmore R, Dumin JVGA. Human energy expenditure. *Physiol Rev* 1955;35:801. Last three entries from Givoni B, Goldman RF. Predicting metabolic energy cost. *J Appl Physiol* 1971;30:429.

[b]The correction factor represents a multiple of the energy expenditure for walking on a paved road or grass track. For example, the energy cost of walking in a plowed field averages 1.5 times the cost of walking on the paved road.

ENERGY EXPENDITURE DURING RUNNING

Terrain, weather, training goals, and the performer's fitness level influence running speed. Running energy expenditure can be quantified in two ways:

1. During performance of the actual activity in the ambient environment
2. On a treadmill in the laboratory, with precise control over running speed, grade, and environmental conditions

Jogging and running represent qualitative terms related to locomotor speed. This difference relates largely to the relative aerobic energy demands required in raising and lowering the body's center of gravity and accelerating and decelerating the limbs. At identical running speeds, a trained distance runner moves at a lower percentage of aerobic capacity than an untrained runner, although for

fyi Strength and Endurance Training Improves Running Economy of Master Runners

For master marathon runners (>40-year-old) who were training 4 to 5 d · wk^{-1} for a total of 50 km · wk^{-1} (slow runs, interval training, and tempo runs), adding a maximal strength training program (2 × week, 4 sets of 3 to 4 repetitions a set for lower and upper body at 85% to 90% of estimated 1RM) increased running economy at marathon pace by a statistically significant 6.2% compared to a similar group of master runners who only participated in regular strength training (2 × week, 3 sets of 10 repetitions at 70% 1RM) and to a control group of master runners who did no strength training.

Source: Piacentini, MF, et al. Concurrent strength and endurance training effects on running economy in master endurance runners. *J Strength Cond Res* 2013;2295:2303.

both the oxygen uptake during the run may be similar. The demarcation between jogging and running depends on the participant's fitness—a jog for one person represents a run for another.

Independent of fitness, it becomes more economical from an energy standpoint to discontinue walking and begin to jog or run at speeds greater than about 6.5 km • h^{-1} *(~4.0 mph;* **Fig. 8.6**).

Running Economy

The data in **Figure 8.6** illustrate an important principle related to running speeds (>5 mph or 8 km • h^{-1}) versus energy expenditure. *Oxygen uptake relates linearly to running speed; thus, the same total caloric cost results when running a given distance at a steady-rate oxygen uptake at a fast or slow pace.* In simple terms, if one runs a mile at a 10-mph pace (16.1 km • h^{-1}), it requires about twice as much energy per minute as a 5-mph pace (8 km • h^{-1}). The runner finishes the mile in 6 minutes, but running at the slower speed requires twice the time or 12 minutes. Consequently, the *net* energy cost for the mile (subtracting out the resting requirement for the same time period) remains about the same regardless of the pace ±10%. A ±10% error, while considerable for research purposes, is usually acceptable for field use.

For horizontal running, the net energy cost excluding the resting requirement per kilogram of body mass per kilometer traveled averages approximately 1 kcal or 1 kcal • kg^{-1} *• km*$^{-1}$. For an individual who weighs 78 kg, for example, the net energy requirement for running 1 km equals about 78 kcal regardless of running speed. Expressed as oxygen uptake, this amounts to 15.6 L of oxygen consumed per kilometer (1 L O_2 = 5 kcal; 5.0 × 15.6).

Energy Cost of Running

Table 8.7 presents values for net energy expended during running for 1 hour at different speeds. The table expresses running speed as kilometers per hour, miles per hour, and number of minutes required to complete 1 mile at a given running speed. The boldface values represent *net* calories expended to run 1 mile for a person of a given body mass, where net calories remain independent of running speed. For a person who weighs 62 kg, running a 26.2-mile marathon requires about 2600 net kcal whether the run takes just over 2 hours or 4 hours or more.

The energy cost per mile increases proportionately with the runner's body mass (refer to column 3). This observation

TABLE 8.7 Net Energy Expenditure per Hour for Horizontal Running Related to Velocity and Body Mass[a,b]

Body Mass		km • h^{-1}	8	9	10	11	12	13	14	15	16
		mph	4.97	5.60	6.20	6.84	7.46	8.08	8.70	9.32	9.94
		min per mile	12:00	10:43	9:41	8:46	8:02	7:26	6:54	6:26	6:02
kg	lb	kcal per mile									
50	110	**80**	400	450	500	550	600	650	700	750	800
54	119	**86**	432	486	540	594	648	702	756	810	864
58	128	**93**	464	522	580	638	696	754	812	870	928
62	137	**99**	496	558	620	682	744	806	868	930	992
66	146	**106**	528	594	660	726	792	858	924	990	1056
70	154	**112**	560	630	700	770	840	910	980	1050	1120
74	163	**118**	592	666	740	814	888	962	1036	1110	1184
78	172	**125**	624	702	780	858	936	1014	1092	1170	1248
82	181	**131**	656	738	820	902	984	1066	1148	1230	1312
86	190	**138**	688	774	860	946	1032	1118	1204	1290	1376
90	199	**144**	720	810	900	990	1080	1170	1260	1350	1440
94	207	**150**	752	846	940	1034	1128	1222	1316	1410	1504
98	216	**157**	784	882	980	1078	1176	1274	1372	1470	1568
102	225	**163**	816	918	1020	1122	1224	1326	1428	1530	1632
106	234	**170**	848	954	1060	1166	1272	1378	1484	1590	1696

[a] Interpret the table as follows: For a 50-kg person, the *net* energy expenditure for running for 1 hour at 8 km • h^{-1} (4.97 mph) equals 400 kcal; this speed represents a 12-minute per mile pace. Thus, 5 miles would be run in 1 hour and 400 kcal would be expended. If the pace increased to 12 km • h^{-1} (7.46 mph), 600 kcal would be expended during the 1-hour run.

[b] Running speeds expressed as kilometers per hour (km • h^{-1}), miles per hour (mph), and minutes required to complete each mile (min per mile). The values in **boldface type** equal *net* calories (resting energy expenditure subtracted) expended to run 1 mile for a given body mass, independent of running speed.

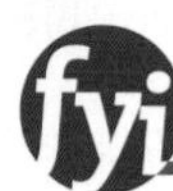

Exercise Economy and Muscle Fiber Type

Muscle fiber type affects economy of cycling effort. During submaximal cycling, economies of trained cyclists varied up to 15%. Differences in muscle fiber types in active muscles account for an important component of this variation. Cyclists who exhibit the most economical cycling pattern possessed greater percentage of slow-twitch (type I) muscle fibers in their legs. Type I fibers probably act with greater mechanical efficiency than faster-acting type II fibers.

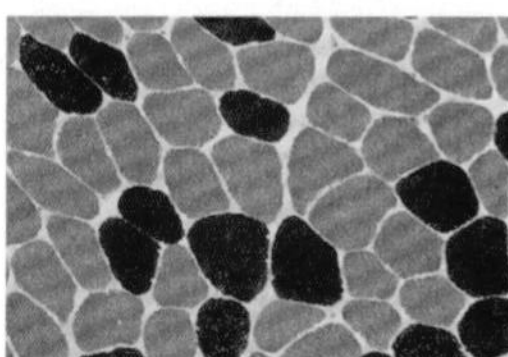

supports the pivotal role of weight-bearing activity as a caloric stress for overweight individuals who wish to increase energy expenditure for weight loss. For example, a 102-kg person who jogs 5 miles daily at any comfortable pace expends about 163 kcal for each mile completed or a total of 815 kcal for the 5-mile run. Increasing or decreasing the speed within the broad range of steady-rate paces simply alters the duration of the activity period required to burn a set number of calories.

Stride Length and Stride Frequency: Effects on Running Speed

Running speed can increase in three ways:

1. Increase step number each minute (stride frequency)
2. Increase distance between steps (stride length)
3. Increase stride length and stride frequency

Intuitively, the third option may seem the obvious way to increase running speed, and several experiments provide objective data concerning this question.

In 1944, researchers studied the stride pattern for a Danish champion in the 5- and 10-km running events. At a running speed of 9.3 $km \cdot h^{-1}$ (5.8 mph), this athlete's stride frequency equaled 160 per minute with a corresponding stride length of 97 cm (38.2 in). When running speed increased 91% to 17.8 $km \cdot h^{-1}$ (11.1 mph), stride frequency increased only 10% to 176 per minute, whereas an 83% increase to 168 cm occurred in stride length. These data illustrate that running speed increased predominantly by lengthening stride length. Only at faster speeds did stride frequency become important.

Optimum Stride Length

An optimum combination of stride length and frequency exists for running at a particular speed. The optimum combination depends largely on the person's "style" of running and cannot be determined from objective body measurements. Running speed chosen by the person incorporates the most economical stride length. Lengthening the stride above the optimum increases oxygen uptake more than a shorter-than-optimum stride length. Urging a runner who shows signs of fatigue to "lengthen stride" to maintain speed proves counterproductive for exercise economy.

Well-trained runners run at a stride length "selected" through years of training. This trial and error method produces the most economical running performance. This dovetails with the principal that the body naturally attempts to achieve a level of "**minimum effort**." No "best" style exists to characterize elite runners. Instead, individual differences in body size, inertia of limb segments, and anatomic development interact to subconsciously vary one's stride to the one most economical.

Effects of Air Resistance

Anyone who has run into a strong headwind knows it requires more energy to maintain a given pace compared with running in calm weather or with the wind at one's back. Three factors influence how air resistance affects energy cost of running:

1. Air density
2. Runner's projected surface area
3. Square of headwind velocity

Depending on running speed, overcoming air resistance accounts for 3% to 9% of the total energy requirement of running in calm weather. Running into a headwind creates an additional energy expense. In one study, running at 15.9 $km \cdot h^{-1}$ (9.9 mph) in calm conditions produced a 2.92 $L \cdot min$ oxygen uptake. This increased by 5.5% to 3.1 $L \cdot min^{-1}$ against a 16 $km \cdot h^{-1}$ (9.9 mph) headwind and to 4.1 $L \cdot min^{-1}$ while running against the strongest wind (41 mph). Running into the strongest wind represents a 40% additional expenditure of energy to maintain running velocity.

Some may argue that the negative effects of running into a headwind counterbalance on one's return with the tailwind. This does not occur because the energy cost of cutting through a headwind exceeds the reduction in oxygen uptake with an equivalent rear wind velocity. Wind tunnel tests show that running performance increases by wearing form-fitting clothing. Even shaving body hair improves aerodynamics and reduces wind resistance effects by up to 6%. In competitive cycling, manufacturers continually modify clothing and helmets to reduce the air resistance effects on energy cost. This includes frame redesign to optimize the rider's body position on the bicycle.

At altitude, wind velocity affects energy expenditure less than at sea level because of reduced air density at higher elevations. Speed skaters experience a lower oxygen requirement while skating at a particular speed at altitude compared with sea level. Overcoming air resistance at altitude only becomes important at the faster skating speeds. An altitude effect also applies to competitive cycling, where the impeding air resistance effect increases at the high speeds these athletes achieve.

Drafting

Athletes use "**drafting**" by following directly behind a competitor to counter the negative effects of air resistance and headwind on energy cost. Running 1 m behind another runner at a speed of 21.6 $km \cdot h^{-1}$ (13.4 mph) decreases total energy expenditure by about 7%. Drafting at this speed could save about 1 second for each 400 m covered during a race. The beneficial aerodynamic effect of drafting on economy of effort also exists for cross-country skiing, speed skating, and cycling. About 90% of the power generated when cycling at 40 km • h^{-1} (24.9 mph) on a calm day goes to overcome air resistance. At this speed, energy expenditure decreases between 26% and 38% when a competitor follows closely behind another cyclist.

Treadmill Versus Track Running

Researchers use the treadmill almost exclusively to evaluate running physiology. One question concerns the association between treadmill running and running performance on a track or road race. For example, in calm weather does it require the same energy to run a given speed or distance on a treadmill and a track? To answer this question, researchers studied distance runners on both a treadmill and track at three submaximal speeds of 10.8, 12.6, and 15.6 km • h^{-1} (6.7, 7.8, and 9.7 mph). They also measured the athletes during a graded exercise test to determine possible differences between treadmill and track running on submaximal and maximal oxygen uptake.

From a practical standpoint, no meaningful differences occurred in aerobic requirements of submaximal running up to 17.2 km • h^{-1} on the treadmill or track or between the $\dot{V}O_{2max}$ measured in both forms under similar environmental conditions. At the faster running speeds of endurance competition, air resistance could negatively impact outdoor running performance and oxygen cost may exceed that of "stationary" treadmill running at the same speed.

Marathon Running

On September 29, 2014 at the Berlin Marathon, Kenyan Dennis Kiprutto Kimetto established a new world record for the fastest marathon run ever at 2 hours:02 minutes:57 seconds—the first man to complete the 26.2-mile course in under 2:03! This blistering pace not only requires a steady-rate oxygen uptake that exceeds the aerobic capacity of most male college students but also demands the marathoner sustain about 90% of $\dot{V}O_{2max}$ for over 2 hours! This represents an extraordinary achievement in human running capacity and raises the possibility of a sub-2-hour run sometime in the near future.

Researchers measured two distance runners during a marathon to assess minute-by-minute and total energy expenditure. They determined oxygen uptake every 3 miles using open-circuit spirometry. Marathon times were 2 hours:36 minutes: 34 seconds ($\dot{V}O_{2max}$ = 70.5 mL • kg^{-1} • min^{-1}) and 2 hours: 39 minutes:28 seconds ($\dot{V}O_{2max}$ = 73.9 mL • kg^{-1} • min^{-1}). The first runner maintained an average speed of 16.2 km • h^{-1} that required an oxygen uptake equal to 80% of his $\dot{V}O_{2max}$. For the second runner, who averaged a slightly slower speed of 16.0 km • h^{-1}, the aerobic component averaged 78.3% of his maximum. For both men, the total energy required to run the marathon ranged between 2300 and 2400 kcal.

ENERGY EXPENDITURE DURING SWIMMING

Swimming differs in several respects from walking and running. The most obvious—swimmers must expend energy to maintain buoyancy while generating horizontal movement at the same time using the arms and legs, either in combination or separately. Other differences include energy requirements for overcoming drag forces that impede movement of an object through a water medium. The amount of drag depends on characteristics of the water medium and the object's size, shape, and velocity. *These factors contribute to a considerably lower economy swimming compared with running. More specifically, it requires about four times more energy to swim a given distance than to run the same distance.* Energy expenditure has been computed from oxygen uptake measured by open-circuit spirometry during swimming (**Fig. 8.7**). In the pool, the researcher walks alongside the swimmer while carrying the portable measurement gas collection equipment.

Energy Cost and Drag

Three components comprise the total drag force that impedes a swimmer's forward movement:

1. **Wave drag** caused by waves that build up in front of and form hollows behind the swimmer moving through water. This component of drag only becomes a significant factor at fast speeds.
2. **Skin friction drag** produced as water slides over the skin's surface. Removal of body hair reduces drag to slightly decrease swimming energy cost and physiologic demands during swimming.
3. **Viscous pressure drag** contributes substantially to counter propulsive efforts of the swimmer at slow velocities. It results from separation of the thin water sheet of water (boundary layer) adjacent to the swimmer. The pressure differential created in front of and behind the swimmer represents viscous pressure drag.

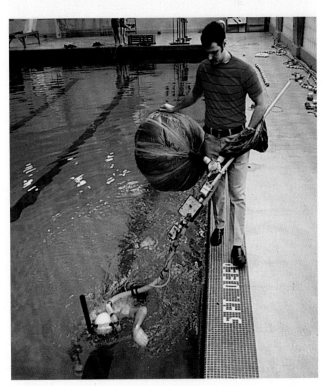

FIGURE 8.7 In this example of open-circuit spirometry, the investigator walks alongside the swimmer to collect expired air for later laboratory analyses for oxygen uptake.

Highly skilled swimmers who "streamline" their stroke reduce this component of total drag. Streamlining with improved stroke mechanics reduces the separation region by moving the separation point closer to the water's trailing edge. This also occurs when an oar slices through the water with the blade parallel rather than perpendicular to water movement.

Differences in total drag force between swimmers can make the difference between winning and losing, particularly in longer distance competitions. Wet suits worn during the swim portion of a triathlon can reduce body drag by 14%. Improved swimming economy largely explains the faster swim times of athletes who wear wet suits. Proponents of the neck-to-body suits worn by pool swimmers maintain that the technology-driven approach to competitive swimming maximizes swimming economy and allows swimmers to achieve approximately 3% faster times than when wearing standard swimsuits. As in running, cross-country skiing, and cycling, drafting in ocean swimming by following closely behind the wake of a lead swimmer reduces energy expenditure. This enables endurance swimmers to conserve energy and possibly improve performance toward the end of competition.

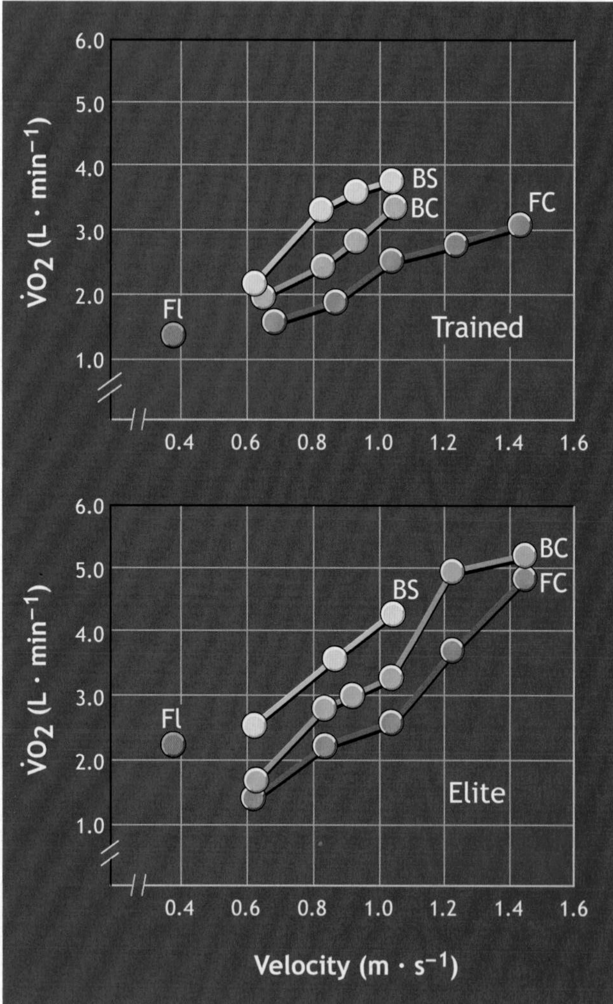

FIGURE 8.8 Oxygen uptake for two elite and two trained swimmers during three competitive strokes. *BS*, Breast stroke; *BC*, Back crawl; *FC*, Front crawl. (Adapted with permission from Holmer I. Oxygen uptake during swimming in man. *J Appl Physiol* 1972;33:502.)

Energy Cost, Swimming Velocity, and Skill

Figure 8.8 presents oxygen uptake measurements for two elite and two trained swimmers during three competitive strokes. Elite swimmers swim a given speed with a lower oxygen uptake than untrained yet skilled swimmers. Swimming the breaststroke "costs" the most at any speed and represents the least economical of the different strokes, followed by backstroke. In terms of calories expended, the front crawl represents the least "expensive" and most economical mode among the three strokes.

Effects of Buoyancy: Men Versus Women

Women of all ages possess, on average, more total body fat than men. Because fat floats and muscle and bone sink, the average woman gains a hydrodynamic lift and floats more easily than the average man. This difference in **buoyancy** can help to explain women's greater swimming economy compared with men. For example, women swim a given distance at a lower energy cost than men; expressed another way, women achieve a higher swimming velocity than men at the same energy expenditure.

Body fat distribution toward the periphery in women causes their legs to float higher in water, making them more horizontal or "streamlined," whereas men's leaner legs tend to swing down in water. Lowering the legs to a deeper position increases body drag, thus reducing swimming economy. The potential hydrodynamic benefits enjoyed by women become noteworthy in longer distances due to better swimming economy and better body insulation from subcutaneous fat. For example, the women's record for swimming the

Some Women Actually Swim Faster Than Men!

In several instances, women actually swim faster than men (see **Table 8.8**). American Gertrude Ederle (1905–2003; **www.nytimes.com/2003/12/01/sports/othersports/01EDER.html?pagewanted=all**) achieved a milestone by becoming the first woman without a life vest to swim the English Channel from Dover to Calais on August 6, 1926, in 14 hours, 31 minutes. Her time was faster by more than 2 hours than British steamship Captain Matthew Webb (1848–1883), the first man to complete the swim without a vest 51 years earlier in 1875 in 21 hours, 45 minutes (**www.bbc.co.uk/shropshire/features/2003/12/captain_webb.shtml**).

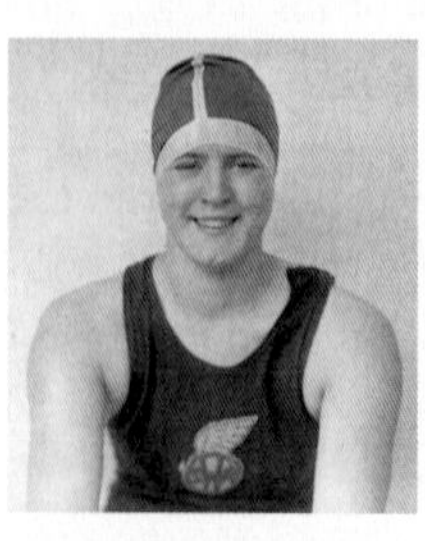

Gertrude Ederle © Corbis

TABLE 8.8 **Comparisons of English Channel World Record Swimming Times Between Men and Women**

English Channel Records (h · min^{-1}): Male Versus Female			
Record	**Male**	**Female**	**% Difference (Male:Female)**
First attempt—one way	21:45 (1875)	14:39 (1926)	34.9
Fastest—one way	07:17 (1994)	7:40 (1978)	−5.26
Youngest—one way	11:54 (11 y, 11 mo; 1988)	15:28 (12 y, 11 mo; 1983)	−29.9
Oldest—one way	18:37 (67 y; 1987)	12:32 (57 y; 1999)	32.69
Fastest—two way	16:10 (1987)	17:14 (1991)	−6.6
Fastest—three way	28:21 (1987)	34:40 (1990)	−22.2

Note that for two records (first attempt, oldest) females exceeded the male record by more than 30%.

21-mile English Channel from England to France is 7 hours, 40 minutes; the men's record, 23 minutes faster, amounts to a faster time of only 5.3% (see **Table 8.8**).

SUMMARY

1. Mechanical efficiency represents the percentage of total chemical energy expended contributing to external work, with the remainder representing lost heat.
2. Exercise economy refers to the relationship between energy input and energy output commonly evaluated by oxygen uptake while exercising at a preset power output or speed.
3. Walking speed relates linearly to oxygen uptake between speeds of 1.9 and 3.1 mph; walking becomes less economical at speeds faster than 4.0 mph.
4. Walking surface impacts energy expenditure; walking on soft sand requires about twice the energy expenditure as walking on hard surfaces.
5. Heavier people have a proportionally larger energy cost of weight-bearing activity.
6. Handheld and ankle weights increase the energy cost of walking to values reported for running.
7. It is more energetically economical to begin to jog-run than to walk at speeds between 6.5 km · h^{-1} (4.0 mph) and 8.0 km · h^{-1} (5.0 mph).
8. The total energy cost for running a given distance remains independent of running speed. For horizontal running, the net energy expenditure averages about 1 kcal · kg^{-1} · km^{-1}.
9. Shortening running stride and increasing stride frequency to maintain a constant running speed requires less energy than lengthening stride and reducing stride frequency.
10. Overcoming air resistance accounts for 3% to 9% of the total energy cost of running in calm weather.
11. Running directly behind a competitor, a favorable aerodynamic technique called "drafting," counters the negative effect of air resistance and headwind on running energy cost.
12. It requires the same amount of energy to run a given distance or speed on a treadmill as on a track under identical environmental conditions.
13. Children run at a preset speed with less economy than adults because they require between 20% and 30% more oxygen per unit of body mass.
14. Swimming requires approximately four times more energy than running the same distance due to greater energy expended to maintain buoyancy and overcome drag forces during movement.
15. Elite swimmers expend fewer calories to swim a given stroke at any velocity.
16. Significant gender differences in swimming exist for body drag, economy, and net oxygen uptake.
17. Compared to men, women expend approximately 30% less energy to swim a given distance.

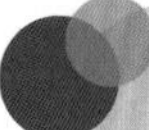

THINK IT THROUGH

1. A 60-kg (132-lb) elite marathoner who trains year round expends about 4000 kcal daily over a 4-year training period before Olympic competition. Assuming the athlete's body mass remains unchanged, and 70% of daily caloric intake comes from carbohydrate and 1.4 g per kg body mass comes from protein, compute the runner's total 4-year calorie intake and total grams consumed from carbohydrate and protein.
2. Respond to this question, "Why do children who run in 10-km races never seem to perform better than adults?"
3. Explain why it is untrue that it burns more total calories to run a given distance faster than at a slower pace. In what way does correcting this misunderstanding contribute to a recommendation for using physical activity for weight loss?
4. An elite 120-lb runner claims she consistently consumes 12,000 kcal daily simply to maintain body weight based on her strenuous training regimen. Using examples of energy expenditures, discuss whether this intake level could reflect a plausible regular energy intake requirement.

5. Discuss practical implications of knowing that children demonstrate lower walking and running economy than adults.
6. Discuss whether swim training improves swimming economy more than run training improves running economy.
7. Give two recommendations for mode-specific aerobic physical activities for training individuals with knee osteoarthritis.

KEY TERMS

Basal metabolic rate (BMR): Rate of energy expenditure at rest in a thermoneutral environment in the postabsorptive state, expressed in kilocalorie per meter squared per hour ($kcal \cdot m^{-2} \cdot h^{-1}$).

Body surface area (BSA): Area of the external surface of the length and width of the body expressed in square meters (m^2).

Buoyancy: Upward force exerted by a fluid that opposes the weight of an immersed object.

Crossover velocity: Juncture where the walking speed versus energy expenditure line of identity crosses the running speed versus energy expenditure line of identity; point at which it becomes more economical to run than walk.

Delta efficiency: A measure of the economy of physical effort when workloads are changed; expressed as a percentage ratio of change in work performed per minute to change in energy expended per minute.

Dietary-induced thermogenesis (DIT or thermic effect of food [TEF]): Increase in metabolism from the energy-requiring processes of digesting, absorbing, and assimilating food nutrients.

Drafting: When a runner, skier, cyclist, or swimmer follows directly behind a competitor to counter the negative effects on energy cost of the drag force imposed by air, headwind, or water resistance.

Economy of human movement: Quantity of energy to perform a steady-rate task, usually measured as $\dot{V}O_2$ in $mL \cdot kg^{-1} \cdot min^{-1}$.

Gross energy expenditure: Energy metabolism for a task of set duration, which *includes* the resting energy expenditure for the same duration.

Gross mechanical efficiency: The percentage of total chemical energy expended that contributes to external work, with the remainder lost as heat; includes energy expended during rest.

Mechanical efficiency (ME): Work Output ÷ Energy Expended × 100; the percentage of chemical energy expended (denominator) that contributes to the external work output (numerator).

Metabolic equivalents (METs): Used to express intensity of effort relative to resting energy expenditure; 1 MET = adult's average seated resting VO_2 or energy expenditure—about 250 $mL\ O_2 \cdot min^{-1}$, 3.5 $mL\ O_2 \cdot kg^{-1} \cdot min^{-1}$, 1 $kcal \cdot kg^{-1} \cdot h^{-1}$, or 0.017 $kcal \cdot kg^{-1} \cdot min^{-1}$ (1 $kcal \cdot kg^{-1} \cdot h^{-1} \div 60\ min \cdot h^{-1} = 0.017$).

Minimum effort: Principal that postulates that animals and humans will naturally use the absolute least amount of effort to perform a specific physical task; choosing the path of least resistance or effort.

Net energy expenditure: Metabolism for a given task for a set duration, which *excludes* resting energy expenditure for the same duration.

Net mechanical efficiency: Total oxygen uptake (excluding resting value) converted to kilocalories using calorific equivalent for oxygen values from RQ minus the resting oxygen uptake in kilocalories for the equivalent physical activity time period as the denominator of the ME ratio.

Non–weight-bearing activity (weight-supported activity): Any activity where total body weight, or part of body weight, is supported as in cycling and swimming.

Physical activity ratio (PAR): System used to rate the "strenuousness" of physical activity expressed in multiples of resting metabolism for light work, heavy work, and maximal work.

Postabsorptive state: No food consumed for a 12-hour minimum.

Resting daily energy expenditure (RDEE): Amount of energy expended by the body for a 24-hour period during resting conditions; usually expressed in kcal.

Resting metabolic rate (RMR): Rate of energy expenditure measured 3 to 4 hours following a light meal without physical activity.

Shivering thermogenesis: Increase in metabolism from uncontrollable shaking or trembling from small, multiple muscular contractions in response to cold exposure.

Total daily energy expenditure (TDEE): Total calories expended by the body during any 24-hour period.

Weight-bearing activity: Any activity where body weight is transported as in walking, jogging, running, or climbing.

SELECTED REFERENCES

Aguirre N, et al. The role of amino acids in skeletal muscle adaptation to exercise. *Nestle Nutr Inst Workshop Ser* 2013;76:85.

Ainsworth BE, et al. Compendium of physical activities: classification of energy costs of human physical activities. *Med Sci Sports Exerc* 1993;25:71.

Alexander RM. Physiology: enhanced: walking made simple. *Science* 2005; 308:58.

Alfonzo-Gonzalez G, et al. Estimation of daily energy needs with the FAO/WHO/UNU 1985 procedures in adults: comparison to whole-body indirect calorimetry measurements. *Eur J Clin Nutr* 2004;58:1125.

Angus SD. Did recent world record marathon runners employ optimal pacing strategies? *J Sports Sci* 2014;32:31.

Ariëns GA, et al. The longitudinal development of running economy in males and females aged between 13 and 27 years: the Amsterdam Growth and Health Study. *Eur J Appl Physiol* 1997;76:214.

Barbosa TM, et al. Energetics and biomechanics as determining factors of swimming performance: updating the state of the art. *J Sci Med Sport* 2010;13:262.

Barbosa TM, et al. Energy cost and intracyclic variation of the velocity of the centre of mass in butterfly stroke. *Eur J Appl Physiol* 2005;93:519.

Bassett DR Jr, et al. Metabolic responses to drafting during front crawl swimming. *Med Sci Sports Exerc* 1991;23:744.

Bellou E, et al. Effect of high-intensity interval exercise on basal triglyceride metabolism in non-obese men. *Appl Physiol Nutr Metab* 2013;38:823.

Berry M, et al. Effects of body mass on exercise efficiency and during steady-state cycling. *Med Sci Sports Exerc* 1993;25:1031.

Bertram JE. Constrained optimization in human walking: cost minimization and gait plasticity. *J Exp Biol* 2005;208:979.

Bilodeau B, et al. Effect of drafting on heart rate in cross country skiing. *Med Sci Sports Exerc* 1994;26:637.

Blanc S, et al. Energy requirements in the eighth decade of life. *Am J Clin Nutr* 2004;79:303.

Bonen A, et al. Maximal oxygen uptake during free, tethered, and flume swimming. *J Appl Physiol* 1980;48:232.

Browning RC, et al. The effects of adding mass to the legs on the energetics and biomechanics of walking. *Med Sci Sports Exerc* 2007;39:515.

Browning RC, et al. Pound for pound: working out how obesity influences the energetics of walking. *J Appl Physiol* 2009;106:1755.

Butte NF, et al. Energy requirements of women of reproductive age. *Am J Clin Nutr* 2003;77:630.

Byrne NM, et al. Metabolic equivalent: one size does not fit all. *J Appl Physiol* 2005;99:1112.

Caird SJ, et al. Biofeedback and relaxation techniques improve running economy in sub-elite long distance runners. *Med Sci Sports Exerc* 1999;31:717.

Cavanagh PR, Kram R. Mechanical and muscular factors affecting the efficiency of human movement. *Med Sci Sports Exerc* 1985;17:326.

Cavanagh PR, Kram R. Stride length in distance running: velocity, body dimensions, and added mass effects. *Med Sci Sports Exerc* 1989;21:467.

Chasan-Taber L, et al. Development and validation of a pregnancy physical activity questionnaire. *Med Sci Sports Exerc* 2004;36:1750.

Chatard J-C, et al. Performance and drag during drafting swimming in highly trained triathletes. *Med Sci Sports Exerc* 1998;30:1276.

Chatard J-C, et al. Drafting distance in swimming. *Med Sci Sports Exerc* 2003;35:1176.

Chatard JC, Wilson B. Effect of fastskin suits on performance, drag, and energy cost of swimming. *Med Sci Sports Exerc* 2008;40:1149.

Clevenger HC, et al. Acute effect of dietary fatty acid composition on postprandial metabolism in women. *Exp Physiol* 2014;99:1182.

Collings PJ, et al. Physical activity intensity, sedentary time, and body composition in preschoolers. *Am J Clin Nutr* 2013;97:1020.

Cortesi MF, et al. Passive drag reduction using full-body swimsuits: the role of body position. *J Strength Cond Res* 2014;28:3164.

Coyle EF. Improved muscular efficiency displayed as Tour de France champion matures. *J Appl Physiol* 2005;98:2191.

Crouter SE, et al. Accuracy of polar S410 heart rate monitor to estimate energy cost of exercise. *Med Sci Sports Exerc* 2004;36:1433.

Cureton KJ, Sparling PB. Distance running performance and metabolic responses to running in men and women with excess weight experimentally equated. *Med Sci Sports Exerc* 1988;12:288.

da Rocha EE, et al. Can measured resting energy expenditure be estimated by formulae in daily clinical nutrition practice? *Curr Opin Clin Nutr Metab Care* 2005;8:319.

Das SK, et al. Energy expenditure is very high in extremely obese women. *J Nutr* 2004;134:1412.

DeLany JP, et al. Energy expenditure in African American and white boys and girls in a 2-y follow-up of the Baton Rouge Children's Study. *Am J Clin Nutr* 2004;79:268.

Delextrat A, et al. Drafting during swimming improves efficiency during subsequent cycling. *Med Sci Sports Exerc* 2003;35:1612.

Di Michele R, Merni F. The concurrent effects of strike pattern and ground-contact time on running economy. *J Sci Med Sport* 2014;17:414.

Doke J, et al. Mechanics and energetics of swinging the human leg. *J Exp Biol* 2005;208:439.

Doma K, Deakin GB. The effects of strength training and endurance training order on running economy and performance. *Appl Physiol Nutr Metab* 2013;38:651.

Donahoo WT, et al. Variability in energy expenditure and its components. *Curr Opin Clin Nutr Metab Care* 2004;7:599.

Duffield R, et al. Energy system contribution to 100-m and 200-m track running events. *J Sci Med Sport* 2004;7:302.

Durnin JVGA, Passmore R. *Energy, Work and Leisure*. London: Heinmann, 1967.

Edwards AG, Byrnes WC. Aerodynamic characteristic as determinants of the drafting effect in cycling. *Med Sci Sports Exerc* 2007;39:170.

Enders H, et al. The effects of preferred and non-preferred running strike patterns on tissue vibration properties. *J Sci Med Sport* 2014;17:218.

Farshchi HR, et al. Decreased thermic effect of food after an irregular compared with a regular meal pattern in healthy lean women. *Int J Obes Relat Metab Disord* 2004;28:653.

Figueiredo P, et al. Changes in arm coordination and stroke parameters on transition through the lactate threshold. *Eur J Appl Physiol* 2013;113:1957.

Figueiredo P, et al. Interplay of biomechanical, energetic, coordinative, and muscular factors in a 200 m front crawl swim. *Biomed Res Int* 2013; 2013:897232.

Flodmark CE. Calculation of resting energy expenditure in obese children. *Acta Paediatr* 2004;93:727.

Franz JR, et al. Metabolic cost of running barefoot versus shod: is lighter better? *Med Sci Sports Exerc* 2012;44:1519.

Frederick EC, et al. Lower oxygen demands of running in soft soled shoes. *Res Q Exerc Sport* 1986;57:174.

Galbraith A, et al. A One-year study of endurance runners: training, laboratory and field tests. *Int J Sports Physiol Perform* 2014;9:1019.

Garet M, et al. Estimating relative physical workload using heart rate monitoring: a validation by whole-body indirect calorimetry. *Eur J Appl Physiol* 2005;94:46.

Gault ML, et al. Cardiovascular responses during downhill treadmill walking at self-selected intensity in older adults. *J Aging Phys Act* 2013;21:335.

Going S, et al. Aging and body composition: biological changes and methodological issues. *Exerc Sport Sci Rev* 1995;23:459.

Gottschall JS, Kram R. Ground reaction forces during downhill and uphill running. *J Biomech* 2005;38:445.

Hagberg JM, Coyle EF. Physiological determinants of endurance performance as studied in competitive race walkers. *Med Sci Sports Exerc* 1983; 15:287.

Hall C, et al. Energy expenditure of walking and running: comparison with prediction equations. *Med Sci Sports Exerc* 2004;36:2128.

Halsey LG, White CR. Comparative energetics of mammalian locomotion: humans are not different. *J Hum Evol* 2012;63:718.

Haugen HA, et al. Variability of resting metabolic rate. *Am J Clin Nutr* 2003;78:1141.

Hausswirth C, et al. Effects of cycling alone or in a sheltered position on subsequent running performance during a triathlon. *Med Sci Sports Exerc* 1999;31:599.

Helseth J, et al. How do low horizontal forces produce disproportionately high torques in human locomotion? *J Biomech* 2008;41:1747.

Hiilloskorpi HK, et al. Use of heart rate to predict energy expenditure from low to high activity levels. *Int J Sports Med* 2003;24:332.

Hoyt RW, et al. Total energy expenditure estimated using foot-ground contact pedometry. *Diabetes Technol Ther* 2004;6:71.

Joyner MJ. Physiological limiting factors and distance running: influence of gender and age on record performance. *Exerc Sport Sci Rev* 1993;21:103.

Keytel LR, et al. Prediction of energy expenditure from heart rate monitoring during submaximal exercise. *J Sports Sci* 2005;23:289.

Kien CL, Ugrasbul F. Prediction of daily energy expenditure during a feeding trial using measurements of resting energy expenditure, fat-free mass, or Harris-Benedict equations. *Am J Clin Nutr* 2004;80:876.

Kinnunen H, et al. Wrist-worn accelerometers in assessment of energy expenditure during intensive training. *Physiol Meas* 2012;33:1841.

Kram R. Muscular force or work: what determines the metabolic energy cost of running? *Exerc Sport Sci Rev* 2000;28:138.

Kyröläinen H, et al. Interrelationships between muscle structure, muscle strength, and running economy. *Med Sci Sports Exerc* 2003;35:45.

Lake MJ, Cavanagh PR. Six weeks of training does not change running mechanics or improve running economy. *Med Sci Sports Exerc* 1996;28:860.

Larsson L, Lindqvist PG. Low-impact exercise during pregnancy study of safety. *Acta Obstet Gynecol Scand* 2005;84:34.

Lätt E, et al. Longitudinal development of physical and performance parameters during biological maturation of young male swimmers. *Percept Mot Skills* 2009;108:297.

Lätt E, et al. Physical development and swimming performance during biological maturation in young female swimmers. *Coll Antropol* 2009;33:117.

Lazzer S, et al. The energetics of ultra-endurance running. *Eur J Appl Physiol* 2012;112:1709.

Lin PH, et al. Estimation of energy requirements in a controlled feeding trial. *Am J Clin Nutr* 2003;77:639.

Lusk G. *The Elements of the Science of Nutrition*. 4th Ed. Philadelphia: WB Saunders, 1928.

Malison ER, et al. Running performance in middle-school runners. *J Sports Med Phys Fitness* 2004;44:383.

Manini TM. Energy expenditure and aging. *Ageing Res Rev* 2010;9:1.

Margaria R, et al. Energy cost of running. *J Appl Physiol* 1963;18:367.

Maron M, et al. Oxygen uptake measurements during competitive marathon running. *J Appl Physiol* 1976;40:836.

McArdle WD, et al. Aerobic capacity, heart rate and estimated energy cost during women's competitive basketball. *Res Q* 1971;42:178.

McArdle WD, Foglia GF. Energy cost and cardiorespiratory stress of isometric and weight training exercise. *J Sports Med Phys Fitness* 1969;9:23.

Mollendorf JC, et al. Effect of swim suit design on passive drag. *Med Sci Sports Exerc* 2004;36:1029.

Mooses M, et al. Dissociation between running and running performance in elite Kenyan distance runners. *J Sports Sci* 2015;33:136.

Morgan DW, et al. Longitudinal stratification of gait economy in young boys and girls: the locomotion energy and growth study. *Eur J Appl Physiol* 2004;91:30.

Morgan DW, et al. Prediction of the aerobic demand of walking in children. *Med Sci Sports Exerc* 2002;34:2097.

Myers J. *ACSM's Resources for Clinical Exercise Physiology*. 2nd Ed. Baltimore: Lippincott Williams & Wilkins, 2010.

Naemi R, Chockalingam N. Mathematical models to assess foot-ground interaction: an overview. *Med Sci Sports Exerc* 2013;45:1524.

Pendergast D, et al. Energy balance of human locomotion in water. *Eur J Appl Physiol* 2003;90:377.
Pendergast D, et al. The influence of drag on human locomotion in water. *Undersea Hyperb Med* 2005;32:45.
Pendergast DR, et al. Evaluation of fins used in underwater swimming. *Undersea Hyperb Med* 2003;30:57.
Perl DP, et al. Effects of footwear and strike type on running economy. *Med Sci Sports Exerc* 2012;44:1335.
Pescatello LS. *ACSM's Guidelines for Exercise Testing and Prescription*. 9th Ed. Baltimore: Lippincott Williams & Wilkins, 2014.
Peyrot N, et al. Why does walking economy improve after weight loss in obese adolescents? *Med Sci Sports Exerc* 2012;44:659.
Piers LS, et al. Is there evidence for an age-related reduction in BMR related to quantitative or qualitative change in components of lean tissue. *J Appl Physiol* 1998;85:2196.
Poehlman ET, et al. Endurance exercise in aging humans: effects on energy metabolism. *Exerc Sport Sci Rev* 1994;22:751.
Pontzer H. A new model predicting locomotor cost from limb length via force production. *J Exp Biol* 2005;208:1513.
Pugh LGCE, Edholm OG. The physiology of channel swimmers. *Lancet* 1955;2:761.
Pugh LGCE. Oxygen uptake in track and treadmill running with observations on the effect of air resistance. *J Physiol* 1970;207:823.
Puthoff ML, et al. The effect of weighted vest walking on metabolic responses and ground reaction forces. *Med Sci Sports Exerc* 2006;38:746.
Ramirez-Marrero FA, et al. Comparison of methods to estimate physical activity and energy expenditure in African American children. *Int J Sports Med* 2005;26:363.
Ratel S, Poujade B. Comparative analysis of the energy cost during front crawl swimming in children and adults. *Eur J Appl Physiol* 2009;105:543.
Ravn AM, et al. Thermic effect of a meal and appetite in adults: an individual participant data meta-analysis of meal-test trials. *Food Nutr Res* 2013;23:57.
Ray AD, et al. Respiratory muscle training reduces the work of breathing at depth. *Eur J Appl Physiol* 2010;108:811.
Reeves KA. Barefoot running improves economy at high intensities and peak treadmill velocity. *J Sports Med Phys Fitness* 2014. [Epub ahead of print].
Reis VM, et al. Examining the accumulated oxygen deficit method in front crawl swimming. *Int J Sports Med* 2010;31:421.
Rosenberger F, et al. Running 8000 m fast or slow: are there differences in energy cost and fat metabolism? *Med Sci Sports Exerc* 2005;37:1789.
Rotstein A, et al. Preferred transition speed between walking and running: effects of training status. *Med Sci Sports Exerc* 2006;37:1864.
Roy J-PR, Stefanyshyn DJ. Shoe midsole longitudinal bending stiffness and running economy, joint energy, and EMG. *Med Sci Sports Exerc* 2006;38:562.
Royer TD, Martin PE. Manipulations of leg mass and moment of inertia: effects on energy cost of walking. *Med Sci Sports Exerc* 2005;37:649.
Sabounchi NS, et al. Best-fitting prediction equations for basal metabolic rate: informing obesity interventions in diverse populations. *Int J Obes (Lond)* 2013;37:1364.
Sarafian D. A standardized approach to study human variability in isometric thermogenesis during low-intensity physical activity. *Front Physiol* 2013;4:155.
Saunders PU, et al. Reliability and variability of running economy in elite distance runners. *Med Sci Sports Exerc* 2004;36:1972.
Sazonov ES, Schuckers S. The energetics of obesity: a review: monitoring energy intake and energy expenditure in humans. *IEEE Eng Med Biol Mag* 2010;29:31. Review.
Schutz Y, et al. Diet-induced thermogenesis measured over a whole day in obese and non-obese women. *Am J Clin Nutr* 1984;40:542.
Scott CB, Devore R. Diet-induced thermogenesis: variations among three isocaloric meal-replacement shakes. *Nutrition* 2005;21:874.
Slawinski JS, Billat VL. Difference in mechanical and energy cost between highly, well, and nontrained runners. *Med Sci Sports Exerc* 2004;36:1440.
Smolander J, et al. Cardiorespiratory strain during walking in snow with boots of differing weights. *Ergonomics* 1989;32:319.
Sobhani S, et al. Rocker shoe, minimalist shoe, and standard running shoe: a comparison of running economy. *J Sci Med Sport* 2014;17:312.
Sousa A, et al. Anaerobic alactic energy assessment in middle distance swimming. *Eur J Appl Physiol* 2013;113:2153.
Speakman JR. Body size, energy metabolism and lifespan. *J Exp Biol* 2005;208:1717.
Srinivasan, M. Optimal speeds for walking and running, and walking on a moving walkway. *Chaos* 2009;19:026112.
Støren, Ø, et al. Maximal strength training improves running economy in distance runners. *Med Sci Sports Exerc* 2008;40:1087.
Stickford A. Lower leg compression, running mechanics and economy in trained distance runners. *Int J Sports Physiol Perform* 2015;10:76.
Taboga P, et al. Energetics and mechanics of running men: the influence of body mass. *Eur J Appl Physiol* 2012;112:4027.
Tam E, et al. Energetics of running in top-level marathon runners from Kenya. *Eur J Appl Physiol* 2012;112:3797.
Tharion WJ, et al. Energy requirements of military personnel. *Appetite* 2005;44:47.
Toussaint HM, et al. The mechanical efficiency of front crawl swimming. *Med Sci Sports Exerc* 1990;22:402.
Trappe TA, et al. Thermal responses to swimming in three water temperatures: influence of a wet suit. *Med Sci Sports Exerc* 1995;27:1014.
Trembly A, et al. Diminished dietary thermogenesis in exercise-trained human subjects. *Eur J Appl Physiol* 1983;52:1.
Unnithan V, et al. Aerobic cost in elite female adolescent swimmers. *Int J Sports Med* 2009;30:194.
Vasconcellos MT, Anjos LA. A simplified method for assessing physical activity level values for a country or study population. *Eur J Clin Nutr* 2003;57:1025.
Vercruyssen F, et al. Cadence selection affects metabolic responses during cycling and subsequent running time to fatigue. *Br J Sports Med* 2005;39:267.
Volpe Ayub B, Bar-Or O. Energy cost of walking in boys who differ in adiposity but are matched for body mass. *Med Sci Sports Exerc* 2003;35:669.
Weissgerber TL, et al. The role of regular physical activity in preeclampsia prevention. *Med Sci Sports Exerc* 2004;36:2024.
Westerterp KR. Physical activity and physical activity induced energy expenditure in humans: measurement, determinants, and effects. *Front Physiol* 2013;4:90.
Weyand PG, Bundle MW. Energetics of high-speed running: integrating classical theory and contemporary observations. *Am J Physiol Regul Integr Comp Physiol* 2005;288:R956.
Williams PT. Greater weight loss from running than walking during a 6.2-yr prospective follow-up. *Med Sci Sports Exerc* 2013;45:76.
Willy RW, Davis IS. Kinematic and kinetic comparison of running in standard and minimalist shoes. *Med Sci Sports Exerc* 2014;46:318.
Zamparo P, et al. How fins affect the economy and efficiency of human swimming. *J Exp Biol* 2002;205:2665.
Zamparo P, et al. The interplay between propelling efficiency, hydrodynamic position and energy cost of front crawl in 8 to 19-year-old swimmers. *Eur J Appl Physiol* 2008;104:689.

SECTION IV

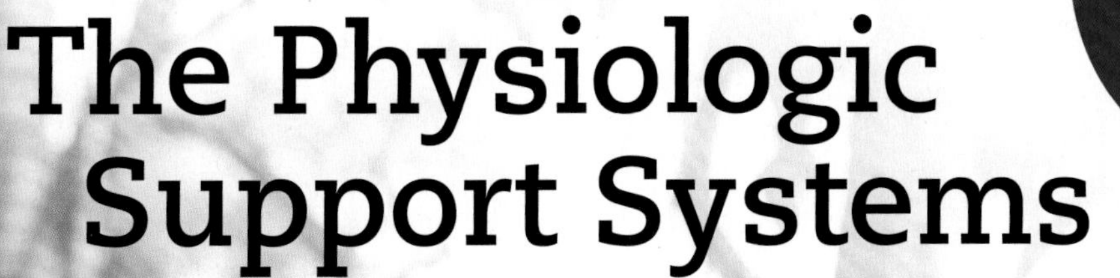

The Physiologic Support Systems

Most sport, recreational, and occupational activities require a moderately intense yet sustained energy release. The aerobic breakdown of carbohydrates, fats, and proteins generates this energy from the phosphorylation of adenosine diphosphate (ADP) to adenosine triphosphate (ATP). Without a *steady rate* between oxidative phosphorylation and the energy requirements of physical activity, an anaerobic-aerobic energy imbalance develops, lactate accumulates, tissue acidity increases, and fatigue quickly ensues. Two factors limit an individual's ability to sustain a high intensity of physical activity without undue, overall body fatigue:

1. Oxygen delivery capacity to active muscle cells
2. Active muscle cells' capacity to generate ATP aerobically

Understanding the roles of the ventilatory, circulatory, muscular, and endocrine systems during physical activity explains the broad range of individual differences in performance capacity. Knowing the energy requirements of physical activity and corresponding physiologic adjustments necessary to meet these requirements helps to formulate an effective physical fitness program to properly evaluate an individual's physiologic and fitness status before and during such a program.

All the problems of the world could be settled easily if men were only willing to think. The trouble is that men very often resort to all sorts of devices in order not to think, because thinking is such hard work.

— Thomas J. Watson,
IBM President, 1924–1952

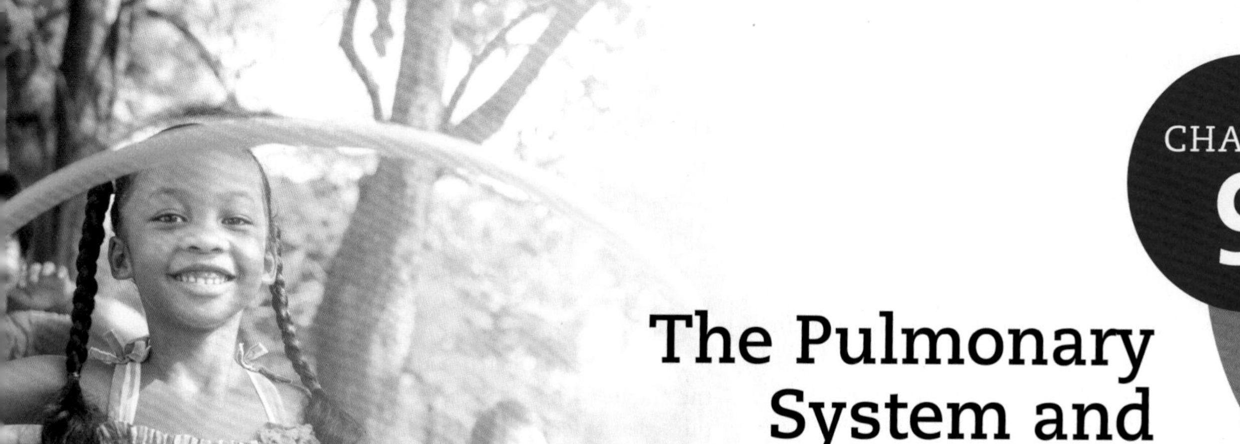

CHAPTER 9

The Pulmonary System and Physical Activity

CHAPTER OBJECTIVES

- Diagram the ventilatory system and label the glottis, larynx, trachea, bronchi, bronchioles, and alveoli.
- Describe the dynamics of inspiration and expiration during rest and physical activity.
- Define and quantify static and dynamic lung function measures and their relation to physical performance.
- Describe the Valsalva maneuver and its physiologic consequences.
- Define minute ventilation, alveolar minute ventilation, ventilation-perfusion ratio, and anatomic and physiologic dead spaces.
- List the partial pressures of respired gases in alveoli, arterial blood, active muscles, and mixed-venous blood during rest and maximal physical activity.
- Discuss two physiologic advantages of oxyhemoglobin's S-shaped dissociation curve.
- Explain the Bohr effect and its major benefit during physical activity.
- Explain what triggers exercise-induced asthma, and identify three factors that affect its severity.
- List and quantify three mechanisms for carbon dioxide transport in blood.
- Identify three major factors that regulate pulmonary ventilation during rest and physical activity.
- Describe how hyperventilation extends breath-holding time.
- Graph relationships among pulmonary ventilation, blood lactate concentrations, and oxygen uptake during incremental physical activity.
- Indicate the demarcation points for the lactate threshold and onset of blood lactate accumulation.
- Explain the rationale for substituting the blood lactate threshold for $\dot{V}O_{2max}$ to predict endurance performance.
- Discuss two pros and two cons to the argument that pulmonary ventilation represents the "weak link" in oxygen supply during maximal physical activity.
- Summarize how chemical and physiologic buffer systems regulate acid-base quality of body fluids during rest and physical activity.

ANCILLARIES AT A GLANCE

Visit **http://thePoint.lww.com/MKKESS5e** to access the following resources.

- References: Chapter 9
- Interactive Question Bank
- Animation: Asthma
- Animation: Gas Exchange in Alveoli
- Animation: Oxygen Transport
- Animation: Pulmonary Ventilation
- Animation: Renal Function
- Animation: Transport of Carbon Dioxide

PART 1 Pulmonary Structure and Function

If oxygen supply depended only on diffusion through the body's multiple skin layers weighing about 8 pounds (3.6 kg) and comprising about 22 square feet (2.2 square meters), it would be impossible to support the basal energy requirement, let alone the 4- to 6-L oxygen uptake needed each minute to sustain a world-class 5 minute per mile marathon pace. The remarkably effective **ventilatory system** meets the body's needs to maintain efficient gas exchange. This system, depicted in **Figure 9.1**, regulates the gaseous state of the "external" environment for aerating fluids of the "internal" environment during rest and physical activity. The three major functions of the ventilatory system are the following:

1. Supply oxygen required in metabolism
2. Eliminate carbon dioxide produced in metabolism
3. Regulate hydrogen ion concentration $[H^+]$ to sustain acid-base balance

ANATOMY OF VENTILATION

The term **pulmonary ventilation** describes how ambient atmospheric air moves into and exchanges with air in the lungs. A distance of about 0.3 m (1 ft) separates ambient air just outside the nose and mouth from the blood flowing through the lungs. Air entering the nose and mouth flows into the conductive portion of the ventilatory system, where it adjusts to body temperature and filtered and humidified as it flows through the trachea. The trachea, a short 1-inch-diameter hollow tube that extends from the larynx (voice box), divides into two tubes of smaller diameter called **bronchi** (from the Greek *brónchos* or windpipe). The bronchi serve as primary conduits within the right and left lungs. They further subdivide into numerous **bronchioles** that conduct inspired air through a narrow route until eventually mixing it with the air in the **alveoli** (from the Latin alveolus or "little cavity"), the respiratory tract's terminal branches.

Lungs

The lungs provide the surface between blood and the external environment. Lung volume varies between 4 and 6 L, the

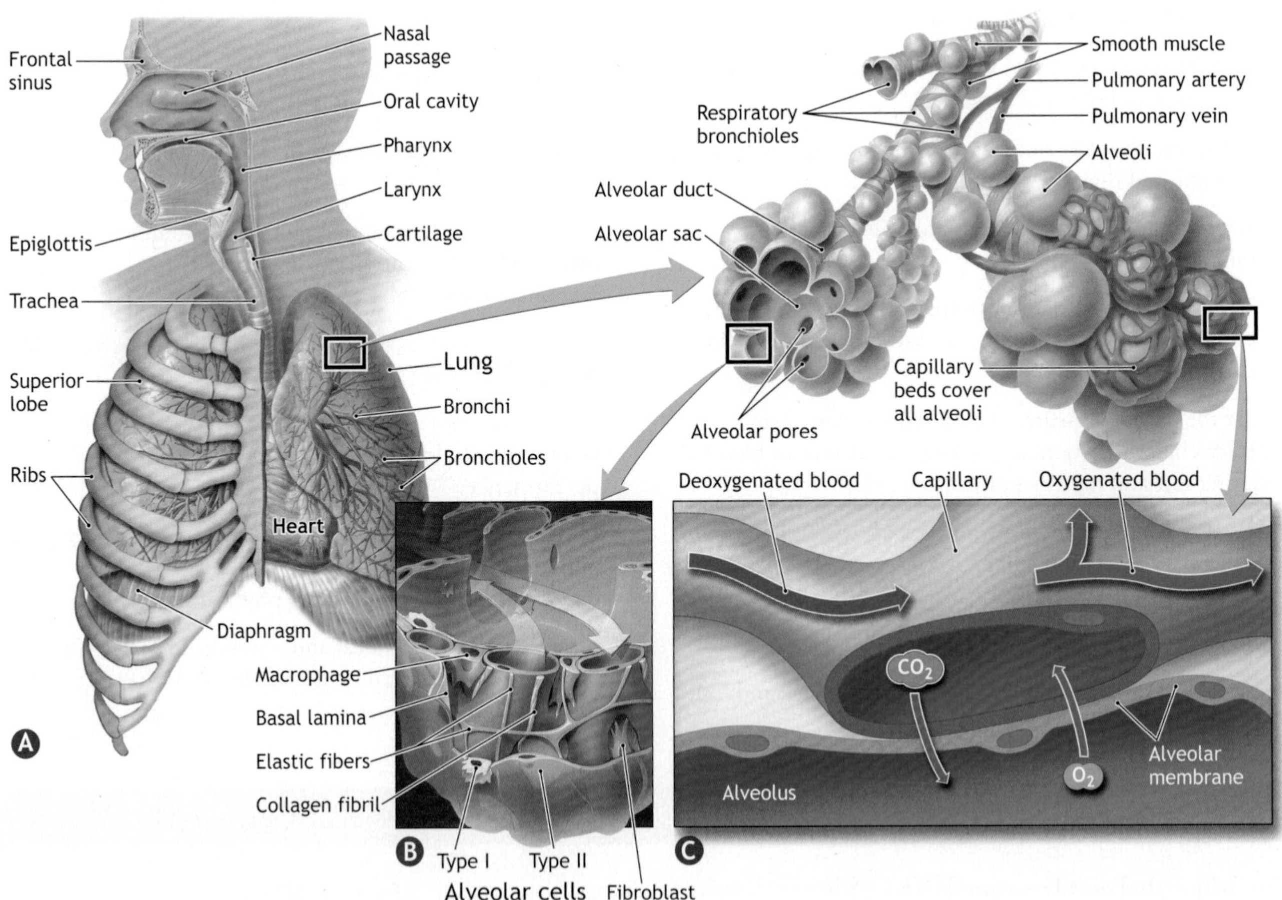

FIGURE 9.1 **A.** Major pulmonary structures within the thoracic cavity including the terminal respiratory tree branches. **B.** Section of lung tissue showing individual alveolus including type I cells that form the structure of the alveolar wall, type II cells that secrete pulmonary surfactant, and macrophages that destroy foreign substances including bacteria. **C.** Alveolar gas exchange function. (Adapted with permission from McArdle WD, Katch FI, Katch VL. *Exercise Physiology: Nutrition, Energy, and Human Performance*. 8th Ed. Baltimore: Wolters Kluwer Health, 2015.)

amount of air in a basketball, and provides an exceptionally large moist surface. The lungs of an average-sized person weigh between 1 and 2 kg, yet if spread out, they would cover a surface of 50 to 100 m^2, about 20 to 50 times the external surface of the person, and almost half the size of a tennis court or an entire badminton court (**Fig. 9.2**). This provides a considerable interface for aeration. During any 1 second of maximal activity, no more than 1 pint of blood flows in the lung tissue's weblike, intricate, and interlaced blood vessel network.

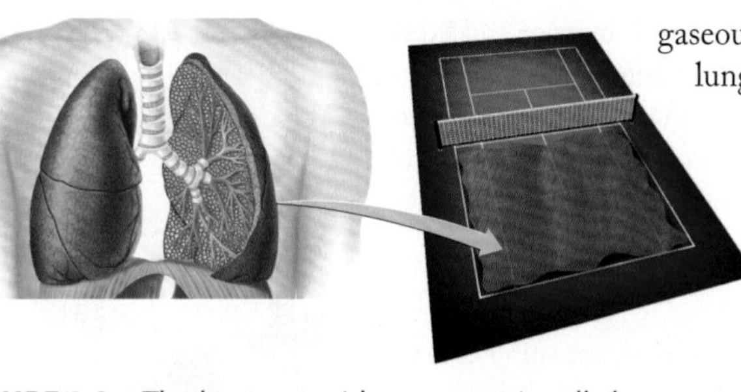

FIGURE 9.2 The lungs provide an exceptionally large surface for gas exchange. (Adapted with permission from McArdle WD, Katch FI, Katch VL. *Exercise Physiology: Nutrition, Energy, and Human Performance*. 8th Ed. Baltimore: Wolters Kluwer Health, 2015.)

Alveoli

Lung tissue contains more than 600 million alveoli. These elastic, thin-walled, membranous sacs provide the vital surface for gas exchange between the lungs and blood. Alveolar tissue has the largest blood supply of any organ. Millions of thin-walled capillaries and alveoli lie adjacent to each other, with air moving on one side and blood on the other. The capillaries form a dense, meshlike cover that encircles the entire outside of each alveolus. This web becomes so dense that blood essentially flows as a sheet over an alveolus. When blood reaches the pulmonary capillaries, only a single-cell barrier, the **respiratory membrane**, separates it from alveolar air. This ultrathin tissue-blood barrier allows for almost instantaneous diffusion between alveolar and blood gases.

During each minute at rest, approximately 250 mL of oxygen *leave* the alveoli and enter the blood, and about 200 mL of carbon dioxide diffuse *into* the alveoli. When trained endurance athletes perform intense activity, about 20 times the resting oxygen uptake each minute transfers across the respiratory membrane into the blood. The primary function of pulmonary ventilation during rest and physical activity attempts to maintain a relatively constant and favorable concentration of oxygen and carbon dioxide in the alveolar chambers. This ensures effective alveolar gaseous exchange before blood exits the lungs for transit throughout the body.

Mechanics of Ventilation

Figure 9.3 depicts the physical principle underlying breathing dynamics. The illustration shows two balloons connected to a jar whose glass bottom has been replaced by a thin elastic membrane. When the membrane lowers, the jar's volume increases, and air pressure within the jar becomes less than air pressure outside the jar. Consequently, air rushes into the balloons and they inflate. Conversely, if the elastic membrane recoils, pressure within the jar temporarily increases and air rushes out. Air exchange occurs within the balloons as distance and rate of descent and ascent of the membrane increases.

Unlike the balloons in our illustration, the lungs are not merely suspended in the chest cavity. Rather, the difference in pressure between the lungs and the lung–chest wall interface

A CLOSER LOOK

Common Symbols Used by Pulmonary Physiologists

Pulmonary Ventilation		External Respiration		Internal Respiration	
$\dot{V}_E$ =	Minute ventilation	$\dot{V}_A$ =	Alveolar minute ventilation	$a\text{-}\bar{v}O_{2diff}$ =	Quantity of oxygen carried in arteries minus amount carried in veins
V_d =	Dead space	P_AO_2 =	Partial pressure of oxygen in alveoli	PaO_2 =	Partial pressure of oxygen in arterial blood
V_T =	Tidal volume	PaO_2 =	Partial pressure of oxygen in arterial blood	$PaCO_2$ =	Partial pressure of carbon dioxide in arterial blood
F =	Breathing frequency	$(A\text{-}a)PO_{2diff}$ =	Oxygen or PO_2 pressure gradient between alveoli and arteries	$PvCO_2$ =	Partial pressure of carbon dioxide in venous blood
V_d/V_T =	Ratio of dead space to tidal volume	$SaO_2\%$ =	Percent saturation of arterial blood with oxygen	$SvO_2\%$ =	Percent saturation of venous blood with oxygen
		P_ACO_2 =	Partial pressure of carbon dioxide in alveoli	PvO_2 =	Partial pressure of oxygen in venous blood

causes the lungs to adhere to the chest wall interior and literally follow its every movement. Any change in thoracic cavity volume produces a corresponding change in lung volume. Ventilatory skeletal musculature action during inspiration and expiration alters thoracic dimensions to change lung volume.

Inspiration

The **diaphragm** (from the Ancient Greek meaning "partition"), a large, dome-shaped sheet of muscle, serves the same purpose as the jar's separating elastic membrane in **Figure 9.3**. The diaphragm muscle makes an airtight separation between the abdominal and thoracic cavities. During **inspiration**, the diaphragm contracts, flattens out, and moves downward up to 10 cm toward the abdominal cavity. This enlarges and elongates the chest cavity. The air in the lungs then expands, reducing its pressure (referred to as **intrapulmonic pressure**) to about 5 mm Hg below atmospheric pressure. *The pressure differential between the lungs and ambient air literally sucks air in through the nose and mouth and the lungs inflate.* Two factors control lung filling:

1. Magnitude of inspiratory movements
2. Pressure gradient between the air inside and outside the lung

Inspiration concludes when thoracic cavity expansion ceases and intrapulmonic pressure increases to equal atmospheric pressure.

fyi A Common Posture After Running

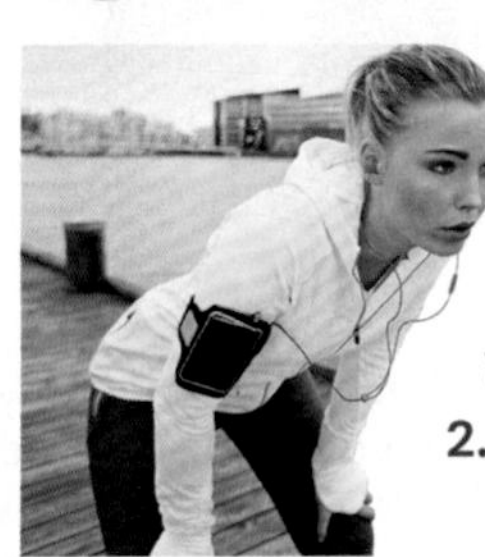

Following intense physical activity, individuals frequently bend forward from the waist to facilitate breathing. This body position accomplishes two purposes:

1. Facilitates blood flow to the heart
2. Minimizes antagonistic effects of gravity on respiratory movements

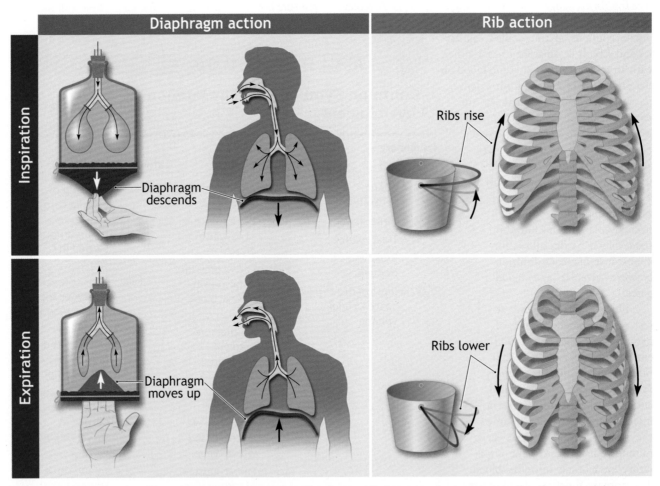

FIGURE 9.3 Mechanics of breathing. During inspiration, the chest cavity increases in size because the ribs rise and the muscular diaphragm lowers. During exhalation, the ribs swing down, and the diaphragm returns to a relaxed position. This reduces the thoracic cavity volume, and air rushes out. The movement of the jar's rubber bottom causes air to enter and leave the two balloons, simulating the diaphragm's action. The movement of the bucket handle simulates rib action. (Reprinted with permission from McArdle WD, Katch FI, Katch VL. *Exercise Physiology: Nutrition, Energy, and Human Performance*. 8th Ed. Baltimore: Wolters Kluwer Health, 2015.)

During physical activity, the scalene and external intercostal muscles between the ribs contract. This causes the ribs to rotate and lift up and away from the body—a subtle but deliberate action similar to the movement of the handle lifted up and away from the side of the bucket at the right in **Figure 9.3**. Three factors cause air to move into the lungs when chest cavity volume increases:

1. Diaphragm descends
2. Ribs lift upward
3. Sternum thrusts outward

Expiration

Expiration, a predominantly passive process, occurs as air moves out of the lungs from the recoil of stretched lung tissue and inspiratory muscle relaxation. This causes the sternum and ribs to swing down while the diaphragm moves toward the thoracic cavity. These movements decrease chest cavity volume and compress alveolar gas, forcing air from the respiratory tract into the atmosphere. During ventilation in moderate-to-intense activity, the internal intercostal muscles and abdominal muscles act powerfully on the ribs and abdominal cavity to produce a rapid and greater exhalation depth. Greater involvement of the pulmonary musculature during progressively intense exertion causes larger pressure differentials and concomitant increases in air movement.

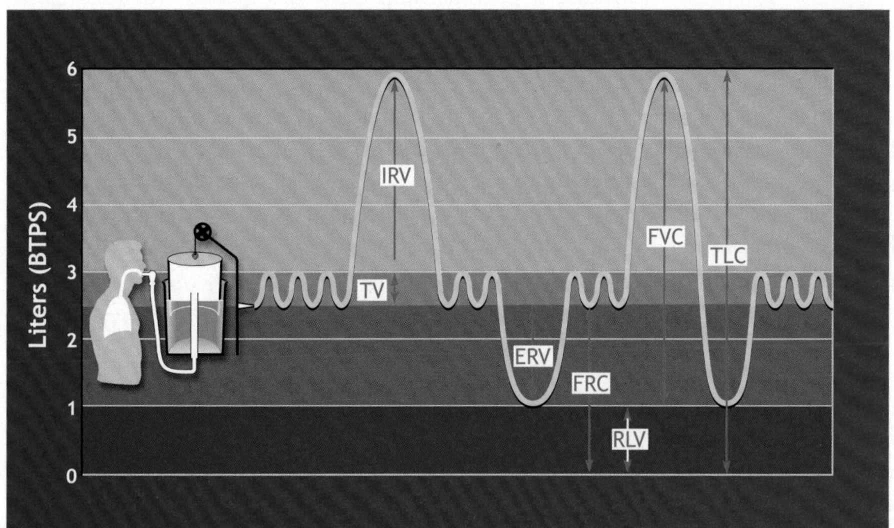

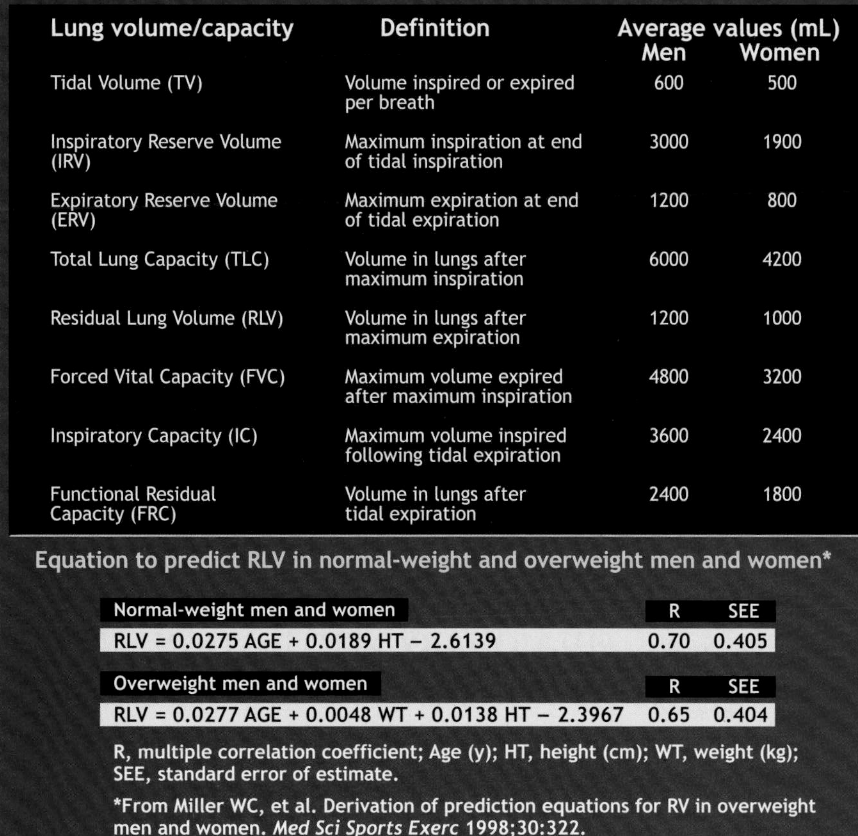

Lung volume/capacity	Definition	Average values (mL) Men	Women
Tidal Volume (TV)	Volume inspired or expired per breath	600	500
Inspiratory Reserve Volume (IRV)	Maximum inspiration at end of tidal inspiration	3000	1900
Expiratory Reserve Volume (ERV)	Maximum expiration at end of tidal expiration	1200	800
Total Lung Capacity (TLC)	Volume in lungs after maximum inspiration	6000	4200
Residual Lung Volume (RLV)	Volume in lungs after maximum expiration	1200	1000
Forced Vital Capacity (FVC)	Maximum volume expired after maximum inspiration	4800	3200
Inspiratory Capacity (IC)	Maximum volume inspired following tidal expiration	3600	2400
Functional Residual Capacity (FRC)	Volume in lungs after tidal expiration	2400	1800

Equation to predict RLV in normal-weight and overweight men and women*

Normal-weight men and women	R	SEE
RLV = 0.0275 AGE + 0.0189 HT − 2.6139	0.70	0.405

Overweight men and women	R	SEE
RLV = 0.0277 AGE + 0.0048 WT + 0.0138 HT − 2.3967	0.65	0.404

R, multiple correlation coefficient; Age (y); HT, height (cm); WT, weight (kg); SEE, standard error of estimate.

*From Miller WC, et al. Derivation of prediction equations for RV in overweight men and women. *Med Sci Sports Exerc* 1998;30:322.

FIGURE 9.4 Static measures of lung volume and capacity. (Adapted with permission from McArdle WD, Katch FI, Katch VL. *Exercise Physiology: Nutrition, Energy, and Human Performance*. 8th Ed. Baltimore: Wolters Kluwer Health, 2015.)

LUNG VOLUMES AND CAPACITIES

Figure 9.4 presents a lung volume tracing with average values for men and women. To obtain these measurements, the subject rebreathes through a water-sealed, volume-displacement spirometer similar to the one described in Chapter 7 for measuring oxygen uptake with closed-circuit spirometry. As with many anatomic and physiologic measures, lung volumes vary with age, gender, and body size and composition but particularly with stature. After the American Civil War, the physicians of that era believed the tallest soldiers were in top physical condition because of their large lung volumes measured by spirometry. In fact, vital capacity was then considered a standard measure of "physical fitness." Beginning in the 1920s, common practice began to evaluate lung volumes by comparing them with established standards from large-scale population surveys that now include age, stature, and body weight.

Two types of measurements, static and dynamic, provide information about lung volume dimensions and capacities.

Static lung volume tests evaluate the *dimensional component* for air movement within the pulmonary tract and impose no time limitation on the individual. In contrast, **dynamic lung volume** measures assess the *power component* of pulmonary performance during different phases of the ventilatory excursion.

Static Lung Volumes

During static lung function measurement, the spirometer bell falls and rises with each inhalation and exhalation to provide a record of ventilatory volume and breathing rate. **Tidal volume (TV)** describes the air moved during either the inspiratory or expiratory phase of each breathing cycle. For healthy men and women, TV under resting conditions ranges between 0.4 and 1.0 L air per breath.

An additional volume of 2.5 to 3.5 L above TV air represents the reserve for inhalation; this is the **inspiratory reserve volume (IRV)**. After recording several representative TVs, the individual inspires normally and then maximally to determine the IRV.

Following the IRV, the normal breathing pattern begins once again. After a normal exhalation, the individual continues to exhale and forces as much air as possible from the lungs. This additional volume, the **expiratory reserve volume (ERV)**, ranges between 1.0 and 1.5 L for an average-size man (10% to 20% lower for women). During physical activity, TV increases considerably from encroachment on IRV and ERV, particularly IRV.

Forced vital capacity (FVC) represents total air volume moved in one breath from full inspiration to maximum expiration or vice versa. FVC varies with body size and body position during measurement; values usually average 4 to 5 L in healthy young men and 3 to 4 L in healthy young women. FVCs of 6 to 7 L are common for tall individuals, and values above 8 L have been reported for some large-size professional basketball, volleyball, and American football players. These large lung volumes probably reflect genetic endowment because training does not appreciably change static lung volumes.

Residual Lung Volume

Following a maximal exhalation, a volume of air remains in the lungs that cannot be exhaled. This volume, called the **residual lung volume (RLV)**, averages between 0.9 and 1.2 L for young adult women and 1.1 and 1.7 L for men.

Aging changes lung volumes due to decreased lung tissue elasticity and reductions in pulmonary muscle power. Nonetheless, these two factors do not entirely result from aging per se. *Sedentary living, rather than true aging, likely determines the largest changes in lung volumes and pulmonary function with advancing age.*

Dynamic Lung Volumes

Dynamic measures of pulmonary ventilation depend on two factors:

1. Maximum air volume expired (FVC)
2. Speed of moving a volume of air

*Airflow speed depends on the pulmonary airways' resistance to smooth air flow and the resistance or "stiffness" presented by chest and lung tissue to changes in their shape during breathing termed **lung compliance**.*

Ratio of Forced Expiratory Volume to Forced Vital Capacity

Normal values for vital capacity occur even in severe lung disease if no time limit exists to expel air. For this reason, a dynamic lung function measure, such as the percentage of **forced expiratory volume (FEV)** expelled in 1 second (**$FEV_{1.0}$**), is more useful for diagnostic purpose than are static lung function measures. The ***forced expiratory volume-to-FVC ratio ($FEV_{1.0}$/FVC)*** *reflects expiratory power and overall resistance to air movement in the lungs.* Normally, the $FEV_{1.0}$/FVC averages about 85%. With severe obstructive pulmonary emphysema and bronchial asthma, the $FEV_{1.0}$/FVC typically decreases below 40% of vital capacity. *The clinical demarcation for airway obstruction represents the point where a person expels less than 70% of FVC in 1 second.*

Maximum Voluntary Ventilation

Another dynamic assessment of ventilatory capacity requires 15 seconds of rapid, deep breathing. Extrapolation of the 15-second volume to the volume breathed for 1 minute represents the **maximum voluntary ventilation (MVV)**. For healthy young men, the MVV ranges between 140 and 180 $L \cdot min^{-1}$; the average for women equals 80 to 120 $L \cdot min^{-1}$. Male members of the US Nordic Ski Team averaged 192 $L \cdot min^{-1}$, with an individual high MVV of 239 $L \cdot min^{-1}$. Patients with obstructive lung disease achieve only about 40% of the MVV predicted normal for their age and stature.

Ventilatory Muscles Respond Positively to Training

Specific ventilatory muscle training improves their strength and endurance and increases inspiratory muscle function and MVV. Ventilatory training in patients with chronic pulmonary disease enhances capacity and reduces physiologic strain. Progressive desensitization to feelings of breathlessness and greater self-control of respiratory symptoms represent important benefits from ventilatory muscle training and regular physical activity for patients with chronic obstructive pulmonary disease (COPD).

PULMONARY VENTILATION

One can view pulmonary ventilation from two perspectives:

1. Volume of air moved into or out of the total respiratory tract each minute
2. Air volume that ventilates only the alveolar chambers each minute

See the animation "Pulmonary Ventilation" on **http://thePoint.lww.com/MKKESS5e** for a demonstration of this process.

TABLE 9.1 **Relationships Among Tidal Volume, Breathing Rate, and Minute and Alveolar Minute Ventilation**

Condition	Tidal Volume (mL)	×	Breathing Rate (breaths · min^{-1})	=	Minute Ventilation (mL · min^{-1})	–	Dead Space Ventilation (mL · min^{-1})	=	Alveolar Ventilation (mL · min^{-1})
Shallow breathing	150		40		6000		(150 mL × 40)		0
Normal breathing	5000		12		6000		(150 mL × 12)		4200
Deep breathing	1000		6		6000		(150 mL × 6)		5100

Minute Ventilation

During quiet breathing at rest, an adult's breathing rate averages 12 breaths a minute, and the TV averages about 0.5 L of air per breath. Under these conditions, the volume of air breathed each minute, termed **minute ventilation**, equals 6 L.

$$\textbf{Minute ventilation } (\dot{V}_E) = \textbf{Breathing rate} \times \textbf{TV}$$

$$\mathbf{6.0\ L \cdot min^{-1} = 12 \times 0.5\ L}$$

An increase in breathing depth or rate both increase minute ventilation. During maximal exertion, the breathing rate of healthy young adults increases to 35 to 45 breaths per minute, while elite athletes often achieve 60 to 70 breaths per minute. During intense physical activity, TV commonly increases to 2.0 L and greater. For adults, this causes exercise minute ventilation to reach 100 L or about 17 times the resting value. In well-trained male endurance athletes, ventilation can increase to 160 L · min^{-1} during maximal effort, with several studies of elite endurance athletes reporting ventilation volumes exceeding 200 L · min^{-1}. *Even with such large minute ventilations, TV rarely exceeds 55% to 65% of vital capacity.*

Alveolar Ventilation

***Alveolar ventilation** refers to the portion of minute ventilation that mixes with air in the alveolar chambers.* A portion of each inspired breath *does not* enter the alveoli and *does not* engage in gaseous exchange with blood. The air that fills the nose, mouth, trachea, and other nondiffusible conducting portions of the respiratory tract constitutes the **anatomic dead space**. In healthy people, this volume equals 150 to 200 mL or about 30% of resting TV. An almost equivalent composition exists between dead space air and ambient air except for dead space air's full saturation with water vapor.

Because of dead space volume, approximately 350 mL of the 500 mL of ambient air inspired in each TV at rest mixes with existing alveolar air. This does not mean that only 350 mL of air enters and leaves the alveoli with each breath. To the contrary, if TV equals 500 mL, then 500 mL of air enters the alveoli but only 350 mL represents fresh air or about one-seventh of the alveoli's total air. This relatively small, seemingly inefficient alveolar ventilation is an evolutionary protective mechanism to prevent drastic changes in alveolar air composition. This ensures a consistency in arterial blood gases throughout the breathing cycle.

Table 9.1 shows that minute ventilation does not always reflect real alveolar ventilation. In the first example of shallow breathing, TV decreases to 150 mL, yet a 6-L per minute ventilation occurs when breathing rate increases to 40 breaths a minute. The same 6-L per minute volume can occur by decreasing breathing rate to 12 breaths a minute and increasing TV to 500 mL. Doubling TV and reducing ventilatory rate by half, as in the example of deep breathing, again produces a 6-L per minute ventilation. Each ventilatory adjustment drastically impacts alveolar ventilation. In the example of shallow breathing, dead space air represents the entire air volume moved, as no alveolar ventilation has taken place. The other examples involve deeper breathing; in this case, a larger portion of each breath mixes with existing alveolar air. *Alveolar ventilation, not dead space ventilation, determines gaseous concentrations at the alveolar-capillary membrane.*

The Gas Laws

Four laws govern gas behavior:

- **Boyle's law** (Discovered in 1662 by Irish chemist Robert Boyle): If temperature remains constant, gas pressure varies inversely with its volume.
  http://video.mit.edu/watch/boyles-law-pressure-vs-volume-8456/
- **Gay-Lussac's law** (named in 1808 to honor its discoverer, French chemist Joseph Louis Gay-Lussac): If gas volume remains constant, its pressure increases proportionally to its absolute temperature.
- **Law of partial pressures** (first described in 1801 by English chemist John Dalton): In a mixture of gases, each gas exerts a partial pressure proportional to its concentration.
- **Henry's law** (formulated in 1803 by English chemist William Henry): If temperature remains constant, the quantity of a gas dissolved in a liquid varies in direct proportion to its partial pressure.

Physiologic Dead Space

Two factors help to explain why some alveoli may not function adequately in gas exchange:

1. Underperfusion of blood
2. Inadequate ventilation relative to alveolar surface area

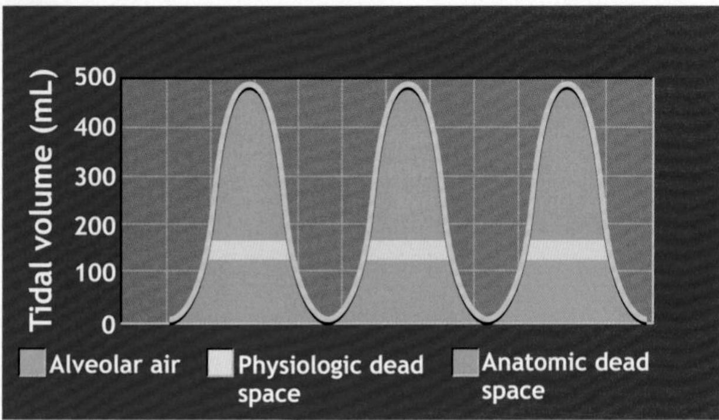

FIGURE 9.5 Distribution of tidal lung volume of a healthy subject at rest. Tidal volume includes about 350 mL of ambient air that mixes with alveolar air, 150 mL of air in the larger air passages (anatomic dead space), and small portion of air distributed to either poorly ventilated or poorly perfused alveoli (physiologic dead space). (Adapted with permission from McArdle WD, Katch FI, Katch VL. *Exercise Physiology: Nutrition, Energy, and Human Performance*. 8th Ed. Baltimore: Wolters Kluwer Health, 2015.)

The term **physiologic dead space** describes the portion of alveolar volume with poor tissue regional perfusion or inadequate ventilation. **Figure 9.5** illustrates that only a negligible physiologic dead space exists in healthy lungs.

Physiologic dead space can increase to 50% of resting TV. This occurs because of two factors:

1. Inadequate perfusion during hemorrhage or an embolism or blood clot that blocks pulmonary circulation
2. Inadequate alveolar ventilation in chronic pulmonary disease

Adequate gas exchange and aeration of blood are impossible when the lung's total dead space exceeds 60% of lung volume.

Breathing Rate Versus Tidal Volume

As intensity of effort increases, adjustments in breathing rate and depth maintain alveolar ventilation. In moderate activity, trained endurance athletes sustain adequate alveolar ventilation by increasing TV and only minimally by increasing breathing rate. With deeper breathing, alveolar ventilation usually increases from 70% of minute ventilation at rest to more than 85% of total exercise ventilation. *This increase occurs because a greater percentage of incoming TV enters the alveoli with deeper breathing.*

Figure 9.6 shows that increasing TV during physical activity results largely from encroachment on IRV, with an accompanying but smaller decrease in end-expiratory level. As intensity increases, TV plateaus at about 60% of vital capacity; further increases in minute ventilation result from increases in breathing rate. These ventilatory adjustments occur unconsciously; each individual develops a "style" of breathing by blending the breathing rate and TV so alveolar ventilation matches alveolar perfusion. *Conscious attempts to modify breathing during running and other general physical activities do not benefit performance. In most instances, conscious manipulation of breathing detracts from the exquisitely regulated ventilatory adjustments to physical activity.* During rest and physical activity, each individual should breathe in the

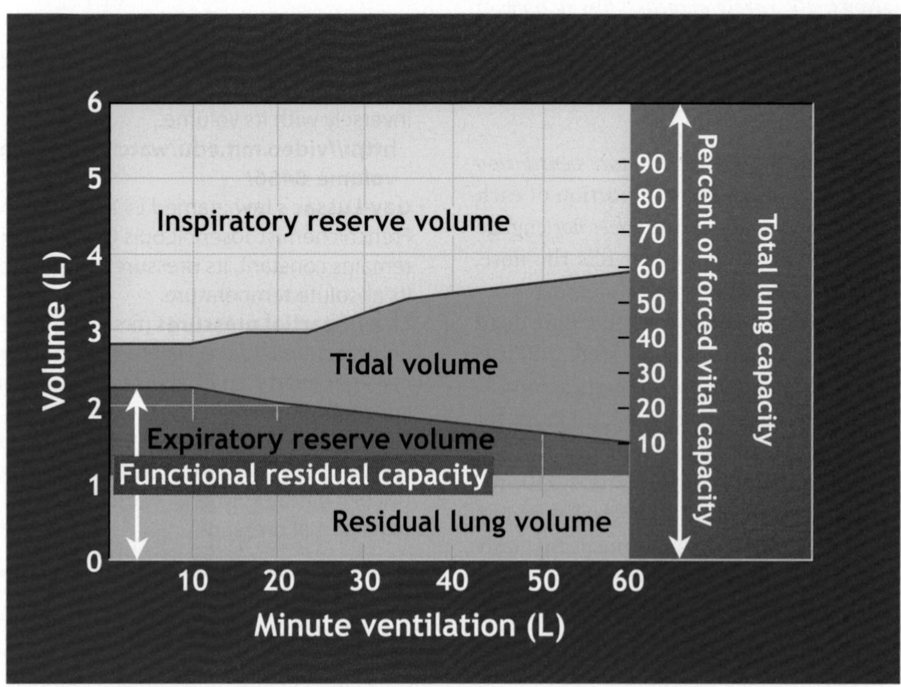

FIGURE 9.6 Tidal volume and subdivisions of pulmonary air during rest and physical activity. (Adapted with permission from McArdle WD, Katch FI, Katch VL. *Exercise Physiology: Nutrition, Energy, and Human Performance*. 8th Ed. Baltimore: Wolters Kluwer Health, 2015.)

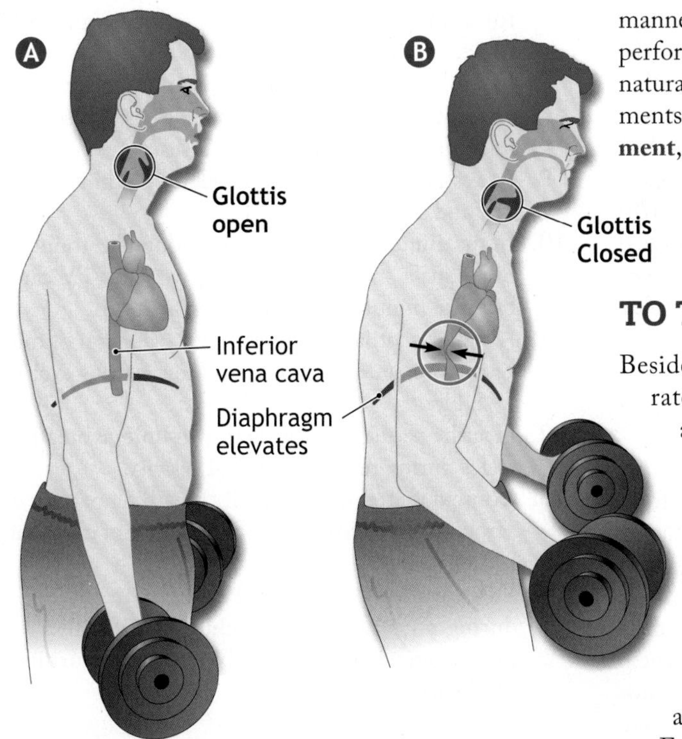

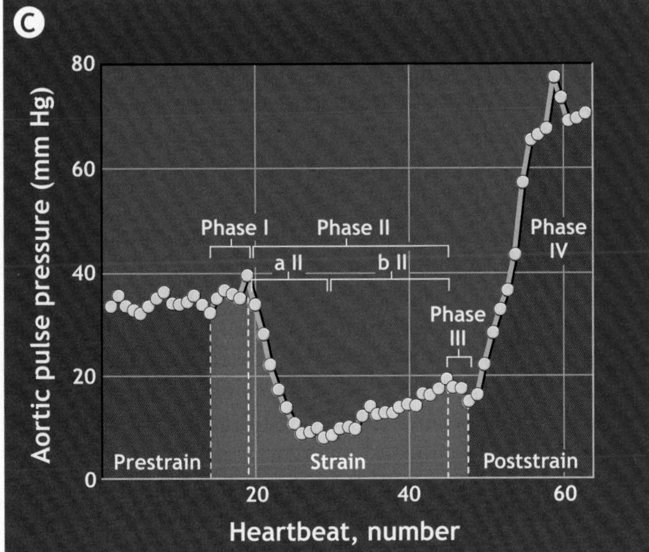

FIGURE 9.7 The Valsalva maneuver reduces blood returning to the heart because increased intrathoracic pressure collapses the inferior vena cava that passes through the chest cavity. **A.** Normal breathing. **B.** Straining exercise with accompanying Valsalva maneuver. **C.** Typical normal response of aortic pulse pressure with a Valsalva maneuver during calibrated muscle strain. The figure illustrates 63 consecutive heartbeats. High-fidelity aortic pressure recordings were obtained at the aortic root level. Pulse pressure represents systolic pressure minus diastolic pressure. (Data from Hébert J-L, et al. Pulse pressure response to the strain of the Valsalva maneuver in humans with preserved systolic function. *J Appl Physiol* 1998;85:817; image adapted with permission from McArdle WD, Katch FI, Katch VL. *Exercise Physiology: Nutrition, Energy, and Human Performance*. 8th Ed. Baltimore: Wolters Kluwer Health, 2015.)

manner that seems "most natural." Most individuals who perform rhythmical walking, running, cycling, and rowing naturally synchronize breathing frequency with limb movements. This breathing pattern, termed **breathing entrainment**, reduces the activity's energy cost.

VALSALVA MANEUVER IMPEDES BLOOD FLOW RETURN TO THE HEART

Besides their normal role in pulmonary ventilation, expiratory muscles assist in coughing and sneezing. They also contribute to stabilizing abdominal and chest cavities during heavy lifting. In quiet breathing, intrapulmonic pressure decreases only about 3 mm Hg during inspiration and rises a similar amount above atmospheric pressure in exhalation (**Fig. 9.7A**). Closing the glottis following a full inspiration while maximally activating the expiratory muscles (**Fig. 9.7B**) generates compressive forces to increase intrathoracic pressure above 150 mm compared to atmospheric pressure. Furthermore, the abdominal cavity experiences even higher pressures during a maximal exhalation against a closed glottis. Forced exhalation against a closed glottis, termed the ***Valsalva maneuver*** (first described in 1704 by Italian anatomist and physician Antonio Maria Valsalva [1666–1723]), commonly occurs in weightlifting and other activities that require a rapid, maximum application of a short-duration force. A voluntary Valsalva stabilizes the abdominal and thoracic cavities to enhance muscle action but not without potential consequences.

Physiologic Consequences of the Valsalva Maneuver

A prolonged Valsalva produces an acute drop in blood pressure. The increased intrathoracic pressure transmits through the thin walls of veins that enter into the thoracic region. The venous blood remains under relatively low pressure, causing the thoracic veins to collapse which reduces blood flow to the heart. Reduced venous return sharply lowers the heart's stroke volume, triggering a fall in blood pressure below the resting level. Performing a prolonged Valsalva maneuver during static or "isometric" straining-type movements dramatically reduces venous return and arterial blood pressure. These two effects diminish the brain's blood supply, often producing dizziness, "spots before the eyes," or fainting. Once the glottis reopens and intrathoracic pressure stabilizes, blood flow re-establishes with an "overshoot" in arterial blood pressure.

Figure 9.7C illustrates four phases of the typical blood pressure in a healthy subject, heartbeat by heartbeat, during the Valsalva maneuver. Aortic pulse pressure increases slightly as the Valsalva begins (phase I), probably from the mechanical effect of elevated intrathoracic pressure that expels blood from the left ventricle into the aorta. A biphasic response occurs within six heartbeats of Valsalva onset. This consists of a large reduction in aortic pulse pressure (phase IIa) followed by a relatively small gradual rise (phase IIb) and secondary decrease (phase III) during the continued Valsalva strain. When the maneuver ceases (strain release), blood pressure rises rapidly and overshoots the resting value (phase IV).

A Common Misconception

During heavy resistance exercise, the Valsalva maneuver does not cause substantial increases in blood pressure. Recall from **Figure 9.7** that blood pressure dramatically *decreases* during a prolonged Valsalva. Confusion arises because a Valsalva maneuver of insufficient duration to lower blood pressure usually accompanies straining muscular efforts common during isometric and dynamic resistance exercise. These activities, with or without Valsalva, greatly increase resistance to blood flow in active muscle with a resulting rise in systolic blood pressure. For example, intramuscular fluid pressure increases linearly with all levels of isometric force to the maximum. Increased peripheral vascular resistance increases the arterial blood pressure and the heart's workload throughout exercise. These responses pose a potential danger to individuals with cardiovascular disease; they form the basis for advising cardiac patients to refrain from heavy resistance training. In contrast, performing rhythmic muscular activity, including moderate-effort weightlifting, promotes a steadier blood flow and only modest increase in blood pressure and work of the heart.

SUMMARY

1. The healthy lung provides a large interface between the body's internal fluid environment and gaseous external environment.
2. No more than 1 pint of blood flows in the pulmonary capillaries during any 1 second.
3. Pulmonary ventilation adjustments maintain favorable concentrations of alveolar oxygen and carbon dioxide to ensure adequate aeration of lung blood flow.
4. Pulmonary airflow depends on small pressure differences between ambient air and air within the lungs.
5. Lung volumes vary with age, gender, body size, and stature and should be evaluated only on norms based on these variables.
6. TV increases during physical activity by encroachment on inspiratory and ERVs.
7. When breathing to vital capacity, RLV remains in the lungs at maximal exhalation, which allows for uninterrupted gas exchange during a breathing cycle.
8. $FEV_{1.0}$ and MVV provide a dynamic assessment of ability to sustain high airflow levels and serve as screening tests to detect lung disease.
9. At rest, minute ventilation equals breathing rate times TV and averages about 6 L.
10. In maximum activity in large, endurance-trained individuals, increased breathing rate and TV can produce minute ventilations above 200 L.
11. Alveolar ventilation represents the portion of minute ventilation entering the alveoli for gaseous exchange with blood.
12. Healthy people exhibit their own unique breathing styles during rest and physical activity.
13. Conscious attempts to modify breathing pattern during aerobic activity confer no physiologic or performance benefits.
14. Disruptions in normal breathing patterns during physical activity include the Valsalva maneuver, which impedes blood flow returning to the heart.

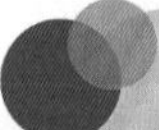

THINK IT THROUGH

1. Advise a track athlete trying to change their breathing pattern in hope of becoming a more economical runner.
2. Explain how a person accelerates breathing rate at rest without disrupting normal alveolar ventilation.
3. Explain how regular resistance and aerobic training can blunt the typical decline in lung function with advancing age.
4. After straining to "squeeze out" a maximum lift in the standing press, the person states: "I feel slightly dizzy and see spots before my eyes." Provide a plausible physiologic explanation, and what can be done to prevent this from happening?

PART 2 Gas Exchange

Oxygen supply depends on oxygen *concentration* in ambient air and its *pressure*. Ambient air composition remains constant: 20.93% oxygen, 79.04% nitrogen (including small quantities of inert gases that behave physiologically like nitrogen), 0.03% carbon dioxide, and small quantities of water vapor. These gas molecules move relatively quickly, exerting a pressure against any surface they contact.

Weather Changes and Barometric Pressure

At sea level, the pressure of air's gas molecules raises a column of mercury to an average height of 760 mm (29.9 in.). Barometric readings vary with changing weather conditions and decrease predictably at increased altitude.

As an example of the influence of changing weather conditions, consider the barometric pressure at the Ann Arbor, MI, municipal airport on December 2, 2014 at 3:00 P.M.—30.24 inches at 32°F and 66% humidity. Only 30 minutes later at the same 32°F temperature but a slightly elevated 69% humidity, barometric pressure decreased slightly to 30.21. By 6:45 P.M., when the temperature decreased to 25°F, the barometric pressure had declined further to 30.16 inches.

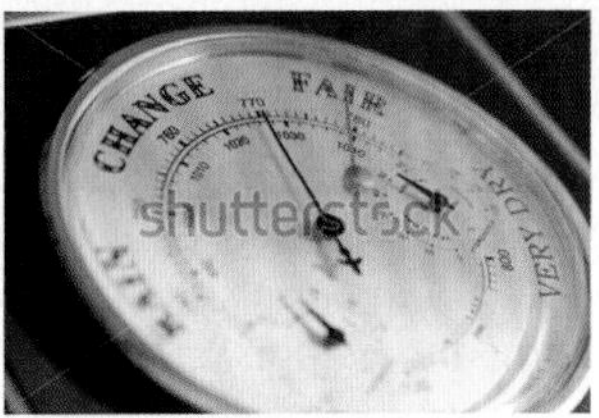

RESPIRED GASES: CONCENTRATIONS AND PARTIAL PRESSURES

Gas concentration differs from gas pressure:

- **Gas concentration** reflects an amount of gas in a given volume determined by the product of gas partial pressure and solubility
- **Gas pressure** represents atomic forces gas molecules exert against a unit of area surfaces they encounter

A mixture's total pressure equals the sum of the **partial pressures** of the individual gases, which computes as follows:

Partial pressure = Percentage concentration × Total gas mixture pressure

Ambient Air

Table 9.2 presents the percentages, partial pressures, and volumes of specific gases in 1 L of dry, ambient air at sea level. The partial pressure of oxygen equals 20.93% of the total 760 mm Hg pressure exerted by the air mixture, or 159 mm Hg (0.2093 × 760 mm Hg); the letter *P* before the gas symbol denotes partial pressure. The random movement of the minute quantity of carbon dioxide exerts a pressure of only 0.2 mm Hg (0.0003 × 760 mm Hg), and nitrogen molecules exert a pressure that raises the mercury in a **manometer** about 600 mm Hg (0.7904 × 760 mm Hg). For sea-level ambient air:

PO_2 = 159 mm Hg; PCO_2 = 0.2 mm Hg; and PN_2 = 600 mm Hg

Tracheal Air

Air entering the nose and mouth passes down the respiratory tract completely saturated with water vapor, which slightly dilutes the inspired air mixture. At body temperature, pressure of water molecules in humidified air equals 47 mm Hg; this leaves 713 mm Hg (760 mm Hg – 47 mm Hg) as the total pressure exerted by inspired dry air molecules at sea level. This decreases the effective tracheal air PO_2 by about 10 mm Hg from its dry ambient value of 159 mm Hg to 149 mm Hg (0.2093 × [760 mm Hg – 47 mm Hg]). Humidification minimally affects inspired PCO_2 because of carbon dioxide's near negligible inspired air concentration.

Alveolar Air

Alveolar air composition differs quantitatively from incoming ambient air because carbon dioxide continually enters the alveoli from blood and oxygen leaves the lungs for transport throughout the body. **Table 9.3** shows that moist alveolar air contains approximately 14.5% oxygen, 5.5% carbon dioxide, and 80.0% nitrogen.

After subtracting water vapor pressure in moist alveolar gas, the average alveolar PO_2 equals 103 mm Hg (0.145 × [760 mm Hg – 47 mm Hg]), and PCO_2 equals 39 mm Hg (0.055 × [760 mm Hg – 47 mm Hg]). These values represent average pressures exerted by oxygen and carbon dioxide molecules against the alveolar side of the respiratory membrane. They do not exist as physiologic constants but vary slightly with ventilation cycle phase and ventilator adequacy in different lung segments.

TABLE 9.2 Percentages, Partial Pressures, and Volumes of Gases in 1 L of Dry Ambient Air at Sea Level

Gas	Percentage	Partial Pressure (at 760 mm Hg)	Volume of Gas ($mL \cdot L^{-1}$)
Oxygen	20.93	159 mm Hg	209.3
Carbon dioxide	0.03	0.2 mm Hg	0.4
Nitrogen	79.04[a]	600 mm Hg	790.3

[a]Includes 0.93% argon and other trace rare gases.

TABLE 9.3 Percentages, Partial Pressures, and Volumes of Gases in 1 L of Moist Alveolar Air at Sea Level (37°C)

Gas	Percentage	Partial Pressure (at 760 – 47 mm Hg)	Volume of Gas ($mL \cdot L^{-1}$)
Oxygen	14.5	103 mm Hg	145
Carbon dioxide	5.5	39 mm Hg	55
Nitrogen	80.00	571 mm Hg	800
Water vapor		47 mm Hg	

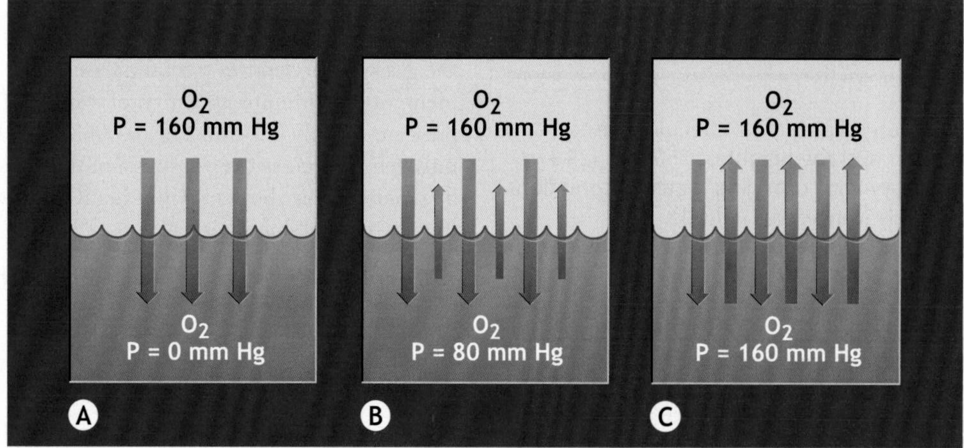

FIGURE 9.8 **A.** Solution of oxygen in water when oxygen first contacts pure water. **B.** Dissolved oxygen halfway to equilibrium with gaseous oxygen. **C.** Equilibrium between oxygen in air and oxygen dissolved in water. (Reprinted with permission from McArdle WD, Katch FI, Katch VL. *Exercise Physiology: Nutrition, Energy, and Human Performance*. 8th Ed. Baltimore: Wolters Kluwer Health, 2015.)

GAS MOVEMENT IN AIR AND FLUIDS

Knowledge of how gases act in air and fluids allows an understanding of the mechanism for gas movement between the external environment and the body's tissues. In accord with Henry's law, the amount of a specific gas dissolved in a fluid depends on two factors:

1. **Pressure differential** between the gas above the fluid and dissolved in the fluid
2. **Solubility** of gas in the fluid

Pressure Differential

Figure 9.8 shows three examples of gas movement between air and fluid. Oxygen molecules continually strike the water surface in each of the three chambers. Pure water in chamber **A** contains no oxygen, allowing a larger number of oxygen molecules to dissolve in water. Some oxygen molecules also leave the water because the dissolved molecules move randomly in continuous motion. In chamber **B**, the pressure gradient between air and water still favors oxygen's net movement or diffusion into the fluid from the gaseous state, yet the quantity of additional oxygen dissolving in the fluid remains less than in chamber **A**. Eventually, the pressures attain equilibrium, and the number of molecules entering and leaving the fluid equalize (chamber **C**). Conversely, if pressure of dissolved oxygen molecules exceeds the air's oxygen pressure, oxygen escapes the fluid until it attains a new pressure equilibrium. These examples illustrate that a gas' net diffusion occurs only when a *difference* exists in gas pressure. A specific gas' partial pressure gradient represents the driving force for its diffusion. Similarly, concentration gradients provide the driving force for diffusion of the nongaseous glucose, sodium, and calcium molecules.

Solubility

Gas solubility or its dissolving power reflects the quantity dissolved in fluid at a particular pressure. A gas with greater solubility has a higher concentration at a specific pressure. For two different gases at identical pressure differentials, the solubility of each gas determines the number of molecules moving into or out of a fluid. *For each unit of pressure favoring diffusion, approximately 25 times more carbon dioxide than oxygen moves into or out of a fluid.*

GAS EXCHANGE IN THE BODY

Exchange of gases between the lungs and blood and gas movement at the tissue level progresses passively by diffusion, depending on their pressure gradients. **Figure 9.9** schematically illustrates the pressure gradients favoring gas transfer in the body.

See the animation "Oxygen Transport" on **http://thePoint.lww.com/MKKESS5e** for a demonstration of this concept.

Gas Exchange in Lungs

The first step in oxygen transport involves oxygen transfer from the alveoli into the blood. Three factors account for the dilution of oxygen in inspired air as it passes into the alveolar chambers:

1. Water vapor saturates relatively dry inspired air.
2. Oxygen continually leaves alveolar air.
3. Carbon dioxide continually enters alveolar air.

Considering these three factors, alveolar Po_2 averages about 100 mm Hg, a value considerably below the 159 mm Hg in dry ambient air. Despite a reduced Po_2, the pressure of oxygen molecules in alveolar air still averages about 60 mm Hg higher than the Po_2 in venous blood that enters pulmonary capillaries. This allows oxygen to diffuse through the alveolar membrane into the blood.

Carbon dioxide exists under slightly greater pressure in returning venous blood than in alveoli, causing carbon dioxide to diffuse from blood to lungs. Only a small pressure gradient of 6 mm Hg exists for carbon dioxide diffusion compared with oxygen, but because of carbon dioxide's high

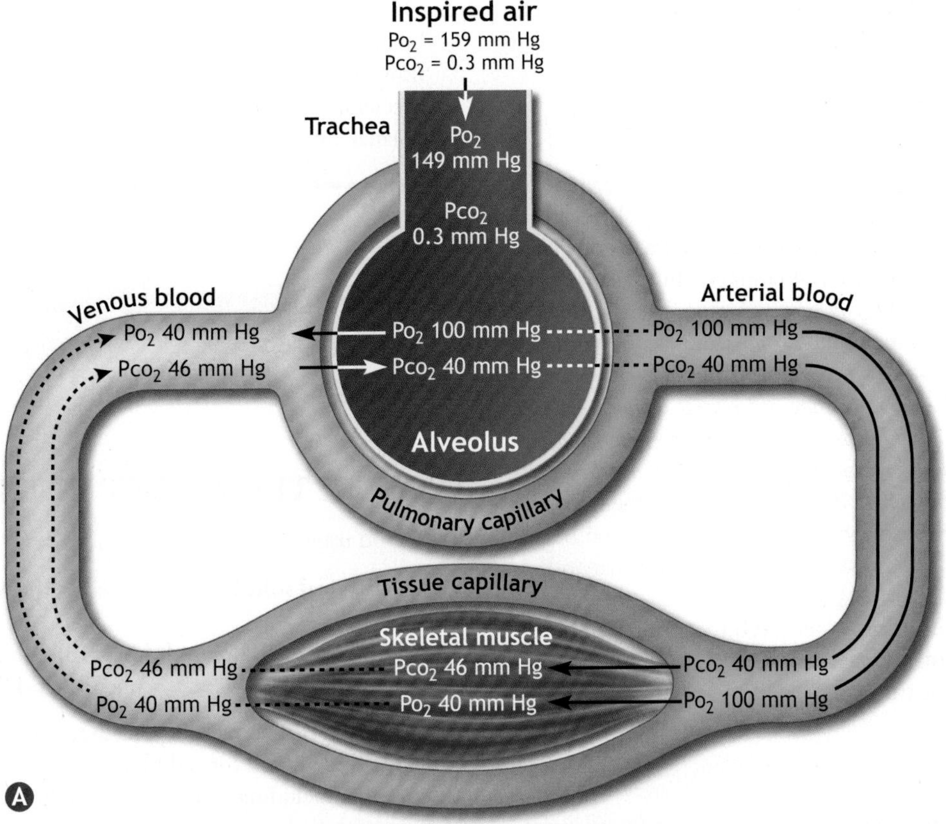

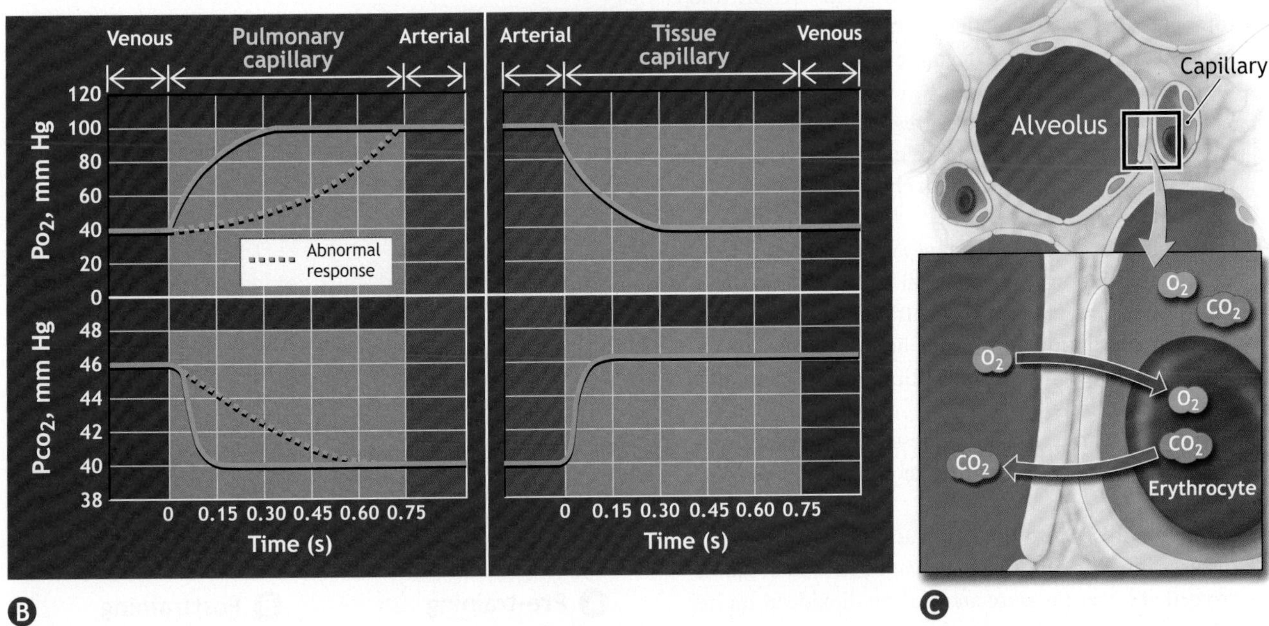

FIGURE 9.9 Gas transfer pressure gradients at rest. **A.** The Po_2 and Pco_2 of ambient, tracheal, and alveolar air and gas pressures in venous and arterial blood and muscle tissue. Gas movement at the alveolar-capillary and tissue-capillary membranes always progresses from an area of higher partial pressure to lower partial pressure. **B.** Time required for gas exchange. At rest, blood remains in the pulmonary and tissue capillaries for about 0.75 seconds. Pulmonary disease (*dashed line*) impairs the rate of gas transfer across the alveolar-capillary membrane, thus prolonging the time for gas equilibration. Blood's transit time through the pulmonary capillaries during maximal exercise decreases to about 0.4 seconds, but this still remains adequate for complete aeration in the healthy lung. **C.** Gas exchange or diffusion between a pulmonary capillary and its adjacent alveolus. (Adapted with permission from McArdle WD, Katch FI, Katch VL. *Exercise Physiology: Nutrition, Energy, and Human Performance*. 8th Ed. Baltimore: Wolters Kluwer Health, 2015.)

solubility, carbon dioxide transfer occurs rapidly. Nitrogen, an inert gas in metabolism, remains relatively unchanged in alveolar-capillary gas.

Gas Exchange in Tissues

Gas pressures differ from arterial blood in tissues where energy metabolism consumes oxygen at a rate about equal to carbon dioxide production (see **Fig. 9.9**). At rest, the average Po_2 within the muscle rarely declines below 40 mm Hg; intracellular Pco_2 averages about 46 mm Hg. Whereas vigorous exercise reduces the pressure of oxygen molecules in active muscle to 3 mm Hg, carbon dioxide pressure approaches 90 mm Hg in vigorous physical activity. *The large pressure differential between gases in plasma and tissues establishes the diffusion gradient—oxygen leaves capillary blood and flows toward metabolizing cells, and carbon dioxide flows from the cell into blood.* Blood then enters the veins and returns to the heart for delivery to the lungs. Diffusion begins when venous blood enters the lung's dense capillary network.

See the animation "Gas Exchange in Alveoli" on **http://thePoint.lww.com/MKKESS5e** for a demonstration of this concept.

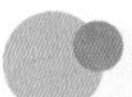

SUMMARY

1. Partial pressure of a specific gas in a gas mixture varies proportionally to its concentration in the mixture and total pressure exerted by the mixture.
2. Pressure and solubility determine the quantity of gas dissolved in a fluid.
3. Carbon dioxide has 25 times greater solubility than oxygen in plasma to allow more carbon dioxide molecules to move down relatively small pressure gradients in body fluids.
4. Gas molecules diffuse in the lungs and tissues down their concentration gradients from higher concentration (higher pressure) to lower concentration (lower pressure).
5. Alveolar ventilation adjusts during intense physical activity so alveolar gas composition remains similar to resting conditions.
6. Alveolar and arterial oxygen pressures equal about 100 mm Hg, and carbon dioxide pressure remains at 40 mm Hg.
7. Oxygen diffuses into the blood and carbon dioxide diffuses into the lungs because venous blood contains oxygen at lower pressure and carbon dioxide at higher pressure than alveolar gas.
8. Tissue diffusion gradients favor oxygen movement from capillaries to tissues and carbon dioxide movement from cells to blood.
9. Physical activity expands diffusion gradients, making oxygen and carbon dioxide diffuse rapidly.

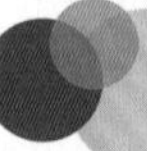

THINK IT THROUGH

1. Discuss the driving forces for respiratory gas exchange in lungs and active muscles.
2. One technique during "natural" childbirth requires rapid breathing to effectively "work with" the normal ebb and flow of uterine contractions. Explain how a person can accelerate resting breathing rate without disrupting normal alveolar ventilation.

PART 3 Oxygen and Carbon Dioxide Transport

OXYGEN TRANSPORT IN THE BLOOD

The blood transports oxygen in two ways:

1. In **physical solution**—dissolved in the blood's fluid portion
2. Combined with **hemoglobin (Hb)**—in loose combination with red blood cells' iron-protein Hb molecules

Figure 9.10A shows the percentage composition of centrifuged whole blood for red blood cells (termed *hematocrit*) and plasma, including representative values for the quantity of oxygen carried in each component.

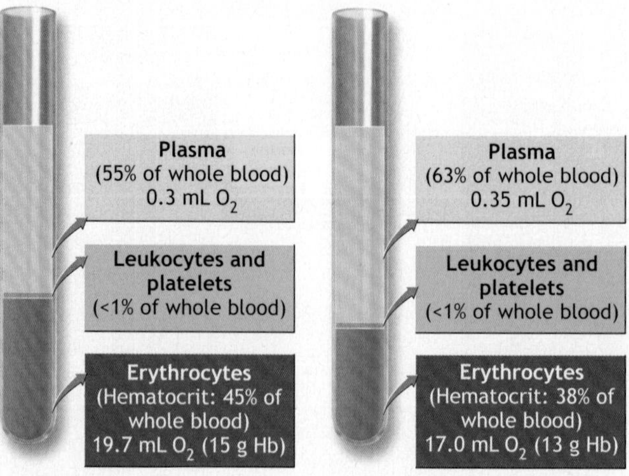

FIGURE 9.10 **A.** Major components of centrifuged whole blood, including the quantity of oxygen carried in each deciliter of blood (Hb, hemoglobin) in an untrained individual. **B.** Changes in whole blood constituents following 4 days of aerobic exercise training. Note the increase in plasma volume or hemodilution early in training decreases erythrocyte concentration toward borderline anemia. Oxygen transport capacity does not decrease with training because the total erythrocyte mass of blood remains constant or increases slightly. (Reprinted with permission from McArdle WD, Katch FI, Katch VL. *Exercise Physiology: Nutrition, Energy, and Human Performance*. 8th Ed. Baltimore: Wolters Kluwer Health, 2015.)

Oxygen Transport in Physical Solution

Oxygen does not dissolve readily in fluids. At an alveolar Po_2 of 100 mm Hg, only about 0.3 mL of gaseous oxygen dissolves in each 100 mL of blood plasma (3 mL · L^{-1}). The average adult's total blood volume equals about 5 L, allowing 15 mL of dissolved oxygen for transport in the blood's fluid portion (3 mL · L^{-1} × 5 = 15 mL). This amount of oxygen would sustain life for about 4 seconds. Viewed somewhat differently, the body would need to circulate 80 L of blood each minute just to supply resting oxygen requirements if oxygen were transported *only* in physical solution.

FIGURE 9.11 The hemoglobin molecule in **(A)** consists of the protein globin composed of four subunit polypeptide chains. Each polypeptide **(B)** contains a single heme group with its single iron atom that acts as an oxygen "magnet." (Adapted with permission from McArdle WD, Katch FI, Katch VL. *Exercise Physiology: Nutrition, Energy, and Human Performance.* 8th Ed. Baltimore: Wolters Kluwer Health, 2015.)

Oxygen Combined With Hemoglobin

The blood of many animal species contains a metallic compound to augment its oxygen-carrying capacity. In humans, the iron-containing protein pigment hemoglobin (Hb), illustrated in **Figure 9.11**, constitutes the main component of the body's 25 trillion red blood cells. *Hb increases the blood's oxygen-carrying capacity 65 to 70 times above that normally dissolved in plasma.* For each liter of blood, Hb temporarily "captures" about 197 mL of oxygen. Each of the four iron atoms in the Hb molecule loosely binds one molecule of oxygen to form oxyhemoglobin in the reversible **oxygenation reaction**:

$$\mathbf{Hb + 4O_2 \rightarrow Hb_4O_8}$$

This reaction requires no enzymes; it progresses without a change in the Fe^{2+} valance as occurs during the more permanent oxidation process. *Oxygen's partial pressure in solution solely determines the Hb oxygenation to oxyhemoglobin.*

An Important Function

Despite its limited quantity, oxygen transported in physical solution serves a vital physiologic function. Dissolved oxygen establishes the Po_2 of the blood and tissue fluids to help regulate breathing and determines the magnitude of Hb loading with oxygen in the lungs and discharging it in the tissues.

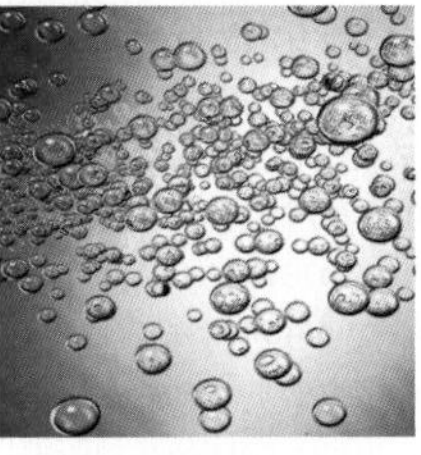

Hemoglobin's Oxygen-Carrying Capacity

In men on average, each 100 mL of blood contains approximately 14 to 16 g of Hb. The value averages 5% to 10% less for women, or about 14 g per 100 mL of blood. The gender difference in Hb concentration contributes to the lower aerobic capacity of women even after adjusting statistically for gender-related differences in body mass and body fat. Hb concentration decreases slightly with aging beginning at age 50.

Each gram of Hb can combine loosely with 1.34 mL of oxygen. Thus, the oxygen-carrying capacity of the blood from its Hb concentration computes as follows:

Oxygen-carrying capacity = Hb (g · 100 mL blood^{-1}) × Hb Oxygen capacity

If the blood's Hb concentration equals 15 g, then approximately 20 mL of oxygen (15 g per 100 mL × 1.34 mL = 20.1) combine with the Hb in each 100 mL of blood if Hb achieves full oxygen saturation (i.e., if all Hb existed as Hb_4O_8).

Po_2 and Hemoglobin Saturation

A discussion of blood's oxygen-carrying capacity assumes that Hb achieves full saturation with oxygen when exposed to alveolar gas. **Figure 9.12A** shows the relationship between percentage saturation of Hb (*left vertical axis*) at various Po_2s under normal resting physiologic conditions (arterial pH 7.4, 37°C) and the effects of changes in pH and temperature (inset curves) on Hb's oxygen affinity. The percentage saturation of Hb computes as follows:

Percentage saturation = (Total O_2 combined with Hb ÷ Hb Oxygen-carrying capacity) × 100

This curve, termed the **oxyhemoglobin dissociation curve**, also quantifies the oxygen carried in each 100 mL of blood related to plasma Po_2 (*right vertical axis,* **Fig. 9.12A**). For example, at a Po_2 of 90 mm Hg (95% Hb saturation), the normal Hb complement in 100 mL of blood carries about 19 mL of oxygen; at a Po_2 of 40 mm Hg (75% Hb saturation), the oxygen quantity decreases to about 15 mL, and the oxygen quantity is only slightly exceeds 2 mL at a Po_2 of 10 mm Hg. These values indicate that at relatively low oxygen partial pressures at the capillary-tissue membrane, oxygen readily dissociates or unloads from Hb for cell use. **Figure 9.12B** shows partial pressure gradients as oxygen moves from ambient air at sea level into mitochondria.

A

Oxyhemoglobin Dissociation Curve

pH 7.40

Po_2	Percentage saturation	Arterial O_2 content ($mL \cdot L^{-1}$)
10	13.3	24.9
20	35.5	66.6
30	58.0	108.8
40	73.9	138.6
44	78.4	147.1
48	82.0	153.8
52	84.9	159.3
56	87.3	163.8
60	89.3	167.5
64	90.9	170.5
68	92.2	173.0
76	94.1	176.5
80	94.9	178.0
90	96.3	180.7
100	97.2	182.4

Effect of temperature: 10°C, 20°C, 38°C, 43°C

Effect of acidity: Low acidity (pH 7.45); High acidity (pH 7.35); Normal arterial acidity (pH 7.40)

Percent saturation

Oxygen content of hemoglobin (mL per dL blood)

Pressure of oxygen in solution (mm Hg)

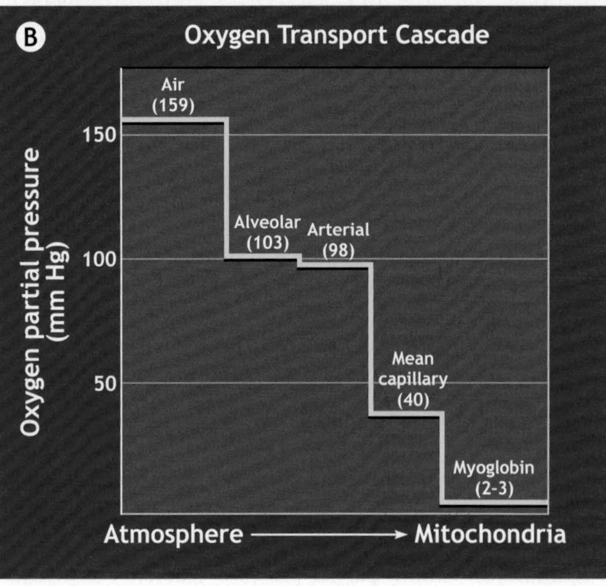

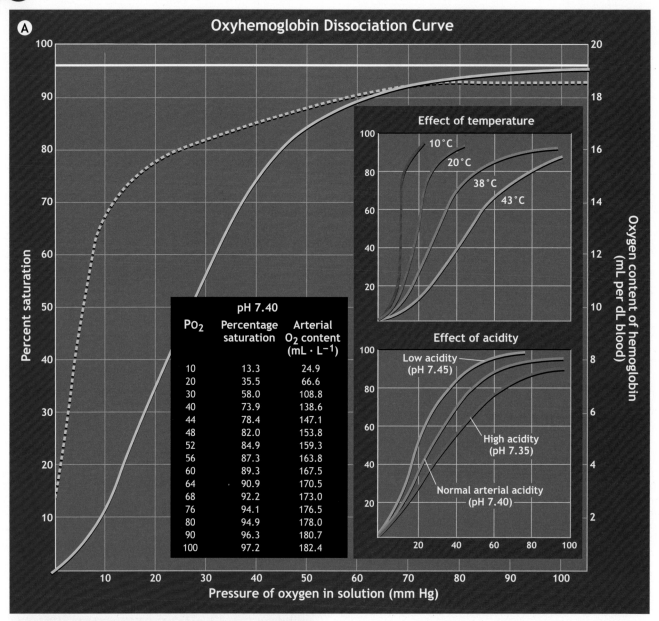

FIGURE 9.12 **A.** Oxyhemoglobin dissociation curve. The *two yellow lines* indicate the percentage saturation of Hb (*solid line*) and myoglobin (*dashed line*) in relation to oxygen pressure. The *right ordinate* shows the quantity of oxygen carried in each deciliter of blood under normal conditions. The *two inset curves* within the figure illustrate the effects of temperature and acidity in altering Hb's affinity for oxygen (Bohr effect). The *black inset box* presents oxyhemoglobin saturation and arterial blood's oxygen-carrying capacity for different Po_2 values with Hb concentration of 14 g $\cdot$ dL^{-1} blood at a pH of 7.40. The *white horizontal line* at the top of the graph indicates percentage saturation of Hb at the average sea-level alveolar Po_2 of 100 mm Hg. **B.** The term oxygen transport cascade characterizes partial pressures as oxygen moves from ambient air at sea level to the mitochondria of maximally active muscle tissue. (Adapted with permission from McArdle WD, Katch FI, Katch VL. *Exercise Physiology: Nutrition, Energy, and Human Performance*. 8th Ed. Baltimore: Wolters Kluwer Health, 2015.)

The "**oxygen transport cascade**" describes downward steps in oxygen partial pressures from ambient air at sea level to maximally active muscle's mitochondria, with progressively lowering of Po_2 to facilitate unloading of oxygen.

Po_2 in the Lungs

At an alveolar-capillary Po_2 of 100 mm Hg, Hb remains 98% saturated with oxygen; under these conditions, Hb in each 100 mL of blood contains about 19.7 mL of oxygen. An additional increase in alveolar Po_2 contributes little to how much oxygen combines with Hb. Each 100 mL of plasma in arterial blood contains about 0.3 mL of oxygen in physical solution. For healthy individuals who breathe sea-level ambient air, 100 mL of arterial blood carries 20.0 mL of oxygen (19.7 mL bound to Hb and 0.3 mL dissolved in plasma).

Careful examination of **Figure 9.12A** shows that Hb saturation changes little until oxygen pressure decreases to about 60 mm Hg. This relatively flat upper portion of the oxyhemoglobin dissociation curve provides a safety margin to ensure near full Hb loading in lungs despite relatively large decreases in alveolar Po_2. Alveolar Po_2 reduction to 75 mm Hg as occurs in certain lung diseases or when one travels to moderate altitude, only decreases arterial Hb saturation by about 6%. In contrast, when Po_2 drops below 60 mm Hg, a sharp decrease occurs in how much oxygen combines with Hb.

Tissue Po_2

The Po_2 in cell fluids at rest averages 40 mm Hg. Dissolved oxygen in arterial plasma (Po_2 = 100 mm Hg) thus readily diffuses across the capillary membrane through tissue fluids into cells. This reduces plasma Po_2 below that in red blood cells, causing Hb to release its oxygen in the reaction $HbO_2 \rightarrow Hb + O_2$. The oxygen then moves from the blood cells through the capillary membrane into the tissues.

At the tissue-capillary Po_2 of 40 mm Hg at rest, Hb holds roughly 75% of its total capacity for oxygen (see *solid line* in **Fig. 9.12A**). Consequently, each 100 mL of blood leaving the resting tissues carries 15 mL of oxygen, with nearly 5 mL released to cells for energy metabolism. The **arteriovenous oxygen difference (a-$\bar{v}o_{2diff}$)** describes this difference in oxygen content between arterial and mixed-venous blood expressed in milliliters per 100 mL blood.

The a-$\bar{v}o_2$ difference at rest averages 5 mL · 100 mL^{-1}. The oxygen still remaining with Hb provides an "automatic" reserve for cells to immediately obtain oxygen if demands increase suddenly. Tissue Po_2 rapidly decreases as the cells' need for oxygen above rest increases with physical activity. This forces Hb to release greater quantities of oxygen to meet metabolic requirements. In vigorous physical activity, tissue Po_2 decreases to 15 mm Hg and Hb retains about 5 mL of oxygen. This expands the tissue a-$\bar{v}o_2$ difference to 15 mL of oxygen per 100 mL of blood. During exhaustive physical activity when active muscles' Po_2 decreases to about 3 mm Hg, Hb releases all of its remaining oxygen to active tissues. Even without any increase in local blood flow, the amount of oxygen released to active muscle increases three times above that supplied at rest by more complete Hb unloading.

Bohr Effect

The inset curves in **Figure 9.12** show that increases in acidity ([H$^+$] and CO_2) and temperature cause the oxyhemoglobin dissociation curve to shift downward and to the right to reflect enhanced unloading. This occurs particularly in the Po_2 range of 20 to 50 mm Hg. This phenomenon, known as the **Bohr effect** results from alterations in Hb's molecular structure from blood chemistry and temperature changes. The Bohr effect was named in honor of its discoverer in 1904, Danish physician and physiologist Christian Bohr (1855–1911; father of 1922 Nobel physicist Niels Bohr [1885–1962; **www.nobelprize.org/nobel_prizes/physics/laureates/1922/**] and distinguished mathematician and Olympian Harold Bohr [1887–1951]).

The Bohr effect becomes particularly important in vigorous activities because increased metabolic heat and acidity in active tissues augments oxygen release. For example, at a Po_2 of 20 mm Hg and normal body temperature of about 37°C, percentage Hb saturation with oxygen equals 35%. At the same Po_2, but with body temperature increased to 43°C, a temperature commonly recorded at the end of a marathon run, Hb's percentage saturation decreases to about 23%. This means that more oxygen unloads from Hb for use in cellular metabolism. Similar effects take place with increased acidity during intense exertion. The lack of a negligible Bohr effect in pulmonary capillary blood at normal alveolar Po_2 means that Hb fully loads with oxygen as blood passes through the lungs, even during maximal effort.

The compound **2,3-diphosphoglycerate (2,3-DPG)**, the anaerobic metabolite produced in red blood cells during glycolysis, also affects Hb's oxygen affinity. 2,3-DPG facilitates oxygen dissociation by combining with Hb subunits to reduce its affinity for oxygen. Individuals with cardiopulmonary disease and inhabitants of altitudes above 12,000 ft (3658 m) have increased levels of this metabolic intermediate compound. Elevated 2,3-DPG for these individuals represents a compensatory adjustment that facilitates oxygen release to the cells. In general, adaptations in 2,3-DPG occur relatively slowly compared with the immediate Bohr effect from increased tissue temperature, acidity, and carbon dioxide.

Myoglobin and Muscle Oxygen Storage

Skeletal and cardiac muscle contain the iron-protein compound **myoglobin**. Myoglobin, similar to Hb, combines reversibly with oxygen. The difference between myoglobin and Hb is that myoglobin contains only 1 iron atom compared to Hb's 4. Myoglobin adds additional oxygen to the muscle in the following reaction:

$$MbO_2 \rightarrow MbO_2$$

Myoglobin facilitates mitochondrial oxygen transfer, notably at the initiation of physical activity and during intense effort when cellular Po_2 decreases considerably. **Figure 9.12A** reveals the dissociation curve for myoglobin (*dashed yellow line*) forms a rectangular hyperbola, not the S-shaped Hb curve. This makes myoglobin bind and retain oxygen at low pressures much more readily than Hb. During rest and moderate activity when cellular Po_2 remains

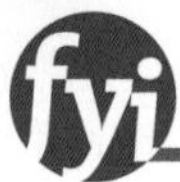

Physical Training and Myoglobin

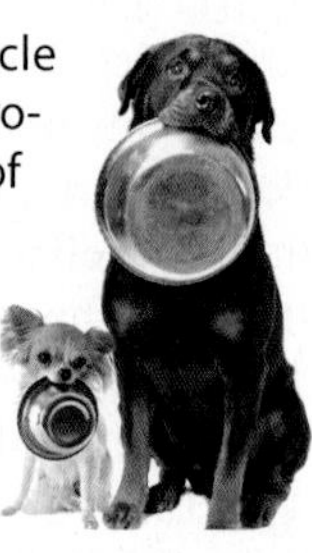

As might be expected, slow-twitch muscle fibers with high capacity to generate ATP aerobically contain relatively large quantities of myoglobin. Among animals, a muscle's myoglobin content relates to their physical activity level. The leg muscles of hunting dogs, for example, contain more myoglobin than do muscles of sedentary house pets; similar findings exist for grazing cattle compared with penned animals.

relatively high, myoglobin remains highly saturated with oxygen. At a Po_2 of 40 mm Hg, for example, myoglobin retains 85% of its oxygen. MbO_2 releases its greatest amount of oxygen when tissue Po_2 decreases to less than 10 mm Hg. Unlike Hb, myoglobin does not exhibit a Bohr effect.

CARBON DIOXIDE TRANSPORT IN BLOOD

Once carbon dioxide forms in cells, diffusion and transport to the lungs in venous blood provides its only means to "escape." **Figure 9.13** illustrates how blood transports carbon dioxide to the lungs in three ways:

1. Physical solution in plasma (7% to 10%)
2. Loose combination with Hb (20%)
3. Combined with water as bicarbonate (70%)

See the animation "Transport of Carbon Doxide" on **http://thePoint.lww.com/MKKESS5e** for a demonstration of this concept.

Carbon Dioxide in Solution

Plasma transports 7% to 10% of carbon dioxide produced in energy metabolism as free carbon dioxide in physical solution. **Figure 9.13** illustrates carbon dioxide transport in blood (**A**), physically dissolved in blood plasma (**B**), and chemically bound to hemoglobin (**C**). The random movement of this relatively small quantity of dissolved carbon dioxide molecules establishes blood's Pco_2.

Carbon Dioxide as Carbamino Compounds

About 20% of carbon dioxide reacts directly with amino acid molecules of blood proteins to form carbamino compounds (**Fig. 9.13B**). The globin portion of Hb carries a significant amount of carbon dioxide in the blood as follows:

$$\underset{\text{Hemoglobin}}{CO_2 + HbNH} \longrightarrow \underset{\text{Carbaminohemoglobin}}{HbNHCOOH}$$

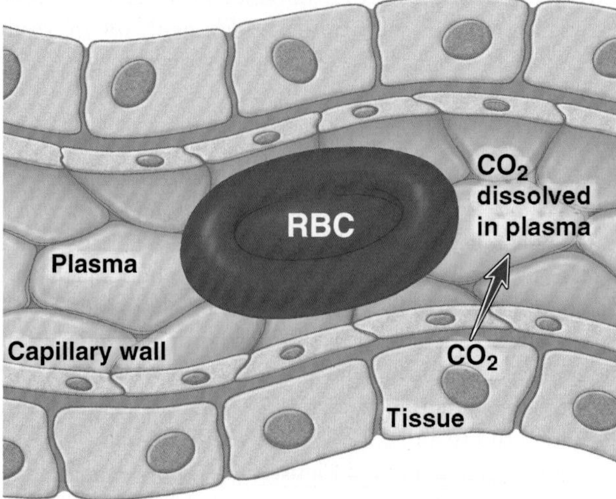

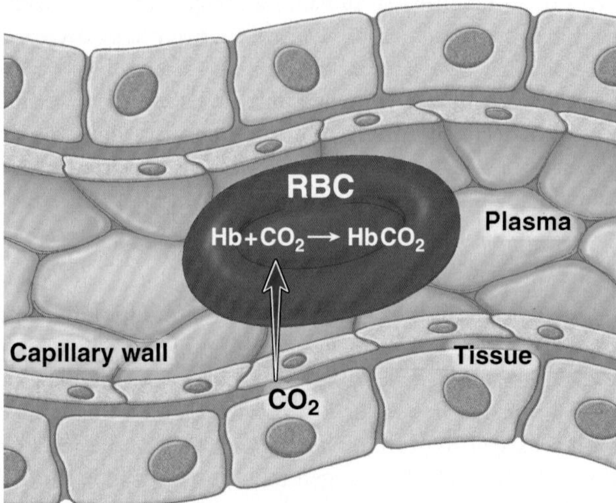

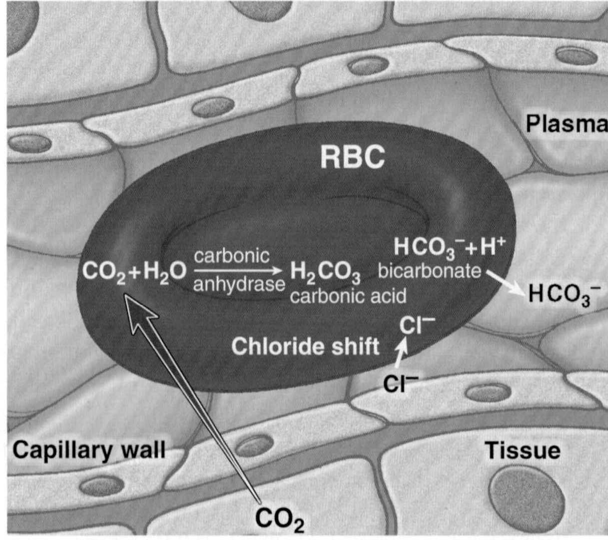

FIGURE 9.13 Carbon dioxide transport in blood. **A.** Physically dissolved in blood plasma. **B.** Chemically bound to hemoglobin (Hb). **C.** Combined with water as bicarbonate.

Formation of carbamino compounds reverses in the lungs as plasma Pco_2 decreases. This moves carbon dioxide into solution for diffusion into the alveoli. Concurrently, Hb's oxygenation reduces its capacity to bind carbon dioxide. The interaction between oxygen loading and carbon dioxide release facilitates the lungs' removal of carbon dioxide. This effect, termed the **Haldane effect**, honors its discoverer, Scottish physiologist John Scott Haldane (1860–1936; **www.giffordlectures.org/Author.asp?AuthorID=73**).

Carbon Dioxide as Bicarbonate

Approximately 70% of carbon dioxide in solution combines with water to form carbonic acid (**Fig. 9.13C**).

$$CO_2 + H_2O \leftrightarrow H_2CO_3^-$$

Based on this reactions slow rate, little carbon dioxide transports in this form without **carbonic anhydrase**, a zinc-containing enzyme within red blood cells. This catalyst accelerates interaction of carbon dioxide and water about 5000 times.

In Tissues

When carbonic acid forms in tissues, most of it ionizes to hydrogen ions (H^+) and bicarbonate ions (HCO_3^-) as follows:

$$CO_2 + H_2O \xrightarrow{\text{Carbonic anhydrase}} H_2CO_3 \rightarrow H^+ + HCO_3^-$$

The protein portion of the Hb molecule then buffers H^+ to maintain blood pH within narrow limits. Bicarbonate's high solubility causes it to diffuse from red blood cells into plasma in exchange for a chloride ion (Cl^-), which then moves into the blood cell to maintain ionic equilibrium. The term *chloride shift* describes exchange of Cl^- for HCO^-; in fact, it accounts for the higher Cl^- content of erythrocytes in venous blood compared with arterial blood.

In Lungs

As tissue Pco_2 increases, carbonic acid forms rapidly. Conversely, in the lungs, carbon dioxide diffuses from plasma into the alveoli; this lowers plasma Pco_2 and disturbs the equilibrium between carbonic acid and bicarbonate ion formation. Carbonic acid reforms from H^+ and HCO_3^-. In turn, carbon dioxide and water reform to allow carbon dioxide to exit through the lungs as follows:

$$H^+ + HCO_3^- \rightarrow H_2CO_3 \xrightarrow{\text{Carbonic anhydrase}} CO_2 + H_2O$$

Plasma bicarbonate concentration decreases in the pulmonary capillaries; this permits Cl^- to move from the red blood cell into plasma.

SUMMARY

1. Hb, the iron-protein pigment in red blood cells, increases oxygen-carrying capacity of whole blood about 65 times compared with the amount dissolved in physical solution in plasma.
2. The small quantity of oxygen dissolved in plasma exerts molecular movement and establishes blood's Po_2.
3. Plasma Po_2 determines Hb loading or oxygenation at the lungs and its unloading or deoxygenation at the tissues.
4. The blood's oxygen transport capacity changes only slightly with normal variations in Hb content.
5. Gender differences in Hb concentration contribute to the lower aerobic capacity of women even after adjusting for gender-related differences in body mass and body fat.
6. The S-shaped nature of the oxyhemoglobin dissociation curve dictates that Hb-oxygen saturation changes little until Po_2 decreases below 60 mm Hg.
7. Oxygen releases rapidly from capillary blood and flows into the cells to meet metabolic demands.
8. About 25% of the blood's total oxygen releases to the tissues at rest; the remaining 75% returns in the venous blood "unused" to the heart.
9. The Bohr effect reflects alterations in the molecular structure of hemoglobin from increased acidity, temperature, carbon dioxide concentration, and red blood cell 2,3-DPG that reduce its effectiveness to hold oxygen; physical activity accentuates these factors to further facilitate oxygen's release to tissues.
10. Myoglobin stores "extra" oxygen in skeletal and cardiac muscle.
11. Myoglobin releases its oxygen only at a low Po_2, thus facilitating oxygen transfer to the mitochondria during strenuous physical activity.
12. About 7% of carbon dioxide dissolves as free carbon dioxide in plasma to establish blood's Pco_2.
13. About 20% of the body's carbon dioxide combines with blood proteins including Hb to form carbamino compounds.
14. Approximately 70% of carbon dioxide combines with water to form bicarbonate, with the reaction reversing in the lungs to allow carbon dioxide to leave blood and diffuse into alveoli.

THINK IT THROUGH

1. Discuss whether it would be advantageous for runners to breathe 100% oxygen immediately before running a marathon to "load-up" the metabolically active tissues with oxygen.
2. Explain why minute amounts of CO_2 and CO impurities in a breathing mixture exert profound physiologic effects.
3. Advise a coach who wants football players to breathe from an oxygen canister during time outs or rest breaks to speed recovery during a game at sea level.

PART 4 Regulation of Pulmonary Ventilation

VENTILATORY CONTROL DURING REST

The body exquisitely regulates breathing rate and depth in response to metabolic needs. During all physical activity intensities in healthy individuals, arterial pressures for oxygen and carbon dioxide, and pH, remain essentially unchanged at resting values. Neural information from higher brain centers, lungs, and mechanical and chemical sensors throughout the body regulates pulmonary ventilation. The gaseous and chemical state of blood that bathes the medulla's respiratory center, including aortic and carotid chemoreceptors, also affect alveolar ventilation. **Figure 9.14** presents the primary factors that influence medullary control of pulmonary ventilation.

Neural Factors

*The normal respiratory cycle comes from inherent, automatic inspiratory neuron activity whose cell bodies reside in the medial **medulla**.* The lungs inflate because neurons activate the diaphragm and intercostal muscles. The inspiratory neurons cease firing from two sources—their own self-limitation and inhibitory influence from the medulla's expiratory neurons. Inflation of lung tissue stimulates bronchiole stretch receptors that inhibit inspiration and stimulate expiration.

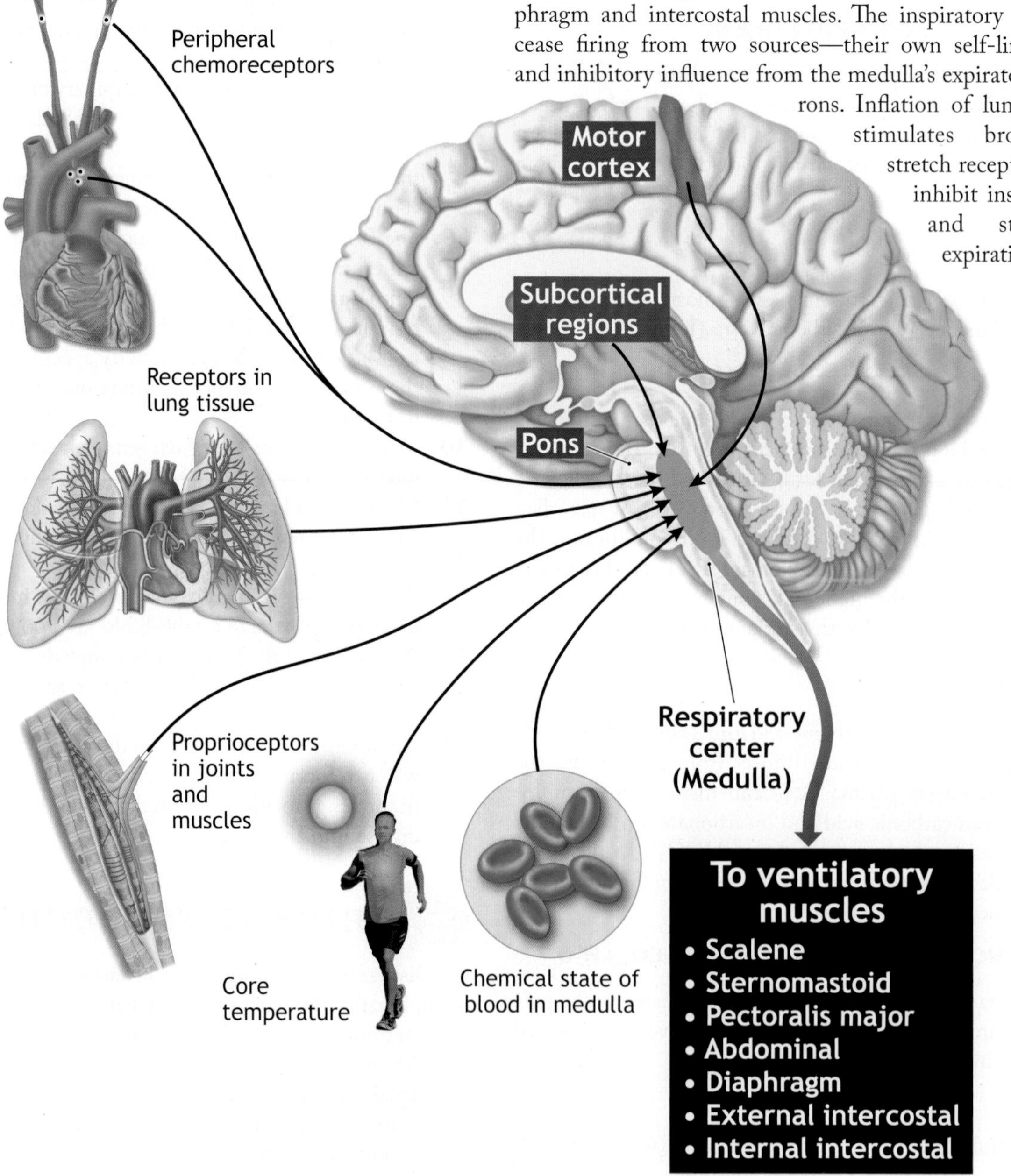

FIGURE 9.14 Schematic representation of factors that affect medullary control of pulmonary ventilation. (Adapted with permission from McArdle WD, Katch FI, Katch VL. *Exercise Physiology: Nutrition, Energy, and Human Performance*. 8th Ed. Baltimore: Wolters Kluwer Health, 2015; portions adapted and reprinted with permission from Moore KL, et al. *Clinically Oriented Anatomy*. 7th Ed. Baltimore: Wolters Kluwer Health, 2013 used with permission from Agur AMR, Dalley AF. *Grant's Atlas of Anatomy*. 13th Ed. Baltimore: Wolters Kluwer Health, 2013.)

When inspiratory muscles relax, exhalation begins by passive recoil of stretched lung tissue and raised ribs. Activation of expiratory neurons and associated muscles that further facilitate expiration synchronizes with this passive phase. As expiration proceeds, the inspiratory center releases again from inhibition and progressively becomes more active.

Humoral Factors

The chemical state of blood largely regulates pulmonary ventilation at rest. Variations in arterial Po_2, Pco_2, acidity, and temperature activate sensitive neural units in the medulla and arterial system to adjust ventilation to maintain arterial blood chemistry within narrow limits.

Plasma Po_2 and Chemoreceptors

Inhaling a gas mixture of 80% oxygen increases alveolar Po_2 and reduces minute ventilation by about 20%. Conversely, reducing the inspired oxygen concentration increases minute ventilation, particularly if alveolar Po_2 decreases below 60 mm Hg. Recall that at 60 mm Hg, Hb's oxygen saturation dramatically decreases. The term **hypoxic threshold** refers to the point at which decreasing arterial Po_2 stimulates ventilation and usually occurs at an arterial Po_2 between 60 and 70 mm Hg.

Sensitivity to reduced arterial oxygen pressure or arterial hypoxia results from stimulation of small structures located outside the central nervous system called **chemoreceptors**. **Figure 9.15** shows these specialized neurons located in the aortic arch (**aortic bodies**) and branching of the carotid arteries (**carotid bodies**) in the neck. Tiny cluster of these chemoreceptor-carotid bodies, about 5 mm in diameter, maintain a strategic position to monitor arterial blood status just before it perfuses brain tissues. Nerve fibers from carotid and aortic bodies activate the brain's respiratory neurons.

Peripheral chemoreceptors provide an "early warning detection system" to alert against reduced oxygen pressure. These structures also stimulate ventilation in response to an increase in carbon dioxide; decrease in blood pressure, temperature, and acidity, and perhaps decline in circulating potassium.

Plasma Pco_2 and H^+ Concentration

At rest, carbon dioxide pressure in arterial plasma provides the most important respiratory stimulus. Small increases in Pco_2 in inspired air stimulate the medulla and peripheral chemoreceptors to initiate large increases in minute ventilation. For example, resting ventilation almost doubles when inspired Pco_2 increases to just 1.7 mm Hg (0.22% CO_2 in inspired air).

Molecular carbon dioxide does not entirely account for CO_2's effect on ventilatory control. Recall that carbonic acid formed from the union of carbon dioxide and water rapidly dissociates to bicarbonate ions and hydrogen ions. The increase in $[H^+]$, which varies directly with the blood's CO_2 content in cerebrospinal fluid bathing respiratory areas, stimulates inspiratory activity. The resulting ventilatory increase eliminates carbon dioxide with subsequent lowering of arterial $[H^+]$.

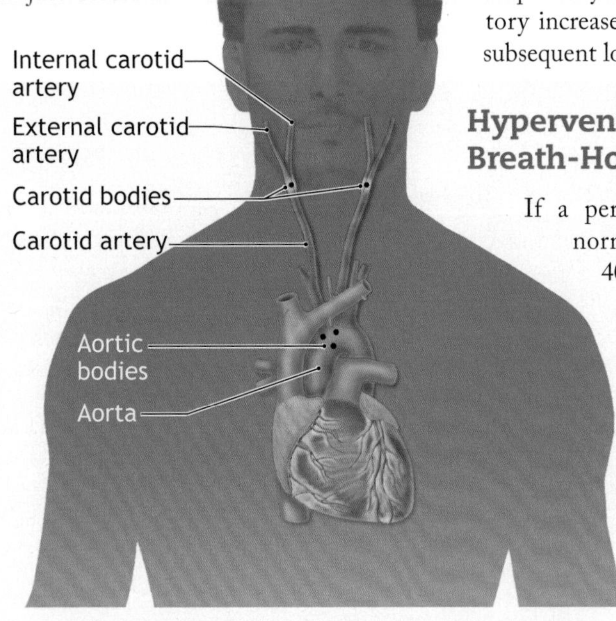

FIGURE 9.15 The aortic arch and bifurcation of carotid arteries contain aortic and carotid cell bodies sensitive to reduced plasma Po_2 and defend against arterial hypoxia. (Adapted with permission from McArdle WD, Katch FI, Katch VL. *Exercise Physiology: Nutrition, Energy, and Human Performance*. 8th Ed. Baltimore: Wolters Kluwer Health, 2015.)

fyi Breath-Holding's Often Tragic Consequences

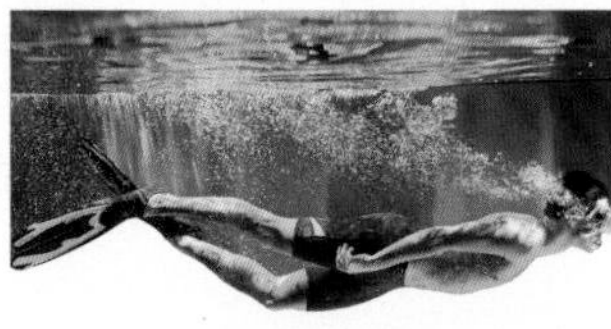

Swimmers and sport divers hyperventilate and breath-hold to improve their physical performance. In sprint swimming, it is biomechanically undesirable to roll the body and turn the head during the stroke's breathing phase. Swimmers hyperventilate on the starting blocks to prolong their breath-hold time during the start of a swim.

Snorkel divers hyperventilate to extend breath-hold time but often with tragic results. As dive length and depth increase, the oxygen content of blood can decrease to critically low values before arterial Pco_2 increases to stimulate breathing and signal the need to ascend to the surface. Reduced arterial Po_2 can cause loss of consciousness before the diver reaches the surface.

Hyperventilation and Breath-Holding

If a person breath-holds following a normal exhalation, it takes about 40 seconds before breathing commences. This urge to breathe results mainly from the stimulating effects of increased arterial Pco_2 and $[H^+]$, not decreased arterial Po_2. *The "break point" for breath-holding generally corresponds to an increase in arterial* Pco_2 *to about 50 mm Hg.*

If this same person consciously increased alveolar ventilation above a normal level before breath-holding, alveolar air composition becomes more similar to ambient air. Alveolar Pco_2

with **hyperventilation** may decrease to 15 mm Hg, creating a considerable diffusion gradient for carbon dioxide runoff from venous blood that enters the pulmonary capillaries. Consequently, a larger than normal amount of carbon dioxide leaves the blood, decreasing arterial Pco_2 below normal levels. Reduced arterial Pco_2 extends the breath-hold until the arterial Pco_2, $[H^+]$, or both increase to a level that stimulates ventilation.

VENTILATORY CONTROL DURING PHYSICAL ACTIVITY

Chemical Factors

Chemical stimuli cannot fully explain increased ventilation or **hyperpnea** during physical activity. For example, manipulating arterial Po_2, Pco_2, and acidity does not increase minute ventilation nearly as much as vigorous physical activity.

Arterial Po_2 during physical activity does not decrease to the point that it stimulates ventilation by chemoreceptor activation. In fact, large breathing volumes during vigorous activity actually increase alveolar and arterial Po_2 above the average resting value of 100 mm Hg. Figure 9.16 illustrates the dynamics of venous and alveolar Pco_2, and alveolar Po_2 related to oxygen uptake in men during a graded exercise test. During light and moderate physical activity ($\dot{V}O_2$ = <2000 mL · min^{-1}), pulmonary ventilation closely couples to oxygen uptake and carbon dioxide production to maintain alveolar Po_2 at about 100 mm Hg and Pco_2 at 40 mm Hg. Increases in acidity and subsequent increases in CO_2 and $[H^+]$ during strenuous effort provide an additional ventilatory stimulus that reduces alveolar Pco_2 to below 40 mm Hg and sometimes to 25 mm Hg. This eliminates carbon dioxide and decreases arterial Pco_2. Concurrently, augmented ventilation slightly increases alveolar Po_2 to facilitate oxygen loading.

Less Breathing During Swimming

Lower ventilatory equivalents from restrictive breathing occur at all levels of energy expenditure during prone swimming. Depressed ventilation may hinder gas exchange during maximal swimming and contribute to the lower $\dot{V}O_{2max}$ when swimming compared with running.

Nonchemical Factors

Ventilation increases so rapidly when vigorous physical activity begins that it occurs almost within the first ventilatory cycle. A plateau lasting about 20 seconds follows the abrupt ventilation increase; thereafter, minute ventilation gradually increases and approaches a steady level relative to metabolic gas exchange demands. When activity stops, ventilation decreases rapidly to about 40% of the final activity value and then slowly returns to resting levels. The rapidity of the ventilatory response at the onset and cessation of activity shows that input other than from changes in arterial Pco_2 and $[H^+]$ mediate these components of physical activity and recovery hyperpnea.

Neurogenic Factors

Cortical and peripheral factors regulate pulmonary ventilation in physical activity:

- **Cortical influence:** Neural outflow from motor cortex regions during physical activity and cortical activation in anticipation of activity stimulate medullary respiratory neurons. When activity begins, cortical outflow

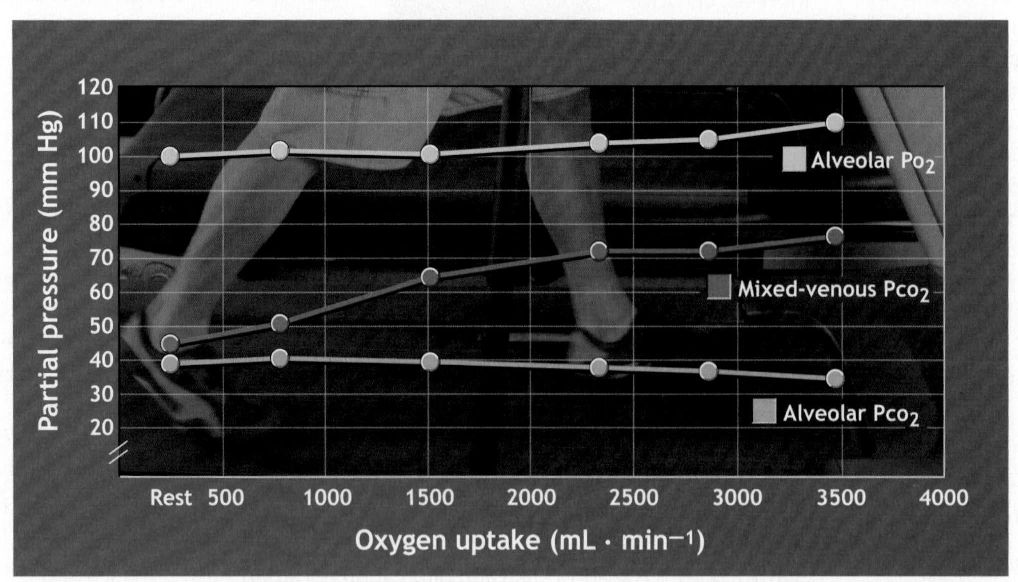

FIGURE 9.16 Values for Pco_2 in mixed-venous blood entering the lungs, and alveolar Po_2 and Pco_2 related to oxygen uptake during graded exercise. Despite increased metabolism with exercise, alveolar Po_2 and Pco_2 remain near resting levels. Increases in mixed-venous Pco_2 result from increased carbon dioxide production in metabolism. (Adapted with permission from McArdle WD, Katch FI, Katch VL. *Exercise Physiology: Nutrition, Energy, and Human Performance*. 8th Ed. Baltimore: Wolters Kluwer Health, 2015; data courtesy of the Laboratory of Applied Physiology, Queens College.)

acting in concert with demands of physical effort abruptly increases ventilation.

- **Peripheral influence:** Sensory input from joints, tendons, and muscles adjusts ventilation during physical activity. The specific peripheral receptors remain unknown, but experiments involving passive limb movements, electrical muscle stimulation, and voluntary physical activity with the muscle's blood flow occluded support the existence of **mechanoreceptors** in peripheral tissues that produce reflex hyperpnea.

Temperature Influence

An increase in body temperature directly excites respiratory center neurons, which likely help to regulate ventilation in prolonged physical effort. The rapidity of ventilatory changes at the onset and end of activity cannot be explained by the relatively *slow* increases in core temperature.

Integrated Regulation

No single factor controls breathing during physical activity; rather, control depends on the combined and simultaneous effects of several chemical and neural stimuli.

During Physical Activity

Figure 9.17 illustrates dynamic phases of minute ventilation during moderate physical activity and recovery. In **phase I ventilation** at the start of activity, neurogenic stimuli from the cerebral cortex or central command, combined with feedback from active limbs, stimulate the medulla to increase ventilation abruptly. Cortical and locomotor peripheral input continues throughout the activity.

After a short plateau of approximately 20 seconds, minute ventilation then rises exponentially in **phase II ventilation** to achieve a steady level related to metabolic gas exchange demands. **Central command** input, including factors intrinsic to neurons of the respiratory control system, regulates this phase of ventilation. Continued respiratory neuron activity in the medulla causes short-term potentiation that augments their responsiveness to the same continuing stimulation. This brings minute ventilation to a new, higher level. In all likelihood, peripheral chemoreceptor input in the carotid bodies also contributes to phase II regulation.

The final **phase III ventilation** control involves fine-tuning of steady-state ventilation through peripheral sensory feedback mechanisms. Central and reflex stimuli from the main by-products of increased muscle metabolism—carbon dioxide and H^+ concentration—modulate alveolar gas pressures in this phase. These factors stimulate chemoreceptor group IV unmyelinated neurons that communicate with the central nervous system to regulate cardiorespiratory function.

An additional stimulus to increase ventilation in strenuous activity occurs from the lactate anion itself, apart from lactic acidosis. Reflexes related to pulmonary blood flow and lung and respiratory muscle mechanical movement also provide regulatory input during physical activity.

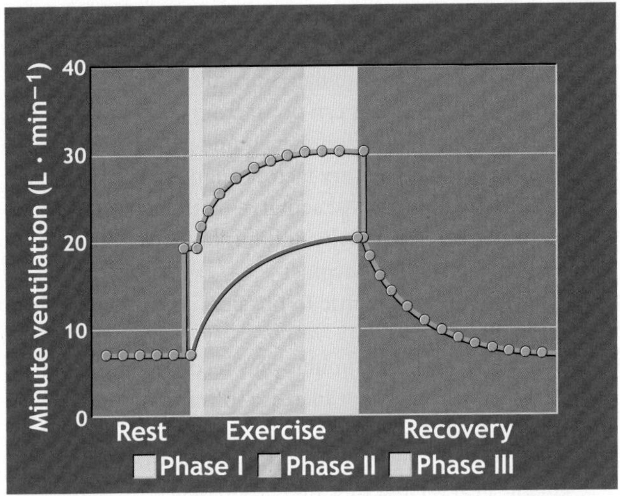

FIGURE 9.17 Three phases of exercise hyperpnea. Phase I: rapid increase from rest and brief plateau from central command drive and input from active muscles. Phase II: slower exponential rise begins approximately 20 seconds following exercise onset. Central command continues, along with feedback from active muscles plus the added effect of short-term potentiation of respiratory neurons. Phase III: major regulatory mechanisms reach stable values; added input from peripheral chemoreceptors fine-tunes the ventilatory response. The lower *red* curve in exercise depicts only the contribution of central neuronal short-term potentiation and rise in arterial H^+ concentration to the total respiratory response. (Reprinted with permission from McArdle WD, Katch FI, Katch VL. *Exercise Physiology: Nutrition, Energy, and Human Performance*. 8th Ed. Baltimore: Wolters Kluwer Health, 2015.)

During Recovery

The abrupt ventilatory decline immediately following physical activity reflects removal of central command drive and sensory input from previously active muscles. More than likely, the slower recovery phase results from two factors:

1. Gradual diminution of short-term potentiation of the respiratory center
2. Re-establishment of a normal cellular metabolic, thermal, and chemical milieu

SUMMARY

1. Inherent medullary neural activity controls the normal respiratory cycle.
2. Neural circuits that relay information from higher brain centers, the lungs themselves, and other sensors throughout the body modulate medullary activity.
3. At rest, arterial P_{CO_2} and acidity [H^+] act directly on the respiratory center or modify its activity reflexly through chemoreceptors to control alveolar ventilation.
4. Peripheral chemoreceptor activation stimulates breathing when arterial P_{O_2} decreases during high-altitude ascent or severe pulmonary disease.

5. Hyperventilation lowers arterial P_{CO_2} and $[H^+]$ to prolong breath-hold time until carbon dioxide and acidity increase to stimulate breathing.
6. Deadly consequences can occur from extended breath-hold by hyperventilation during underwater swimming.
7. Nonchemical regulatory factors augment ventilatory adjustments to physical activity—cortical activation in anticipation of activity and outflow from the motor cortex when activity begins.
8. The ventilatory response to physical activity occurs in three phases.
9. In phase I, cortical stimulus plus feedback from active limbs causes an abrupt increase in ventilation as activity begins.
10. Phase II ventilation rises exponentially to reach a steady level related to activity demands.
11. Phase III ventilation fine-tunes steady-state breathing through peripheral sensory feedback mechanisms.

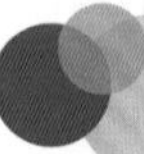

THINK IT THROUGH

1. Outline the mechanism of how hyperventilation extends breath-hold duration.
2. Explain why individuals should not hyperventilate during breath-hold diving.

PART 5 Pulmonary Ventilation During Physical Activity

PULMONARY VENTILATION AND ENERGY DEMANDS

Physical activity increases oxygen uptake and carbon dioxide production more than any other physiologic stress. During activity, considerable oxygen diffuses from the alveoli into the blood for return to the lungs. Conversely, considerable carbon dioxide moves from the blood into the alveoli. Concurrently, increases in pulmonary ventilation maintain stable alveolar gas concentrations to enable oxygen and carbon dioxide exchange to proceed unimpeded. **Figure 9.18** illustrates the relationship among minute pulmonary ventilation, blood lactate concentration, and oxygen uptake through the range of steady-rate and non–steady-rate physical activity levels to $\dot{V}O_{2max}$.

Ventilation During Steady-Rate Physical Activity

During light and moderate physical effort ($\dot{V}O_2 < 2.5\ L \cdot min^{-1}$ in this example), pulmonary ventilation increases linearly with oxygen uptake, mainly by increases in TV.

The **ventilatory equivalent for oxygen** ($\dot{V}_E/\dot{V}O_2$) represents the ratio of minute ventilation to oxygen uptake. This index indicates **breathing economy** because it reflects the quantity of air breathed per amount of oxygen consumed. Healthy young adults usually maintain $\dot{V}_E/\dot{V}O_2$ at about 25, which equals about 25-L air breathed per L oxygen consumed, during submaximal activity up to approximately 55% of $\dot{V}O_{2max}$. Higher ventilatory equivalents occur in children, averaging about 32 in 6-year-old children. Despite variations in ventilatory equivalents among healthy individuals, complete aeration of blood takes place because of two factors:

1. Alveolar P_{O_2} and P_{CO_2} remain at near-resting values.
2. Transit time for blood flowing through the pulmonary capillaries proceeds slowly enough to allow complete gas exchange.

During steady-rate physical activity, the ventilatory equivalent for carbon dioxide ($\dot{V}_E/\dot{V}CO_2$) also remains relatively constant because pulmonary ventilation eliminates the carbon dioxide produced during cellular respiration.

Ventilation During Non–Steady-Rate Physical Activity

Ventilatory Threshold

Note in **Figure 9.18** that as oxygen uptake increases, minute ventilation eventually increases disproportionately to the increase in oxygen uptake. This changes the ventilatory equivalent above the steady-rate value to reach as high as 35 or 40 during maximal effort. The point at which pulmonary ventilation increases disproportionately with oxygen uptake during graded activity is called **ventilatory threshold (Tvent)**. At this effort level, pulmonary ventilation no longer links tightly to oxygen demand at the cellular level. Rather, "excess" ventilation relates directly to carbon dioxide's increased output from the buffering of lactate that begins to accumulate from anaerobic metabolism.

Recall that sodium bicarbonate in blood buffers lactate generated during anaerobic metabolism in the following reaction:

$$\text{Lactate} + NaHCO_3 \rightarrow \text{Na lactate} + H_2CO_3 \rightarrow H_2O + CO_2$$

Excess, nonmetabolic carbon dioxide liberated in this buffering reaction stimulates pulmonary ventilation that disproportionately increases $\dot{V}_E/\dot{V}O_2$. The respiratory exchange ratio ($\dot{V}CO_2/\dot{V}O_2$) exceeds 1.00 when acid buffering triggers additional exhalation of carbon dioxide.

The term ***anaerobic threshold*** originally defined the abrupt increase in ventilatory equivalent caused by nonmetabolic carbon dioxide production from lactate buffering. Some researchers believed this point signaled the body's shift to anaerobic metabolism. They proposed the anaerobic threshold as a noninvasive ventilatory measure of anaerobiosis onset. Subsequent research showed that the ratios of $\dot{V}_E/\dot{V}O_2$ or $\dot{V}CO_2/\dot{V}O_2$ did not necessarily link in a *causal* manner with lactate production or its accumulation during physical activity.

Even if the association between ventilatory dynamics and cellular metabolic events remains noncausal, useful information about performance comes from applying these indirect

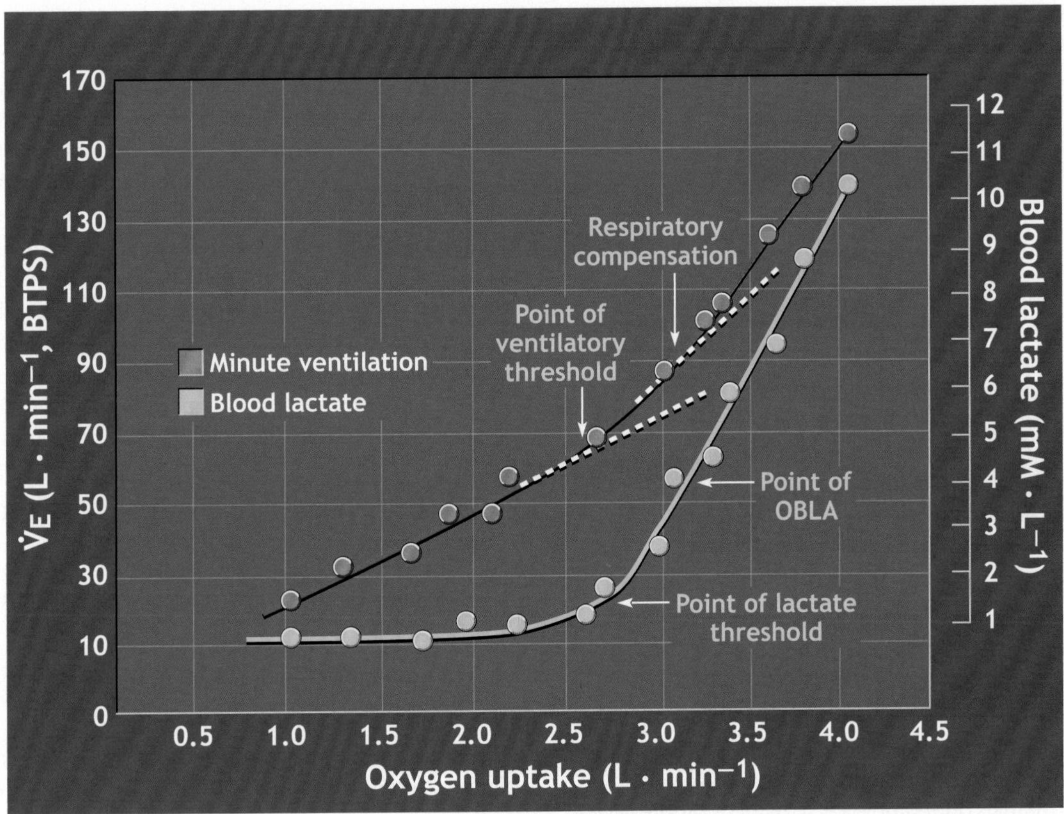

FIGURE 9.18 Pulmonary ventilation, blood lactate concentration, and oxygen uptake during graded exercise to maximum. The *lower dashed white line* extrapolates the linear relationship between $\dot{V}_E/\dot{V}O_2$ during submaximal effort. The lactate threshold, not necessarily the threshold for anaerobic metabolism, represents the highest exercise intensity or oxygen uptake not associated with elevated blood lactate concentration. It occurs at the point where the relation between $\dot{V}_E/\dot{V}O_2$ deviates from linearity, indicated as the point of ventilatory threshold. OBLA represents the point of lactate increase just above a 4.0-mM baseline. Respiratory compensation represents a further disproportionate increase in ventilation indicated by deviation from *the upper dashed white line* to counter the plasma pH decrease in intense physical activity. (Reprinted with permission from McArdle WD, Katch FI, Katch VL. *Exercise Physiology: Nutrition, Energy, and Human Performance*. 8th Ed. Baltimore: Wolters Kluwer Health, 2015.)

procedures. **Figure 9.19** outlines possible underlying factors that relate to anaerobic threshold detected from pulmonary gas exchange dynamics during graded physical activity levels.

Onset of Blood Lactate Accumulation

Steady-rate physical activity reveals oxygen supply and utilization satisfy the energy requirements of muscular effort. When this occurs, lactate production does *not* exceed its removal, and blood lactate does not accumulate. The term **lactate threshold** describes the highest oxygen uptake or exercise intensity achieved with less than a 1.0-mM increase in blood lactate concentration above the pre-exercise level. **Figure 9.18** showed that exercise intensity or oxygen uptake where blood lactate begins to increase above a baseline level of about 4 $mM \cdot L^{-1}$ indicates the point of **onset of blood lactate accumulation (OBLA)**. OBLA normally occurs between 55% and 65% of $\dot{V}O_{2max}$ in healthy, untrained subjects and often equals more than 80% $\dot{V}O_{2max}$ in highly trained endurance athletes.

Added Breathing Stimulus

Lactate produced during intense physical activity places an added demand on pulmonary ventilation, causing "overbreathing" due to the buffering of lactate to the weaker carbonic acid. In the lungs, carbonic acid splits into water and carbon dioxide components; this "nonmetabolic" carbon dioxide provides an added stimulus to pulmonary ventilation.

Possible Causes of Onset of Blood Lactate Accumulation

The exact cause of OBLA remains controversial. Some believe it represents the point of muscle hypoxia or inadequate oxygen and therefore anaerobiosis. Others contend that muscle lactate accumulation does not necessarily coincide with hypoxia because lactate forms even in the presence of adequate muscle oxygenation. OBLA does imply an imbalance between rate of blood lactate appearance and disappearance. The imbalance may not result from muscle hypoxia, but rather from decreased total lactate clearance or increased lactate production only in specific muscle fibers. Practitioners should cautiously interpret the specific metabolic significance of OBLA and its possible relationship to tissue hypoxia.

Onset of Blood Lactate Accumulation and Endurance Performance

Figure 9.20 depicts major variables that contribute to oxygen transport and use. They ultimately determine maximum effort intensity a person can maintain in prolonged physical

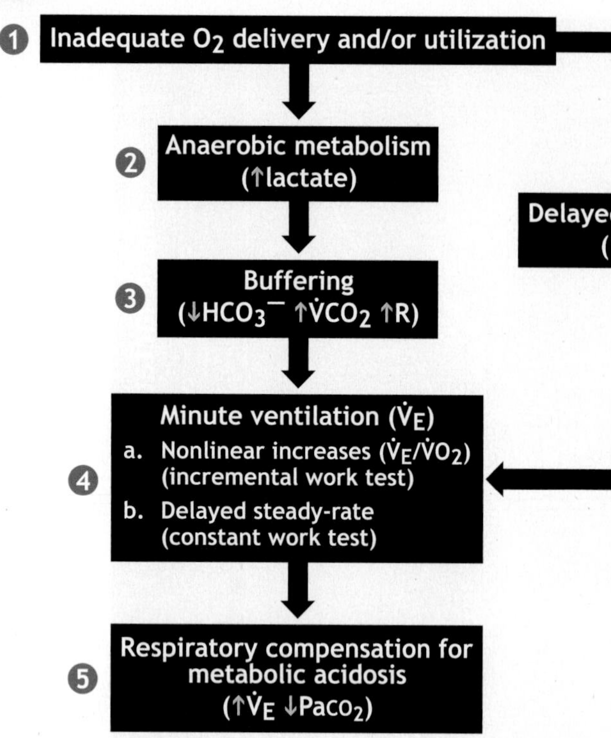

FIGURE 9.19 Five possible underlying factors that relate to detecting the lactate threshold from pulmonary gas exchange dynamics during physical activity of progressively increasing intensity.

activity. Two important factors influence endurance performance in a specific activity mode:

1. Maximum capacity to consume oxygen ($\dot{V}O_{2max}$)
2. Maximum level for steady-rate physical activity (OBLA)

Aerobic training increases OBLA, often without an accompanying $\dot{V}O_{2max}$ increase. Traditionally, exercise physiologists have applied $\dot{V}O_{2max}$ as the main yardstick to gauge capacity for endurance physical activity. This measure generally relates to long-duration physical performance but does not fully explain all aspects of success. Experienced distance athletes generally compete at an intensity slightly above the point of OBLA. Intensity of effort at OBLA has emerged as a consistent and powerful predictor of aerobic performance. *Changes in endurance performance with training often relate more closely to training-induced changes in the exercise-induced level for OBLA (peripheral adaptations) than to changes in* $\dot{V}O_{2max}$ *(central circulatory adaptations).*

DOES VENTILATION LIMIT AEROBIC CAPACITY FOR THE AVERAGE PERSON?

With inadequate breathing capacity, the line relating pulmonary ventilation and oxygen uptake in **Figure 9.18** would not curve upward during intense effort; instead, it would level off or slope downward to the right to reflect a decrease in the ventilatory equivalent. Such a response would indicate a *failure* for ventilation to keep pace with increasing oxygen demands; in this case, a person truly would "run out of wind." Actually, healthy individuals tend to overbreathe relative to oxygen uptake with increasing intensity of effort. **Figure 9.16** demonstrated that the ventilatory adjustment to strenuous physical activity decreases alveolar Pco_2 concomitant with small increases in alveolar Po_2. For most individuals, arterial Po_2 and Hb oxygen saturation remain at near-resting values during intense activity. This means that pulmonary function *does not* represent the "weak link" in the oxygen transport system of healthy individuals with average to moderately high aerobic capacities.

Energy Requirements (Work) of Breathing

Two major factors determine energy requirements of breathing:

1. **Compliance** of lungs and thorax
2. Resistance of airways to smooth flow of air

Lung and thorax compliance refers to how "easily" these tissues stretch. The radius of the bronchi primarily establishes airflow resistance. More specifically, airflow resistance varies inversely with a vessel's radius raised to the fourth power in accordance with Poiseuille law. Reducing airway radius by half causes airway resistance to increase 16 times. Normally, bronchi and bronchiole dimensions do not impede smooth air flow, and breathing requires relatively little energy. In some lung diseases airways constrict or lung tissues themselves lose compliance and impose considerable resistance to airflow. Trying to breathe through a drinking straw gives some appreciation of the breathing difficulties associated with severe obstructive lung disease.

A healthy person rarely senses the breathing effort even during moderate physical activity. In contrast, respiratory disease often makes the work of breathing during activity exhausting. For patients with **chronic obstructive pulmonary disease (COPD)** such as asthma or emphysema, breathing effort at rest can reach three times that of healthy individuals. In severe pulmonary disease, breathing's energy requirement may easily reach 40% of the total exercise oxygen uptake. This obviously encroaches on the oxygen available to active, nonrespiratory muscles and seriously limits these patients' physical capacity.

Figure 9.21 specifies the oxygen cost of breathing during whole-body graded physical activity to maximum. The top insert illustrates effects of increasing minute ventilation on oxygen cost of breathing, expressed as a percentage of total exercise oxygen uptake. The bottom insert illustrates the influence of increasing minute ventilation on oxygen cost per liter of air breathed each minute. The oxygen requirement of breathing remains relatively small at rest and during light-to-moderate activity, with no differences observed between nonobese women and men. For ventilations up to about 100 $L \cdot min^{-1}$, oxygen cost averaged between 1.5 and 2.0

mL per liter of air breathed per minute. This represented from 3% to 5% of the total oxygen uptake in moderate activity and 8% to 11% for minute ventilations at $\dot{V}O_{2max}$ values typical for most individuals. Among highly trained endurance athletes with maximum minute ventilations of 150 L · min^{-1} and higher, the cost of exercise hyperpnea can exceed 15% of total oxygen uptake. At this level, inspiratory muscles operate at 40% to 60% of maximum capacity to generate force. The rate of blood flow to these muscles may equal that of limb locomotor muscles.

During maximal effort, up to 15% of total blood flow sustains the respiratory muscle's metabolic demands. Evidence from healthy, fit individuals indicates a "competition" during intense activity between respiratory and locomotor muscle control for blood flow and oxygen. For example, altering respiratory muscle work during maximal effort to increase the energy cost of breathing constricts locomotor muscle vasculature. Redirection of cardiac output to the respiratory musculature compromises perfusion to active, nonrespiratory muscles. This reduces the total percentage of $\dot{V}O_{2max}$ used by the active locomotor muscles. Conversely, easing the work of breathing during maximal effort with an assist ventilator elicited a corresponding increase in the active leg muscle's oxygen uptake.

In COPD, the added expiratory resistance often triples the normal cost of breathing at rest; during light activity, ventilatory cost may reach 10 mL of oxygen for each liter of air breathed. Competition between the oxygen–blood flow needs of locomotor and respiratory muscles encroaches on the oxygen available to active, nonrespiratory muscle mass. In COPD, the increased cost of breathing severely limits the exercise capacity of individuals with this debilitating medical condition. Unfortunately, exercise training produces only small improvements in pulmonary function parameters or disease status. Regular physical activity improves capacity, reduces dyspnea, decreases ventilatory equivalents for oxygen, improves respiratory and peripheral muscle function, and enhances psychological state.

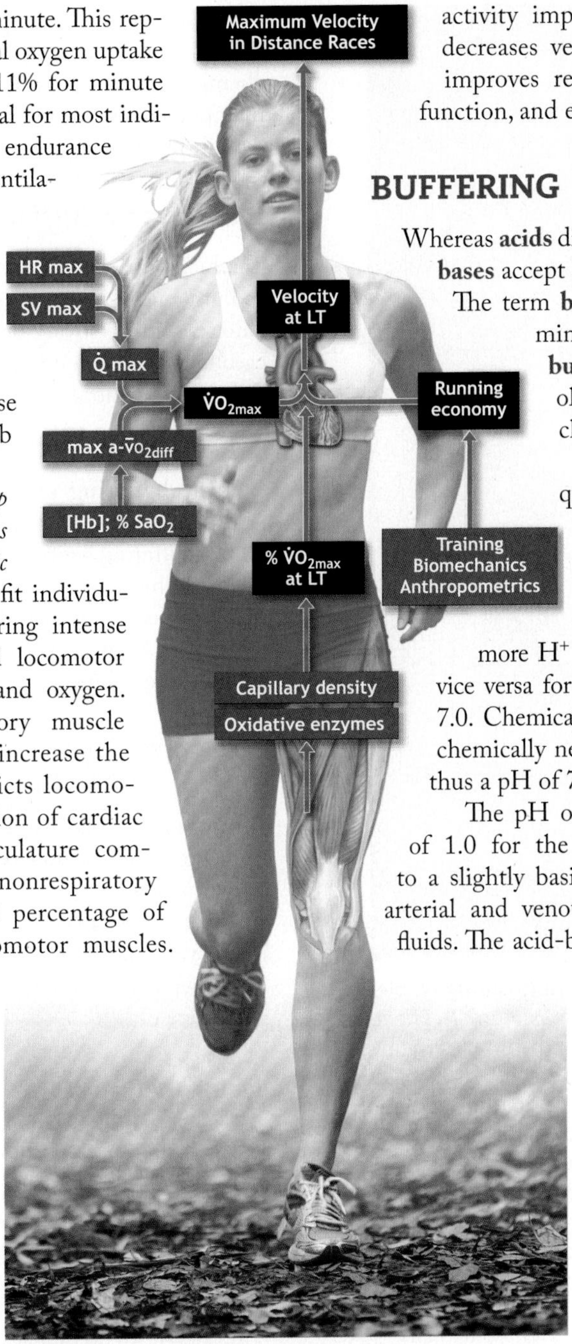

FIGURE 9.20 Major variables related to maximal oxygen uptake, onset of blood lactate accumulation, and maximal running velocity during endurance exercise. $\dot{Q}$, cardiac output; [Hb], hemoglobin concentration; % Sa_{O_2}, percentage saturation with oxygen; max a-$\bar{v}O_{2diff}$, maximum arteriovenous oxygen difference; LT, lactate threshold. (Adapted from Bassett DR Jr, Howley ET. Maximal oxygen uptake: "classical" versus "contemporary" viewpoints. *Med Sci Sports Exerc* 1997;29:591.) (Reprinted with permission from McArdle WD, Katch FI, Katch VL. *Exercise Physiology: Nutrition, Energy, and Human Performance*. 8th Ed. Baltimore: Wolters Kluwer Health, 2015; portions modified and reprinted with permission from Moore KL, et al. *Clinically Oriented Anatomy*. 7th Ed. Baltimore: Wolters Kluwer Health, 2013, as used with permission from Agur AMR, Dalley AF. *Grant's Atlas of Anatomy*. 13th Ed. Baltimore: Wolters Kluwer Health, 2013.)

BUFFERING

Whereas **acids** dissociate in solution and release H^+, **bases** accept H^+ to form hydroxide ions (OH^-). The term **buffering** designates reactions that minimize changes in H^+ concentration; **buffers** refer to chemical and physiologic mechanisms that prevent this change.

The symbol **pH** designates a quantitative measure of acidity or alkalinity (basicity) of a liquid solution. Specifically, pH refers to the concentration of protons or H^+. Acid solutions have more H^+ than OH^- at a pH below 7.0 and vice versa for basic solutions whose pH exceeds 7.0. Chemically pure distilled water, considered chemically neutral, has equal H^+ and OH^- and thus a pH of 7.0.

The pH of bodily fluids ranges from a low of 1.0 for the digestive acid hydrochloric acid to a slightly basic pH between 7.35 and 7.45 for arterial and venous blood and most other bodily fluids. The acid-base characteristics of bodily fluids fluctuate within narrow tolerance limits because metabolism remains highly sensitive to H^+ concentrations in the reacting medium. Three mechanisms regulate the pH of the internal environment:

1. Chemical buffers
2. Pulmonary ventilation
3. Renal function

Chemical Buffers

The chemical buffering system consists of a weak acid and salt of that acid. Bicarbonate buffer, for example, consists of the weak acid carbonic acid and its salt, sodium bicarbonate. Carbonic acid forms when bicarbonate binds H^+. With H^+ concentration elevated, the reaction produces the weak acid because excess H^+ ions bind in accord with the general reaction:

$$H^+ + \text{Buffer} \rightarrow \text{H-Buffer}$$

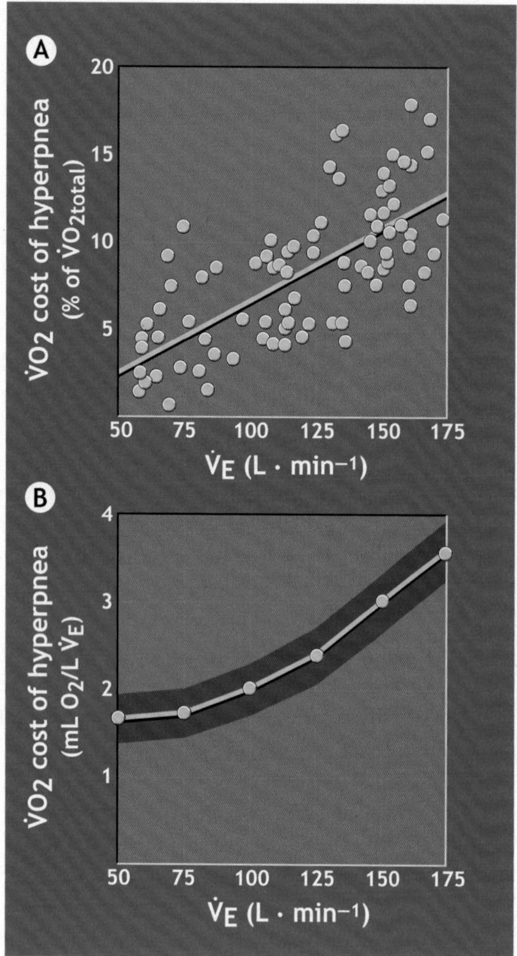

FIGURE 9.21 Oxygen cost of breathing during whole-body graded physical activity up to maximum. **A.** Effects of increasing minute ventilation ($\dot{V}_E$) on the total oxygen cost of breathing expressed as a percentage of total exercise oxygen uptake. **B.** Effects of increasing minute ventilation on the oxygen cost per liter air breathed per minute. (Reprinted with permission from McArdle WD, Katch FI, Katch VL. *Exercise Physiology: Nutrition, Energy, and Human Performance*. 8th Ed. Baltimore: Wolters Kluwer Health, 2015, as adapted with permission from Dempsey JA, et al. Respiratory muscle perfusion and energetics during exercise. *Med Sci Sports Exerc* 1996;28:1123.)

In contrast, H^+ concentration decreases when the buffering reaction moves in the opposite direction and releases H^+ as follows:

$$\mathbf{H^+ + Buffer \leftarrow H\text{-}Buffer}$$

During hyperventilation, plasma carbonic acid declines because carbon dioxide leaves the blood and exits the lungs.

Most of the carbon dioxide generated in energy metabolism reacts with water to form the relatively weak carbonic acid that dissociates into H^+ and HCO_3^-. Likewise, the stronger lactic acid reacts with sodium bicarbonate to form sodium lactate and carbonic acid; in turn, carbonic acid dissociates and increases the extracellular fluids' H^+ concentration. Other organic acids such as fatty acids dissociate and liberate H^+, as do sulfuric and phosphoric acids generated during protein catabolism. Bicarbonate, phosphate, and protein chemical buffers provide the rapid first line of defense to maintain consistency in the internal environment's acid-base equilibrium.

Bicarbonate Buffer

The bicarbonate buffer system consists of carbonic acid and sodium bicarbonate in solution. During buffering, hydrochloric acid (a strong acid) converts to the much weaker carbonic acid by combining with sodium bicarbonate in the following reaction:

$$\mathbf{HCl + NaHCO_3 \rightarrow NaCl + H_2CO_3 \leftrightarrow H^+ + HCO_3^-}$$

The buffering of hydrochloric acid produces only a slightly reduced pH. Sodium bicarbonate in plasma exerts a strong buffering action on lactic acid to form sodium lactate and carbonic acid. Any additional increase in H^+ concentration from carbonic acid dissociation causes the dissociation reaction to move in the opposite direction to release carbon dioxide into solution.

Result of Acidosis

$$\mathbf{H_2O + CO_2 \leftarrow H_2CO_3 \leftarrow H^+ + HCO_3^-}$$

An increase in plasma carbon dioxide or H^+ concentration immediately stimulates ventilation to eliminate "excess" carbon dioxide.

Conversely, a decrease in plasma H^+ concentration inhibits the ventilatory drive and retains carbon dioxide that then combines with water to increase acidity (carbonic acid) and normalize pH.

Result of Alkalosis

$$\mathbf{H_2O + CO_2 \rightarrow H_2CO_3 \rightarrow H^+ + HCO_3^-}$$

Phosphate Buffer

The phosphate buffering system consists of phosphoric acid and sodium phosphate. These chemicals act similarly to bicarbonate buffers. Phosphate buffers exert an important effect on acid-base balance in the kidney tubules and intracellular fluids where phosphate concentration remains high.

Protein Buffer

Venous blood buffers the H^+ released from dissociation of the relatively weak carbonic acid produced from H_2O + CO_2. *By far, Hb provides the most important H^+ acceptor for this buffering function.* Hb is almost six times more potent in regulating acidity than the other plasma proteins. Hb's oxygen release to cells makes Hb a weaker acid, thereby increasing its affinity to bind H^+. The H^+ generated when carbonic acid forms in the erythrocyte combines readily with deoxygenated Hb or Hb^- in the following reaction:

$$\mathbf{H^+ + Hb^- (Protein) \rightarrow HHb}$$

Intracellular tissue proteins also regulate plasma pH. Some amino acids possess free acidic radicals. When dissociated, they form OH^-, which reacts with H^+ to form water.

Physiologic Buffers

The pulmonary and renal systems present the second line of defense in acid-base regulation. Their buffering function occurs only with a previously existing change in pH.

Ventilatory Buffer

When the quantity of free H^+ in extracellular fluid and plasma increases, it directly stimulates the respiratory center to immediately increase alveolar ventilation. This rapid adjustment reduces alveolar Pco_2 and causes carbon dioxide to be "blown off" from the blood. Reduced plasma carbon dioxide levels accelerate the recombination of H^+ and HCO_3^-, lowering free H^+ concentration in plasma. For example, doubling alveolar ventilation by hyperventilation at rest increases blood alkalinity and pH by 0.23 units from 7.40 to 7.63. Conversely, reducing normal alveolar ventilation or hypoventilation by half increases blood acidity by approximately 0.23 pH units. The potential magnitude of ventilatory buffering equals twice the combined effect of all the body's chemical buffers.

Renal Buffer

Chemical buffers only temporarily impact excess acid buildup. Relatively slow kidney excretion of H^+ provides an important longer-term defense to maintain the body's buffer reserve, known as **alkaline reserve.** To this end, the kidneys stand as final guardians to preserve normal function. The renal tubules regulate acidity through complex chemical reactions that secrete ammonia and H^+ into the urine and then reabsorb alkali, chloride, and bicarbonate.

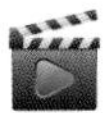
See the animation "Renal Function" on **http://thePoint.lww.com/MKKESS5e** for a demonstration of this concept.

A CLOSER LOOK

Exercise-Induced Asthma (EIA)

Asthma, a **chronic obstructive pulmonary disease (COPD)**, affects more than 25 million individuals in the United States, and the most common chronic children's disease (**http://www.who.int/mediacentre/factsheets/fs307/en/index.html**). A public health problem not just for high-income countries, asthma occurs in all countries regardless of the level of development. Unfortunately, most asthma-related deaths occur in low- and lower-middle-income economies grouped by world region (**http://data.worldbank.org/about/country-and-lending-groups#MENA**). Asthma is underdiagnosed and undertreated and often restricts individuals' activities for a lifetime.

A high fitness level does not confer immunity from this ailment. Pulmonary airway hyperirritability usually manifests by coughing, wheezing, and shortness of breath, all characteristic of an asthmatic condition.

With physical activity, catecholamines released from the sympathetic nervous system produce a relaxation effect on smooth muscle that lines the pulmonary airways. Everyone experiences initial bronchodilation with physical activity. For people with asthma, in contrast, bronchospasm and exertion cause mucous secretion following normal bronchodilation. An acute episode of airway obstruction often occurs 10 minutes after physical activity; recovery usually occurs spontaneously within 30 to 90 minutes. One technique for diagnosing EIA uses progressive increments of treadmill or bicycle ergometer activity. During a 10- to 20-minute recovery following each activity bout, spirometric testing assesses $FEV_{1.0}/FVC$. A 15% reduction in pre-exercise values confirms the EIA diagnosis.

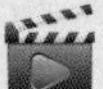
See the animation "Asthma" on **http://thePoint.lww.com/MKKESS5e** for a demonstration of the effects of asthma on the pulmonary system.

Sensitivity to Thermal Gradients

An attractive theory to explain EIA relates to the rate and magnitude of pulmonary heat exchange alterations as ventilation increases with physical activity. As the incoming breath of air moves down the pulmonary pathways, air warms and humidifies as heat and water transfer from the respiratory tract. This form of "air conditioning" both cools and dries the respiratory mucosa, allowing for an abrupt airway rewarming during recovery. The thermal gradient from cooling and subsequent rewarming and loss of water from mucosal tissue stimulates proinflammatory chemical mediators that cause bronchospasm.

Environment Makes a Difference

Physical activity in a humid environment diminishes the EIA response regardless of ambient air temperature. This is perplexing because conventional belief maintains that a dry climate best suits people with asthma. In fact, inhaling ambient air fully saturated with water vapor in physically active patients often abolishes the bronchospastic response. This also explains why people with asthma tolerate walking or jogging on a warm, humid day, or swimming in an indoor pool, yet outdoor winter sports usually trigger an asthmatic attack. People with asthma should perform 15 to 30 minutes of continuous warm-up activity because it initiates a "refractory period" that minimizes the severity of a bronchoconstrictive response during subsequent, more intense physical activity.

Currently, medications offer considerable relief from bronchoconstriction without affecting performance in individuals who want to be active on a regular basis. Exercise training cannot "cure" the asthmatic condition, but it can increase airway reserve and reduce the work of breathing during all modes of physical activity.

Even Physically Fit Athletes Can Have Asthma

Champion athletes are not immune from asthma. One of the most famous examples, 1984 Olympic marathon champion Joan Benoit Samuelson (1957–), experienced breathing problems during several races in 1991 that led to the discovery of her asthmatic condition (**www.joanbenoitsamuelson.com**). Despite experiencing breathing difficulties during the 1991 New York Marathon, she finished with a time of 2 hours:33 minutes:40 seconds!

Intense Physical Activity Effects

Increased H^+ concentration from carbon dioxide production and lactate formation during intense physical activity makes pH regulation progressively more difficult. Acid-base regulation becomes exceedingly difficult during repeated, brief bouts of all-out effort that elevate blood lactate values to 30 mM (270 mg of lactate per dL of blood) or higher. **Figure 9.22** illustrates the inverse linear relationship between blood lactate concentration and blood pH. Blood lactate concentration varied between a pH of 7.43 at rest and 6.80 during exhaustive physical effort. This response indicates that highly trained, top athletes can *temporarily* tolerate pronounced disturbances in acid-base balance during maximal exertion at least to a blood pH of 6.80. This occurs rarely during maximal treadmill activity in which athletes push beyond their usual end point when in a "zone state," surpassing the point at which pain and discomfort terminate most maximal effort tests. A plasma pH below 7.00 has potentially serious medical consequences including coma and cardiac arrhythmias; prior to blackout or collapse, symptoms can include nausea, headache, and dizziness in addition to pain within active muscles that ranges from mild to severely debilitating.

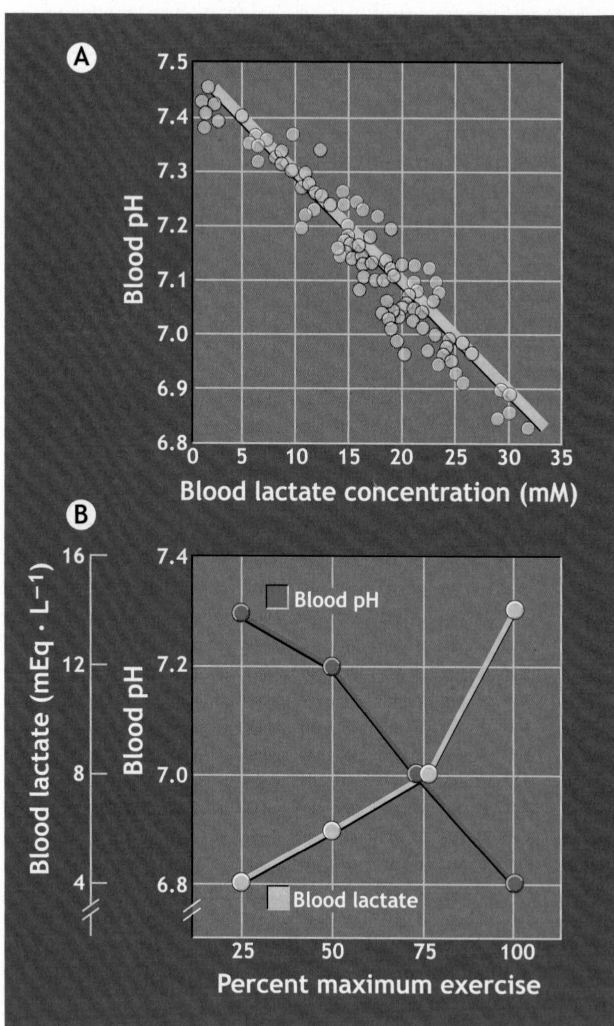

FIGURE 9.22 **A.** Relationship between blood pH and blood lactate concentration during rest and increasing intensities of short-duration physical effort to maximum. **B.** Blood pH and blood lactate concentration related to exercise intensity expressed as a percentage of maximum. Decreases in blood pH accompany increases in blood lactate concentration. (Adapted with permission from McArdle WD, Katch FI, Katch VL. *Exercise Physiology: Nutrition, Energy, and Human Performance*. 8th Ed. Baltimore: Wolters Kluwer Health, 2015, as adapted with permission from Osnes JB, Hermansen L. Acid-base balance after maximal exercise of short duration. *J Appl Physiol* 1972;32:59.)

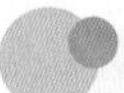

SUMMARY

1. Pulmonary ventilation increases linearly with oxygen uptake during light and moderate physical activity.
2. The ventilatory equivalent during light and moderate physical activity averages 20 to 25 L of air breathed per liter of oxygen consumed.
3. In non–steady-rate physical activity, pulmonary ventilation increases disproportionately with increases in oxygen uptake, and the ventilatory equivalent may attain 35 or 40.
4. The eventual sharp upswing in pulmonary ventilation related to oxygen uptake during incremental physical activity indicates the point of OBLA.
5. OBLA effectively predicts endurance performance and is measured without significant metabolic acidosis or cardiovascular strain.
6. Breathing normally requires a relatively small oxygen cost even during physical activity.
7. In respiratory disease, the work of breathing becomes excessive and exercise alveolar ventilation often becomes inadequate.
8. For individuals of average aerobic fitness, maximal physical activity does not tax pulmonary ventilation to a point that limits optimal alveolar gas exchange and arterial saturation.
9. Buffers consist of a weak acid and the salt of that acid, which regulate the acid-base balance of bodily fluids.
10. Buffering during acidosis converts a strong acid to a weaker acid and neutral salt.
11. The bicarbonate, phosphate, and protein chemical buffers provide the first line of defense to maintain a narrow range for acid-base regulation.
12. The lungs contribute to pH regulation. Changes in alveolar ventilation alter the extracellular fluids' free H^+ concentration.
13. The renal tubules act as a final buffering defense mechanism by secreting H^+ into urine and reabsorbing bicarbonate.
14. Anaerobic physical activity increases buffering demand making pH regulation progressively more difficult.
15. EIA represents a common obstructive lung disorder associated with rate and magnitude of airway cooling, drying, and subsequent rewarming.
16. Breathing humidified air during physical activity often eliminates the consequences of EIA.

THINK IT THROUGH

1. How would the relationship change between $\dot{V}_E$ / $\dot{V}O_2$ under the following two conditions:
   a. An aging person who remains sedentary versus an aging person who performs regular aerobic activities
   b. During transition from adolescence to young adulthood
2. Present two arguments to justify why pulmonary ventilation does not limit aerobic exercise performance for most healthy people.
3. Explain how the terms *lactate threshold* and *OBLA* are biochemically more precise than *anaerobic threshold*?
4. Explain the biochemical rationale for measuring oxygen uptake and carbon dioxide production during physical activity to infer the onset of metabolic anaerobiosis or lactate accumulation.

KEY TERMS

2,3-Diphosphoglycerate (2,3-DPG): Produced in red blood cells during glycolysis and binds loosely with subunits of the hemoglobin molecule to reduce its oxygen affinity.

Acids: Substances that dissociate in solution to release H^+.

Alkaline reserve: Any additional amount of buffer compound, particularly sodium bicarbonate, that the body maintains as a buffer reserve to increase its defense against a decrease in pH.

Alveolar ventilation: That portion of inspired air that reaches the alveoli and participates in gas exchange.

Alveoli: More than 600 million thin-walled sacs that represent the final branching of the respiratory tree; represent the surface for gas exchange between lung tissue and blood.

Anaerobic threshold: The abrupt increase in ventilatory equivalent caused by nonmetabolic carbon dioxide production from lactate buffering; believed by some to be a noninvasive ventilatory measure to signal the body's shift to anaerobic metabolism.

Anatomic dead space: Air that fills the mouth, nasal passages, nasopharynx, larynx, and other nondiffusible conducting portions of the respiratory tract, which do not participate in gas exchange.

Aortic bodies: Small structures of neural tissue that attach to a branch of the aorta near its arch that contain chemoreceptors that respond primarily to decreases in blood oxygen concentration and trigger an increased respiratory rate.

Arteriovenous oxygen difference ($a\text{-}\bar{v}O_{2diff}$): Difference between the oxygen content of arterial and mixed-venous blood.

Bases: Substances that in aqueous solution accept H^+ to form hydroxide ions (OH^-).

Bohr effect: Inverse relationship between hemoglobin's oxygen binding affinity and plasma acidity (pH), temperature, and concentration of carbon dioxide in plasma.

Breathing economy: Quantity of air breathed per amount of oxygen consumed.

Breathing entrainment: Coordination of breathing frequency to the rhythm of locomotion.

Bronchi: Either of two main airway passages, which function as primary conduits into each lung.

Bronchioles: Subdivisions of the bronchi, which conduct inspired air through a winding, narrow route until it mixes with existing air in alveolar ducts.

Buffering: Physiologic mechanisms or chemical reactions to minimize changes in H^+ concentration.

Buffers: Chemical and physiologic mechanisms that resist changes in pH.

Carbonic anhydrase: Zinc-containing enzyme within red blood cells that greatly accelerates the union of carbon dioxide and water to form carbonic acid, a primary transport method for carbon dioxide to travel from tissues to lungs.

Carotid bodies: Chemoreceptors located in the branching of carotid arteries in the right and left sides of the neck to monitor the state of arterial blood (O_2, CO_2, pH) before it enters the brain.

Central command: Centrally mediated integration of multiple chemical and neural signals involving feedback mechanisms to control cardiovascular response prior to, during, and in recovery from physical activity.

Chemoreceptors: Specialized neurons located in the aortic arch and branching of carotid arteries to detect arterial hypoxia, increased carbon dioxide, and decreased pH to reflexly initiate a ventilatory response.

Chronic obstructive pulmonary disease (COPD): Several respiratory tract diseases (e.g., emphysema, asthma, chronic bronchitis) that obstruct airflow and compromise breathing effort.

Compliance (lung): Resistance of respiratory passages to smooth flow of air; includes "stiffness" imposed by chest and lung tissue properties to a change in shape during breathing.

Cortical influence: In relation to pulmonary physiology describes neural outflow from motor cortex regions during physical activity and cortical activation in anticipation of activity stimulates medullary respiratory neurons.

Diaphragm: Large dome-shaped sheet of muscle separating the thoracic cavity from the abdominal cavity; contraction increases thoracic cavity volume, drawing air into the lungs.

Dynamic lung volume: Lung volume that depends rate of airflow into or out of the lungs.

Expiration: Airflow out of the lungs initiated by muscles that compress the thoracic cavity.

Expiratory reserve volume (ERV): Maximum expired air volume at the end of tidal expiration.

$FEV_{1.0}$: Maximum amount of air expired after maximum inspiration over a 1-second period.

Forced expiratory volume (FEV): Dynamic lung function measure indicating the volume of air moved over a period of time, usually 1 second ($FEV_{1.0}$) following a maximal inspiration.

Forced expiratory volume-to-FVC ratio ($FEV_{1.0}$/FVC): Percentage of forced vital capacity expelled in 1 second; reflects pulmonary expiratory power and overall resistance to air movement upstream in the lungs.

Forced vital capacity (FVC): Maximum expiration volume following a full inspiration.

Gas concentration: Amount of a gas in a given volume determined by the product of gas partial pressure and solubility.

Gas pressure: Force exerted by gas molecules against surfaces they encounter.

Gas solubility: Dissolving power of a gas reflecting the quantity of a gas dissolved in fluid at a particular pressure.

Haldane effect: Interaction between oxygen loading and carbon dioxide release, such that oxygenation of hemoglobin in the lungs reduces its ability to bind carbon dioxide and facilitates the lung's removal of carbon dioxide.

Hemoglobin (Hb): Iron-containing globular protein pigment carried within red blood cells that loosely combines with oxygen to carry 65 to 70 times more oxygen than normally dissolves in plasma.

Hyperpnea: Increased breathing required to meet metabolic demands during physical activity or when the body lacks oxygen as in high-altitude exposure.

Hyperventilation: Increase in alveolar ventilation that exceeds the oxygen uptake and carbon dioxide elimination needs of metabolism.

Hypoxic threshold: Point at which decreasing arterial Po_2 detected by carotid bodies stimulates ventilation; usually occurs at a Po_2 between 60 and 70 mm Hg.

Inspiration: Airflow into the lungs initiated by muscles that expand the thoracic cavity.

Inspiratory reserve volume (IRV): Maximum inspired air volume following tidal inspiration.

Intrapulmonic pressure: Gas pressure maintained within lung tissue and its passages.

Lactate threshold: Highest oxygen uptake or exercise intensity achieved with less than a 1.0 mmol increase in blood lactate concentration above the pre-exercise level.

Lung compliance: Measure of the lung's ability to stretch and expand.

Manometer: Sensitive instrument to measure the pressure of a gas or vapor indicated by the difference from a control level within the calibrated instrument to a new level with the gas present.

Maximum voluntary ventilation (MVV): Maximum air volume breathed over a specified period of time, usually extrapolated to a 1-minute value.

Mechanoreceptors: Sensory receptors in peripheral tissue that respond to mechanical pressure or distortion and provide information to the central nervous system about touch, pressure, vibration, and cutaneous tension.

Medulla: Lower half of the brainstem that controls the autonomic functions as breathing, digestion, and heart and blood vessel function; helps to transfer neural signals between the brain and spinal cord.

Minute ventilation: Volume of air inhaled or exhaled each minute.

Myoglobin: Iron-containing globular protein in skeletal and cardiac muscle fibers with about 240 times greater affinity for oxygen than hemoglobin; provides intramuscular oxygen storage for release at low tissue Po_2.

Onset of blood lactate accumulation (OBLA): Point at which blood lactate concentration rises to 4.0 mmol during physical activity.

Oxygen transport cascade: Depicts oxygen partial pressure as it moves from sea-level ambient air to maximally active skeletal muscle mitochondria.

Oxygenation reaction: Four iron atoms in the hemoglobin molecule each loosely bind one oxygen molecule without requiring enzymes.

Oxyhemoglobin dissociation curve: Illustrates hemoglobin saturation with oxygen at various Po_2 values; shows how readily hemoglobin acquires and releases oxygen molecules into the fluid surrounding it.

Partial pressures: Pressure exerted by each specific gas in a mixture of gases.

Peripheral influence: In relation to pulmonary physiology refers to sensory input from joints, tendons, and muscles that adjusts ventilation during physical activity.

pH: Quantitative measure of the acidity or basicity of aqueous or other liquid solutions reflected by the molar concentration of hydrogen ions in the solution.

Phase I ventilation: At the start of physical activity, neurogenic stimuli from the cerebral cortex combined with feedback from the active limbs, stimulate the medulla to abruptly increase ventilation.

Phase II ventilation: Slower exponential rise in pulmonary ventilation that begins approximately 20 seconds following physical activity onset; central command continues input along with feedback from active muscles plus the added effect of short-term potentiation of respiratory neurons.

Phase III ventilation: Final phase of ventilatory response to physical activity that involves fine-tuning of steady-state ventilation through peripheral sensory feedback mechanisms.

Physical solution: Amount of a gas dissolved in a liquid.

Physiologic dead space: Portion of the alveolar volume with a ventilation-perfusion ratio that approaches zero; portion of the alveolar volume with poor tissue regional perfusion or inadequate ventilation.

Pressure differential: As related to gas movement into and out of a fluid refers to the difference in pressure between the gas above the fluid and dissolved in the fluid.

Pulmonary ventilation: Total volume of gas breathed (inspired or expired) each minute.

Residual lung volume (RLV): Air volume remaining in the lungs following maximal exhalation.

Respiratory membrane: Alveolar and capillary walls comprised of two layers of simple squamous epithelium and their basement membranes for purposes of gas exchange.

Solubility: Dissolving power of a gas that reflects the quantity dissolved in fluid at a particular pressure.

Static lung volume: Lung volume that remains unaffected by the rate air enters or exits the lungs.

Tidal volume (TV): Under resting conditions, the air volume moved during the inspiratory or expiratory phase of each breathing cycle.

Valsalva maneuver: Forced exhalation against a closed glottis following a full inspiration.

Ventilatory equivalent for oxygen: Symbolized $\dot{V}_E/\dot{V}O_2$ and describes the ratio of minute ventilation to oxygen uptake.

Ventilatory system: Specific organs and structures involved in the intake and exchange of oxygen and carbon dioxide between the body and environment; primarily functions to supply oxygen to the blood for delivery throughout the body.

Ventilatory threshold (Tvent): Point where pulmonary ventilation increases disproportionately relative to increases in oxygen uptake.

SELECTED REFERENCES

Ainslie PN, Duffin J. Integration of cerebrovascular CO_2 reactivity and chemoreflex control of breathing: mechanisms of regulation, measurement, and interpretation. *Am J Physiol Regul Integr Comp Physiol* 2009;265:R1473.

Andrianopoulos V, et al. Six-minute walk distance in patients with chronic obstructive pulmonary disease: which reference equations should we use? *Chron Respir Dis* 2015;12:111.

Auersperger I, et al. The effects of 8 weeks of endurance running on hepcidin concentrations, inflammatory parameters, and iron status in female runners. *Int J Sport Nutr Exerc Metab* 2012;22:55.

Babb TG, et al. Short- and long-term modulation of exercise ventilatory response. *Med Sci Sports Exerc* 2010;42:1691.

Bassett DR Jr, Howley ET. Limiting factors for maximum oxygen uptake and determinants of endurance performance. *Med Sci Sports Exerc* 2000;32:270.

Beck KC, et al. Ventilation-perfusion distribution in normal subjects. *J Appl Physiol* 2012;113:872.

Cannon DT, et al. On the determination of ventilatory threshold and respiratory compensation point via respiratory frequency. *Int J Sports Med* 2009; 30:157.

Clanton TL, et al. Regulation of cellular gas exchange, oxygen sensing, and metabolic control. *Compr Physiol* 2013;3:1135.

Coyle EF. Integration of the physiological factors determining endurance performance in athletes. *Exerc Sport Sci Rev* 1995;23:25.

Crocker GH, et al. Combined effects of inspired oxygen, carbon dioxide and carbon monoxide on oxygen transport and aerobic capacity. *J Appl Physiol* 2013;115:643.

Degens H, et al. Diffusion capacity of the lung in young and old endurance athletes. *Int J Sports Med* 2013;34:1051.

Del Coso J, et al. Respiratory compensation and blood pH regulation during variable intensity exercise in trained and untrained subjects. *Eur J Appl Physiol* 2009;107:83.

DellaValle DM, Haas JD. Impact of iron depletion without anemia on performance in trained endurance athletes at the beginning of a training season: a study of female collegiate rowers. *Int J Sport Nutr Exerc Metab* 2011;2:501.

Dempsey JA, et al. Respiratory system determinants of peripheral fatigue and endurance performance. *Med Sci Sports Exerc* 2008;40:457.

Dempsey JA. Challenges for future research in exercise physiology as applied to the respiratory system. *Exerc Sport Sci Rev* 2006;34:92.

Farkas GA, et al. Contractility of the ventilatory pump muscles. *Med Sci Sports Exerc* 1996;28:1106.

Faude O, et al. Lactate threshold concepts: how valid are they? *Sports Med* 2009;39:469.

Gläser S, et al. Influence of smoking and obesity on alveolar-arterial gas pressure differences and dead space ventilation at rest and peak exercise in healthy men and women. *Respir Med* 2013;107:919.

Gold DR, et al. Effects of cigarette smoking on lung function in adolescent boys and girls. *N Engl J Med* 1996;331:335.

Hackett DA, et al. Respiratory muscle adaptations: a comparison between bodybuilders and endurance athletes. *J Sports Med Phys Fitness* 2013;53:139.

Harms CA, Rosenkranz S. Sex differences in pulmonary function during exercise. *Med Sci Sports Exerc* 2008;40:664.

Ito K, et al. Electrically stimulated ventilation feedback improves the ventilation pattern in patients with COPD. *J Phys Ther Sci* 2015;27:325.

Legrand R, et al. O_2 arterial desaturation in endurance athletes increases muscle deoxygenation. *Med Sci Sports Exerc* 2005;36:782.

Lorenzo S, Babb TG. Oxygen cost of breathing and breathlessness during exercise in nonobese women and men. *Med Sci Sports Exerc* 2012;44:1043.

Louvaris Z, et al. Intensity of daily physical activity is associated with central hemodynamic and leg muscle oxygen availability in COPD. *J Appl Physiol* 2013;115:794.

Mann T, et al. Methods of prescribing relative exercise intensity: physiological and practical considerations. *Sports Med* 2013;43:613.

McClaran SR, et al. Smaller lungs in women affect exercise hyperpnea. *J Appl Physiol* 1998;84:1872.

Miller JD, et al. Skeletal muscle pump versus respiratory muscle pump: modulation of venous return from the locomotor limb in humans. *J Physiol* 2005;563:925.

Nybo L, Rasmussen O. Inadequate cerebral oxygen delivery and central fatigue during strenuous exercise. *Exerc Sport Sci Rev* 2007;35:110.

Ramponi S, et al. Pulmonary rehabilitation improves cardiovascular response to exercise in COPD. *Respiration* 2013;86:17.

Richardson RS. Oxygen transport: air to muscle cell. *Med Sci Sports Exerc* 1998;30:53.

Simões RP, et al. Lactate and heart rate variability threshold during resistance exercise in the young and elderly. *Int J Sports Med* 2013;34:991.

Spires J, et al. Distinguishing the effects of convective and diffusive O_2 delivery on VO2 on-kinetics in skeletal muscle contracting at moderate intensity. *Am J Physiol Regul Integr Comp Physiol* 2013;305:R512.

Stickland MK, et al. Pulmonary gas exchange and acid-base balance during exercise. *Compr Physiol* 2013;3:693.

Strickland MK, Lovering AT. Exercise-induced intrapulmonary arteriovenous shunting and pulmonary gas exchange. *Exerc Sport Sci Rev* 2006;34:99.

Torchio R, et al. Mechanical effects of obesity on airway responsiveness in otherwise healthy humans. *J Appl Physiol* 2009;107:408.

Wagner PD. Why doesn't exercise grow the lungs when other factors do? *Exerc Sport Sci Rev* 2005;33:3.

West JB. Fragility of pulmonary capillaries. *J Appl Physiol* 2013;115:1.

Weston A, et al. African runners exhibit greater fatigue resistance, lower lactate accumulation, and higher oxidative enzyme activity. *J Appl Physiol* 1999;86:915.

Zebrowska A, et al. Cardiovascular effects of the valsalva maneuver during static arm exercise in elite power lifting athletes. *Adv Exp Med Biol* 2013;755:335.

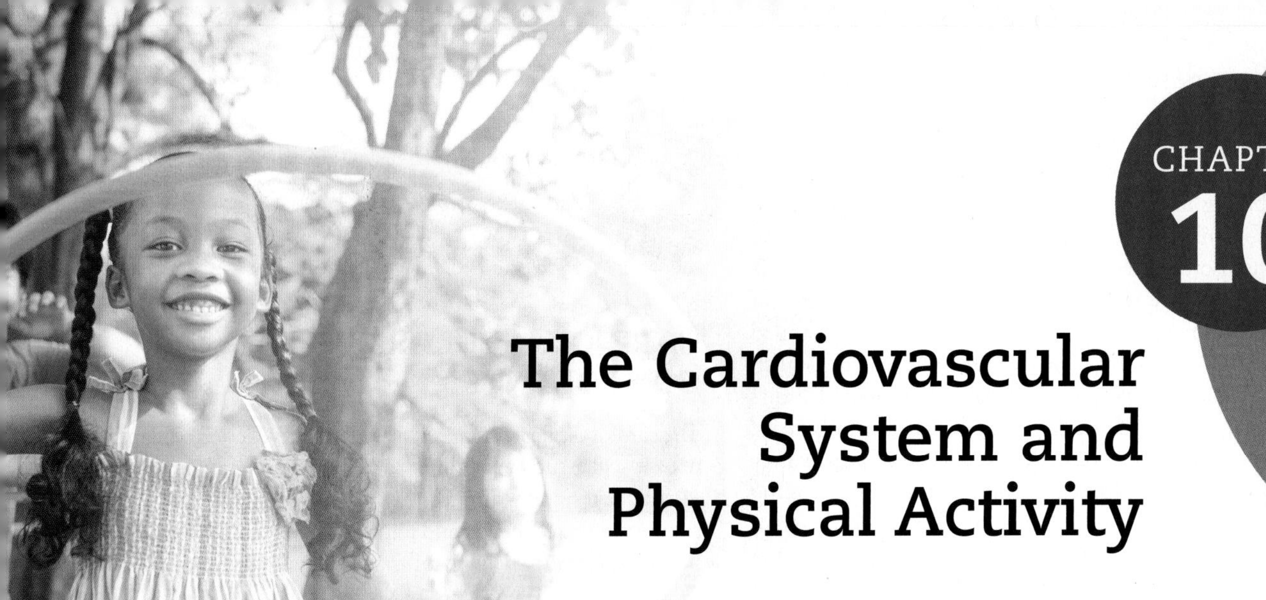

CHAPTER 10

The Cardiovascular System and Physical Activity

CHAPTER OBJECTIVES

- List four important functions of the cardiovascular system.
- Describe how to use the auscultatory method to measure blood pressure, and give average values for systolic and diastolic blood pressure during rest and moderate aerobic physical activity.
- Describe the blood pressure response during resistance exercise, upper-body activity, and inverted (head down) position.
- State three potential benefits of aerobic activity for treating moderate hypertension.
- Identify two intrinsic and extrinsic factors that regulate heart rate during rest and physical activity.
- Identify two neural and local metabolic factors that regulate blood flow during rest and physical activity.
- Compare average values of cardiac output during rest and maximal exertion for an endurance-trained male and female athlete and a male and female sedentary person.
- Explain three physiologic mechanisms that affect the heart's stroke volume.
- Describe the relationship between maximal cardiac output and maximal oxygen uptake among individuals with varied aerobic fitness levels.

ANCILLARIES AT A GLANCE

Visit **http://thePoint.lww.com/MKKESS5e** to access the following resources.

- References: Chapter 10
- Interactive Question Bank
- Animation: Blood Circulation
- Animation: Blood Flow
- Animation: Cardiac Cycle
- Animation: Fick Principle
- Animation: Hypertension
- Animation: Myocardial Blood Flow
- Animation: Perform a Basic 12-Lead Electrocardiogram
- Animation: Renal Function

Galen (A.D. 131–201), a Greek physician of antiquity (see Chapter 1), theorized that blood flowed like ocean tides, surging and abating into arteries, away from the heart and back again. In Galen's view, fluid carried with it "humors," good and evil that determined well-being. If a person became ill, the standard practice required "blood-letting"—draining off the diseased humors to restore health. This theory prevailed for almost 2000 years until the 17th century when English physician William Harvey (see Chapter 1) proposed a different theory of blood flow. Experimenting with frogs, cats, and dogs, Harvey demonstrated the existence of heart valves that provided one-way blood flow through the body, a finding incompatible with Galen's "ebb-and-flow" view. In a set of ingenious experiments, Harvey measured the volume of the heart's chambers and counted the number of times the heart contracted in 1 hour. He concluded that if the heart emptied only half of its volume with each beat, the body's total blood volume would be pumped in minutes. This finding led Harvey to hypothesize that blood *circulated* within a closed system in a circular, unidirectional pattern throughout the body. Harvey, of course, was correct; the heart pumps the entire 5-L blood volume in 1 minute. Harvey's experiments changed medical science forever, yet it would take nearly 200 more years for his theories to play important roles in physiology and medicine.

From Harvey's early experiments to sophisticated research at the dawn of the 21st century, we know that the highly efficient ventilatory system described in Chapter 9 complements a rapid blood transport and delivery system comprising blood, the heart, and more than 60,000 miles (100,000 km) of blood vessels, equivalent to 2.5 times around the Earth, that integrate the body as a unit. The circulatory system serves five important functions during physical activity:

1. Delivers oxygen to active tissues
2. Aerates blood returned to the lungs
3. Transports heat, a by-product of cellular metabolism, from the body's core to the skin
4. Delivers fuel nutrients to active tissues
5. Transports hormones, the body's sophisticated chemical messengers

PART 1 The Cardiovascular System

CARDIOVASCULAR SYSTEM COMPONENTS

The cardiovascular system consists of an interconnected, continuous vascular circuit containing a pump (heart), a high-pressure distribution system (arteries), exchange vessels (capillaries), and a low-pressure collection and return system (veins). **Figure 10.1** presents a schematic view of the cardiovascular system.

The Heart

The heart provides the force to propel blood throughout the vascular circuit. This fist-sized, four-chambered organ beats at rest an average of 70 b · min^{-1}, 100,800 times a day, and 36.8 million times a year. For the average 70-year-old, this represents over 2.5 billion beats in a lifetime, the equivalent of about 1 million barrels of blood or enough to fill more than 3 super tankers, literally without skipping a beat until death! Even for a healthy person of average fitness, maximum output of blood from this extraordinary organ exceeds fluid output from a household faucet turned wide open. Even more remarkable is that in just one day, the blood travels a total of about 12,000 miles (19,000 km), nearly equal to five, nonstop trips from New York City's Empire State Building to Ceaser's Palace in Las Vegas!

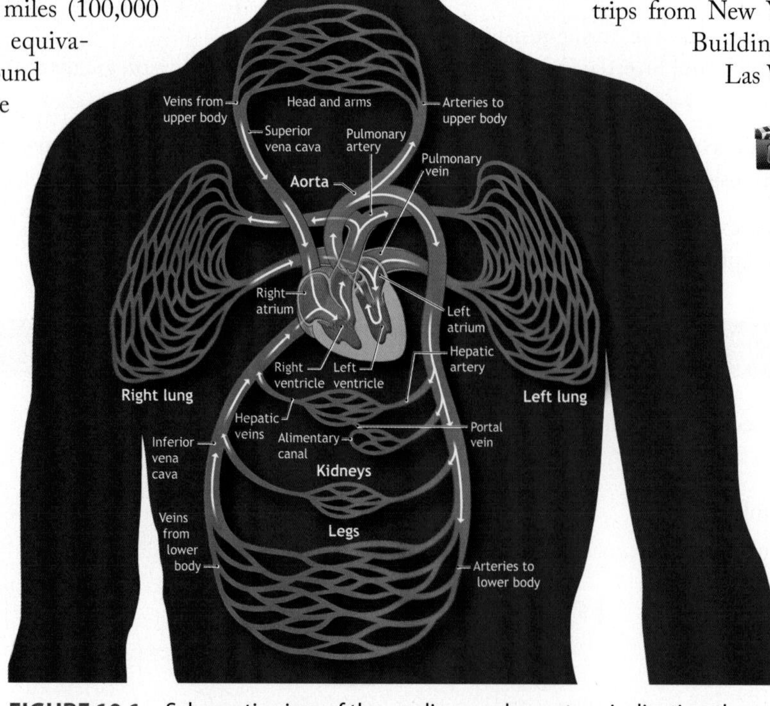

FIGURE 10.1 Schematic view of the cardiovascular system indicating the heart and pulmonary and systemic vascular circuits. *Red shading* depicts oxygen-rich arterial blood; *blue shading* denotes deoxygenated venous blood. The situation reverses in the pulmonary circuit; oxygenated blood returns to the heart in the right and left pulmonary veins. (Adapted with permission from McArdle WD, Katch FI, Katch VL. *Exercise Physiology: Nutrition, Energy, and Human Performance*. 8th Ed. Baltimore: Wolters Kluwer Health, 2015.)

See the animation "Blood Circulation" on **http://thePoint.lww.com/MKKESS5e** for a demonstration of this process.

The heart muscle or **myocardium** consists of striated muscle similar to skeletal muscle. Unlike skeletal muscle, individual fibers interconnect in latticework fashion. As a result, stimulation or depolarization of one myocardial cell spreads an action potential throughout the myocardium, causing the heart to function as a unit. **Figure 10.2** details the heart's pumping

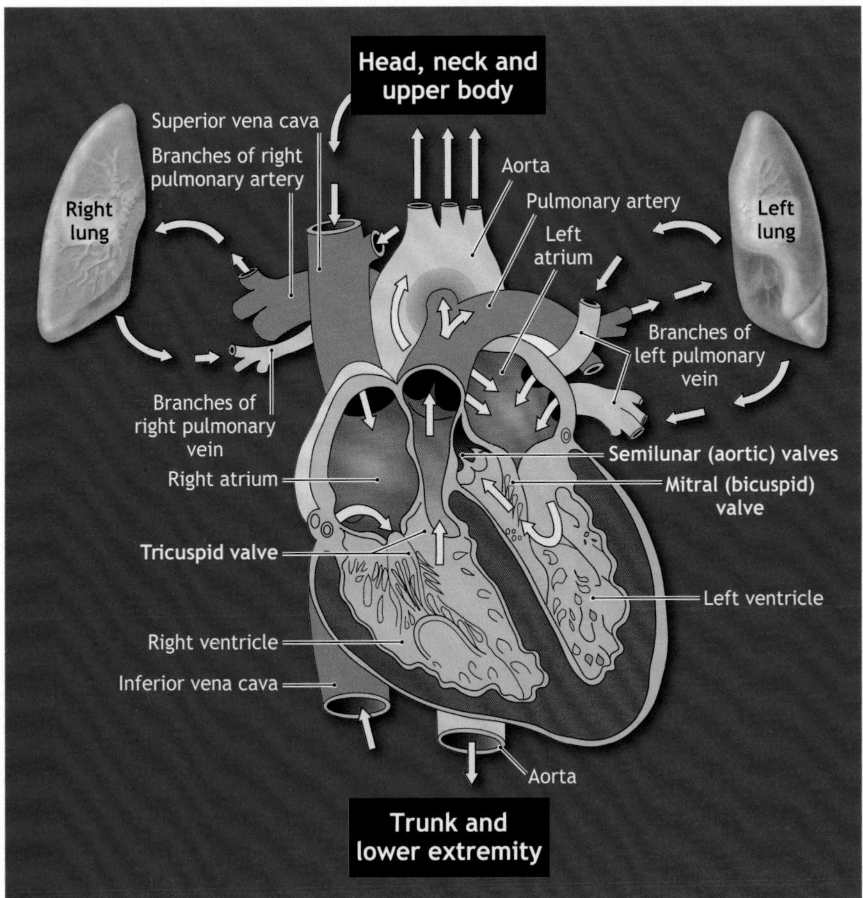

FIGURE 10.2 The heart's valves provide for the one-way flow of blood indicated by the *yellow arrows.*

action. Functionally, the heart consists of two separate pumps.

The hollow chambers of the *right heart pump* perform two crucial functions:

1. Receive deoxygenated blood returning from all body areas
2. Pump blood to the lungs for aeration via the **pulmonary circulation**

The chambers of the *left heart pump* also perform two crucial functions:

1. Receive oxygenated blood from the lungs
2. Pump blood into the thick-walled, muscular aorta for distribution throughout the body in the **systemic circulation**

A thick, solid muscular septum separates the heart's left and right sides. The **atrioventricular valves** situated within the heart direct one-way blood flow from the right atrium to the right ventricle (**tricuspid valve**) and from the left atrium to the left ventricle (**mitral valve** or bicuspid valve). **Semilunar valves** located in the arterial wall just outside the heart prevent blood from seeping back or regurgitating into the heart between ventricular contractions.

The relatively thin-walled, saclike atrial chambers receive and store blood returning from the lungs and body during ventricular contraction. About 70% of blood returning to the atria flows directly into the ventricles before the atria contract. Simultaneous atrial contractions force the remaining blood into the respective ventricles directly below. Almost immediately after atrial contraction, the ventricles contract and force blood into the arterial systems. To learn more, visit **www.pbs.org/wgbh/nova/eheart/human.html**, to view important aspects of heart function.

Arteries

The **arteries** serve as high-pressure tubing that delivers oxygen-rich blood to the tissues. **Figure 10.3** illustrates how the arteries are composed of layers of connective tissue and smooth muscle. Because of their thickness, no gaseous exchange takes place between arterial blood and surrounding tissues.

Blood pumped from the left ventricle into the highly muscular yet elastic **aorta** circulates throughout the body via a network of arteries and **arterioles or smaller arterial branches**. *The arteriole walls contain circular layers of smooth muscle that either constrict or relax to regulate peripheral blood flow.* The arterioles' redistribution function becomes important during physical activity because blood diverts to active muscles from areas that can temporarily compromise their blood supply.

Capillaries

The arterioles branch and form smaller and less muscular vessels called *metarterioles*. These tiny vessels merge into **capillaries** (see bottom of **Fig. 10.3**), a network of microscopic blood vessels so thin they provide only enough room for blood cells to squeeze through in single file. Capillaries contain about 5% of the body's total blood volume at any time. Gases, nutrients, and waste products rapidly transfer across the thin, porous capillary walls. A ring of smooth muscle called the **precapillary sphincter** encircles the capillary at its origin to control the vessel's internal diameter. This sphincter provides a local means to regulate capillary blood flow within a specific tissue to meet metabolic requirements that change rapidly and dramatically in physical activity. In essence, when the sphincter opens, more blood flows, and when it narrows, flow reduces.

Capillary branching increases the total cross-sectional area of the microcirculation 800 times more than that of the 1-inch diameter aorta. Blood flow velocity relates inversely to the vasculature's total cross section, making velocity progressively decrease as blood moves toward and into the capillaries.

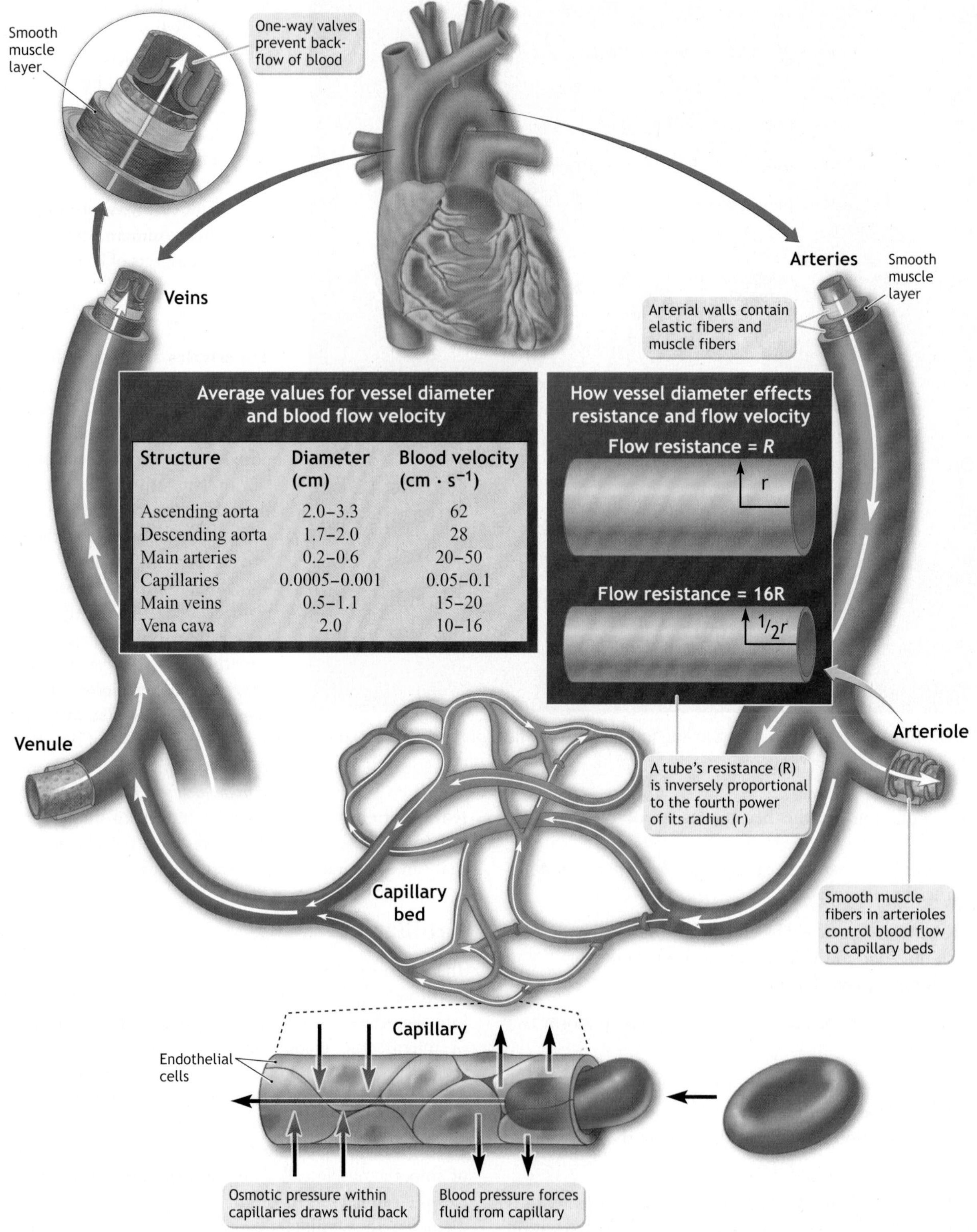

Average values for vessel diameter and blood flow velocity

Structure	Diameter (cm)	Blood velocity ($cm \cdot s^{-1}$)
Ascending aorta	2.0–3.3	62
Descending aorta	1.7–2.0	28
Main arteries	0.2–0.6	20–50
Capillaries	0.0005–0.001	0.05–0.1
Main veins	0.5–1.1	15–20
Vena cava	2.0	10–16

FIGURE 10.3 The structure of blood vessel walls. A single layer of endothelial cells lines each vessel. Fibrous tissue wrapped in several layers of smooth muscle surrounds the arterial walls. A single layer of muscle cells sheaths the arterioles; capillaries consist of only one layer of rolled-up endothelial cells, often less than 1 micron (μm) thick, with a flat surface area of 300 to 1200 μm^2. In the venule, fibrous tissue encases the endothelial cells; veins also possess a layer of smooth muscle. The *inset table* displays the average values for vessel diameter and corresponding values for blood flow velocity. A vessel's resistance (*R*) to flow depends on its radius. Decreasing vessel radius (*r*) by one-half increases resistance 16-fold. (Reprinted with permission from McArdle WD, Katch FI, Katch VL. *Exercise Physiology: Nutrition, Energy, and Human Performance*. 8th Ed. Baltimore: Wolters Kluwer Health, 2015.)

Veins

The vascular system maintains continuity of blood flow as capillaries feed deoxygenated blood at almost a trickle into the small veins or **venules** (Fig. 10.3). Blood flow then increases slightly because the venous system's cross-sectional area becomes less than that of the capillary system. The lower body's smaller veins eventually empty into the largest vein, the **inferior vena cava**, which travels through the abdominal and thoracic cavities toward the heart. Venous blood draining the head, neck, and shoulder regions empties into the **superior vena cava** and moves downward to join the inferior vena cava at heart level. The mixture of blood from the upper and lower body, called **mixed-venous blood**, then enters the **right atrium** and descends into the **right ventricle** for delivery through the pulmonary artery to the lungs. Gas exchange takes place in the lungs' alveolar-capillary network, where pulmonary veins return oxygenated blood to the left heart pump, and the journey through the body resumes.

Venous Return

A unique characteristic of veins solves a potential problem related to venous bloods' low pressure. Figure 10.4 shows that thin, membranous, flaplike valves spaced at short intervals within veins permit one-way blood flow back to the heart. With low venous blood pressure, veins compress from muscular contractions or minor pressure changes within the chest cavity during breathing. Alternate venous compression and relaxation, combined with one-way valve action, provide a "milking" effect similar to the heart's action. Whereas venous compression imparts considerable energy for blood flow, "diastole" or relaxation allows these vessels to refill as blood moves toward the heart. Without valves, blood would stagnate or congregate as it sometimes does in extremity veins. With pooling of blood and little way to make the blood proceed upward toward the heart, a person would faint every time they stood up because of severely diminished blood reaching the brain.

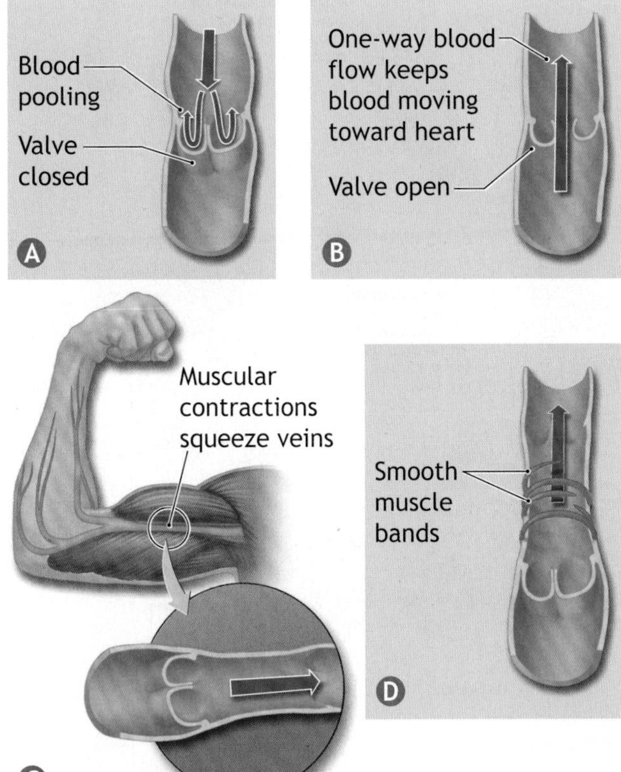

FIGURE 10.4 The valves in veins **(A)** prevent the backflow of blood, but **(B)** do not hinder the normal one-way flow of blood. **C.** Blood moves through veins by the action of nearby active muscle (muscle pump) or **(D)** contraction of smooth muscle bands within the veins. (Reprinted with permission from McArdle WD, Katch FI, Katch VL. *Exercise Physiology: Nutrition, Energy, and Human Performance*. 8th Ed. Baltimore: Wolters Kluwer Health, 2015.)

Mechanical Compression

In sedentary older individuals, and individuals with compromised cardiovascular function who drive long distances or take frequent airline flights, wearing full-length leg "support" compression stockings compresses the vessels to minimize blood pooling and also to prevent blood clot formation. During surgical operations and for three to four days into recovery, mechanical pneumatic cuffs worn around the lower limbs alternately compress and relax lower limb musculature to mechanically provide the "milking" action and to prevent blood pooling and chances of blood clot or deep vein thrombosis (DVT) in those limbs.

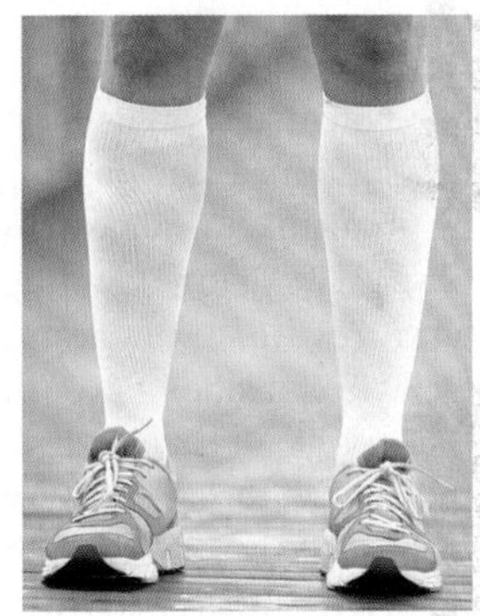

A Significant Blood Reservoir

Veins do not merely function as passive conduits. At rest, the venous system normally contains about 65% of total blood volume; hence, veins serve as capacitance vessels or blood reservoirs. A slight increase in tension or tone by the veins' smooth muscle layer alters venous tree diameter. A generalized increase in **venous tone** rapidly redistributes blood from peripheral veins toward the central blood volume returning to the heart. *In this manner, the venous system serves as an active blood reservoir to either retard or enhance blood flow to the systemic circulation.*

Venous Pooling

The fact that people faint when forced to maintain an upright posture without movement (e.g., standing at attention for a prolonged period as in graduation ceremonies) demonstrates the importance of a contracting muscle to augment venous return. Changing from a horizontal to a vertical (standing) position also affects the dynamics of venous return and triggers predictable physiologic responses. If a person suddenly rises and remains erect without movement, an uninterrupted column of blood exists from heart level to the toes, creating a hydrostatic force of 80 to 100 mm Hg. Swelling (edema) occurs from blood stagnating in the lower extremities and creates "back pressure" that forces fluid from the capillary bed into surrounding tissues. Concurrently, impaired venous

The Physiology of Crucifixion

In ancient Rome, suspending people from a patibulum (crossbar) with rope or with nails that punctured the ends of the extremities to keep the body on the stipes (upright post) was the ultimate punishment. Death occurred mainly from blood pooling in the lower extremities, called *hypovolemic shock*, with accompanying pulmonary edema that resulted in asphyxia, not by excruciating physical torture as often assumed.

return decreases blood pressure; at the same time, heart rate accelerates and venous tone increases to counter the hypotensive condition. Maintaining an upright position without movement can lead to dizziness and eventual fainting from insufficient cerebral blood supply. Resuming a horizontal or head-down position restores circulation and consciousness.

Active Cool-Down

The potential for venous pooling justifies continued slow jogging or walking immediately following strenuous physical activity. **"Cooling down"** with rhythmic physical activity facilitates blood flow through the vascular circuit, including the heart, during recovery. An "active recovery" of light-to-moderate physical activity also speeds the blood's removal of lactate (see Chapter 6). The pressurized suits worn by test pilots retard hydrostatic blood shifts to lower extremity veins when in the upright position. A similar supportive effect occurs in upright activity in a swimming pool because the water's external support facilitates venous return.

BLOOD PRESSURE

With each left ventricular contraction, a surge of blood enters the aorta, distending the vessel and creating pressure within it. The aortic wall's stretch and subsequent recoil propagates as a wave through the entire arterial system. The pressure wave readily appears as a pulse in the following areas: superficial radial artery on the thumb side of the wrist, temporal artery on the side of the head at the temple, and carotid artery adjacent to the trachea. In healthy persons, pulse rate equals heart rate.

Determinants of Blood Pressure and Total Peripheral Resistance

Arterial blood pressure relates to arterial blood flow per minute (**cardiac output**) and peripheral vascular resistance to blood flow in the following relationships:

Blood pressure = Cardiac output × Total peripheral resistance

Rearranging terms:

Total peripheral resistance = Blood pressure ÷ Cardiac output

A CLOSER LOOK

Understanding Hypertension: Effect on Bodily Systems

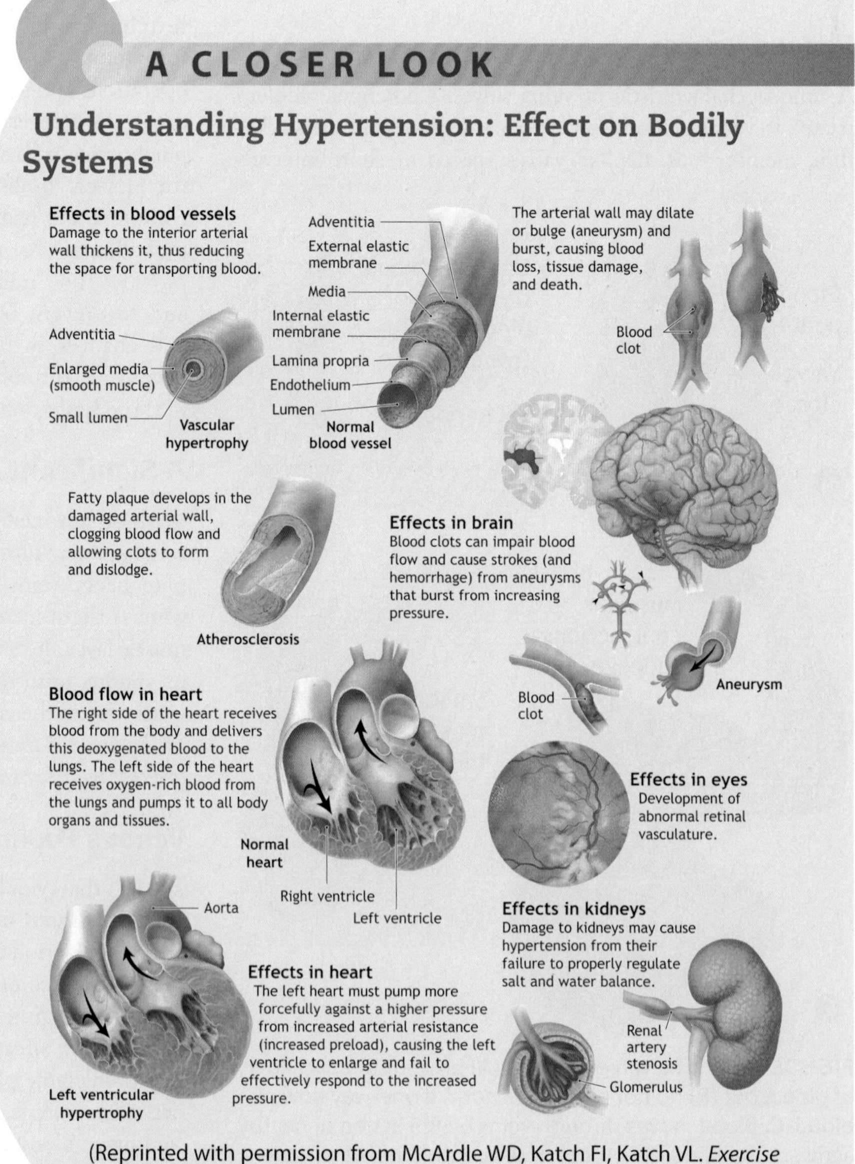

Effects in blood vessels
Damage to the interior arterial wall thickens it, thus reducing the space for transporting blood.
Adventitia
External elastic membrane
Media
Internal elastic membrane
Lamina propria
Endothelium
Lumen
Normal blood vessel
Adventitia
Enlarged media (smooth muscle)
Small lumen
Vascular hypertrophy
The arterial wall may dilate or bulge (aneurysm) and burst, causing blood loss, tissue damage, and death.
Blood clot
Fatty plaque develops in the damaged arterial wall, clogging blood flow and allowing clots to form and dislodge.
Atherosclerosis
Effects in brain
Blood clots can impair blood flow and cause strokes (and hemorrhage) from aneurysms that burst from increasing pressure.
Blood clot
Aneurysm
Blood flow in heart
The right side of the heart receives blood from the body and delivers this deoxygenated blood to the lungs. The left side of the heart receives oxygen-rich blood from the lungs and pumps it to all body organs and tissues.
Normal heart
Right ventricle
Left ventricle
Aorta
Effects in eyes
Development of abnormal retinal vasculature.
Effects in heart
The left heart must pump more forcefully against a higher pressure from increased arterial resistance (increased preload), causing the left ventricle to enlarge and fail to effectively respond to the increased pressure.
Left ventricular hypertrophy
Effects in kidneys
Damage to kidneys may cause hypertension from their failure to properly regulate salt and water balance.
Renal artery stenosis
Glomerulus

(Reprinted with permission from McArdle WD, Katch FI, Katch VL. *Exercise Physiology: Nutrition, Energy, and Human Performance*. 8th ed. Baltimore: Wolters Kluwer Health, 2015.)

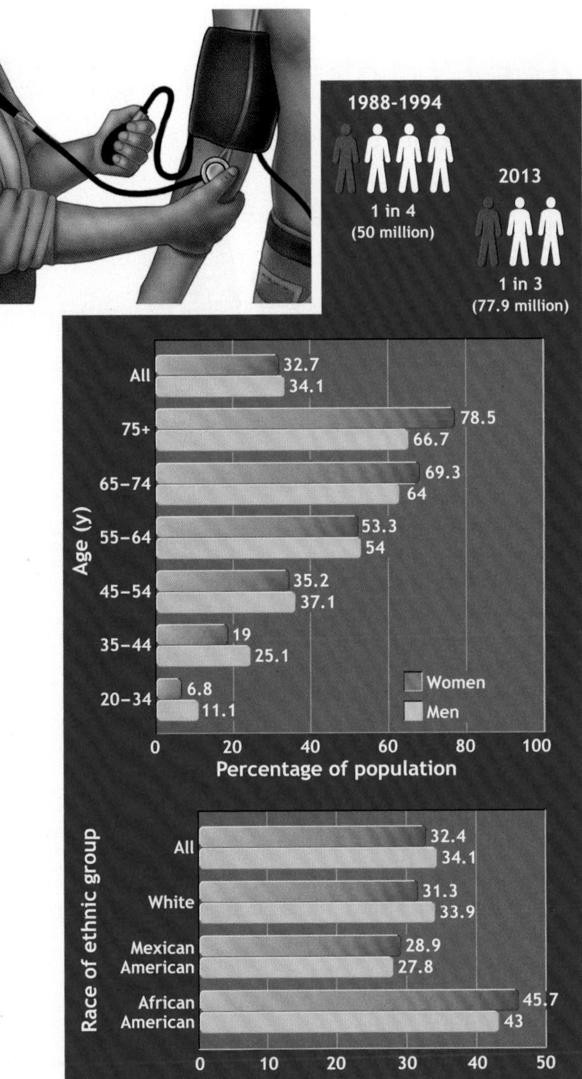

FIGURE 10.5 **(Top)** Prevalence of hypertension in adults in the United States by age and gender. Blood pressure levels vary by age, and women are about as likely as men to develop hypertension during their lifetimes. For people under age 45, hypertension affects more males than females; after age 65 or older, hypertension affects more women than men. **(Bottom)** Prevalence of hypertension in adults in the United States by race and ethnicity. Blacks develop hypertension more often, and at an earlier age, than whites and Hispanics. More black women than men have hypertension. (Adapted with permission from McArdle WD, Katch FI, Katch VL. *Exercise Physiology: Nutrition, Energy, and Human Performance*. 8th Ed. Baltimore: Wolters Kluwer Health, 2015; updated data from Centers for Disease Control and Prevention (CDC); National Center for Health Statistics (NCHS) High Blood Pressure: **http://www.cdc.gov/bloodpressure/facts.htm**; Mozzafarian D, et al. Heart Disease and Stroke Statistics—2015 Update: a report from the American Heart Association. *Circulation*. 2015;e29-322; and James PA, et al. Evidence-Based Guideline for the Management of High Blood Pressure in Adults: Report From the Panel Members Appointed to the Eighth Joint National Committee (JNC 8) Special Communication. *JAMA* 2014;311(5):507. doi:10.1001/jama.2013.284427.)

See the animation "Hypertension" on **http://thePoint.lww.com/MKKESS5e** for a demonstration of this process.

Figure 10.5 shows the percentages of the United States population with hypertension, where systolic pressure exceeds 140 mm Hg and diastolic pressure exceeds 90 mm Hg

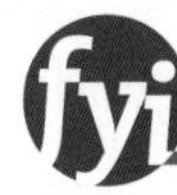

Lifestyle Choices That Lower Blood Pressure

Advice	Details	Decrease in Systolic Blood Pressure (mm Hg)
Lose excess weight	For every 20 lb you lose	5–20
Follow the DASH[a] diet	Consume a lower fat diet rich in vegetables, fruits, and low-fat dairy foods	8–14
Exercise daily	Do 30 minutes of daily aerobic activity (e.g., brisk walking)	4–9
Limit sodium	Consume no more than 2400 mg a day (1500 mg is better)	2–8
Limit alcohol	Consume no more than 2 drinks a day for men or 1 drink daily for women (*1 drink = 12 oz beer, 5 oz wine, or 1.5 oz 80-proof liquor*)	2–4

[a]DASH, Dietary Approaches to Stop Hypertension; **www.nhlbi.nih.gov/health/public/heart/hbp/dash/new_dash.pdf**.

Source: The Seventh Report of the Joint National Committee on Prevention, Detection, Evaluation, and Treatment of High Blood Pressure (**www.nhlbi.nih.gov/guidelines/hypertension**).

for individuals less than 60 years of age and 150 mm Hg systolic; 90 mm Hg diastolic for those over age 60. The Centers for Disease Control and prevention estimated that as of 2015 about 70 million American adults (29%) have high blood pressure—1 of every 3 adults! Fifty-two percent of people with hypertension have their condition under control. The risk of becoming hypertensive increases with age, with the lifetime risk exceeding 80%. Hypertension costs the US over $46 billion each year in health-care services, medications to treat hypertension, and missed days of work.

Blood Pressure at Rest

The highest pressure generated by left ventricular contraction or **systole** to move blood through a healthy, resilient arterial system at rest usually reaches 120 mm Hg. As the heart relaxes in **diastole** and the aortic valves snap shut, the aorta and other arteries' natural elastic recoil provides a continuous pressure head to move blood into the periphery until the next surge from ventricular systole. During the cardiac cycle's diastole, arterial blood pressure decreases to 70 to 80 mm Hg. Arteries "hardened" by mineral and fatty deposits within their walls, or arteries with excessive peripheral resistance to blood flow from kidney malfunction, can induce systolic pressures in excess of 300 mm Hg and diastolic pressures above 120 mm Hg.

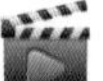

See the animation "Cardiac Cycle" on **http://thePoint.lww.com/MKKESS5e** for a demonstration of this process.

High blood pressure or **hypertension** imposes a chronic strain on normal cardiovascular function. If left untreated, severe hypertension leads to heart failure as the heart muscle weakens and becomes unable to maintain its normal pumping ability. Degenerating, brittle vessels can obstruct blood flow or can burst in a hypertensive state, shutting off vital blood flow to brain tissue to precipitate a stroke.

A CLOSER LOOK

How to Measure Blood Pressure

Blood pressure represents the force exerted by blood against the arterial walls during a cardiac cycle. Systolic blood pressure (SBP), the higher of the two pressure measurements, occurs during ventricular contraction (systole) as the heart propels 70 to 100 mL of blood into the aorta. Following systole, the ventricles relax (diastole), the arteries recoil, and arterial pressure continually declines as blood flows into the periphery and the heart refills with blood. The lowest pressure attained during ventricular relaxation represents diastolic blood pressure (DPB). Pulse pressure refers to the difference between systolic and diastolic pressures. SBP in a typical adult varies between 110 and 140 mm Hg; DBP varies between 60 and 90 mm Hg, with slightly lower values among females.

Elevated systolic or diastolic blood pressure (termed hypertension) refers to a resting SBP above 140 mm Hg and DBP exceeding 90 mm Hg. Blood pressure readings that fall in the prehypertension range should be treated with lifestyle changes that include reducing excess weight, exercising more, quitting smoking, cutting back on salt, having no more than one or two alcoholic drinks daily, and eating more fruits, vegetables, and low-fat dairy products.

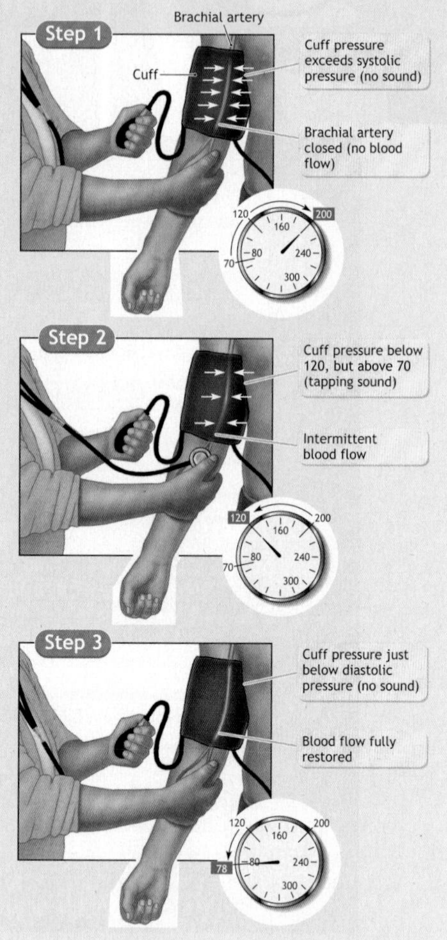

Blood Pressure Measurement Procedures

Different measurement procedures to record blood pressure are used, depending on the situation. It is common in hospitals to use automated blood pressure devices for convenience, speed, and consistency of measurement. Most, but not all devices, have been subjected to scientifically credible validity studies. The auscultation method (listening to sounds; first described in 1902 by Russian vascular surgeon Nikolai S. Korotkoff, 1874–1920; see, for example,

Blood Pressure During Physical Activity

Rhythmic Steady-Rate Activity

During rhythmic brisk walking, hiking, jogging, swimming, and bicycling, dilation of the active muscles' blood vessels increases the vascular area for blood flow. The alternate, rhythmic contraction and relaxation of skeletal muscles force blood through the vessels and returns it to the heart. In the first few minutes during moderate activity, increased blood flow raises the systolic pressure, which then levels off usually between 140 and 160 mm Hg. Diastolic pressure remains relatively unchanged.

http://circ.ahajournals.org/content/94/2!116.full) is considered the gold standard for measuring blood pressure. This technique makes use of a stethoscope and a sphygmomanometer, that consists of a blood pressure cuff and either an aneroid or a mercury column pressure gauge. A typical measurement sequence occurs as follows:

1. Seat the subject in a quiet room and have the subject expose the upper right arm.
2. Locate the brachial artery at the inner side of the subject's upper arm, approximately 1 inch above the bend in the elbow.
3. Take the free end of the cuff, gently slide it through the metal loop (or wrap over exposed Velcro) and flap it back over so the cuff wraps around the upper arm at heart level. Align the arrows on the cuff with the brachial artery. Secure the Velcro parts of the cuff. To obtain accurate readings, fit the sphygmomanometer cuff snugly (but not tightly). Use appropriate-sized cuffs for children and obese persons.
4. Place the stethoscope bell below the antecubital space over the brachial artery.
5. Confirm that the connecting tube from the sphygmomanometer bulb and gauge exits the cuff toward the arm.
6. Before inflating the cuff, ensure that the air release switch remains closed (turn the knob clockwise).
7. Inflate the cuff with quick, even pumps to 180 to 200 mm Hg, as observed on the manometer.
8. Gradually release cuff pressure (about 3 to 5 mm per s) by slowly opening the air release knob (counterclockwise turn) and note the pressure when you hear the first sound. Turbulence from the sudden rush of blood produces the sound as the formerly closed artery briefly opens during the highest pressure in the cardiac cycle. The first appearance of sound represents SBP.

Reference

Sims AJ, et al. Automated non-invasive blood pressure devices: are they suitable for use? *Blood Press Monit* 2005;10(5):275.

Figure 10.6 reveals the general pattern for systolic and diastolic blood pressures during continuous, graded treadmill activity. After an initial rapid increase from the resting level, SBP increases linearly with effort intensity, and DBP remains stable or decreases slightly at the higher physical activity levels. Healthy, sedentary, and endurance-trained subjects demonstrate similar blood pressure responses. During maximum exertion by healthy, fit men and women, SBP may increase to 200 mm Hg or higher despite reduced total peripheral resistance. This level of arterial blood pressure most likely reflects the heart's large cardiac output during maximal effort in individuals with high aerobic capacity.

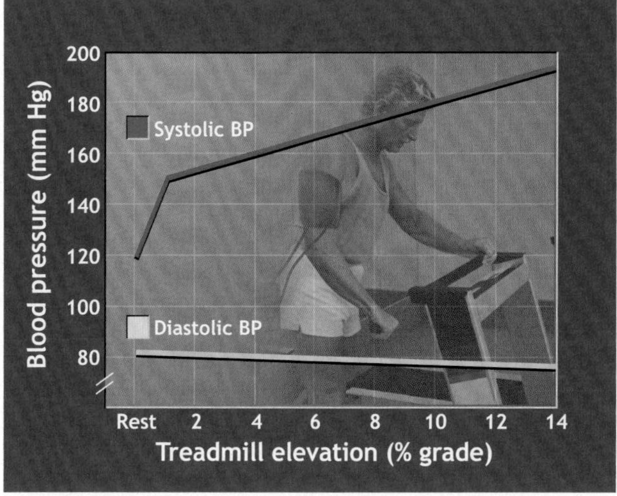

FIGURE 10.6 Generalized response for systolic and diastolic blood pressures during continuous, graded treadmill exercise up to maximum. (Reprinted with permission from McArdle WD, Katch FI, Katch VL. *Exercise Physiology: Nutrition, Energy, and Human Performance*. 8th Ed. Baltimore: Wolters Kluwer Health, 2015.)

Resistance Exercise

Figure 10.7 contrasts the blood pressure responses during rhythmic aerobic physical activity and intense resistance exercises that engage small and large amounts of muscle mass. Straining-type activity (e.g., heavy resistance physical activity, shoveling wet snow) increases blood pressure dramatically because sustained muscular force compresses peripheral arterioles, considerably increasing the resistance to blood flow. The heart's additional workload from acute elevations in blood

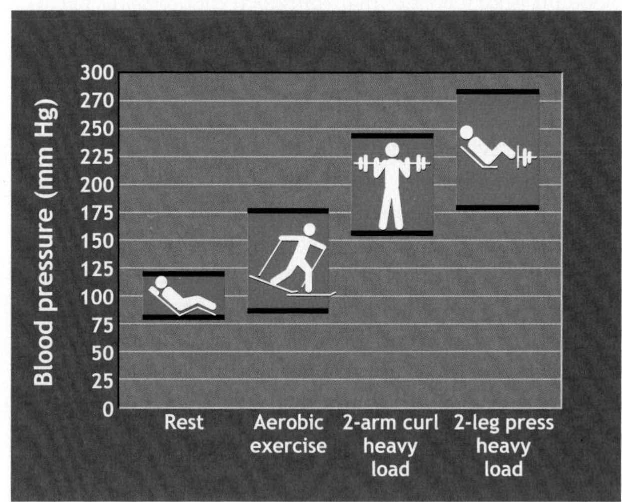

FIGURE 10.7 Heavy-resistance exercise magnifies the exercise blood pressure response (higher with legs than arms) compared with rhythmic, continuous aerobic exercise. The height of the bar indicates pulse pressure. (Reprinted with permission from McArdle WD, Katch FI, Katch VL. *Exercise Physiology: Nutrition, Energy, and Human Performance*. 8th Ed. Baltimore: Wolters Kluwer Health, 2015.)

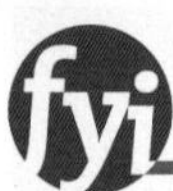

Record Blood Pressure in Both Arms—Maybe?

It may be a good idea to obtain SBP in both arms because a difference in readings acts as an independent heart disease risk factor. About 4400 healthy individuals (56% female) aged 40 and older from the Framingham Heart Study were followed over an average of 13 years. During this period, 598 participants suffered a first heart attack, stroke, or other cardiovascular complication. Of those individuals, more than 25% had a between-arm difference in SBP of 10 mm Hg or greater, a difference that increased the risk of a cardiac event by nearly 40%. The increased risk was independent of age, cholesterol level, body mass index, hypertension, or other known cardiovascular risk factors. Studies have linked subclavian artery stenosis, which supplies blood to the upper arm, to the differences in interarm blood pressure. In this regard, a systolic interarm blood pressure difference that exceeds 15 mm Hg may serve as an upper limit cutoff to indicate significant valvular disease risk and subsequent death.

Sources: Clark CE, et al. Association of a difference in systolic blood pressure between arms with vascular disease and mortality: a systematic review and meta-analysis. *Lancet* 2012;379:905.

Weinberg I, et al. The systolic blood pressure difference between arms and cardiovascular disease in the *Framingham Heart Study*. *Am J Med* 2014;127:209.

pressure increases the risk for individuals with existing hypertension or coronary heart disease. In such cases, rhythmic forms of moderate physical activity provide less risk and more positive health outcomes. On a more optimistic note, those who regularly engage in resistance training show less dramatic blood pressure increases than untrained counterparts, particularly when each exerts the same absolute muscle force.

Upper-Body Activity

Physical activity at a given percentage of $\dot{V}O_{2max}$ increases systolic and diastolic blood pressures substantially more in rhythmic arm (upper body) compared with rhythmic leg (lower body) physical activity. The smaller arm muscle mass and vasculature offer greater resistance to blood flow than the larger and more vascularized lower-body regions. This means that blood flow to the arms during activity requires a much larger systolic pressure head and accompanying increase in myocardial workload and vascular strain. For individuals with cardiovascular dysfunction, more prudent activity involves larger muscle groups, as in walking, running, bicycling, and stair climbing, rather than unregulated activities of a limited muscle mass in shoveling, overhead hammering, or even arm-crank ergometry.

Blood Pressure During Recovery

Following a bout of sustained light- to moderate-intensity physical activity, SBP temporarily decreases below pre-exercise levels for up to 12 hours in normal and hypertensive subjects. Blood pooling in the visceral organs and lower limbs during recovery reduces central blood volume, which contributes to lower blood pressure. This **hypotensive recovery response** further supports physical activity as an important nonpharmacologic hypertension therapy—*an effective approach spreads several bouts of moderate physical activity throughout the day.*

MYOCARDIAL BLOOD SUPPLY

Nearly 2000 gallons of blood flow from the heart each day, but none of its oxygen or nutrients pass directly to the myocardium from the heart's chambers. The myocardium maintains its own elaborate circulatory system. **Figure 10.8** illustrates the **coronary circulation** as a visible, crownlike network that arises from the top of the heart.

The openings of the left and right coronary arteries emerge from the aorta just above the semilunar valves where oxygenated blood leaves the left ventricle. The arteries then curl around the heart's surface. The **right coronary artery** supplies predominantly the right atrium and ventricle; the greatest blood volume flows in the **left coronary artery** to the left atrium and ventricle and smaller portion of the right ventricle. These vessels divide to eventually form a dense capillary network within the myocardium. Blood leaves the tissues of the left ventricle through the coronary sinus; blood from the right ventricle exits through the anterior cardiac veins and empties directly into the right atrium.

Myocardial Oxygen Use

The heart muscle's oxygen use remains high relative to its blood flow. At rest, the myocardium extracts 70% to 80% of the oxygen from blood flowing in the coronary vessels. In contrast, most other tissues at rest use only about 25% of the blood's available oxygen. Because near-maximum oxygen extraction occurs in the myocardium at rest, increases in coronary blood flow provide the main way to fulfill physical activity's myocardial oxygen demands. Coronary blood flow increases four to six times above resting levels during vigorous physical activity from elevated myocardial metabolism and increased aortic pressure.

Profuse myocardial vascularization supplies each muscle fiber with at least one capillary. Adequate oxygenation becomes so crucial that impairment in coronary blood flow triggers chest discomfort and pain, a condition termed **angina pectoris**. The pain increases during physical activity when myocardial oxygen demand rises considerably with supply remaining limited. A blood clot or **thrombus** lodged in one of the coronary vessels can severely impair normal heart function (**Fig. 10.9**). This form of "heart attack," termed **myocardial infarction**, injures the myocardium. Depending on the severity of the attack, severe and irreversible muscle damage can occur that often ends in death.

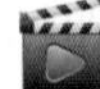

See the animation "Myocardial Blood Flow" on **http://thePoint.lww.com/MKKESS5e** for a demonstration of this process.

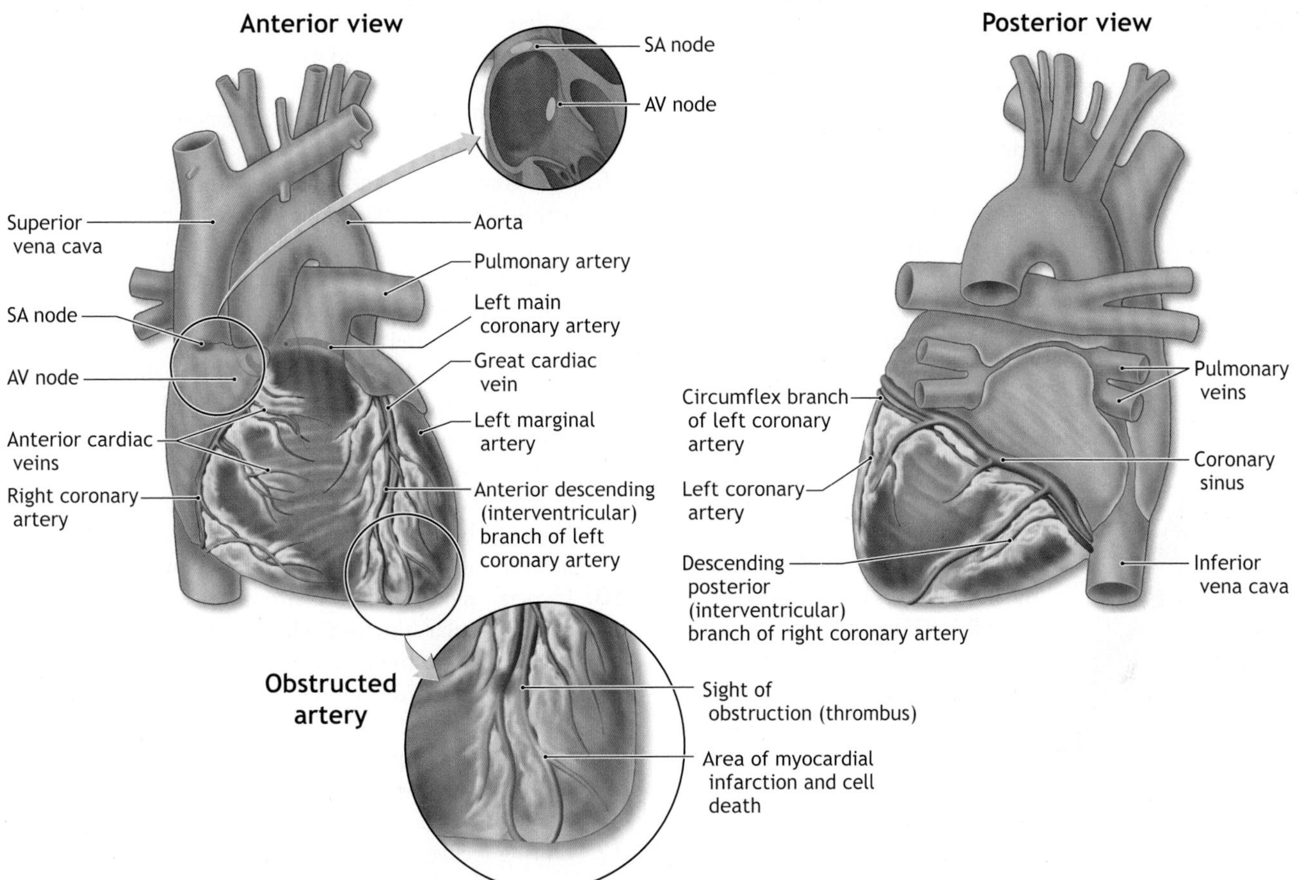

FIGURE 10.8 Anterior and posterior views of the coronary circulation including the SA and AV nodes (*upper inset*). Arteries are shaded *red* and veins *blue*, with the exception of the pulmonary circulation where colors reverse. The *lower inset* illustrates a myocardial infarction from the blockage of a coronary vessel. (Reprinted with permission from McArdle WD, Katch FI, Katch VL. *Exercise Physiology: Nutrition, Energy, and Human Performance*. 8th Ed. Baltimore: Wolters Kluwer Health, 2015.)

Rate Pressure Product: Estimate of Myocardial Work

Three important mechanical factors determine myocardial oxygen uptake:

1. Tension development within the myocardium
2. Myocardial contractility
3. Heart rate

When physical activity increases each of these three factors, myocardial blood flow adjusts to balance oxygen supply with demand. The product of SBP (measured at the brachial artery) and heart rate (HR) provides a convenient estimate of myocardial workload or its oxygen uptake. This index of *relative* cardiac work, called the double product or **rate pressure product (RPP)**, closely reflects directly measured myocardial oxygen uptake and coronary blood flow in healthy subjects over a range of intensities. RPP computes as:

$$\mathbf{RPP = SBP \times HR}$$

Studies of people with coronary heart disease link RPP to the onset of angina or electrocardiographic (ECG) abnormalities. RPP also has assessed various clinical, surgical, and physical activity interventions for their effects on cardiac performance. Reductions in heart rate and SBP at a specific level of submaximal effort with endurance training improve cardiac patients' physical activity capacity before angina onset from reduced myocardial oxygen requirement. In addition, aerobic training increases RPP of patients before they experience onset of heart disease symptoms. In nine patients followed over 7 years of training, RPP increased 11.5% before ischemic abnormalities appeared. These important findings provide indirect evidence for training-induced improvements in myocardial oxygenation, perhaps from greater coronary vascularization, reduced obstruction, or a combination of both factors. Typical values for RPP range from 6000 at rest (HR, 50 b · min^{-1}; SBP, 120 mm Hg) to 40,000 during intense activity (HR, 200 b · min^{-1}; SBP, 200 mm Hg). Changes in heart rate and blood pressure contribute equally to RPP changes.

The Heart's Energy Supply

The myocardium relies almost exclusively on energy released from aerobic reactions; not surprisingly, myocardial tissue has a threefold higher oxidative capacity than skeletal muscle. Of all body tissues, myocardial muscle fibers contain the greatest mitochondrial concentration. They have exceptional capacity for long-chain fatty acid catabolism as a primary way to resynthesize adenosine triphosphate (ATP).

Glucose, fatty acids, and lactate formed from glycolysis in skeletal muscle all provide energy for myocardial functioning. At rest, these three substrates contribute to ATP resynthesis, with the majority of energy (60% to 70%) coming from free fatty acid breakdown. Following a meal, glucose becomes the heart's preferred energy substrate. In essence, the heart uses for energy whatever substrate it "sees" on a physiologic level.

During intense physical activity, the heart derives its major energy by oxidizing circulating lactate when lactate efflux from active skeletal muscle into the blood increases dramatically. In more moderate activity, equal amounts of fat and carbohydrate provide the energy fuel. In prolonged submaximal effort, myocardial metabolism of free fatty acids increases to almost 80% of the total energy requirement. Trained and untrained individuals have similar patterns of myocardial metabolism. An endurance-trained person in submaximal activity demonstrates considerably greater myocardial reliance on fat catabolism. This difference, similar to the effect for skeletal muscle, illustrates the "carbohydrate-sparing effect" of aerobic training.

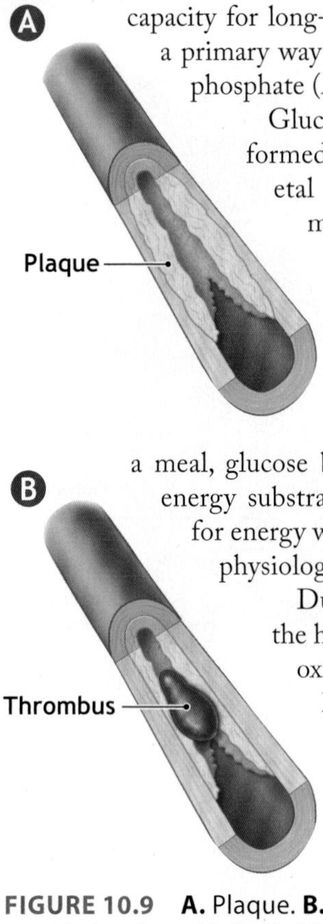

A

Plaque

B

Thrombus

FIGURE 10.9 **A.** Plaque. **B.** Thrombus. (Reprinted with permission from McArdle WD, Katch FI, Katch VL. *Exercise Physiology: Nutrition, Energy, and Human Performance*. 8th Ed. Baltimore: Wolters Kluwer Health, 2015; as adapted with permission from Moore KL, Dalley AF, Agur AMR. *Clinically Oriented Anatomy*. 7th Ed., as adapted with permission from Willis MC. *Medical Terminology: The Language of Health Care*. Baltimore: Lippincott Williams & Wilkins, 1995.)

SUMMARY

1. The heart functions as two separate pumps: one pump receives blood from the body and pumps it to the lungs for aeration (pulmonary circulation) and the other pump accepts oxygenated blood from the lungs and pumps it throughout the body (systemic circulation).
2. Pressure changes during the cardiac cycle act on the heart's valves to provide one-way blood flow through the vascular circuit.
3. A dense capillary network provides a large, effective surface for nutrient and molecular exchange between blood and tissues.
4. Capillaries adjust blood flow in response to a tissue's metabolic activity.
5. Vein compression and relaxation through muscle actions impart considerable energy for venous return.
6. "Muscle pump" action justifies use of active recovery from vigorous physical activity.
7. Nerves and hormones constrict or stiffen the smooth muscle layer in venous walls, as alterations in venous tone profoundly affect total blood volume redistribution.
8. Systolic blood pressure represents the highest pressure generated during the cardiac cycle.
9. Diastolic blood pressure describes the lowest pressure prior to the next ventricular contraction.
10. Hypertension imposes a chronic stress on cardiovascular function, while regular aerobic training modestly reduces systolic and diastolic blood pressures during rest and submaximal physical activity.
11. During graded physical activity, SBP increases in proportion to oxygen uptake and cardiac output, but DBP remains essentially unchanged.
12. During recovery from light–to-moderate physical activity, blood pressure decreases below preactivity levels, called a hypotensive response, and remains lower for up to 12 hours.
13. Peak systolic and diastolic blood pressures mirror the hypertensive state during resistance exercises.
14. Inordinately high blood pressure and RPP during resistance exercise poses a risk to individuals with hypertension and coronary heart disease.
15. Resistance exercise training blunts the hypertensive response to straining-type physical activity.
16. At rest, the myocardium extracts about 80% of the oxygen from coronary blood flow.
17. Physical activity's increased myocardial oxygen demands depend on proportionate increases in coronary blood flow.
18. Impaired coronary blood flow causes chest discomfort and pain called angina pectoris, and blockage of a coronary artery or myocardial infarction can irreversibly damage the myocardium and pose an increased health risk.
19. Clinicians use the product of heart rate and SBP (RPP) to estimate relative myocardial workload to study physical activity training effects on cardiac performance in heart disease patients.
20. Glucose, fatty acids, and lactate represent the heart's main substrates for energy metabolism, and their percentage utilization varies with nutritional status and physical activity intensity and duration.

THINK IT THROUGH

1. What advantage does a "closed" circulatory system provide to a physically active individual?
2. The ancient Romans executed individuals by tying their arms and legs to a crossbar mounted in the vertical position. What physiologic outcomes cause death under these circumstances?

PART 2 Cardiovascular Regulation and Integration

At rest in a comfortable environment, the skin receives 250 mL or approximately 5% of the 5 L of blood pumped from the heart each minute. In contrast, when exercising in a hot, humid environment, 20% of total cardiac output flows to the body's surface for heat dissipation. A rapid redistribution or "shunting" of blood occurs to meet metabolic and physiologic requirements with appropriate blood pressure regulation. This tightly regulated adjustment requires a closed circulatory system with both central and local control of pump output and vascular dimensions.

HEART RATE REGULATION

Cardiac muscle possesses intrinsic rhythmicity. Without extrinsic stimuli, the adult heart would beat steadily about 100 times each minute. Within the body, cardiac nerves that directly supply the myocardium and specialized chemical regulators within the blood rapidly adjust heart rate. Extrinsic control of cardiac function causes the heart to speed up in "anticipation" even before physical activity begins. To a large extent, extrinsic regulation can adjust heart rate to as slow as 35 to 40 b · min^{-1} at rest in endurance athletes; during maximum physical effort, the rate can increase to 220 b · min^{-1}.

Intrinsic Regulation

A mass of specialized muscle tissue, the **sinoatrial (SA) node**, lies within the right atrium's posterior wall. The SA node spontaneously depolarizes and repolarizes to provide an "innate" stimulus to the heart. For this reason, the term "**pacemaker**" describes the SA node. **Figure 10.10A** shows the normal route for myocardial impulse transmission.

The Heart's Electrical Impulse

The myocardium's electrical activity creates an electrical field throughout the body. The salty bodily fluids provide an excellent conducting medium, so electrodes placed on the skin's surface detect voltage changes from the sequence of electrical events before and during each cardiac cycle.

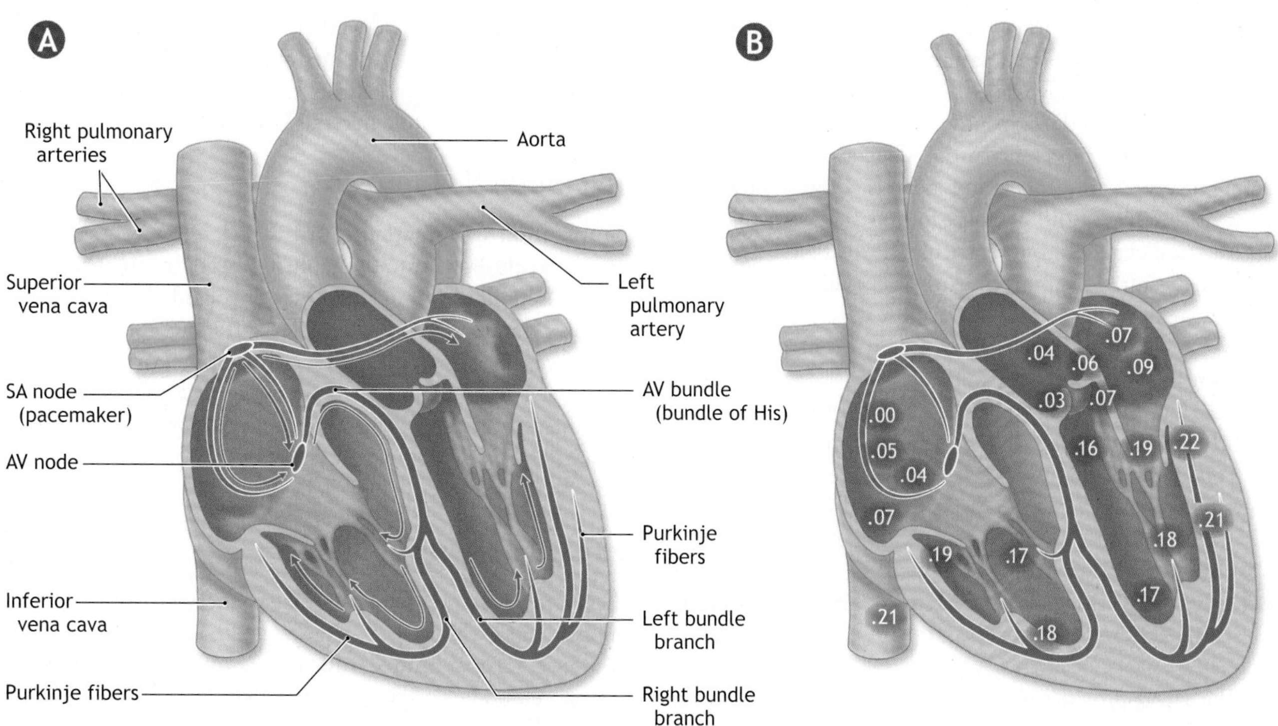

FIGURE 10.10 **A.** The *red arrows* denote the normal route for excitation and conduction of the cardiac impulse. The impulse originates at the SA node, travels to the AV node, and then spreads throughout the ventricular mass. **B.** Time sequence in seconds for electrical impulse transmission from the SA node throughout the myocardium. Walter Gaskell (1847–1914) first demonstrated the specialized muscle fibers joining the atria and ventricles. (Reprinted with permission from McArdle WD, Katch FI, Katch VL. *Exercise Physiology: Nutrition, Energy, and Human Performance*. 8th Ed. Baltimore: Wolters Kluwer Health, 2015.)

Figure 10.10B illustrates the time sequence of electrical impulse propagation from the SA node throughout the myocardium. Rhythms originating at the SA node spread across the atria to the **atrioventricular (AV) node**, another small knot of tissue. This node or impulse barrier delays the impulse about 0.10 seconds to provide sufficient time for the atria to contract and force blood into the ventricles. The AV node gives rise to the AV bundle (called **bundle of His**), which speeds the impulse rapidly through the ventricles over specialized conducting fibers called the **Purkinje system**. Purkinje fibers form distinct branches that penetrate the right and left ventricles. Each ventricular cell becomes stimulated within 0.06 seconds from passage of the impulse into the ventricles; this causes both ventricles to contract simultaneously. Cardiac impulse transmission progresses as follows:

SA node → Atria → AV node →
AV bundle (Purkinje fibers) → Ventricles

See the animation "Cardiac Cycle" on **http://thePoint.lww.com/MKKESS5e** to view this process.

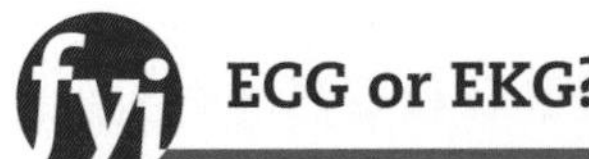

ECG or EKG?

ECG sometimes appears abbreviated as EKG. The "K" comes from the German spelling of the word for *electrocardiograph*. In 1895, Dutch physiologist at Leiden University, Holland, Wilhelm Einthoven (1860–1927), 1924 Noble Prize winner in physiology or medicine for his pioneering work in myocardial electrophysiology, made the first tracings of the heart's electrical activity. He used his invention of a 500-lb string galvanometer consisting of a thin quartz wire in a magnetic field to record the heart's electrical activity. The device had electrodes attached to both hands; the hands and one foot were immersed in a salt water solution.

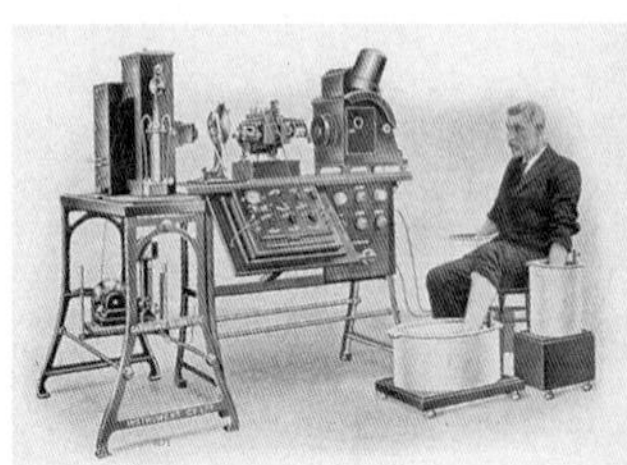

Electrocardiography

The electrical activity generated by the myocardium creates an electrical field throughout the body, which is readily detected at the skin's surface during each cardiac cycle. **Figure 10.11A** outlines the conduction pathway of the electrical impulse as it spreads throughout the myocardium to produce the heart muscle's rhythmic contraction and relaxation. **Figure 10.11B** graphically displays the heart's normal cycle of electrical activity as recorded by an **electrocardiogram (ECG)**. Its important patterns of electrical deflection are referred to as P, QRS, and T waves, including P-R and Q-T intervals and S-T segment.

The P wave represents atrial depolarization. It lasts approximately 0.15 seconds and heralds atrial contraction. The relatively large QRS complex follows the P wave; it signals electrical changes from ventricular depolarization. At this point, the ventricles contract. Atrial repolarization follows the P wave; it produces a small wave usually obscured by the large QRS complex. The T wave represents ventricular repolarization that occurs during ventricular diastole. The heart's relatively long depolarization period of 0.20 to 0.30 seconds prevents initiation of the next myocardial impulse and subsequent contraction. This rest or brief time-out **refractory period** allows sufficient time between beats for ventricular filling.

See the animation "Perform a Basic 12-Lead Electrocardiogram" on **http://thePoint.lww.com/MKKESS5e** for a demonstration of this process.

The ECG provides a way to monitor heart rate during physical activity. Radiotelemetry allows ECG transmission while a person freely performs a variety of physical activities—football, weight lifting, basketball, ice hockey, volleyball, ballroom and disco dancing, mountain climbing, roller derby, motocross, parachuting, cross-country and downhill skiing, gymnastic tumbling, skydiving, and swimming. The ECG can uncover four categories of heart function abnormalities:

1. Cardiac rhythm
2. Electrical conduction
3. Myocardial oxygen supply
4. Myocardial tissue damage

Extrinsic Regulation

Neural impulses override inherent myocardial rhythmicity. The signals originate in the medulla, the cardiovascular regulatory center, and travel through the sympathetic and parasympathetic autonomic nervous system.

Sympathetic Influence

Stimulation of sympathetic cardioaccelerator nerves releases the **catecholamines** epinephrine and norepinephrine. These neural hormones increase myocardial contractility and accelerate SA node depolarization to increase heart rate, a response termed **tachycardia**. Epinephrine, released from the medullary section of the adrenal glands in response to general sympathetic activation, also produces a similar though slower acting effect on overall cardiac function.

Parasympathetic Influence

Acetylcholine, the parasympathetic nervous system hormone, retards the sinus discharge rate to slow the heart. This response, termed **bradycardia**, comes from the **vagus nerve** whose cell bodies originate in the medulla's cardioinhibitory region. Vagal stimulation does not affect myocardial contractility. **Table 10.1** summarizes autonomic nervous system effects on cardiovascular function.

Vascular smooth muscles also contract and relax in response to chemical substances released by endothelium

A

Cardiac Conduction

Repeating electrical impulses travel through the heart to control the heart muscle's rhythmic contraction and dilation.

1. The impulse originates from the sinoatrial (SA) node located in the right atrium and spreads across the atria causing them to contract.
2. The impulse then passes to the atrioventricular (AV) node, travels along the atrioventricular bundle into its' two branches, the right and left crus, and spreads into the ventricles causing them to contract.
3. Dissipation of the impulse causes the atria and ventricles to relax or dilate.

1. Sinoatrial (SA) node
2. Interatrial septum
3. Atrioventricular (AV) node
4. Atrioventricular bundle (bundle of His)
5. Right crus
6. Left crus
7. Interventricular septum
8. Purkinje fibers

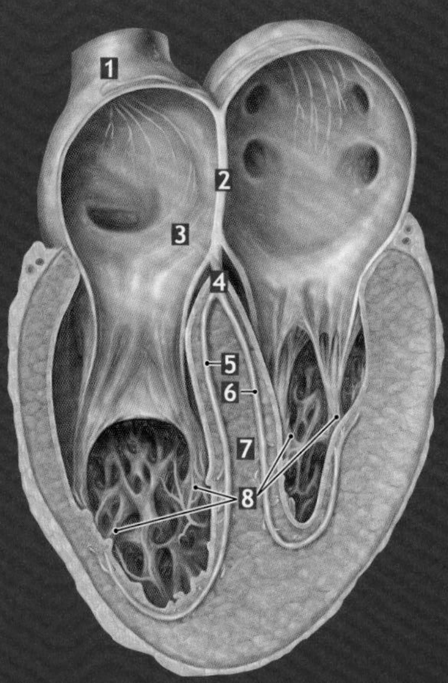

B

Atrial Depolarization (P wave)

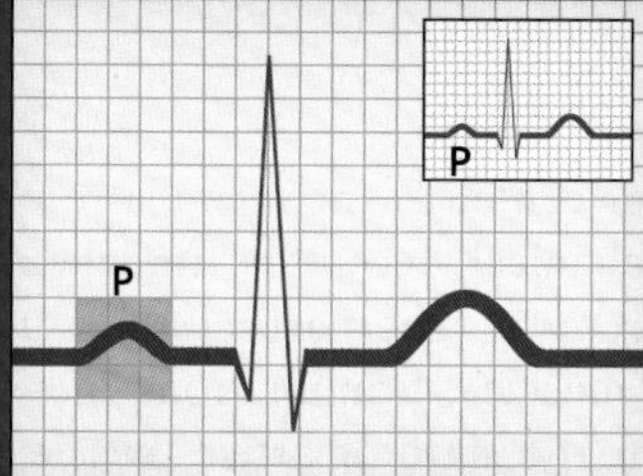

P wave, the first ECG deflection, represents depolarization of both atria.

P-R Interval

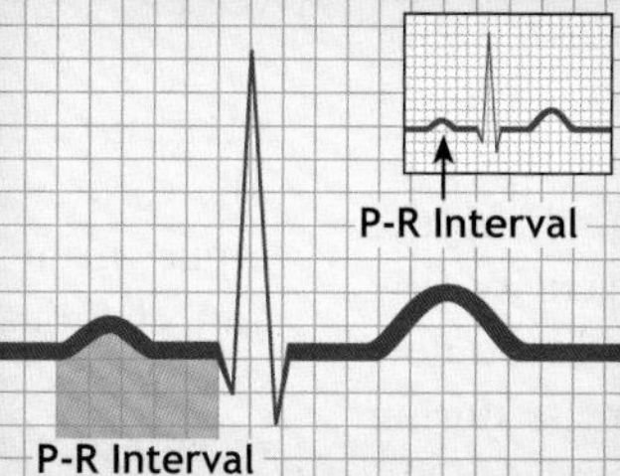

The electrical transmission from atria to ventricles includes the P wave and P-R segment.

Ventricular Depolarization (QRS)

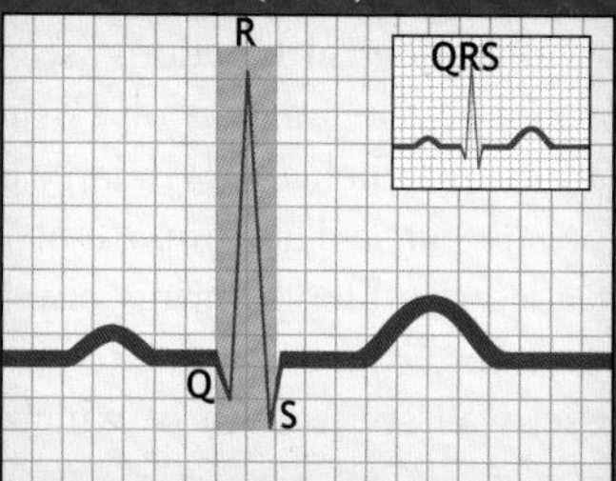

QRS complex indiates ventricular depolarization; R wave indicates the initial positive deflection; Q wave the negative deflection before the R wave; S wave the negative deflection following the R wave.

Ventricular Repolarization (S-T Segment)

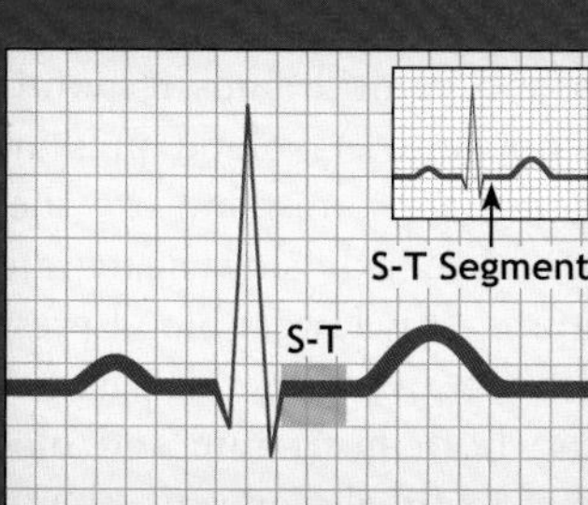

Earlier phase repolarization extends from end of the QRS to start of the T wave. The J (junction) point represents where S-T segment joins the beginning of the T wave.

Ventricular Repolarization (T wave)

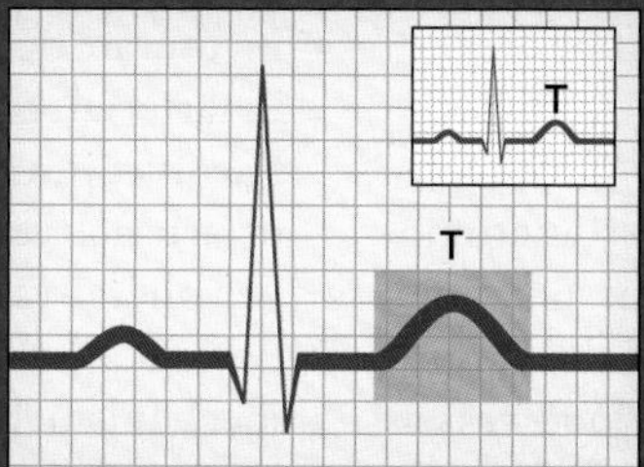

T wave represents repolarization of both ventricles; S-T segment and T wave provide sensitive indicators of the ventricular myocardium's oxygen demand-oxygen supply status.

Ventricular Depolarization and Repolarization (Q-T Interval)

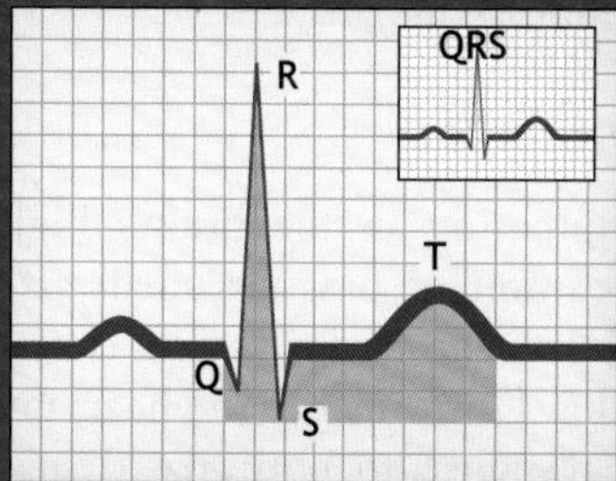

Q-T interval includes the QRS complex, S-T segment, and T wave.

FIGURE 10.11 **A.** Normal transmission of the electrical impulse through the myocardium. **B.** Different phases of the normal ECG from atrial depolarization (*upper left*) to ventricular repolarization (*lower middle*). (Reprinted with permission from McArdle WD, Katch FI, Katch VL. *Exercise Physiology: Nutrition, Energy, and Human Performance*. 8th Ed. Baltimore: Wolters Kluwer Health, 2015; **A**, adapted with permission from Anatomical Chart Company.)

TABLE 10.1 The Autonomic Nervous System and Cardiovascular Function

Sympathetic Influence	Parasympathetic Influence
Increase heart rate	Decrease heart rate
Increase myocardial contraction force	Decrease myocardial contraction force
Dilate coronary blood vessels	Constrict coronary blood vessels
Constrict pulmonary blood vessels	Dilate pulmonary blood vessels
Constrict blood vessels in abdomen, muscle, skin, and kidneys	Dilate blood vessels in abdomen, muscle, skin, and kidneys

tissue consisting of cells from blood vessel's interior lining. Nitric oxide, a biologically reactive molecule with a short half-life, has the chemical formula NO. This important signaling molecule represents the most potent relaxing factor with many physiological functions (see A Closer Look: "Nitric Oxide and Autoregulation of Tissue Blood Flow"). NO released from endothelial cells in large arteries that supply muscle appears particularly important in supplying the muscles with adequate blood during physical activity. The endothelium releases NO in response to pulsatile blood flow and blood vessel wall stress, both of which increase during exertion.

Endurance training creates an imbalance between sympathetic accelerator and parasympathetic depressor activity to favor greater vagal parasympathetic dominance. The effect occurs primarily from increased parasympathetic activity, with some decrease in sympathetic discharge. Training also can depress the SA node's intrinsic firing rate. These adaptations account for the bradycardia frequently observed among highly conditioned endurance athletes and sedentary individuals who undertake aerobic training.

Cortical Influence

Impulses originating in the brain's higher somatomotor **central command** pass via small afferent nerves to directly modulate the cardiovascular center in the ventrolateral medulla. This provides the heart and blood vessels' coordinated response to optimize tissue perfusion and maintain central blood pressure related to motor cortex involvement. *Central command provides the greatest control over heart rate.* It exerts its effect not only during all facets of physical activity but also at rest and during the immediate preactivity period. Thus, variation in one's current emotional state can considerably affect cardiovascular responses, often masking "true" heart rate and blood pressure resting values. Cortical input also causes heart rate to increase rapidly in anticipation of exertion. The combined effects of an increase in sympathetic discharge and reduced vagal tone produce the **anticipatory heart rate**, which becomes apparent just prior to all-out physical effort.

The heart "turns on" for physical activity from three sources:

1. Increased sympathetic activity
2. Decreased parasympathetic activity combined with input from the brain's central command
3. Feedback information from activation of joint and muscle receptors as effort begins

Even for nonsprint events, the heart rate reaches 180 b · min^{-1} within 30 seconds of 1- and 2-mile runs. Further heart rate increases progress gradually, with plateaus attained several times during the runs.

Figure 10.12 depicts major factors that control heart rate and myocardial contractility. The medulla receives continual input about blood pressure from baroreceptors within the carotid arteries and aorta. The medulla also acts as an integrating and coordinating center, receiving stimuli from the cortex and peripheral tissues and directing an appropriate response to the heart and blood vessels.

Peripheral Input

The cardiovascular center in the medulla receives sensory input from mechanical receptors (**mechanoreceptors**) and chemical receptors (**chemoreceptors**) in blood vessels, joints, and muscles. Stimuli from these peripheral receptors monitor the state of active muscle; they modify vagal or sympathetic outflow to create an appropriate cardiovascular response. Reflex neural input from active muscle, termed the **exercise pressor reflex**, in conjunction with output originating in the brain's higher motor areas, assesses the type of movement, its intensity, and quantity of muscle recruited.

During dynamic activity, input from mechanoreceptors provides important feedback for central nervous system blood flow and blood pressure regulation. Receptors in the aortic arch and carotid sinus respond to changes in arterial blood pressure. As blood pressure increases, **baroreceptors** immediately respond to the stretching of arterial vessels, and reflexly slow heart rate and dilate peripheral vasculature. This lowers blood pressure toward normal. Physical activity overrides this particular feedback mechanism because both heart rate and blood pressure increase. Baroreceptors likely prevent abnormally high physical activity blood pressure levels.

Carotid Artery Palpation

For healthy adults and cardiac patients, **carotid artery palpation** has little effect on heart rate during rest, physical activity, and recovery. Exerting strong external pressure against the carotid artery slows heart rate, probably from direct carotid artery baroreceptor stimulation.

Accurate heart rate measurement provides the basis to establish "target heart rates" during physical training (see Chapter 13). If heart rate measurement is consistently

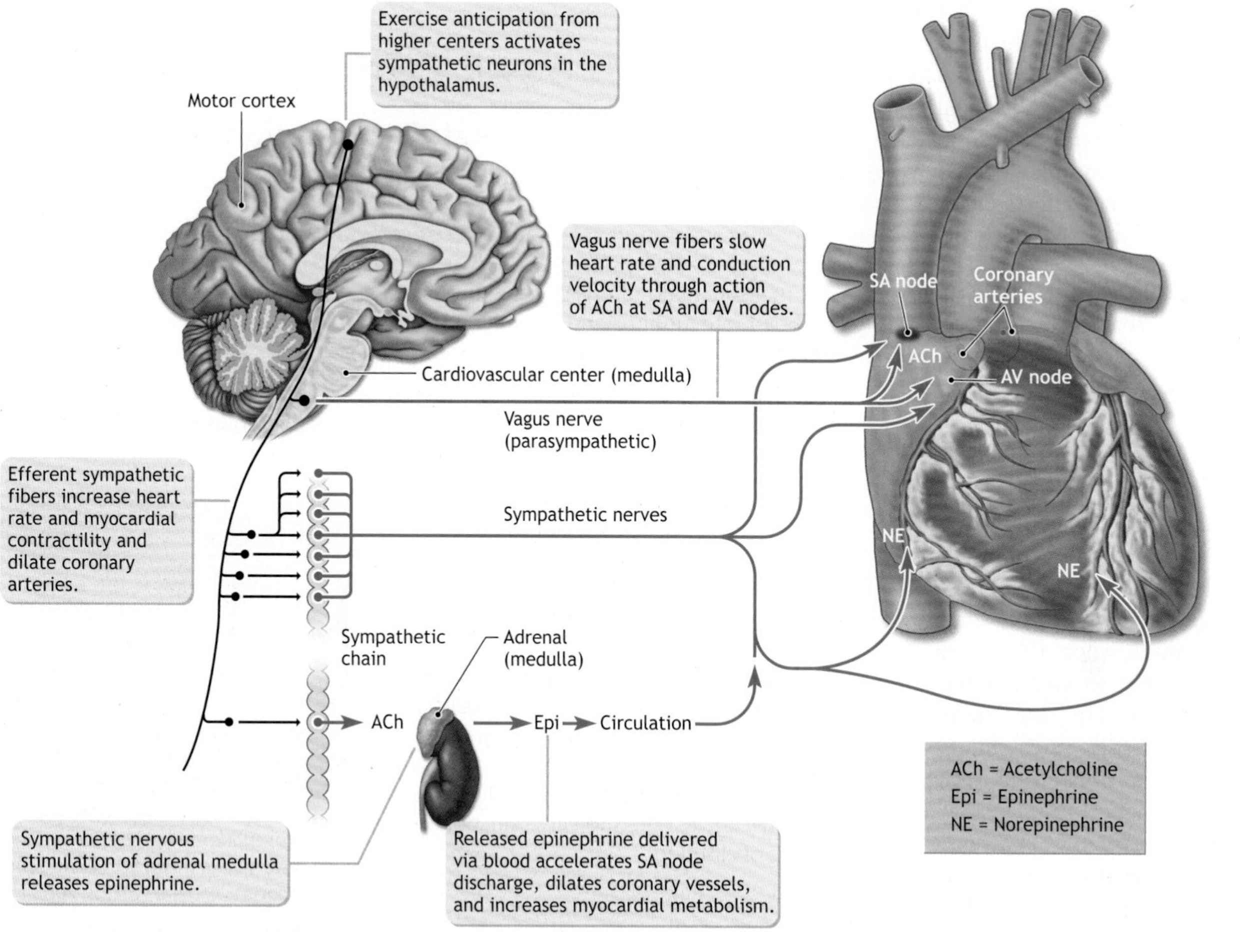

Exercise anticipation from higher centers activates sympathetic neurons in the hypothalamus.
Motor cortex
Vagus nerve fibers slow heart rate and conduction velocity through action of ACh at SA and AV nodes.
SA node
Coronary arteries
ACh
AV node
Cardiovascular center (medulla)
Vagus nerve (parasympathetic)
Efferent sympathetic fibers increase heart rate and myocardial contractility and dilate coronary arteries.
Sympathetic nerves
NE
NE
Sympathetic chain
Adrenal (medulla)
ACh
Epi
Circulation
ACh = Acetylcholine
Epi = Epinephrine
NE = Norepinephrine
Sympathetic nervous stimulation of adrenal medulla releases epinephrine.
Released epinephrine delivered via blood accelerates SA node discharge, dilates coronary vessels, and increases myocardial metabolism.

FIGURE 10.12 Heart rate regulation under normal conditions. Heart transplantation produces cardiac denervation by removing vagal and sympathetic efferent stimulation to the myocardium. Under these conditions, epinephrine from the adrenal medulla provides the primary mechanism to regulate exercise heart rate. (Reprinted with permission from McArdle WD, Katch FI, Katch VL. *Exercise Physiology: Nutrition, Energy, and Human Performance*. 8th Ed. Baltimore: Wolters Kluwer Health, 2015.)

underestimated, a person would exercise at higher levels than prescribed, an undesirable effect when prescribing physical activity for cardiac patients. An excellent substitute method to increase accuracy of this critical measurement involves determining pulse rate at the radial or temporal arteries because palpation at these sites does not alter the heart rate (see A Closer Look: "Assessing Heart Rate by Palpation and Auscultation Methods").

Arrhythmias

Exquisite heart rate regulation by intrinsic and extrinsic mechanisms generally progresses unnoticed for a lifetime and without adverse consequence. ECG and heart rate irregularities do occur and can herald myocardial disease. The term **arrhythmia** describes heart rhythm irregularities.

Heart Rhythm Irregularities

Interruption of regular heart rate pattern often occurs as extra beats or **extrasystoles**. Parts of the atria can become prematurely electrically active and depolarize spontaneously before SA node excitation, a condition called **premature atrial contraction (PAC)**. Premature ventricle excitation (**premature ventricular contraction [PVC]**) also

Automated External Defibrillator

Automated and semiautomated portable defibrillators are now commonplace in airports, subway systems, sports stadiums, hotels, casinos, restaurants, shopping centers, ambulances, fitness centers, and other high traffic public and governmental office buildings (with automated models also available for home use).

Although paramedics, nurses, and hospital medical staff receive formal training with defibrillation techniques, including CPR, all physical activity and fitness specialists need to be CPR certified and recertified yearly. The American Red Cross maintains CPR testing and appropriate certification programs (**www.redcross.org/**; **depts.washington.edu/learncpr/**).

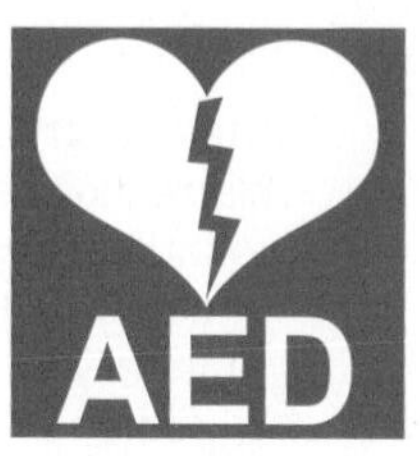

occurs in the interval between two regular beats. Occasional extrasystoles appear during rest and usually progress unnoticed. Psychological stress, anxiety, and caffeine consumption can trigger extrasystoles, probably from catecholamines' effects on the rate of change of the SA node's membrane potential. Removal of such stimuli usually reestablishes normal heart rhythm. If this fails, medication blocking norepinephrine's action on the beta-receptors of atrial cells (**beta-blockers**) effectively treats this condition. Atrial arrhythmias do not compromise the heart's pumping ability because atrial contraction contributes little to ventricular filling. A potentially dangerous situation arises when PACs link successively to create **atrial fibrillation**. In the most serious cardiac arrhythmia, **ventricular fibrillation**, foci of stimulation continually, affect different ventricle parts rather than the normal single stimulus from the AV node. *Portions of the ventricle contract in an uncoordinated manner with repetitive PVCs, thus negating the ventricle's ability to pump blood. Cardiac output and blood pressure decrease, and the person rapidly losses consciousness.*

Resuscitation takes two forms:

1. Reestablish normal heart pumping action to restore blood pressure and blood flow
2. Halt fibrillation and reestablish normal electrical rhythm

Cardiopulmonary resuscitation (CPR) mechanically simulates the heart's pumping action and often reverses fibrillation. If this fails, an automated or semi-automated defibrillator supplies a strong burst of electric current across the entire myocardium (see FYI, Automated External Defibrillator). This depolarizes the heart so the SA node upon repolarization can initiate a normal rhythm.

A CLOSER LOOK

Assessing Heart Rate by Palpation and Auscultation Methods

The cardiac cycle rate (i.e., heart rate) provides a fundamental tool to establish physical activity intensity and assess changes with training. Four methods can measure heart rate: (1) by ear (auscultation), (2) by touch (palpation), (3) with a heart rate monitor, and (4) with an ECG recorder. The auscultation and palpation methods are practical and useful.

Heart Rate by Auscultation

The auscultation method uses a stethoscope to amplify sound waves, thus bringing the ear of the listener closer to the source of the heart sounds.

Using the Stethoscope

1. With the ear tips of the stethoscope pointing forward, insert them directly into each of your ear canals.
2. Gently tap the diaphragm of the stethoscope to verify you can hear the sound.
3. Position the stethoscope just below the subject's left breast at the pectoralis major muscle over the third intercostal space to the left of the sternum.
4. Hold the diaphragm of the stethoscope firmly against the subject's skin, not on top of clothing.

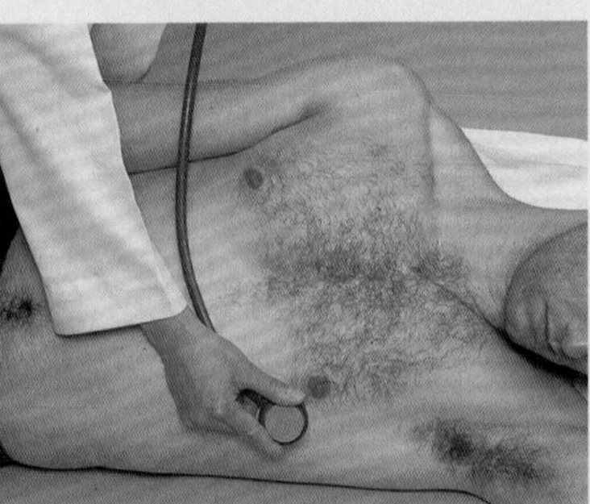

(Reprinted with permission from Bickely LS. *Bate's Guide to Physical Examination and History Taking*. 8th Ed. Philadelphia: Lippincott Williams & Wilkins, 2003.)

Heart Rate by Palpation

1. The pulse wave generated by blood pumping through the arteries is mostly measured with a finger or hand over the radial or carotid arteries.
2. Use the tip of the middle and index fingers; do not use the thumb because it has a pulse of its own.
3. Press lightly to avoid obstructing blood flow.
4. An apical beat (vibration pulse) generated by the left ventricle hitting the chest wall near the left fifth rib becomes prominent immediately following physical activity in lean individuals. To palpate an apical beat, position the entire hand over the left side of the chest at heart level.

Location for the Palpation Method

Four common palpation sites are as follows:

1. Temporal artery: At the temple around the hairline of the head (Figure A)
2. Carotid artery: Just lateral to the larynx (do not apply excessive pressure at this site because it may trigger a reflex that slows the heart rate) (Figure B)
3. Radial artery: Anterolateral aspect of the wrist directly in line with the base of the thumb (Figure C)
4. Brachial artery: Anteromedial aspect of the arm below the belly of the biceps brachii, 2 to 3 cm (1 in) above the antecubital fossa

Counting Heart Rate

Record the heart rate as a rate per minute (e.g., 150 b · min^{-1}). Two common approaches for counting heart rate include the timed heart rate method and the 30-beat heart rate method.

Timed Heart Rate Method

This method counts the number of pulses in a specific duration. Usually, pulse counts are taken for 6, 10, or 15 seconds. If palpating the pulse for 6 seconds, multiply by 10 to express as a per-minute rate; for a 10-second palpation, multiply by 6; and if palpating for 15 seconds, multiply the pulse count by 4. Table 1 presents the heart rate conversion for each of the above 6-, 10-, or 15-second multiplications. The 6-second count produces the least accurate pulse count.

TABLE 1 Heart Rate (in Beats Per Minute; BPM) Conversion. Find the Number of Pulse Counts for 6, 10, or 15 Seconds; Read Across for the BPM

6-s Count	Per Min Rate	10-s Count	Per Min Rate	15-s Count	Per Min Rate
4	40	7	42	10	40
5	50	8	48	11	44
6	60	9	54	12	48
7	70	10	60	13	52
8	80	11	66	14	56
9	90	12	72	15	60
10	100	13	78	16	64
11	110	14	84	17	68
12	120	15	90	18	72
13	130	16	96	19	76
14	140	17	102	20	80
15	150	18	108	21	84
16	160	19	114	22	88
17	170	20	120	23	92
18	180	21	126	24	96
19	190	22	132	25	100
20	200	23	138	26	104
21	210	24	144	27	108
22	220	25	150	28	112
		26	156	29	116
		27	162	30	120
		28	168	31	124
		29	174	32	128
		30	180	33	132
		31	186	34	136
		32	192	35	140
		33	198	36	144
		34	204	37	148
		35	210	38	152
		36	216	39	156
		37	222	40	160
				41	164
				42	168
				43	172
				44	176
				45	180
				46	184
				47	188
				48	192
				49	196
				50	200
				51	204
				52	208
				53	212
				54	216
				55	220

A Carotid

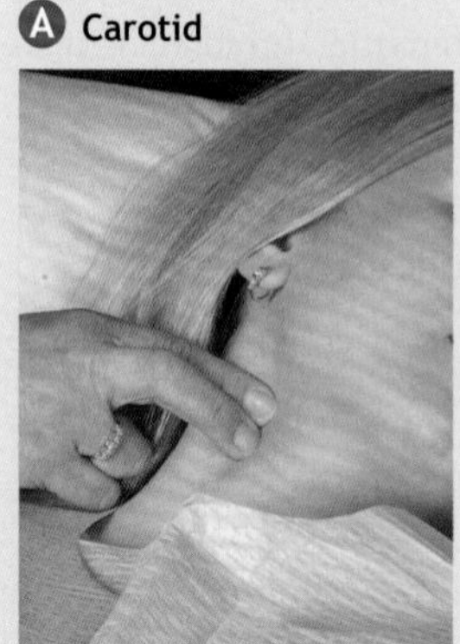

B Brachial

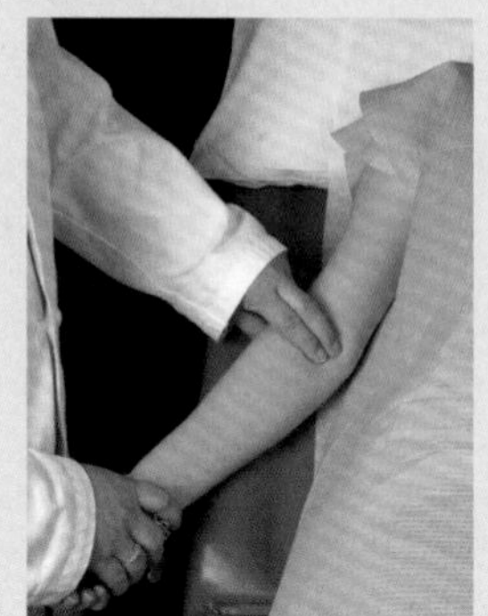

C Radial

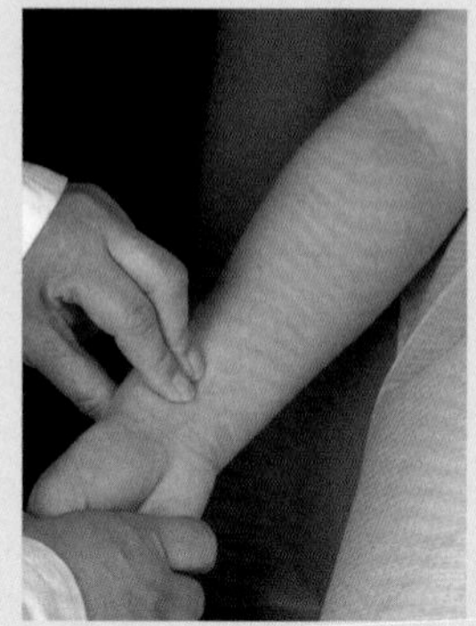

Three typical locations for palpating pulse: (**A**) Carotid, (**B**) brachial, and (**C**) radial arteries.

(*Continues on next page*)

A CLOSER LOOK *(Continued)*

Thirty-Beat Heart Rate Method

This method counts the time in seconds (s) for 30 pulse beats to occur. Count the first beat as "zero" and simultaneously begin to record the time to count 30-pulse beats. The computational formula for computing heart rate in beats per min (bpm) follows:

$$\text{HR (bpm)} = 30\ \text{b} \div \text{Time (s)} \times 60\ \text{s} \div 1\ \text{min}$$

For example, if 30 beats (b) occur in 20 seconds:

$$\begin{aligned}\text{HR (bpm)} &= 30\ \text{b} \div \text{time (s)} \times 60\ \text{s} \div 1\ \text{min}\\ &= 30\ \text{b} \div 20\ \text{s} \times 60\ \text{s} \div 1\ \text{min}\\ &= 1.5 \times 60\\ &= 90\ \text{bpm}\end{aligned}$$

Table 2 presents a conversion chart for the above method, with heart rate rounded to the nearest whole number. Find the time for recording 30 beats and the corresponding heart rate (bpm).

TABLE 2 Conversion Chart for 30-Beat Heart Rate Method

Time for 30 Beats, s	HR, BPM	Time for 30 Beats, s	HR, BPM	Time for 30 Beats, s	HR, BPM
8	225	21	86	34	53
9	200	22	82	35	51
10	180	23	78	36	50
11	164	24	75	37	49
12	150	25	72	38	47
13	138	26	69	39	46
14	129	27	67	40	45
15	120	28	64	41	44
16	113	29	62	42	43
17	106	30	60	43	42
18	100	31	58	44	41
19	95	32	56	45	40
20	90	33	55		

BLOOD DISTRIBUTION

If fully dilated, the body's 60 thousand miles (100,000 km) of blood vessels could hold approximately 20 L of blood, four times more than an average individual's 5 L total blood volume. Thus, maintenance of blood flow and blood pressure, particularly during physical activity, requires a finely regulated balance between vascular dilation and vascular constriction. *The capacity of large portions of the vasculature to constrict or dilate provides rapid blood redistribution to meet metabolic requirements. It also optimizes blood pressure within the vascular circuit.*

Effects of Physical Activity

Increased energy expenditure requires rapid readjustments in blood flow that affect the entire cardiovascular system. For example, nerves and local metabolic conditions act on the smooth muscle bands of arteriole walls, causing them to alter their internal diameter almost instantaneously. Concurrently, neural stimulation of venous capacitance vessels causes them to "stiffen," moving blood from peripheral veins into the central circulation.

During physical activity, the vascular portion of active muscles increases through local arteriole dilatation; at the same time, other vessels constrict to "shut down" blood flow to tissues, which can temporarily compromise blood supply. Kidney function vividly illustrates the body's regulatory capacity for adjusting regional blood flow. Renal circulation at rest normally averages 1100 mL · min^{-1} or about 20% of total cardiac output. In maximal effort, renal blood flow decreases to 250 mL · min^{-1} or only 1% of a 25-L physical activity cardiac output.

See the animation "Renal Function" on **http://thePoint.lww.com/MKKESS5e** for a review of this process.

Blood Flow Regulation

Pressure differentials and resistances determine fluid movement through a vessel. Resistance varies directly with the length of the vessel and inversely with its diameter; greater driving force increases flow, and increased resistance impedes flow. The interaction between pressure, resistance, and fluid flow is expressed as:

$$\text{Flow} = \text{Pressure} \div \text{Resistance}$$

Three factors determine resistance to blood flow:

1. Blood thickness or viscosity
2. Conducting tube length
3. Blood vessel radius

The following equation, referred to as **Poiseuille law**, named after French physician, physicist, and physiologist Jean Leonard Marie Poiseuille (1797 to 1869) expresses the relationship among pressure differential (gradient), resistance, and flow in a cylindrical vessel:

$$\text{Flow} = \text{Pressure gradient} \times \text{Vessel radius}^4 \div \text{Vessel length} \times \text{Fluid viscosity}$$

Blood viscosity and transport vessel length in the body remain relatively constant. Consequently, blood vessel radius represents the most important factor affecting blood flow. Reducing a vessel's radius by half decreases flow by a factor of 16; conversely, doubling the radius increases volume 16-fold. This means that a relatively small degree of vasoconstriction or vasodilation dramatically impacts regional blood flow.

Local Factors

In muscle tissue at rest, one of every 30 to 40 capillaries actually remains open. Thus, the opening of large numbers of "dormant" capillaries with physical activity serves three important functions:

1. Increases muscle blood flow
2. Only a small increase in velocity accompanies an increase in blood flow volume
3. Increases effective surface for gas and nutrient exchange between blood and individual muscle fibers

A decrease in tissue oxygen supply stimulates local vasodilation in skeletal and cardiac muscle. Local increases in temperature, carbon dioxide, acidity, adenosine, nitric oxide (NO), and magnesium (Mg) and potassium (K) ions also enhance regional blood flow. These autoregulatory mechanisms for blood flow make sense physiologically because they reflect elevated tissue metabolism and increased oxygen need. *Rapid, local vasodilation provides the most effective, immediate step to increase a tissue's oxygen supply.*

Neural Factors

Central vascular control via sympathetic and parasympathetic portions of the autonomic nervous system overrides vasoregulation assisted by local factors. For example, muscles contain small sensory nerve fibers highly sensitive to chemical substances released in active muscle during physical activity. Such fiber stimulation provides central nervous system input to dictate appropriate cardiovascular responses. With central regulation, blood flow in one area cannot dominate when a concurrent oxygen need exists in other, more "needy" tissues.

A CLOSER LOOK

Nitric Oxide and Autoregulation of Tissue Blood Flow

Nitric oxide (NO) serves as an important signaling molecule that dilates blood vessels and decreases vascular resistance. This gas is a common, unstable industrial and automotive air pollutant formed when nitrogen burns.

Most living organisms naturally produce this vascular gatekeeper from its precursor L-arginine. Stimuli from diverse signal chemicals increase blood flow. These stimuli include neurotransmitters, sheering stress, and vessel stretch through the vessel lumen which provoke NO synthesis and release by the vascular endothelium. NO was formerly termed *endothelium-derived relaxing factor* by pharmacologist Robert F. Furchgott (1916–2009; 1998 Nobel Prize in Physiology or Medicine corecipient for discovering NO as a signaling molecule in the cardiovascular system along with his colleagues Louis Ignarro and Ferid Murad [**www.nobelprize.org/nobel_prizes/medicine/laureates/1998/furchgott-bio.html**]). NO rapidly spreads through underlying cell membranes to smooth muscle cells within the arterial wall, where it binds with and activates guanylyl cyclase, an enzyme important in cellular communication and signal transduction. This initiates a cascade of reactions that attenuate sympathetic vasoconstriction and induce arterial smooth muscle relaxation to increase blood flow in neighboring blood vessels. NO exerts its potent vasodilator effect on skeletal muscle including the diaphragm, sponge-like vascular tissues, skin, and myocardial tissue (see Figure).

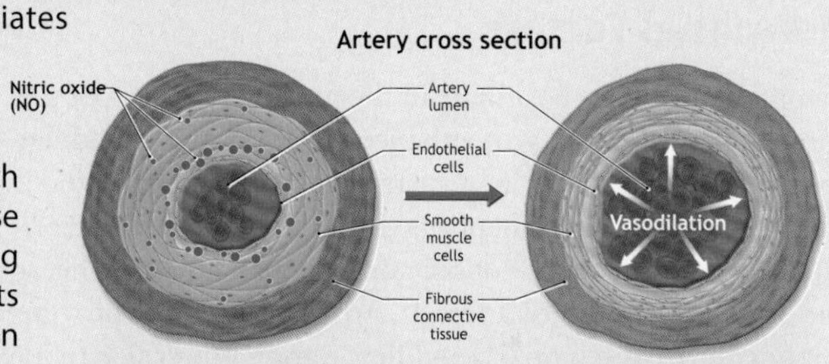

Artery cross section

Role of Nitric Oxide

- Endothelial cells within blood vessels release nitric oxide (NO) gas, which initiates a cascade of events that attenuate sympathetic vasoconstriction and induce arterial smooth muscle relaxation to increase blood flow
- NO is either released by autonomic neurons and synthesized by the vascular endothelium or from drugs like Viagra or nitroglycerin (and related heart drugs), which cause vasodilation by stimulating NO gas release.
- Vasodilation occurs when NO penetrates smooth muscle cells.

Mechanism for how nitric oxide regulates local blood flow. (Reprinted with permission from McArdle WD, Katch FI, Katch VL. *Exercise Physiology: Nutrition, Energy, and Human Performance*. 8th Ed. Baltimore: Wolters Kluwer Health, 2015.)

NO mediates bodily functions as diverse as olfaction, inhibition of blood clot formation, and enhanced immune response regulation, and acts as an interneuron or signaling messenger. It also contributes to cutaneous active vasodilation during heat stress and rapidly dilates the coronary vasculature as an early adaptation to moderate training. Vascular wall receptors for NO contribute to blood pressure regulation in response to central cardiovascular stimulation during emotionally stressful situations including physical activity.

Racial differences in resting blood pressure relate to a lower sensitivity to NO's dilating action in blacks than in whites. In coronary artery disease, the endothelium produces less NO. Reduced NO bioavailability explains the potent beneficial effect of exogenous nitroglycerin treatment (which releases NO gas) to reverse angina pectoris from inadequate oxygen delivery induced by coronary vessel disease.

Sympathetic nerve fibers end in the muscular layers of small arteries, arterioles, and precapillary sphincters. Norepinephrine acts as a general vasoconstrictor released at certain sympathetic nerve endings (**adrenergic fibers**). Other sympathetic neurons in skeletal and heart muscle release acetylcholine, allowing these **cholinergic fibers** to dilate blood vessels. Continual sympathetic constrictor neuron activity maintains a relative state of vasoconstriction termed **vasomotor tone**. Blood vessel dilatation regulated by adrenergic neurons

TABLE 10.2 Summary of Integrated Chemical, Neural, and Hormonal Adjustments Before and During Physical Activity

Condition	Activator	Response
Preactivity "anticipatory" response	Activation of motor cortex and higher areas of brain increases sympathetic outflow and reciprocal inhibition of parasympathetic activity	Heart rate acceleration; increased myocardial contractility; vasodilation in skeletal and heart muscle (cholinergic fibers); vasoconstriction in skin, gut, spleen, liver, and kidneys (adrenergic fibers); arterial blood pressure increase
Activity	Continued sympathetic cholinergic outflow; alterations in local metabolic conditions due to hypoxia (↓pH, ↑P_{CO_2}, ↑ADP, ↑Mg^{2+}, ↑Ca^{2+}, ↑NO, ↑temperature)	Further muscle vasculature dilation
	Continued adrenal medulla sympathetic adrenergic outflow with epinephrine and norepinephrine	Concomitant vasculature constriction in inactive tissues to maintain adequate arterial system perfusion pressure Venous vessels stiffen to reduce their capacity Venoconstriction facilitates venous return to maintain central blood volume

results more from reduced vasomotor tone than increased sympathetic or parasympathetic dilator fiber activity.

Hormonal Factors

Sympathetic nerves terminate in the medullary region of the adrenal glands. Upon sympathetic activation, this glandular tissue releases relatively large quantities of epinephrine and a small amount of norepinephrine into the blood. These hormones cause a general constrictor response *except* in heart and skeletal muscle blood vessels. Adrenal hormones provide minor control of regional blood flow during physical activity compared with local sympathetic neural drive.

INTEGRATIVE RESPONSE DURING PHYSICAL ACTIVITY

Table 10.2 summarizes the integrated chemical, neural, and hormonal adjustments immediately before and during physical activity.

At initiation of physical activity or even slightly before activity begins, nerve centers above the medullary region activate cardiovascular activity. The adjustments increase the heart's rate and pumping strength and alter regional blood flow in direct proportion to exertion level. As activity becomes more intense, sympathetic cholinergic outflow plus local metabolic factors act on chemosensitive nerves to directly dilate active musculature's resistance vessels. Reduced peripheral resistance permits muscle tissue to accommodate greater blood flow. Constrictor adjustments in less active tissues maintain adequate perfusion pressure despite dilatation of the muscle's vasculature. During physical activity, vasoconstriction in the less active kidneys and the gastrointestinal tract also promotes blood redistribution to meet specific tissues' metabolic needs.

Venous Return Important

Factors that affect venous return are as important as those that regulate arterial blood flow. Muscle and ventilatory pump actions, combined with visceral vasoconstriction, return blood to the right ventricle when activity begins and continue to facilitate venous return with further increases in cardiac output. These adjustments balance venous return with cardiac output. In upright physical activity, gravity impedes blood from returning from the extremities, emphasizing the importance of venous blood flow regulation.

SUMMARY

1. The cardiovascular system regulates heart rate and distributes blood while maintaining blood pressure in response to physical activity's increased metabolic and physiologic demands.
2. The cardiac impulse originates at the SA node, where it travels across the atria to the AV node, and then spreads rapidly across the large ventricular mass.
3. With a normal conduction pattern, atria and ventricles contract efficiently to provide the impetus for blood flow.
4. The ECG displays the sequence of myocardial electrical events during a cardiac cycle.
5. The majority of heart rhythm irregularities or arrhythmias involve extra beats or extrasystoles.
6. Atrial arrhythmias generally do not compromise the heart's pumping ability.
7. Ventricular fibrillation, the most serious arrhythmia, results from repetitive, spontaneous ventricular discharge.
8. Epinephrine and norepinephrine accelerate heart rate and increase myocardial contractility.
9. Acetylcholine, a parasympathetic neurotransmitter, slows heart rate via the vagus cranial nerve.
10. Increases in temperature, carbon dioxide, acidity, adenosine, nitrous oxide, and magnesium and potassium ions provide potent stimuli to autoregulate blood flow in active tissues.
11. Nitric oxide (NO), an extraordinarily important and potent endothelium-derived relaxing factor, facilitates blood vessel dilation and decreases vascular resistance.

12. In transition from rest to physical activity, increased sympathetic and decreased parasympathetic activity turns the heart "on."
13. Neural and hormonal extrinsic factors modify the heart's inherent rhythmicity.
14. The heart accelerates rapidly in anticipation of activity; in maximum effort, it can exceed 200 b · min^{-1}.
15. Carotid artery palpation accurately measures heart rate during and immediately following physical activity. However, in certain medical conditions, pressure against the carotid artery reflexly slows the heart, which results in underestimating the heart rate during physical activity.
16. Cortical stimulation immediately before and during the initial stages of physical activity substantially adjusts heart rate response to physical effort.
17. Blood flow regulation occurs when nerves, hormones, and local metabolic factors alter the internal diameter of smooth muscle bands in blood vessels.
18. Adrenergic sympathetic fibers release norepinephrine to induce vasoconstriction.
19. Cholinergic sympathetic neurons secrete acetylcholine and trigger vasodilation.
20. During physical activity, the kidneys and splanchnic regions dramatically compromise their blood flow to augment blood flow to tissues in need.

THINK IT THROUGH

1. Give a physiologic rationale for biofeedback and relaxation techniques to treat hypertension and stress-related disorders.
2. If heart transplantation surgically removes all nerves to the myocardium, explain why heart rate for these patients increases during physical activity.
3. Explain the following statement: Task-specific, regular aerobic physical activity not only trains the cardiovascular system but also "trains" the neuromuscular system to facilitate physiologic adjustments specific to the activity mode.

PART 3 Cardiovascular Dynamics during Physical Activity

CARDIAC OUTPUT

Cardiac output provides the most important indicator of the circulatory system's functional capacity to meet physical activity's demands. As with any pump, the rate of pumping (**heart rate**) and quantity of blood ejected with each stroke (**stroke volume**) determine the heart's output of blood:

$$\textbf{Cardiac output} = \textbf{Heart rate} \times \textbf{Stroke volume}$$

The relationship among cardiac output, oxygen uptake, and difference between the oxygen content of arterial and mixed-venous blood (a-$\bar{v}O_2$ **difference**) embodies the principle discovered in 1870 by German physiologist Adolph Fick (1829–1901).

$$\text{Cardiac output, mL}\cdot\text{min}^{-1} = [\dot{V}O_2, \text{mL}\cdot\text{min}^{-1} \div \text{a-}\bar{v}O_{2\text{diff}}, \text{mL}\cdot\text{dL blood}^{-1}] \times 100$$

See the animations "Blood Flow" and "Fick Principle" on **http://thePoint.lww.com/MKKESS5e** for a demonstration of this process.

RESTING CARDIAC OUTPUT: UNTRAINED VERSUS TRAINED

The left ventricle of an average-sized man ejects his entire 5-L blood volume every minute. This value pertains to most individuals, but stroke volume and heart rate vary considerably depending on cardiovascular fitness status. A heart rate of about 70 b · min^{-1} adequately sustains the average adult's 5-L (5000 mL) resting cardiac output. Substituting this heart rate value in the cardiac output equation (Cardiac output = Stroke volume × Heart rate; Stroke volume = Cardiac output ÷ Heart rate) yields a calculated stroke volume of 71 mL · b^{-1}.

An endurance athlete's resting heart rate averages about 50 b · min^{-1} (although it can be as low as 35 to 40 b · min^{-1}), resting cardiac output averages 5 L · min^{-1} as blood circulates with a proportionately larger stroke volume of 100 mL per beat (5000 mL ÷ 50 b). Stroke volumes for women typically average 25% below values for men with equivalent training. The smaller body size of the average woman chiefly accounts for this apparent gender difference.

Table 10.3 summarizes average values for cardiac output, heart rate, and stroke volume for endurance-trained and untrained men at rest.

The underlying mechanisms remain unclear for the heart rate and stroke volume differences between trained and untrained individuals. The following two factors probably interact as aerobic fitness improves:

1. Increased vagal tone slows the heart, allowing more time for ventricular filling
2. Enlarged ventricular volume and more powerful myocardium eject a larger blood volume with each systole

PHYSICAL ACTIVITY CARDIAC OUTPUT: UNTRAINED VERSUS TRAINED

For both trained and untrained individuals, blood flow from the heart increases in direct proportion to physical activity intensity. From rest to steady-rate activity, cardiac output increases rapidly, followed by a more gradual increase until it plateaus as blood flow matches an activity's metabolic requirements.

TABLE 10.3 Average Values for Cardiac Output, Heart Rate, and Stroke Volume for Endurance-Trained and Untrained Men at Rest and During Maximal Effort

	Cardiac Output ($mL \cdot min^{-1}$)	Heart Rate ($b \cdot min^{-1}$)	Stroke Volume ($mL \cdot b^{-1}$)
At Rest			
Untrained	5000	70	71
Trained	5000	50	100
At Maximal Effort			
Untrained	22,000	195	113
Trained	35,000	195	179

In sedentary, college-age men, cardiac output in maximal aerobic activity increases about four times the resting level to an average 22 L maximum of blood circulated per minute. Maximum heart rate (HR_{max}) for these young adults averages 195 $b \cdot min^{-1}$. Consequently, stroke volume averages 113 mL of blood per beat during physical activity (22,000 mL ÷ 195 b). In contrast, world-class endurance athletes generate maximum cardiac outputs of 35 $L \cdot min^{-1}$, with a similar or slightly lower maximum heart rate than untrained counterparts. The difference between maximum cardiac outputs of both individuals relates *solely* to differences in stroke volume. **Table 10.3** summarizes average values for cardiac output, heart rate, and stroke volume of endurance-trained and untrained men during maximal exertion.

PHYSICAL ACTIVITY STROKE VOLUME

Figure 10.13 relates stroke volume and percentage $\dot{V}O_{2max}$ (to better equate effort intensity among subjects) for eight healthy college-age men during graded physical activity on a cycle ergometer. Stroke volume increases progressively with effort to about 50% $\dot{V}O_{2max}$ and then gradually stabilizes until the effort terminates. For several subjects, stroke volume decreased slightly at near-maximal intensities.

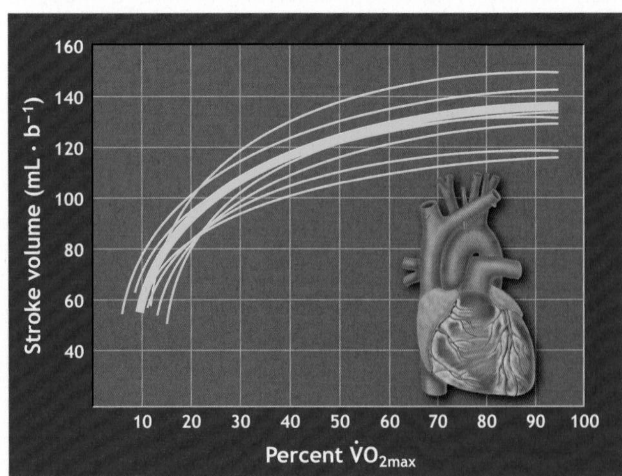

FIGURE 10.13 Stroke volume ($mL \cdot b^{-1}$) related to increasing exercise intensity (percent maximal oxygen uptake [$\dot{V}O_{2max}$]) for eight healthy male subjects. (Data from the Applied Physiology Laboratory, University of Michigan.)

Stroke Volume and $\dot{V}O_{2max}$

Stroke volume clearly differentiates people with high and low $\dot{V}O_{2max}$. For example, three groups of subjects were studied: (1) patients with mitral stenosis, a valvular disease that causes inadequate left ventricle emptying; (2) healthy but sedentary men; and (3) endurance athletes. Differences in $\dot{V}O_{2max}$ among groups closely paralleled differences in maximal stroke volume (SV_{max}). In mitral stenosis patients, $\dot{V}O_{2max}$ and SV_{max} averaged half the values of sedentary subjects. This close linkage also emerges in comparisons among healthy subjects; a 60% larger SV_{max} in endurance athletes compared with sedentary men paralleled the 62% larger $\dot{V}O_{2max}$. All groups showed fairly similar HR_{max}; thus, SV_{max} differences accounted for the between-group variations in maximum cardiac output and $\dot{V}O_{2max}$.

Stroke Volume Changes During Rest and Physical Activity

Three physiologic mechanisms increase the heart's stroke volume during physical activity:

1. Enhanced cardiac filling in diastole followed by a forceful systolic contraction
2. Neurohormonal influence, which involves normal ventricular filling with a subsequent forceful ejection and emptying during systole.
3. Training-induced expansion of blood volume and reduced resistance to blood flow in peripheral tissues

Greater Systolic Emptying Versus Enhanced Diastolic Filling

During the cardiac cycle, greater ventricular filling occurs in diastole through any factor that increases venous return (**preload**) or slows heart rate. An increase in end-diastolic volume stretches myocardial fibers, which causes a powerful ejection stroke as the heart contracts. This expels the normal stroke volume plus the additional blood that entered the ventricles and stretched the myocardium.

German physiologist Otto Frank (1865–1944) and British colleague Ernest H. Starling (1866–1927) conducted animal experiments in the early 1900s dealing with relationships between muscle force and resting fiber length. Improved contractility of stretched muscle within a limited range probably relates to a more optimum arrangement of intracellular myofilaments as muscle fibers stretch.

Frank-Starling Law of the Heart describes this phenomenon as applied to the myocardium. For many years, physiologists taught the Frank-Starling mechanism as the main cause of increases in stroke volume during physical activity. They believed that enhanced venous return during activity caused greater cardiac filling, which stretched the ventricles in diastole to produce a more forceful ejection.

Body position affects circulatory dynamics. In a horizontal position, cardiac output and stroke volume reach the highest and most stable levels. *Near-maximal stroke volume occurs at rest in a horizontal position and increases only slightly during physical activity.* In contrast, gravity's effect in the upright position counters venous return to lower stroke volume. This postural dynamic at rest remains prominent when comparing circulatory dynamics in upright and supine positions. As upright effort intensity increases, stroke volume also increases to approach the supine position's maximum value.

In most forms of upright activity, the heart does not fill to an extent that increases cardiac volume to values observed in the recumbent position. The increase in stroke volume during physical activity likely results from the *combined effects* of enhanced diastolic filling *and* more complete systolic emptying. In both recumbent and upright positions, the heart's stroke volume increases in physical activity despite resistance to flow, called **afterload**, from increased systolic pressure.

At rest in the upright position, 40% to 50% of total end-diastolic blood volume remains in the left ventricle following systole; this **functional residual heart volume** amounts to 50 to 70 mL of blood. Epinephrine and norepinephrine increase myocardial stroke power and systolic emptying during physical activity to reduce the heart's residual blood volume from enhanced systolic ejection.

fyi Watson Supercomputer Seeks to Predict Genetic Heart Dangers

Sudden cardiac arrest kills a man or women in the United States every 5 seconds. Scientists at the Lawrence Livermore National Laboratory in California and colleagues (**www.lbl.gov/research-areas**) have turned to Watson, IBM's famous supercomputer (**www.ibm.com/smarterplanet/us/en/ibmwatson/**), to quantify the genetic predisposition behind the condition of sudden cardiac arrest. Watson uses detailed CT and MRI 3D computer heart models to help identify risk factors leading to fatal heart arrhythmia. The simulations mimic actual heart function from heart gross anatomy to ultrastructural details at the cellular level. Researchers are then able to recreate pathologic conditions that cause underlying problems, including scenarios to simulate effects on heart cells from various antiarrhythmic drugs. The novelty of this approach addresses the important issue of genetic susceptibility to disease. Adding the speed and capacity of the Watson computer to tap into the world literature facilitates discovery of interactions between specific genes and possible factors that contribute to sudden cardiac arrest. The ultimate plan is to combine 3D scanning with clinical assessment of the heart's electrical conduction patterns and gene sequence data to predict risk of sudden cardiac arrest and ultimately prescribe life-saving targeted medications.

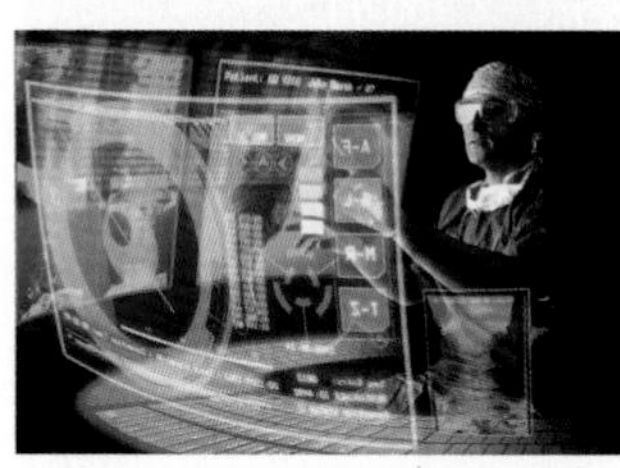

Ejection Fraction: A Measure of Ventricular Function

Clinicians use ventricular ejection fraction to assess the heart's pumping ability and subsequent prognosis for cardiovascular health; individuals with significantly reduced ejection fractions typically have poorer prognosis.

Ejection fraction refers to the fraction of blood pumped from the left ventricle relative to its end-diastolic volume. For example, if the ventricular end-diastolic volume equals 110 mL of blood, and the heart's stroke volume equals 70 mL, the ejection fraction computes as 70 mL ÷ 110 or 0.64 or 64%. Healthy individuals usually have ejection fractions that range between 50% and 70%. A depressed ejection fraction often accompanies poor left-ventricular function.

Cardiovascular Drift: Reduced Stroke Volume and Increased Heart Rate During Prolonged Physical Activity

Submaximal physical activity lasting more than 15 minutes, particularly in the heat, produces progressive water loss through sweating and a fluid shift from plasma to tissues. A rise in core temperature also causes blood redistribution to the periphery for body cooling. At the same time, the progressive decrease in plasma volume decreases central venous cardiac filling pressure, which reduces stroke volume. A reduced stroke volume initiates a compensatory heart rate increase to maintain a nearly constant cardiac output as activity progresses. The term **cardiovascular drift** describes this gradual time-dependent downward "drift" in several cardiovascular responses, most notably stroke volume with concomitant heart rate increase during prolonged steady-rate effort. Under these circumstances, a person usually must exercise at a lower intensity than if cardiovascular drift did not occur.

One explanation for cardiovascular drift suggests that a stroke volume decline during prolonged activity in a thermoneutral environment relates to an increased activity heart rate and not increased cutaneous blood flow. More than likely, the progressive heart rate increase with cardiovascular drift decreases end-diastolic volume to subsequently reduce the heart's stroke volume.

HEART RATE DURING PHYSICAL ACTIVITY

Graded Physical Activity

Figure 10.14 depicts the relationship for endurance-trained individuals and their sedentary counterparts between heart rate and oxygen uptake during increasing intensity graded physical activity to maximum. Heart rate for untrained individuals accelerates rapidly with increasing physical activity demands; trained individuals have a smaller increase in heart rate. Trained individuals achieve a higher level of oxygen uptake at a given submaximal

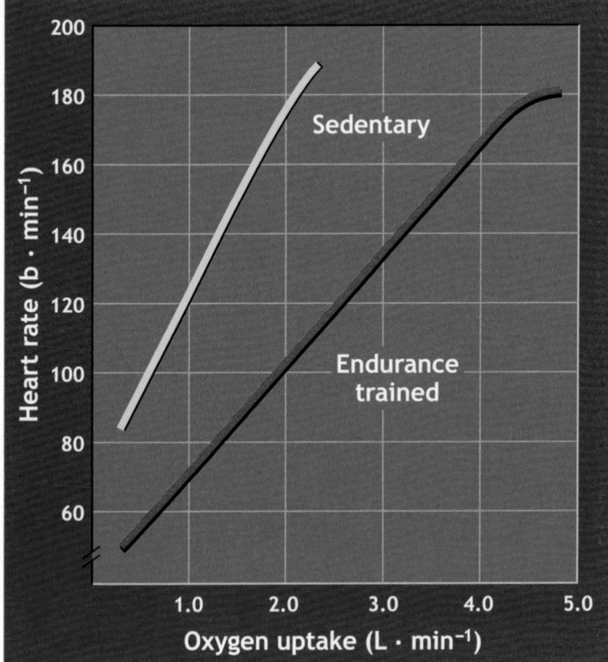

FIGURE 10.14 Generalized response for heart rate in relation to oxygen uptake during exercise for endurance-trained individuals (*red line*) and sedentary counterparts (*green line*).

heart rate than their sedentary counterparts. Maximum heart rate and the heart rate–oxygen uptake relationship remain fairly consistent intra-day and day-to-day for a particular individual, although with aerobic training, the slope of the relationship decreases considerably from increases in stroke volume.

Submaximum Physical Activity

Heart rate increases rapidly and levels off within several minutes during submaximal steady-rate activity. A subsequent increase in effort intensity accelerates heart rate to a new plateau as the body attempts to match the cardiovascular response to the new metabolic demands. Each increment in intensity requires progressively more time to achieve heart rate stabilization.

CARDIAC OUTPUT DISTRIBUTION

Blood flow to specific tissues increases in proportion to their metabolic demands.

At Rest

Figure 10.15A shows the approximate distribution of a 5-L cardiac output at rest. More than one-fourth of the cardiac output flows to the liver, one-fifth flows to the kidneys and muscles, and the remainder diverts to the heart, skin, brain, and other tissues.

During Physical Activity

Figure 10.15B illustrates the distribution of cardiac output to various tissues during intense aerobic activity. *Regional blood flow varies considerably depending on environmental conditions, level of fatigue, and activity mode, yet active muscles receive a disproportionately large distribution of cardiac output.* During rest, each 100 g of muscle receives 4 to 7 mL of blood per minute. Muscle blood flow increases steadily during activity to reach a maximum of between 50 to 75 mL per 100 g of active muscle tissue.

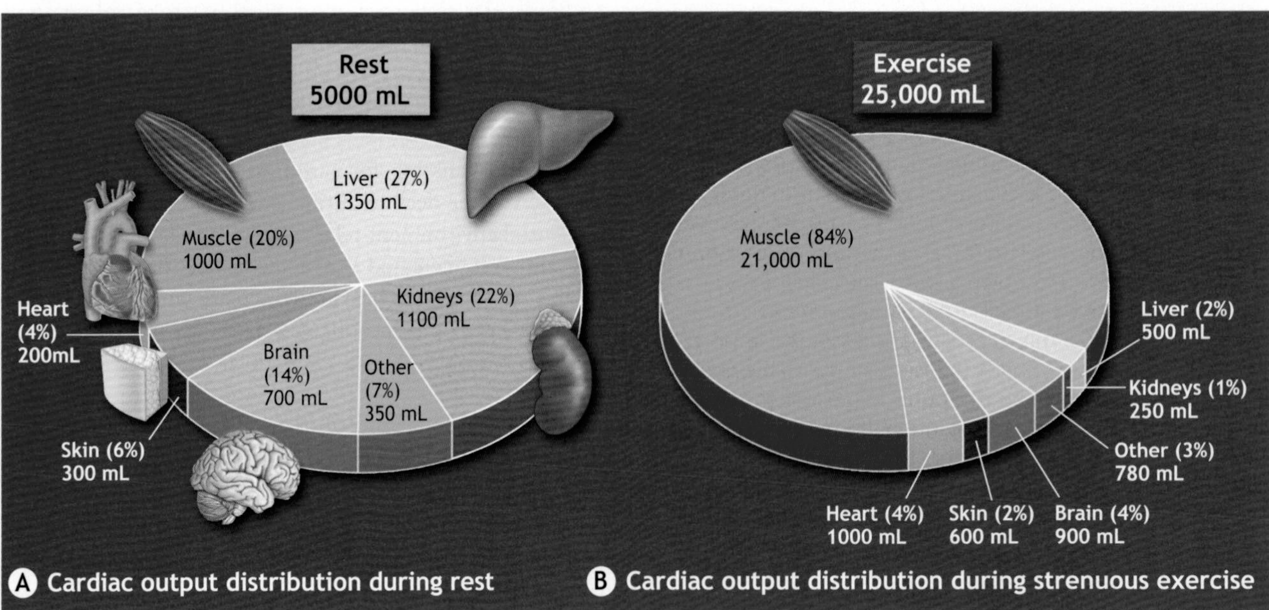

FIGURE 10.15 Relative distribution of cardiac output during rest **(A)** and strenuous endurance exercise **(B)**. The number in parentheses indicates percentage of the total cardiac output. The large absolute mass of muscle tissue at rest receives about the same quantity of blood as the much smaller kidneys. In strenuous physical activity, approximately 84% of the cardiac output diverts to the active musculature. (Reprinted with permission from McArdle WD, Katch FI, Katch VL. *Exercise Physiology: Nutrition, Energy, and Human Performance.* 8th Ed. Baltimore: Wolters Kluwer Health, 2015.)

Blood Flow Redistribution

The increase in muscle blood flow with physical activity comes largely from increased cardiac output. Neural and hormonal vascular regulation, including local metabolic conditions within muscles, moves blood through active muscles from areas that can temporarily tolerate compromised blood flow. Shunting of blood away from specific tissues occurs primarily during intense physical effort. Blood flow to the skin increases during light and moderate activity, so metabolic heat generated in muscle can dissipate at the skin's surface. In contrast, during intense but short duration effort, cutaneous blood flow decreases even when exercising in a hot environment.

In some tissues, blood flow during physical activity decreases to four-fifths the normal resting flow. At rest, the kidneys and splanchnic tissues use only 10% to 25% of oxygen available in their blood supply. Consequently, these tissues tolerate reduced blood flow before oxygen demand exceeds supply and disrupts organ function. With reduced blood flow, increased oxygen extraction from available blood maintains the tissue's oxygen needs. During intense activity, the visceral organs can tolerate reduced blood flow for more than 1 hour, "freeing" as much as 600 mL each minute of oxygen for use by active musculature.

Heart and Brain Blood Flow

The myocardium and brain cannot compromise their blood supplies. At rest, the myocardium normally uses 75% of the oxygen in the blood flowing through the coronary circulation. With such a limited "safety margin," increased coronary blood flow primarily meets the heart's oxygen demands. Cerebral blood flow increases up to 30% with physical activity compared with rest; the largest portion of any "extra" blood probably diverts to areas related to motor functions.

See the animation "Myocardial Blood Flow" on **http://thePoint.lww.com/MKKESS5e** for further insights about this process.

CARDIAC OUTPUT AND OXYGEN TRANSPORT

At Rest

At sea level, each 100 mL (deciliter [dL]) of arterial blood normally carries about 20 mL of oxygen or 200 mL of oxygen per liter of blood (see Chapter 9). Trained and untrained adults circulate about L of blood each minute at rest, so potentially 1000 mL of oxygen becomes available during 1 minute (5 L blood × 200 mL O_2). Resting oxygen uptake averages only about 250 mL · min^{-1}; this means 750 mL of oxygen returns "unused" to the heart. This does not represent an unnecessary waste of cardiac output. To the contrary, extra oxygen in the blood above the resting requirement maintains oxygen in reserve—a margin of safety for immediate use if the need arises like in a last second sprint to catch a bus.

During Physical Activity

A person with a maximum heart rate of 200 b · min^{-1} and stroke volume of 80 mL per beat generates a maximum cardiac output of 16 L (200 b · min^{-1} × 0.080 L). Even during maximum effort, hemoglobin remains fully saturated with oxygen, so each liter of arterial blood carries about 200 mL of oxygen. Consequently, 3200 mL of oxygen circulate each minute via a 16-L cardiac output (16 L × 200 mL O_2). If the body extracted all of the oxygen delivered in a 16-L cardiac output, $\dot{V}O_{2max}$ would equal 3200 mL. This represents the theoretical upper limit for this person since certain tissue's oxygen needs, like the brain for example, do not increase greatly with physical activity yet require an uninterrupted blood supply.

An increase in maximum cardiac output directly improves a person's capacity to circulate oxygen and profoundly impacts maximal oxygen uptake. If the heart's stroke volume increased from 80 to 200 mL while the maximum heart rate remained unchanged at 200 b · min^{-1}, the maximum cardiac output would dramatically increase to 40 L · min^{-1}. This means that the amount of oxygen circulated in maximum exertion each minute increases approximately 2.5 times from 3200 to 8000 mL (40 L × 200 mL O_2).

Maximum Cardiac Output and $\dot{V}O_{2max}$

Figure 10.16 displays the relationship between maximum cardiac output and $\dot{V}O_{2max}$ and includes values representative of sedentary individuals and elite endurance athletes. An unmistakable relationship emerges. Whereas a low aerobic capacity links closely to a low maximum cardiac output, a 30- to 40-L cardiac output always accompanies a 5- or 6-L $\dot{V}O_{2max}$.

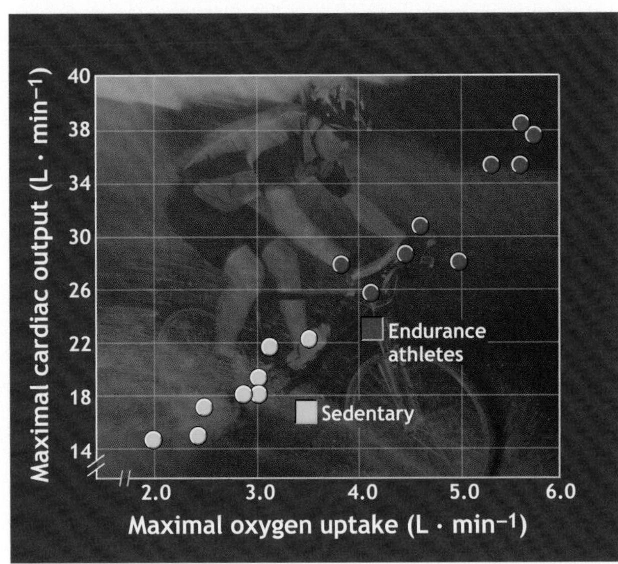

FIGURE 10.16 Relationship between maximal cardiac output and maximal oxygen uptake ($\dot{V}O_{2max}$) in endurance trained and untrained individuals. Maximal cardiac output relates to $\dot{V}O_{2max}$ in the ratio of about 6:1. (Reprinted with permission from McArdle WD, Katch FI, Katch VL. *Exercise Physiology: Nutrition, Energy, and Human Performance*. 8th Ed. Baltimore: Wolters Kluwer Health, 2015.)

Cardiac Output Differences Among Men, Women, and Children

Cardiac output and oxygen uptake for boys and girls and men and women remain linearly related during graded (progressively more intense) physical activity. Teenage and adult females generally exercise at any level of submaximal oxygen uptake with a 5% to 10% larger cardiac output than males. Any apparent gender difference in submaximal cardiac output most likely results from the 10% lower hemoglobin concentration in women compared to men. A proportionate increase in submaximal cardiac output compensates for this small gender-related decrease in the blood's oxygen-carrying capacity.

In children, higher heart rates during submaximal treadmill and cycle ergometer activity do not fully compensate for their smaller stroke volume. This produces a smaller cardiac output at a given submaximal physical activity oxygen uptake. Consequently, the a-$\bar{v}o_2$ difference expands to satisfy the oxygen requirements. The biologic significance of this difference in central circulatory function between children and adults remains unclear.

EXTRACTION OF OXYGEN: THE a-$\bar{v}o_2$ DIFFERENCE

If blood flow were the only means to increase a tissue's oxygen supply, cardiac output would need to increase from 5 L · min^{-1} at rest to 100 L in maximum exertion to achieve a 20-fold increase in oxygen uptake, an oxygen uptake increase common among endurance athletes. Fortunately, intense physical effort does not require such a large cardiac output because hemoglobin releases its "extra" oxygen from blood perfusing active tissues.

Two mechanisms for oxygen supply increase a person's oxygen uptake capacity:

1. Increased tissue blood flow
2. Use of the relatively large quantity of oxygen remaining unused by tissues at rest (i.e., expanded a-$\bar{v}o_2$ difference)

The following rearrangement of the Fick equation summarizes the important relationship between maximum cardiac output, maximum **a-$\bar{v}o_2$ difference**, and $\dot{V}O_{2max}$:

$$\dot{V}O_{2max} = \text{Maximum cardiac output} \times \text{Maximum a-}\bar{v}o_2 \text{ difference}$$

Rest and Physical Activity a-$\bar{v}o_2$ Difference

Figure 10.17 shows a representative pattern for changes in a-$\bar{v}o_2$ difference from rest to maximum effort for physically active men. A similar pattern emerges for women except that the arterial oxygen content averages 5% to 10% lower because of lower hemoglobin concentrations. The figure includes values for the oxygen content of arterial blood and mixed-venous blood during different intensities of physical activity. Arterial blood oxygen content varies little from its value of 20 mL · dL^{-1} at rest throughout the full intensity range. In contrast, mixed-venous oxygen content varies between 12 and 15 mL · dL^{-1} at rest to a low of 2 to 4 mL · dL^{-1} during maximum physical activity. The difference between arterial and mixed-venous blood oxygen content or a-$\bar{v}o_2$ difference at any time represents oxygen extraction from blood as it circulates through the body's tissues. At rest, for example, the a-$\bar{v}o_2$ difference equals 5 mL of oxygen, which represents only 25% of the blood's oxygen content (5 ÷ 20 mL × 100); 75% of the oxygen bound to hemoglobin returns "unused" to the heart.

The progressive expansion of a-$\bar{v}o_2$ difference to at least three times resting values occurs from a reduced venous oxygen content, which in maximal effort approaches 20 mL in active muscle with all the oxygen extracted. The oxygen content of a true mixed-venous sample from the pulmonary artery rarely falls below 2 to 4 mL · dL^{-1} because blood returning from active tissues mixes with oxygen-rich venous blood from metabolically less active regions.

Figure 10.17 also indicates that the capacity of each dL of arterial blood to carry oxygen actually *increases* during physical activity. Two factors explain why increased RBC concentration, called *hemoconcentration*, occurs from progressive fluid movement from the plasma to interstitial spaces:

1. Increases in capillary hydrostatic pressure as blood pressure increases
2. Metabolic by-products of exercise metabolism create an osmotic pressure gradient that draws fluid from plasma into tissue spaces, thus increasing RBC concentration.

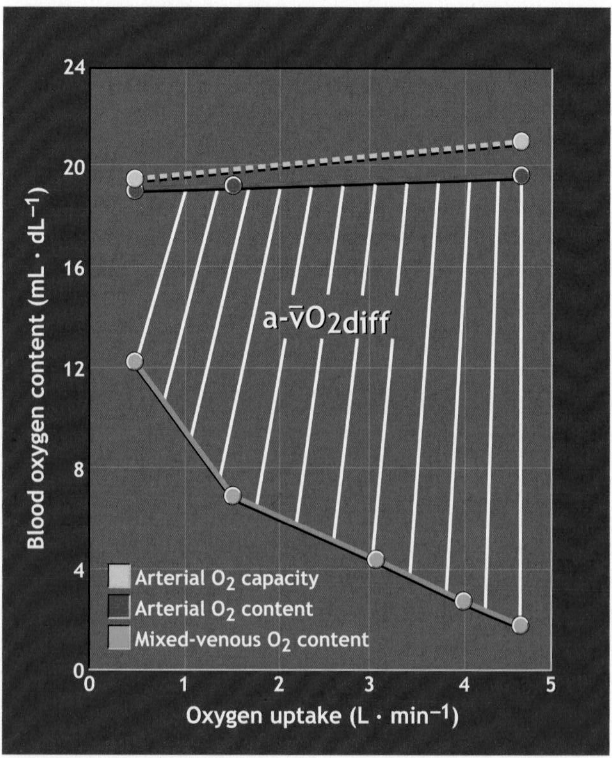

FIGURE 10.17 Changes in a-$\bar{v}o_2$ difference from rest to maximal exercise in physically active men. (Reprinted with permission from McArdle WD, Katch FI, Katch VL. *Exercise Physiology: Nutrition, Energy, and Human Performance*. 8th Ed. Baltimore: Wolters Kluwer Health, 2015.)

FACTORS THAT AFFECT a-$\bar{v}O_2$ DIFFERENCE DURING PHYSICAL ACTIVITY

Central and peripheral factors interact to increase oxygen extraction in active tissue during physical activity. Diverting a large portion of the cardiac output to active muscles influences the magnitude of a-$\bar{v}O_2$ difference during maximal effort. As mentioned previously, some tissues temporarily compromise blood supply during physical activity by redistributing blood to make more oxygen available for muscle metabolism. Physical activity training, for example, facilitates central circulation redirection to more active musculature.

Increases in the size and number of mitochondria and augmented aerobic enzyme activity improve muscle's metabolic capacity during physical activity. Increases in skeletal muscle microcirculation with endurance training also increase tissue oxygen extraction. Muscle biopsy specimens from the quadriceps femoris in individuals who exhibit large a-$\bar{v}O_2$ differences during intense exertion show a relatively large capillary-to-muscle fiber ratio. An increase in this ratio reflects a positive training adaptation that promotes a large interface for nutrient and gas exchange. Another important factor involves individual muscle cells' ability to generate energy aerobically.

CARDIOVASCULAR ADJUSTMENTS TO UPPER-BODY PHYSICAL ACTIVITY

The highest oxygen uptake during upper-body physical activity generally averages 70% to 80% of $\dot{V}O_{2max}$ assessed in bicycle and treadmill testing. Similarly, HR_{max} and pulmonary ventilation remain lower in arm physical activity. The relatively smaller muscle mass of the upper body largely accounts for these physiologic differences. The lower maximal heart rate in exercise that activates a smaller muscle mass likely results from the following two factors:

1. Reduced output stimulation from the motor cortex central command to the cardiovascular center in the medulla from less feedforward stimulation.
2. Reduced feedback stimulation to the medulla from the smaller active musculature.

During submaximal physical activity, a reversal occurs in metabolic and cardiovascular response patterns between upper- and lower-body activities. **Figure 10.18** illustrates that any level of submaximal power output produces a higher oxygen uptake with arm than with leg physical activity. This difference remains small during light physical activity but becomes larger as intensity of effort increases. Lower economy of effort during arm cranking probably results from static muscle actions that do not produce external work but consume extra oxygen. In addition, the extra musculature activated to stabilize the torso during most forms of arm physical activity adds to the activity's oxygen requirement. Upper-body activity also produces greater physiologic demand in heart rate, blood pressure, pulmonary ventilation, and perception of physical effort for any level of oxygen uptake or percentage of $\dot{V}O_{2max}$ than lower-body leg physical activity.

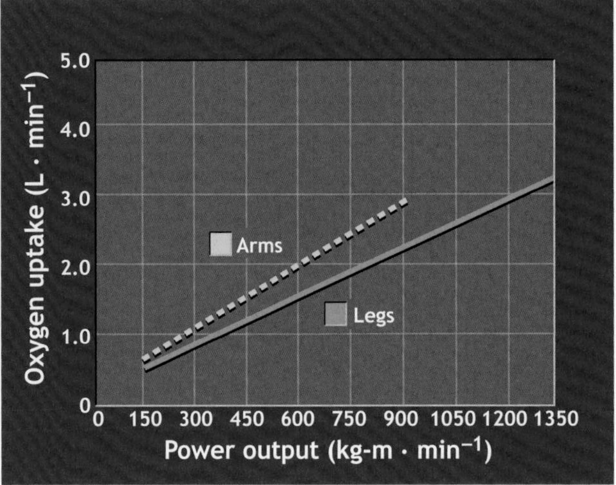

FIGURE 10.18 Arm exercise requires greater oxygen uptake than leg exercise at any submaximal power output throughout the comparison range. The largest differences occur during intense exertion. Data represent averages for men and women. (Reprinted with permission from McArdle WD, Katch FI, Katch VL. *Exercise Physiology: Nutrition, Energy, and Human Performance*. 8th Ed. Baltimore: Wolters Kluwer Health, 2015. Data from Laboratory of Applied Physiology, Queens College, Flushing.)

The health care professional and physical activity specialist should appreciate the differences in physiologic response between upper- and lower-body physical activities so they can create prudent activity programs using both activity modes. A standard intensity load based on power output or $\dot{V}O_2$ produces greater physiologic strain with the arms. Thus, physical activity prescriptions based on running and bicycling *should not* be applied to upper-body activity. Also, $\dot{V}O_{2max}$ for arm activity does not strongly correlate or relate with leg activity $\dot{V}O_{2max}$. Stated somewhat differently, one cannot accurately predict $\dot{V}O_{2max}$ for arm activity from a test using the legs and vice versa. *Such findings continue to validate the concept of aerobic fitness specificity.*

SUMMARY

1. Heart rate and stroke volume determine the heart's output capacity in the following relationship: Cardiac output = Heart rate × Stroke volume.
2. Cardiac output increases proportionately with effort intensity, starting from approximately 5 L · min^{-1} at rest to a maximum of 20 to 25 L · min^{-1} in untrained college-age men and to 35 to 40 L · min^{-1} in elite male endurance athletes.
3. Differences in maximum cardiac output primarily relate to individual differences in the heart's maximum stroke volume.
4. During upright physical activity, stroke volume increases during the transition from rest to moderate activity, reaching maximum at about 50% $\dot{V}O_{2max}$. Thereafter, increases in heart rate produce increases in cardiac output.

5. Stroke volume increases in upright physical activity generally result from interactions between greater ventricular filling during diastole and more complete emptying during systole.
6. Sympathetic hormones that augment myocardial force generated during systole produce larger stroke volumes.
7. Training adaptations that expand blood volume and reduce peripheral tissue resistance to blood flow also contribute to enhanced stroke volume.
8. In trained and untrained individuals, heart rate and oxygen uptake relate linearly throughout the major portion of an activity's intensity range.
9. Improved stroke volume with endurance training shifts the heart rate–oxygen uptake line to the right.
10. Local metabolism generally determines blood flow in specific limb and trunk tissues because it can divert cardiac output to more active muscles during physical activity.
11. Kidneys and splanchnic regions temporarily compromise their blood supplies to redirect blood to active muscles.
12. Maximum cardiac output and maximum a-$\bar{v}O_2$ difference determine $\dot{V}O_{2max}$ in the following relationship: $\dot{V}O_{2max}$ = Maximum cardiac output × Maximum a-$\bar{v}O_2$ difference.
13. Large cardiac outputs clearly differentiate endurance athletes from untrained counterparts. Training also expands the maximum a-$\bar{v}O_2$ difference.
14. Upper-body arm cranking activity generates about a 25% lower $\dot{V}O_{2max}$ than lower-body running or cycling.
15. Arm activity produces greater physiologic demand than lower-body activity for any level of submaximal power output or oxygen uptake.

THINK IT THROUGH

1. In what way does the Fick equation fully explain the physiologic components that determine $\dot{V}O_{2max}$?
2. Explain which component of the maximal oxygen uptake equation, oxygen delivery or oxygen utilization, becomes the limiting factor in $\dot{V}O_{2max}$.
3. How would factors that influence a-$\bar{v}O_2$ difference in maximal effort explain the specificity of $\dot{V}O_{2max}$ improvement with different aerobic training modes?

KEY TERMS

Adrenergic fibers: Nerve fibers whose neurotransmitter is adrenaline (epinephrine), noradrenaline, or dopamine.

Afterload: Increased resistance to blood flow in the arterial circuit from elevated aortic blood pressure and left ventricular wall tension developed during systole.

Angina pectoris: Chest pain related to impaired coronary blood flow caused by coronary vessel spasm or obstruction.

Anticipatory heart rate: Abrupt increase in heart rate in anticipation of a muscular performance such as a sprint race or other intense competition before the activity begins.

Aorta: Largest artery in the body; originates from the left ventricle and descends through the abdominal cavity where it splits into two smaller common iliac arteries.

Arrhythmia: Abnormal cardiac rhythm involving altered electrical impulse transmission within the myocardium.

Arteries: High-pressure blood vessels composed of multiple layers of connective tissue and smooth muscle that propel blood away from the heart to cells, tissues, and organs.

Arterioles or smaller arterial branches: "Resistance vessels" that constrict or relax to regulate peripheral blood flow.

Atrial fibrillation: Type of abnormal irregular and rapid heart rate caused by a chaotic and irregular beating of the two atria.

Atrioventricular (AV) node: Specialized myocardial fibers of the heart's electrical conduction system that connect atrial and ventricular chambers through the bundle of His.

Atrioventricular valves: Heart valves that provide one-way blood flow from the right atrium through the tricuspid valve to the right ventricle and from the left atrium through the mitral valve to the left ventricle.

a-$\bar{v}O_2$ difference: Difference between the oxygen content of arterial blood and mixed-venous blood; averages 5 mL of oxygen at rest to 15 to 17 mL of oxygen during intense physical activity.

Baroreceptors: Pressure sensitive receptors located within the aortic arch and carotid sinus that respond to arterial wall stretching.

Beta-blockers: Class of drugs commonly prescribed for hypertension; act by blocking the effects of epinephrine.

Bradycardia: Relatively slow heart rate, usually below 60 beats a minute at rest.

Bundle of His: Specialized heart muscle cells that transmit electrical impulses from the atrioventricular node through the ventricles over specialized Purkinje system conduction fibers.

Capillaries: Meshwork of microscopically small blood vessels consisting of a layer of endothelial cells, interfaced between red blood cells and adjacent tissues for passage of water, oxygen, carbon dioxide, and diverse nutrients and waste products.

Cardiac output: Volume of blood pumped by the heart each minute; computed as the product of heart rate and stroke volume.

Cardiopulmonary resuscitation (CPR): Emergency procedure to restore normal breathing and heart rate by assisted breathing and rhythmic chest compression overlying the heart.

Cardiovascular drift: Gradual time-dependent downward "drift" in stroke volume with concomitant heart rate increase during prolonged steady-rate physical activity, particularly in the heat.

Carotid artery palpation: Heart rate measurement by applying gentle external pressure with the fingertips against the carotid artery.

Catecholamines: Neurotransmitters and hormones including dopamine, epinephrine, and norepinephrine; produced from phenylalanine and tyrosine and synthesized and released by nerve tissue and adrenal glands.

Central command: Impulses that originate in the brain's higher somatomotor center that continually modulate medullary action; coordinate heart and blood vessel rapid adjustments to optimize tissue perfusion and maintain blood pressure prior to and during physical activity.

Chemoreceptors: Peripheral receptors that provide sensory feedback to the cardiovascular center relative to the blood's chemical state.

Cholinergic fibers: Nerve fibers that transmit impulses to other nerve cells, muscle fibers, or gland cells that respond to acetylcholine.

Cooling down: Easy physical activity (slow jog, walk, stretching) following more intense activity so heart rate gradually returns to its preactivity resting state.

Coronary circulation: Visible, crownlike vascular network that arises from the top portion of the heart; functions as the heart's intricate circulatory network to deliver oxygen-rich blood to the myocardium.

Diastole: Ventricular relaxation as the heart refills with blood.

Ejection fraction: Measurement of how much blood the left ventricle pumps out with each heart contraction; an ejection fraction of 60% means that 60% of the total amount of blood in the left ventricle is pushed out with each heartbeat. A normal heart's ejection fraction may be between 55% and 70%.

Electrocardiogram (ECG): Recording of the heart's electrical activity by systematically tracking the conduction pathway of electrical impulses as they propagate the myocardium during rhythmic contraction and relaxation.

Exercise pressor reflex: Neurological reflex activated during muscle contraction via stimulation of receptors within muscle that respond to either mechanical distortion or metabolic by-products of active muscle.

Extrasystoles: Premature heart contraction independent of the normal rhythm in response to a heart impulse other than originating from the sinoatrial node.

Frank-Starling law of the heart: The relationship between contractile force (stroke volume) and myocardial fibers' resting length (end-diastolic volume); within physiologic limits.

Functional residual heart volume: Amount of blood remaining in the ventricles following systole.

Heart rate: Rate the heart beats per unit time, usually expressed as a 1-minute rate.

Hypertension: Persistently high blood pressure, which chronically strains cardiovascular system functions, and over time, leads to arteriosclerosis, heart disease, stroke, and kidney failure.

Hypotensive recovery response: Temporary decline in blood pressure below pre-exercise levels in normotensive and hypertensive individuals following a single bout of low- or moderate-intensity physical activity.

Inferior vena cava: Largest vein in the body; returns blood to the right atrium from abdominal, pelvis, and lower extremity structures.

Left coronary artery: Artery that arises from the aorta above the left cusp of the aortic valve, feeding blood to the left side of the myocardium, and then bifurcating into the anterior interventricular artery and left circumflex artery.

Mechanoreceptors: Sensory receptors responsive to mechanical pressure and distortion that relay their signals to the central nervous system.

Mitral valve: Dual-flap heart valve between the left atrium and left ventricle.

Mixed-venous blood: Mixture of venous blood that drains all regions of the upper and lower body.

Myocardial infarction: Commonly termed a heart attack; occurs when the myocardium receives inadequate blood flow resulting in myocardial injury from oxygen deprivation.

Myocardium: Spontaneously contracting cardiac muscle representing a homogenous form of involuntary striated muscle with high capillary density and abundant mitochondria.

Nitric oxide: Important biological signaling molecule that dilates blood vessels and decreases vascular resistance.

Pacemaker: Common term to describe the sinoatrial (SA) node consisting of specialized cells within myocardium that create rhythmical impulses to directly control heart rate.

Poiseuille law: Velocity of the steady fluid flow through a cylindrical vessel varies directly as the pressure and fourth power of the radius of the tube and inversely as tube length and coefficient of viscosity in the formula: Flow = Pressure gradient × Vessel radius^4 ÷ Vessel length × Fluid viscosity.

Precapillary sphincter: Ring of smooth muscle encircling a capillary at its origin; controls capillary diameter to regulate tissue blood flow to meet metabolic requirements.

Preload: Any factor that increases venous return or slows the heart rate; produces greater ventricular filling during the cardiac cycle's diastolic phase.

Premature atrial contraction (PAC): A cardiac dysrhythmia characterized by premature heartbeats originating in a region of the atria that depolarizes before the sinoatrial node triggers depolarization.

Premature ventricular contraction (PVC): Heartbeat initiated by the ventricle's Purkinje fibers, rather than impulses originating in the sinoatrial node.

Pulmonary circulation: Portion of the cardiovascular system that delivers deoxygenated blood to the lungs for oxygenation and returns it to the heart.

Purkinje system: Specialized conducting fibers that penetrate the right and left ventricles and transmit the impulse throughout the ventricular wall to allow unified and simultaneous ventricular contractions.

Rate pressure product (RPP): Also known as double product; estimates relative myocardial workload (energy demand) computed from the product of heart rate and systolic blood pressure.

Refractory period: Heart's relatively long depolarization interval, which delays initiation of the next myocardial impulse and subsequent contraction.

Right atrium: Heart chamber that receives deoxygenated blood from the superior and inferior venae cava, coronary sinus, and small cardiac vein from the heart wall (cardiac sinus), and propels it through the tricuspid valve into the right ventricle.

Right coronary artery: Arises above the aortic valve's right cusp and travels toward the crux of the heart, then splits into acute marginal arteries and right posterior coronary artery.

Right ventricle: Heart's lower right chamber that receives deoxygenated blood via the tricuspid valve from the right atrium and pumps it under low pressure through the pulmonary valve into the lungs via the pulmonary artery.

Semilunar valves: Either of two valves, one located at the opening of the aorta and the other at the opening of the pulmonary artery, which prevents blood flowing back into the heart between contractions.

Sinoatrial (SA) node: Specialized mass of tissue situated within the right atrium's posterior wall, which spontaneously depolarizes and repolarizes to provide the innate stimulus for heart action.

Stroke volume: Quantity of blood ejected by the heart's left ventricle with each contraction.

Superior vena: Conducts blood from tributary vessels in the head, neck, upper extremities, and thorax to join the inferior vena cava at heart level.

Systemic circulation: Portion of the cardiovascular system that receives oxygenated blood from the lungs and pumps it into the aorta for transport throughout the body.

Systole: Ventricular contraction forces blood forward within the myocardial chambers with each heartbeat.

Tachycardia: Faster than normal heart rate at rest; usually greater than 100 beats a minute.

Thrombus: Solid mass of platelets and/or fibrin, which forms in a vessel and restricts or blocks blood flow.

Tricuspid valve: Right atrioventricular valve between the right atrium and right ventricle.

Vagus nerve: Tenth pair of cranial nerves, which extends from the brain stem to the abdomen via the heart, esophagus, and lungs.

Vasomotor tone: Blood vessels that always exhibit a relative state of constriction.

Venous tone: Venous system characteristic that reflects venous resistance and pressure; degree of venous constriction relative to its maximally dilated state.

Ventricular fibrillation: Life-threatening cardiac rhythm disturbance characterized by uncoordinated, chaotic ventricular contraction, where ventricles flutter rather than beat, making them highly ineffective to pump blood.

Venules: Small veins that merge with larger veins as blood returns toward the heart.

SELECTED REFERENCES

ACSM position stand: exercise and hypertension. *Med Sci Sports Exerc* 2004;36:533.

Beckett N, et al. Treatment of hypertension in patients 80 years of age or older. *N Engl J Med* 2008;358:1887.

Bhammar DM, et al. Effects of fractionized and continuous exercise on 24-h ambulatory blood pressure. *Med Sci Sports Exerc* 2012;44:2270.

Buckwalter JB, et al. Role of nitric oxide in exercise sympatholysis. *J Appl Physiol* 2004;97:417.

Calbet JA, Lundby C. Skeletal muscle vasodilatation during maximal exercise in health and disease. *J Physiol* 2012;590:6285.

Clark CE, et al. Association of a difference in systolic blood pressure between arms with vascular disease and mortality: a systematic review and meta-analysis. *Lancet* 2012;379:905.

Colakoglu M, et al. Shorter intervals at peak SV vs.VO_{2max} may yield high SV with less physiological stress. *Eur J Sport Sci* 2014:1.

Coyle EF, González-Alonso J. Cardiovascular drift during prolonged exercise: new perspectives. *Exer Sport Sci Rev* 2001;28:88.

Currie KD, et al. Effects of resistance training combined with moderate-intensity endurance or low-volume high-intensity interval exercise on cardiovascular risk factors in patients with coronary artery disease. *J Sci Med Sport* 2014. (In Press as of 06.13.15.)

DeVan AE, et al. Acute effects of resistance exercise on arterial compliance. *J Appl Physiol* 2005;98:2287.

Dujic Z, et al. Postexercise hypotension in moderately trained athletes after maximal exercise. *Med Sci Sports Exerc* 2006;38:318.

Edwards WD, et al. On the physical death of Jesus Christ. *JAMA* 1986;255:1455.

Franklin BA, et al. Exercise-based cardiac rehabilitation and improvements in cardiorespiratory fitness: implications regarding patient benefit. *Mayo Clin Proc* 2013;88:431.

Gillespie C, et al. Vital signs: prevalence, treatment, and control of hypertension—United States, 1999–2002 and 2005–2008. *MMWR Morb Mortal Wkly Rep* 2011;60:103.

Goldring N, et al. The effects of isometric wall squat exercise on heart rate and blood pressure in a normotensive population. *J Sports Sci* 2013;32:129.

González-Alonso J. Point:Counterpoint: stroke volume does/does not decline during exercise at maximal effort in healthy individuals. *J Appl Physiol* 2008;104:275.

Gorman MW, Feigl EO. Control of coronary blood flow during exercise. *Exerc Sport Sci Rev* 2012;40:37.

Heinonen I, et al. Role of adenosine in regulating the heterogeneity of skeletal muscle blood flow during exercise in humans. *J Appl Physiol* 2007; 103:2042.

Izquierdo M, et al. Effects of combined resistance and cardiovascular training on strength, power, muscle cross-sectional area, and endurance markers in middle-aged men. *Eur J Appl Physiol* 2005;94:70.

Lackland DT, Voeks JH. Metabolic syndrome and hypertension: regular exercise as part of lifestyle management. *Curr Hypertens Rep* 2014;16:492.

Lafrenz AJ, et al. Effect of ambient temperature on cardiovascular drift and maximal oxygen uptake. *Med Sci Sports Exerc* 2008;40:1065.

Lakin R, et al. Effects of moderate-intensity aerobic cycling and swim exercise on post-exertional blood pressure in healthy young untrained and triathlon-trained men and women. *Clin Sci (Lond)* 2013;125:543.

Lee JF, et al. Warm skin alters cardiovascular responses to cycling after preheating and precooling. *Med Sci Sports Exerc* 2015;47:1168.

Li Y, et al. Aerobic, resistance and combined exercise training on arterial stiffness in normotensive and hypertensive adults: a review. *Eur J Sport Sci* 2014:1.

Liu S, et al. Blood pressure responses to acute and chronic exercise are related to prehypertension. *Med Sci Sports Exerc* 2012;44:1644.

Lockwood JM, et al. Postexercise hypotension is not explained by a prostaglandin-dependent peripheral vasodilation. *J Appl Physiol* 2005;98:447.

Mattsson CM, et al. Reversed drift in heart rate but increased oxygen uptake at fixed work rate during 24 h ultra-endurance exercise. *Scand J Med Sci Sports* 2010;20:298.

Mortensen SP, et al. Limitations to systemic and locomotor limb muscle oxygen delivery and uptake during maximal exercise in humans. *J Physiol* 2005; 566:273.

Neves VJ, et al. Exercise training in hypertension: role of microRNAs. *World J Cardiol* 2014;6:713.

Pearson TA, et al. American Heart Association guide for improving cardiovascular health at the community level, 2013 update: a scientific statement for public health practitioners, healthcare providers, and health policy makers. American Heart Association Council on Epidemiology and Prevention. *Circulation* 2013;127:1730.

Perry BG, et al. Hemodynamic response to upright resistance exercise: effect of load and repetition. *Med Sci Sports Exerc* 2013;46:479.

Pricher MP, et al. Regional hemodynamics during postexercise hypotension. I. Splanchnic and renal circulations. *J Appl Physiol* 2004;97:2065.

Rankinen T, et al. Cardiorespiratory fitness, BMI, and risk of hypertension: the HYPGENE Study. *Med Sci Sports Exerc* 2007;39:1687.

Rodrigues B, et al. Role of exercise training on autonomic changes and inflammatory profile induced by myocardial infarction. *Mediators Inflamm* 2014;2014:702473.

Roof SR, et al. Neuronal nitric oxide synthase is indispensable for the cardiac adaptive effects of exercise. *Basic Res Cardiol* 2013;108:332.

Rowell LB, et al. Integration of cardiovascular control systems in dynamic exercises. In: Rowell LB, Shepard J, eds. *Handbook of Physiology*. New York: Oxford University Press, 1996.

Swain DP, Franklin BA. Comparison of cardioprotective benefits of vigorous versus moderate intensity aerobic exercise. *Am J Cardiol* 2006;97:141.

Thomas GD, Segal SS. Neural control of muscle blood flow during exercise. *J Appl Physiol* 2004;97:731.

Tordi N, et al. Intermittent versus constant aerobic exercise: effects on arterial stiffness. *Eur J Appl Physiol* 2010;108:801.

Vieira GM, et al. Intraocular pressure during weight lifting. *Arch Ophthalmol* 2006;124:1251.

Walther C, et al. The effect of exercise training on endothelial function in cardiovascular disease in humans. *Exerc Sport Sci Rev* 2004;32:129.

Weinberg I, et al. The systolic blood pressure difference between arms and cardiovascular disease in the Framingham Heart Study. *Am J Med* 2014;127:209.

Williams PT, Franklin B. Vigorous exercise and diabetic, hypertensive, and hypercholesterolemia medication use. *Med Sci Sports Exerc* 2007;39:1933.

Wing RR, et al.; Look AHEAD Research Group. Cardiovascular effects of intensive lifestyle intervention in type 2 diabetes. *N Engl J Med* 2013;369:145.

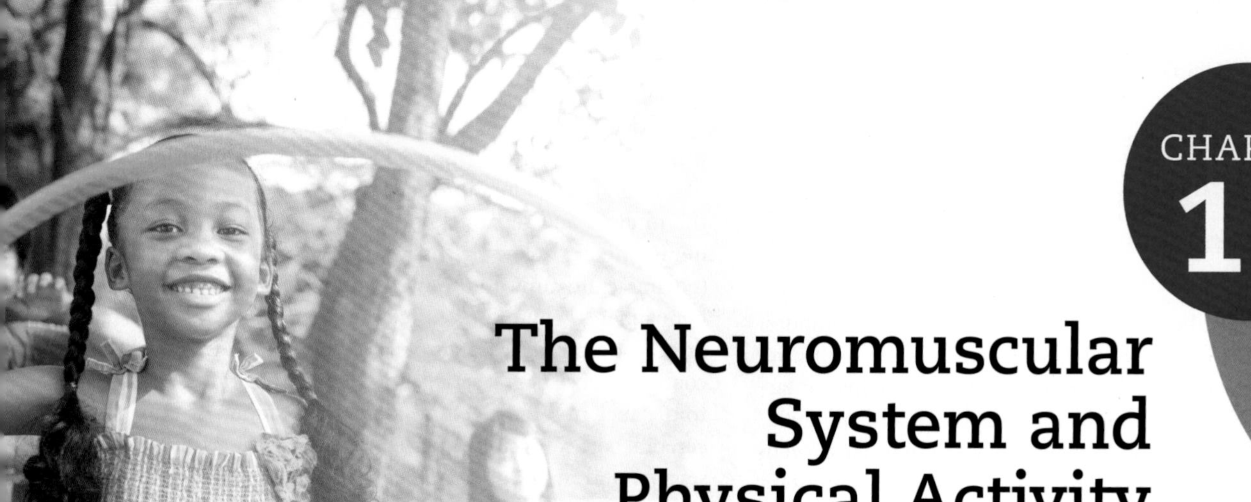

CHAPTER

11

The Neuromuscular System and Physical Activity

CHAPTER OBJECTIVES

- Identify three major structural components of the central nervous system that control human movement.
- Diagram the anterior motor neuron and discuss its role in human movement.
- Draw and label the basic components of a reflex arc.
- Define *motor unit*, *neuromuscular junction*, *autonomic nervous system*, *excitatory postsynaptic potential*, and *inhibitory postsynaptic potential*.
- Explain three factors associated with neuromuscular fatigue.
- Describe the main function of muscle spindles and Golgi tendon organs.
- Draw and label a skeletal muscle fiber's ultrastructural components.
- Describe the sequence of chemical and mechanical events during skeletal muscle contraction and relaxation.
- Contrast slow- and fast-twitch muscle fiber characteristics, including subdivisions.
- Outline muscle fiber–type distribution patterns among diverse groups of elite athletes.
- Explain how exercise training modifies muscle fibers and fiber types.

ANCILLARIES AT A GLANCE

Visit **http://thePoint.lww.com/MKKESS5e** to access the following resources.

- References: Chapter 11
- Interactive Question Bank
- Appendix SR-6: Additional Video Links
- Appendix SR-7: Nervous System Control, Sports Medicine Injuries, and Biomechanics
- Animation: Action Potential
- Animation: Fatigue Mechanism
- Animation: Lactic Acid Accumulation
- Animation: Muscle Contraction
- Animation: Nerve Synapse
- Animation: Neural Control of CV System
- Animation: Patella Tendon Stretch
- Animation: Proprioceptors: How Do They Work
- Animation: Sliding Filament Theory

PART 1 Neural Control of Human Movement

Similarities exist between the most advanced supercomputer and the brain's highly sophisticated and intricate multilayer system of neurons and their interconnections to diverse target tissues. Not surprisingly, the integrative and organizational complexity of the human nervous system far exceeds the capacity of many clusters of dedicated supercomputers, including the tremendous processing capacity of all public, private, and hybrid "cloud" processing power worldwide!

Interactive neural control mechanisms selectively process bits of sensory input in response to ever-changing internal and external stimuli. Human movements that require little force, and sophisticated movements that require large force, depend on the coordinated reception and integration of sensory neural input to transmit and coordinate signals to the effector organs—the muscles. For example, the effective application of force during a complex tennis serve, shot put, golf swing, or back somersault off a diving board requires a series of precise, coordinated neuromuscular movements patterns—not simply the strength of the muscles activated during the movement.

This chapter describes the neural control of human movement including the following:

1. Structural organization of the neuromotor system, with emphasis on the central and peripheral nervous systems
2. Neuromuscular transmission
3. Sensory input for muscular activity
4. Motor unit type, function, and activation

HUMAN NEUROMOTOR SYSTEM ORGANIZATION

The human nervous system consists of two major components:

1. **Central nervous system (CNS)**: includes the brain and spinal cord.
2. **Peripheral nervous system (PNS)**: composed of 12 cranial nerves and 31 pairs of spinal nerves (8 cervical, 12 thoracic, 5 lumbar, 5 sacral, 1 coccygeal), with each pair connecting to a specific body region.

Figure 11.1 presents an overview of these two components of the human nervous system.

Central Nervous System: The Brain

Figure 11.2A illustrates a lateral view of the brain's six main divisions:

1. Medulla oblongata
2. Pons
3. Midbrain
4. Cerebellum
5. Diencephalon
6. Telencephalon

Each of the 12 cranial nerves originates in one of these anatomic areas. **Figure 11.2B** shows a superior view of the brain. The longitudinal fissure or groove runs down the midline and separates the brain's right and left sides or **hemispheres**. Below the fissure, a large tract of nerve fibers (**corpus callosum**, not shown) connects the right and left hemispheres. The brain's outer portion, the **cerebral cortex** or **gray matter** (gray because nerve fibers lack a white myelin coating), consists of a series of folded convolutions. The bottom panel in **Figure 11.2C** depicts the four lobes of the cerebral cortex (occipital, parietal, temporal, and frontal) and sensory and motor areas and cerebellum (sometimes known as "little brain"). The **cerebellum** contains about 50% of the brain's total neurons, yet only 10% of cranial volume. It is involved in four crucial functions:

1. Balance and posture
2. Coordination of voluntary movements
3. Motor learning (coordinating and fine-tuning motor programs for "recall" to make accurate muscle movements)
4. Cognition (language)

The bony skull and a composite of four tough membranes called *meninges,* which contain a jellylike cushioning substance, surround the brain to protect it when an external force injures the brain, as occurs in sports-related **traumatic brain injury (TBI)**. This all too common sports injury, prevalent in contact sports at all ages and competitive levels, occurs approximately 300,000 times annually; most of these injuries classify as mild-to-moderate severity **concussions** (**www.headinjury.com/sports.htm**; **www.traumatic-braininjury.com**). Intracranial injuries also can occur from a bump, blow, or jolt to the head in vehicle accidents, violent physical confrontations, slips and falls, and military combat.

Central Nervous System—The Spinal Cord

The spinal cord (**Fig. 11.3A**) is about 45 cm long and 1 cm in diameter. It is encased by 33 vertebrae—7 cervical, 12 thoracic, 5 lumbar, 5 sacral, and 4 coccygeal. The 12 pairs of peripheral nerves, grouped into cervical, thoracic, lumbar, and sacral sections according to their location along the spine, exit the spinal cord through a small hole or foramen at the juncture between each pair of vertebrae (**Fig. 11.3C**).

The spinal cord's unique anatomical design allows extreme vertebral movement without affecting spinal nerve function. Twenty-four fibrocartilage **intervertebral discs** separate adjacent vertebrae and, under normal circumstances, provide cushioning and act as a shock absorber protective mechanism. Unfortunately, a disc can bulge into the space occupied by that segment's spinal nerve (**Fig. 11.4**), compressing it and causing pain. **Figure 11.4** shows a normal lumbar disc (left) and a **herniated disc**. In the latter, a portion of the nucleus pulposus consisting of gel-like structures moves out of its normal enclosure to impinge on a spinal nerve, compressing it and causing referred or radiating pain "downstream" in areas the nerve innervates (e.g., lower back, buttocks, back of the

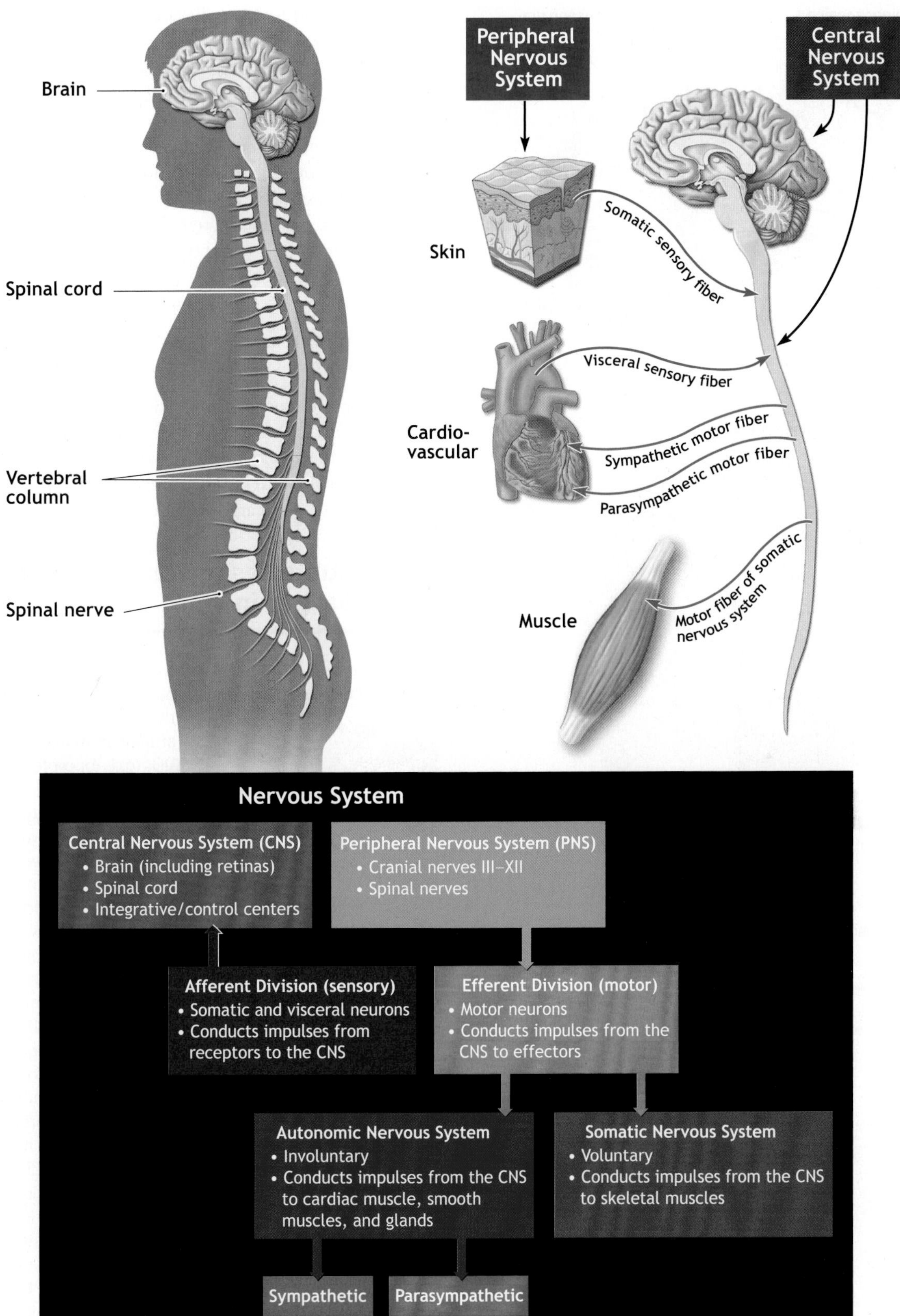

FIGURE 11.1 Two main divisions of the human nervous system. The central nervous system (CNS) contains the brain including the retinas, spinal cord, and integrating and control centers; the peripheral nervous system (PNS) consists of 12 cranial nerves and 31 pairs of spinal nerves, with each pair connecting to a specific body region (8 cervical, 12 thoracic, 5 lumbar, 5 sacral, 1 coccygeal). The PNS further subdivides into the afferent (sensory) and efferent (motor) divisions. The efferent division consists of the somatic nervous system and autonomic nervous system (sympathetic and parasympathetic divisions). (Adapted with permission from McArdle WD, Katch FI, Katch VL. *Exercise Physiology: Nutrition, Energy, and Human Performance*. 8th Ed. Baltimore: Wolters Kluwer Health, 2015.)

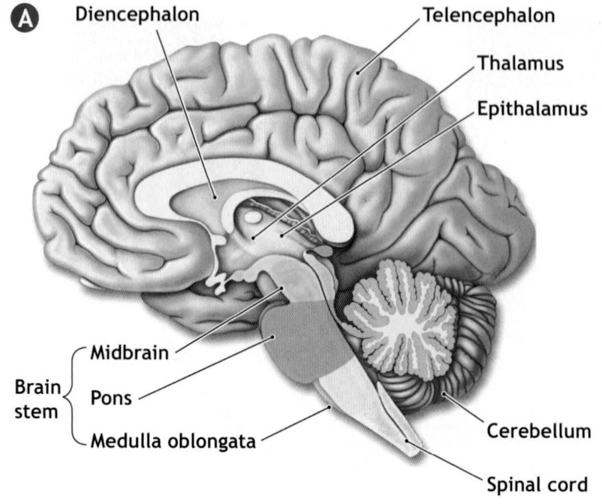

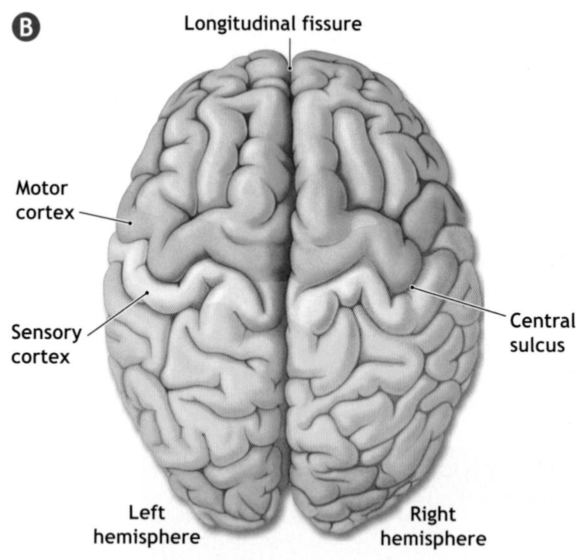

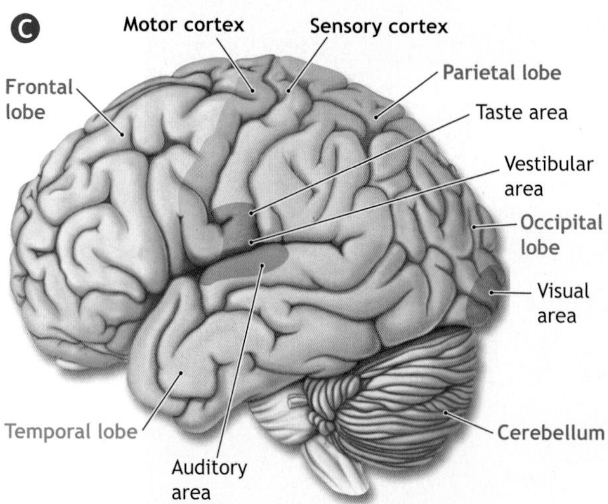

FIGURE 11.2 **A.** Principal six divisions of the brain, lateral view. **B.** Superior view of the brain. **C.** Four lobes of the cerebral cortex including the cerebellum shown in darker blue. (Reprinted with permission from McArdle WD, Katch FI, Katch VL. *Exercise Physiology: Nutrition, Energy, and Human Performance*. 8th Ed. Baltimore: Wolters Kluwer Health, 2015.)

leg [sciatica], and heel into the foot). This cascade of events can disrupt motor control. If the condition persists with significant muscle weakness (e.g., inability to raise and lower the body vertically off the ball of one foot, or numbness in the leg and foot area), surgical repair or removal of the offending herniated disc may be needed to relieve the pressure and pain, although it is not a foolproof solution.

In cross-section (**Fig. 11.3B**), the spinal cord shows its H-shaped core of gray matter. The limbs of this core, the ventral (anterior) and dorsal (posterior) horns, contain principally three types of nerves:

1. Interneurons
2. Sensory neurons
3. Motor neurons

Motor efferent neurons conduct impulses outward from the brain or spinal cord. They exit the cord through the ventral root to supply extrafusal and intrafusal skeletal muscle fibers. **Sensory afferent neurons** enter the spinal cord via the dorsal root and carry impulses from sensory receptors

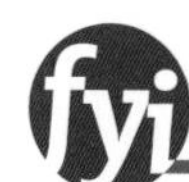

Strategies to Relieve Lower Back Pain

For the one in four Americans who during their lifetime experiences some form of lower back pain, the first attempt at pain relief includes nonsteroidal anti-inflammatory drugs or NSAIDs (e.g., ibuprofen [Motrin, Advil], aspirin [Ascriptin], naproxen [Aleve, Naprosyn]). NSAIDs stop cyclooxygenase enzymes, commonly referred as COX enzymes, from working. COX enzymes accelerate production of the hormonelike molecule prostaglandin, which causes pain sensations by irritating sensitive nerve endings. Tylenol (acetaminophen), not an NSAID, is a common alternative pain reliever. Most popular prescription-only NSAIDs include Celebrex (celecoxib), Voltaren (dislofenac), Mobic (meloxicarn), and Relafen (nabumetone. Reliance on long-term NSAID use has undesirable side effects. Other pain relief strategies include muscle relaxants like Flexeril, and Zanaflex, and oral corticosteroids (Medrol [methylprednisolone]). Although opioids and narcotic drugs provide relief for long-lasting chronic pain conditions, these drugs act in part to suppress pain receptor activity in brain and neural cells. Corticosteroid medications injected into the level of spinal nerve roots or facet joints also relieve pain. If drug relief is unsuccessful, minimally invasive surgical discectomy (removal of herniated disc substances pressing on a spinal nerve root) or laminectomy (removal of a section of vertebral bone lamina, the spongy tissue between spine discs) may be required. A "live" minimally invasive lumbar discectomy to relieve the source of recurrent lower back pain when the alternative drug interventions no longer provided relief can be viewed at **www.orlive.com/baptisthealth/videos/minimally-invasive-lumbar-discectomy?view=displayPageNLM**.

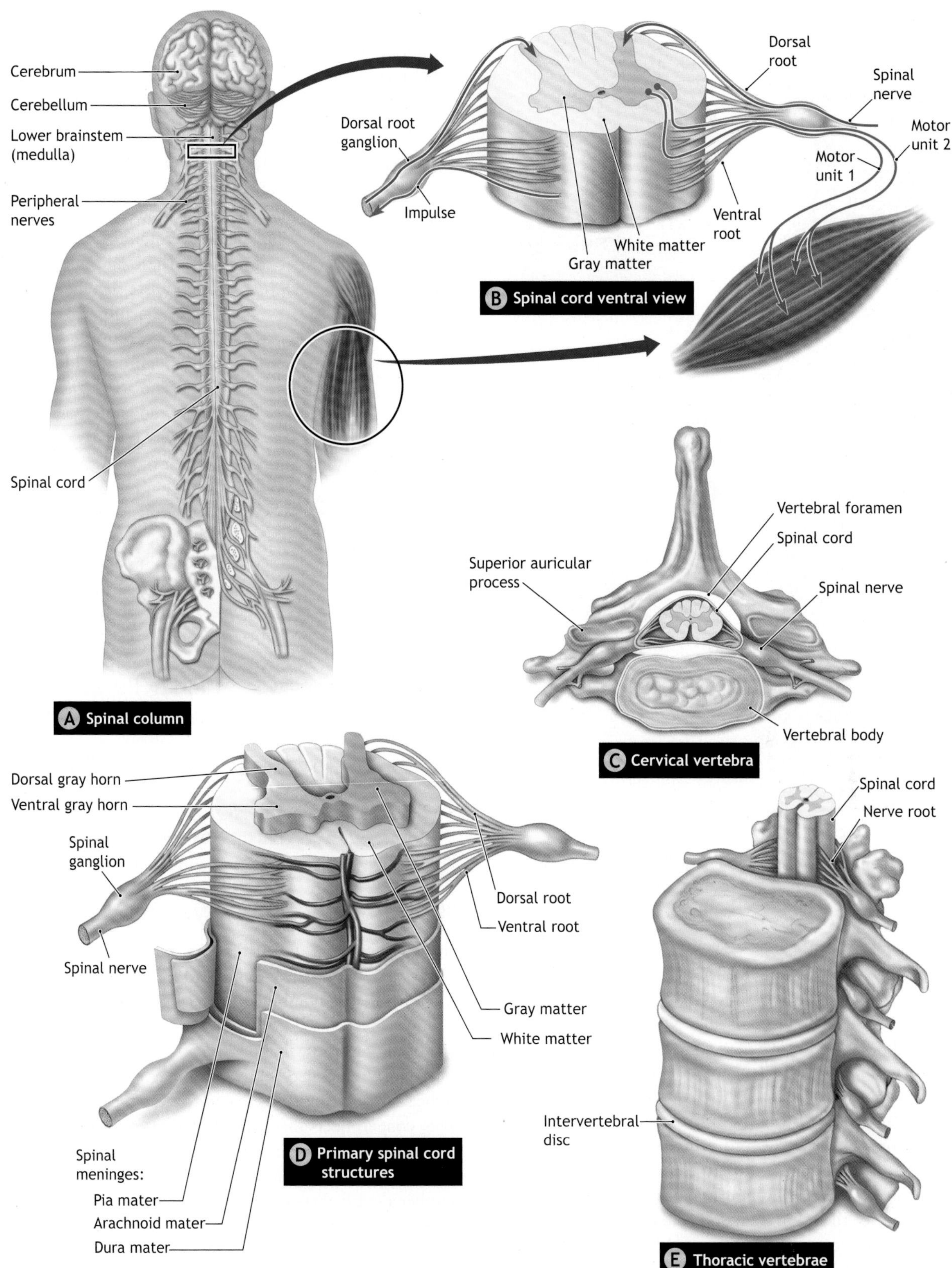

FIGURE 11.3 **A.** Human spinal cord showing the peripheral nerves. **B.** Ventral view of a spinal cord section to illustrate dorsal and ventral root neural pathways and nerve impulse direction. **C.** Junction of two lumbar vertebral bodies and a cross-section through one cervical vertebra. **D.** Primary spinal cord structures. **E.** Enlarged view of the junction of three thoracic vertebral bodies. (Adapted with permission from McArdle WD, Katch FI, Katch VL. *Exercise Physiology: Nutrition, Energy, and Human Performance*. 8th Ed. Baltimore: Wolters Kluwer Health, 2015.)

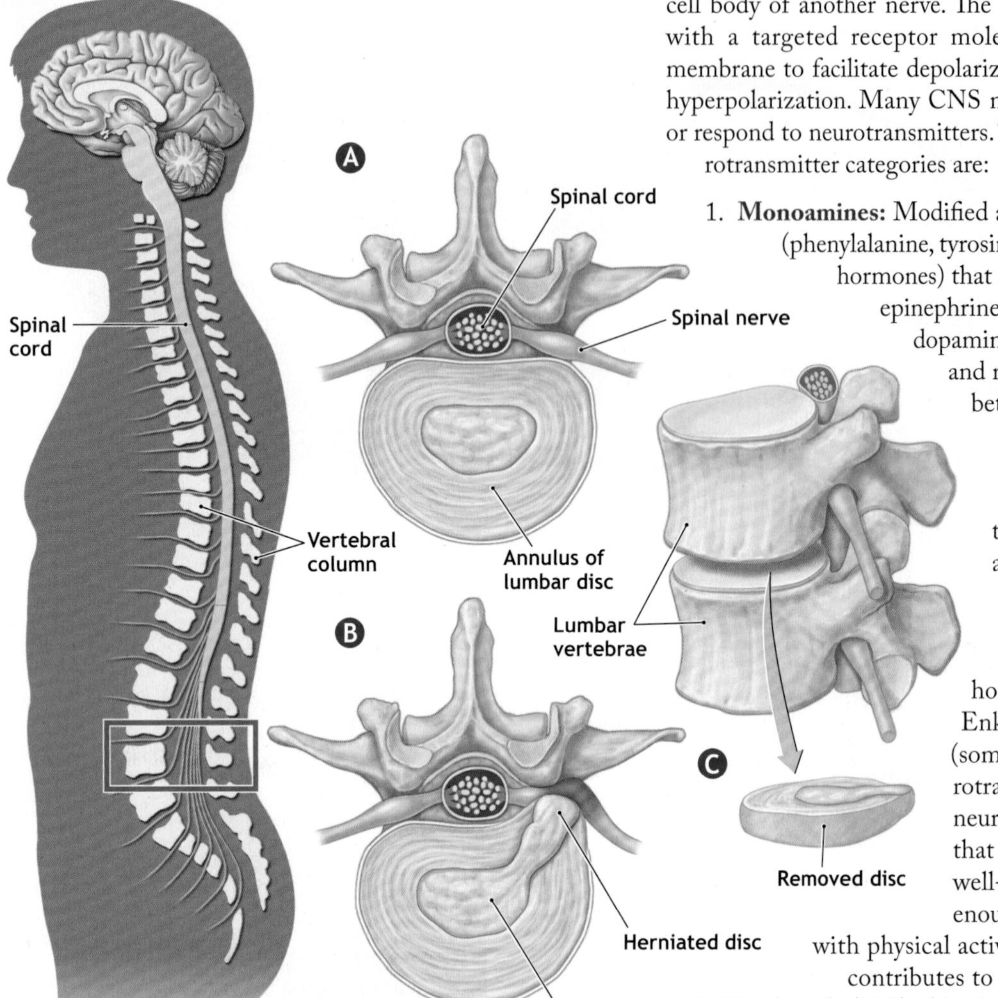

FIGURE 11.4 **A.** Normal lumbar disc. **B.** Herniated disc impinging on a spinal nerve. **C.** Surgically removed disc.

toward the CNS. An area of white matter with ascending and descending nerve tracts within the cord surrounds the gray core. The ascending nerve tracts within the spinal cord transmit sensory information from peripheral sensory receptors to the brain. Tracts of nerve tissue descend from the brain and terminate at neurons in the spinal cord. An important set of nerve fibers, the **pyramidal tract**, transmits impulses downward within the spinal cord. By direct routes and interconnecting spinal cord neurons, these nerves eventually excite motor neurons that control skeletal muscles. **Extrapyramidal tract** neurons originate in the primary upper motor cortex of the brain stem and connect at all spinal cord levels. These neurons control posture and provide a continual background level of neuromuscular tone in contrast to discrete movements stimulated by pyramidal tract nerves.

Brain Neurotransmitters

Nerves communicate by releasing at their terminal ends chemical messengers called **neurotransmitters** that diffuse across the **synapse** or junction between one nerve end and the cell body of another nerve. The neurotransmitter combines with a targeted receptor molecule on the postsynaptic membrane to facilitate depolarization or, in some instances, hyperpolarization. Many CNS neurons in the brain release or respond to neurotransmitters. Three important brain neurotransmitter categories are:

1. **Monoamines:** Modified aromatic amino acids (phenylalanine, tyrosine, tryptophan, thyroid hormones) that include epinephrine, norepinephrine, serotonin, histamine, and dopamine. These substances amplify and modulate signaling patterns between neurons to increase their effectiveness.
2. **Neuropeptides:** Short amino acid sequences that modulate synaptic activity from larger precursor molecules include arginine, vasopressin, and angiotensin II (also act as hormones [see Chapter 12]). Enkephalins and endorphins (sometimes called opioid neurotransmitters) represent other neuronal signaling molecules that produce a general sense of well-being. Release of endogenous opioid neurotransmitters with physical activity likely contributes to the exercise "high."
3. **Nitric oxide (NO):** Also known as nitrogen monoxide (one oxygen atom in NO). Neurons in the CNS and other cell types contain NO receptors that serve as cardiovascular system signaling molecules.

Peripheral Nervous System

The PNS consists of 31 pairs of spinal nerves (8 cervical, 12 thoracic, 5 lumbar, 5 sacral, and 1 coccygeal) and 12 pairs of cranial nerves numbered I through XII (**Fig 11.5**).

Note that CI is the first nerve from the cervical region, and it and CII serve visual and olfactory functions and belong to the CNS. Cranial nerves emerge through foramina or fissures in the skull or cranium. These nerves, as do their spinal counterparts, contain fibers that transmit sensory and/or motor information. Their neurons innervate muscles or glands or transmit impulses from sensory areas into the brain. A specific letter and number identify these nerves (e.g., C-I, first nerve from the cervical region; T-IV, fourth nerve in the thoracic region).

The exact location of the spinal nerves is traced by mapping the tissues they innervate. An injury to a specific area of the cord produces predictable neurologic damage. For example, quadriplegia almost always results from damage to the upper thoracic vertebra and corresponding descending nerve tract.

The PNS includes afferent nerves that relay sensory information from muscles, joints, skin, and bones *toward* the brain and efferent nerves that transmit information *away* from

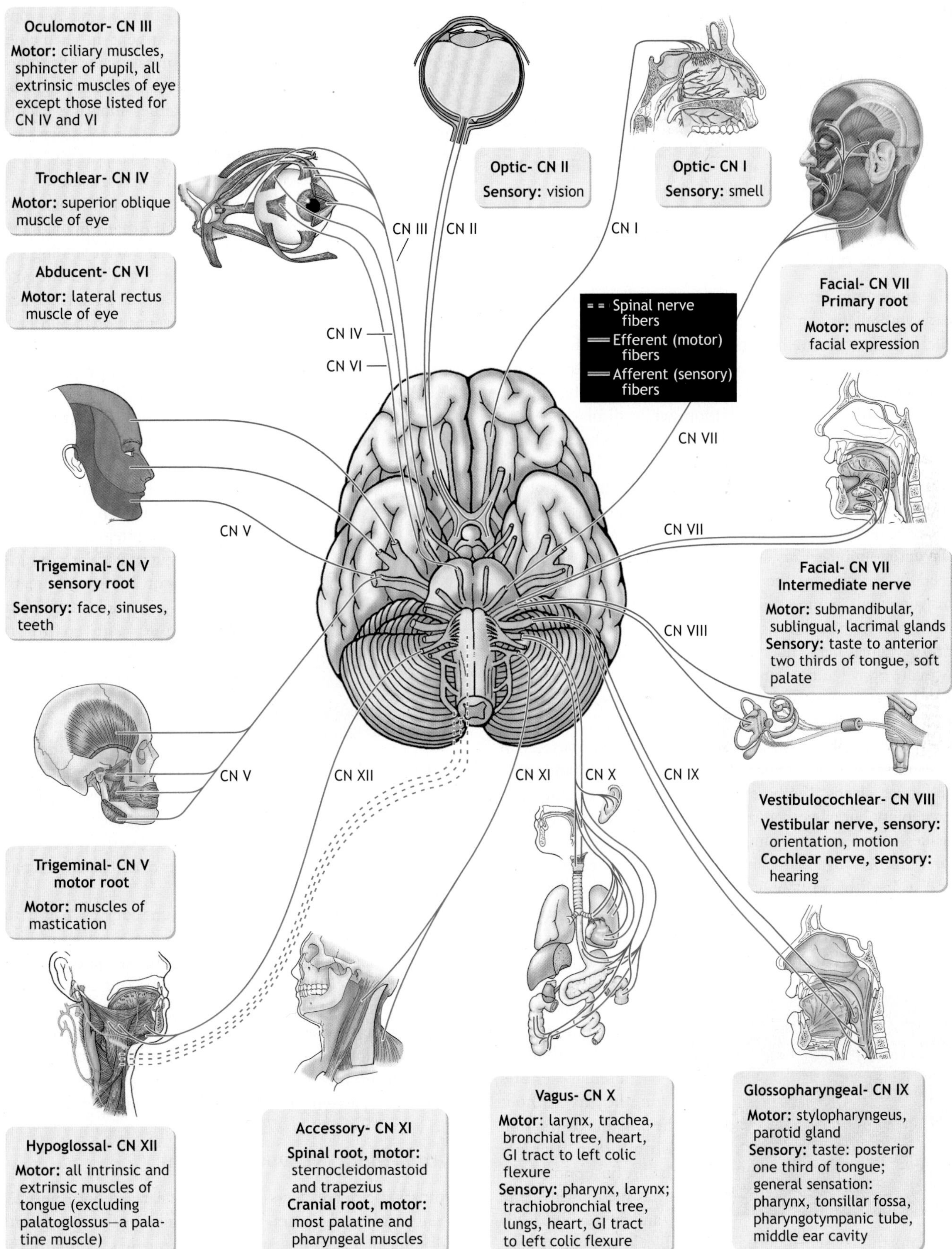

FIGURE 11.5 Distribution of the 12 cranial nerves. (Reprinted with permission from Moore KL, et al., eds. *Clinically Oriented Anatomy*. 7th Ed. Baltimore: Lippincott Williams & Wilkins, 2013.)

the brain to glands and muscles. The somatic and autonomic nervous systems consist of efferent neurons (**Fig 11.5**).

Somatic Nervous System

The **somatic nervous system**, a component of the PNS, innervates voluntary skeletal muscle. Somatic efferent nerve firing excites muscle activation; autonomic nerve firing (discussed in the next section) either excites or inhibits activation.

Sympathetic and Parasympathetic Nervous Systems

The autonomic nervous system consists of sympathetic and parasympathetic components. These neurons operate in parallel but use structurally distinct pathways and differ in their transmitter systems. The two systems operate independently in some functions and interact cooperatively in others.

Sympathetic fiber distribution, while displaying some overlap with parasympathetic fibers, supplies the heart, smooth muscle, sweat glands, and viscera. Parasympathetic nervous system fibers leave the brainstem and sacral segments of the spinal cord to supply the thorax, abdomen, and pelvic regions.

Regions of the medulla, pons, and diencephalon control the autonomic nervous system. Fibers that originate in the medullary region of the lower brainstem control variables instrumental in prescribing fitness training programs for most people (blood pressure, heart rate, pulmonary ventilation), whereas nerve fibers of the upper hypothalamic origin regulate body temperature.

Efferent nerves of the autonomic nervous system activate viscera and other tissues on a subconscious level. Autonomic nerves innervate smooth muscle (involuntary muscle) in intestines, sweat and salivary glands, myocardium, and some endocrine glands. The heart and intestines display automatic excitability, but one can also exert conscious control over these tissues under some circumstances. For example, individuals who practice yoga or meditation can modify their heart rate and regional blood flow on command. In hypnosis (from an ancient word for "trance"), a state of heightened awareness and focused concentration can manipulate pain perception, access repressed material, and "reprogram" some behaviors. Some champion weightlifters apply self-hypnosis before attempting heavy lifts to focus all their muscular efforts on the lift without the possible distraction of discomfort in attempting the lift (just prior to the lift as the muscles tense and prepare for an all-out effort). This self-induced "trance" blocks out superfluous neural input that might interfere with a maximal effort.

See the animation "Neural Control of CV System" on **http://thePoint.lww.com/MKKESS5e** for a demonstration of this process.

Conscious modulation of aspects of autonomic nervous system function offers alternative treatment in medicine, such as control of hypertension and stress-related disorders through biofeedback techniques applicable to certain sports. Competitors in archery and other target-shooting events consciously modify their cardiovascular and respiratory patterns, so normal breathing and pulse rate temporarily "stop" during the crucial steadying phase of the performance.

For example, an archer attempts to minimize postural sway preceding the arrow release (called the moment of loose). The time interval is important to control between holding the breath and the first finger movement to initiate loose. The goal is to release the arrow in the middle phase of the normal cardiac cycle, with the body held in a precise position to optimize the release phase. Once the archer sets in the shooting position, the bowstring is pulled back to the neck region just under the chin. For men who weigh 130 to 150 lb, the draw weight equals 30 to 40 lb; for larger men who exceed 180 lb, the draw weight increases to 60 to 70 lb. Draw weight values for women average about 10 to 20 lb less. In essence, not only must posture be maintained under exquisite neuromuscular control but also a strength component must integrate with the neuromuscular component. The idea of breath hold and heart rate control is to "unteather" or negate any influence these variables might negatively impinge neuromuscular and strength components. This allows the archer to concentrate on precisely hitting a 48-inch diameter target 86.4 yards away with a 4.8-inch center ring standing 51.4 inches above the ground! This ultimate test of neuromuscular control with considerable parasympathetic involvement takes years of dedicated practice and refinement.

The autonomic nervous system functions as a unit to maintain constancy in the internal environment. **Figure 11.6** illustrates the autonomic nervous system's **sympathetic** and **parasympathetic** divisions. Sympathetic nerve fibers mediate excitation, and parasympathetic activation inhibits excitation except for vagal parasympathetic excitation of gastrointestinal motility and tone and pancreatic insulin secretion. In contrast to the somatic nervous system, some cell bodies or ganglia of sympathetic and parasympathetic neurons exist outside the CNS.

Sympathetic Nervous System

Sympathetic nerve fibers supply the heart, smooth muscle, sweat glands, and viscera. These neurons exit the spinal cord and enter a series of ganglia near the cord's **sympathetic chain**. The nerves terminate relatively far from the target organ in **adrenergic fiber** endings that release norepinephrine. Sympathetic nervous system excitation occurs during fight-or-flight situations that require whole-body arousal for emergencies. Autonomic sympathetic stimulation accelerates

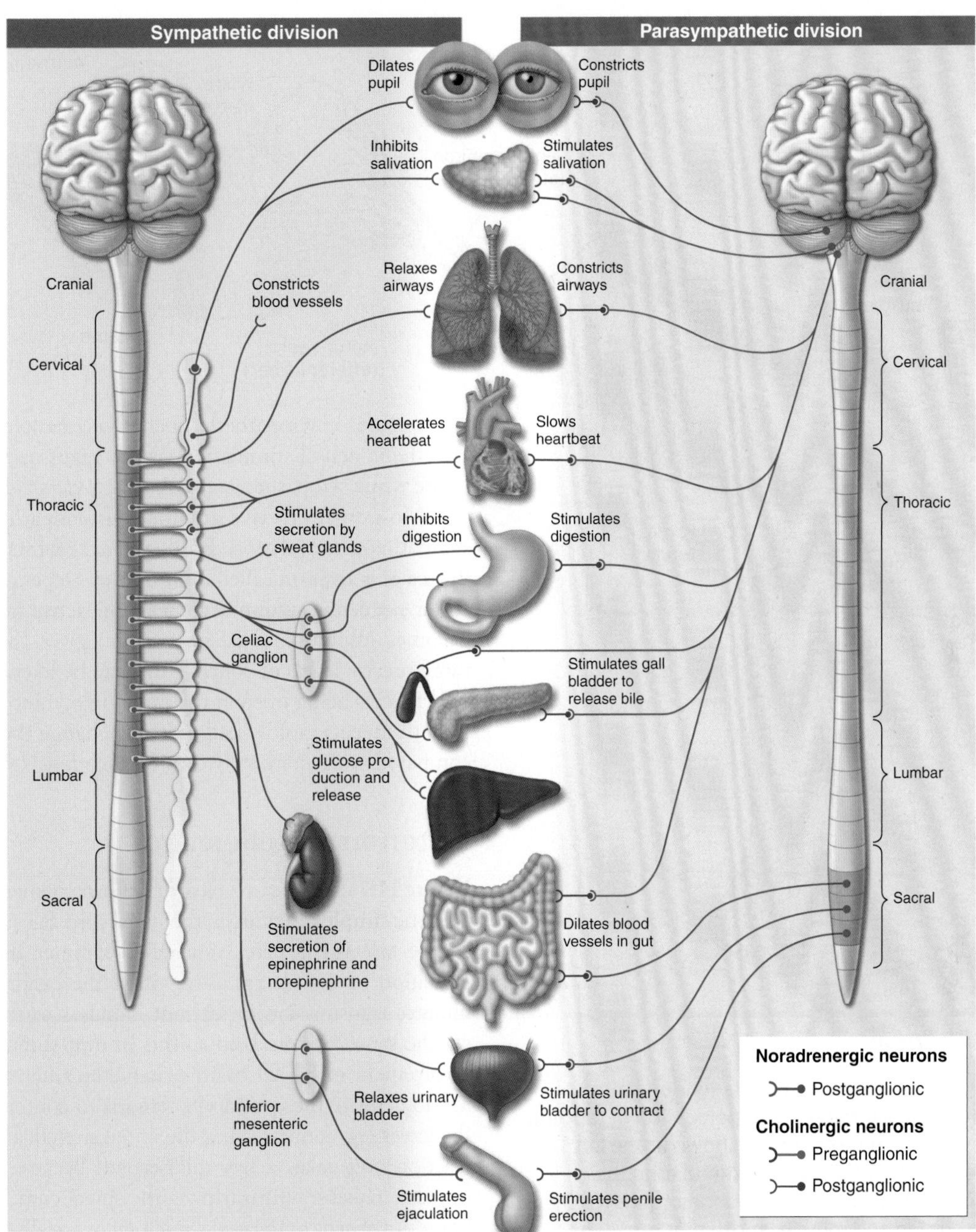

Comparison of effects of sympathetic and parasympathetic activation on end organs		
End organ	**Sympathetic effects**	**Parasympathetic effects**
Skeletal muscle	Increase blood flow	Decrease blood flow
Ventilation	Increase	Decrease
Sweat glands	Increase perspiration	No effect
Heart	Increase force and contraction rate	Decrease force and contraction rate
GI tract motility	Decrease	Increase
Eyes	Dilate pupils	Constrict pupils
Secretion of digestive juices	Decrease	Increase
Blood pressure	Increase mean pressure	Decrease mean pressure
Airways	Increase diameter	Decrease diameter

FIGURE 11.6 The sympathetic and parasympathetic divisions of the autonomic nervous system: comparisons of effects of activation of each. The preganglionic inputs of both divisions use acetylcholine (ACh; *colored red*) as a neurotransmitter. The postganglionic parasympathetic innervation of the visceral organs also uses ACh, but postganglionic sympathetic innervation uses norepinephrine (NE; *colored blue*), with the exception of innervation of the sweat glands, which use ACh. The adrenal medulla receives preganglionic sympathetic innervation and secretes epinephrine into the bloodstream when activated. In general, sympathetic stimulation produces catabolic effects that prepare the body to "fight" or "flee," and parasympathetic stimulation produces anabolic responses that promote normal function and conserve energy. (Adapted with permission from Bear MF, et al. *Neuroscience: Exploring the Brain*. 3rd Ed. Baltimore: Lippincott Williams & Wilkins, 2006.)

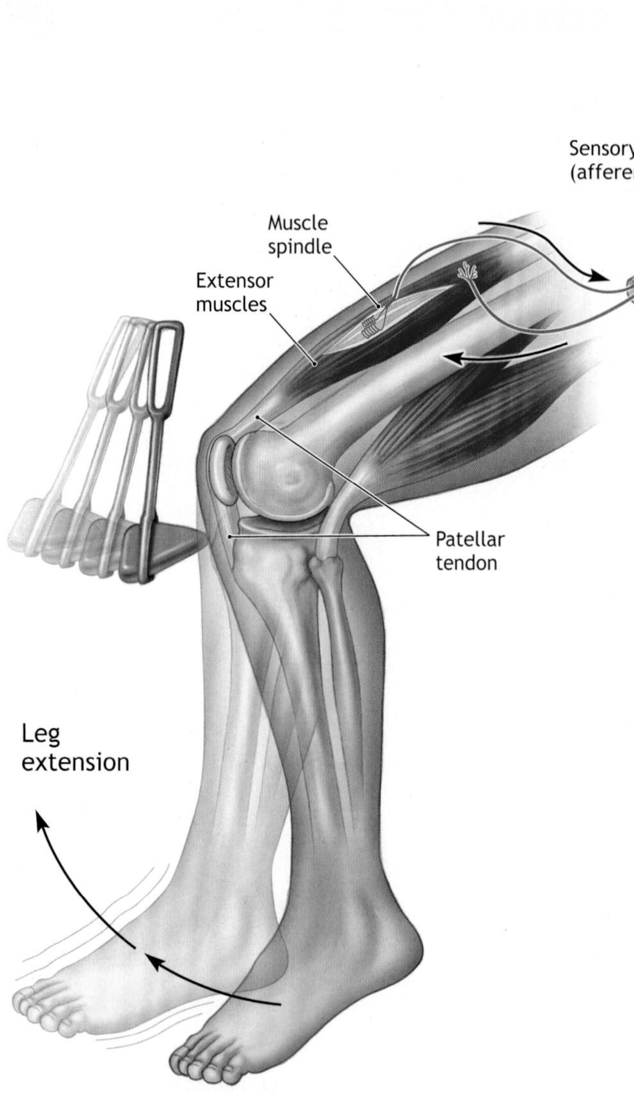

FIGURE 11.7 Schematic of the patella tendon stretch reflex (also called patellar reflex). Firm percussion or tapping of the patellar with the reflex hammer shown at the left draws the patella momentarily down, stimulating the muscle spindles' afferents and Golgi tendon organs (GTOs) by altering the stretch and muscle length that provokes a preprogrammed reflex contraction. The diagram only shows one side of the spinal nerve complex. (Reprinted with permission from McArdle WD, Katch FI, Katch VL. *Exercise Physiology: Nutrition, Energy, and Human Performance*. 8th Ed. Baltimore: Wolters Kluwer Health, 2015.)

breathing and heart rate almost instantaneously; pupils of the eye dilate, and blood flows from the skin to deeper tissues in anticipation of a perceived bodily challenge.

Parasympathetic Nervous System

Parasympathetic nerve fibers exit the brainstem and sacral segments of the spinal cord to supply the thorax, abdomen, and pelvic regions. Parasympathetic nerve endings release the neurotransmitter acetylcholine (**ACh; cholinergic fibers**). The postganglionic parasympathetic nerve fibers are located close to the organs they innervate and produce effects *opposite* those of sympathetic fibers. For example, parasympathetic neural stimulation via the vagus nerve *slows* heart rate while sympathetic stimulation *accelerates* heart rate.

Most organs receive simultaneous sympathetic and parasympathetic stimulation. Both systems maintain a constant degree of activation called **neural tone**. Depending on physiologic need, one system becomes more active while the other becomes inhibited. Dual innervation gives the end organs more precise levels of control. This can be likened to hot and cold faucets being open at the same time; minor adjustments in both faucets rapidly and precisely change the temperature compared with alternately turning each faucet on or off.

Autonomic Reflex Arc

Figure 11.7 illustrates a typical neural arrangement for a monosynaptic **simple reflex arc** in the spinal cord. Sensory input (e.g., a knee tap with a percussion reflex hammer and subsequent excitation of muscle spindles within the quadriceps muscle) initiates transmission of afferent impulses to the spinal cord via the sensory (dorsal) root. This in turn stimulates, without involvement of higher brain centers, the anterior motor neuron to activate the quadriceps femoris to contract and extend the lower leg, counteracting the initial stretch. The "knee-jerk" reaction only takes a few milliseconds because the triggered impulse makes a return trip via the spinal cord, bypassing the brain. An absent or delayed stretch reflex usually indicates possible neurologic or neuromuscular dysfunction to spinal nerves and their innervations, or injuries to the knee and leg.

A **polysynaptic reflex arc** refers to the neural synapses in either the spinal cord or the brain interfacing through about 100 billion **interneurons**. This reflex arc excludes other parts of the PNS that distribute or relay information to various cord levels. The interneurons "fire" from releasing the excitatory neurotransmitter glutamate that helps to initiate a reflex response. The impulse then passes over the motor root pathway through anterior motor neurons to the effector organ. Interneurons also can release the abundant inhibitory neurotransmitter **GABA (gamma-aminobutyric acid)** at synapses to reduce or stop a particular tissue from responding as, for example, a muscle in a reflex action.

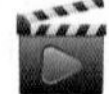
See the animation "Nerve Synapse" on **http://thePoint.lww.com/MKKESS5e** for a review of this process.

Types of Motor Neurons

The large diameters of anterior motor neurons, termed type A or α fibers, range between 8 and 20 μm (1 μm = one-millionth [0.000001] of a meter). Diameters of other smaller type A fibers (γ efferent motor neurons) do not exceed 10 μm. Their conduction velocities equal about half of α fibers. γ-Efferent fibers connect with proprioceptors (special stretch sensors) in skeletal muscle to detect minute changes in muscle fiber length.

Source: Image excerpted with permission from McArdle WD, Katch FI, Katch VL. *Exercise Physiology: Nutrition, Energy, and Human Performance*. 8th Ed. Baltimore: Wolters Kluwer Health, 2015.

Another example of a simple reflex arc occurs when a person accidentally touches a hot object. Stimulation of pain receptors in the fingers fires sensory information over afferent fibers to the spinal cord to activate efferent motor fibers to remove the hand from the hot object. Concurrently, the signal transmits via interneurons up the cord to the sensory area in the brain that actually "feels" the pain. The various operational levels for sensory input, processing, and motor output, including the reflex action just described, explain how the hand withdraws from the hot object *before* the person perceives pain. Reflex actions in the spinal cord and other subconscious areas of the CNS control many muscle functions. These reflex actions even operate for people who have spinal cords severed above the level required for the reflex.

Complex Reflexes

Complex spinal reflexes involve multiple synapses and muscle groups. Consider the situation of stepping on a tack with the left foot. Almost simultaneously as the tack pierces the skin, the right leg straightens to remove weight from the injured foot, which lifts off the ground. **Figure 11.8** illustrates the neural and motor pathways activated in this complex, five-step sequence termed the **crossed-extensor reflex**:

Step 1. The tack stimulates pain receptors in the skin. The receptors transmit the message to the spinal cord via the sensory nerve.

Step 2. Sensory neurons branch to each side of the cord to activate interneurons in the gray matter.

Step 3. Interneurons synapse with motor neurons, innervating both flexor and extensor muscles in each leg.

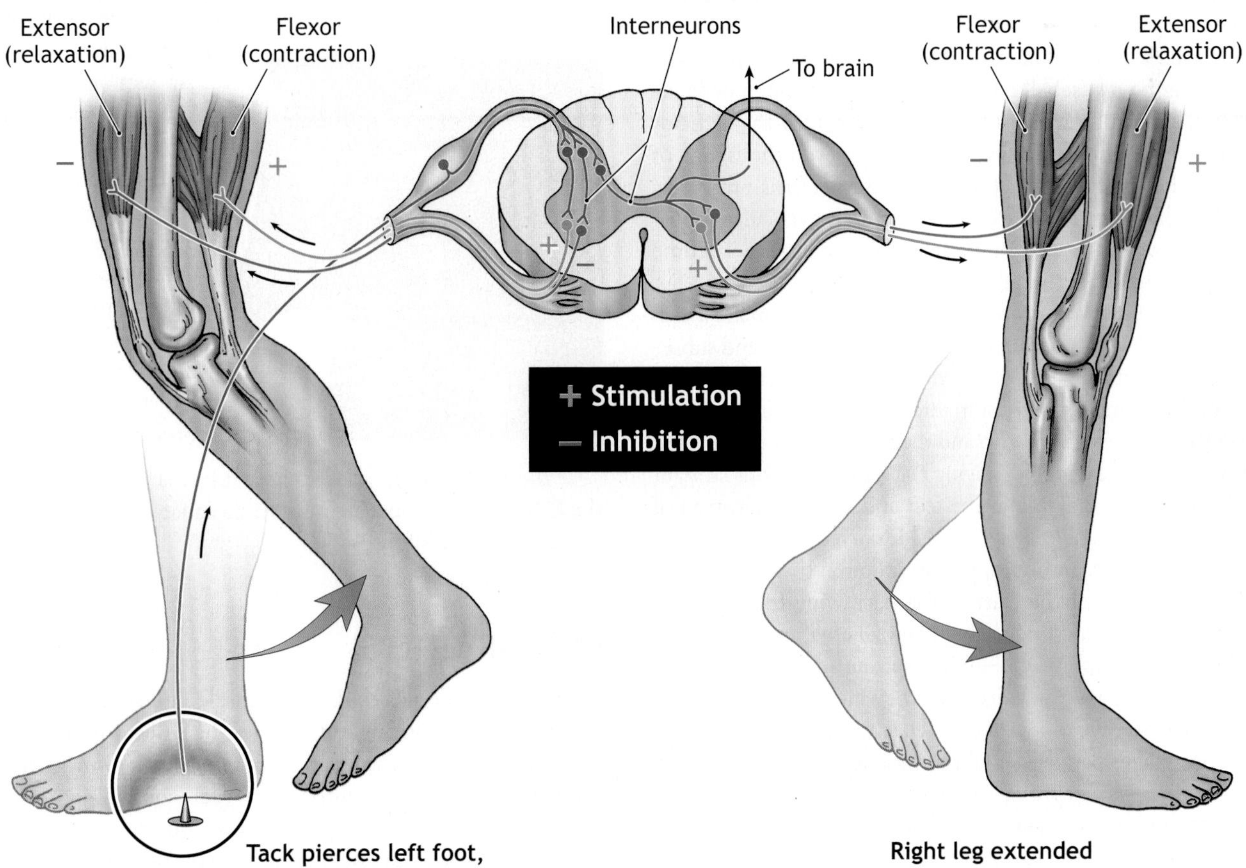

FIGURE 11.8 Crossed-extensor reflex in both legs represents complex reflex with multiple synapses and muscle groups.

Step 4. Inhibition and stimulation of appropriate leg flexor and extensor muscles cause concurrent rapid extension of the uninjured limb and flexion to remove the injured limb.

Step 5. Interneuron connections simultaneously activate neural pathways to transmit information to appropriate sensory areas of the brain where the pain is "felt."

Learned Reflexes

The knee-jerk and crossed-extensor reflexes occur automatically and require no learning. Practice facilitates other more complex reflex patterns as in most sport performances and occupational tasks. Consider a trained office worker who types 90 words a minute. At an average of five letters per word, this requires six to eight keystrokes per second. The sight of a word to type initiates a series of rapid hand and finger movements that require little conscious effort. A beginning typist, in contrast, proceeds slowly since thought must be directed to the position of each key along the keyboard and proper execution and sequencing of wrist and finger movements. As neuromuscular pathways become "ingrained" through proper or meaningful practice, the typing movements progressively become reflex actions as the beginner approaches expert status. People who routinely send text messages have mastered the proper sequencing of finger and hand movements, so the desired outcome occurs essentially automatically.

Improving a Sports Skill—Perfect Practice Produces Perfect Performance

Improving a sports skill, no matter how simple it appears—like swinging a baseball bat to contact a "fast" pitch or kicking a soccer ball with just the right speed into the right or left side of the net—requires hundreds or even thousands of practice hours to *engrain* the movement patterns until they become flawless in execution. Practicing a particular motor task "grooves" the neuromuscular movements to become automatic, no longer requiring conscious control.

Unfortunately, improper practice also can automate a task to produce less than optimal neuromuscular actions and subsequent poor performance. Most individuals who practice the golf swing, for example, do so by reinforcing poor neuromuscular actions. It starts with the grip and the first 6 inches of the takeaway in the backswing by moving the hands and arms straight back along a parallel line to the feet and shoulders, instead of starting the movement along an inside curved path. Setting up in the stance with an improper grip followed by a rapid cocking of the wrists at the start of the backswing fuels a recipe for disaster. Instead of pounding one ball after another on the range—often hours on end—both aspiring and advanced golfers should purposely practice correct swing mechanics, hopefully under the eye of a proficient coach or teacher. The adage "practice makes perfect" should be amended to this five-word mnemonic—"*perfect practice produces perfect performance.*" If one practices an incorrect movement pattern, no matter how simple or complex, that movement pattern becomes "learned"—in essence, perfecting poor mechanics and grooving improper movement sequencing produce a poor movement outcome!

Nerve Supply to Muscle

The terminal branches of each neuron innervate at least one of the body's approximately 250 million muscle fibers. The typical individual possesses about 420,000 motor neurons so a single nerve usually supplies many individual muscle fibers. In general, the branches of a nerve within a muscle pass to specific localized groups of motor units. In multiple group muscles, for example, the quadriceps, four separate muscles act in concert to perform the main muscle action, with no single muscle responsible for the full movement. *The number of muscle fibers per motor neuron, termed the* ***innervation ratio****, generally relates to a muscle's particular movement function.* The finger contains 120 motor units that control 41,000 muscle fibers, while the medial gastrocnemius muscle (calf) has 580 motor units that innervate 1.03 million fibers. The ratio of muscle fibers per motor unit averages 340:1 for finger muscles, 1800:1 for the gastrocnemius muscle, and only 10:1 for the precise movement functions of the eye muscles. The ratio in the larynx is an even lower 1:1. Muscles with a low innervation ratio can produce very delicate movements because each neuron only has to produce a small increment in force. In contrast when the innervation ratio is relatively large, the neuron can create a substantially large force output as in more general, gross motor movements. Consequently, motor neuron size impacts motor unit force capacity. Stated somewhat differently, the largest axons supply more muscle fibers than the smallest axons, and there is a strong relation between motor unit force and the size of the motor neuron. This is an important principle because the smooth force gradation during muscle action depends on the orderly and systematic recruitment of more forceful motor units and their rate of recruitment. During any muscular activity, the spinal cord represents the major processing and distribution center for motor control.

The next sections address how information processed in the CNS activates specific muscles to cause appropriate, specialized motor responses.

MOTOR UNITS

A **motor unit** describes skeletal muscle fibers and their corresponding, innervating **anterior (alpha) motor neuron**. *The motor unit thus represents movement's functional unit.* A whole muscle contains many motor units, each containing a single motor neuron and its composite muscle fibers.

The muscle fibers belonging to a particular motor unit are scattered over subregions of the muscle; fibers from one motor unit intersperse among fibers of other motor units.

To minimize mechanical stress, the consequence of dispersion allows forces to spread over a larger muscle area.

Motor Unit Anatomy

Anterior Motor Neuron

Figure 11.9 illustrates an anterior (alpha) motor neuron with its three main parts: cell body, axon, and dendrites. The cell's unique architectural design permits the transmission of electrochemical impulses from the spinal cord to muscle. The **cell body**, located within the spinal cord's gray matter, houses the **control center**, the structures involved in replicating and transmitting the genetic code. The **axon** extends from the cord and delivers an impulse to the muscle fibers it innervates. Short neural branches called **dendrites** receive impulses through numerous spinal cord connections and conduct them to the cell body. The two longest nerves in the body, about one meter (3 feet) in length, include the sciatic nerve and its branches and median and ulnar nerves. Some anatomists argue that because the sciatic nerve divides at about knee level into common peroneal and tibial branches, it no longer qualifies as a "one-piece" full sciatic nerve.

Nerve cells conduct impulses *in one direction only*, akin to a one-way street, down the axon away from the stimulation point. As the axon approaches the muscle, it branches with each terminal branch to innervate a single muscle fiber. A whole muscle contains numerous motor units, each with a single motor neuron and its complement of muscle fibers.

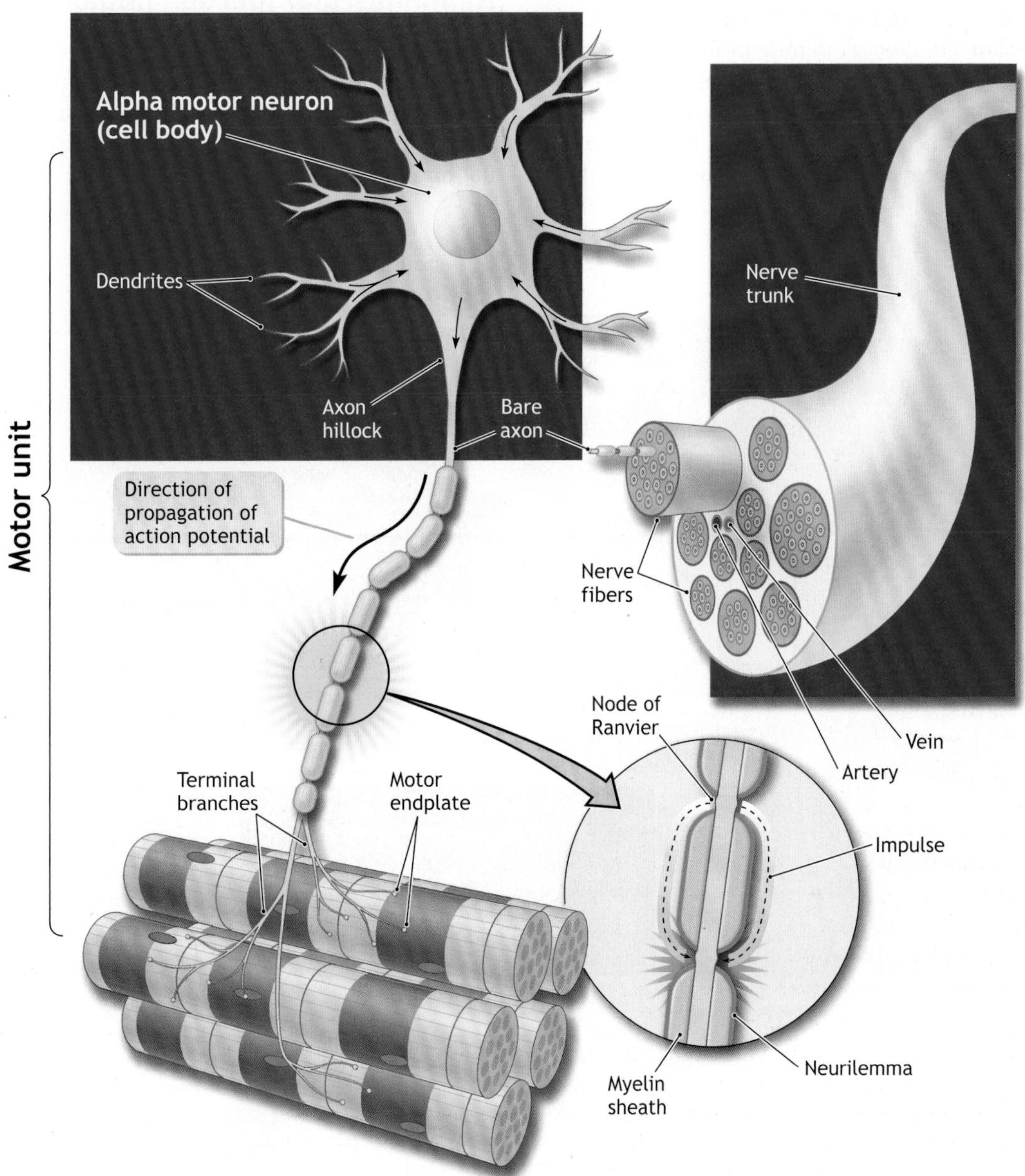

FIGURE 11.9 The anterior α-motor neuron consists of a cell body, axons, and dendrites. The *round inset* at the bottom right illustrates a node of Ranvier that permits impulses to jump from one node to the next as the electrical current travels toward the terminal branches at the motor end plate. (Reprinted with permission from McArdle WD, Katch FI, Katch VL. *Exercise Physiology: Nutrition, Energy, and Human Performance*. 8th Ed. Baltimore: Wolters Kluwer Health, 2015.)

The lipid-rich **myelin sheath** encircles the axon of nerve fibers that are either long in length or large in diameter. Portions of the sheath act as an electrical insulator that envelops the axon akin to plastic coating surrounding a copper electrical wire. The lipid-protein membrane myelin consists of approximately 75% lipids (cholesterol and phospholipid) and 25% proteins. Myelin's main function increases the speed of neural impulses along the myelinated fiber. This occurs because myelin increases electrical resistance across the cell membrane by a factor of 5000 and decreases capacitance by 10-fold this number. Fiber myelination thus keeps the electrical current from leaving the exposed axon while at the same time allowing a high signal transmission speed. The fat-containing molecules inhibit the propagation of electricity to make the signals jump from one section of myelin to the next. In the PNS, specialized **Schwann cells** encase the bare axon and then spiral around it. Myelin forms a large part of this sheath to insulate the axon. A thinner membrane, the **neurilemma**, covers the myelin sheath. **Nodes of Ranvier** interrupt the Schwann cells and myelin every 1 or 2 mm along the axon's length. Whereas myelin insulates the axon to the flow of ions, the nodes of Ranvier permit depolarization of the axon. The alternating sequence of myelin sheath and node of Ranvier allows impulses to "jump" from node to node (termed *saltatory conduction*), similar to signals progressing from one cellphone tower to the next, as electrical current travels toward terminal branches at the motor end plate. Nerve conduction in this manner accounts for the higher transmission velocity in myelinated compared with unmyelinated fibers. Degeneration of the myelin sheath produces peripheral neuropathy and disease. In multiple sclerosis, an autoimmune disease that affects approximately 200 people each week in the United States (**www.nationalmssociety.org**), destruction of the myelin sheath surrounding nerve fibers adversely affects neural pathways to the brain, spinal cord, and optic nerves. This interferes with vision, sensation, and body movements.

Neuromuscular Junction (Motor End Plate)

Figure 11.10 highlights the microanatomy of the **neuromuscular junction or motor end plate**, which provides interface between the end of a myelinated motor neuron and a muscle fiber (**http://thebrain.mcgill.ca/flash/i/i_06/i_06_m/i_06_m_mou/i_06_m_mou.html**). The neuromuscular

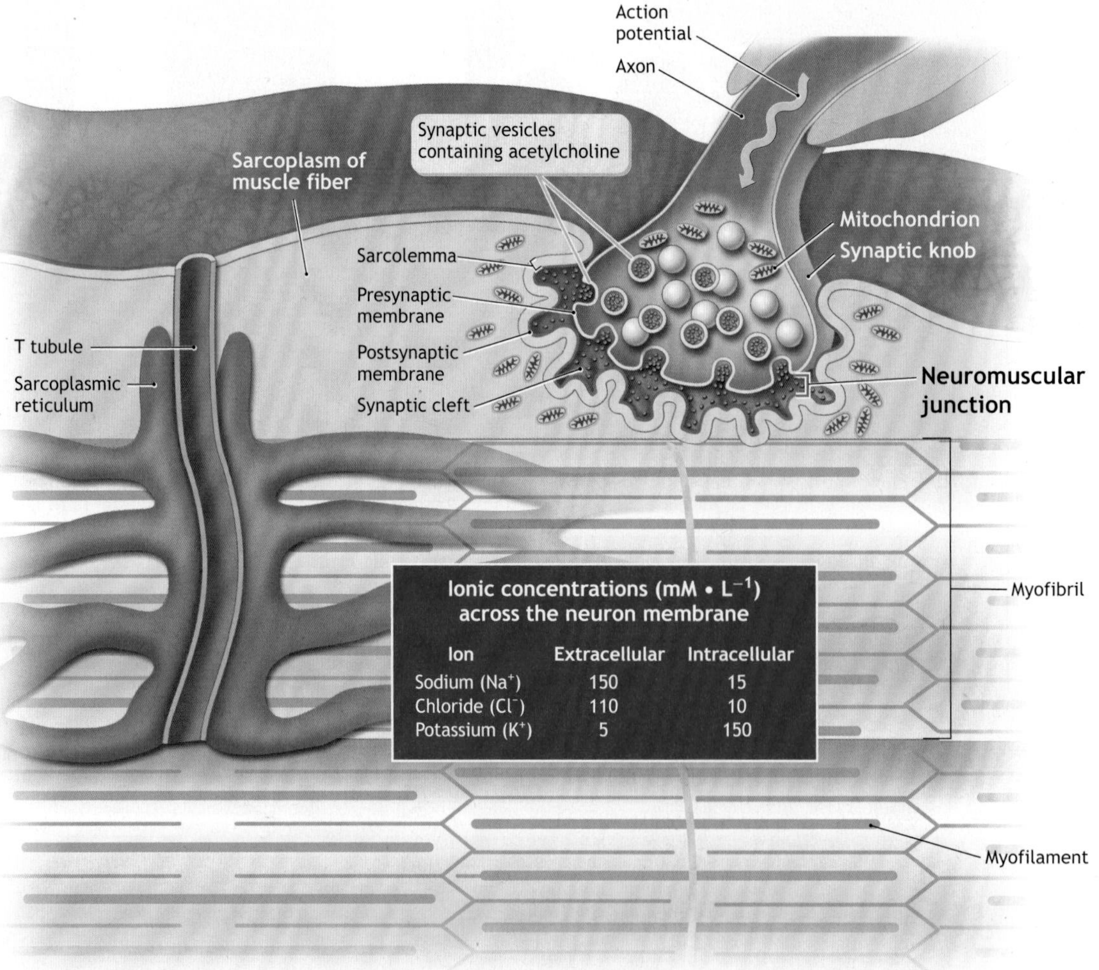

Ionic concentrations ($mM \cdot L^{-1}$) across the neuron membrane

Ion	Extracellular	Intracellular
Sodium (Na^+)	150	15
Chloride (Cl^-)	110	10
Potassium (K^+)	5	150

FIGURE 11.10 Microanatomy of the neuromuscular junction, including details of the presynaptic and postsynaptic contact area between the motor neuron and the muscle fiber it innervates. The *inset table* shows representative values for ionic concentrations across the motor neuron membrane. (Reprinted with permission from McArdle WD, Katch FI, Katch VL. *Exercise Physiology: Nutrition, Energy, and Human Performance*. 8th Ed. Baltimore: Wolters Kluwer Health, 2015.)

junction functions to transmit nerve impulses to muscle fibers. Each muscle fiber usually has one neuromuscular junction. The inset table in **Figure 11.10** lists representative values for ionic concentrations across the motor neuron membrane.

The axon's terminal portion forms several smaller axon branches whose endings, called **presynaptic terminals**, lie close to but not in contact with the muscle fiber's plasma membrane or sarcolemma. The **synaptic gutter**, the region of the postsynaptic membrane, contains infoldings that tremendously increase its surface area. The **synaptic cleft** lies between the synaptic gutter and the axon's presynaptic terminal, the region where neural impulse transmission occurs.

Excitation

Excitation normally occurs only at the neuromuscular junction. The neurotransmitter **acetylcholine (ACh)** provides the chemical stimulus to change an electrical neural impulse at the motor end plate into a chemical stimulus. Acetylcholine, released from small, saclike vesicles within the terminal axon, increases the postsynaptic membrane's permeability to sodium and potassium ions. This spreads the impulse over the entire muscle fiber as a distinct depolarization wave. As depolarization progresses, the muscle fiber's contractile machinery primes for its major function—to contract or shorten.

The enzyme **cholinesterase** catalyzes the hydrolysis of acetylcholine into choline and acetic acid to allow the return of a cholinergic neuron to the resting state following its activation. German pharmacologist Otto Loewi (1873–1961; **www.nobelprize.org/nobel_prizes/medicine/laureates/1936/loewi-bio.html**) and English physiologist and pharmacologist Sir Henry Hallet Dale (1875–1968; **www.nobelprize.org/nobel_prizes/medicine/laureates/1936/dale-bio.html**) purified and crystallized the enzyme concentrated at the borders of the synaptic cleft from electric eels. They received the 1936 Nobel Prize in Physiology or Medicine for their discovery. Cholinesterase degrades acetylcholine within 5 ms of its release from the synaptic vesicles. This action immediately repolarizes the postsynaptic membrane. The axon then resynthesizes acetylcholine from its constituent acetic acid and choline, so the entire process can repeat with the arrival of successive nerve impulses.

Facilitation

A motor neuron generates an action potential when its microvoltage decreases sufficiently to reach its excitation threshold. With a subthreshold action potential, the neuron does not discharge, but its resting membrane potential still lowers, temporarily increasing its "tendency" to fire. A neuron fires when many subthreshold excitatory impulses arrive in rapid succession, a condition termed **temporal summation**. **Spatial summation** refers to simultaneous stimulation of different presynaptic terminals on the same neuron. The "summing" of each excitatory effect often initiates an **action potential**.

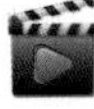

See the animation "Action Potential" on **http://thePoint.lww.com/MKKESS5e** for a demonstration of this process.

Removing inhibitory neural influences achieves importance under certain physical activity conditions. In an all-out maximal bench press or a vertical jump leap, for example, disinhibition and maximal activation of all motor neurons required for a movement enhance performance.

Joe Rollino—Coney Island Strongman and Superhuman Feats of Strength

Joe Rollino (1905–2010), weighing only 150 lb and 5′5″ in height, performed many superhuman feats of strength before he was accidentally killed in a car accident at age 104. His most famous feat of strength was lifting 635 lb (288 kg) with only his fingers and 3200 lb (1450 kg) with his back.

In their book on strength training, Zatsiorsky and Kraemer describe three broad factors that limit an athlete's lifting potential. The highest potential, called *absolute strength,* represents the theoretical maximum force that the combined interacting effects of muscle fibers, tendons, and bony structures can develop under neuromuscular-controlled, precise movement patterns as Rollino had apparently perfected. This value can never be exceeded and is rarely reached. The lowest maximum force value, termed *maximum strength*, represents the most one can lift under typical conditions that involve conscious effort, which equals about two thirds of an individual's theoretical absolute strength. For experienced strongmen like Joe Rollino who routinely trained close to maximum during his workouts, his maximum lift capacity exceeded the two thirds typical limit and reached about 80% before his muscular system would experience undue strain.

The third type of lifting potential occurs when weightlifters set a world record in competition or when heroic efforts are performed under extreme duress. The latter includes men and women lifting automobiles off individuals unexpectedly pinned under an auto or other heavy objects to save their lives. These are examples of how neuronal facilitation supercharges CNS excitation under conditions of extreme stress. Other physiologic mechanisms, besides conscious control, come into play; the most notable is the "fight-or-flight" arousal response that immediately precedes and accompanies an emotionally charged condition (**http://learn.genetics.utah.edu/content/begin/cells/fight_flight/**). See also Appendix SR-6, which provides a link to an interview with Joe Rollino.

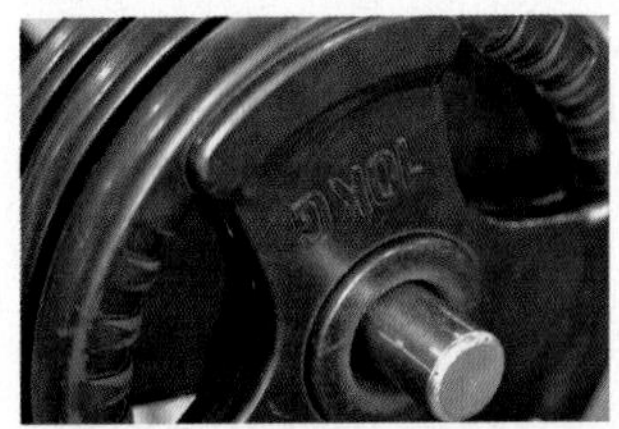

Sources: Zatsiorsky VM, Kraemer W. *Science and Practice of Strength Training*. 2nd Ed. Champaign: Human Kinetics, 2006.

Henneman E, Mendell LM. Functional organization of the motoneurone pool and its outputs. In: Brooks VB, ed. *Handbook of Physiology, Section 1, The Nervous System*, Vol. I. Bethesda: American Physiological Society, 1981:423.

Rafuse VF, et al. Innervation ratio and motor unit force in large muscles: a study of chronically stimulated cat medial gastrocnemius. *J Physiol* 1997;499:809.

TABLE 11.1 Characteristics and Correspondence Between Motor Units and Muscle Fiber Types

Motor Unit Designation	Force Production	Contraction Speed	Fatigue Resistance[a]	SAG[b]	Motor Unit Muscle Fiber Type
Fast fatigable (FF)	High	Fast	Low	Yes	Fast glycolytic (FG)
Fast fatigue-resistance (FR)	Moderate	Fast	Moderate	Yes	Fast-oxidative-glycolytic (FOG)
Slow (S)	Low	Slow	High	No	Slow-oxidative (SO)

[a]How much the muscle tension declined with repetitive stimulation.

[b]Under repetitive stimuli, some motor units respond smoothly with a systematic increase in tension, but others first increase tension and then decrease or "sag" slightly in response to the same tetanic stimulus. These sag characteristics can classify the different motor units. Only the slow (S) motor units do not exhibit sag, which probably relates more to their lower force-generating capabilities than their fatigue characteristics.

Modified with permission from Lieber RL. *Skeletal Muscle Structure, Function, and Plasticity*. 3rd Ed. Baltimore: Lippincott Williams & Wilkins, 2010.

Effective disinhibition fully activates muscle groups during maximal lifting, an effect that accounts for the rapid, highly specific strength increases observed during the first few days and weeks of resistance training. Enhanced neuromuscular activation accounts for considerable improvements in muscular strength *without* concurrent increases in muscle size. CNS excitation, also called "neuronal facilitation," explains why intense concentration or "psyching" can substantially "supercharge" activities requiring feats of strength and power not possible under normal conditions.

Inhibition

Some presynaptic terminals generate inhibitory impulses by releasing chemicals that increase postsynaptic membrane permeability to potassium and chloride ions. The efflux of positively charged potassium ions or influx of negatively charged chloride ions increases the membrane's resting electrical potential to create an **inhibitory postsynaptic potential (IPSP)**, making the neuron more difficult to fire. No action potential occurs when a motor neuron encounters excitatory and inhibitory influences or encounters a large IPSP. For example, one can usually override or inhibit the reflex to pull the hand away when removing a splinter.

The neurotransmitter gamma-aminobutyric acid (GABA; **www.med.nyu.edu/content?ChunkIID=222543**) and glycine exert inhibitory effects, causing nerves to "calm down." Neural inhibition serves protective functions and reduces the input of unwanted stimuli to produce smooth, purposeful responses.

Motor Unit Physiology

Identifying Muscle Fibers With Motor Units

A whole muscle contains many possible motor units, each containing a single motor neuron; thus, it is difficult to identify which fibers belong to which motor unit. The classic motor unit physiology experiments were performed in the late 1960s and early 1970s. Researchers used isolated cat hind limb motor units and intracellular motor neuron stimulation to measure different electrophysiologic properties of the motor neuron and mechanical properties of the motor units within the whole muscle. This research strategy, still used today, describes motor unit differences based on the physiologic properties of the respective muscle fibers innervated. **Table 11.1** and **Figure 11.11** present the three physiologic and mechanical properties of motor units and the muscle fibers they innervate:

1. Twitch (speed of contraction) characteristics
2. Tension-generating (force) characteristics
3. Neuromuscular fatigability

Motor Unit Twitch Characteristics

Early studies of motor unit characteristics revealed that some units developed high-twitch tensions but others developed "relatively" low-twitch tensions in response to a single electrical impulse, whereas still others generated intermediate tension. The differences between motor units were judged on a relative rather than absolute basis, sometimes making comparisons between studies difficult. Motor units with low-twitch tensions also tended to have "slower" contraction times; those with higher tensions tended to have "faster" contraction times.

Tension-Generating Characteristics

Different motor units and the muscles they innervate can develop different amounts of tension based on many factors. For example, fast motor units and their corresponding fast muscle fibers generate more tension than slow motor units and their corresponding slower muscle fibers. Alternatively, perhaps fast and slow fibers generate the same tension, but fast motor units simply innervate a greater number of fibers than slow motor units. Or, fast and slow units have the same number of fibers of equal intrinsic strength, but fast fibers are larger and therefore generate more tension. Each of these possibilities is supported by research, with fast and slow muscle fibers within a motor unit having about the same specific tension capacity. Fiber size and innervation differ among motor unit types. Three factors govern differences in tension generation:

1. All-or-none principle
2. Graduation of force principle
3. Level of motor unit recruitment patterns.

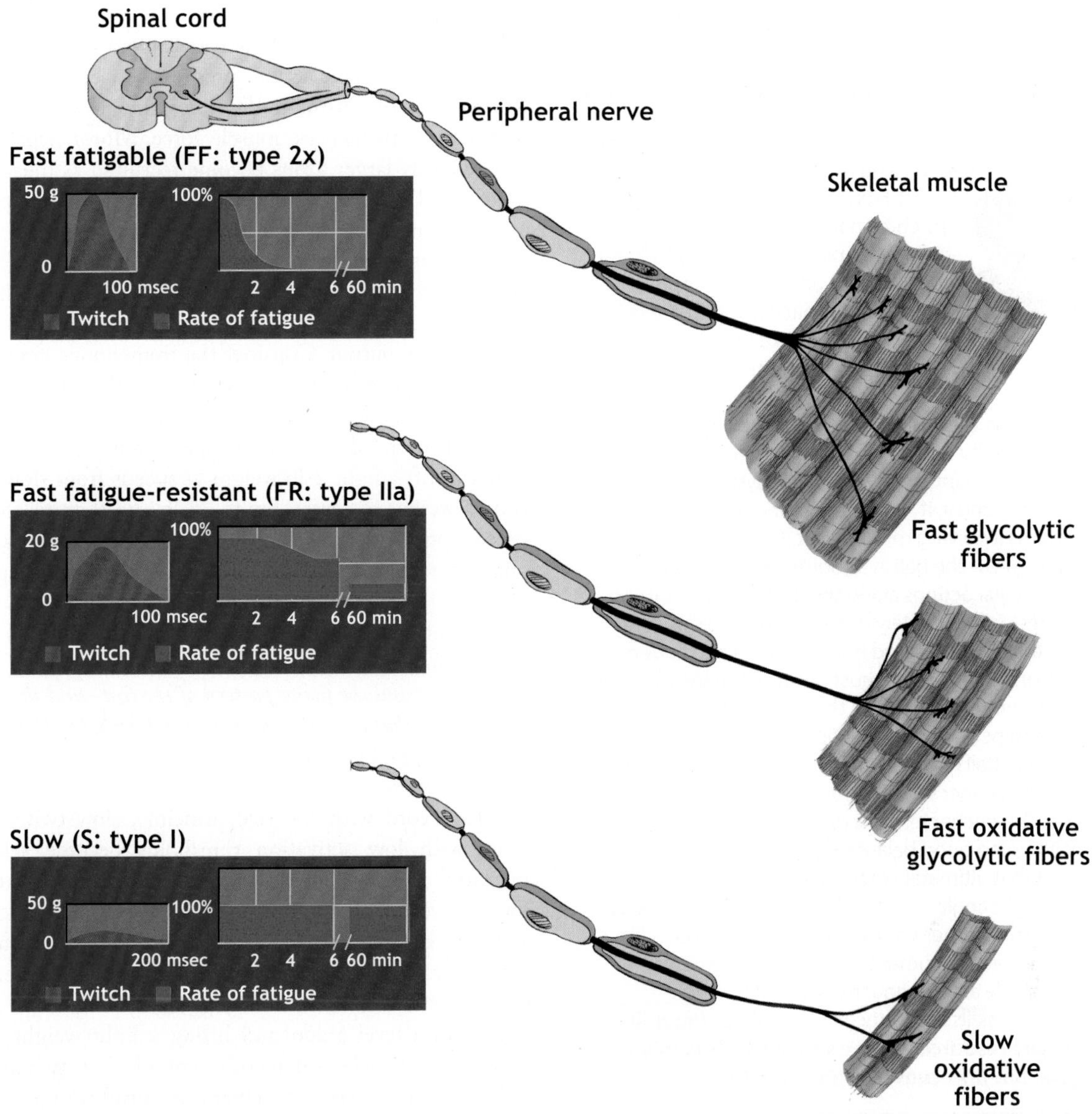

FIGURE 11.11 Schematic representation of the anatomic, physiologic, and histochemical properties of the three motor unit types. Fast fatigable (FF) motor units **(top)** have large axons that innervate many large muscle fibers. The units generate large tensions but fatigue rapidly (see the tension and fatigue graphs to the left). Fast-fatigue-resistant (FR) units **(middle)** have moderately sized axons that innervate many muscle fibers. The units generate moderate tensions and do not fatigue much. Slow units (S) **(bottom)** composed of small axons innervate few small fibers. These units generate low forces but maintain force for a prolonged time period. (Reprinted with permission from McArdle WD, Katch FI, Katch VL. *Exercise Physiology: Nutrition, Energy, and Human Performance*. 8th Ed. Baltimore: Wolters Kluwer Health, 2015.)

All-or-None Principle

All of the accompanying muscle fibers contract synchronously when a stimulus triggers an action potential in the motor neuron. A single motor unit cannot generate strong and weak actions; either the impulse elicits an action or it does not. Once the neuron fires and the impulse reaches the neuromuscular junction, the muscle cells always act to the fullest extent in accord with the **all-or-none principle** first described in 1871 by Henry Pickering Bowditch (1840–1911), a renowned American physiologist at Harvard's Medical School and Department of Anatomy, Physiology, and Physical Training (see Chapter 1, "Origins of Exercise Physiology").

Gradation of Force Principle

The force of muscle action varies from slight to maximal by blending two mechanisms:

1. Increasing the *number* of motor units recruited
2. Increasing the *frequency* of motor unit discharge

Activation of all motor units in a muscle generates considerable force compared with activating only a few units. Total tension also increases if repetitive stimuli reach a muscle before it relaxes. Blending recruitment of motor units and their firing rate permits a wide variety of graded muscle actions. These range from the delicate touch of an eye surgeon repairing a retinal blood vessel to the maximal effort in throwing a baseball "fast."

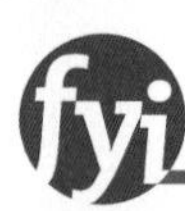

Sports Science and Baseball Pitching Speed

In the 1980s, major and minor league baseball began using radar guns to track pitching speed. From 1997 to 2010, only eight pitchers had thrown 102 mph or higher; one pitch was clocked at 103 mph in 1995 and one at 104.8 mph by Detroit Tigers pitcher Joel Zumaya in 2010. That record was shattered later in the same year when a left-handed pitcher for the Cincinnati Reds, Aroldis Chapman, was clocked at 105 mph. Why is baseball pitching speed of interest in a chapter on the nervous system? First and foremost, it signals the tremendous complexity in neural patterns involving millions of "bits" of information required to just throw the ball in a coordinated manner, initiated by muscular actions along the body's chain: starting at the ankles, moving to the legs, hips, shoulders, arms, and ending when the ball is released from the hand and fingers tenths of a second later. This all must occur simultaneously with just the right amount of force from the fingers gripping the ball, to how fast hips and shoulders open and rotate during the motion leading to ball release. Other coordinated movements must occur in the proper sequence and with proper timing of the sequence. The pitcher remains upright while falling forward, maintaining good balance despite unleashing a maximal effort that ultimately gets the arm to release the ball at just the right angle so the ball flies at maximal velocity and ends up in the catcher's glove. High-speed sports analysis systems have documented important elements in successful muscle action sequences in athletes with exceptional motor skills in a particular sport (**http://m.mlb.com/pitchsmart/resources/; www.somaxsports.com/video.php?analysis=tim-lincecum-97mph-fastball**).

The golf swing provides an example of force gradation, guided closely under neural control to execute a complex human movement with high efficiency. Tension in the fingers, hands, arms, and legs continually adjusts during the backswing, swing initiation and acceleration, club-ball contact, and follow-through. For example, tour PGA players rotate their hips 0.07 of a second before the golf club starts down from the top of the backswing. Most top tour players begin hip rotation even sooner, a characteristic of an optimal neural firing sequence separating the "best" players from the rest.

Similarly, the seemingly simple task of writing with a pen involves innumerable highly complex and coordinated neuromuscular forces and actions, but in a much different way than throwing a baseball fast. In a nonsports example, think about picking up a grape and bringing it to your mouth. Without exquisite neuromuscular control, the fingers would literally crush the grape, and your hand and arm, without exhibiting precise control and coordination over their movements, might thrust what remains of the grape forcibly into your nose or eye, totally missing your mouth!

Motor Unit Recruitment

Low-force muscle actions activate only a few motor units, whereas higher force actions progressively enlist more units. **Motor unit recruitment** describes the process of adding motor units to increase muscle force. Motor neurons with progressively larger axons become recruited as muscle force increases. This response, termed the **size principle**, provides an anatomic basis for the orderly recruitment of specific motor units to produce a smooth muscle action.

All of a muscle's motor units do not fire at the same time. If they did, it would be virtually impossible to control muscle force output. Consider the tremendous gradation of forces and speeds that muscles generate. When lifting a barbell, for example, specific muscles act to move the limb at a particular speed under a set rate of tension development. One can lift a light 2-lb weight at speeds from slow to fast. But as weight increases, say to 25 lb and then to 75 lb, the speed options decrease accordingly. When lifting a pencil, one generates just enough force to lift the pencil regardless of how fast or slowly the arm moves. When lifting the heaviest weight possible, all of the available motor units require activation. *From the standpoint of neuromotor control, selective recruitment and the firing pattern of the fast- and slow-twitch motor units that control movement (and perhaps other stabilizing regions) provide the mechanism to produce the desired coordinated response.*

In accord with the size principle, slow-twitch motor units with low activation thresholds become selectively recruited during light-to-moderate effort. Activation of more powerful, higher threshold, fast-twitch units progresses as force requirements increase. **Figure 11.12** illustrates the general relationship among motor unit type and intensity of effort. Sustained, submaximal jogging, cycling, cross-country skiing on a level grade, and lifting a light weight at slow speed involve selective recruitment of slow-twitch motor units. Rapid, powerful movements in sprint running, cycling, and swimming progressively activate fast-twitch, fatigue-resistant motor units up through the fast-twitch fatigable units at peak force.

The differential control of the motor unit firing pattern distinguishes skilled from unskilled performers. Weightlifters, for example, generally demonstrate a synchronous pattern of motor-unit firing (i.e., many motor units recruited simultaneously during a lift). Endurance athletes generally exhibit an asynchronous firing pattern (i.e., some motor units fire while others recover). The synchronous firing of fast-twitch motor units allows the weightlifter to generate high force quickly for the desired lift. In contrast, for endurance athletes, the asynchronous firing of predominantly slow-twitch, fatigue-resistant motor units serves as a built-in recuperative period so performance continues with minimal fatigue. This becomes possible because motor units share the burden of "cooperation" during multiple movements and changing intensities.

See the animation "Fatigue Mechanism" on **http://thePoint.lww.com/MKKESS5e** for a demonstration of this process.

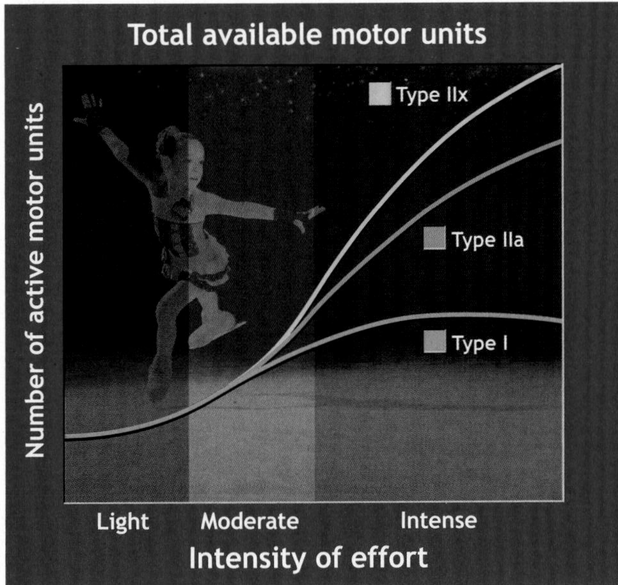

FIGURE 11.12 Recruitment of slow-twitch (type I) and fast-twitch (type IIa and IIx) muscle fibers (motor units) relative to exercise intensity. More intense physical activity progressively recruits more fast-twitch fibers. (Reprinted with permission from McArdle WD, Katch FI, Katch VL. *Exercise Physiology: Nutrition, Energy, and Human Performance*. 8th Ed. Baltimore: Wolters Kluwer Health, 2015.)

Neuromuscular Fatigability

Neuromuscular fatigability represents the decline in muscle tension or force capacity with repeated stimulation per unit time. Resistance to fatigue, defined as maintaining muscle tension with repeated stimulation represents another important quality to distinguish differences in motor units.

Four factors decrease a muscle's force-generating capacity:

1. Exercise-induced alterations in CNS neurotransmitters serotonin, 5-hydroxytryptamine (5-HT), dopamine, and ACh, including neuromodulators ammonia and cytokines secreted by immune cells. The latter alter one's psychic or perceptual state to disrupt ability to exercise.
2. Reduced glycogen content in active muscle fibers during prolonged physical activity. Such "nutrient-related fatigue" occurs despite the sufficient oxygen and fatty acid substrate availability for adenosine triphosphate (ATP) regeneration through aerobic metabolic pathways. Phosphocreatine (PCr) depletion and decline in total adenine nucleotide pool (ATP + adenosine diphosphate [ADP] + adenosine monophosphate [AMP]) accompany the fatigue state during prolonged submaximal effort.
3. Diminished oxygen and increased concentrations of blood and muscle lactate relate to muscle fatigue in short-term, maximal exertion. The dramatic increase in $[H^+]$ in the active muscle disrupts the intracellular environment and energy transfer process.
4. Neuromuscular junction fatigue disallows the action potential to travel from the motor neuron to the muscle fiber.

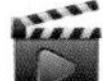 See the animation "Lactic Acid Accumulation" on **http://thePoint.lww.com/MKKESS5e** for a demonstration of this process.

If muscle function declines during prolonged submaximal physical activity, additional motor unit recruitment occurs to maintain crucial force output necessary to sustain a constant performance level. During maximal physical activity that presumably activates the available number of motor units, fatigue occurs when accompanied by an objectively measured neural activity decline to those motor units. Similar to the dimming of a light bulb, reduced neural activity probably indicates that failure in neural or myoneural transmission produces fatigue in activities that involve maximal effort muscle actions.

PROPRIOCEPTORS IN MUSCLES, JOINTS, AND TENDONS

Muscles, joints, and tendons contain specialized sensory receptors sensitive to stretch, tension, and pressure. These **proprioceptor** end organs almost instantaneously relay critical information about muscular dynamics, limb position, and kinesthesia and proprioception to conscious and subconscious portions of the CNS. Proprioception allows continual monitoring of the progress of any movement or sequence of movements and can modify subsequent motor actions. Individuals with chronic low back pain, or individuals who have undergone successful low back surgery, often temporarily lose full proprioception in the ankles, predisposing them to possible balance issues (e.g., an inability to easily balance with the eyes open or closed on one leg without swaying for more than 3 to 5 seconds).

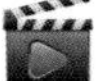 See the animation "Proprioceptors: How Do They Work" on **http://thePoint.lww.com/MKKESS5e** for a demonstration of this process.

thePoint® **See Appendix SR-6: Additional Video Links, for information on stretching techniques.**

Muscle Spindles

The muscle spindles, named for their similar shape to the spindle on a spinning wheel, provide mechanosensory information about changes in muscle fiber length and tension. They primarily respond to any muscle stretch through a reflex response that initiates a stronger muscle action to counteract this stretch.

Structural Organization

Figure 11.13 illustrates the general location of the fusiform-shaped muscle spindle attached in parallel to regular muscle fibers called **extrafusal fibers.** Any muscle elongation stretches the spindle. The number of spindles per gram of muscle varies depending on the muscle group. More spindles exist in muscles that routinely perform complex movements. The spindle contains two types of specialized fibers with contractile capabilities called **intrafusal fibers**.

Two afferent (sensory) and one efferent (motor) nerve fibers innervate the spindles. The motor spindles consist of thin γ (gamma) efferent fibers that innervate the contractile, striated ends of intrafusal fibers. These fibers, activated by higher brain centers, maintain the spindle at peak operation at all muscle lengths.

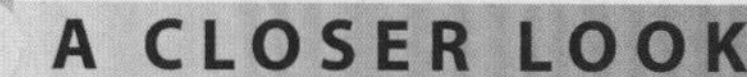

Proprioceptive Neuromuscular Facilitation Stretching

The four static stretching techniques are

1. Passive: relaxation of all voluntary and reflex muscular resistance followed by passive assistance from another person or device during voluntary movement
2. Active assistive: involves assistance from another person as the segment moves through its normal range of motion (ROM)
3. Active: a muscle or joint actively moves through its ROM
4. **Proprioceptive neuromuscular facilitation (PNF)**: inverse stretch reflex induces relaxation in a muscle prior to its being stretched, allowing for increased stretch.

Proprioceptive Neuromuscular Facilitation Stretching

PNF stretching increases ROM by augmenting prior muscle relaxation through spinal reflex mechanisms using these techniques:

1. **Contract-relax stretch (hold-relax stretch).** Involves a prior isometric action of the muscle group to be stretched followed by a slow, static stretch (relaxation phase).
2. **Contract-relax-contract stretch (hold-relax-contract stretch)**, also referred to as the **contract–relax with agonist contraction (CRAC)** technique. Involves an isometric action of the muscle group to be stretched; the relax stretching phase is accompanied by a submaximal action of the opposing (agonist) muscle group.

Both PNF techniques use **reciprocal inhibition**, the isometric action of antagonist muscle group being stretched to induce a reflex facilitation and agonist contraction. Reciprocal inhibition that suppresses contractile activity in the antagonist muscle during the slow static stretch phase allows for greater antagonist stretch.

Performing PNF Stretches

1. Stretch the target muscle group by moving the joint to the end of its ROM (Fig. A).
2. Isometrically contract the prestretched muscle group against an immovable resistance (e.g., partner) for 5 to 6 seconds.

Stretch Reflex

Muscle spindles lodged in parallel with the main fibers in the muscle belly detect, respond to, and modulate changes in extrafusal muscle fiber length. This provides an important regulatory control function for total body movement and maintenance of posture. Postural muscles continuously receive neural input to sustain their readiness to respond to conscious or voluntary movements. These muscles require continual subconscious activity to adjust to gravity's downward pull in upright posture. Without this monitoring and feedback mechanism, the body would literally collapse into a heap from the absence of tension in the antigravity neck muscles, spinal muscles, hip flexors, abdominal muscles, and large leg musculature. The patella tendon **stretch reflex** illustrated in **Figure 11.7** serves as a fundamental controlling mechanism in human movement. The stretch reflex consists of three main components:

1. Muscle spindle that responds to stretch
2. Afferent nerve fiber that delivers the sensory impulse from the spindle to the spinal cord
3. Efferent spinal cord motor neuron that activates the stretched muscle fibers

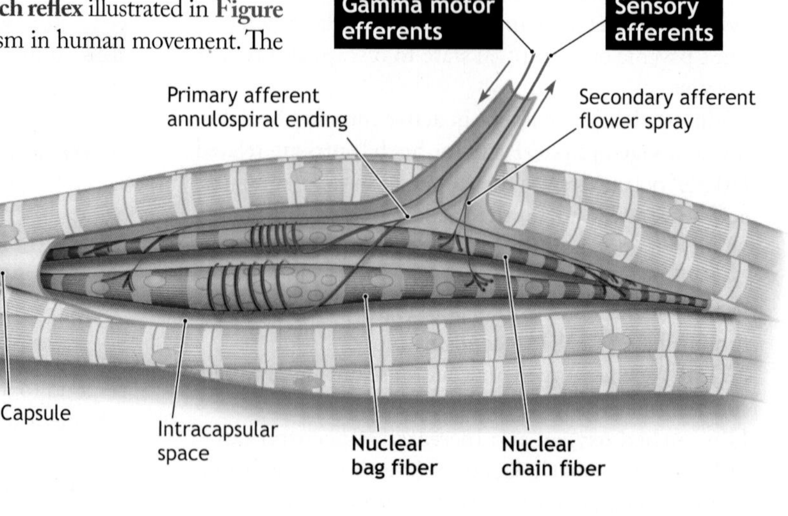

3. Relax the contracted muscle group as the partner stretches the muscle group to a new, increased ROM (Fig. B). With CRAC, the opposing muscle group (agonist) contracts submaximally for 5 to 6 seconds to facilitate relaxation and produce further stretching of the muscle group.

PNF Example: To stretch the hamstring and lower back muscles, the individual sits on the floor with the arms extended forward along the side of the legs (Fig. A). The person contracts the lower back muscle isometrically as the partner offers resistance to horizontal extension. After the isometric action, the partner stretches the hamstrings to a new increased ROM (Fig. B).

Guidelines for Proper PNF Stretching

1. Determine the appropriate posture or position to ensure proper position and alignment.
2. Emphasize proper breathing. Inhale through the nose and exhale during the stretch through pursed lips with the eyes closed to increase concentration and awareness of the stretch.
3. Hold end points progressively for 30 to 90 seconds followed by another deep breath.
4. Exhale and feel the muscle being stretched and relaxed to achieve further ROM.
5. Do *not* bounce or spring during stretching.
6. Do *not* force a stretch during breath-holding.
7. Increasing stretching range during exhalation encourages full-body relaxation.
8. Slowly reposition from the stretch posture and allow the muscles to recover to their natural resting length.

Sources: Kay AD, Blazevich AJ. Effect of acute static stretch on maximal muscle performance: a systematic review. *Med Sci Sports Exerc* 2015;44:154.

Peck E, et al. The effects of stretching on performance. *Curr Sports Med Rep* 2014;13:179. doi: 10.1249/JSR.0000000000000052.

Fasen JM, et al. A randomized controlled trial of hamstring stretch: comparison of fur techniques. *J Strength Cond Res* 2009;23:660.

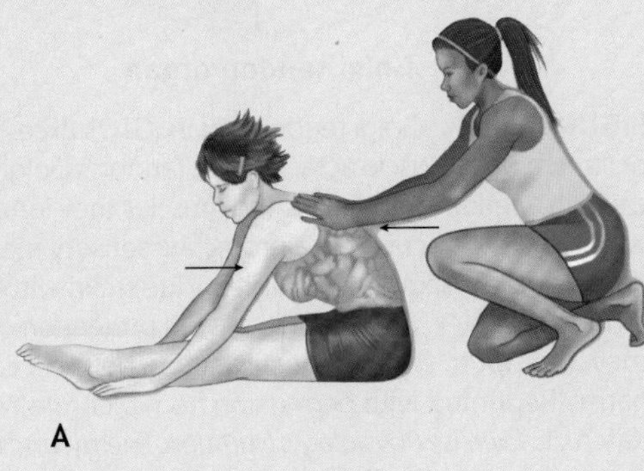

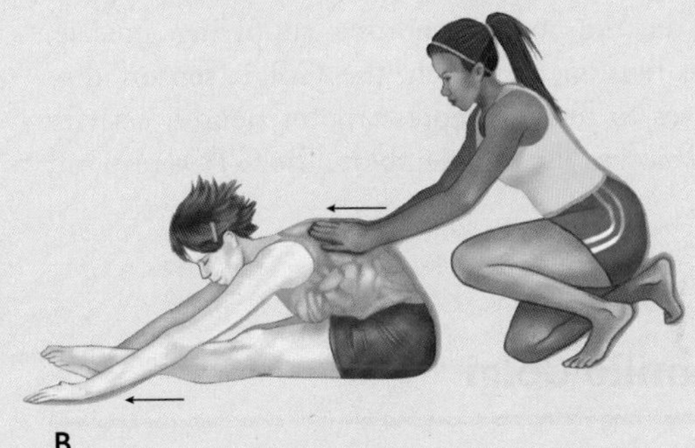

See the animation "Patella Tendon Stretch" on **http://thePoint.lww.com/MKKESS5e** for a demonstration of this process.

This simplest autonomic monosynaptic reflex arc involves only one synapse. Spindles lie parallel to the extrafusal fibers and stretch when these fibers elongate as the reflex hammer strikes the patellar tendon. The spindle's sensory receptors fire when its intrafusal fibers stretch, directing impulses through the dorsal root into the spinal cord to directly activate anterior motor neurons. The gray matter contains neuron cell bodies; the white matter carries longitudinal columns of nerve fibers. Stimulation of a single α-motor neuron affects up to 3000 muscle fibers. The reflex also activates interneurons within the spinal cord to augment an appropriate motor response. For example, excitatory impulses activate synergistic muscles that support the desired movement, and inhibitory impulses flow to motor units that normally counter the movement. In this way, the stretch reflex acts as a self-regulating, compensating mechanism. This salient feature allows the muscle to adjust automatically to differences in load and length without requiring immediate information processing through higher CNS centers. Humans are fortunate to have this checks and balance CNS system. Without it, an individual could not perform relatively "simple" muscular movements like touching the tip of the index finger to the tip of the thumb, let alone the highly complex, coordinated movement patterns such as

FIGURE 11.13 Structural organization of the muscle spindle with an enlarged view of the spindle's equatorial region. Each spindle usually contains four to five nuclear chain fibers. The intrafusal fibers ends contain actin and myosin filaments and exhibit shortening capability. Two sensory afferent fibers and one motor efferent fiber innervate the spindles. A primary afferent nerve fiber, the annulospiral nerve fiber, composed of a set of rings in spiral configuration, entwines the bag fiber's midregion. (Adapted with permission from McArdle WD, Katch FI, Katch VL. *Exercise Physiology: Nutrition, Energy, and Human Performance*. 8th Ed. Baltimore: Wolters Kluwer Health, 2015.)

smashing a volleyball over a net or diving outstretched into the end zone to score a touchdown.

Golgi Tendon Organs

Golgi tendon organs (GTOs), named for Italian physician Camillo Golgi (1843–1926), who first identified these proprioceptors in 1898, connect in series to as many as 25 extrafusal fibers in contrast to muscle spindles that lie parallel to extrafusal muscle fibers. These tiny sensory receptors, also located in ligaments of joints, primarily detect differences in muscle tension rather than length. **Figure 11.14** shows details of the GTOs that respond as a feedback monitor to discharge impulses when muscle shortens or stretches.

When activated by excessive muscle tension or stretch, Golgi receptors immediately transmit signals to cause reflex inhibition of the muscles they supply. This occurs because of the overriding influence of inhibitory spinal interneurons on the motor neurons supplying muscle. With extreme tension or stretch, the Golgi "sensor" discharge increases to further depress motor neuron activity and reduce tension in the muscle fibers. The GTOs respond as a feedback monitor to discharge impulses under either of two conditions:

1. Tension created in the muscle when it shortens
2. Tension created when the muscle stretches passively

Ultimately, the GTOs protect muscle and its connective tissue harness from injury by sudden, excessive load or stretch.

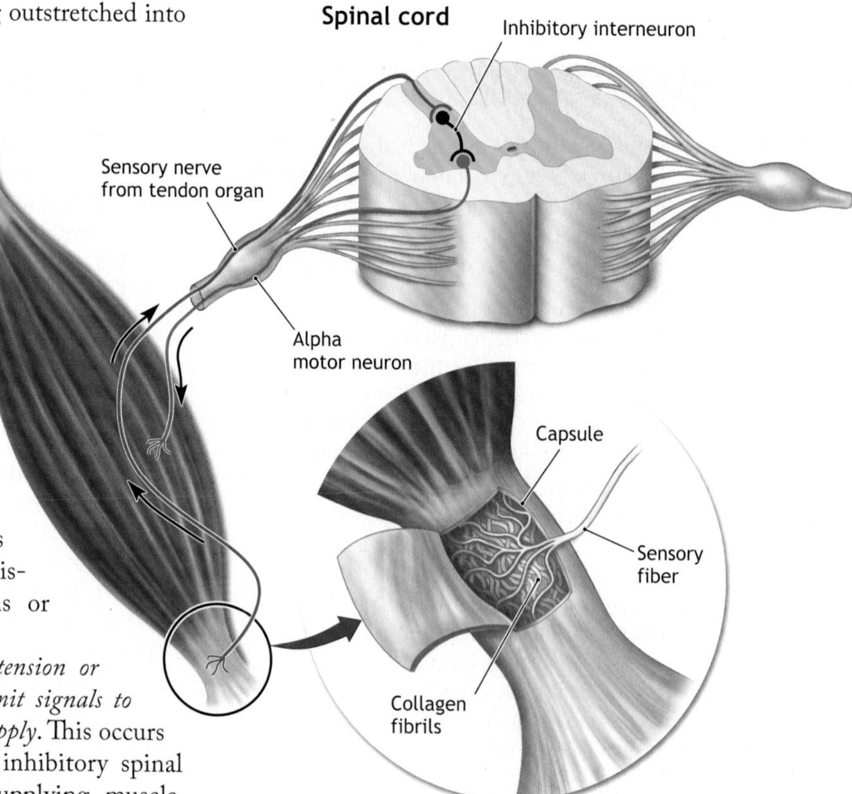

FIGURE 11.14 Golgi tendon organ (GTO). Excessive tension or stretch on a muscle activates the tendon's Golgi receptors, causing a reflex inhibition of the muscles they innervate. In this way, the GTO functions as a protective sensory mechanism to detect and subsequently inhibit undue strain within the muscle-tendon complex. Think of GTOs as FBI protection officers—they attempt to thwart a hostile action before it can cause any harm! (Reprinted with permission from McArdle WD, Katch FI, Katch VL. *Exercise Physiology: Nutrition, Energy, and Human Performance*. 8th Ed. Baltimore: Wolters Kluwer Health, 2015.)

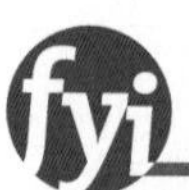

Camillo Golgi

In 1878, Camillo Golgi (1843–1926), an Italian neurohistochemist, discovered the minute tendon organs that now bear his name, using a silver nitrate stain described in his masterful text, *On the Fine Anatomy of the Nervous System*. Golgi received the Nobel Prize in Physiology or Medicine in 1906 with Santiago Ramón y Cajal (1852–1934; **www.nobelprize.org/nobel_prizes/medicine/laureates/1906/golgi-bio.html**) for their insightful contributions about nervous system structures. One of Golgi's greatest contributions was his creative method of staining individual nerve and cell structures using a weak solution of silver nitrate (**www.nobelprize.org/nobel_prizes/medicine/laureates/1906/golgi-lecture.pdf**). This invaluable method traced the outlines of intricate cell structures. The image below shows a silver nitrate–stained spinal cord neuron.

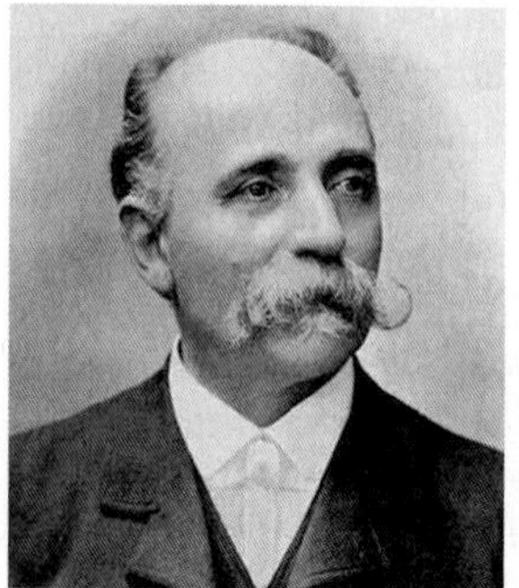

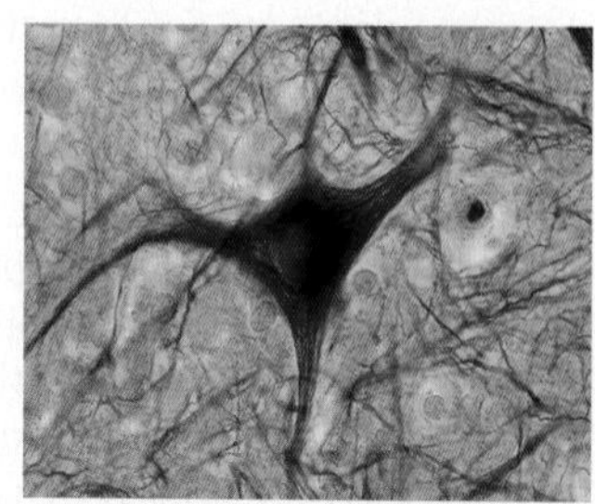

Pacinian Corpuscles

Pacinian corpuscles, named after their discoverer Italian anatomist Filippo Pacini (1812–1883), are small, ellipsoidal bodies located close to the GTOs and embedded in a single, unmyelinated nerve fiber. They are positioned in the following four, general anatomic locations:

1. Subcutaneous tissues on the nerves of the soles of the feet and palms of the hands
2. Mucous membranes
3. Male and female genital organs
4. Close proximity with the nerves of joints

A sensitive receptor membrane covers the ends of the corpuscles, whose sodium channels open with any membrane deformation or vibration. Several concentric capsules of connective tissue with a viscous gel between them surround each corpuscle; these attach to and enclose the end of a single nerve fiber.

These sensitive sensory receptors respond to quick movement and deep pressure. Deformation or compression of the onionlike capsule by any mechanical stimulus transmits pressure to the sensory nerve ending within its core; this changes the sensory nerve ending's electric potential. If this generator potential achieves sufficient magnitude, a sensory signal propagates down the myelinated axon that leaves the corpuscle and enters the spinal cord. Think of Pacinian corpuscles as fast-adapting mechanical sensors. They discharge a few impulses at the onset of a steady stimulus and then remain electrically silent, or discharge another volley of impulses when the stimulus ceases. Pacinian corpuscles detect *changes* in movement or pressure rather than the magnitude of movement or amount of applied pressure.

thePoint® See Appendix SR-7: Nervous System Control, Sports Medicine Injuries, and Biomechanics, at **http://www.thePoint.lww.com/MKKESS5e**, for a list of reliable web-based information sources.

SUMMARY

1. CNS neural control mechanisms finely regulate human movement.
2. In response to internal and external stimuli, bits of sensory input are automatically and rapidly routed, organized, and retransmitted to muscles.
3. The cerebellum serves as the primary center for comparing, evaluating, and integrating stimuli to fine-tune muscular activity.
4. The spinal cord and other subconscious areas of the CNS control numerous muscular functions.
5. The reflex arc processes and initiates automatic (subconscious) muscular movements and responses.
6. The number of muscle fibers in a motor unit depends on the muscle's movement function.
7. Intricate movement patterns require a relatively small fiber-to-neuron ratio, but for gross movements, a single neuron may innervate several thousand muscle fibers.
8. The anterior motor neuron (cell body, axon, and dendrites) transmits the electrochemical neural impulse from the spinal cord to the muscle.
9. Dendrites receive impulses and conduct them toward the cell body; the axon transmits the impulse in one direction only—down the axon to the muscle.
10. The neuromuscular junction provides the interface between the motor neuron and its muscle fibers, with ACh release at this junction activating the muscle.
11. Excitatory and inhibitory impulses continually bombard synaptic junctions between neurons to alter a neuron's threshold for excitation by increasing or decreasing its tendency to fire.
12. In all-out, high-power output physical activity, a large degree of disinhibition benefits performance because it allows for maximal activation of a muscle's motor units.
13. Gradation of muscle force results from an interaction of factors that regulate the number and type of motor units recruited and their discharge frequency.
14. In accordance with the size principle, light physical activity predominantly recruits slow-twitch motor units followed by activation of fast-twitch units when force output requirements increase.
15. Sensory receptors in muscles, tendons, and joints relay information about muscular dynamics and limb movement to specific CNS locations.
16. Golgi tendon organ receptors are neurological structures located within the tendon that sense changes in muscle tension.
17. Pacinian corpuscles detect changes in movement or pressure.

THINK IT THROUGH

1. Discuss why fatigue may not relate to "only" muscular factors.
2. Present two factors to explain why some individuals are "faster learners" of certain movement-oriented tasks.
3. How do neurotransmitter-type drugs mimic physiology and performance during physical activity?

PART 2 Muscular System: Organization and Activation

Skeletal muscles transform chemical energy within ATP molecules into mechanical energy of motion. Part 2 presents the architectural organization of skeletal muscle and focuses on its gross and microscopic structure. The discussion includes the sequence of chemical and mechanical events in muscular action and relaxation, including differences in muscle fiber characteristics among elite performers in diverse sports.

COMPARISON OF SKELETAL, CARDIAC, AND SMOOTH MUSCLE

Humans possess three muscle types—cardiac, smooth, and skeletal—each with functional and anatomical differences. Only the heart contains cardiac muscle. It shares several common features with skeletal muscle: both appear striated or striped under microscopic examination and contract or shorten in a similar manner. Smooth muscle lacks a striated appearance but shares cardiac muscle's characteristic of nonconscious or inherent regulation. **Table 11.2** contrasts the structural and functional characteristics of the three human muscle types.

How Skeletal Muscles Develop

Skeletal muscle tissue develops from specialized embryonic mesodermal cells called **myoblasts**. These cells undergo cell

TABLE 11.2 Characteristics of the Three Types of Human Muscle

Characteristics	Type of Muscle		
	Skeletal	Cardiac	Smooth
Location	Attached to bones	Heart only	Part of blood vessel structure: surrounds many internal hollow organs
Function	Movement	Pumps blood	Constricts blood vessels; moves contents of internal organs
Anatomical description	Large cylindrical, multinucleated cells arranged in parallel	Quadrangular cells	Small, spindle-shaped cells with long axis oriented in the same direction
Striated	Yes	Yes	No
Initiation of action potential	By neuron only	Spontaneous (pacemaker cells)	Spontaneous
Duration of electrical activity	Short (1–2 ms)	Long (~200 ms)	Very long, slow (~300 ms)
Energy source	Anaerobic, aerobic	Aerobic	Aerobic
Energy efficiency	Low	Moderate	High
Fatigue resistance	Low to high	Low	Very low
Rate of shortening	Fast	Moderate	Very slow
Duration of action	As brief as 100 ms; prolonged tetanus	Short (~300 ms); summation and tetanus not possible	Very long; may be sustained indefinitely

division to increase their size (hypertrophy) and number (hyperplasia). Further development occurs when myoblasts fuse together to form another intermediate structure, the **myotube**, which then matures and develops into a muscle fiber. Newly formed fibers begin to exhibit reflexive, contractile properties during early fetal development at about week 7, which continues in a head-to-toe direction, and proximally to distally. The early origins of cardiac and smooth muscle follow a slightly different developmental path than skeletal muscle (myotubes form gap junctions instead of fusing; **https://embryology.med.unsw.edu.au/embryology/index.php/Musculoskeletal_System_-_Muscle_Development**).

GROSS STRUCTURE OF SKELETAL MUSCLE

Each of the body's approximately 600-plus skeletal muscles contains various wrappings of fibrous connective tissue. **Figure 11.15** shows a cross-section of skeletal muscle structures and arrangement of connective tissue wrappings, including the thousands of cylindrical cells called fibers. Their number largely becomes fixed by the second trimester of fetal development. These long, slender multinucleated fibers lie parallel to each other, with the force of action directed mainly along the fiber's long axis. Individual fiber length varies from a few mm in the eye muscles to nearly 30 cm in the large antigravity leg muscles with fiber width reaching 0.15 mm.

Levels of Organization

As shown in **Figure 11.15A**, a fine layer of connective tissue, the **endomysium**, wraps each muscle fiber and separates it from neighboring fibers. Another layer of connective tissue, the **perimysium**, surrounds a bundle of up to 150 muscle fibers to form a **fasciculus**. The **epimysium** surrounds the entire muscle with a fascia of fibrous **connective tissue**. This protective sheath tapers at its distal end as it blends into and joins the intramuscular tissue sheaths to form the dense, strong connective tissue of **tendons**. Tendons connect each end of the muscle to the **periosteum**, the bone's outermost covering. The force of muscle action transmits directly from the muscle's connective tissue harness to the tendons at their bony points of attachment. **Figure 11.15B** presents a cross-sectional view of the sarcoplasmic reticulum and T-tubule system.

Figure 11.15C shows that the tissues of the tendon intermesh with the collagenous fibers within bone. This forms a powerful link between muscle and bone that remains inseparable except during severe stress when the tendon can sever or literally pull away from the bone. When the tendon attaches to the end of a long bone, the bone adapts by enlarging at that end to create a more stable union. Depending on bone size, the term *tubercle*, *tuberosity*, or *trochanter* describes this overgrowth.

The force of muscle action transmits directly from the connective tissue harness to the tendons, which then pull on the bone at their attachment point. Forces exerted on the tendinous attachments under muscular exertion range from 20 to 50 N (197 to 492 kg) per cm^2 of cross-sectional area—forces often larger than the muscle fibers themselves can tolerate.

Medical Problems with Tendons

Tendinitis, a condition of tendon inflammation, most commonly occurs from trauma at the patellar tendon of the knee (common in basketball and volleyball athletes)

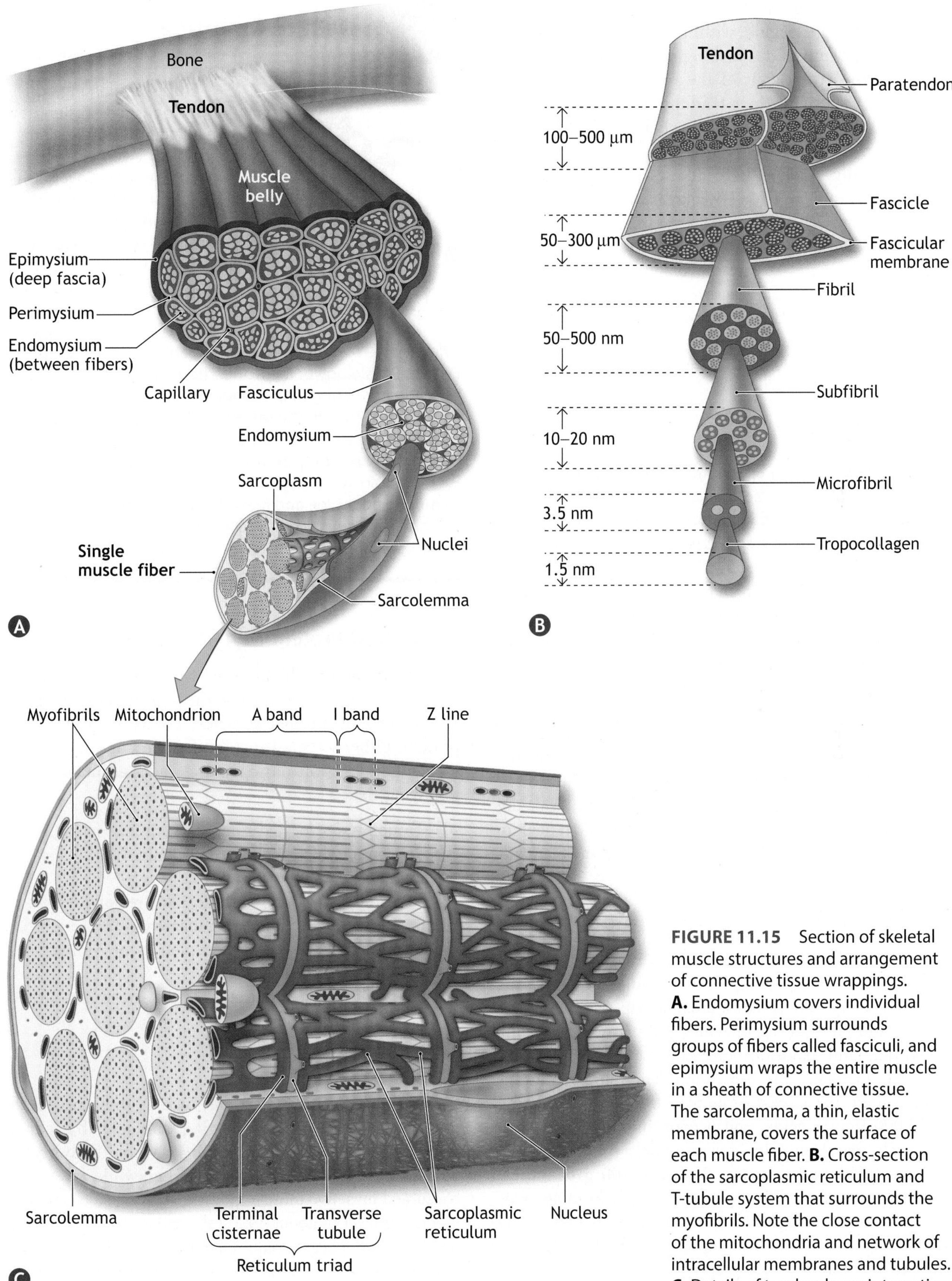

FIGURE 11.15 Section of skeletal muscle structures and arrangement of connective tissue wrappings. **A.** Endomysium covers individual fibers. Perimysium surrounds groups of fibers called fasciculi, and epimysium wraps the entire muscle in a sheath of connective tissue. The sarcolemma, a thin, elastic membrane, covers the surface of each muscle fiber. **B.** Cross-section of the sarcoplasmic reticulum and T-tubule system that surrounds the myofibrils. Note the close contact of the mitochondria and network of intracellular membranes and tubules. **C.** Details of tendon-bone interaction.

and other body regions. Common trauma sites include the ankle's Achilles region, with injury common in sports requiring high impact during lunging and jumping activities, or at the attachment of the rotator cuff muscles, a group of muscles and their tendons that act to stabilize the shoulder as in high-velocity baseball pitching, shotput, or discuss throwing. These injuries usually take months to heal, especially in older individuals. Tendinitis also can occur from chronic overuse ("weekend warrior syndrome," where an individual may try to do too much without sufficient, gradual and systematic training workouts), and putting limbs through extreme movements that exceed the joints' normal ROM. In less severe tendon trauma, common therapies include nonsteroidal anti-inflammatory medicines (NSAIDs; **www.nsaids-list.com**), immobilization, ice, and rest, with gradual return to normal physical activities.

Sarcolemma

The **sarcolemma**, a thin elastic membrane that encloses the fiber's cellular contents, lies beneath the endomysium and surrounds each muscle fiber. **Sarcoplasm**, the fiber's aqueous protoplasm, contains enzymes, fat and glycogen particles, and nuclei (approximately 250 per mm of fiber length) that contain the genes, mitochondria, and other specialized organelles. The sarcoplasm includes an extensive interconnecting network of tubular channels and vesicles called the **sarcoplasmic reticulum**. This highly specialized system enhances the cell's structural integrity. It allows the depolarization wave to spread rapidly from the fiber's outer surface to its inner environment through the T-tubule system to initiate muscle action. The sarcoplasmic reticulum that surrounds each myofibril contains biologic "pumps" that take up Ca^{2+} from the fiber's sarcoplasm. This produces a calcium concentration gradient between the sarcoplasmic reticulum (higher Ca^{2+}) and the sarcoplasm surrounding the filaments (lower Ca^{2+}).

Muscles' Chemical Composition

Skeletal muscle mass contains about 75% water and 20% protein, with the remaining 5% containing inorganic salts and high-energy phosphates, urea, lactate, calcium, magnesium, and phosphorus; enzymes and pigments; sodium, potassium, and chloride ions; and amino acids, fats, and carbohydrates. The most abundant muscle proteins include **titin**, the largest protein in the body (consisting of 27,000 amino acids, and accounting for about 10% of muscle mass), myosin (approximately 60% of muscle protein), actin, and tropomyosin. Each 100 g of muscle tissue contains about 700 mg of the oxygen-binding, conjugated protein **myoglobin** (see the accompanying 3-D model). Myoglobin was first reported in 1958 by English biochemist and crystallographer John Cowdery Kendrew (1917–1997), who shared the 1962 Nobel Prize in Chemistry with Austrian scientist Max Ferdinand Perutz (1914–2002) for the discovery of myoglobin and the globular protein hemoglobin.

fyi A Debt of Gratitude

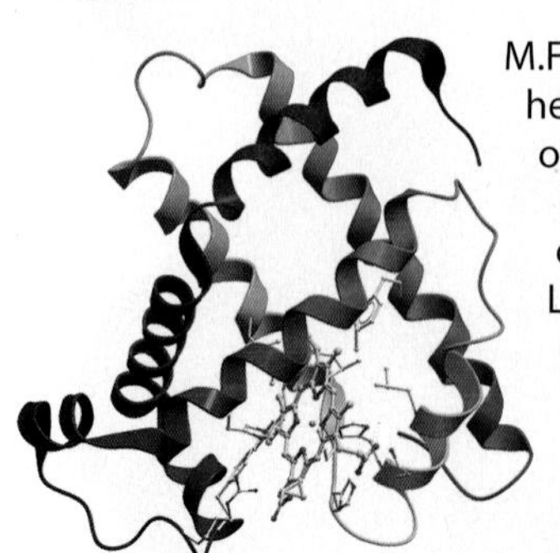

M.F. Perutz was working on hemoglobin and J.C. Kendrew on myoglobin. Interestingly, Kendrew's work grew out of the same Cavendish Laboratory at the University of Cambridge (founded in 1874; **www.phy.cam.ac.uk**) that produced the discoverers of DNA's helical structure in 1953—James Watson (1928–) and Francis Crick (1916–2004)—who jointly shared the 1962 Nobel Prize in Physiology or Medicine. These four researcher-colleagues working in the Cavendish laboratory received their Nobel Prizes in the same year. Exercise physiologists owe a debt of gratitude to these Nobel Prize winners, who paved the way for future studies in exercise biochemistry (hemoglobin and myoglobin and their correlates related to muscle fiber type and maximal oxygen uptake) and exercise molecular biology (DNA and RNA structures and the genetics of almost all related fields in medicine).

Additional Protein Myofilaments

The **myofilaments** chiefly consist of ordered assemblages of the proteins actin and myosin that account for about 85% of the myofibrillar complex. Twelve to fifteen other proteins either serve a structural function or affect protein filament interaction during muscle action, including the following six:

1. Tropomyosin, located along the actin filaments (5%)
2. Troponin (which consists of troponin-1, T, C), located in the actin filaments (3%)
3. α-actinin, distributed in the Z-band region (7%)
4. β-actinin, found in the actin filaments (1%)
5. M protein, identified in the region of the M lines within the sarcomere (<1%)
6. C protein, which contributes to the sarcomere's structural integrity (<1%)

Blood Supply

Intense dynamic muscle actions, such as those needed for sprinting up a steep hill or jogging with a 45-lb backpack over uneven terrain, often require a whole-body oxygen uptake of 4000 $mL \cdot min^{-1}$ and higher, while the oxygen consumed by active muscle increases at least 70 times above its resting level to about 3400 $mL \cdot min^{-1}$. To accommodate the increased oxygen requirement, the local vascular bed redirects blood flow through active tissues similar to a traffic officer rerouting congested traffic. In continuous, rhythmic running, swimming, and cycling, muscle blood flow fluctuates; it decreases during the shortening action and increases during muscle relaxation. Alternating muscle contraction and relaxation provide a "milking action" to propel blood through the muscles for return to the heart. Concurrently, the rapid dilation of previously dormant capillaries complements the pulsatile blood flow. Between 200 and 500 capillaries deliver blood to each square millimeter of active muscle cross-section, with up to four capillaries directly contacting each fiber. The situation differs for endurance athletes; they may have five to seven capillaries surrounding each fiber to ensure greater local blood flow and adequate tissue oxygenation when needed, an adaptation that occurs when genetic predisposition combines with many years of endurance-type training.

Straining-type activities such as trying to lift a heavy object present a somewhat different picture. When a muscle acts at about 60% of its force-generating capacity, elevated intramuscular pressure begins to restrict the muscle's blood supply. The muscle's compressive force with a maximal isometric action literally retards blood flow. This changes the energy dynamics so the breakdown of stored intramuscular phosphagens and anaerobic glycolytic reactions now provide the continuous energy stream to sustain muscular effort.

Muscle Capillarization

Capillary microcirculation expedites removal of heat and metabolic byproducts from active tissues. A rich network of these tiny exchange vessels provides a large surface area to exchange not only metabolically generated heat but fluids, electrolytes, gases, and macromolecules as well. In contracting muscles, micro-vessels immediately after stimulation exhibit increased flow of blood and perfused capillary surface area transport. In regards to exercise training, electron microscopy reveals that the total number of capillaries per muscle (and capillaries per mm^2 of muscle tissue) averages about 40% higher in endurance-trained athletes than untrained counterparts. A positive association also exists between maximal oxygen uptake and average number of muscle capillaries. Enhanced vascularization on the capillary level proves particularly beneficial during physical activity that requires a high level of steady-rate aerobic metabolism.

ULTRASTRUCTURE OF SKELETAL MUSCLE

Electron microscopy, laser diffraction, and histochemical staining techniques have revealed the ultrastructure of skeletal muscle (**http://muscle.ucsd.edu/musintro/jump.shtml**). **Figure 11.16A–F** shows the gross and subcellular microscopic organization of skeletal muscle.

Each muscle fiber contains smaller functional units that lie parallel to the fiber's long axis. These **myofibrils**, approximately 1 μm in diameter, contain even smaller subunits called myofilaments that also run parallel to the myofibril's long axis. The myofilaments consist mainly of the proteins **actin** and **myosin** that constitute about 85% of the myofibrillar complex.

Sarcomeres: Functional Units of Muscle Cells

At low magnification under a light microscope, the alternating light and dark bands along the length of the skeletal muscle fiber appear **striated**. **Figure 11.17** illustrates the structural details of the myofibril's cross-striation pattern. In the resting state, the length of each sarcomere averages 2.5 μm. Thus, a myofibril 15 mm long contains about 6000 sarcomeres joined end to end. The length of the sarcomere largely determines a muscle's functional properties.

The **I band** represents the lighter area and the **A band** represents the darker area. The **Z line** bisects the I band and adheres to the sarcolemma to stabilize the entire structure. *The* ***sarcomere****, the repeating unit between two Z lines, comprises the functional unit of the muscle cell.* The actin and myosin filaments within a sarcomere provide the mechanical mechanism for muscle action (i.e., contraction and relaxation). Optical properties denote the specific bands. When polarized light passes through the I band, it moves at the same velocity in all directions, while light passing through the A band

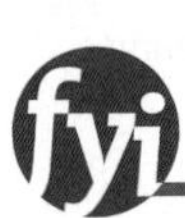

Subcellular Systems and Muscle Function

According to researchers in the Department of Bioengineering and Orthopaedic Surgery at the University of California, San Diego (**http://iem.ucsd.edu/centers/center-for-musculoskeletal-research**), skeletal muscle function depends on efficient coordination patterns established among subcellular systems. A subset of tightly regulated genes encodes these protein-mediated systems. Even slightly altering system regulation can lead to disease, injury, and dysfunction.

The researchers identified nine biologic networks critical to "normal" muscle function, which begin via the expression of proteins necessary to optimize neuromuscular junction function to initiate the muscle cell's action potential. That signal, transmitted to specialized proteins involved in excitation–contraction coupling, enables Ca^{2+} release, which activates contractile proteins to support actin and myosin crossbridge cycling. The forces generated by crossbridge action are then transmitted by cytoskeletal proteins through the sarcolemma to critical proteins that support the muscle extracellular matrix. Ultimately, muscle action requires "turning on" target-specific proteins that regulate energy metabolism. Inflammation, a common response to muscle injury, can alter many pathways within muscle. Muscle also possesses multiple pathways that regulate its mass through diminished size (*atrophy*) or enhanced size (*hypertrophy*). Different isoforms associated with "fast" muscle fibers and corresponding isoforms in "slow" muscle fibers perform highly specific functions. The different networks represent critical biological systems that affect skeletal muscle function. Analogous to a modern computer network, combining high-throughput systems analysis with advanced networking software can potentially study the interrelationships among network systems and muscle function.

Source: Smith LR, et al. Systems analysis of biological networks in skeletal muscle function. *Wiley Interdiscip Rev Syst Biol Med* 2013;5:55.

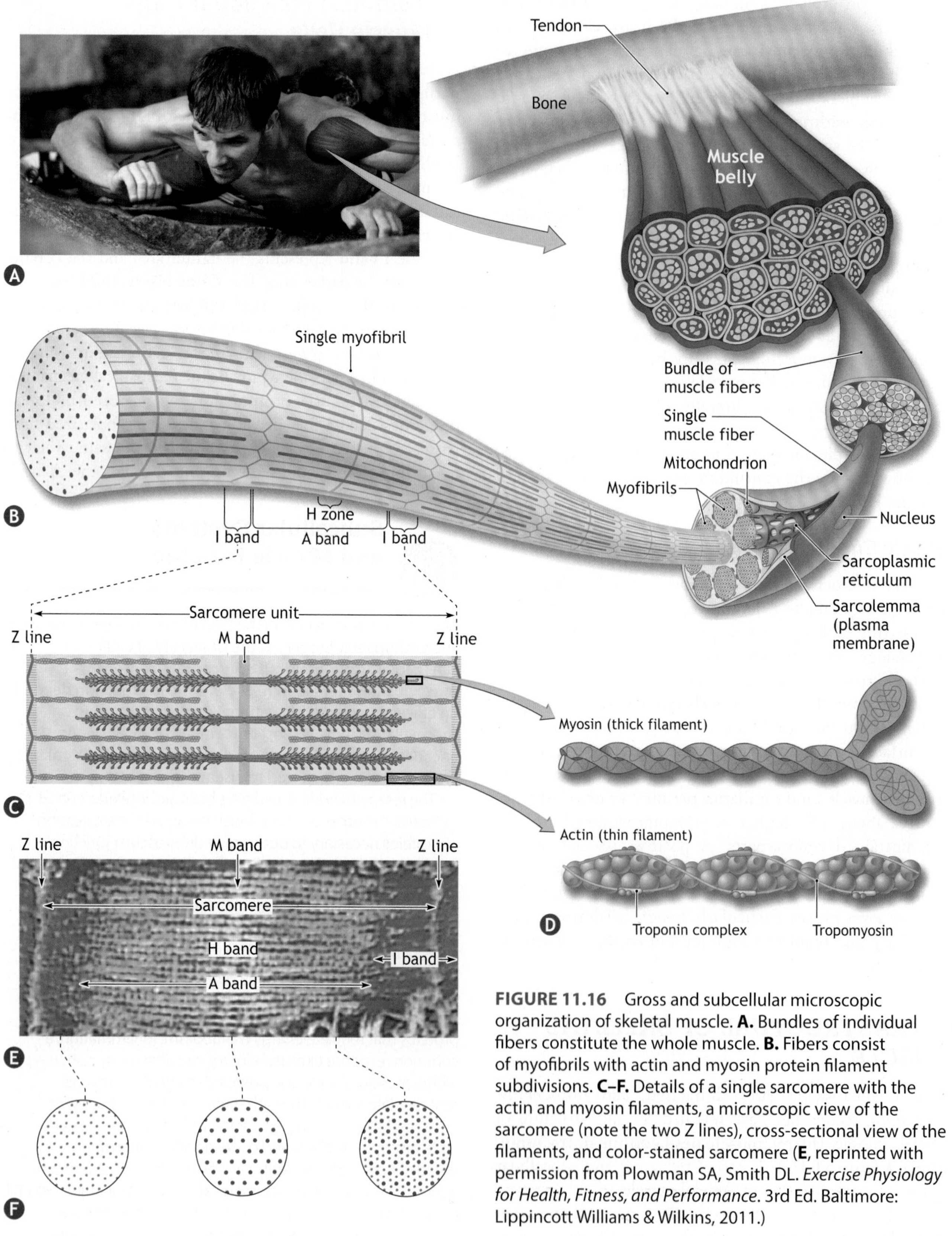

FIGURE 11.16 Gross and subcellular microscopic organization of skeletal muscle. **A.** Bundles of individual fibers constitute the whole muscle. **B.** Fibers consist of myofibrils with actin and myosin protein filament subdivisions. **C–F.** Details of a single sarcomere with the actin and myosin filaments, a microscopic view of the sarcomere (note the two Z lines), cross-sectional view of the filaments, and color-stained sarcomere (**E**, reprinted with permission from Plowman SA, Smith DL. *Exercise Physiology for Health, Fitness, and Performance*. 3rd Ed. Baltimore: Lippincott Williams & Wilkins, 2011.)

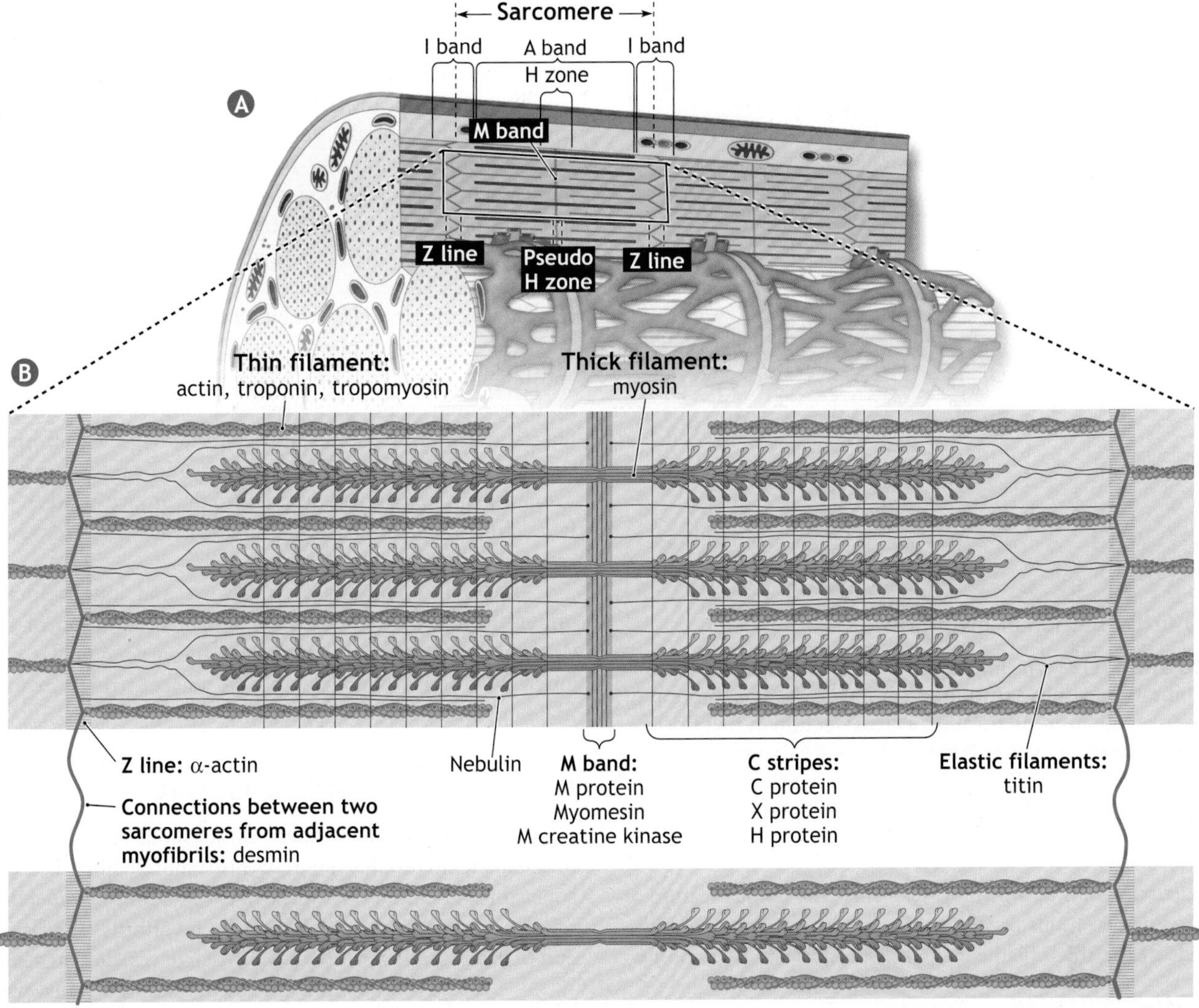

FIGURE 11.17 **A.** Structural position of the filaments in a sarcomere. The Z line bounds a sarcomere at both ends. **B.** Detailed view of a sarcomere, including the additional proteins nebulin (major regulator of force production with three subunits that lie in the groove of each actin filament that block myosin's binding site in the absence of ionic calcium) and titin (closely associated with the myosin molecule, it appears to anchor the myosin network to the actin network).

does not scatter equally. The letter Z indicates "between" (from German, *zwischenscheibe*); the letter M (*mittelscheibe*) denotes "middle"; and the letter H (*hellerscheibe*) denotes "a clear disk or zone." The position of the sarcomere's thin actin and thicker myosin proteins overlaps the two filaments. The center of the A band contains the **H zone**, a region of lower optical density because of the absence of actin filaments in this region. The **M line** bisects the central portion of the H zone and delineates the sarcomere's center. The M line contains the protein structures that support the arrangement of myosin filaments.

Actin-Myosin Orientation

Thousands of myosin filaments lie along the line of actin filaments in a muscle fiber. **Figure 11.18** illustrates the ultrastructure of actin–myosin orientation within a sarcomere at resting length. Six thin actin filaments, each about 50 angstroms (Å; 1 Å = 100 millionths of a centimeter) in diameter and 1 μm long, surround a thicker myosin filament (150 Å in diameter and 1.5 μm long). This forms an impressive muscular substructure. For example, a myofibril 1 μm in diameter contains about 450 thick filaments in the center of the sarcomere and 900 thin filaments at each end. Consequently, a single muscle fiber 100 μm in diameter and 1 cm long contains about 8000 myofibrils, each with 4500 sarcomeres. In a single muscle fiber, this translates to a total of 16 billion thick and 64 billion thin filaments in a single muscle fiber!

Figure 11.19 details the spatial orientation of various proteins that form the contractile filaments. Projections or **crossbridges** spiral around the myosin filament in the region where the actin and myosin filaments overlap. Crossbridges repeat at intervals of 450 Å along the filament. Their globular, "lollipoplike" heads extend perpendicularly to latch onto the thinner, double-twisted actin strands to create structural and

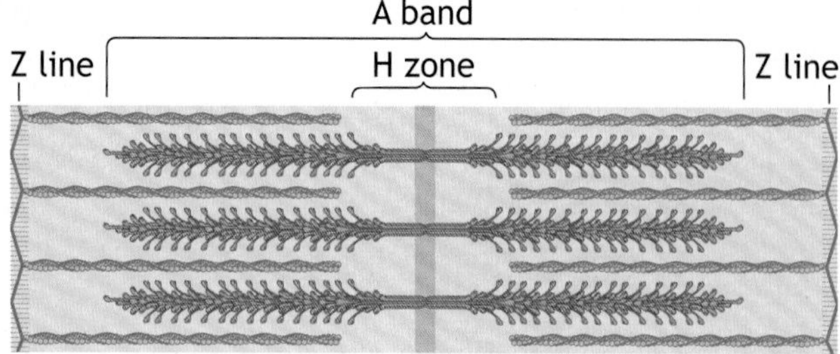

A Resting sarcomere

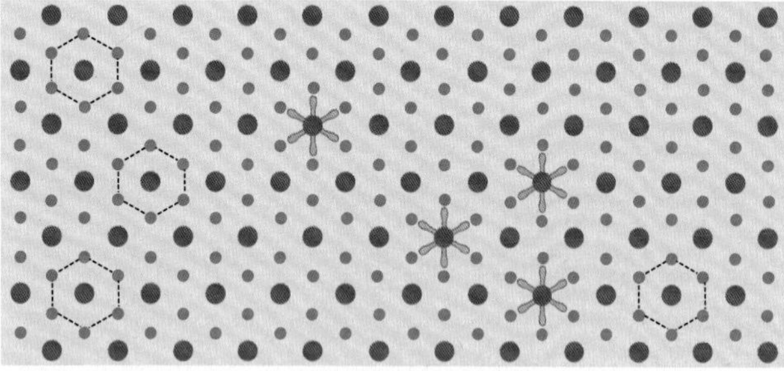

B Cross-section of myofibrils

FIGURE 11.18 **A.** Ultrastructure of actin–myosin orientation within a resting sarcomere. **B.** Representation of electron micrograph through a cross-section of myofibrils in a single muscle fiber. Note the hexagonal orientation of the smaller actin and larger myosin filaments, including crossbridges that extend from a thick to thin filament.

functional links between myofilaments. The unique feature of myosin's two heads concerns their opposite orientation at the ends of the thick filament. ATP hydrolysis activates the two heads, placing them in an optimal orientation to bind actin's active sites. This pulls the thin filaments and Z lines of the sarcomere toward the middle.

Tropomyosin and **troponin**, the two most important core constituents of the actin helix structure, regulate the make-and-break contacts between myofilaments during muscle action. Tropomyosin distributes along the length of the actin filament in a groove formed by the double helix. It inhibits actin and myosin coupling to prevent their permanent bonding. Troponin, which embeds at fairly regular intervals along actin strands, exhibits a high affinity for calcium ions (Ca^{2+}). Troponin plays a crucial role in muscle function and fatigue. The action of Ca^{2+} and troponin triggers myofibrils to interact and slide past each other. During muscle fiber stimulation, troponin molecules undergo a conformational change that "tugs" on tropomyosin protein strands. Tropomyosin then moves deeper into the groove between the two actin strands, "uncovering" actin's active sites so muscle action proceeds.

The *M* line consists of transverse and longitudinally oriented proteins that maintain proper orientation of the thick filament within a sarcomere. The perpendicular oriented M-bridges connect with six adjacent thick myosin filaments in a hexagonal pattern.

Intracellular Tubule Systems

Figure 11.20 illustrates a three-dimensional representation of the intricate tubule system within a muscle fiber. The sarcoplasmic reticulum's complex network of interconnecting tubular channels runs parallel to the myofibrils. The lateral end of each tubule terminates in a saclike vesicle that stores Ca^{2+}. Another network of tubules, the transverse-tubule system or **T-tubule system**, runs perpendicular to the myofibril. The T tubules lie between the lateral-most portions of two sarcoplasmic channels; the vesicles of these structures abut the T tubule. The repeating pattern of two vesicles and T tubules in the region of each Z line forms a **triad**. Each sarcomere contains two triads; this pattern repeats regularly throughout the myofibril's length.

The T tubules pass through the fiber and open externally from the inside of the muscle cell. *The triad and T-tubule system function as a microtransportation or plumbing network to spread the action potential or wave of depolarization from the fiber's outer membrane inward to the deeper cell regions.* The triad sacs release Ca^{2+} during depolarization; this diffuses a relatively short distance to activate the actin filaments. Muscle action begins when the myosin filaments' crossbridges interact with the active sites on actin filaments. When electrical excitation ceases, cytoplasmic free Ca^{2+} concentration decreases and the muscle relaxes.

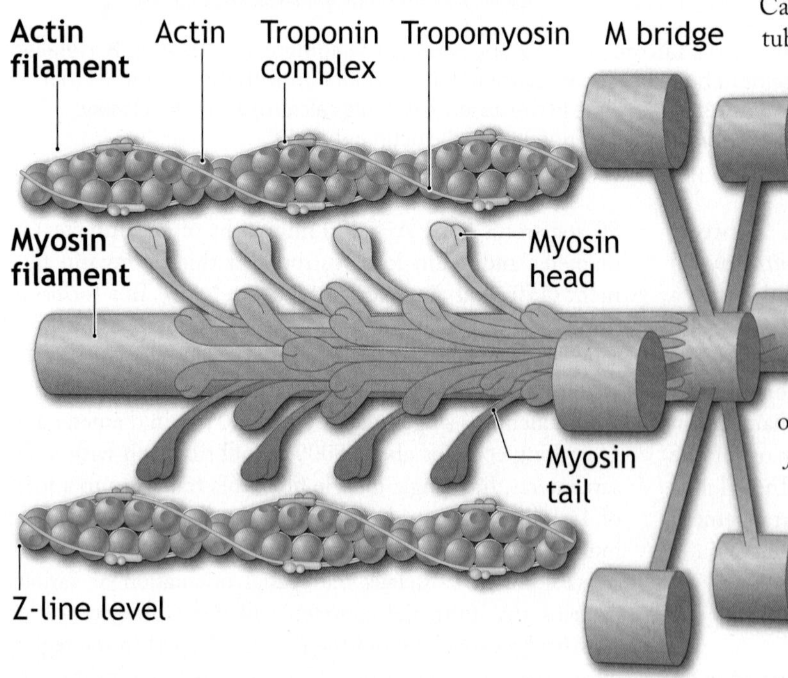

FIGURE 11.19 Details of the thick and thin protein filaments, including tropomyosin, troponin complex, and M bridge. The globular heads of myosin contain myosin ATPase; these "active" heads free the energy from adenosine triphosphate (ATP) to power muscle actions.

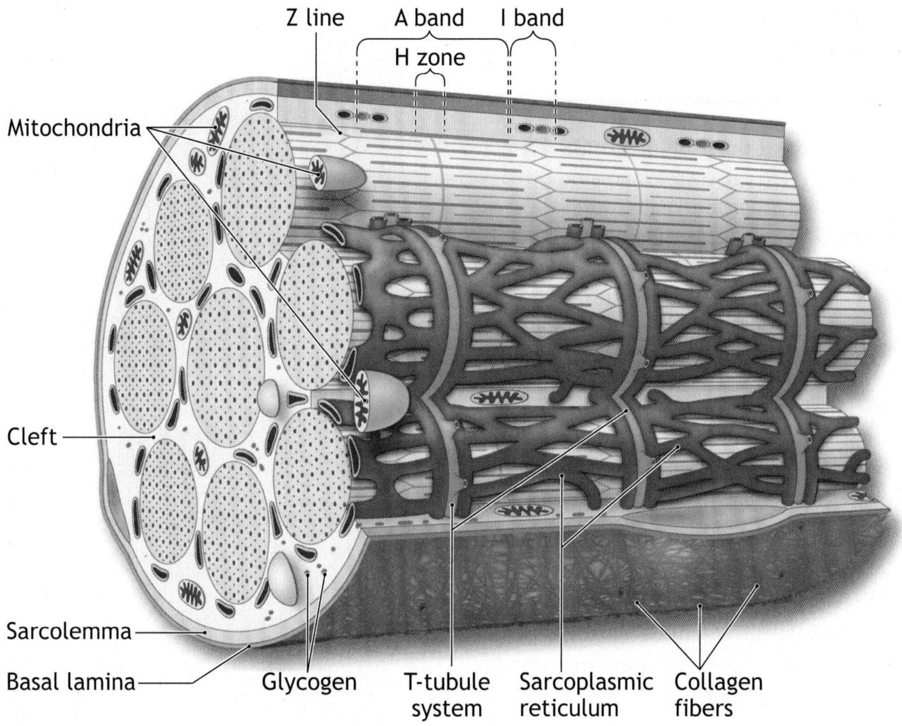

FIGURE 11.20 Three-dimensional representation of the sarcoplasmic reticulum and interlocking mesh T-tubule system within a muscle fiber.

CHEMICAL AND MECHANICAL EVENTS DURING MUSCLE ACTION AND RELAXATION

Sliding-Filament Model

Two British physiologists with the same last name, Hugh Huxley (1924–2013) and Sir Andrew Fielding Huxley (1917–2012), unrelated and working independently in the early 1950s, received the 1963 Nobel Prize in Physiology or Medicine for work on ionic mechanisms involved in excitation and inhibition in the peripheral and central portions of the nerve cell membrane. Their breakthrough scientific experiments led to a proposed **sliding-filament model of muscle action**.

The sliding-filament model proposes that muscle fibers shorten or lengthen because thick and thin myofilaments glide past each other without the filaments themselves changing length. The myosin crossbridges, which cyclically attach, rotate, and detach from the actin filaments with energy from ATP hydrolysis, provide the ***molecular motor*** *to drive fiber shortening* (**http://muscle.ucsd.edu/musintro/Bridge.shtml**). Muscle action changes the relative size of the sarcomere's various zones and bands. **Figure 11.21** shows structural rearrangement of actin and myosin filaments as the thin actin myofilaments slide past the myosin myofilaments and move into the region of the A band during muscle action and move out in relaxation.

thePoint® Appendix SR-6, available online at **http://thePoint.lww.com/MKKESS5e**, provides a link to a video lecture by Dr. Hugh Huxley on the sliding filament model of muscle action as well as other muscle action videos.

See the animation "Sliding Filament Theory" on **http://thePoint.lww.com/MKKESS5e** for a demonstration of this process.

The major structural rearrangement during muscle action occurs in the I band region. The I band decreases markedly in size as the Z bands become pulled toward each

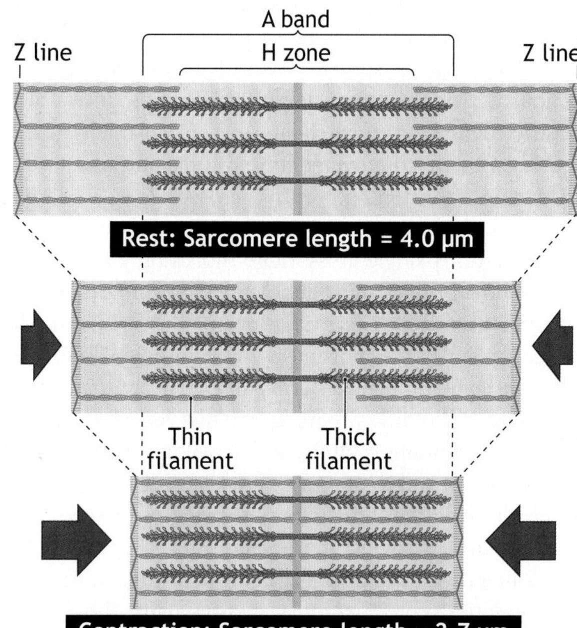

FIGURE 11.21 Structural rearrangement of actin and myosin filaments at rest (sarcomere length, 4.0 μm) and during muscle shortening (contracted sarcomere length, 2.7 μm).

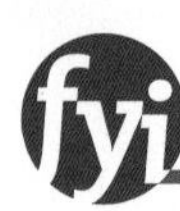

Muscular Contraction or Muscular Action?

During the previous 50 years or so, the term ***muscular contraction*** commonly referred to processes involving generation of muscular tension associated with muscle shortening. In striated muscle, three types of actions can occur during muscle tension: (1) the muscle can shorten *(concentric action)*, (2) it can remain the same length *(static action)*, or (3) it can lengthen *(eccentric action)*. Thus, the term ***muscular action*** seems preferable to refer to tension development in skeletal muscle. In this text, we use the terms "contraction" and "action" interchangeably to refer to the same event.

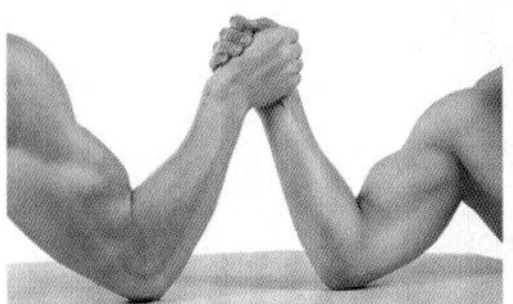

sarcomere's center. No change occurs in A band width, although the H zone can disappear when the actin filaments contact at the center of the sarcomere. An isometric muscle action generates force, but the fiber's length remains relatively unchanged. In this situation, the relative spacing of I and A bands remains constant to allow the same molecular groups to repeatedly interact with each other. The A band widens when a muscle generates force while lengthening in an eccentric action.

Mechanical Action of Crossbridges

Myosin plays a dual enzymatic and structural role in muscle action. *The globular head of the myosin crossbridge provides the mechanical power stroke for actin and myosin filaments to glide past each other.* **Figure 11.22** shows that the oscillating to-and-fro motion of crossbridges powered by ATP hydrolysis; the crossbridges move like oars knifing through water. Unlike oars, however, crossbridges do not move synchronously. If they did, muscle action would produce a series of uneven and jerky movements instead of finely graded, smoothly modulated movements and force outputs.

During shortening, each crossbridge undergoes repeated but independent cycles of attachment and detachment to actin. A single crossbridge moves only a short distance, so crossbridges must attach, produce movement, and detach thousands of times to shorten the sarcomere. The process resembles the movement of an individual climbing a rope, with the individual's arms and legs representing the crossbridges. Climbing progresses by first reaching with the arms; then grabbing, pulling, and breaking contact while the legs extend; and then repeating this procedure throughout the climb as the individual traverses from one point to the next point and so on. Only about 50% of the crossbridges make contact with the actin filaments at any instant to form the contractile protein complex **actomyosin**; the remaining crossbridges maintain some other position during their vibrating cycle. The biochemical technique of *in vitro* motility assay quantifies the behavior of actin and myosin molecules (**www.umass.edu/musclebiophy/techniques%20-%20in%20vitro%20motility%20assay.html**).

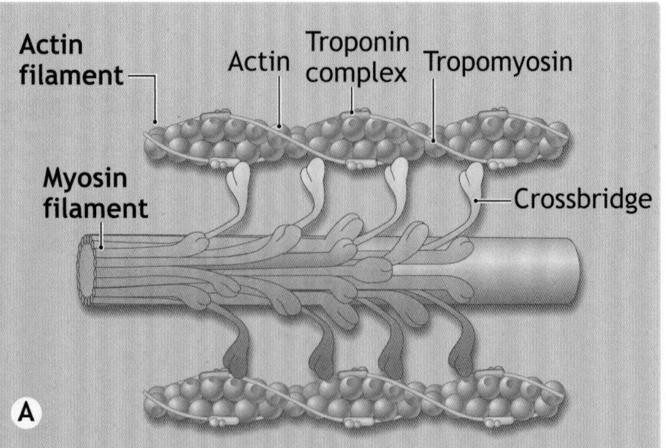

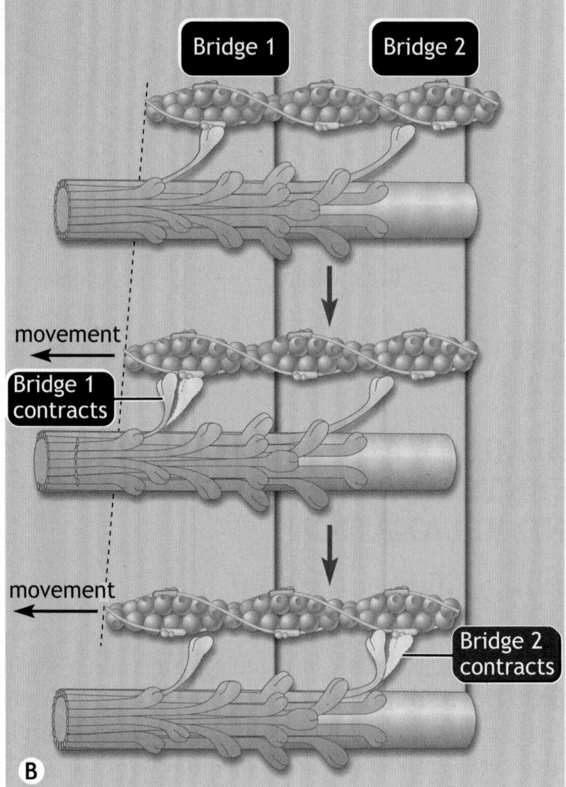

FIGURE 11.22 **A.** Relative positioning of actin and myosin filaments during the oscillating to-and-fro action of the crossbridges. **B.** Each crossbridge action contributes a small displacement of movement. For clarity, we show only one actin strand.

Linking of Actin, Myosin, and Adenosine Triphosphate

The interaction and movement of the protein filaments during a muscle action require the myosin crossbridges to continually oscillate by combining, detaching, and recombining to new sites along the actin strands (or the same sites in a static action). When an ATP molecule interacts with the actomyosin complex, it detaches the myosin crossbridges from the actin filament. This chemical reaction allows the myosin crossbridge to return to its original state so it can again bind to a new active actin site. The dissociation of actomyosin occurs in the following reaction:

Actomyosin + ATP → Actin + Myosin − ATP + Force

ATP serves an important function in muscle action. *Splitting the terminal phosphate from ATP provides energy*

Like a Cocked Spring

Before the muscle action the elongated, flexible myosin head literally bends around the ATP molecule and becomes cocked, almost like a spring. Myosin then interacts with the adjacent action filament, producing a sliding motion that initiates muscle shortening.

for crossbridge movement. One of the reacting sites on the globular head of the myosin crossbridge binds to an actin reactive site. The other myosin active site acts as the enzyme myofibrillar adenosine triphosphatase (**myosin-ATPase**) that splits ATP to release its energy for subsequent force production. ATP splits "slowly" if myosin and actin remain apart; when joined, the ATP hydrolysis rate increases tremendously. Energy released from ATP changes the shape of the globular head of the myosin crossbridge so it interacts and oscillates with the appropriate actin molecule.

Excitation-Contraction Coupling

Excitation-contraction coupling *serves as the physiologic mechanism so an electrical discharge at the muscle initiates chemical events responsible for activation.* An inactive muscle's Ca^{2+} concentration remains relatively low. When stimulated to contract, the action potential's arrival at the transverse tubules releases Ca^{2+} from the sarcoplasmic reticulum's lateral sacs to dramatically increase intracellular Ca^{2+} levels. The rapid binding of Ca^{2+} to troponin in actin filaments releases troponin's inhibition of actin-myosin interaction. In essence, the muscle "turns on," preparing for action.

Myosin–ATPase splits ATP when the active sites of actin and myosin join together. Energy transfer from ATP breakdown moves the myosin crossbridges, allowing the muscle to generate tension as follows:

$$\textbf{Actin + Myosin ATPase} \rightarrow \textbf{Actomyosin ATPase}$$

Joining active sites on actin and myosin activates myosin ATPase to split ATP. The energy generated causes myosin crossbridge movement to produce muscle tension.

$$\textbf{Actomyosin – ATPase} \rightarrow \textbf{Actomyosin + ADP + Pi + Energy}$$

Crossbridges uncouple from actin when ATP binds to the myosin crossbridge. Coupling and uncoupling continue as long as Ca^{2+} concentration remains high enough to inhibit the troponin–tropomyosin system. When neural stimulation ceases, Ca^{2+} moves back into the lateral sacs of the sarcoplasmic reticulum. This restores the inhibitory action of troponin-tropomyosin, and actin and myosin stay apart, provided ATP concentration remains adequate.

Figure 11.23 illustrates the interaction among actin and myosin filaments, Ca^{2+}, and ATP in relaxed and contracted skeletal muscle fibers. In essence, the magnitude and duration of muscle action relates directly to calcium's presence. Muscle

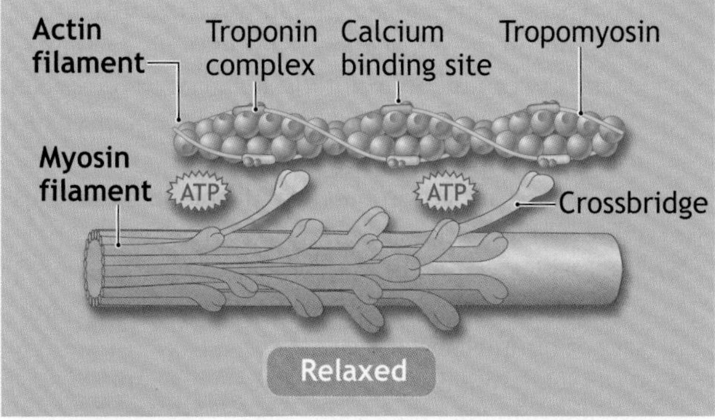

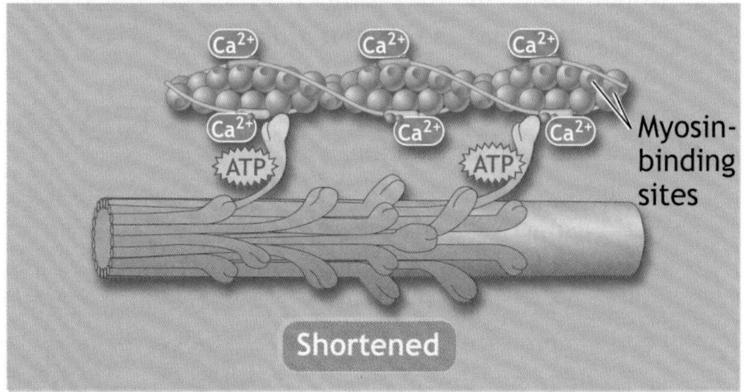

FIGURE 11.23 Interaction among actin-myosin filaments, Ca^{2+}, and ATP in relaxed and contracted muscle. In the relaxed state, troponin and tropomyosin interact with actin, preventing the myosin crossbridge from coupling to actin. During muscle action, the crossbridge couples with actin from Ca^{2+} binding with troponin–tropomyosin.

action ceases and relaxation begins when calcium moves back into the sarcoplasmic reticulum, allowing the troponin-tropomyosin complex to inhibit myosin and actin interaction.

Relaxation

When muscle stimulation ceases, Ca^{2+} flow stops and troponin frees up to inhibit actin-myosin interaction. Recovery involves actively pumping Ca^{2+} into the sarcoplasmic reticulum, where it concentrates in lateral vesicles. Calcium's retrieval from the troponin-tropomyosin protein complex "turns off" active sites on actin's filament. This deactivation serves two purposes:

1. Prevents any mechanical link between myosin crossbridges and actin filaments
2. Inhibits myosin ATPase activity to curtail ATP splitting

Muscle relaxation occurs when actin and myosin filaments return to their original states.

Sequence of Events in Muscle Action and Relaxation

Figure 11.24 summarizes the main events in muscle activation, action, and relaxation. The sequencing begins with initiation of a motor nerve action potential. The impulse then propagates over the entire fiber surface or sarcolemma as it depolarizes. The following nine steps correspond to the numbered sequence in **Figure 11.24**:

Step 1: Generation of an action potential in the motor neuron causes the small, saclike vesicles within the terminal axon to release ACh. ACh diffuses across the synaptic cleft and attaches to specialized ACh receptors on the sarcolemma. Almost perfect symmetry exists between the "imprint" of the presynaptic vesicles that contain ACh and the "imprint" of the postsynaptic receptors that capture ACh.

Step 2: The muscle action potential depolarizes the transverse tubules at the sarcomere's A–I junction.

Step 3: Depolarization of the T-tubule system causes Ca^{2+} release from the sarcoplasmic reticulum's lateral sacs or terminal cisternae.

Step 4: Ca^{2+} binds to troponin—tropomyosin in the actin filaments. This releases the inhibition that prevented actin from combining with myosin.

Step 5: During muscle action, actin combines with myosin-ATP. Actin also activates the enzyme myosin ATPase, which then splits ATP. The reaction's energy produces myosin crossbridge movement and creates tension.

Step 6: ATP binds to the myosin crossbridge; this breaks the actin–myosin bond and allows the crossbridge to dissociate from actin. The thick and thin filaments then slide past each other, and the muscle shortens.

Step 7: Crossbridge activation continues when Ca^{2+} concentration remains high enough from membrane depolarization to inhibit the troponin–tropomyosin system.

Step 8: When muscle stimulation ceases, intracellular Ca^{2+} concentration rapidly decreases as Ca^{2+} moves back into the sarcoplasmic reticulum's lateral sacs through active transport, which requires ATP hydrolysis.

Step 9: Ca^{2+} removal restores the inhibitory action of troponin–tropomyosin. In the presence of ATP, actin and myosin remain in the dissociated, relaxed state.

See the animation "Muscle Contraction" on **http://thePoint.lww.com/MKKESS5e** for a demons

MUSCLE FIBER TYPES

Through the years, different researchers have devised different schemes to classify skeletal muscle fiber types (see A Closer Look: "Histochemical Staining Assays"). Moreover, different researchers have applied different nomenclature

A CLOSER LOOK

Histochemical Staining Assays

Many schemes classify skeletal muscle histochemical, physiologic, and morphologic properties. The most relevant schemes rely on physiologic, biochemical, and histochemical experiments and methodologies combined to develop an iterative and unified understanding of human skeletal muscle types.

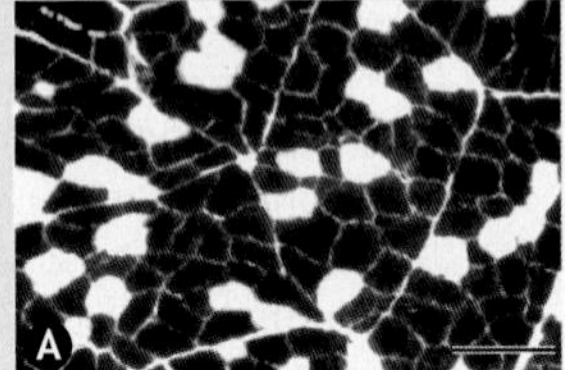

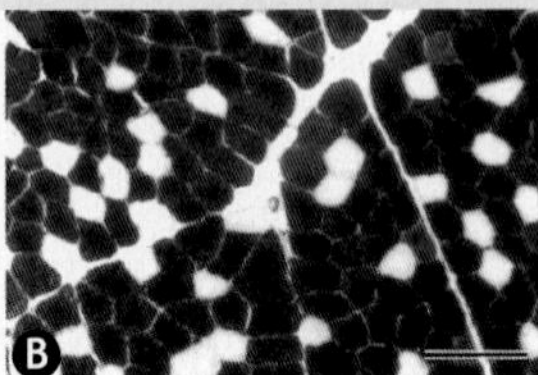

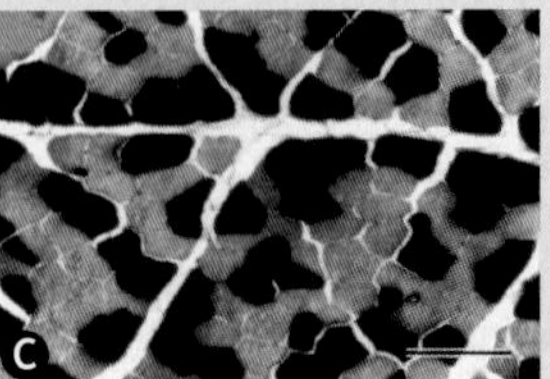

Light micrographs of the vastus lateralis **(A)**, vastus medialis **(B)**, and rectus femoris muscles **(C)**. All micrographs were taken at the same magnification. Fast fibers appear dark, and slow fibers appear light. Calibration bars = 100 µm. (From Lieber RL. *Skeletal Muscle Structure, Function, and Plasticity: The Physiological Basis of Rehabilitation*. 3rd Ed. Baltimore: Lippincott Williams & Wilkins, 2010.)

The term "histochemical" (histo = tissue) implies that the chemical reaction occurs in the tissue itself rather than in a test tube. The three main assays include the myosin ATPase (mATPase) assay, the succinate dehydrogenase (SDH) assay, and the α-glycerophosphate dehydrogenase (α-GPD) assay. These assays rely on the premise that enzymes located in carefully biopsied, thin frozen sections of muscle fibers (6 to 8 µm; [1000 µm = 1 mm thick]) react when treated chemically to allow the researcher to visualize the extent of enzyme activity. The biochemical assay methods rely on the following three basic requirements:

1. Introduction of a biological fuel to serve as one of many enzymes for analyses
2. Addition of an energy source to activate the enzyme so it joins with the substrate
3. Formation of a reaction product to link to another product to form a precipitate for final microscopic assessment

Histochemical methods identify muscle fibers as fast or slow, oxidative or nonoxidative, and glycolytic or nonglycolytic. If a muscle fiber stains for all three properties, any of eight (2^3) fiber types could theoretically occur. However, more than 95% of human muscle classify into one of three categories.

Human Fiber Type by Histochemical Assay

Fiber Type	ATPase Activity (Fast or Slow)	SDH Activity	α-GPD Activity
Fast-glycolytic (FG)	High	Low	High
Fast-glycolytic-oxidative (FOG)	High	High	High
Slow-oxidative (SO)	Low	High	Low

GPD, glycerophosphate dehydrogenase; SDH, succinate dehydrogenase.

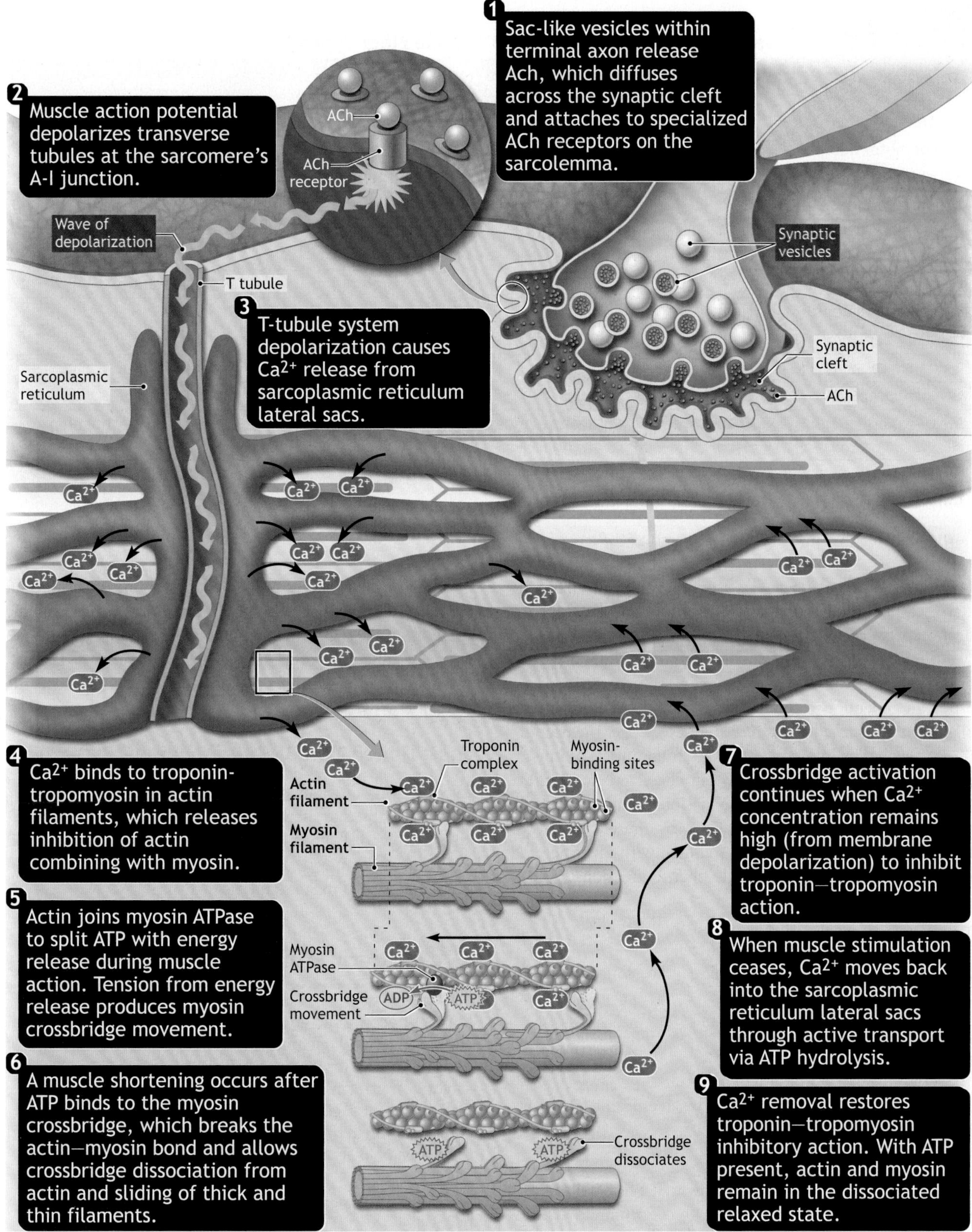

1 Sac-like vesicles within terminal axon release Ach, which diffuses across the synaptic cleft and attaches to specialized ACh receptors on the sarcolemma.
2 Muscle action potential depolarizes transverse tubules at the sarcomere's A-I junction.
ACh
ACh receptor
Wave of depolarization
T tubule
Synaptic vesicles
3 T-tubule system depolarization causes Ca2+ release from sarcoplasmic reticulum lateral sacs.
Sarcoplasmic reticulum
Synaptic cleft
ACh
Ca2+
4 Ca2+ binds to troponin-tropomyosin in actin filaments, which releases inhibition of actin combining with myosin.
Troponin complex
Myosin-binding sites
Actin filament
Myosin filament
5 Actin joins myosin ATPase to split ATP with energy release during muscle action. Tension from energy release produces myosin crossbridge movement.
Myosin ATPase
Crossbridge movement
ADP
ATP
6 A muscle shortening occurs after ATP binds to the myosin crossbridge, which breaks the actin–myosin bond and allows crossbridge dissociation from actin and sliding of thick and thin filaments.
Crossbridge dissociates
7 Crossbridge activation continues when Ca2+ concentration remains high (from membrane depolarization) to inhibit troponin–tropomyosin action.
8 When muscle stimulation ceases, Ca2+ moves back into the sarcoplasmic reticulum lateral sacs through active transport via ATP hydrolysis.
9 Ca2+ removal restores troponin–tropomyosin inhibitory action. With ATP present, actin and myosin remain in the dissociated relaxed state.

FIGURE 11.24 Schematic view of the nine main events in muscle contraction and relaxation. Numbers correspond to the sequence of nine steps outlined in the section "Sequence of Events in Muscle Action and Relaxation." The neurotransmitter acetylcholine (ACh), released from saclike vesicles within the terminal axon, initiates transmission at the myoneural junction where the electrochemical signal "jumps" across the 0.05-μm cleft between neuron and muscle fiber. The electrical impulse traveling at a velocity of $1\ m \cdot s^{-1}$ or faster, spreads through the fiber's architecturally elegant tubule transportation system to the myofibril's inner contractile "machinery."

TABLE 11.3 Classification of Human Skeletal Muscle Fiber Types

Fiber Type	Type I Fibers	Type IIa Fibers	Type IIx Fibers	Type IIb Fibers
Contraction time	Slow	Moderately fast	Fast	Very fast
Size of motor neuron	Small	Medium	Large	Very large
Resistance to fatigue	High	Fairly high	Intermediate	Low
Activity used for	Aerobic	Long-term anaerobic	Short-term anaerobic	Short-term anaerobic
Maximum duration of use	Hours	30 minutes	5 minutes	1 minute
Force production	Low	Medium	High	Very high
Mitochondrial density	High	High	Medium	Low
Capillary density	High	Intermediate	Low	Low
Oxidative capacity	High	High	Intermediate	Low
Glycolytic capacity	Low	High	High	High
Major storage fuel	Triacylglycerol	Creatine phosphate, glycogen	Creatine phosphate, glycogen	Creatine phosphate, glycogen
Myosin heavy chains, human genes	MYH7[a]	MYH2	MYH1	MYH4

[a]MYH7 is also known as myosin or myosin heavy chain 4.

to describe different fibers. To date, the so-called metabolic classification emerges as the most useful to make the connection between fiber type and function.

Skeletal muscle does not simply contain a homogeneous group of fibers with similar metabolic and contractile properties. In general, two distinct fiber types have emerged for classification, termed *fast twitch* and *slow twitch*. The proportions of each type of muscle fiber vary from muscle to muscle and person to person. **Table 11.3** lists characteristics of these fiber types and their different subdivisions, and **Figure 11.25** shows serial cross-sections obtained by muscle biopsy of human vastus lateralis muscle (A and B) with identification of type I and type IIa, IIx, and IIc fiber subdivisions (C–F).

Fast-Twitch Muscle Fibers

Fast-twitch muscle fibers exhibit the following four characteristics:

1. High capability for electrochemical transmission of action potentials
2. High myosin ATPase activity
3. Rapid Ca^{2+} release and uptake by an efficient sarcoplasmic reticulum
4. High crossbridge turnover rate

These four qualities indicate how well a fast-twitch fiber rapidly transfers energy for quick, forceful muscle actions. Recall that myosin-ATPase splits ATP to provide energy for muscle action (force generation). Fast-twitch fiber's intrinsic speed of action and tension development averages two to three times the speed of fibers classified as slow twitch.

Fast-twitch fibers rely on a well-developed, short-term glycolytic system for energy transfer and force production. Labeled as *FG fibers*, they signify fast glycogenolytic capabilities. Short-term, high-power output activities and other forceful muscular actions that depend almost entirely on anaerobic metabolism for energy activate fast-twitch fibers. Stop-and-go or change-of-pace sports like basketball, soccer, rugby, lacrosse, and field hockey also require rapid energy from anaerobic pathways in fast-twitch fibers.

Fast-Twitch Type II Subdivisions

Type II fibers distribute in three primary subtypes: types IIa, IIx, and IIb. Studies show that human skeletal muscle contains types I, IIa, and IIx fibers (previously referred to as type IIb) and a new type IIb subtype. Types IIa, IIx, and IIb fibers appear in skeletal muscle of rodents and cats.

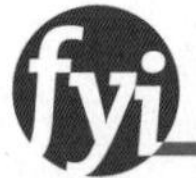

Rigor Mortis

Muscles become stiff and rigid about 3 hours after death, a condition termed *rigor mortis* (Latin *mors*, ***mortis*** meaning "of death"). This occurs because ATP no longer functions in the sarcoplasmic reticulum's membrane to pump calcium ions into the terminal cisternae. When Ca^{2+} diffuses from a higher concentration in the terminal cisternae and extracellular fluid to an area of lower concentration in the sarcomere, it binds with troponin to allow crossbridging between the actin and myosin proteins. In essence, without ATP, the myosin crossbridges and actin remain attached so the muscle cannot return to a relaxed state.

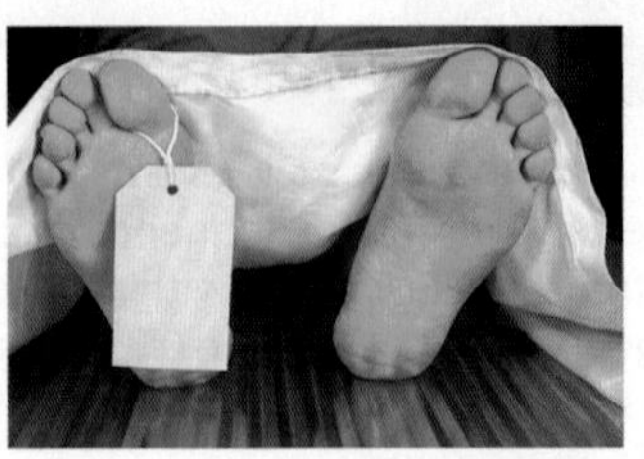

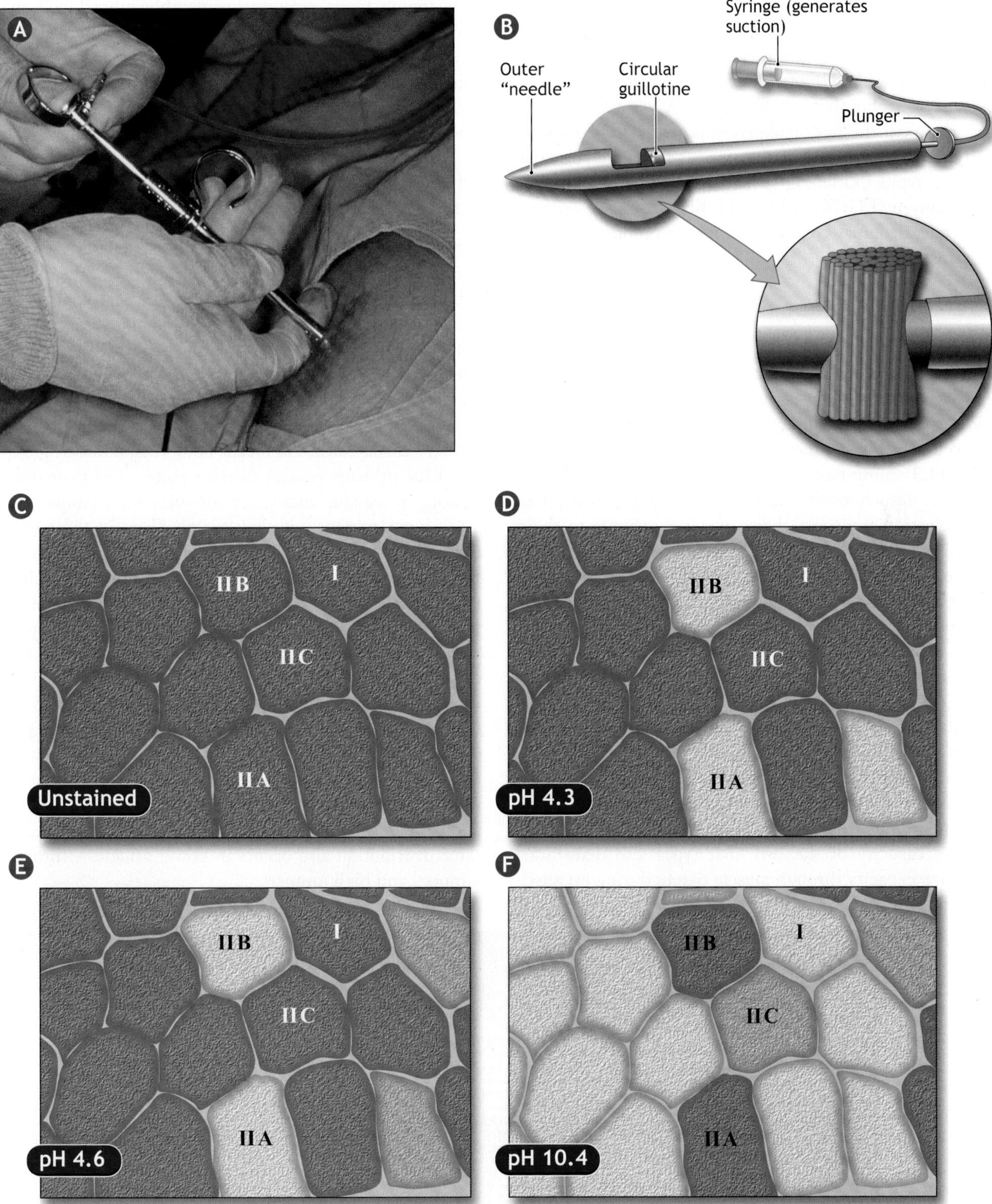

FIGURE 11.25 Serial cross-sections obtained by muscle biopsy of human vastus lateralis muscle (**A** and **B**) with identification of type I and type IIA, X, and C fiber subdivisions. **C.** Thick unstained section (40–50 μm) where all fibers appear similar. *Three other panels* indicate same fibers stained for myosin–ATPase activity at a preincubation pH of 4.3 (highly acidic) **(D)**, 4.6 (intermediate acidity) **(E)**, and **(F)** 10.4 (alkaline). (**A**, reprinted with permission from Plowman SA, Smith DL. *Exercise Physiology for Health, Fitness, and Performance*. 3rd Ed. Baltimore: Lippincott Williams & Wilkins, 2011.)

Muscle type IIa fiber exhibits fast shortening speed and a moderately well-developed capacity for energy transfer from both aerobic (high level of aerobic enzyme succinic dehydrogenase [SDH]) and anaerobic (high level of anaerobic enzyme phosphofructokinase [PFK]) sources. These fibers represent the **fast-oxidative-glycolytic (FOG) fibers.** The **type IIx fiber** possesses the greatest anaerobic potential and most rapid shortening velocity; it represents the "true" **fast-glycolytic (FG) fiber.** A **type IIc fiber,** normally rare and undifferentiated, may contribute to reinnervation and motor unit transformation.

Slow-Twitch Muscle Fibers (Type 1)

Slow-twitch, type 1 muscle fibers generate energy for ATP resynthesis predominantly by aerobic energy transfer. They possess a low activity level of myosin ATPase, a slow speed of muscle action, and a glycolytic capacity less well developed than their fast-twitch counterparts (**Table 11.3**). Slow-twitch fibers contain relatively large and numerous mitochondria and iron-containing cytochromes of the electron transport chain, which contribute to their red appearance. A high concentration of mitochondrial enzymes supports this fiber's enhanced aerobic metabolic machinery. Consequently, slow-twitch fibers resist fatigue and power prolonged aerobic exercise. These fibers are labeled **slow-oxidative (SO) fibers,** which describe their slow contraction speed and predominant reliance on oxidative metabolism.

Studies of muscle glycogen depletion patterns indicate that slow-twitch muscle fibers exclusively power prolonged, moderate intensity physical activity. Even after 12 hours of physical activity, the limited but still available glycogen exists in the unused fast-twitch fibers. Differences in the oxidative capacity of the two fiber types also determine blood flow capacity through muscle tissues during exercise; slow-twitch fibers receive considerably more blood than fast-twitch neighbors. Activity at near-maximum aerobic and anaerobic levels like middle-distance running, swimming, or multiple-sprint sports like field hockey, lacrosse, basketball, ice hockey, and soccer, activates both muscle fiber types.

Muscle Fiber Type Differences Among Athletic Groups

Interesting observations concern muscle fiber type variation among individuals and sport categories and the possible influence of specific exercise training on fiber composition and metabolic capacity. On average, sedentary children and adults possess about 50% slow-twitch fibers. The percentage of fast-twitch fibers probably distributes equally between subdivisions, yet fiber-type distribution varies considerably among individuals. Generally, one's muscle fiber–type distribution remains consistent for the body's major muscle groups.

Elite athletes possess distinct patterns of fiber distribution. Successful endurance athletes, for example, possess a predominance of slow-twitch fibers in the muscles routinely activated in their sport; the fast-twitch muscle fiber predominates for sprint athletes. **Figure 11.26** illustrates sport-specific tendencies for muscle fiber type distribution for top Nordic competitors in different sports. Athletic groups with the highest endurance capacities (e.g., distance runners and cross-country skiers) possess the highest percentage of slow-twitch fibers, often 90% to 95% in their gastrocnemius muscle. Weightlifters, ice hockey players, and sprinters have more fast-twitch fibers and relatively lower aerobic capacities. As might be expected, men and women who perform in middle-distance events display approximately equal percentages of the two fiber types. The same distribution also occurs in power athletes—throwers, jumpers, and high jumpers.

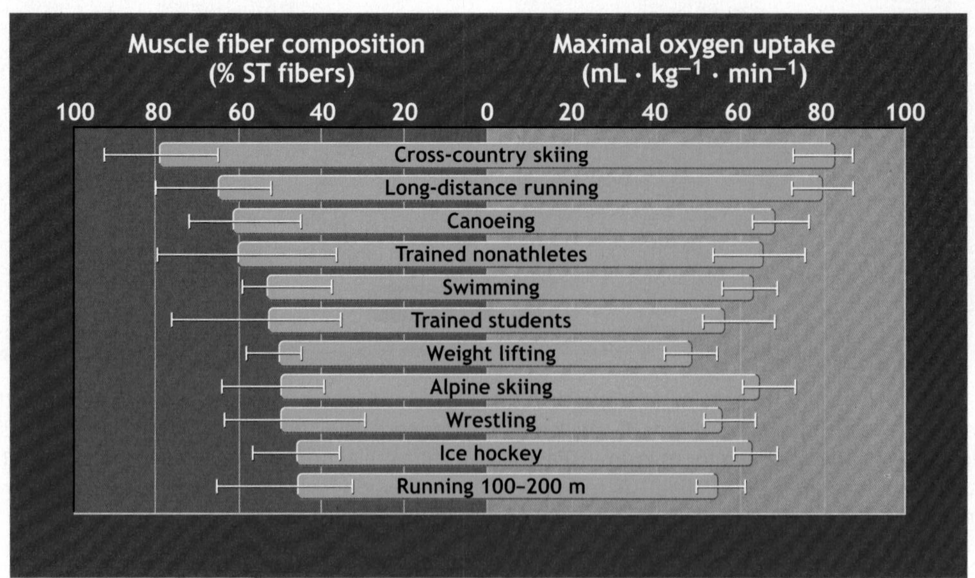

FIGURE 11.26 Muscle fiber composition (percentage slow-twitch fibers, **left side**) and maximal oxygen uptake **(right side)** in athletes representing different sports. The outer *white bars* denote the range. (From Bergh U, et al. Maximal oxygen uptake and muscle fiber types in trained and untrained humans. *Med Sci Sports* 1978;10:151.)

Muscle Fiber Training Specificity

Why do some highly trained athletes who switch to a sport requiring a different neural activation of somewhat similar muscle groups or the activation of totally different muscle groups feel essentially untrained for the new activity, such as a downhill Alpine skier trying to perfect water skiing or an endurance swimmer attempting a distance run? The answer is fairly straightforward—only the specific fibers activated in training adapt metabolically, physiologically, and neurologically to the specific exercise regimen. In the case of Alpine skiing and water skiing, training involves a differing pattern of neurological activation. In swimming, the emphasis falls upon the upper-body musculature while running emphasizes specific lower limb muscle action patterns. Thus, swimmers do not necessarily transfer their predominantly upper-body muscle action "fitness" to a running sport unless they specifically train the muscles required for that sport.

The relatively clear-cut distinctions between exercise performance and muscle fiber composition pertain mainly to elite athletes with prominence in a sport category. Even among this group, muscle fiber composition does not solely determine performance success. This seems reasonable because successful performance reflects the blending of many physiologic, biochemical, neurologic, and biomechanical "support systems," not simply the single factor of muscle fiber type. Endurance athletes have relatively normal-sized muscle fibers with a tendency toward enlarged slow twitch fibers. Conversely, weightlifters and other power athletes show definite enlargement in both fiber types, particularly fast-twitch fibers. These fibers may exceed by 45% those of endurance athletes or sedentary persons of the same age. Strength and power training induce enlargement of the fiber's contractile apparatus—specifically actin and myosin filaments—and total glycogen content. Larger muscle fibers in male athletes and a larger total muscle mass in male athletes characterize the principal gender differences in muscle morphology.

SUMMARY

1. Various connective tissue wrappings that encase skeletal muscle eventually blend into and join the tendinous attachment to bone.
2. Muscles act on the bony levers to transform ATP's chemical energy into mechanical energy and motion.
3. Skeletal muscle contains approximately 75% water and 20% protein, with the remaining 5% containing inorganic salts, enzymes, minerals, pigments, fats, proteins, and carbohydrates.
4. Vigorous aerobic physical activity increases the active muscle's oxygen uptake nearly 70 times above its resting level.
5. Aerobic training augments a muscle's oxygen supply by increasing capillary density up to 40%.
6. The sarcomere contains the contractile proteins actin and myosin, the muscle fiber's functional unit.
7. An average-sized muscle fiber contains about 4500 sarcomeres and a total of 16 billion thick (myosin) and 64 billion thin (actin) filaments.
8. The actin and myosin filaments within the sarcomere provide the mechanical mechanism for muscle action.
9. Crossbridge projections link thin and thick contractile filaments. The globular head of the myosin crossbridge provides the mechanical power stroke for actin and myosin filaments to slide past each other.
10. Tropomyosin and troponin, two core myofibrillar proteins, regulate the make-and-break contacts between filaments during muscle action.
11. Tropomyosin inhibits actin and myosin interaction; troponin with calcium triggers the myofibrils to interact and glide past each other.
12. The triad and T-tubule microtransportation system network spreads the action potential from the fiber's outer membrane inward to deeper cell regions.
13. Muscle action occurs when calcium activates actin, attaching the myosin crossbridges to active sites on the actin filaments. Relaxation occurs when calcium concentration decreases.
14. The sliding-filament model proposes that a muscle fiber shortens or lengthens because its protein filaments slide past each other without changing length.
15. Excitation-contraction coupling initiates an electrical discharge that triggers the chemical events for muscle action.
16. Two types of muscle fibers are classified according to contractile and metabolic characteristics: (1) fast-twitch fibers (type II), which predominantly generate energy anaerobically for quick, powerful contractions; and (2) slow-twitch fibers (type I), which contract at relatively slow speeds and generate energy for ATP resynthesis largely by aerobic metabolism.
17. Muscle fiber–type distribution differs among individuals. A person's genetic code largely determines his or her predominant fiber type.
18. Specific exercise training improves the energy-generating capacity of each fiber type.

THINK IT THROUGH

1. Show how knowledge about neuromuscular exercise physiology can enhance an athlete's (1) muscular strength and power and (2) sports skill performance.
2. In terms of neuromuscular physiology, discuss the validity of the adage "practice makes perfect."
3. Discuss the meaning of *molecular motor* to describe how the myofilament crossbridges contribute to muscle fiber action.

KEY TERMS

A band: Dark band along the length of the skeletal muscle fiber.

Acetylcholine (ACh): Chemical stimulus that changes an electrical neural impulse at the motor end plate into a chemical stimulus.

Ach; cholinergic fibers: Parasympathetic, cholinergic nerve endings that release the neurotransmitter acetylcholine.

Actin: A globular multi-functional protein that forms the muscle fiber's myofilaments; the proteins actin and myosin constitute about 85% of the myofibrillar complex.

Action potential: Electrical potential change between the inside and outside of stimulated nerve or muscle fibers while transmitting nerve impulses.

Actomyosin: Contractile protein complex formed by 50% of the crossbridges that contact the actin filaments at any instant.

Adrenergic fiber: Autonomic nervous system neuron that releases norepinephrine and dopamine.

All-or-none principle: Muscle cells always contract to the fullest extent once the neuron fires and the impulse reaches the neuromuscular junction.

Anterior (alpha) motor neuron: Large brainstem and spinal cord motor neurons; innervate extrafusal muscle fibers of skeletal muscle to directly initiate their contraction.

Axon: Portion of neuron extending from the spinal cord to transmit an impulse to the muscle fibers it innervates.

Cell body: Portion of neuron located within the spinal cord's gray matter.

Central nervous system (CNS): Includes the brain and spinal cord, the main "processing center" for the nervous system that integrates information it receives and coordinates and influences the body's activities.

Cerebellum: Latin for "little brain." Located at the base of the brain, just above the brain stem; composed of two hemispheres; receives information from the sensory system, spinal cord, and other brain areas to regulate motor movements.

Cerebral cortex: Brain's neural tissue covering the surface of each cerebral hemisphere (occipital, parietal, temporal, and frontal) with a series of folded convolutions.

Cholinesterase: Enzyme that degrades acetylcholine within 5 ms of its release from synaptic vesicles, which immediately repolarizes the postsynaptic membrane to receive another stimulus.

Concussion: Most common form of traumatic brain injury resulting from external trauma to the head as occurs in contact sports, vehicle accidents, violence, slips and falls, and military combat.

Connective tissue: Cellular material made up of fibers forming a framework and support structure for body tissues and organs; examples include adipose tissue, cartilage, bone, tendons, and blood.

Contract–relax with agonist contraction (CRAC): Isometric action of the muscle group to be stretched; submaximal action of the opposing muscle group.

Control center: Cell body structure involved in replicating and transmitting its genetic code.

Corpus callosum: Large tract of nerve tissue that connects the brain's right and left hemispheres.

Crossbridges: Projections within a muscle fiber that repeat at intervals of 450 Å around the myosin filament in the region where the actin and myosin filaments overlap their globular, "lollipoplike" heads; extend perpendicularly to latch onto the thinner, double-twisted actin strands to create structural and functional links between myofilaments.

Crossed-extensor reflex: Withdrawal reflex when the flexor muscles contract in the withdrawing limb and extensor muscles relax, with the reverse occurring in the opposite limb.

Dendrites: Short neural branches that receive impulses through spinal cord connections and conduct them to the cell body.

Endomysium: Fine layer of connective tissue that wraps each muscle fiber and separates it from neighboring fibers.

Epimysium: Surrounds the entire muscle with a fascia of fibrous connective tissue.

Excitation-contraction coupling: Provides the physiologic mechanism so an electrical discharge at the muscle initiates chemical events responsible for muscle activation.

Extrafusal fibers: Standard muscle fibers that, when innervated by alpha motor neurons, generate tension to allow skeletal movement.

Extrapyramidal tract: Nerve bundle originating in the primary upper motor cortex of the brain stem and connecting at all spinal cord levels.

Fasciculus: Bundle of up to 150 muscle fibers.

Fast-glycolytic (FG) fibers: Represent "true" fast-glycolytic (FG) fibers; exhibit tendencies of IIa fiber for fast shortening speed and capacity for energy transfer from both SDH (aerobic) and PFK (anaerobic) sources.

GABA (gamma-aminobutyric acid): Inhibitory neurotransmitter that stops a particular tissue from acting.

Golgi tendon organs (GTOs): Tiny sensory receptors connected in series to as many as 25 extrafusal fibers; located near the tendon's junction to the muscle that primarily detect differences in muscle tension rather than length.

Gray matter: Thin outer layer of the brain's neural tissue; appears grey because nerve fibers lack a white myelin coating.

H zone: Center of the muscle fiber's A band; a region of lower optical density because of the absence of actin filaments in this region.

Hemispheres: Longitudinal fissure or groove down the brain's midline, which separates the brain's right and left sides.

Herniated disc: Occurs when a portion of the gel-like nucleus pulposus moves out of its normal enclosure, impinges on a spinal nerve, and causes pain in the neck region, trunk, lower back, or leg and foot.

I band: Light bands along the length of the skeletal muscle fiber.

Inhibitory postsynaptic potential (IPSP): Efflux of positively charged potassium ions or influx of negatively charged chloride ions that increases the membrane's resting electrical potential, making it more difficult to fire.

Innervation ratio: Number of muscle fibers innervated by one motor neuron.

Interneuron: Nerve that distributes or relays information to various levels of the brain and spinal cord; usually conveys information between a motor and sensory neuron.

Intervertebral discs: Twenty-four fibrocartilage structures that separate adjacent vertebrae to provide a cushioning surface and shock absorber protective mechanism.

Intrafusal fibers: Skeletal muscle fibers that serve as proprioceptors to detect the amount and rate of change in muscle length.

M line: Bisects the central portion of the muscle fiber's H zone and delineates the sarcomere's center.

Molecular motor: Refers to the myosin crossbridges, which cyclically attach, rotate, and detach from the actin filaments with energy from ATP hydrolysis to drive muscle fiber shortening.

Monoamines: Modified amino acids that amplify and modulate signaling patterns between neurons to increase their effectiveness.

Motor efferent neurons: Conduct impulses outward from the brain or spinal cord.

Motor unit: Skeletal muscle fibers and their corresponding, innervating anterior (alpha) motor neuron

Motor unit recruitment: Process of adding motor units to increase muscle force.

Muscle type IIa fiber: Muscle fibers that exhibit fast shortening speed and a moderately well-developed capacity for energy transfer from both aerobic (high level of aerobic enzyme succinic dehydrogenase [SDH]) and anaerobic (high level of anaerobic enzyme phosphofructokinase [PFK]) sources.

Muscular action: Refers to tension development in skeletal muscle; preferred term to muscular contraction.

Muscular contraction: Process that involves generation of muscular tension associated with muscle shortening.

Myelin sheath: Lipid-rich tissue cover, either long in length or large in diameter; surrounds the axon and acts as an electrical insulator to speed neural conduction along the fiber.

Myoblasts: Specialized embryonic mesodermal cells that give rise to muscle cells.

Myofibrils: Slender cylindrical threads of a muscle fiber composed of the long proteins actin, myosin, and titin, and other proteins that hold them together.

Myofilaments: Small subunits of myofibrils consisting chiefly of actin and myosin that lie parallel to the myofibril's long axis.

Myoglobin: An iron-containing and oxygen-binding conjugated protein within muscle.

Myosin: A large family of motor proteins that slide along actin filaments, while hydrolyzing ATP.

Myosin–ATPase: Enzyme myofibrillar adenosine triphosphatase that splits ATP to release its energy for muscle force production.

Myotube: Fusing of myoblasts to form a "pre"muscle fiber with a tubular appearance.

Neural tone: Constant degree of activation in the parasympathetic and sympathetic nervous systems.

Neurilemma: Myelin sheath's thin membranous covering.

Neuromuscular fatigability: Decline in muscle tension or force capacity with repeated stimulation per unit time.

Neuromuscular junction or motor end-plate: Interface between the end of a myelinated motor neuron and the muscle fiber it innervates; transmits the neural impulse to initiate muscle action.

Neuropeptides: Short amino acid sequences from larger precursor molecules that serve as neuronal signaling molecules to modulate brain activity.

Neurotransmitters: Chemical messenger molecules that diffuse across the junction between one nerve end and the cell body of another nerve to facilitate depolarization (inhibitory) or hyperpolarization (excitatory) effects.

Nitric oxide (NO): Important cellular signaling molecule involved in many physiological and pathological processes; serves as a powerful vasodilator.

Nodes of Ranvier: Neural tissue that interrupts the Schwann cells and myelin every 1 or 2 mm along an axon's length.

Pacinian corpuscles: Small, ellipsoidal mechanoreceptor structures located close to the Golgi tendon organs and embedded in a single, unmyelinated nerve fiber; detect changes in movement or pressure rather than the magnitude of movement or amount of applied pressure.

Parasympathetic: One of the two divisions of the autonomic nervous system; activation inhibits excitation except for vagal parasympathetic excitation of gastrointestinal motility and tone and pancreatic insulin secretion.

Perimysium: Surrounds a bundle of up to 150 muscle fibers.

Periosteum: Bone's outermost covering.

Peripheral nervous system (PNS): Consists of the nerves and ganglia outside of the brain and spinal cord; comprised of 12 cranial and 31 pairs of spinal nerves.

Polysynaptic reflex arc: Neural synapses in either the spinal cord or brain interface through about 100 billion interneurons.

Presynaptic terminals: Distal terminations of an axon's smaller branches, which lie close to the muscle fiber's plasma membrane.

Proprioceptive neuromuscular facilitation (PNF): Inverse stretch reflex induces relaxation in a muscle prior to a stretch to allow for increased range of motion and further stretch.

Proprioceptor: Specialized sensory receptors sensitive to stretch, tension, and pressure in muscles, joints, and tendons.

Pyramidal tract: Consists of nerve fibers that transmit impulses downward through the spinal cord.

Reciprocal inhibition: Isometric action of antagonist muscle group being stretched to induce a reflex facilitation and agonist contraction.

Sarcolemma: Thin, elastic membrane that encloses a muscle fiber's cellular contents; lays beneath the endomysium and surrounds each muscle fiber.

Sarcomere: Repeating unit between two Z lines; comprises the muscle fiber's functional unit.

Sarcoplasm: Muscle fiber's aqueous protoplasm, which contains enzymes, fat, and glycogen particles, and nuclei that contain the genes.

Sarcoplasmic reticulum: Extensive interconnecting intracellular network of tubular channels and vesicles within muscle fiber.

Schwann cells: PNS specialized cells encasing the bare axon and spiraling around it.

Sensory afferent neurons: Conduct impulses from sensory receptors toward the CNS.

Simple reflex arc: Muscle spindle excitation initiates transmission of afferent impulses to the spinal cord via the sensory (dorsal) root to produce a reflex action without cerebral control.

Size principle: Motor neurons with progressively larger axons become recruited as muscle force increases.

Sliding-filament model of muscle action: Theory of muscle contraction that proposes muscle fibers shorten or lengthen because thick and thin myofilaments glide past each other without the filaments themselves changing length.

Slow-oxidative (SO) fibers: Resist fatigue and power prolonged submaximal aerobic exercise.

Somatic nervous system: Component of the peripheral nervous system that innervates voluntary skeletal muscle.

Spatial summation: Simultaneous repetitive stimulation of different presynaptic terminals on the same neuron.

Stretch reflex: Consists of a muscle spindle that responds to stretch, an afferent nerve fiber that delivers the sensory impulse from the spindle to the spinal cord, and an efferent spinal cord motor neuron that activates stretched muscle fibers to contract.

Striated: Striped alternating light and dark bands along the length of the skeletal muscle fiber.

Sympathetic: One of the autonomic nervous system's two divisions; serves to accelerate heart rate, constrict blood vessels, and raise blood pressure via the fight or flight response.

Sympathetic chain: Neurons that exit the spinal cord and enter a series of ganglia, with the nerves terminating relatively far from the target organ.

Synapse: Junction between the presynaptic end of one nerve cell that interfaces with the postsynaptic membrane of another nerve cell to excite, inhibit, or modulate neural activity.

Synaptic cleft: Space between the synaptic gutter and an axon's presynaptic terminal; region where neural impulse transmission occurs.

Synaptic gutter: Invaginated membrane that forms a space for the synaptic end bulbs to interface with the muscle fiber sarcolemma; infoldings tremendously increase its surface area.

Temporal summation: Arrival of many rapid, successive subthreshold excitatory impulses to fire a neuron.

Tendons: Connect each end of a muscle to its boney attachment.

Titin: Largest protein in the body consisting of 27,000 amino acids, and accounting for about 10% of muscle mass.

Traumatic brain injury (TBI): Mild to severe intracranial injury when an external force traumatically injures the brain, usually from contact sports, vehicle accidents, violence, slips and falls, and military combat.

Triad: Repeating pattern of two vesicles and T tubule in the region of each muscle fiber's Z line.

Tropomyosin: Distributes along the length of the actin filament in a groove formed by the double helix to inhibit actin and myosin coupling to prevent their permanent bonding.

Troponin: Embedded at fairly regular intervals along the actin strands that exhibits a high affinity for calcium ions action and troponin; triggers myofibrils to interact and slide past each other.

T-tubule system: Runs perpendicular to the myofibril, lying between the lateral-most portions of two sarcoplasmic channels; functions as part of the muscle fiber's microtransportation network by spreading the action potential from the outer membrane inward to the deeper cell regions.

Type IIc fiber: Normally rare and undifferentiated fiber that may contribute to re-innervation and motor unit transformation.

Type IIx fiber: Possesses the greatest anaerobic potential and most rapid shortening velocity.

Z line: Bisects the intracellular I band and adheres to the sarcolemma to stabilize the entire structure of the muscle fiber.

SELECTED REFERENCES

Armstrong RB. Muscle fiber recruitment patterns and their metabolic correlates. In: Horton ES, Terjung RL, eds. *Exercise, Nutrition, and Energy Metabolism*. New York: Macmillan, 1988.

Asmussen E. Muscle fatigue. *Med Sci Sports Exerc* 1993;25:412.

Asp S, et al. Muscle glycogen accumulation after a marathon: roles of fiber type and pro- and macroglycogen. *J Appl Physiol* 1999;86:474.

Baldwin J, et al. Muscle IMP accumulation during fatiguing submaximal exercise in endurance trained and untrained men. *Am J Physiol* 1999;277:R295.

Barash IA, et al. Rapid muscle-specific gene expression changes after a single bout of eccentric contractions in the mouse. *Am J Physiol Cell Physiol* 2004;286:C355.

Baron B, et al. The eccentric muscle loading influences the pacing strategies during repeated downhill sprint intervals. *Eur J Appl Physiol* 2009;105:749.

Basmajian JV, Deluca CJ. *Muscles Alive. Their Functions Revealed by Electromyography*. 5th Ed. Baltimore: Williams & Wilkins, 1985.

Bassett DR. Scientific contributions of A.V. Hill: exercise physiology pioneer. *J Appl Physiol* 2002;93:1567.

Billeter R, Hoppler H. Muscular basis of strength. In: Komi P, ed. *Strength and Power in Sport*. London: Blackwell Scientific Publications, 1992.

Boe SG, et al. Decomposition-based quantitative electromyography: effect of force on motor unit potentials and motor unit number estimates. *Muscle Nerve* 2005;31:365.

Booth FW, et al. Viewpoint: gold standards for scientists who are conducting animal-based exercise studies. *J Appl Physiol* 2010;108:219.

Boudreau SA, Falla D. Chronic neck pain alters muscle activation patterns to sudden movements. *Exp Brain Res* 2014;232:2011.

Caiozzo VJ, et al. MHC polymorphism in rodent plantaris muscle: effects of mechanical overload and hypothyroidism. *Am J Physiol Cell Physiol* 2000;278:C709.

Caiozzo VJ, et al. Single-fiber myosin heavy chain polymorphism: how many patterns and what proportions? *Am J Physiol Regul Integr Comp Physiol* 2003;285:R570.

Carins SP, et al. Role of extracellular [Ca^{2+}] in fatigue of isolated mammalian skeletal muscle. *J Appl Physiol* 1998;84:1395.

Chaillou T, et al. Identification of a conserved set of upregulated genes in mouse skeletal muscle hypertrophy and regrowth. *J Appl Physiol* 2015;118:86.

Chidnok W, et al. Muscle metabolic responses during high-intensity intermittent exercise measured by (31)P-MRS: relationship to the critical power concept. *Am J Physiol Regul Integr Comp Physiol* 2013;305:R1085.

Crew JR, et al. Muscle fiber type specific induction of slow myosin heavy chain 2 gene expression by electrical stimulation. *Exp Cell Res* 2010;316:1039.

Davis JM, Bailey SP. Possible mechanisms of central nervous system fatigue during exercise. *Med Sci Sports Exerc* 1997;29:45.

Dawson B, et al. Changes in performance, muscle metabolites, enzymes and fiber types after short sprint training. *Eur J Appl Physiol* 1998;78:163.

Delbono O, et al. Loss of skeletal muscle strength by ablation of the sarcoplasmic reticulum protein JP45. *Proc Natl Acad Sci U S A* 2007;104:20108.

Demirel HA, et al. Exercise induced alterations in skeletal muscle myosin heavy chain phenotype: dose-response relationship. *J Appl Physiol* 1999;86:1002.

Dideriksen JL, et al. Physiological recruitment of motor units by high-frequency electrical stimulation of afferent pathways. *J Appl Physiol* 2015;118(3):365.

Edgerton RA, et al. The effects of constant vs. variable workload cycling on performance and perception. *Sports Med Phys Fitness* 2014. In Press as of 12.07.14.

Ennion S, et al. Characterization of human skeletal muscle fibers according to the myosin heavy chain they express. *J Muscle Res Cell Motil* 1995;16:35.

Farina D, et al. Spike-triggered average torque and muscle fiber conduction velocity of low-threshold motor units following submaximal endurance contractions. *J Appl Physiol* 2005;98:1495.

Fisher S, et al. Structural mechanism of the recovery stroke in the myosin molecular motor. *Proc Natl Acad Sci* 2005;102:6873.

Fong AJ, et al. Recovery of control of posture and locomotion after a spinal cord injury: solutions staring us in the face [review]. *Prog Brain Res* 2009;175:393.

Fontes EB, et al. Brain activity and perceived exertion during cycling exercise: an fMRI study. *Br J Sports Med* 2015;49(8):556.

Fowles JR, Green HJ. Coexistence of potentiation and low-frequency fatigue during voluntary exercise in human skeletal muscle. *Can J Physiol Pharmacol* 2003;81:1092.

Gordon T, et al. The resilience of the size principle in the organization of motor unit properties in normal and reinnervated adult skeletal muscles. *Can J Physiol Pharmacol* 2004;82:645.

Green H, et al. Regulation of fiber size, oxidative potential, and capillarization in human muscle by resistance exercise. *Am J Physiol* 1999;276:R591.

Green HJ, et al. Malleability of human skeletal muscle Na^+-K^+-ATPase pump with short-term training. *J Appl Physiol* 2004;97:143.

Green HJ, et al. Reversal of muscle fatigue during 16-h of heavy intermittent cycle exercise. *J Appl Physiol* 2004;97:2166.

Gregory CM, Bickel CS. Recruitment patterns in human skeletal muscle during electrical stimulation. *Phys Ther* 2005;85:358.

Halson SL. Sleep and the elite athlete. *Sports Sci Exchange* 2013;113:1.

Halson SL, Martin DT. Lying to win—placebo and sport science. *Int J Sports Physiol Performance* 2013;8:597.

Hawke TJ. Muscle stem cells and exercise training. *Med Sci Sports Exerc* 2005;33:63.

Heckmann CJ, et al. Persistent inward currents in motor neuron dendrites: implications for motor output. *Muscle Nerve* 2005;31:135.

Hintz CS, et al. Comparison of muscle fiber typing by quantitative enzyme assays and by myosin ATPase staining. *J Histochem Cytochem* 1984;32:655.

Hochachka PW. *Muscles as Molecular and Metabolic Machines*. Boca Raton: CRC Press, 1994.

Holloszy JO, Coyle EF. Adaptations of skeletal muscle to endurance training and their metabolic consequences. *J Appl Physiol* 1984;56:831.

Huxley HE. The fine structure of striated muscle and its functional significance. *Harvey Lect* 1966;60:85.

Huxley HE, Kress M. Crossbridge behaviour during muscle contraction. *J Muscle Res Cell Motil* 1985;6:153.

Iwayama K, et al. Transient energy deficit induced by exercise increases 24-h fat oxidation in young trained men. *J Appl Physiol* 2015;118:80.

Keenan KG, et al. Influence of amplitude cancellation on the simulated surface electromyogram. *J Appl Physiol* 2005;98:120.

Keller P, et al. Using systems biology to define the essential biological networks responsible for adaptation to endurance exercise training. *Biochem Soc Trans* 2007;35:1306.

Kernell D. Principles of force gradation in skeletal muscles. *Neural Plast* 2003;10:69.

Kraus WE, et al. Skeletal muscle adaptation to chronic low-frequency motor nerve stimulation. *Med Sci Sports Exerc* 1994;22:313.

Lambert EV, et al. Complex systems model of fatigue: integrative homeostatic control of peripheral physiological systems during exercise in humans. *Br J Sports Med* 2005;39:52.

Lewis SF, Fulco CS. A new approach to studying muscle fatigue and factors affecting performance during dynamic exercise in humans. *Exerc Sport Sci Rev* 1998;26:91.

Lieber RL. *Skeletal Muscle Structure, Function, and Plasticity: The Physiological Basis of Rehabilitation*. 3rd Ed. Baltimore: Williams & Wilkins, 2010.

Lieber RL, et al. Biomechanical properties of the brachioradialis muscle: implications for surgical tendon transfer. *J Hand Surg [Am]* 2005;30:273.

Lin J, et al. Transcriptional co-activator PGC-1 alpha drives the formation of slow-twitch muscle fibers. *Nature* 2002;418:797.

Lucas CA, et al. Monospecific antibodies against the three mammalian fast limb myosin heavy chains. *Biochem Biophys Res Commun* 2000;272:303.

Lutz GJ, Lieber RL. Skeletal muscle myosin II structure and function. *Exerc Sport Sci Rev* 1999;27:63.

Mottram CJ, et al. Motor-unit activity differs with load type during a fatiguing contraction. *J Neurophysiol* 2005;93:1381.

Muzykewicz DA, et al. The effect of intrinsic loading and reconstruction upon grip capacity and finger extension kinematics. *J Hand Surg [Am]* 2015;40(1):96.

Nielsen OB, Clausen T. The Na/K-pump protects muscle excitability and contractility during exercise. *Med Sci Sports Exerc* 2000;28:159.

Noakes TD. Challenging beliefs: ex Africa semper aliquid novi. *Med Sci Sports Exerc* 1997;29:571.

Noakes TD. Fatigue is a brain-derived emotion that regulates the exercise behavior to ensure the protection of whole body homeostasis. *Front Physiol* 2012;3:82.

Noakes TD, et al. From catastrophe to complexity: a novel model of integrative central neural regulation of effort and fatigue during exercise in humans: summary and conclusions. *Br J Sports Med* 2005;39:120.

Otten E. Concepts and models of functional architecture in skeletal muscle. In: Pandolf KB, ed. *Exercise and Sport Sciences Reviews*. Vol. 16. New York: Macmillan, 1988.

Patel TJ, Lieber RL. Force transmission in skeletal muscle: from actomyosin to external tendons. *Med Sci Sports Exerc* 1997;25:321.

Roach M, et al. Elastic energy storage in the shoulder and the evolution of high-speed throwing in Homo. *Nature* 2013;7455:483.

Roy RR, et al. Modulation of myonuclear number in functionally overloaded and exercised rat plantaris fibers. *J Appl Physiol* 1999;87:634.

Russell AP, et al. Endurance training in humans leads to fiber type-specific increases in levels of peroxisome proliferator activated receptor-gamma coactivator-1 and peroxisome proliferator-activated receptor-alpha in skeletal muscle. *Diabetes* 2003;52:2874–2881.

Sartori M, et al. Hybrid neuromusculoskeletal modeling to best track joint moments using a balance between muscle excitations derived from electromyograms and optimization. *J Biomech* 2014;47:3613.

Schunk K, et al. Contributions of dynamic phosphorus-31 magnetic resonance spectroscopy to the analysis of muscle fiber distribution. *Invest Radiol* 1999;34:348.

Sieck GC. Neural control of movement. *J Appl Physiol* 2004;96:1247.

Skiba PF, et al. Effect of work and recovery durations on W′ reconstitution during intermittent exercises. *Med Sci Sports Exerc* 2014;46:1433.

Skiba PF, et al. Intramuscular determinants of the ability to recover work capacity above critical power. *Eur J Appl Physiol* 2015;115:703.

Smerdu V, et al. Type IIx myosin heavy chain transcripts are expressed in type IIb fibers of human skeletal muscle. *Am J Physiol Cell Physiol* 1994;267:C1723.

Smith MF. The role of physiology in the development of golf performance. *Sports Med* 2010;40:635.

Sweeney LJ, et al. An introductory biology lab that uses enzyme histochemistry to teach students about skeletal muscle fiber types. *Adv Physiol Educ* 2004;28:23.

Ward SR, et al. Are current measurements of lower extremity muscle architecture accurate? *Clin Orthop Relat Res* 2009;467:1074.

Weston AR, et al. African runners exhibit greater fatigue resistance, lower lactate accumulation, and higher oxidative enzyme activity. *J Appl Physiol* 1999;86:915.

Wickham JB, Brown JM. Muscles within muscles: the neuromotor control of intra-muscular segments. *Eur J Appl Physiol* 1998;78:219.

Young KW, et al. Polarization gating enables sarcomere length measurements by laser diffraction in fibrotic muscle. *J Biomed Opt* 2014;19:117009.

Young KW, et al. Resonant reflection spectroscopy of biomolecular arrays in muscle. *Biophys J* 2014;107:235.

Zawadowska B, et al. Characteristics of myosin profile in human vastus lateralis muscle in relation to training background. *Folia Histochem Cytobiol* 2004;42:181.

Zhou P, Rymer WZ. An evaluation of the utility and limitations of counting motor unit action potentials in the surface electromyogram. *J Neural Eng* 2004;1:238.

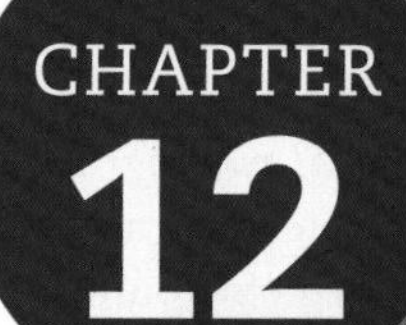

CHAPTER 12

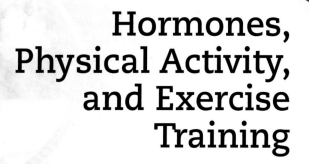

Hormones, Physical Activity, and Exercise Training

CHAPTER OBJECTIVES

- Draw the location of the body's endocrine glands.
- Describe how hormones alter cellular reaction rates of specific target cells.
- Describe how hormonal, humoral, and neural factors stimulate endocrine glands.
- List the hormones secreted by the anterior and posterior pituitary glands, and explain how acute and chronic physical activity affect their release.
- List the thyroid gland hormones, their functions, and how acute and chronic physical activity affects their release.
- List the hormones of the adrenal medulla and adrenal cortex, their functions, and how acute and chronic physical activity affects their release.
- List the hormones released by the pancreatic α and β cells, their functions, and how acute and chronic physical activity affects their release.
- Define type 1 diabetes mellitus (T1DM) and type 2 diabetes mellitus (T2DM), and give three differences between these two diabetes subdivisions.
- List five risk factors for T2DM.
- Outline five benefits of regular physical activity for a type 2 diabetic.
- Explain three general training effects on endocrine function.
- Characterize two functions of opioid peptides, their response to physical activity, and their possible role in the "exercise high."

ANCILLARIES AT A GLANCE

Visit **http://thePoint.lww.com/MKKESS5e** to access the following resources.

- References: Chapter 12
- Interactive Question Bank
- Animation: Diabetes
- Animation: Endocrine Gland Stimulation
- Animation: Hormonal Control
- Animation: Insulin Functions

The **endocrine system** (endocrine *means hormone secreting*) *consists of a host organ or gland, minute quantities of hormone chemical messengers, and a target or receptor organ.* This system integrates and regulates body functions to stabilize the internal environment. Endocrine gland **hormones** affect all aspects of human function; they regulate growth, metabolism, and reproduction, with heightened acute and chronic response to physical and psychological stress. Hormones maintain internal homeostasis by modulating electrolyte and acid-base balance and adjust energy metabolism to power all forms of human biologic work.

The endocrine system operates in synchrony with the nervous system to provide hormonal secretions as needed throughout the body. The endocrine hormones serve as "chemical messengers" in the bloodstream, and the nervous system serves as the "electrical" conduit system. The nervous system essentially performs instantaneously with short-lived results, while the endocrine system hormones act relatively more slowly and often with longer lasting effects.

This chapter reviews important aspects of the endocrine system, including its functions during rest and physical activity and response to acute and chronic exertion.

ENDOCRINE SYSTEM OVERVIEW

Figure 12.1 locates the major endocrine organs—pituitary, thyroid, parathyroid, adrenal, pineal, and thymus glands. Several organs contain discrete areas of endocrine tissue that also produce hormones. These include the pancreas, gonads (ovaries and testes), and hypothalamus; the hypothalamus is also a major organ of the nervous system.

Table 12.1 lists the different endocrine glands and nonglandular endocrine cells and their major hormonal secretions, target tissue(s), and main bodily effects.

ENDOCRINE SYSTEM ORGANIZATION

Three components characterize the endocrine system:

1. Host gland
2. Hormones
3. Target (receptor) cells or organs

Glands classify as endocrine, exocrine, or both. **Endocrine glands** secrete hormones; they lack ducts (referred to as *ductless*) and discharge their substances directly into the extracellular space surrounding the gland. **Figure 12.2** illustrates how hormones diffuse into the blood for transport to target tissues throughout the body. For the kidney shown in the figure, note the receptor structure in gold and the target cell with the hormone molecule (shown as elongated brown triangles) binding to the receptor. Similar to neuromuscular responses, hormone secretion adjusts rapidly to changing bodily functions. For this reason, many hormone secretions occur in a pulsatile or changing rhythmic manner rather than at a constant rate.

See the animation "Endocrine Gland Stimulation" on **http://thePoint.lww.com/MKKESS5e** for a demonstration of this vital endocrine gland function.

Exocrine glands include sweat glands and glands of the upper digestive tract; they contain secretory ducts that lead directly to the specific compartment or surface that requires the hormone. The nervous system controls most exocrine glands.

What Makes a Chemical a Hormone?

The term *hormone* was coined from the Greek word meaning "impetus." An accepted operational definition describes a hormone as *a chemical, usually a peptide or a steroid secreted by a cell or group of cells into blood for transport to a distant target, where it exerts its effect at relatively low concentrations.* Recent findings suggest this may be too broad a definition because many different nonhormone substances also function as chemical messengers.

Must Hormones Be Transported to Distant Targets?

Physiologists have questioned whether a chemical must be transported to a distant target to classify as a hormone. For example, the different hypothalamic-regulating hormones, the trophic chemical messengers that include releasing and release-inhibiting chemicals, and the different "growth factors" seem to lack widespread distribution in the circulation. Nevertheless, they meet the other qualifications for hormone classification. In fact, one hormone secretion can trigger the release of another hormone with a different function. For example, LH (luteinizing hormone) acts on Leydig cells in testes to stimulate testosterone production; **ACTH (adrenocorticotropic hormone)** floods the inner zone of the adrenal gland cortex (zona fasciculata) to stimulate cortisol production; **TSH (thyroid stimulating hormone)** stimulates thyroid gland tissue to release **triiodothyronine (T_3)** and **thyroxine (T_4)**.

Hormones Exert Effects at Low Concentrations

With the discovery of new signal molecules and receptors, the boundary between hormone and nonhormone molecules becomes blurred, particularly at physiologically effective concentrations. Some hormones act at concentrations in the nanomolar (10^{-9} M) to picomolar (10^{-12} M) range, while other chemicals transported in the blood exist in higher concentrations before they exert their effect. For example, **cytokines** (derived from the Greek "cyto" for cell and "kinos" for movement), refer to a group of regulatory, small protein signaling molecules that control cell development and differentiation, including immune response to inflammation and infection, particularly via action of interleukin and interferon. They act on

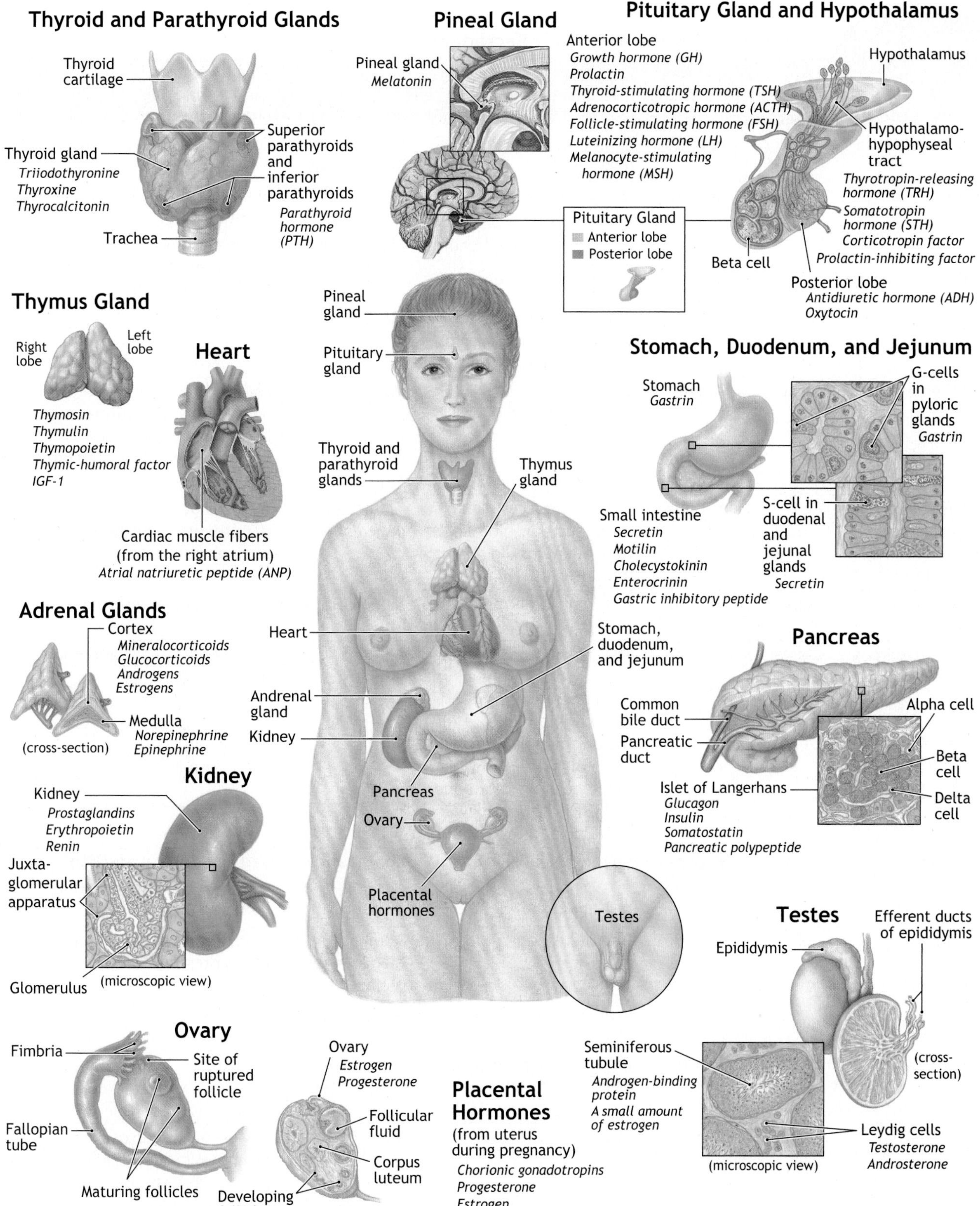
Thyroid and Parathyroid Glands
Thyroid cartilage
Thyroid gland
Triiodothyronine
Thyroxine
Thyrocalcitonin
Trachea
Superior parathyroids and inferior parathyroids
Parathyroid hormone (PTH)
Pineal Gland
Pineal gland
Melatonin
Pituitary Gland and Hypothalamus
Anterior lobe
Growth hormone (GH)
Prolactin
Thyroid-stimulating hormone (TSH)
Adrenocorticotropic hormone (ACTH)
Follicle-stimulating hormone (FSH)
Luteinizing hormone (LH)
Melanocyte-stimulating hormone (MSH)
Hypothalamus
Hypothalamo-hypophyseal tract
Thyrotropin-releasing hormone (TRH)
Somatotropin hormone (STH)
Corticotropin factor
Prolactin-inhibiting factor
Pituitary Gland
Anterior lobe
Posterior lobe
Beta cell
Posterior lobe
Antidiuretic hormone (ADH)
Oxytocin
Thymus Gland
Right lobe
Left lobe
Thymosin
Thymulin
Thymopoietin
Thymic-humoral factor
IGF-1
Heart
Cardiac muscle fibers (from the right atrium)
Atrial natriuretic peptide (ANP)
Pineal gland
Pituitary gland
Thyroid and parathyroid glands
Thymus gland
Heart
Andrenal gland
Kidney
Pancreas
Ovary
Placental hormones
Testes
Stomach, duodenum, and jejunum
Stomach, Duodenum, and Jejunum
Stomach
Gastrin
G-cells in pyloric glands
Gastrin
Small intestine
Secretin
Motilin
Cholecystokinin
Enterocrinin
Gastric inhibitory peptide
S-cell in duodenal and jejunal glands
Secretin
Adrenal Glands
Cortex
Mineralocorticoids
Glucocorticoids
Androgens
Estrogens
Medulla
Norepinephrine
Epinephrine
(cross-section)
Kidney
Kidney
Prostaglandins
Erythropoietin
Renin
Juxta-glomerular apparatus
Glomerulus
(microscopic view)
Pancreas
Common bile duct
Pancreatic duct
Islet of Langerhans
Glucagon
Insulin
Somatostatin
Pancreatic polypeptide
Alpha cell
Beta cell
Delta cell
Testes
Epididymis
Efferent ducts of epididymis
Seminiferous tubule
Androgen-binding protein
A small amount of estrogen
(microscopic view)
(cross-section)
Leydig cells
Testosterone
Androsterone
Ovary
Fimbria
Site of ruptured follicle
Fallopian tube
Maturing follicles
Ovary
Estrogen
Progesterone
Follicular fluid
Corpus luteum
Developing follicles
(cross-section)
Placental Hormones
(from uterus during pregnancy)
Chorionic gonadotropins
Progesterone
Estrogen
Relaxin

FIGURE 12.1 Location of and hormones produced by endocrine system glands. (Adapted with permission from Anatomical Chart Company. The Endocrine System. © 2000 Anatomical Chart Company, a division of Springhouse Corporation.)

TABLE 12.1 Endocrine Organs and Their Secretions

Location	Gland or Cell	Chemical Type	Hormone	Target	Main Effect
Adipose tissue	Cells	Peptide	Leptin; adiponectin (resistin)	Hypothalamus, other tissues	Food intake, metabolism, reproduction
Adrenal cortex	Gland	Steroid	Mineralocorticoids (aldosterone)	Kidney	Stimulates Na^+ resorption and K^+ secretion
			Glucocorticoids (cortisol; corticosterone)	Many tissues	Promotes protein and fat catabolism; raises blood glucose levels; adapts body to stress
			Androgens (androstenedione; dehydroepiandrosterone [DHEA]; estrone)	Many tissues	Promotes sex drive
Adrenal medulla	Gland	Amine	Epinephrine, norepinephrine	Many tissues	Facilitates sympathetic activity; increases cardiac output; regulates blood vessels; increases glycogen catabolism and fatty acid release
Gastrointestinal tract (stomach and small intestine)	Cells	Peptide	Gastrin; cholecystokinin (CCK); secretin; glucose-dependent insulinotropic peptide (GIP)	GI tract and pancreas	Assists digestion and absorption of nutrients; regulates gastrointestinal motility
Heart	Cells	Peptide	Atrial natriuretic peptide (ANP)	Kidney tubules	Inhibits sodium resorption
Hypothalamus	Clusters of neurons	Peptide	Trophic hormones (releasing and release-inhibiting hormones: corticotrophin-releasing hormone [CHR]; thyrotropin-releasing hormone [TRH]; growth hormone–releasing hormone [GHRH]; gonadotropin-releasing hormone [GnRH])	Anterior pituitary	Releases or inhibits anterior pituitary hormones
Kidney	Cells	Peptide	Erythropoietin (EPO)	Bone marrow	Red blood cell production
		Steroid	1,25 Dihydroxyvitamin D_3 (calciferol)	Intestine	Increase calcium absorption
Liver	Cells	Peptide	Angiotensinogen	Adrenal cortex, blood vessels, brain	Aldosterone secretion; increase blood pressure
			Insulinlike growth factors (IGF-1)	Many tissues	Growth
Muscle	Cells	Peptide	Insulinlike growth factors (IGF-1, IGF-II); myogenic regulatory factors (MRFs)	Many tissues	Growth
Pancreas	Gland	Peptide	Insulin	Many tissues	Lowers blood glucose levels; promotes protein, lipid, and glycogen synthesis
			Glucagon	Many tissues	Raises blood glucose levels; promotes glycogenolysis and gluconeogenesis
			Somatostatin (SS)	Many tissues	Inhibits secretion of pancreatic hormones; regulates digestion and absorption of nutrients by GI system

TABLE 12.1 Endocrine Organs and Their Secretions (Continued)

Location	Gland or Cell	Chemical Type	Hormone	Target	Main Effect
Parathyroid	Gland	Peptide	Parathyroid hormone (PTH)	Bone, kidney	Promotes Ca^{2+} release from bone, Ca^{2+} absorption by intestine and Ca^{2+} resorption by kidney; raises blood Ca^{2+} levels; stimulates vitamin D_3 synthesis
Pineal gland	Gland	Amine	Melatonin	Unknown	Controls circadian rhythms
Pituitary-anterior	Gland	Peptides	Growth hormone (GH)	Many tissues	Growth; stimulates bone and soft tissue growth; regulates protein, lipid, and CHO metabolism
			Adrenocorticotropic hormone (ACTH)	Adrenal cortex	Stimulates glucocorticoid secretion
			Thyroid-stimulating hormone (TSH)	Thyroid gland	Stimulates secretion of thyroid hormones
			Prolactin	Breast	Milk secretion
			Follicle-stimulating hormone (FSH)	Gonads	Females: stimulates growth and development of ovarian follicles and estrogen secretion; Males: sperm production by testis
			Luteinizing hormone (LH)	Gonads	Females: stimulates ovulation, secretion of estrogen and progesterone; Males: testosterone secretion by testis
Pituitary-posterior	Extension of hypothalamic neurons	Peptide	Oxytocin (OT)	Breast and uterus	Females: stimulates uterine contractions and milk ejection by mammary glands; Males: unknown function
			Antidiuretic hormone (ADH or vasopressin)	Kidney	Decreases urine output by kidneys; promotes blood vessel (arterioles) constriction
Placenta (pregnant female)	Gland	Steroid	Estrogens and progesterone	Many tissues	Fetal and maternal development
		Peptide	Chorionic somatomammotropin (CS)		Metabolism
			Chorionic gonadotropin (CG)		Hormone secretion
Skin	Cells	Steroid	Vitamin D_3	Intermediate form of hormone	Precursor of 1,25 dihydroxyvitamin D_3
Ovaries (female)	Glands	Steroid	Estrogens (estradiol)	Many tissues	Egg production; secondary sex characteristics
			Progestins (progesterone)	Uterus	Promotes endometrial growth to prepare uterus for pregnancy
Testes (male)	Glands	Peptide	Ovarian inhibin	Anterior pituitary	Inhibits FSH secretion
		Steroid	Androgen	Many tissues	Sperm production; secondary sex characteristics
		Peptide	Inhibin	Anterior pituitary	Inhibit FSH secretion
Thymus	Gland	Peptide	Thymosin, thymopoietin	Lymphocytes	Stimulates proliferation and function of T lymphocytes
Thyroid	Gland	Iodinated amines	Triiodothyronine (T_3); thyroxine (T_4)	Many tissues	Increases metabolic rate; normal physical development
		Peptide	Calcitonin (CT)	Bone	Promotes calcium deposition in bone; lowers blood calcium levels

target cells at higher concentrations than a typical hormone. **Erythropoietin**, a **glycoprotein** molecule that stimulates red blood cell synthesis, classifies as a hormone but functionally behaves as a cytokine. Hormone secretion also occurs in response to varying levels of circulating ions and nutrients. For example, decreased blood levels of Ca^{2+} impact parathyroid gland activity by increasing its parathyroid hormone release.

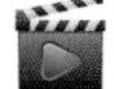

See the animation "Hormonal Control" on **http://thePoint.lww.com/MKKESS5e** for a review of hormone activity.

Hormones Bind to Receptors

Hormone-receptor binding serves as the first step in initiating hormone action. Three factors determine the extent of a target cell's activation by a hormone:

1. Hormone concentration in the blood
2. Number of target cell receptors for the hormone
3. Sensitivity or strength of the union between hormone and receptor

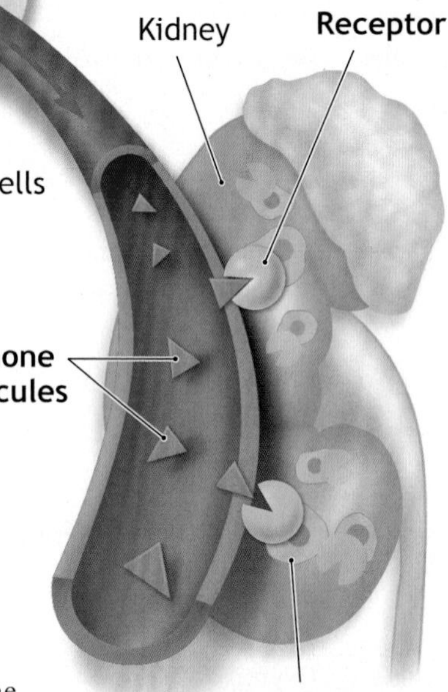

FIGURE 12.2 Hormones secreted from endocrine glands travel in the bloodstream to exert influence on body tissues.

All hormones bind to target cell receptors and initiate biochemical responses. Although this characteristic varies among different hormones and tissues, some hormones act on multiple tissues differently or have little or no effect at different times. Insulin, for example, exhibits varied effects depending on the target tissue; in muscle and adipose cells, insulin alters glucose and protein transport and enzymes for glucose metabolism. In the liver, insulin modulates enzyme activity without directly affecting glucose and protein transport, while in brain tissue, glucose metabolism does not require insulin.

Hormone Classification

Hormones typically classify according to several different systems: their sources, their receptor type, or their chemical structure, which represents the most common classification scheme. Three different chemical structures or hormones exist:

1. *Peptide/protein hormones* composed of linked amino acids
2. *Steroid hormones* derived from cholesterol and amine hormones
3. *Amine hormones* derived from a single-type amino acid.

Peptide/Protein Hormones

Peptide hormones, encoded by a specific gene, range from small peptides consisting of only three amino acids to huge proteins and glycoproteins with hundreds of amino acids. These water-soluble hormones dissolve easily for transport in the body's extracellular fluids. The half-life of activity for peptide hormones ranges in minutes; thus, if a peptide hormone's response requires maintenance beyond several minutes, the hormone secretion must continue. Hormonal clearance rate is typically expressed in two ways:

1. *Metabolic clearance rate (MCR)*—refers to the time to completely remove a hormone from the blood, usually expressed in milliliters per hour or mL · hr^{-1}. Hormones remove faster from the blood when the MCR is a larger number (i.e., a hormone with an MCR = 75 mL · min^{-1} removes faster than a hormone with an MCR = 30 mL · min^{-1})
2. *Circulating half-life (CHL)*—refers to the time to remove 50% of the hormone's initial concentration from the circulation (referred to as $T_{1/2}$). The rate of hormone decline, influenced by its clearance, also is affected by the hormone's rate of synthesis, as hormone production does not remain static but continually occurs. A hormone's half-life depends on its molecular structure. The $T_{1/2}$ for small peptides ranges from 4 to 42 minutes, 15 minutes to 3 hours for large proteins like TSH and LH, and 5 minutes to 2 hours for steroid hormones. The $T_{1/2}$ for hCG (human chorionic gonadotropin, produced during pregnancy) is 6 hours. Interestingly, a tiny fraction of intact hormone (<0.8%) escapes degradation and passes in the urine. The liver and kidneys account for the fate of most hormone breakdown.

The peptide hormones typically bind to surface membrane receptors and act through a second messenger. Tissues respond rapidly to peptide hormones compared with the response times engendered by other hormones. The binding of one peptide hormone molecule can trigger a 1000-fold response!

Steroid Hormones

All steroid hormones have a similar chemical structure because of their derivation from cholesterol. But unlike

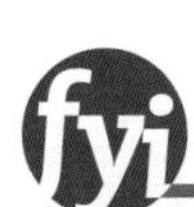

Astronaut Immune Function Compromised During Prolonged Spaceflight

Persistent immune dysregulation can substantially impact clinical risks for astronaut crew members participating in long-duration space missions, particularly in year-long trips to Mars and return to Earth. Plasma cytokine levels were used as a biomarker for immune status in 28 crew members (21 males, 7 females) during various onboard International Space Station missions. Immunoassay techniques assessed plasma concentrations of 22 cytokines monitored three times before flight, three to five times during typical mission durations of 6 months, at landing, and 30 days after landing. Time points were taken during early and later flight adaptation phases to allow kinetic assessment of an entire mission. The salient findings showed a pattern of cytokine dysregulation (e.g., tumor necrosis factor-α, IL-8, IL-1ra, thrombopoietin, vascular endothelial growth factor, C-C motif chemokine ligand 2). The researchers concluded that variable patterns of response in immune and hormonal regulation suggest persistent multiple physiological adaptations during flight, including inflammation, leukocyte recruitment, angiogenesis, and thrombocyte regulation. They suggested: "As future studies continue to characterize in-flight immune alterations, the development of countermeasures to enable exploration missions to be conducted safely may be warranted."

Sources: Crucian B, Sams C. Immune system dysregulation during spaceflight: clinical risk for exploration-class missions. *J Leukoc Biol* 2009;86:1017.

Crucian B, et al. Immune system dysregulation occurs during short duration spaceflight on board the space shuttle. *J Clin Immunol* 2013;33:456.

Crucian BE, et al. Plasma cytokine concentrations indicate that in vivo hormonal regulation of immunity is altered during long-duration spaceflight. *J Interferon Cytokine Res* 2014;34:778.

peptide hormones made in different tissues, only the adrenal cortex, gonads, and placenta (during pregnancy) produce steroid hormones. Steroid hormones readily diffuse across cell membranes, both out of the parent cell and into their target tissue. Steroid-secreting cells cannot store hormones; instead, they synthesize their hormones as needed. Steroid hormones move out of the secreting cell by simple diffusion. These hormones, minimally soluble in plasma and other body fluids, bind to protein carrier molecules in the blood. To produce an effect on a target, the hormones must unbind from their protein carriers.

Amine Hormones

Small molecules created from one or two amino acids comprise the amine hormones. The amino acids tyrosine and tryptophan principally construct the amine hormones. The amine neurohormones, epinephrine and norepinephrine, bind to cell membrane receptors in a manner similar to peptide hormones. Tryptophan serves as the precursor for the hormone serotonin (synthesized in the small intestine's mucosal lining and the larger bronchi), while also serving as an important central nervous system neurotransmitter.

How Hormones Function

Most hormones do not directly affect cellular activity but rather combine with a specific receptor molecule on the cell surface. The cell then discharges a second chemical that initiates a cascade of cellular events. **Figure 12.3** schematically shows a nonsteroid hormone (displayed as a triangle) as it binds to its receptor and penetrates the intracellular space through the bilayer plasma membrane. The binding hormone acts as *"first messenger"* to react with the enzyme **adenyl cyclase** in the plasma membrane to form **cyclic 3,5-adenosine monophosphate (cyclic-AMP).** This compound then acts as *"second messenger"* or mediator. It influences cellular function by initiating a predictable series of actions within the target cell by one of four mechanisms:

1. Change intracellular proteins synthesis rate
2. Alter enzyme activity rate
3. Modify cell membrane transport
4. Influence secretory activity

A target cell's response to a hormone depends on specific protein receptors on its membrane or in its interior.

Three factors determine a hormone's plasma concentration:

1. Sum of synthesis and release by the host gland
2. Rate of receptor tissue uptake
3. Rate of removal from the blood by the liver and kidneys

In most cases, the hormone removal rate, which is usually quantified in the urine, equals the release rate.

Table 12.2 compares the storage, synthesis, release mechanism, transport medium, receptor location and receptor-ligand binding, and target organ response of the peptide, steroid, and amine hormones.

Caffeine Stimulates Lipolysis

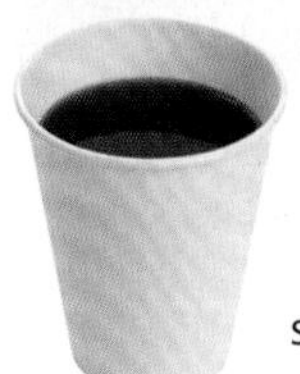

Caffeine augments cyclic-AMP activity in fat cells; cyclic-AMP activates hormone-sensitive lipases to promote lipolysis and release free fatty acids into the plasma. Increased plasma free fatty acid levels stimulate fat oxidation, thus conserving liver and muscle glycogen.

TABLE 12.2 Storage, Synthesis, Release Mechanism, Transport Medium, Receptor Location and Receptor-Ligand Binding, and Target Organ Response for the Peptide, Steroid, and Amine Hormones

	Peptide Hormones	Steroid Hormones	Amine Hormones	
			Catecholamines	Thyroid Hormones
Examples	Insulin, glucagons, leptin, IGF-1	Androgens, DHEA, cortisol	Epinephrine, norepinephrine	Thyroxine (T_4)
Synthesis and storage	Made in advance; stored in secretory vesicles	Synthesized on demand from precursors	Made in advance; stored in secretory vesicles	Made in advance; precursor stored in secretory vesicles
Release from parent cell	Exocytosis[a]	Simple diffusion	Exocytosis	Simple diffusion
Transport medium	Dissolved in plasma	Bound to carrier proteins	Dissolved in plasma	Bound to carrier proteins
Life span (half-life[b])	Short	Long	Short	Long
Receptor location	On cell membrane	Cytoplasm or nucleus; some have membrane receptors	On cell membrane	Nucleus
Response to receptor-ligand binding[c]	Activation of second messenger systems; may activate genes	Activate genes for transcription and translation; may have nongenomic actions	Activation of second messenger systems	Activate genes for transcription and translation
General target response	Modification of existing proteins and induction of new protein synthesis	Induction of new protein synthesis	Modification of existing proteins	Induction of new protein synthesis

[a]Process in which intracellular vesicles fuse with the cell membrane and release their contents into the extracellular fluid.

[b]Amount of time required to reduce hormone concentration by one half.

[c]A ligand (the molecule that binds to a receptor) binds to a membrane protein, which triggers endocytosis (process by which a cell brings molecules into the cytoplasm in vesicles formed from the cell membrane).

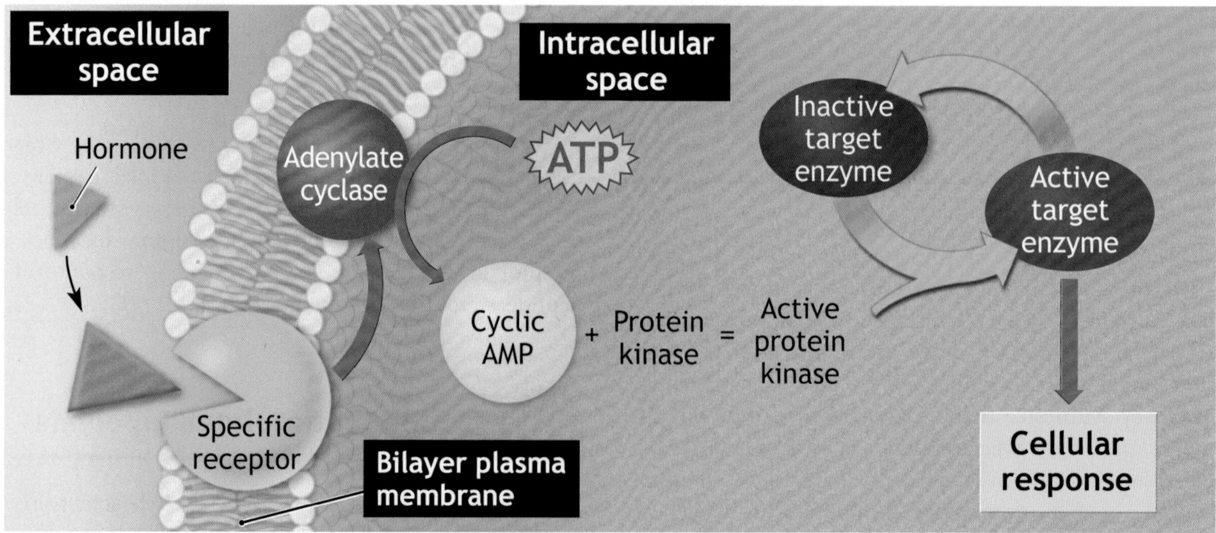

FIGURE 12.3 Action of nonsteroid hormones. Circulating hormone (first messenger) binds to a specific receptor in the cell's plasma membrane to trigger production of cyclic AMP from ATP catalyzed by adenylate cyclase. Cyclic AMP then acts as second messenger to activate a protein kinase within the cell. This in turn activates a target enzyme to elicit the cellular response. (Adapted with permission from McArdle WD, Katch FI, Katch VL. *Exercise Physiology: Nutrition, Energy, and Human Performance*. 8th Ed. Baltimore: Wolters Kluwer Health, 2015.)

Target Cell Activation

The activation of a target cell by hormone-receptor interaction depends on three factors:

1. Blood levels of the specific hormone
2. Relative number of target cell receptors for that hormone
3. Affinity or strength of the union between hormone and receptor

Hormone Effects on Enzymes

Alteration of enzymatic activity and enzyme-mediated membrane transport constitute the major mechanisms of hormone action. Hormones affect enzyme activity in one of three ways:

1. Stimulate enzyme synthesis
2. Combine with the enzyme to change its shape through allosteric modulation, which increases or decreases the enzyme's ability to interact with a substrate
3. Activate many inactive enzyme forms to increase total enzyme activity

In addition to altering enzyme activity, hormones either facilitate or inhibit transport of substances into cells. Insulin, for example, promotes glucose uptake through the cell's plasma membrane. In contrast, the hormone epinephrine inhibits the cell's glucose uptake.

Control of Hormone Secretion

Hormonal, humoral, or neural mechanisms stimulate endocrine gland function. Each of these stimulation methods functions as a reflex pathway, singly or in combination, to ultimately trigger and regulate a specific hormone secretion. All reflex pathways exhibit five similar components:

1. Stimulus
2. Input signal
3. Signal integration
4. Output signal
5. Response

In endocrine reflexes, the output signal represents a hormone or **neurohormone**.

Figure 12.4 illustrates a negative feedback system that turns off hormone release. In this example, an increase in blood glucose concentration following a meal initiates insulin secretion; insulin then travels in the blood to its target tissues to increase glucose uptake and metabolism. The resultant decrease in blood glucose concentration provides a negative feedback signal and turns off the reflex, ending insulin's further release. **Figure 12.4** also shows insulin secretion triggered by nervous system input signals.

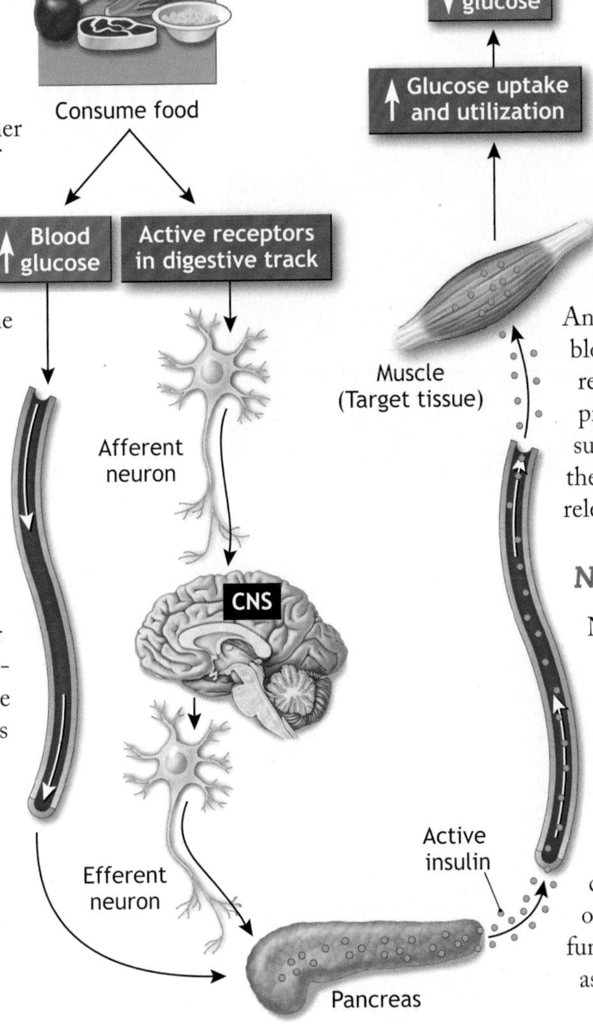

FIGURE 12.4 Multiple stimuli for insulin secretion. Insulin release is triggered by an increase in blood glucose levels or through nervous stimulation triggered by ingestion of a meal.

Hormonal Stimulation

Hormones often influence other hormone secretions. For example, hormones from hypothalamic trophic-releasing and -inhibiting hormones (see **Table 12.1**) induce discharge of most anterior pituitary hormones. The anterior pituitary hormones, in turn, stimulate other "target gland" endocrine organs to release their hormones into the circulation. Increased blood levels of these hormones provide feedback to inhibit release of anterior pituitary hormones; this ultimately inhibits target gland secretion.

Humoral Stimulation

Fluctuating blood levels of ions, nutrients, and bile stimulate hormone release. The term *humoral* denotes these stimuli to distinguish them from "fluid-borne" hormonal stimuli. An increase in the humoral agent blood glucose stimulates insulin release from the pancreas. Insulin promotes glucose entry so blood sugar levels decline to terminate the humoral initiative for insulin release.

Neural Stimulation

Nerve fibers impact hormone release. During stress, for example, sympathetic nervous system activation of the adrenal medulla initiates release of epinephrine and norepinephrine. In this case, the nervous system augments normal endocrine control to maintain homeostasis or stability of internal physiologic functioning. Neurohormones serve as chemical signals when neurons release them into the blood. The nervous system produces three major groups of neurohormones:

1. Catecholamines synthesized by modified neurons in the adrenal medulla
2. Hypothalamic neurohormones secreted from the posterior pituitary
3. Hypothalamic neurohormones that control hormone release from the anterior pituitary

Hormone-Hormone Interactions

Multiple hormones present at the same time control many cells and tissues. Three types of interactions of diverse hormones exist:

1. **Synergism:** Different hormones act together to augment the effect on specific tissues. For example, the pancreatic hormone glucagon in concert with cortisol and epinephrine acts synergistically to elevate blood glucose levels. When two or more hormones interact, the combined effect on the target often exceeds the additive effect of each hormone separately.
2. **Permissiveness:** One hormone cannot exert its full effect without the presence of a second hormone or a greater concentration of the first hormone. For example, thyroid hormone increases the number of receptors available for epinephrine at its target cells, thereby augmenting epinephrine's effect at those cells.
3. **Antagonism:** Some hormones oppose the action of another hormone to diminish the first hormone's effectiveness. Glucagon and growth hormone, for example, both raise blood glucose concentration to counter insulin's glucose-lowering effect.

Skeletal Muscle as an Endocrine Organ

In 2003, scientists discovered small proteins that serve as messengers between cells; they named these substances cytokines. Cytokines were first identified from contracting muscle cells that produced and released substances exhibiting strong metabolic effects. This discovery of contracting muscle as a cytokine-producing organ opened a new paradigm that views skeletal muscle as a hormone-secreting endocrine organ that influences metabolism in other tissues and organs. These muscle-secreted cytokines (referred to as ***myokines***) and other peptides produced, expressed, and released by muscle fibers exert **autocrine, paracrine**, or endocrine signaling effects. Further research now supports muscle as an active endocrine organ with the capacity to produce and express cytokines that belong to distinctly different families. A muscle's contractile activity helps regulate cytokine expression.

Both type I and type II muscle fibers express the myokine ***interleukin (IL)-6***, which exerts its effects locally within the specific muscle through activation of AMP-activated protein kinase [AMPK]). Its release in pulsatile fashion also acts peripherally when released into the circulation. Within skeletal muscle, IL-6 functions in an autocrine or paracrine manner to increase glucose uptake and fat oxidation. During physical activity, its peripheral effect increases glucose production by the liver and lipolysis when transported to adipose tissue. In essence, the myokines help to regulate not only skeletal muscle itself but also other organs a distance away. **Figure 12.5** illustrates the proposed biological role for interleukin (IL)-6R in adipose tissue.

PATTERNS OF HORMONE RELEASE

Most hormones respond to peripheral stimuli on an as-needed basis, but others release at regular intervals during a 24-hour cycle, referred to as *diurnal variation*. Some secretory cycles span several weeks,

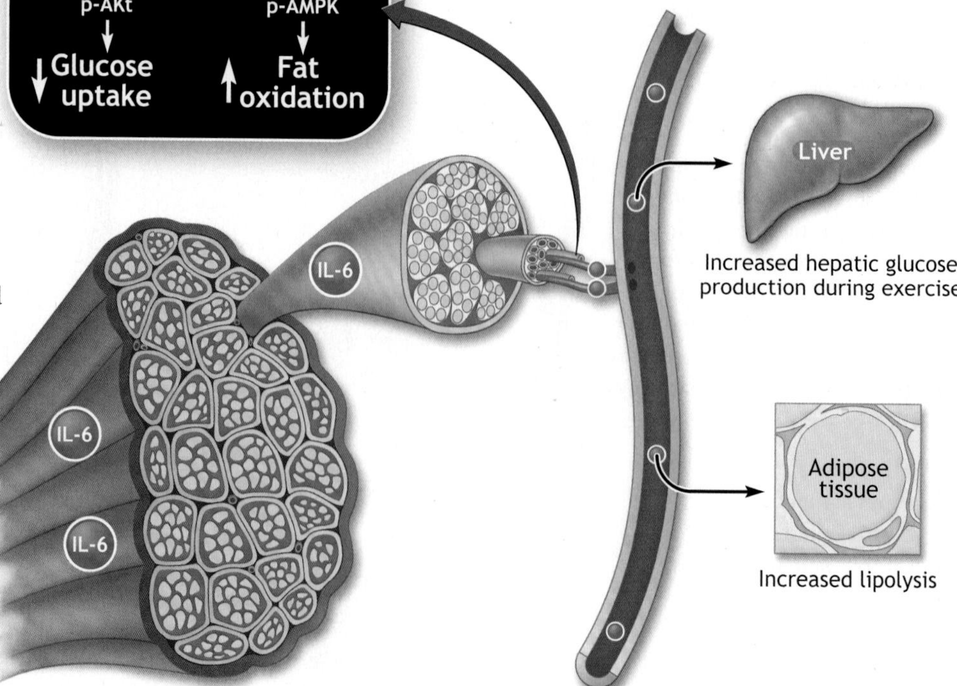

FIGURE 12.5 Proposed biological role for interleukin (IL)-6R. (Adapted with permission from McArdle WD, Katch FI, Katch VL. *Exercise Physiology: Nutrition, Energy, and Human Performance*. 8th Ed. Baltimore: Wolters Kluwer Health, 2015.)

and others follow daily cycles. These cycling patterns do not pertain to just one hormone category.

Assessing pulsatile hormone release patterns reveals information not available from a single blood sample. Patterns of release, amplitude, and frequency of discharge provide more meaningful information about hormone dynamics than a hormone's concentration examined at a single time period.

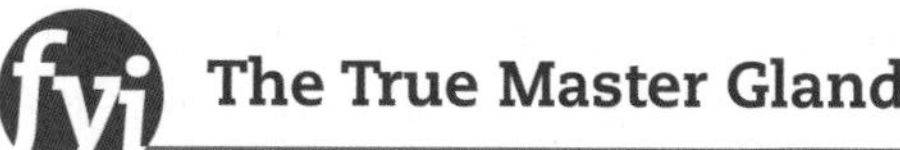

fyi The True Master Gland

The early Greek physicians, including Galen (131–201 AD), described the pituitary gland in their many treatises on health and disease. Galen mistakenly proposed that its role was to drain the phlegm from the brain to the nasopharynx. Over the next 19 centuries, the pituitary gland was considered the body's master gland. In reality, the hypothalamus controls anterior pituitary activity, making it the true *master gland*.

RESTING AND EXERCISE-INDUCED ENDOCRINE SECRETIONS

The following sections review important hormones, their functions during rest and physical activity, and specific host-gland-hormone responses to training.

ANTERIOR PITUITARY HORMONES

Figure 12.6 illustrates the **pituitary gland (hypophysis)**, its secretions and various target glands, and target gland hormone secretions. The pituitary gland consists of distinct anterior and posterior lobes, each with different hormone secretions. The gland attaches to the hypothalamus by neural elements that innervate the posterior pituitary. This nerve bundle (**hypophyseal stalk**) serves as a conduit for hormone movement from its site of synthesis in the hypothalamus to storage in the pituitary. Located beneath the base of the brain, the **anterior pituitary** secretes at least six different polypeptide hormones and influences the secretion of several others.

The **posterior pituitary**, an extension of hypothalamic neurons, secretes the hormone oxytocin, which acts on breasts and the uterus to stimulate milk production and induce labor and delivery, and vasopressin (antidiuretic hormone [ADH]), which acts on the kidneys to decrease urine output and control fluid balance.

Growth Hormone

Human growth hormone (GH or somatotropin) promotes cell division and proliferation throughout the body. This hormone facilitates protein synthesis in three ways:

1. Increases amino acid transport through plasma membranes
2. Stimulates RNA formation
3. Activates cellular ribosomes that increase protein synthesis

GH release depresses carbohydrate utilization while increasing fat use for energy. Insufficient GH secretion early in life blunts skeletal growth (*dwarfism*; **www.webmd.com/**

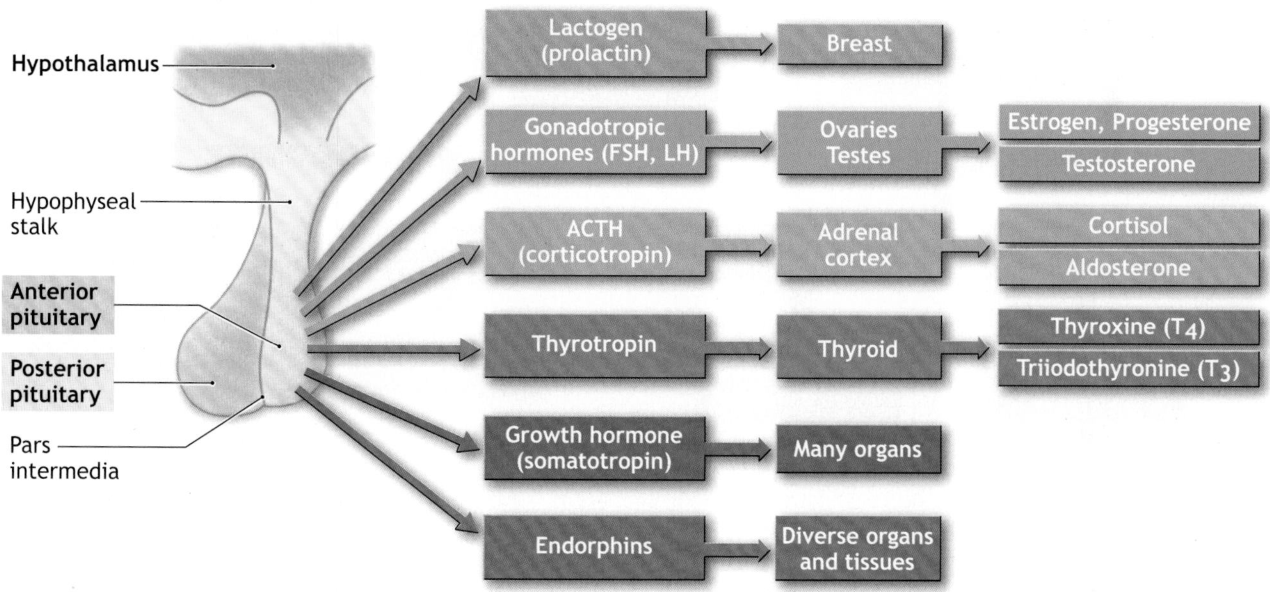

FIGURE 12.6 The pituitary gland, its secretions and various target glands, and their hormone secretions. (Reprinted with permission from McArdle WD, Katch FI, Katch VL. *Exercise Physiology: Nutrition, Energy, and Human Performance*. 8th Ed. Baltimore: Wolters Kluwer Health, 2015.)

children/dwarfism-causes-treatments), and excess production produces extreme growth (***gigantism***; **http://pituitary.ucla.edu/body.cfm?id=83#GigantismPhysiology**). Excessive GH secretion after puberty causes continued soft tissue growth and bone thickening, a condition termed **acromegaly**. Many of the growth-promoting effects of GH arise from intermediary chemical messengers on different target tissues rather than a direct action of GH itself. These peptide messengers, produced in the liver, are termed somatomedins or **insulin-like growth factors (IGFs)** based on their structural similarity to insulin. Two IGFs have been identified, IGF-1 and IGF-2; the liver directly releases them under the stimulatory effects of GH. These factors exert potent peripheral effects on motor units.

Hypothalamic secretion of GH-releasing hormone stimulates the anterior pituitary gland's GH production. Another hormone, hypothalamic **somatostatin,** inhibits GH release. *Each primary pituitary hormone has its own hypothalamic releasing factor.* Anxiety, stress, and physical activity provide neural input to the hypothalamus, causing it to discharge releasing hormones.

Physical Activity, Growth Hormone, and Tissue Synthesis

GH secretion increases a few minutes following initiation of physical activity. Higher intensity activity increases GH production and its total secretion. Moreover, GH secretion relates more closely to peak effort intensity than activity duration or total activity volume.

The exact stimulus for GH release with physical activity remains unknown; neural factors most likely provide primary control. One hypothesis maintains that physical activity directly activates GH secretion that in turn stimulates anabolic processes. For example, activity doubles GH pulse frequency and amplitude. Physical exertion also stimulates endogenous opiate release; these hormones facilitate GH discharge by inhibiting the liver's production of somatostatin, a hormone that blunts GH release.

Figure 12.7 illustrates the actions and regulation of GH. Elevated plasma GH stimulates triacylglycerol release from adipose tissue while inhibiting cellular glucose uptake, known

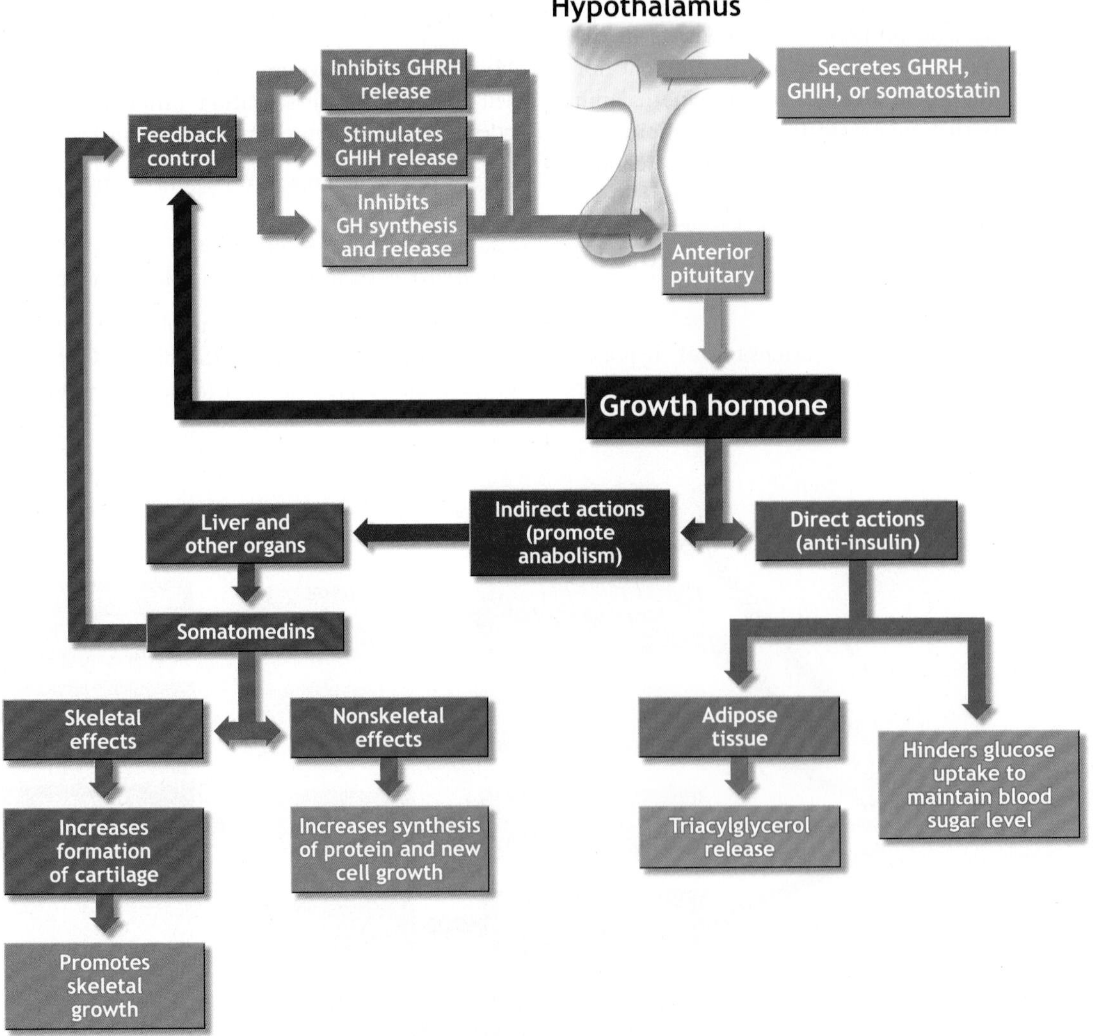

FIGURE 12.7 Overview of growth hormone (GH) actions. GH stimulates breakdown and release of triacylglycerols from adipose tissue and hinders cellular glucose uptake (anti-insulin effect) to maintain a relatively high blood glucose level. Somatomedins mediate the indirect anabolic effects of GH. Elevated GH levels and somatomedins provide feedback to promote GH-inhibiting hormone (GHIH) release and depress hypothalamic release of GH-releasing hormone (GHRH); this further inhibits GH release by the anterior pituitary gland. (Reprinted with permission from McArdle WD, Katch FI, Katch VL. *Exercise Physiology: Nutrition, Energy, and Human Performance*. 8th Ed. Baltimore: Wolters Kluwer Health, 2015.)

as the anti-insulin effect. Inhibiting carbohydrate catabolism while maintaining blood glucose levels sustains prolonged exertion. Concurrently, GH promotes its anabolic, tissue-building effects mediated via somatomedins on diverse tissues that include bone and skeletal muscle. Elevated GH and somatomedins trigger the hypothalamus to release more GH-inhibiting hormone. This action depresses the release of GH-releasing hormone, thus inhibiting anterior pituitary release of GH.

Thyrotropin

Thyrotropin (thyroid-stimulating hormone [TSH]) maintains growth and thyroid gland development, including hormone output regulation from thyroid cells. The thyroid gland plays an important role in controlling cellular metabolism. Physical activity usually increases anterior pituitary TSH output.

Corticotropin

The hypothalamus secretes corticotropin-releasing hormone (CRH) into the hypothalamic-hypophyseal portal system. CRH, transported to the anterior pituitary, stimulates the release of **corticotropin (adrenocorticotropic hormone [ACTH])**. ACTH in turn acts on the adrenal cortex to promote cortisol synthesis and release similar to how TSH controls thyroid secretions. ACTH directly enhances triacylglycerol mobilization from adipose tissue, increases the rate of gluconeogenesis, and stimulates protein catabolism. ACTH concentrations increase with physical activity duration if effort intensity exceeds 25% of aerobic capacity.

Gonadotropic Hormones

The gonadotropic hormones include **follicle-stimulating hormone (FSH)** and **luteinizing hormone (LH)**. In women, FSH initiates follicle growth in ovaries and stimulates ovarian secretion of estrogens, one type of female sex hormone. The combination of LH and FSH stimulates estrogen secretion and initiates follicle rupture to allow the ovum to pass through the fallopian tube for fertilization. In men, FSH stimulates germinal epithelial growth in the testes to promote sperm development. LH stimulates the testes to secrete testosterone.

The nature of gonadotropin release confounds interpretation of any physical activity-associated alterations in FSH and LH. LH normally releases in a pulsatile manner so it becomes difficult to separate any specific activity-related change from the normal secretory pattern. Anxiety affects LH levels via action of the "stress" hormone norepinephrine; thus, LH increases in anticipation of physical effort and reaches its peak during recovery.

Prolactin

Prolactin (PRL) governs milk secretion from the mammary glands. PRL levels increase with higher effort intensities and return toward baseline within 45 minutes of recovery. PRL plays an important role in female sexual function: repeated exercise-induced PRL release can inhibit the ovaries and disrupt the normal menstrual cycle, an effect often observed among athletic women.

POSTERIOR PITUITARY HORMONES

Figure 12.6 depicts the posterior pituitary gland (neurohypophysis) formed as an outgrowth of the hypothalamus. This gland stores two hormones, **antidiuretic hormone (ADH or vasopressin)** and **oxytocin**. The posterior pituitary does not synthesize its hormones. Instead, it receives them from the hypothalamus for release to the general circulation via neural stimulation.

ADH primarily limits how much urine the kidneys produce. Oxytocin stimulates uterine muscle activity and milk ejection from the breasts during lactation; thus, oxytocin contributes importantly to birthing and nursing.

Moderate physical activity provides a potent stimulus for ADH secretion. This secretion increases kidney tubule water resorption during and following physical activity. ADH release stimulated by sweating preserves body fluids, particularly in hot weather activity accompanied by dehydration. Excessive fluid intake inhibits ADH release, with urine volume increasing proportionately.

THYROID HORMONES

The butterfly-shaped thyroid gland shown in **Figure 12.8** weighs approximately 15 to 20 g and is located just below the larynx at the base of the throat. This larger endocrine gland

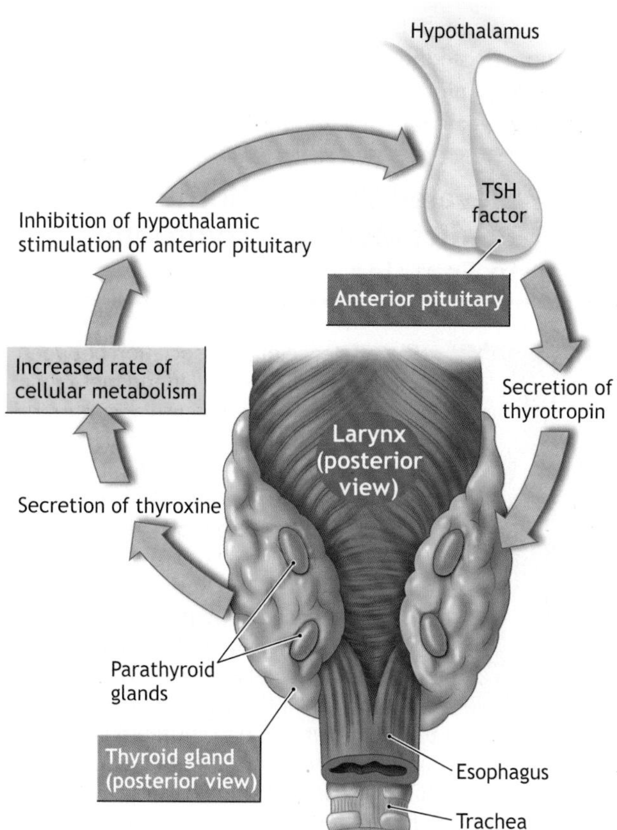

FIGURE 12.8 Feedback system that controls thyroid hormone release. (Adapted with permission from McArdle WD, Katch FI, Katch VL. *Exercise Physiology: Nutrition, Energy, and Human Performance*. 8th Ed. Baltimore: Wolters Kluwer Health, 2015.)

has two distinct endocrine cell types that secrete **calcitonin,** a calcium-regulating hormone, and two protein-iodine bound hormones, T_4 and T_3, often referred to as *major metabolic hormones*. TSH release by the anterior pituitary gland stimulates the thyroid gland to release its hormones.

Thyroid Hormones Affect Quality of Life

Thyroid hormones are not directly essential for life but they do affect its quality. In children, full expression of GH requires thyroid activity. Thyroid hormones provide essential stimulation for normal growth and development, especially of nerve tissue.

Hypersecretion of thyroid hormones (**hyperthyroidism**) has four effects:

1. Increases oxygen uptake and metabolic heat production during rest (heat intolerance a common complaint)
2. Increases protein catabolism to cause subsequent muscle weakness and weight loss
3. Heightens reflex activity and psychological disturbances that range from irritability and insomnia to psychosis
4. Causes an abnormally rapid resting heart rate (**tachycardia**)

Hyposecretion of thyroid hormones (**hypothyroidism**) produces four effects:

1. Reduces metabolic rate, leading to cold intolerance from reduced internal heat production
2. Decreases protein synthesis, resulting in brittle nails; thinning hair; and dry, thin skin

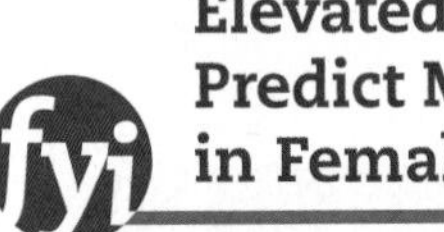

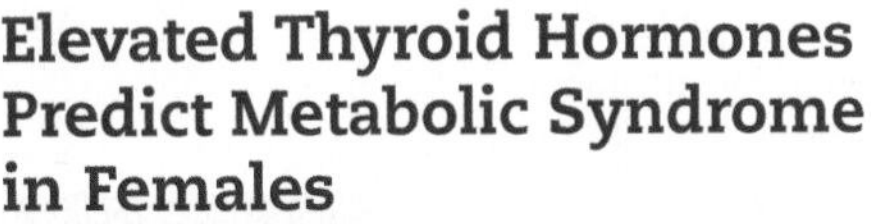

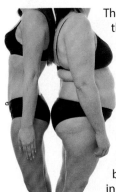

Elevated Thyroid Hormones Predict Metabolic Syndrome in Females

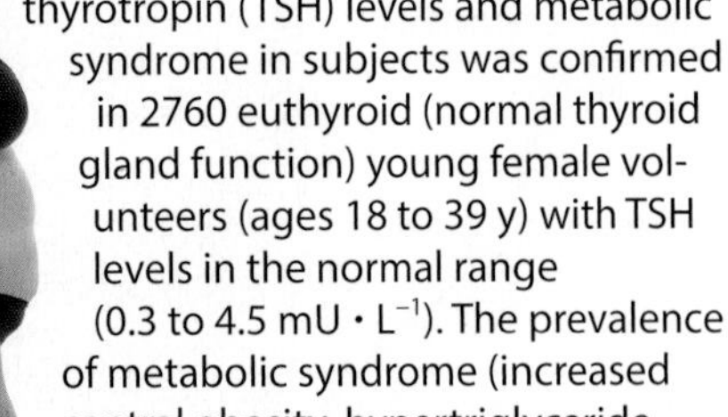

The existence of an association between thyrotropin (TSH) levels and metabolic syndrome in subjects was confirmed in 2760 euthyroid (normal thyroid gland function) young female volunteers (ages 18 to 39 y) with TSH levels in the normal range (0.3 to 4.5 mU · L^{-1}). The prevalence of metabolic syndrome (increased central obesity, hypertriglyceridemia, elevated systolic and diastolic blood pressure) was twofold greater in subjects with higher TSH levels (>2.5 mU · L^{-1}) compared to counterparts with lower TSH levels (<2.5 mU · L^{-1}). Healthy young women with TSH levels greater than 2.5 mU · L^{-1} should be assessed for metabolic syndrome, even if their TSH levels fall within normal range.

Source: Oh JY, et al. Elevated thyroid stimulating hormone levels are associated with metabolic syndrome in euthyroid young women. *Korean J Intern Med* 2013;28:180.

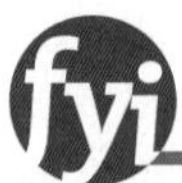

Don't Blame the Hormones

Depressed thyroid production blunts the basal metabolic rate (BMR), which usually leads to gains in body weight and body fat. Nevertheless, fewer than 3% of obese persons present with abnormal thyroid functions. Depressed thyroid activity, therefore, cannot explain excessive body fat gain in more than 60% of adults in the U.S. population.

3. Depresses reflex activity, slows speech and thought processes, and causes feelings of fatigue; in infancy, causes cretinism marked by diminished mental capacity
4. Causes abnormally slow resting heart rate (**bradycardia**)

Blood levels of free T_4 not bound to plasma protein increase during physical activity. This could result from core temperature increases with exertion that alter protein binding of several hormones, including T_4. The importance of these transient alterations in hormone levels remains unknown.

PARATHYROID HORMONE

Four small sections of tissue comprise the **parathyroid gland** within thyroid tissue (see **Fig. 12.8**). This gland secretes the calcium-regulating parathyroid peptide hormone (**parathyroid hormone [PTH]** or parathormone) to increase plasma calcium (Ca^{2+}) concentration. PTH increases plasma Ca^{2+} concentrations in three ways:

1. Mobilizes Ca^{2+} from bone
2. Enhances renal Ca^{2+} resorption
3. Indirectly increases intestinal Ca^{2+} absorption by its influence on vitamin D_3

ADRENAL HORMONES

Figure 12.9 shows the flattened, caplike **adrenal glands** located just above each kidney. The glands form two distinct parts: the **adrenal medulla** in the inner portion and **adrenal cortex** in the outer portion. Each portion secretes a different type of hormone.

Adrenal Medulla Hormones

The adrenal medulla forms part of the sympathetic nervous system. It prolongs and augments sympathetic neural effects by secreting two hormones, **epinephrine** and **norepinephrine,** collectively termed **catecholamines.** Neural outflow from the hypothalamus directly influences adrenal medulla secretions (80% as epinephrine), which affect the heart, blood vessels, and glands in the same but slower way as does direct sympathetic nervous system stimulation.

Physical activity intensity directly governs the quantity of adrenal medulla secretion. For example, norepinephrine levels increase two to six times throughout physical activity

the most physiologically important of these hormones, comprises almost 95% of all mineralocorticoids.

Aldosterone regulates the kidneys' distal tubules sodium resorption. Increased aldosterone secretion moves sodium ions that also draw fluid from the renal filtrate back into the blood, with little sodium passing into urine. Conservation of fluid via sodium resorption increases plasma volume, often with concomitant increases in cardiac output and arterial blood pressure. In contrast, when aldosterone secretion ceases, sodium and fluid literally pour into urine for excretion.

The kidneys exchange either a potassium or hydrogen ion for each reabsorbed sodium ion, enabling aldosterone to indirectly stabilize serum potassium and whole-body pH. Mineral balance preserves nerve transmission and muscle function; neuromuscular activity would cease without proper regulation of sodium and potassium.

Outflow from sympathetic nerve fibers during physical activity constricts kidney blood vessels. Reduced renal blood flow stimulates the kidneys to release the enzyme **renin** into the blood. Renin in turn stimulates the production of the protein **angiotensin**, a potent vasoconstrictor that also activates aldosterone secretion from the adrenal cortex. Aldosterone secretion increases progressively during physical activity, with peak plasma levels as high as six times the resting value. The **renin-angiotensin mechanism** during rest controls aldosterone secretion related to changes in blood pressure in kidneys' afferent arterioles.

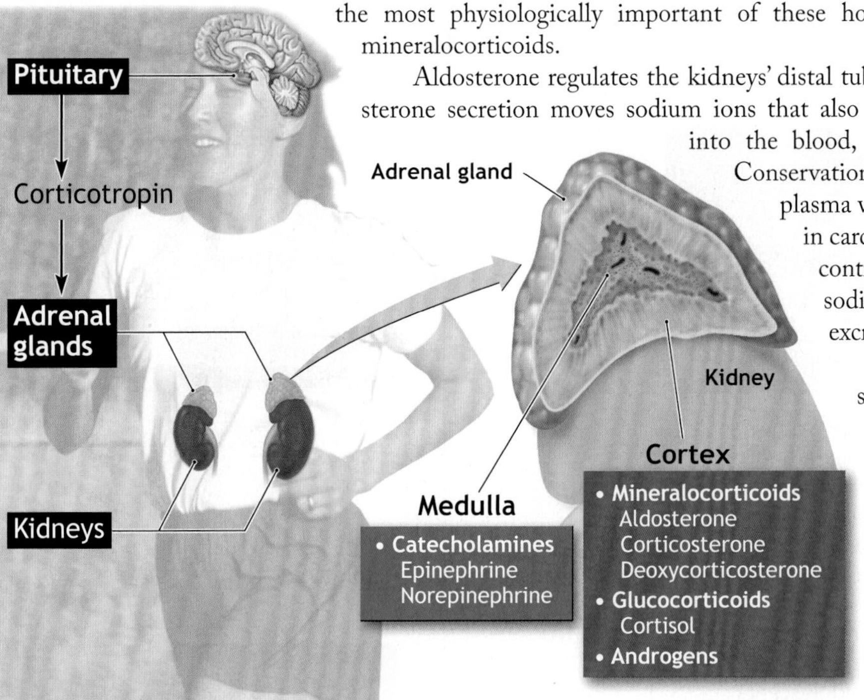

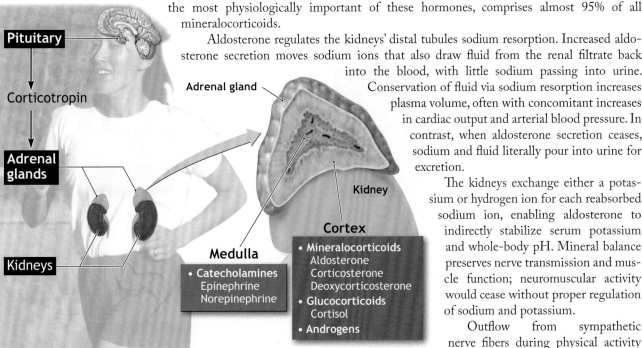

FIGURE 12.9 Adrenal gland and its secretions. (Reprinted with permission from McArdle WD, Katch FI, Katch VL. *Exercise Physiology: Nutrition, Energy, and Human Performance*. 8th Ed. Baltimore: Wolters Kluwer Health, 2015.)

gradations from light to maximum. Duration also influences catecholamine response as revealed by a direct relationship between plasma epinephrine and norepinephrine levels and mileage run. Athletes involved in sprint-power training show greater sympathoadrenergic activation during maximal physical activity than counterparts trained in aerobic activities. This difference relates to higher anaerobic contributions to maximal energy output during sprint-power activities. Other factors that determine catecholamine response to physical activity include age (greater catecholamine secretion in older subjects at an absolute intensity) and gender (greater epinephrine secretion in men than women at the same relative intensity).

Adrenal Cortex Hormones

The adrenal cortex secretes **adrenocortical hormones** in response to ACTH stimulation from the pituitary gland. These steroid hormones are categorized by function into one of three groups, each produced in a different adrenal cortex zone or layer:

1. **Mineralocorticoids**
2. **Glucocorticoids**
3. **Androgens**

Mineralocorticoids

Mineralocorticoids regulate the mineral salts sodium and potassium in the extracellular fluid space. **Aldosterone,**

A Cause for Hypertension

Chronic reduction in renal blood flow at rest, perhaps from abnormal sympathetic stimulation, activates the renin-angiotensin mechanism. Hypertension occurs from the prolonged over response of this mechanism with resulting excess aldosterone output. High blood pressure associated with increased aldosterone production often occurs in obese teenagers and is related to three factors:

1. Decreased salt sensitivity with increased water retention
2. Increased sodium intake
3. Decreased sensitivity to effects of insulin (*hyperinsulinemia*)

Glucocorticoids

Figure 12.10 lists factors that affect **cortisol (hydrocortisone)** secretion, the major steroid glucocorticoid of the adrenal cortex, and its actions on target tissues. Cortisol secretes with a strong diurnal rhythm; secretion normally peaks in the morning and diminishes at night. Cortisol secretion also increases with stress; thus, it is sometimes called the "stress hormone." The catabolic hormone cortisol counters hypoglycemia, which makes it essential for life.

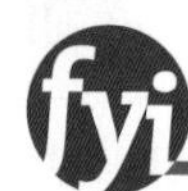

Cardiovascular Health Status of U.S. Adolescents

The most recent estimates of the cardiovascular health of U.S. adolescents come from the 2005–2010 National Health and Nutrition Examination Prevalence Estimates Surveys representing approximately 33.2 million adolescents ages 12 to 19 years.

Population prevalence of individual cardiovascular health behaviors and factors was estimated according to American Heart Association criteria for poor, intermediate, and ideal levels. Ideal blood pressure was most prevalent (males, 78%; females, 90%), whereas a dramatically low prevalence of ideal Healthy Diet Score was observed (males and females, <1%). Females exhibited a lower prevalence of ideal total cholesterol than males (65% vs. 72%, respectively) and ideal physical activity levels (44% vs. 67%, respectively), yet a higher prevalence of ideal blood glucose (89% vs. 74%, respectively). Approximately two thirds of adolescents exhibited ideal body mass index (males, 66%; females, 67%) and ideal smoking status (males, 66%; females, 70%). Less than 50% of the combined group exhibited five or more (total cholesterol, physical activity levels, blood glucose, body mass index) of the ideal cardiovascular health components (45%, males; 50%, females). Prevalence estimates according to sex were consistent across race/ethnic groups.

The low prevalence of ideal cardiovascular health behaviors in U.S. adolescents, particularly physical activity and dietary intake, will likely contribute to a worsening prevalence of obesity, hypertension, hypercholesterolemia, and dysglycemia as the current U.S. adolescent population reaches adulthood.

Source: Shay CM, et al. Status of cardiovascular health in us adolescents: prevalence estimates from the National Health and Nutrition Examination Surveys (NHANES) 2005–2010. *Circulation* 2013;127:1369.

Animals whose adrenal glands have been removed do not survive when exposed to significant environmental stressors. Cortisol, required for full glucagon and catecholamines activity, exerts a *permissive effect* on those hormones.

Cortisol exhibits six main effects:

1. Promotes liver gluconeogenesis
2. Degrades skeletal muscle proteins for gluconeogenic substrate
3. Enhances lipolysis (fat breakdown) during low energy intake and prolonged, moderate physical activity
4. Suppresses immune system function
5. Promotes negative calcium balance
6. Influences brain function, including mood changes and alterations in memory and learning

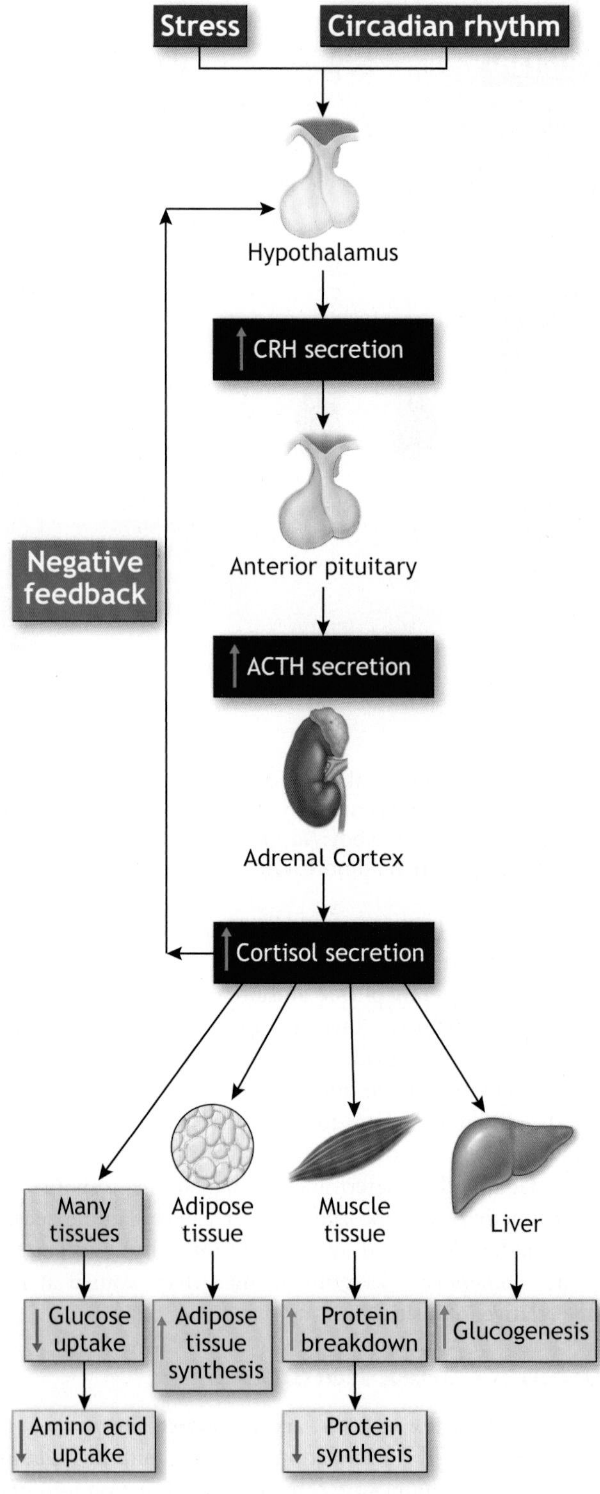

FIGURE 12.10 Factors that affect cortisol secretion and its actions on target tissues. CRH, corticotropic-releasing hormone; ACTH, adrenocorticotropic hormone. (Reprinted with permission from McArdle WD, Katch FI, Katch VL. *Exercise Physiology: Nutrition, Energy, and Human Performance*. 8th Ed. Baltimore: Wolters Kluwer Health, 2015.)

Physical activity intensity and duration, fitness level, nutritional status, and even circadian rhythm determine cortisol production. Cortisol output increases with activity intensity. High cortisol levels occur in prolonged marathon running, long-duration cycling, and hiking. Plasma cortisol also increases at relatively low levels of sustained activity and remains elevated for up to 2 hours during recovery.

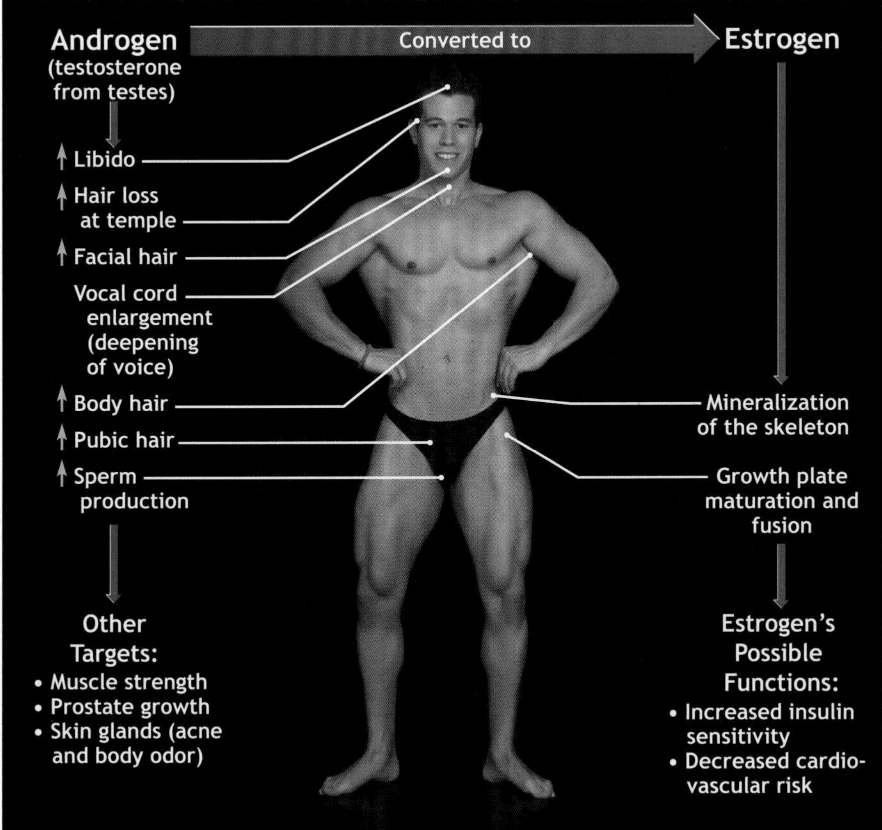

FIGURE 12.11 Androgen's effects in men. Binding with special receptor sites in muscle and various other tissues, androgen (testosterone) contributes to male secondary sex characteristics and sex differences in muscle mass and strength that develop at puberty onset. Some androgen converts to estrogen in peripheral tissues and gives males a considerable edge over females in maintaining bone mass throughout life. (Reprinted with permission from McArdle WD, Katch FI, Katch VL. *Exercise Physiology: Nutrition, Energy, and Human Performance*. 8th Ed. Baltimore: Wolters Kluwer Health, 2015.)

Androgens

The adrenal glands and ovaries (in females) and testes (in males) produce sex steroid hormones collectively termed androgens. These endocrine gland hormones promote sex-specific physical characteristics and initiate and maintain reproductive function. No distinctly "male" or "female" hormones exist; rather, androgens exhibit general differences in hormone concentrations between the sexes. Specifically, ovaries provide the primary source of **estradiol (estrogen)** and luteal phase **progesterone**; the adrenal glands in males and females synthesize **dehydroepiandrosterone (DHEA)** and its sulfate, DHEAS. The testes produce **testosterone**, also secreted in small amounts by the ovaries; conversely, testosterone converts to estrogen in peripheral tissues.

Figure 12.11 shows that testosterone, among its many functions, initiates sperm production and stimulates development of male secondary sex characteristics, mainly an increase in facial, pubic, and body hair; vocal cord enlargement; and deepening of the voice. Testosterone's anabolic, tissue-building role contributes to male-female phenotypic differences (dimorphism) in muscle mass and strength that emerge at puberty onset. Testosterone conversion to estrogen in peripheral tissues, under control of the enzyme aromatase, protects male bone structure throughout life. The ovaries provide the primary source of estrogens.

Plasma testosterone concentration in females, about one tenth the level of males, increases with physical activity (as does concentration of estradiol and progesterone). Resistance exercise and moderate aerobic physical activity increase serum and free testosterone levels after about 15 to 20 minutes in untrained men. Testosterone decreases below resting values during longer duration, intense aerobic activity.

PANCREATIC HORMONES

The pancreas, about 14 cm long and weighing 60 g, lies in the abdominal cavity below the stomach. **Figure 12.12** illustrates its location and its different endocrine cells. In 1868, German microscopic anatomist and physician Paul Langerhans (1847–1888; **www.ncbi.nlm.nih.gov/pmc/articles/PMC1769627/**) first described the clusters of cells within the pancreas. These accumulations of cells, numbering close to 1 million, were later named **islets of Langerhans** in his honor. They contain four distinct cell types, each associated with a different peptide hormone. About three quarters of islet cells are **β cells** that produce **insulin** and a peptide called **amylin**; another 20% are **α cells** that secrete **glucagon**. The remaining cells include somatostatin-secreting D cells and those that produce **pancreatic polypeptide (PP)**.

Insulin and glucagon act in antagonistic fashion to modulate plasma glucose levels. The blood usually contains both hormones; the ratio of these hormones determines which hormone and its action dominate.

In the post–absorptive-fed condition, insulin dominates, and the body remains in a net anabolic state. Ingested glucose provides substrate for energy metabolism; any excess stores as glycogen or synthesizes to fat and protein. In the fasting state, in contrast, glucagon dominates to prevent low plasma glucose concentrations, called **hypoglycemia**.

Insulin Secretion

Five factors influence insulin release following a meal:

1. **Increased blood glucose concentrations:** Plasma glucose concentrations greater than 100 mg · dL^{-1} represent the main stimulus to insulin secretion.

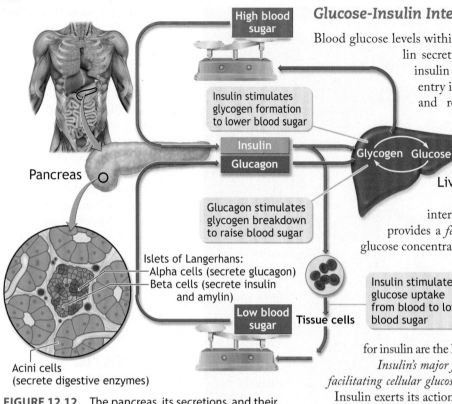

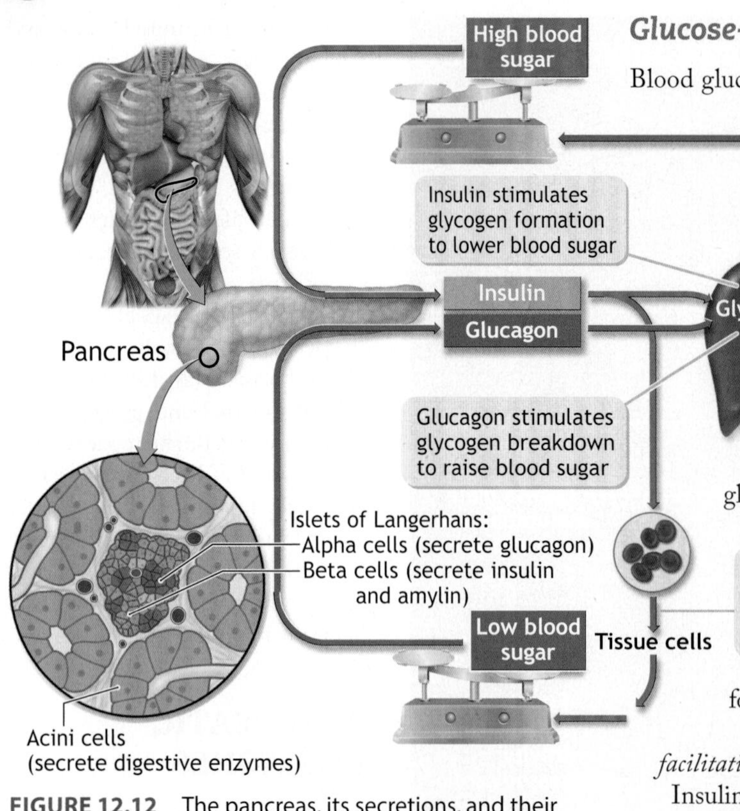

FIGURE 12.12 The pancreas, its secretions, and their actions. (Reprinted with permission from McArdle WD, Katch FI, Katch VL. *Exercise Physiology: Nutrition, Energy, and Human Performance*. 8th Ed. Baltimore: Wolters Kluwer Health, 2015.)

Glucose absorbed from the small intestine travels in the bloodstream to the pancreas' β cells, where a transporter (glucose transporter 2 [GLUT2]) initiates insulin release.

2. **Increased blood amino acid concentrations:** Increased plasma amino acid concentration, which typically occurs after a meal, triggers insulin release.
3. **Gastrointestinal tract hormones:** Several hormones released from the intestinal tract after a meal travel in the circulation to the β cells to stimulate insulin release. Two of the most important of these hormones are glucagonlike peptide-1 (GLP-1) and glucose-dependent insulinotropic peptide (GIP). Both hormones trigger insulin release even before glucose reaches the β cells.
4. **Parasympathetic nervous system stimulation:** During and following a meal, an increase in parasympathetic stimulation of the intestinal region and pancreas directly promotes insulin release.
5. **Sympathetic nervous system stimulation:** Increased sympathetic activity inhibits insulin secretion. During relatively intense physical activity, potentially a stress point, sympathetic input to the pancreas increases to inhibit insulin secretion and stimulate gluconeogenesis; this provides extra glucose fuel for the nervous system and skeletal musculature.

Glucose-Insulin Interaction

Blood glucose levels within the pancreas directly control insulin secretion. Elevated blood glucose triggers insulin release. This in turn induces glucose entry into cells thus lowering blood glucose and removing the stimulus for insulin release. In contrast, a decrease in blood glucose concentration dramatically lowers blood insulin levels to provide a favorable milieu for increasing blood glucose. The interaction between glucose and insulin provides a *feedback mechanism* to maintain blood glucose concentration within narrow limits. Rising levels of plasma amino acids also increase insulin secretion.

Insulin's Functions

The three primary target tissues for insulin are the liver, adipose tissue, and skeletal muscle. *Insulin's major function regulates glucose metabolism by facilitating cellular glucose uptake in all tissues except the brain.* Insulin exerts its action on glucose in four ways:

1. **Increases glucose transport into most, but not all, insulin-sensitive cells:** Adipose tissue and resting skeletal muscle do require insulin for glucose uptake during rest. Active skeletal muscle does *not* depend on insulin for its glucose uptake. When muscles become active, GLUT-4 transporters within cells activate without insulin stimulation to increase glucose uptake. The intracellular signal for this uncoupling appears to be Ca^{2+} and inorganic phosphate (P_i).
2. **Enhances glucose cellular utilization and storage:** Insulin activates enzymes for glucose utilization (glycolysis) and glycogen and fat synthesis (glycogenesis and lipogenesis). Insulin simultaneously inhibits enzymes for glycogen breakdown (glycogenolysis), glucose synthesis (gluconeogenesis), and fat breakdown (lipolysis) to ensure that metabolism moves toward anabolism. Consuming more glucose than needed for energy metabolism converts the excess to glycogen or fatty acids.
3. **Enhances utilization of amino acids:** Insulin activates enzymes for protein synthesis and inhibits enzymes that promote protein breakdown.
4. **Promotes fat synthesis:** Insulin inhibits fatty acid β-oxidation, which instead promotes conversion of excess glucose or amino acids into triacylglycerols via lipogenesis.

Figure 12.13 illustrates how insulin's anabolic functions promote glycogen, protein, and fat synthesis. With insulin deficiency, the action of glucagon predominates, and cells engage in catabolic activity.

See the animation "Insulin Functions" on **http://thePoint.lww.com/MKKESS5e** for a demonstration of insulin's activity.

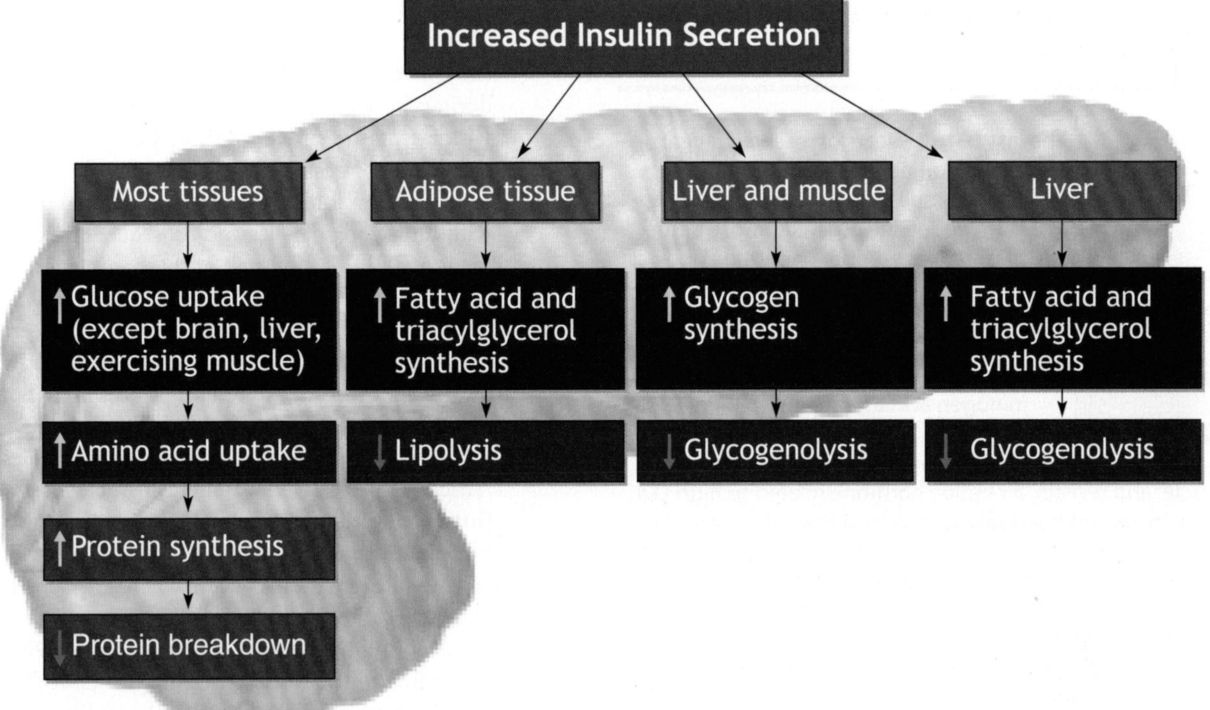

FIGURE 12.13 Increased insulin promotes glycogen, protein, and fat synthesis. (Adapted with permission from McArdle WD, Katch FI, Katch VL. *Exercise Physiology: Nutrition, Energy, and Human Performance*. 8th Ed. Baltimore: Wolters Kluwer Health, 2015.)

Glucagon Secretion

The islets of Langerhans' α cells secrete glucagon, the "insulin antagonist" hormone. In contrast to insulin, glucagon increases blood glucose levels and stimulates liver glycogenolysis, gluconeogenesis, and lipid catabolism.

The blood glucose level regulates glucagon release. A decline in plasma glucose concentration below 100 mg · dL^{-1} stimulates the α cells to release glucagon, resulting in the liver's near-instantaneous glucose release. Glucagon contributes to blood glucose regulation during endurance activity and a considerably reduced caloric intake (semistarvation); both conditions markedly decrease blood glucose and glycogen reserves.

Plasma amino acids also stimulate glucagon release. This pathway prevents hypoglycemia after a person ingests a meal with a very high protein content. If a meal contains protein without carbohydrate, amino acids in the food trigger insulin secretion. Even though no glucose has been absorbed, insulin-stimulated glucose uptake increases, and plasma glucose concentration decreases. Co-secretion of glucagon in this situation prevents hypoglycemia by stimulating hepatic glucose output. When consuming protein (amino acids), peripheral tissues absorb both glucose and amino acids.

Glucagon's Functions

Figure 12.14 illustrates that when glucagon action predominates, cells engage in catabolic activity. The liver represents glucagon's primary target tissue, stimulating glycogenolysis and gluconeogenesis to increase glucose output. During an overnight fast, 75% of the glucose produced by the liver comes from its glycogen stores, with the remaining 25% produced from gluconeogenic reactions. Glucagon also exerts a catabolic effect on adipose tissue throughout the body.

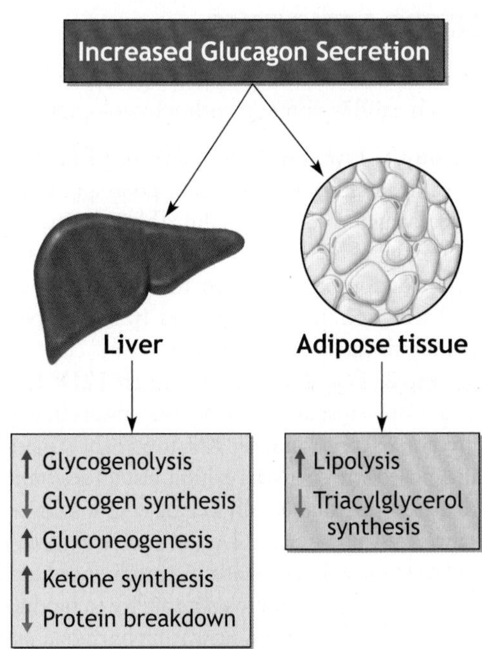

FIGURE 12.14 Glucagon secretion and its actions on target tissues. (Adapted with permission from McArdle WD, Katch FI, Katch VL. *Exercise Physiology: Nutrition, Energy, and Human Performance*. 8th Ed. Baltimore: Wolters Kluwer Health, 2015.)

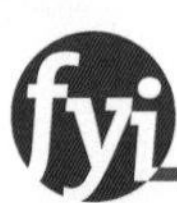

Adipose Tissue as an Endocrine Organ

The last 10 to 15 years of research reveals that, in addition to energy storage, adipose tissue functions as an important endocrine organ. Adipose tissue secretes a number of peptide hormones, including leptin, which influences appetite; several cytokines; adipsin and acylation-stimulating protein (ASP); angiotensinogen; plasminogen activator inhibitor-1 (PAI-1); adiponectin, which increases insulin sensitivity and fatty acid oxidation in muscle; and resistin, a peptide hormone related to high LDL levels, increased heart disease risk, and links obesity to diabetes. Adipose tissue also produces steroid hormones. This adipose tissue secretory function has shifted the view about adipose tissue to one at the heart of a complex network that influences energy balance, glucose and lipid metabolism, vascular homeostasis, immune response, and reproduction function. Most known adipose secreted proteins become dysregulated when "normal" levels of body fat become markedly altered—either increased in the overfat (obese) state or decreased in the underfat (lipoatrophy) state.

Sources: Boscaro M, et al. Visceral adipose tissue: emerging role of glucocorticoid and mineralocorticoid hormones in the setting of cardiometabolic alterations. *Ann N Y Acad Sci* 2012;1264:87.

Guerre-Millo M. Adipose tissue hormones. *J Endocrinol Invest* 2002;25:855.

DIABETES MELLITUS

Diabetes mellitus consists of four subgroups of disorders, each of which exhibit different pathophysiologies:

Subgroup 1. Type 1 diabetes mellitus (T1DM) develops when pancreatic cells no longer function effectively to produce insulin. This liability, initiated or mediated by the body's immune system, severely limits or completely eliminates insulin production and secretion. Between 5% and 10% of diabetics belong to the type 1 subgroup.

Subgroup 2. Type 2 diabetes mellitus (T2DM) refers to a relative insulin deficiency that results in hyperglycemia. Approximately 90% to 95% of Americans diagnosed with diabetes exhibit insulin resistance. This diabetes subgroup usually begins with insulin resistance, in which muscle, liver, and adipose tissue cells fail to use insulin efficiently. As insulin need increases, the pancreas gradually loses its ability to produce sufficient quantities of this regulating hormone. Insulin resistance, as opposed to β-cell dysfunction, differs among individuals; some people have primarily insulin resistance and only a minor insulin secretion defect, while others exhibit only slight insulin resistance but have primarily defective insulin secretion.

Subgroup 3. Gestational diabetes affects as many as 9% of all pregnant women or about 300,000 cases in the US yearly. This condition is typically diagnosed during the second or third trimester of pregnancy. Risk factors are similar to those for T2DM. The occurrence of gestational diabetes itself is a risk factor for developing recurrent gestational diabetes with future pregnancies and subsequent development of T2DM. Children of these women may be at heightened risk of developing obesity and diabetes. Treatment includes dietary restraint for certain food categories, increased regular physical activity, or exogenous insulin to reduce problems for both mother and fetus. Since 1991, the highest prevalence has been in Asians, followed by Hispanics, African Americans, and non-Hispanic whites (**http://care.diabetesjournals.org/content/30/Supplement_2/S141.full**).

Subgroup 4. Prediabetes occurs when a person's blood glucose level reaches higher-than-normal values but is not high enough for diagnosis as T2DM. According to the National Center for Chronic Disease Prevention and Health Promotion 2014 Statistics Report, this condition afflicts an estimated 29.1 million Americans.

Clinicians have discontinued the use of the terms **insulin-dependent diabetes mellitus (T1DM; IDDM; type 1)** and **non–insulin-dependent diabetes mellitus (T2DM; NIDDM; type 2)** because these diseases often require treatments that overlap and vary rather than reflect the underlying pathogenesis (**Table 12.3**).

TABLE 12.3 Differences Between the Two Major Forms of Diabetes Mellitus

	Type 1 (T1DM)	Type 2 (T2DM)
Other names	Type 1-IDDM Juvenile-onset Ketosis-prone Brittle	Type II-NIDDM Adult-onset Ketosis-resistant Stable
Age of onset	<20 y (mean = 12 y) <40 y in some cases	>40 y; increasingly prevalent in youth
Other condition	Viral infection	Obesity
Insulin required	Yes	Sometimes
Insulin receptors	Normal	Low or normal
Symptoms	Relatively severe	Relatively moderate
Prevalence in diabetic population	5%–10%	90%–95%

A Disease of Epidemic Proportions

Table 12.4 presents the latest diabetes statistics in America (report released June, 2014). The United States now ranks third with the largest number of confirmed diabetes cases in the world (China ranks first, India second). Based on these data, diabetes ranks as the seventh leading cause of death; a number that may be underreported. According to the Centers for Disease Control and Prevention, early diagnosis and intervention are major public health initiatives.

Diabetes Signs and Symptoms

Diabetes often progresses undiagnosed because many of its symptoms seem harmless and are rarely noticed. Importantly, early detection of the signs and symptoms of diabetes and subsequent treatment decrease the chance of developing the more serious diabetes complications.

Signs and symptoms of diabetes include:

1. Elevated blood glucose (hyperglycemia)
2. Frequent urination (polyuria)

TABLE 12.4 Diabetes and Prediabetes Statistics

Prevalence	• In 2012, 29.1 million (9.3% of population) (In 2010, 25.8 million [8.3% of population])
Undiagnosed	• 8.1 million (In 2010, 7 million)
Prevalence in seniors (65+ y)	• 11.8 million (25.9%) (In 2010, 26.9%)
New cases of diabetes	• 1.7 million (In 2010, 1.9 million)
Prediabetes	• 86 million age 20 and older (In 2012, 79 million)
Deaths	• In 2012, seventh leading cause
Diabetes in youth	• 208,000 Americans under age 20 diagnosed (25% of that population)
Diabetes by race/ethnicity	• 7.6% of non-Hispanic whites • 9.0% of Asian Americans • 12.8% of Hispanics • 13.2% of non-Hispanic blacks • 15.9% of American Indians/Alaskan Natives
Complications/comorbid conditions	• **Hypoglycemia:** In 2011, 282,000 emergency room visits for adults aged 18 y or older with hypoglycemia • **Hypertension:** In 2009–2012, of adults aged 18 y or older with diagnosed diabetes, 71% had blood pressure ≥140/90 mm of mercury, or used prescription medications to lower high blood pressure. • **Dyslipidemia:** In 2009–2012, of adults aged 18 y or older with diagnosed diabetes, 65% had blood LDL cholesterol ≥100 mg/dL or used cholesterol-lowering medications. • **CVD death rates**: In 2003–2006, after adjusting for population age differences, cardiovascular disease death rates were about 1.7 times higher among adults aged 18 y or older with diagnosed diabetes. • **Heart attack rates:** In 2010, after adjusting for population age differences, hospitalization rates for heart attack were 1.8 times higher among adults aged 20 y or older with diagnosed diabetes. • **Stroke:** In 2010, after adjusting for population age differences, hospitalization rates for stroke were 1.5 times higher among adults with diagnosed diabetes aged 20 y or older. • **Blindness and eye problems**: In 2005–2008, of adults with diabetes aged 40 y or older, 4.2 million (28.5%) people had diabetic retinopathy, which may result in loss of vision. • **Kidney disease**: In 2011, diabetes was listed as the primary cause of kidney failure in 44% of all new cases. • **Amputations**: In 2010, about 73,000 nontraumatic lowerlimb amputations were performed in adults aged 20 y or older with diagnosed diabetes. About 60% of nontraumatic lower limb amputations among people aged 20 y or older occur in people with diagnosed diabetes.
Costs	• $245 billion: Total costs of diagnosed diabetes in the United States in 2012 • $176 billion for direct medical costs • $69 billion in reduced productivity • After adjusting for population age and sex differences, average medical expenditures among people with diagnosed diabetes were 2.3 times higher than what expenditures would be in the absence of diabetes.

Source: Data from the National Diabetes Statistics Report, Atlanta, GA: Division of Diabetes Translation, National Center for Chronic Disease Prevention and Health Promotion, Centers for Disease Control and Prevention. Available at: **www.cdc.gov/diabetes/pubs/statsreport14/national-diabetes-report-web.pdf**

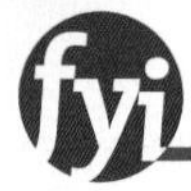

Are You at Risk for T2DM?

ARE YOU AT RISK FOR

TYPE 2 DIABETES?

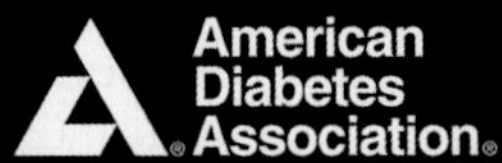

Diabetes Risk Test

Write your score in the box.

1. **How old are you?**
   Less than 40 years (0 points)
   40—49 years (1 point)
   50—59 years (2 points)
   60 years or older (3 points)

2. **Are you a man or a woman?**
   Man (1 point) Woman (0 points)

3. **If you are a woman, have you ever been diagnosed with gestational diabetes?**
   Yes (1 point) No (0 points)

4. **Do you have a mother, father, sister, or brother with diabetes?**
   Yes (1 point) No (0 points)

5. **Have you ever been diagnosed with high blood pressure?**
   Yes (1 point) No (0 points)

6. **Are you physically active?**
   Yes (0 points) No (1 point)

7. **What is your weight status?**
   (see chart at right)

Add up your score.

If you scored 5 or higher:
You are at increased risk for having type 2 diabetes. However, only your doctor can tell for sure if you do have type 2 diabetes or prediabetes (a condition that precedes type 2 diabetes in which blood glucose levels are higher than normal). Talk to your doctor to see if additional testing is needed.

Height	Weight (lbs.)		
4′ 10″	119-142	143-190	191+
4′ 11″	124-147	148-197	198+
5′ 0″	128-152	153-203	204+
5′ 1″	132-157	158-210	211+
5′ 2″	136-163	164-217	218+
5′ 3″	141-168	169-224	225+
5′ 4″	145-173	174-231	232+
5′ 5″	150-179	180-239	240+
5′ 6″	155-185	186-246	247+
5′ 7″	159-190	191-254	255+
5′ 8″	164-196	197-261	262+
5′ 9″	169-202	203-269	270+
5′ 10″	174-208	209-277	278+
5′ 11″	179-214	215-285	286+
6′ 0″	184-220	221-293	294+
6′ 1″	189-226	227-301	302+
6′ 2″	194-232	233-310	311+
6′ 3″	200-239	240-318	319+
6′ 4″	205-245	246-327	328+
	(1 Point)	(2 Points)	(3 Points)

You weigh less than the amount in the left column (0 points)

Adapted from Bang et al., Ann Intern Med 151:775-783, 2009.
Original algorithm was validated without gestational diabetes as part of the model.

3. Excessive thirst (polydipsia)
4. Extreme hunger (polyphagia)
5. High levels of blood ketones from reliance on excessive fat catabolism
6. Unexplained weight loss
7. Increased fatigue
8. Irritability
9. Blurry vision
10. Numbness or tingling in the extremities (hands, feet)
11. Slow-healing wounds or sores
12. Abnormally high frequency of infection

See the animation "Diabetes" on **http://thePoint.lww.com/MKKESS5e** for an explanation of this disorder and its causes.

Genetics of Diabetes

A simple pattern of inherited characteristics does not fully explain the risk of contracting diabetes. Two factors predispose a person to diabetes:

1. Inherited genetic predisposition
2. Environment factors trigger activation

Type 1 Diabetes

Most type 1 diabetics inherit risk factors from both parents, with inherited traits more common in whites than blacks or Asians. The most prominent "environmental triggers" include cold weather exposure (develops more often in winter than summer and more frequently in places with cold climates), viral infection, and early dietary patterns (less common in those who were breast-fed and in those who first ate solid foods at a later age). Disease onset can occur at any age, but peak age for diagnosis occurs in the mid-teens. In Western populations, each child has a 0.3% to 0.4% risk of developing diabetes by age 20; the risk increases 15-fold in siblings of an affected child (**www.diapedia.org/type-1-diabetes-mellitus/genetics-of-type-1-diabetes**). Genes in the human leukocyte antigen (HLA) region on chromosome 6 account for approximately 50% of the genetic risk of type 1 diabetes. Research has shown that chromosome 11, located at a specific region of the insulin gene, contributes about 10% of genetic susceptibility; 40 additional genes make only a minor contribution to T1DM.

Type 2 Diabetes

T2DM has a stronger genetic basis than T1DM, yet its occurrence depends more on environmental and behavioral factors. A family history of T2DM represents one of the strongest risk factors for the disease but *only* for people living a typical Western lifestyle, which consists of a high-fat diet, low intake of complex carbohydrates and fiber, and inadequate physical activity. Overfatness provides a considerable T2DM risk factor. Diabetes-prone individuals possess a gene that directs synthesis of three mitogen-activated protein kinases that inhibit insulin's action in cellular glucose transport. The peak age of T2DM onset usually occurs later than T1DM. African Americans, Mexican Americans, and Pima Indians have the highest risk for developing T2DM. The disease results from five complex physiologic processes:

1. Pancreatic β cells
2. Peripheral glucose uptake by muscle
3. Adipocyte release of multiple cytokines and hormone-like molecules
4. Hepatic glucose production
5. Central nervous system

Three factors can produce high blood glucose levels in T2DM:

1. Inability of the pancreas to produce sufficient insulin to control blood sugar known as **relative insulin deficiency**
2. Decreased insulin effects on peripheral tissue, particularly skeletal muscle, known as **insulin resistance**
3. Combined effect of factors 1 and 2

Tests for Diabetes

Several tests diagnose diabetes. The American Diabetes Association (**www.diabetes.org/home.jsp**) recommends the **fasting plasma glucose (FPG) test** rather than the popular **oral glucose tolerance test**. The latter evaluates blood sugar levels 5 times over a 3-hour period after drinking a glucose-containing solution. The FPG test measures plasma glucose following an 8-hour fast.

The current value for suspected diabetes (FPG >126 mg · dL^{-1}) is now lower than the previous 140 mg · dL^{-1} standard; this acknowledges that patients can remain asymptomatic with microvascular small blood vessel damage with FPG values in the low-to-mid 120 mg · dL^{-1} range. The impaired range represents a transition between normal and T2DM at which the body no longer responds properly to insulin or fails to secrete adequate amounts. These prediabetic individuals require close monitoring because they run a high risk of developing full-blown T2DM.

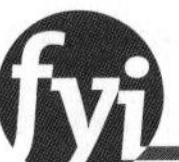

The Hemoglobin A1c Test

The test to determine blood glucose status over a more prolonged time period, the glycosylated hemoglobin test or A1c test (also known as Hb1c), quantifies how much hemoglobin has been coated (glycosylated) by glucose. In other words, the A1c test measures the amount of glucose attached to hemoglobin in red blood cells. In practical terms, as blood sugar increases, more hemoglobin becomes glycosylated, and this effect remains relatively stable until new red blood cells form in about 2 to 3 months. Thus, the A1c test reflects an individual's average blood glucose status for 2 to 3 months prior to the test. The results, reported as a percentage, would mean that someone with a higher percentage (usually above 5.7%) had an undesirable blood glucose level. The A1c cutoffs for diagnosing prediabetes range between 5.7% and 6.4%, and above 6.5% for diagnosing T2DM. As a frame of comparison, A1c test results have been compared to standard blood glucose values. For a 6% A1c, an average glucose reading would correspond to 126 mg · dL^{-1}; (7% = 154 mg · dL^{-1}; 8% = 183 mg · dL^{-1}; 9% = 212 mg · dL^{-1}, with higher values of 10% [240 mg · dL^{-1}, 11% = 269 mg · dL^{-1}, and 12% = 298 mg · dL^{-1}]). The National Glycohemoglobin Standardization Program (NGSP; **www.ngsp.org**) certifies that manufacturers of A1c tests provide results consistent with established criterion standards.

Individuals with higher than normal A1c are at increased risk of developing T2DM, heart disease, and stroke. Studies of individuals at high risk for diabetes show that lifestyle intervention that resulted in weight loss and increased physical activity can prevent or delay T2DM; in some cases, blood glucose levels have returned to the normal range. In 2009–2012, based on fasting glucose or A1c levels, 37% of U.S. adults age 20 years or older had prediabetes (51% of those aged 65 y or older). Applying this percentage to the entire U.S. population in 2012 yielded an estimated 86 million Americans age 20 years or older with prediabetes.

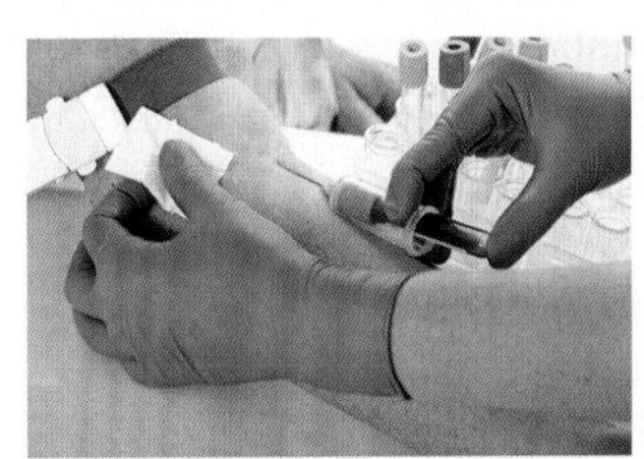

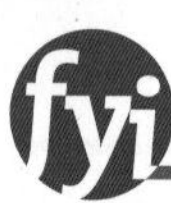

Combining Five Healthy Lifestyle Changes to Reduce Diabetes Risk

1. Engage in 30 to 60 minutes or more of daily physical activity over and above normal daily routines.
2. Keep alcohol consumption at the light-to-moderate level.
3. Do not smoke.
4. Maintain body mass index less than 25 and waist size less than 34.6 inches for women and 36.2 inches for men.
5. Consume a healthy diet with above-average daily fiber intake (>25 g), a positive ratio of polyunsaturated fat to saturated fat, low *trans*-fat, and food with a relatively low glycemic index (see below for dietary suggestions).

Instead of this:	Consume this:
Soft drinks, fruit drinks, fruit juice	Water, unsweetened coffee or tea
Saturated fat, trans fat (margarine, cream, pies, cake frostings, French fries)	Unsaturated fats (vegetable oils, nuts)
Refined grains and sweets	Whole grains
Red meats, especially processed meats (bacon, sausage, ham, hot dogs)	Seafood, poultry, beans, soy foods

METABOLIC SYNDROME

Metabolic syndrome represents a multifaceted grouping of coronary artery disease risks defined with three or more of the criteria listed in **Table 12.5**. This "disease of modern civilization" affects millions of adults in Western industrialized countries and is more common in men than women. Disease occurrence relates to genetic, hormonal, and lifestyle factors (i.e., obesity, physical inactivity, and nutrient excesses, including higher than desirable intakes of saturated and *trans* fatty acids). The clustering of insulin resistance and hyperinsulinemia characterizes metabolic syndrome. Individuals with these prominent characteristics remain at higher risk for coronary artery disease and should receive appropriate attention and treatment.

TABLE 12.5 Identifying the Metabolic Syndrome

Risk Factor	Defining Level
Abdominal fatness (waist girth)[a]	
Men	>102 cm (>40 in.)
Women	>88 cm (>35 in.)
Triacylglycerols	≥150 mg/dL
High-density lipoprotein	
Men	<40 mg/dL
Women	<50 mg/dL
Blood pressure	≥130/≥85 mm Hg
Fasting glucose	≥110 mg/dL

[a]Overweight and overfatness associate with insulin resistance and metabolic syndrome. The presence of abnormal obesity more highly correlates with metabolic risk factors than elevated body mass index (BMI). We recommend waist girth to identify the body weight component of the metabolic syndrome.

DIABETES AND PHYSICAL ACTIVITY

Hypoglycemia during physical activity represents the most common disturbance of glucose homeostasis in T1DM. During prolonged moderate effort, hepatic glucose release does not keep pace with active muscle's increased glucose utilization. Severely reduced plasma glucose becomes of concern in patients who require intensive insulin therapy throughout the day to normalize their glucose levels. Sedentary lifestyle and excessive body fat reduce exercise tolerance in individuals with T1DM or T2DM independent of blood glucose regulation.

Physical Training Among Diabetics

The clinical use of exercise before training to control glucose in T1DM remains complex despite the clear association between regular physical activity and improved insulin sensitivity by peripheral tissues. Individuals with T1DM must remain cautious about how much physical activity they undertake because increased insulin sensitivity of muscle and fast delivery of injected insulin via rapid circulation accelerate glucose removal from plasma, which can induce serious hypoglycemia and diabetic shock.

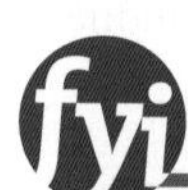

Resistance Training Reduces T2DM Risk

Resistance training, either alone or combined with aerobic activity, lowers diabetes risk in men. Training for at least 30 minutes daily, five times a week reduced the chance of developing type 2 diabetes up to 34%. Combining resistance training with diverse aerobic activities for a weekly total of 150 minutes reduced risk by as much as 59%. A dose-response relationship emerged between an increasing amount of time spent on resistance training or aerobic activity and lower diabetes risk.

Source: Grøntved A, et al. A prospective study of weight training and risk of type 2 diabetes mellitus in men. *Arch Intern Med* 2012;172:1306.

A CLOSER LOOK

Metabolic Syndrome: Organs Affected, Common Characteristics, Associated Medical Conditions, and Treatment

What is Metabolic Syndrome?

Metabolic syndrome afflicts 25% of adult Americans. This common condition includes **obesity, high blood pressure, high blood glucose ("blood sugar")**, and an **abnormal cholesterol profile (dyslipidemia)**. The chance of developing **coronary heart disease**, stroke, and diabetes increases when these risk factors cluster together significantly more than when risk factors develop independently.

Medical Conditions Associated with Metabolic Syndrome

Left untreated, metabolic syndrome increases risk of coronary heart disease, stroke, and type 2 diabetes.

A Stroke

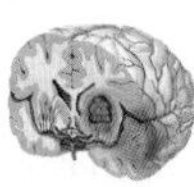

The term stroke refers to the sudden death of brain tissue from lack of oxygen. In ischemic stroke, blocked or reduced blood flow occurs in brain tissues. This blockage may result from atherosclerosis and blood clot formation.

B Coronary Heart Disease

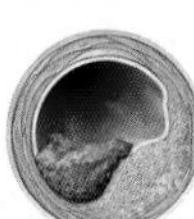

Narrowing of the coronary arteries can lead to a heart attack. Atherosclerosis, the buildup of plaque in the lining of the arteries, causes arterial narrowing; all of the metabolic syndrome risk factors can induce atherosclerosis. Heart attacks occur when blood fails to flow through narrowed coronary vessels, which results in ischemic myocardial tissue.

C Type 2 Diabetes

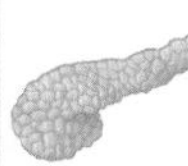

In type 2 diabetes, the pancreas produces little or no insulin and/or the body loses the ability to respond normally to insulin (called insulin resistance). Insulin transports glucose into the cells for use as energy; without insulin, body tissues have less access to essential nutrients for energy and storage. Diabetes requires proper management, and if left untreated, can lead to complications that impact the eyes, mouth, cardiovascular system, kidneys, nerves, and extremities.

Organs Affected by Untreated Metabolic Syndrome
A Brain
B Heart
C Pancreas
Fibrous plaque (atherosclerosis)

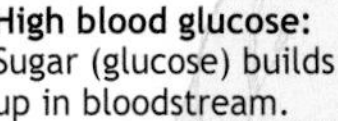
High blood glucose: Sugar (glucose) builds up in bloodstream.

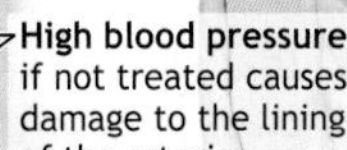
High blood pressure, if not treated causes damage to the lining of the arteries.

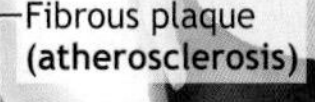

Common Characteristics

- Insulin resistance
- Glucose intolerance
- Dyslipidemia (high triglycerol, low HDL, high LDL)
- Stroke
- Upper-body obesity
- Type 2 diabetes
- Hypertension
- Coronary artery disease
- Reduced ability to dissolve blood clots

Treating Metabolic Syndrome

Metabolic syndrome requires long-term management of each risk factor. Poor nutrition and reduced physical activity represent underlying causes of these risk factors. Regular monitoring of blood pressure, cholesterol, and glucose are important for detecting the syndrome, even if an individual fails to experience outward disease symptoms.

- **Weight loss:** A weight loss of 5 to 10% of body weight improves insulin sensitivity.
- **Increased physical activity:** Increased physical activity reverses insulin resistance, reduces blood pressure, lowers "bad" cholesterol, raises "good" cholesterol, and reduces overall type 2 diabetes risk.
- **Eat a heart healthy diet:** Reduce saturated fat, cholesterol, and salt intake. Increase intake of high fiber fruits, vegetables, and grains.

Adapted with permission from McArdle WD, Katch FI, Katch VL. *Exercise Physiology: Nutrition, Energy, and Human Performance*. 8th Ed. Baltimore: Wolters Kluwer Health, 2015.

As a consequence of obesity and possibly poor diet, many "normal" overweight men and women experience reduced glucose tolerance from generalized insulin resistance; this malady triggers excessive insulin output from the pancreas with resulting hyperinsulinemia. For individuals who eventually develop T2DM, physical activity often reduces fasting plasma insulin levels and lowers insulin output, thus indicating improved insulin sensitivity.

Physical Activity Benefits for Type 2 Diabetics

Regular physical activity provides important nonpharmacologic therapy for individuals with T2DM (see **http://journals.lww.com/acsm-msse/pages/collectiondetails.aspx?TopicalCollectionId=1** for the American College of Sports Medicine's position stand on physical activity and T2DM). Individuals at greatest risk for T2DM due to obesity, hypertension, family history, and sedentary lifestyle gain the greatest benefit from increased physical activity. Regular physical activity for people with T2DM improves glycemic control, cardiovascular function, body composition, and psychological profile and reduces a broad array of heart disease risks. Some patients with T1DM improve their blood glucose control with lower daily insulin requirements with regular activity, but the results are less consistent than for type 2 patients. Despite this limitation, people with T1DM and T2DM benefit medically and physically from regular physical activity participation.

Glycemic Control

An acute bout of resistance or endurance training or both abruptly decrease plasma glucose levels in type 2 diabetics. Extending the duration of weekly physical activity by nearly 50% from 115 to 170 minutes produces the greatest increase in insulin

A CLOSER LOOK

Overweight Adults With Type 2 Diabetes Suffer Deleterious Effects

Individuals with T2DM suffer different disorders related to organ metabolic rate, heretofore unrecognized. One study was the first to assess differences in lean body mass (LBM), skeletal muscle mass, and mass of specific high metabolic rate organs (e.g., liver, kidneys, spleen, heart) in biracial adult men ($n = 33$ Caucasian; $n = 6$ African Americans) and women ($n = 28$ Caucasian; $n = 28$ African Americans) with T2DM compared with 76 nondiabetic male and female Caucasian and African American controls. No between-group differences emerged for age, height, sex, and race distribution. The researchers also examined whether differences in tissue and organ masses between T2DM and controls exhibited race and sex dependency. Body composition techniques (dual-energy x-ray absorptiometry [DXA], described in Chapter 16) assessed total body fat and fat-free mass. LBM was computed as fat-free mass minus bone mineral mass, with whole-body MRI assessing the latter, including organ mass for liver, kidney, and spleen, and left ventricular volume. The salient findings were as follows:

1. Males and females with T2DM possessed less skeletal muscle mass and LBM than nondiabetic controls.
2. Nondiabetic males and females had lower kidney, liver, and spleen masses than counterparts with T2DM.
3. Only Caucasians with T2DM had larger liver and spleen masses.
4. Compared with controls, males with T2DM had smaller left ventricular volumes.
5. In general, type 2 diabetics had lower muscle mass, LBM, and total skeletal mass than did sex-, race-, age-, weight-, and height-matched nondiabetic controls.
6. Liver size correlates positively with A1c levels in diabetics, suggesting that an enlarged and fatty liver associates with inadequate glucose control and other metabolic complications including poor organ blood flow (hemorheology).
7. In Caucasians but not in African Americans, diabetes-dependent differences occurred in liver and spleen masses. The authors suggested such differences might impact caloric expenditure (but without needed data on metabolic rates of the organs to better understand this possibility).
8. In view of the role that regular "additional" physical activity has played to ameliorate the deleterious effects of T2DM by reversing the trend of attenuated muscle mass and LBM, type 2 diabetics should employ physical activity training to preserve and/or enhance muscle mass and thus avoid further T2DM. complications

Additional data analysis, displayed in Table 1, highlights differences in body composition variables by sex and race. African American females with T2DM (AAFT2DM) and males with T2DM (AFMT2DM) had significantly greater total body fat, LBM, and skeletal mass than Caucasian females with T2DM (CFT2DM) and males with T2DM (CMT2DM).

TABLE 1 Body Composition Differences in Total Fat, LBM, and Skeletal Mass by Race and Sex[a]

	Total Fat, kg		LBM, kg		Skeletal Mass, kg	
Group	**Mean**	**SD**	**Mean**	**SD**	**Mean**	**SD**
CMT2DM	30.1	6.42	61.9	6.57	30.8	4.12
CFT2DM	26.6	9.87	42.5	6.23	20.6	4.21
AFMT2DM	33.3	5.49	63.2	5.65	32.4	2.83
AAFT2DM	33.7	6.31	43.9	5.93	20.7	3.23

[a]Data courtesy of Lance E. Davidson. Department of Exercise Sciences. Brigham Young University Provo, UT.

Source: Davidson LE, et al. Skeletal muscle and organ masses differ in overweight adults with type 2 diabetes. *J Appl Physiol* 2014;117:377.

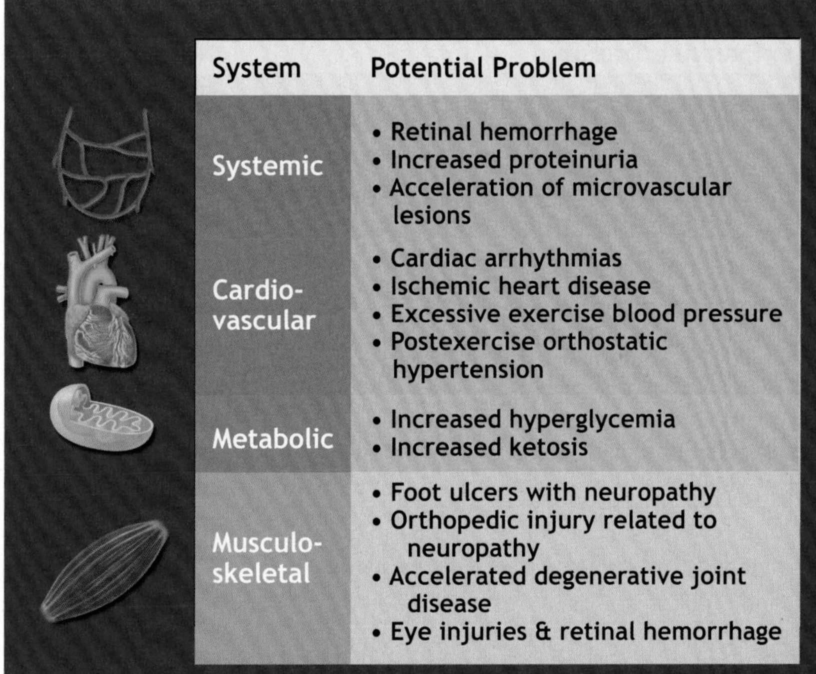

System
Potential Problem
Systemic
• Retinal hemorrhage
• Increased proteinuria
• Acceleration of microvascular lesions
Cardio-vascular
• Cardiac arrhythmias
• Ischemic heart disease
• Excessive exercise blood pressure
• Postexercise orthostatic hypertension
Metabolic
• Increased hyperglycemia
• Increased ketosis
Musculo-skeletal
• Foot ulcers with neuropathy
• Orthopedic injury related to neuropathy
• Accelerated degenerative joint disease
• Eye injuries & retinal hemorrhage

FIGURE 12.15 Potential physical and physiologic problems for individuals with type 2 diabetes who begin an exercise program. (Reprinted with permission from McArdle WD, Katch FI, Katch VL. *Exercise Physiology: Nutrition, Energy, and Human Performance*. 8th Ed. Baltimore: Wolters Kluwer Health, 2015.)

sensitivity. Improved glucose regulation with acute exertion may persist for hours to days because of the muscles' increased insulin sensitivity. Improved longer-term glycemic control in physically active people with diabetes probably occurs from the cumulative effects of *each* acute activity session rather than from changes in physical fitness per se. Consequently, patients with hyperinsulinemia show the greatest benefit from regular physical activity participation, a response consistent with the notion that physical activity reverses insulin resistance (i.e., increases insulin sensitivity). *Improved insulin sensitivity with regular physical activity provides type 2 diabetics with important "therapy" that ultimately lowers their insulin requirements. Improvements in blood glucose homeostasis with regular physical activity rapidly decrease when training ceases and completely dissipate within several weeks of inactivity.*

Cardiovascular Effects

Increases in disease state and mortality in T2DM occur from coronary heart disease, stroke, and peripheral vascular and nerve disease related to accelerated atherosclerosis and elevated blood glucose levels. In this regard, increased regular physical activity favorably modifies plasma lipoproteins, hyperinsulinemia, hyperglycemia, some blood coagulation parameters, local vascularization, and blood pressure.

Weight Loss

Physical activity without diet therapy only moderately reduces body weight among type 2 diabetics. This moderate effect should not be underestimated, however, because small changes in body weight with regular physical activity may not reflect more favorable changes in overall body composition, that is, a lean tissue mass increase may accompany the body fat loss. For both diabetic and nondiabetic individuals, body fat loss occurs most effectively by combining diet *plus* regular, moderate-intensity physical activity.

Psychological Benefits

Regular, moderate-intensity physical activity for diabetics and nondiabetics decreases anxiety, improves mood and self-esteem, increases sense of well-being, and enhances overall quality of life.

Physical Activity Risks for Diabetics

The potential complications of physical activity for diabetics can be minimized through proper patient screening before diabetic individuals undertake a physical activity program; any such program must be carefully monitored. **Figure 12.15** lists 13 potential adverse effects of physical activity for diabetics.

ENDURANCE TRAINING AND ENDOCRINE FUNCTION

Few studies have evaluated changes in hormonal response to systematic alterations in the frequency, intensity, and duration of physical activity. Most of what researchers know about changes in hormonal dynamics with training comes from studies in which hormone assessment occurred secondarily to other variables. Nevertheless, a picture has emerged of the integrated response of different hormones to training, particularly fluid balance, energy modulation, glycemic control, cardiovascular dynamics, and growth and development. **Table 12.6** lists selected endocrine hormones and their general responses to regular physical activity. Limited research exists concerning multiple hormone secretions and chronic physical activity adaptations.

Endurance training generally decreases the magnitude of hormonal response to a standard activity level. Physical activity at a particular absolute intensity produces a lower hormonal response in trained subjects than in untrained counterparts. Adjusting intensity to the same percentage of each person's maximum capacity (i.e., same relative intensity) eliminates the training-related difference in hormonal response. With maximal effort, trained subjects have a similar or slightly higher catecholamine and pituitary hormonal response than untrained subjects.

TABLE 12.6 Hormonal Response to Exercise Training

Hormone	Training Response
Hypothalamus-Pituitary Hormones	
GH	Resting values increased: trained tend to have less dramatic rise during exercise
TSH	No known training effect
ACTH	Trained persons have increased exercise values
PRL	Some evidence that training lowers resting values
FSH, LB, and testosterone	Trained females have depressed values; testosterone levels may increase in males with long-term strength training
Posterior Pituitary Hormones	
Vasopressin (ADH)	Some evidence that training slightly reduces ADH at a given workload
Oxytocin	Limited human research available
Thyroid Hormones	
Thyroxine (T_4)	Reduced concentration of total T_3 and increased free thyroxine at rest
Triiodothyronine (T_3)	Increased turnover of T_3 and T_4 during exercise
Adrenal Hormones	
Aldosterone	No significant training adaptation
Cortisol	Trained exhibit slight elevations during exercise
Epinephrine	Decrease in secretion at rest and same absolute exercise intensity after training
Norepinephrine	
Pancreatic Hormones	
Insulin	Training increases sensitivity to insulin; normal decrease in insulin during exercise is greatly reduced
Glucagon	Smaller increase in glucose levels during exercise at both absolute and relative workloads
Kidney Hormones	
Renin (enzyme)	No apparent training effect
Angiotensin	

Anterior Pituitary Hormones

Growth Hormone and Long-Term Exercise Training

Most research regarding GH involves responses to a single physical activity session. Less information exists on GH levels during a prolonged training period. Understanding the dynamics of GH secretions with chronic physical activity takes on significance because of the causal relationship between GH availability and maintenance of fat-free body mass (FFM) with aging and weight loss.

Figure 12.16A illustrates the training-induced depression of GH response of a representative subject from a group of six men during 20 minutes of constant-load, intense effort before and after 3 and 6 weeks of endurance training. Integrated GH concentrations during physical activity plus recovery for the group averaged 45% lower than pretraining values at both training measures. Responses for plasma catecholamines (**Fig. 12.16B** and **C**) and blood lactate (**Fig. 12.16D**) paralleled the GH decrease. The constant-load test represented less physiologic demand after training (reflected by lower catecholamine and lactate levels), so a similar GH release following training probably would require higher absolute intensity. The effect of training on GH release also may occur under nonactivity conditions.

Corticotropin

ACTH stimulates the adrenal cortex and increases fat mobilization for energy. Training increases ACTH levels during physical activity. Enhanced fatty acid oxidation from ACTH spares muscle glycogen to benefit prolonged intense exercise performance.

Prolactin

It remains unclear whether long-term training alters PRL release other than the training-induced changes mediated by sympathetic activity or other multiple hormone interactions. It does appear that resting PRL levels of male runners average below values for sedentary nonrunners.

Follicle-Stimulating Hormone, Luteinizing Hormone, and Testosterone

Regular physical activity depresses reproductive hormone responses in women and men. Women with a history of exercise participation

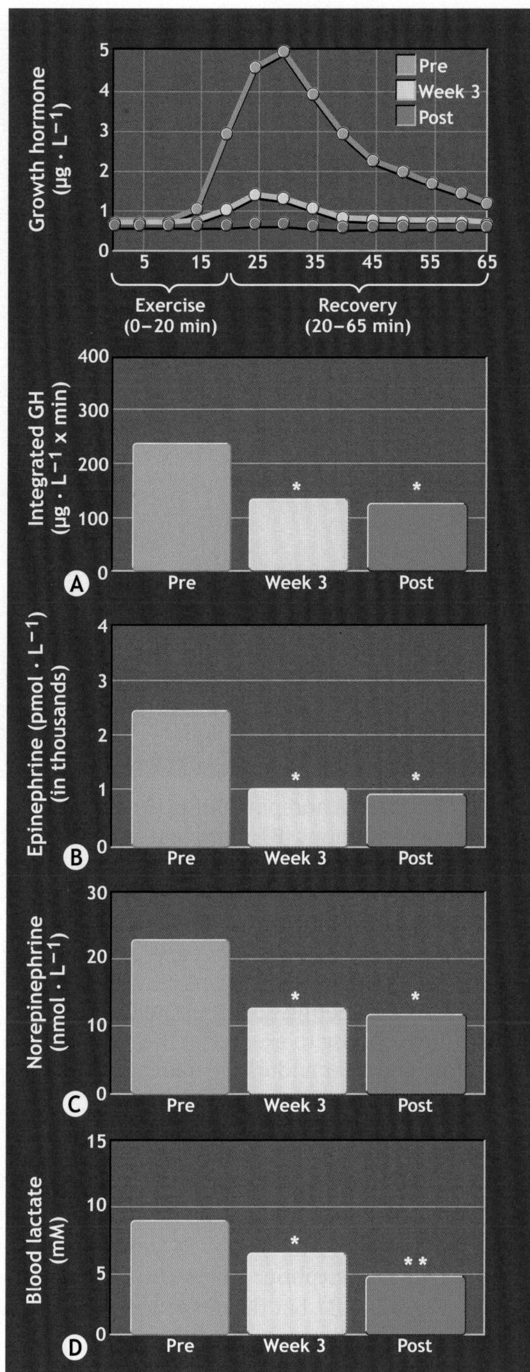

FIGURE 12.16 **Top.** Serum growth hormone (GH) concentrations in a representative subject during 20 minutes of constant-load exercise and 45 minutes of recovery at pretraining, after 3 weeks of training, and after 6 weeks of training. **Bottom.** Effects of 6 weeks of training on integrated GH concentration **(A)**, and end-of-exercise concentrations of epinephrine **(B)**, norepinephrine **(C)**, and blood lactate **(D)** in response to constant-load cycle ergometry (n = 6, mean). Pre, before training; Week 3, after 3 weeks of training; Post, after 6 weeks of training. *p <0.05 versus pretraining; **p <0.05 versus week 3. (Reprinted with permission from McArdle WD, Katch FI, Katch VL. *Exercise Physiology: Nutrition, Energy, and Human Performance.* 8th Ed. Baltimore: Wolters Kluwer Health, 2015; as adapted with permission from Weltman A, et al. Exercise training decreases the growth hormone (GH) response to acute constant-load exercise. *Med Sci Sports Exerc* 1997;29:669.)

have altered FSH and LH levels at different menstrual cycle phases. These hormone alterations often relate to menstrual dysfunction. FSH levels decrease in trained women throughout an abbreviated anovulatory menstrual cycle, whereas LH and progesterone concentrations increase in the cycle's follicular phase. Five factors other than acute and long-term physical activity also can alter reproductive function in women athletes:

1. Weight loss
2. Dietary changes
3. Changes in the body's lean-to-fat ratio
4. Emotional stress of training and competition
5. Altered clearance rates of gonadal steroid hormones

Endurance training in men affects pituitary-gonadal function, including testosterone and PRL concentrations. In comparisons of testosterone, LH, and FSH levels among 46 male runners (64 km average weekly running distance) and 18 nonrunners matched for age, stature, and body mass, runners had depressed testosterone levels with no difference in LH and FSH compared with nonrunners. Reduced testosterone concentration, both increased clearance and decreased production, in endurance-trained men parallels the sex steroid reductions in women who undergo endurance training and associated lower body fat levels. Because LH and FSH do not differ between trained and untrained persons, impaired gonadotropin release from the anterior pituitary does not explain reduced testosterone levels in the trained state. Resistance training presents a different situation because elite resistance-trained male athletes have elevated levels of serum testosterone, LH, and FSH.

Researchers studied the effects of a supraphysiologic dose of exogenous testosterone in healthy, untrained men randomly assigned to one of four groups: placebo without physical activity, testosterone without physical activity, placebo plus physical activity, and testosterone plus physical activity. The men received injections of 600 mg of testosterone or placebo weekly for 10 weeks. The physical activity groups performed standardized weight lifting for the arms and legs three times weekly. Measurements before and after the treatment period included FFM determined by underwater weighing, muscle size determined by magnetic resonance imaging, and arm and leg strength determined with bench-press and squatting exercises. For the no-physical activity groups, men given testosterone experienced a 14% increase in arm muscle size compared with the placebo group and a 9% increase in arm strength. Similar results occurred for the lower body. Men assigned to testosterone and physical activity showed greater increases in FFM and muscle size of the arms and legs compared with the testosterone without physical activity group. Neither mood nor behavior changed in any of the groups during training. These data support the conclusion that a supraphysiologic dose of testosterone, especially when combined with resistance training, increases FFM and muscle size and strength in healthy men.

Parathyroid Hormone

Endurance training enhances physical activity-related increases in PTH in young and elderly adults.

Posterior Pituitary Hormones

Antidiuretic Hormone

Maximal exhaustive physical activity or prolonged submaximal physical activity at the same relative intensity produces no difference in ADH response in trained and untrained individuals. ADH concentration decreases with training in response to submaximal physical activity at the same absolute intensity.

Oxytocin

Oxytocin combined with arginine vasopressin (AVP) increase following prolonged intense endurance physical activity.

Thyroid Hormones

Exercise training coordinates a pituitary-thyroid response that increases turnover of thyroid hormones, a response usually associated with excessive hormonal action that leads to hyperthyroidism. No evidence indicates that hyperthyroidism develops in highly trained individuals. BMR and resting core temperature remain normal with training. The increased T_4 turnover that accompanies chronic physical activity occurs through a mechanism that differs from this hormone's normal dynamics.

Research with endurance-trained women reveals that training 48 km a week mildly depressed thyroid function reflected by *decreased* T_3 and T_4 levels. Extending training distance to 80 km a week *increased* these hormone levels. The changes in body composition that accompany a high training volume may contribute to discrepancies in an exercise-induced change in female thyroid function.

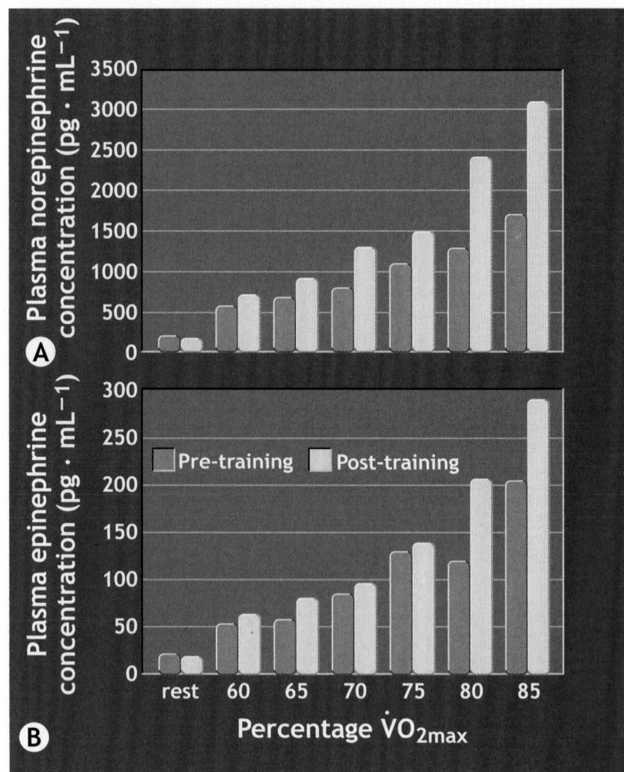

FIGURE 12.17 Plasma norepinephrine **(A)** and epinephrine concentrations **(B)** at rest and after 15 minutes of exercise at the same relative exercise intensity (%$\dot{V}O_{2max}$) before and after 10 weeks of endurance exercise training. (Reprinted with permission from McArdle WD, Katch FI, Katch VL. *Exercise Physiology: Nutrition, Energy, and Human Performance*. 8th Ed. Baltimore: Wolters Kluwer Health, 2015; as adapted with permission from Greiwe JS, et al. Norepinephrine response to exercise at the same relative intensity before and after endurance training. *J Appl Physiol* 1999;86:531.)

Adrenal Hormones

Aldosterone

The renin-angiotensin-aldosterone system contributes to homeostatic control of body fluid volumes, electrolytes, and blood pressure, but physical training does not affect resting levels of these compounds or their normal response to physical activity.

Cortisol

Plasma cortisol levels increase less in trained than in sedentary subjects at the same (*absolute*) moderate physical activity levels. Greater cortisol output among untrained individuals may partly result from heightened psychological stress experienced during exercise testing. Elevated cortisol levels promote fatty acid and protein catabolism to provide fuel for energy and substrates for tissue repair following exertion.

Epinephrine and Norepinephrine

An important aspect of the catecholamine response to physical activity and exercise training involves the **sympathoadrenal response** rather than the typical adrenal gland response. **Figure 12.17A** and **B** illustrates norepinephrine and epinephrine response during physical activity at intensities that ranged between 60% and 85% of aerobic capacity by three adult men and six women prior to and following 10 weeks of aerobic training that increased $\dot{V}O_{2max}$ by 20%. Plasma norepinephrine levels (**Fig. 12.17A**) increased progressively with intensity before and after training. Training produced higher plasma norepinephrine levels, particularly at higher intensities. Consistently, higher epinephrine values also emerged following training (**Fig. 12.17B**), but the differences did not achieve statistical significance.

For equivalent *relative* intensities, a *higher* sympathoadrenal response occurs following aerobic training. This training response reflects three factors that require greater sympathetic nervous system activation from increased activity:

1. Greater absolute demand for substrate use via glycogenolysis and lipolysis
2. Increased overall cardiovascular response via cardiac output
3. Larger muscle mass activation

Pancreatic Hormones

Insulin and Glucagon

Endurance training maintains plasma insulin and glucagon levels in physical activity similar to values at rest.

In essence, the trained state requires less insulin at any stage from rest through light to moderately intense activity. Two mechanisms help to explain the reduced hormonal response with training:

1. **Increased muscle and fat tissue sensitivity to insulin.** Training reduces the insulin requirement to regulate blood glucose. Improved insulin sensitivity most likely occurs from improved insulin-binding capacity to receptor sites on individual muscle fibers and adipocytes. Liver cells also increase their insulin sensitivity.
2. **Increased percentage contribution of fat catabolism for fuel during submaximal activity**. Decreased carbohydrate metabolism lowers the insulin requirement.

Pancreatic Enzymes

Lipase, Amylase, Protease

In addition to the pancreas's important role as an endocrine gland that provides pancreatic hormones, the pancreas also plays a crucial part in the digestive process. Under normal, nonmedical conditions, the pancreas, in addition to secreting hormones, typically generates almost 2 L or roughly eight cups of pancreatic secretions daily into the duodenum. This pancreatic juice contains three main enzymes—lipase, amylase, and protease—that break down fat, protein, and carbohydrate molecules before they enter the small intestine. With bile from the liver, lipase splits apart the structure of fat molecules for their absorption by the small intestine. Amylase (also present in saliva where the digestive process begins) splits apart complex carbohydrate (starch) molecules into simple sugars. The protease enzyme catabolizes the large protein structures into their simpler components. If there is any blockage of the usually inactive enzymes so they cannot pass unimpeded through the pancreatic duct to the small intestines, they back up within the organ and become prematurely activated, significantly raising their concentration and potentially damaging this gland. The end result can range from an inflamed pancreas termed acute pancreatitis (associated with bloating, abdominal swelling and discomfort, and back pain) to chronic pancreatitis with potentially life-threatening consequences from bleeding and organ failure (**www.webmd.com/digestive-disorders/digestive-diseases-pancreatitis**). Acute pancreatitis is usually triggered by gallstones (hardened deposits of digestive fluid that pass from the gallbladder), other minute particles (inelegantly termed "sludge") that travel from the liver or gall bladder into the common bile duct, or adverse drug side effects.

Resistance Training and Endocrine Function

The large variation among individuals in muscular strength and gains in hypertrophy with similar resistance-training programs suggests considerable individual differences in endocrine dynamics with chronic muscle overload. Muscle remodeling with resistance training reflects a complex process that involves cell receptor interaction with specific hormones, which stimulates DNA synthesis of contractile proteins. The magnitude of the change links to the configuration of the physical activity stimulus (e.g., frequency, intensity, volume, and mode) and more than likely a genetically influenced hormonal response. **Figure 12.18** proposes how heavy resistance training improves overall muscular size, strength, and power. Three hormonal

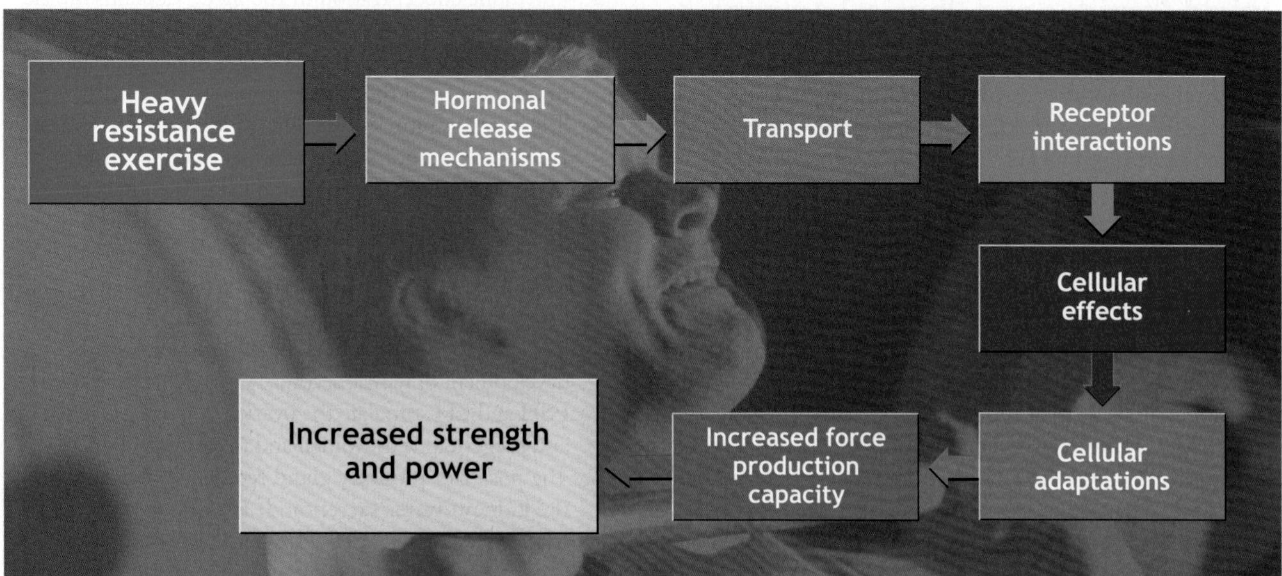

FIGURE 12.18 Schematic model of how heavy resistance training produces favorable adaptations in muscle structure and maximal strength performance. (Reprinted with permission from McArdle WD, Katch FI, Katch VL. *Exercise Physiology: Nutrition, Energy, and Human Performance*. 8th Ed. Baltimore: Wolters Kluwer Health, 2015; as adapted with permission from Kraemer WJ. Endocrine responses and adaptations to strength training. In: Komi PV, ed. *Strength and Power in Sport*. London: Blackwell Scientific, 1992.)

factors trigger training-induced changes in muscle size and function:

1. Changes in hepatic and extrahepatic hormone clearance rates
2. Differential rates of hormone secretion with accompanying fluid shifts around the receptor sites
3. Altered receptor-site activation via neurohumoral control

Early-phase adaptations to resistance training reflect a hormonal response that mediates neuromuscular system adaptations that improve muscle strength.

In general, resistance training increases testosterone and GH secretion frequency and amplitude, thereby contributing to hypertrophic effects on muscles. Testosterone augments GH release and interacts with nervous system dynamics to increase muscle force production. The importance of these functions may exceed any direct anabolic effect of testosterone on muscle structure and function. A single session of resistance training generally elicits a short-term increase in serum testosterone and decrease in cortisol, with a greater response in men than women. Catecholamine release from the adrenal medulla also increases with the acute stress of high-force and high-power exercise protocols.

Resistance training in men increases frequency and amplitude of testosterone and GH secretion, thereby creating a favorable hormonal environment for muscle growth. In contrast, most studies fail to demonstrate changes in testosterone and GH concentrations with such training in women. Gender differences in hormone output with resistance training may ultimately explain variations in responsiveness of muscle strength and size to prolonged muscular overload.

Opioid Peptides and Physical Activity

Researchers in the 1970s isolated and purified two opioid pentapeptides, methionine and leucine enkephalin (Greek "in the head"). These breakthrough discoveries provided the first direct evidence that endogenous substances behaved like opiates. By the early 1980s, researchers discovered groups of endogenous opioid compounds now generically termed "endorphins" that bind to families of receptors. By definition, the term **endorphin** characterizes a group of endogenous peptides whose pharmacologic action mimics those of opium and its analogs. Opioid substances include β-lipotropin, β-endorphin, and dynorphin, the most potent opioid peptide. Endorphins regulate menstruation and modulate the response of GH, ACTH, PRL, catecholamines, and cortisol. Endorphins also regulate other hormones including ACTH, the catecholamines, and cortisol.

Serum concentrations of β-endorphin and/or β-lipotropin generally increase similarly with physical activity in men and women, although the response varies among individuals and varies inversely with activity intensity. Physical activity increases β-endorphin up to five times the resting level and probably even more in the brain itself, particularly region-specific effects involved with mood states. With resistance exercise, β-endorphin release varies with the activity protocol; longer duration (lighter resistance) and longer intraset rest intervals elicit the greatest response.

Evidence now links physical activity with decreases in mental depression, mediated through the endocannabinoid system's action on neurotrophins, such as brain-derived neurotrophic factor (BDNF). BDNF is considered a major candidate molecule for exercise-induced brain plasticity.

Several noteworthy effects emerge concerning the postulated opioid effect in triggering the **exercise "high,"** a state described as euphoria and exhilaration as the duration of moderate-to-intense aerobic activity increases. Endorphin secretion also may increase pain tolerance, improve appetite control, and reduce anxiety, tension, anger, and confusion. Interestingly, these effects generally reflect the documented psychologic benefits of regular physical activity.

The effect of training on endorphin response remains controversial. One study reported no significant change in β-endorphin response to prolonged effort following 8 weeks of endurance training. Contrasting research showed that general physical conditioning augmented β-endorphin and β-lipotropin release during physical activity.

SUMMARY

1. The endocrine system consists of a host organ, a hormone, and a target or receptor organ. Hormones exist as either steroids or amino acid (polypeptide) derivatives.
2. Hormones alter rates of cellular reactions by acting at specific receptor sites to enhance or inhibit enzyme function.
3. Hormone concentration in the blood depends on the amount of hormone synthesized, the amount released, the amount taken up by the target organ, and its rate of removal from the blood.
4. The anterior pituitary secretes at least six hormones: PRL, the gonadotropic hormones FSH and LH, corticotropin, thyrotropin, and GH. The anterior pituitary also releases endorphins.
5. GH promotes cell division and cellular proliferation; TSH controls the amount of hormone secreted by the thyroid gland; ACTH regulates the output of the hormones of the adrenal cortex; PRL affects reproduction and development of female secondary sex characteristics; and FSH and LH stimulate the ovaries to secrete estrogen and progesterone in women and testosterone in men.
6. The posterior pituitary gland secretes ADH to control the kidneys' water excretion. It also secretes oxytocin, which is important in birthing and milk secretion.
7. Thyroxine elevates the metabolic rate in all cells and increases carbohydrate and fat breakdown in energy metabolism.
8. The inner medulla and outer cortex components of the adrenal gland secrete two different types of hormones—epinephrine and norepinephrine.

9. The adrenal cortex secretes mineralocorticoids that regulate extracellular sodium and potassium, glucocorticoids that stimulate gluconeogenesis and serve as an insulin antagonist, and androgens that control secondary sex characteristics.
10. Insulin secreted by pancreatic β cells increases glucose transport into cells to control the body's rate of carbohydrate metabolism. Pancreatic α cells secrete glucagon, an insulin antagonist that increases blood sugar.
11. Type 1 diabetes mellitus (T1DM) causes insulin deficiency by destroying the pancreas' insulin-producing β cells. Type 2 diabetes mellitus (T2DM) generally occurs in overweight, sedentary, middle-aged individuals with a family history of the disease.
12. T2DM arises mainly from insulin resistance (body tissues require greater than normal insulin for glucose regulation), so even a large insulin output fails to properly regulate blood sugar.
13. The increase in T2DM in children and adults has reached epidemic proportions worldwide. More than one third of all new cases occur in children younger than age 16 years.
14. Metabolic syndrome reflects a common condition in which obesity, high blood pressure, high blood glucose, and dyslipidemia cluster together to increase the individual's risk of developing coronary heart disease, stroke, and T2DM.
15. Training exerts differential effects on resting and exercise-induced hormone production and release.
16. Training elevates hormone response during physical activity for ACTH and cortisol and depresses GH, PRL, FSH, LH, testosterone, ADH, T_4, and insulin; no known training response occurs for aldosterone and angiotensin.
17. Exercise-induced elevation of β-endorphins coincides with euphoria, increased pain tolerance, the "exercise high," and menstrual dysfunction.

THINK IT THROUGH

1. Visit a local health food store and list the supplements that claim to enhance physical performance. Identify the ingredients and their alleged effects. Which supplements purport to simulate hormonal release? Based on your knowledge of hormonal regulation and function, can any of these products deliver on their claims?
2. Discuss how hormones act as silent messengers to integrate the body as a unit.
3. Give two specific examples of why *more* is not necessarily *better* regarding how hormones play crucial roles in regulating normal growth and development and physiologic function.
4. Explain the sweet-smelling breath of individuals who suffer from poorly regulated diabetes mellitus or malnutrition from starvation.

KEY TERMS

Acromegaly: Condition resulting from excessive growth hormone production following growth cessation; produces an irreversible disorder that presents as enlarged hands, feet, and facial features.

ACTH (adrenocorticotropic hormone): Polypeptide hormone, also known as corticotropin, released by the anterior pituitary gland; often produced in response to stress.

Adenyl cyclase: Enzyme in cell's plasma membrane; reacts with hormone to form the compound cycle 3′5′-adenosine monophosphate (cyclic AMP) to activate a specific protein kinase, which then activates a target enzyme to initiate cellular response.

Adrenal cortex: Outer portion of the adrenal gland that secretes the mineralocorticoids, glucocorticoids, and androgens.

Adrenal glands: Flattened, caplike glandular tissues situated above each kidney. The glands have two distinct parts: medulla (inner portion that secretes the catecholamines) and cortex (outer portion that secretes the mineralocorticoids, glucocorticoids, and androgens).

Adrenal medulla: Inner portion of the adrenal gland that secretes the catecholamines epinephrine and norepinephrine.

Adrenocortical hormone: Secreted by posterior pituitary gland; provides potent stimulation of adrenal cortex to increase free fatty acid mobilization for energy.

Aldosterone: Adrenal cortex secretion that controls total sodium concentration and extracellular fluid volume; stimulates sodium ion resorption with fluid in the kidneys' distal tubules by increasing sodium transporter protein synthesis.

α cells: Cells of the islets of Langerhans of pancreas; serve an exocrine function and secrete digestive enzymes.

Amylin: Peptide hormone secreted with insulin from the pancreatic β cells; contributes to glycemic regulation by slowing gastric emptying and promoting satiety.

Androgens: Hormone group that includes testosterone and androstenedione; play important roles in male traits and reproductive activity.

Angiotensin: Peptide hormone produced by the kidneys that causes vasoconstriction and subsequent increase in blood pressure.

Anterior pituitary: Front portion of the pituitary gland whose secreted hormones influence growth, sexual development, skin pigmentation, and thyroid and adrenocortical function.

Antidiuretic hormone (ADH or vasopressin): Posterior pituitary gland hormone that inhibits water excretion by the kidneys; also acts as a vasoconstrictor.

Autocrine signaling: Form of signaling in which a cell secretes a hormone (autocrine agent) that binds to autocrine receptors on the same cell, leading to cell changes.

β cells: Cells of the islets of Langerhans of pancreas; secrete insulin and amylin peptide.

Bradycardia: Abnormally slow resting heart rate of less than 60 beats per minute.

Calcitonin: Calcium-regulating thyroid gland hormone that promotes calcium deposition in bone and lowers blood calcium levels.

Catecholamines: Collective term to describe the hormones epinephrine and norepinephrine.

Corticotropin (adrenocorticotropic hormone [ACTH]): Anterior pituitary gland hormone that functions as part of the hypothalamic-pituitary-adrenal axis to regulate adrenal cortex output, enhance fatty acid mobilization from adipose tissue, increase gluconeogenesis, and stimulate protein catabolism.

Cortisol (hydrocortisone): Adrenal cortex major glucocorticoid known as the "stress" hormone; promotes protein and fat catabolism, raises blood glucose levels, and supports body's adaptation to stressors.

Cyclic 3,5-adenosine monophosphate (cyclic-AMP): Ubiquitous second messenger to activate a specific protein kinase, which then activates a target enzyme to alter cellular response.

Cytokines: Small proteins that serve as messengers between cells; function in immune responses and stimulate the movement of cells toward sites of inflammation, infection, and trauma.

Dehydroepiandrosterone (DHEA): Adrenal cortex hormone; acts similarly to testosterone.

Dwarfism: Genetic mutation (inherited or spontaneous); includes metabolic and hormonal disorder (growth hormone deficiency) leading to reduced adult stature of 4 feet 10 inches or less (average 4 feet).

Endocrine glands: Possess no ducts (referred to as ductless glands); secrete substances directly into extracellular spaces around the gland.

Endocrine system: Consists of a host organ (gland), minute quantities of chemical messengers (hormones), and a target or receptor organ.

Endorphin: Group of endogenous peptides whose pharmacologic action mimics those of opium and its analogs.

Epinephrine: Sympathetic nervous system hormone and neurotransmitter produced in some neurons of the nervous system and secreted by the adrenal medulla; represents 80% of adrenal medulla secretions. Facilitates sympathetic activity; increases cardiac output; regulates blood vessel diameter; and increases glycogen catabolism and fatty acid release.

Erythropoietin: Glycoprotein hormone that controls red blood cell production.

Estradiol (estrogen): Ovarian hormone that regulates ovulation, menstruation, and physiologic adjustments during pregnancy.

Exercise "high": Endorphin secretion related to a state of euphoria and exhilaration as the duration of moderate-to-intense aerobic activity increases; also may increase pain tolerance, improve appetite control, and reduce anxiety, tension, anger, and confusion.

Exocrine glands: Contain secretory ducts that carry substances directly to a specific body compartment or surface.

Fasting plasma glucose (FPG) test: Measure of plasma glucose following an 8-hour fast; recommended as the first test for suspected type 2 diabetes.

Follicle-stimulating hormone (FSH): Anterior pituitary gland hormone that initiates follicle growth in the ovaries and stimulates these organs to secrete estrogen; in males, FSH stimulates germinal epithelium growth in the testes to promote sperm development.

Gestational diabetes: Condition of pregnancy in which blood sugar rises to levels that signify the diabetic condition; prevalence among pregnant women in U.S. is as high as 9.2%.

Gigantism: Excessively high linear growth from overproduction of insulinlike growth factor I (IGF-I) induced by growth hormone excess during childhood.

Glucagon: Hormone secreted by pancreatic α cells; termed "insulin antagonist" because it primarily stimulates liver glycogenolysis and gluconeogenesis and increases lipid catabolism.

Glucocorticoids: Adrenal cortex secretions of steroid hormones, which promote protein and fat catabolism, raise blood glucose levels, and adapt body to stress.

Glycoprotein: Carbohydrate group (oligosaccharide chain) covalently attached to a protein side chain.

Hormones: Chemical messengers produced by endocrine glands affecting all aspects of human function.

Human growth hormone (GH or somatotropin): Family of related polypeptides with widespread physiologic activity that promote cell division and cellular proliferation.

Hyperthyroidism: Excessive secretion of thyroid hormones; promotes increased metabolism, protein catabolism, muscle weakness, weight loss, heightened reflex activity, and tachycardia.

Hypoglycemia: Condition characterized by abnormally low blood glucose levels, usually less than 70 $mg \cdot dL^{-1}$.

Hypophyseal stalk: Funnel-shaped structure that anatomically connects the pituitary gland with the hypothalamus.

Hypothyroidism: Blunted thyroid hormone secretion; effects include reduced metabolism and cold intolerance, decreased protein synthesis, depressed reflex activity and fatigue, and bradycardia.

Insulin: Peptide hormone released by pancreatic β cells; lowers blood glucose levels and promotes protein, lipid, and glycogen synthesis.

Insulin resistance: Depressed insulin effects on peripheral tissue, particularly skeletal muscle.

Insulin-dependent diabetes mellitus (T1DM; IDDM; type 1 diabetes): Form of diabetes representing an autoimmune response, possibly from a single protein that renders the β cells incapable of producing insulin and other pancreatic hormones.

Insulin-like growth factors (IGFs): Proteins, similar to insulin (also called somatomedin C), that mediate many of growth hormone's potent effects as chemical messengers.

Interleukin (IL)-6: Family of pro-inflammatory cytokines and anti-inflammatory myokines secreted by T cells and macrophages to stimulate immune response to trauma.

Islets of Langerhans: Cluster of pancreatic cells; islets consist of 20% α cells (secrete glucagon) and 75% β cells (secrete insulin and peptide amylin).

Luteinizing hormone (LH): Anterior pituitary gland hormone; complements FSH action to initiate estrogen secretion and rupture the egg follicle, allowing the ovum to pass through the fallopian tube for fertilization. Also stimulates testes to secrete testosterone.

Metabolic syndrome: Increasingly common cluster of unhealthy conditions (obesity, high blood pressure, high blood glucose, dyslipidemia) that increase a person's risk of developing coronary heart disease, stroke, and T2DM.

Mineralocorticoids: Steroid hormones produced by the adrenal cortex to regulate sodium and potassium salts in the extracellular fluid.

Myokines: Cytokines and other peptides produced and released by muscle that exert autocrine, paracrine, or endocrine effects; contractile activity regulates the expression of these cytokines in skeletal muscle.

Neurohormone: Any hormone produced and released by neuroendocrine or neurosecretory cells.

Non–insulin-dependent diabetes mellitus (T2DM; NIDDM; type 2 diabetes): Diabetes form related to relative insulin resistance and/or deficiency; usually associated with obesity, poor diet, and sedentary lifestyle.

Norepinephrine: Adrenal medulla sympathetic nervous system hormone; facilitates sympathetic activity, increases cardiac output, regulates blood vessel diameter, and increases glycogen catabolism and fatty acid release.

Oral glucose tolerance test: Evaluates blood sugar levels 5 times over a 3-hour period after drinking a concentrated glucose-containing solution.

Oxytocin: Posterior pituitary gland hormone; targets breast and uterus tissues and stimulates uterine contractions and mammary gland milk secretion.

Pancreatic polypeptide (PP): Pancreatic hormone that self-regulates pancreatic secretion activities.

Paracrine signaling: Form of cell-to-cell communication in which a cell produces a signal to induce changes in nearby cells, thereby altering those cells.

Parathyroid gland: Four small glands embedded in the posterior aspect of the thyroid gland; secretes parathyroid hormone (PTH) to promote calcium balance.

Parathyroid hormone (PTH): Regulates blood calcium balance, and promotes calcium release from bone, absorption from intestine, resorption by the kidneys, and stimulates vitamin D_3 synthesis.

Pituitary gland (hypophysis): Endocrine gland comprised of anterior and posterior portions; forms a protrusion from bottom of the hypothalamus at the base of the brain.

Posterior pituitary: Glandular tissue formed from the extension of hypothalamic neurons; secretes the peptide hormones oxytocin and antidiuretic hormone.

Prediabetes: Borderline condition (fasting blood glucose level between 110 and 125 mg · dL^{-1}) that increases risk of developing type 2 diabetes.

Progesterone: Ovarian hormone that promotes endometrial growth to prepare uterus for pregnancy; contributes specific regulatory input to the female reproductive cycle, uterine smooth muscle action, and lactation.

Prolactin (PRL): Anterior pituitary gland hormone; initiates and supports mammary gland milk secretion.

Relative insulin deficiency: Condition of inadequate pancreatic insulin production to control blood sugar.

Renin: Kidney enzyme that catabolizes protein, which produces rise in blood pressure via the renin-angiotensin mechanism.

Renin-angiotensin mechanism: Diminished renal blood flow that stimulates the kidneys to release renin into the blood, which stimulates production of the renal hormones angiotensin II and angiotensin III.

Somatostatin: Polypeptide hormone secreted by the delta cells of the islets of Langerhans to inhibit *thyrotropin*, *somatotropin*, and *corticotropin* secretion; regulates gastrointestinal digestion and nutrient absorption.

Sympathoadrenal response: Increased sympathetic activity involving the sympathetic nervous system and adrenal glands, which causes increased epinephrine secretion from the adrenal medulla and norepinephrine from postganglionic sympathetic nerve endings.

Tachycardia: Resting heart rate that exceeds 100 beats per minute.

Testosterone: Principal male sex hormone; anabolic steroid secreted primarily by the male testis and female ovaries.

Thyroxine (T_4): Thyroid gland hormone; exerts stimulating effect on enzyme activity, increases metabolic rate, and promotes normal physical development.

Triiodothyronine (T_3): Most powerful active form of thyroid hormone; significantly impacts tissue growth, body temperature, and heart rate.

TSH (thyroid stimulating hormone): Anterior pituitary gland hormone that controls thyroid gland hormone secretion; maintains thyroid gland growth and development, and increases thyroid gland metabolism.

Type 1 diabetes mellitus (T1DM): Most often diagnosed in children and young adults and previously known as juvenile diabetes or insulin-dependent diabetes; a chronic condition in which the pancreas produces little or no insulin. *See Insulin-dependent diabetes mellitus.*

Type 2 diabetes mellitus (T2DM): Most common form of diabetes, affecting 90% to 95% of the 26 million diabetic Americans; a metabolic disorder characterized by hyperglycemia from insulin resistance, a relative lack of insulin, or a combination of both factors. *See Non–insulin-dependent diabetes mellitus.*

SELECTED REFERENCES

The Action to Control Cardiovascular Risk in Diabetes Study Group. Effects of intensive glucose lowering in type 2 diabetes. *N Engl J Med* 2008;358:2545.

Adolfsson P, et al. Hormonal response during physical exercise of different intensities in adolescents with type 1 diabetes and healthy controls. *Pediatr Diabetes* 2012;13:587.

Ahtiainen JP, et al. Acute hormonal responses to heavy resistance exercise in strength athletes versus nonathletes. *Can J Appl Physiol* 2004;29:527.

American College of Sports Medicine: Position Stand. Exercise and type 2 diabetes. *Med Sci Sports Exerc* 2000;32:1345.

Baylor LS, Hackney AC. Resting thyroid and leptin changes following intense, prolonged exercise training. *Eur J Appl Physiol* 2003;88:480.

Bertoli A, et al. Lipid profile, BMI, body fat distribution, and aerobic fitness in men with metabolic syndrome. *Acta Diabetol* 2003;40:S130.

Bunprajun T, et al. Lifelong physical activity prevents aging-associated insulin resistance in human skeletal muscle myotubes via increased glucose transporter expression. *PLoS One* 2013;8:e66628.

Cadore EL, et al. Correlations between serum hormones, strength and endurance in healthy elderly South-American men. *J Sports Med Phys Fitness* 2013;53:255.

Cadore EL, et al. Neuromuscular, hormonal and metabolic responses to different plyometric training volumes in rugby players. *J Strength Cond Res* 2013;27:3001.

Boecker H, et al. The runner's high: opioidergic mechanisms in the human brain. *Cereb Cortex* 2008;18:2523.

Bruce CR, Hawley JA. Improvements in insulin resistance with aerobic exercise training: a lipocentric approach. *Med Sci Sports Exerc* 2004;36:1196.

Charro MA, et al. Hormonal, metabolic and perceptual responses to different resistance training systems. *J Sports Med Phys Fitness* 2010;50:229.

Chwalbinska-Moneta J, et al. Early effects of short-term endurance training on hormonal responses to graded exercise. *J Physiol Pharmacol* 2005;56:87.

Cox AJ, et al. Cytokine responses to treadmill running in healthy and illness-prone athletes. *Med Sci Sports Exerc* 2007;39:1918.

Daly W, et al. Relationship between stress hormones and testosterone with prolonged endurance exercise. *Eur J Appl Physiol* 2005;93:375.

Di Luigi L, et al. Heredity and pituitary response to exercise-related stress in trained men. *Int J Sports Med* 2003;24:551.

Di Luigi L, et al. Andrological aspects of physical exercise and sport medicine. *Endocrine* 2012;42:278.

Dittrich N, et al. Continuous and intermittent running to exhaustion at maximal lactate steady state: neuromuscular, biochemical and endocrinal responses. *J Sci Med Sport* 2013;16:545.

Dobrosielski DA, et al. Effect of exercise on blood pressure in type 2 diabetes: a randomized controlled trial. *J Gen Intern Med* 2012;27:1453.

Eliakim A, Nemet D. Interval training and the GH-IGF-I axis—a new look into an old training regimen. *J Pediatr Endocrinol Metab* 2012;25:815.

Ford ES, et al. Prevalence of the metabolic syndrome among US adults: findings from the third National Health and Nutrition Examination Survey. *JAMA* 2002;287:356.

Garnett SP, et al. Optimal macronutrient content of the diet for adolescents with prediabetes; RESIST a randomised control trial. *J Clin Endocrinol Metab* 2013;98:2116.

Gerson LS, Braun B. Effect of high cardiorespiratory fitness and high body fat on insulin resistance. *Med Sci Sports Exerc* 2006;38:1709.

Gleeson M. Immune function in sport and exercise [invited review]. *J Appl Physiol* 2007;103:963.

Gleeson M, et al. Sex differences in immune variables and respiratory infection incidence in an athletic population. *Exerc Immunol Rev* 2011;17:122.

Gleeson M. Nutritional support to maintain proper immune status during intense training. *Nestle Nutr Inst Workshop Ser* 2013;75:85.

Hackney AC, et al. Testosterone responses to intensive interval versus steady-state endurance exercise. *J Endocrinol Invest* 2012;35:947.

Healy ML, et al. High dose growth hormone exerts an anabolic effect at rest and during exercise in endurance-trained athletes. *J Clin Endocrinol Metab* 2003;88:5221.

Hew-Butler T, et al. Acute changes in endocrine and fluid balance markers during high-intensity, steady-state, and prolonged endurance running: unexpected increases in oxytocin and brain natriuretic peptide during exercise. *Eur J Endocrinol* 2008;15:729.

Holloszy JO. "Deficiency" of mitochondria in muscle does not cause insulin resistance. *Diabetes* 2013;62:1036.

Holmes B, Dohm GL. Regulation of GLUT 4 gene expression during exercise. *Med Sci Sports Exerc* 2004;36:1202.

Houmard JA, et al. Effect of the volume and intensity of exercise training on insulin sensitivity. *J Appl Physiol* 2004;96:101.

Huovinen HT, et al. Body composition and power performance improved after weight reduction in male athletes without hampering hormonal balance. *J Strength Cond Res* 2015;29:29.

Huang WS, et al. Effect of treadmill exercise on circulating thyroid hormone measurements. *Med Princ Pract* 2004;13:15.

Iizuka K, et al. Skeletal muscle is an endocrine organ. *J Pharmacol Sci* 2014;125:125.

Ivy JL. Muscle insulin resistance amended with exercise training: role of GLUT4 expression. *Med Sci Sports Exerc* 2004;36:1207.

Jurca R, et al. Associations of muscle strength and aerobic fitness with metabolic syndrome in men. *Med Sci Sports Exerc* 2004;36:1301.

Kasa-Vubu JZ, et al. Differences in endocrine function with varying fitness capacity in postpubertal females across the weight spectrum. *Arch Pediatr Adolesc Med* 2004;158:333.

Kochańska-Dziurowicz AA, et al. The effect of maximal physical exercise on relationships between the growth hormone (GH) and insulin growth factor 1 (IGF-1) and transcriptional activity of CYP1A2 in young ice hockey players. *J Sports Med Phys Fitness* 2015;55:158.

Kraemer RR, et al. Estrogen mediation of hormone responses to exercise. *Metabolism* 2012;61:1337.

Kraemer WJ, et al. Cortisol supplementation reduces serum cortisol responses to physical stress. *Metabolism* 2005;54:657.

Kraemer WJ, Ratamess NA. Hormonal responses and adaptations to resistance exercise and training. *Sports Med* 2005;35:339.

Kriska AM, et al. Physical activity and the prevention of type II diabetes. *Curr Sports Med Rep* 2008;7:182.

Lane AR, et al. Influence of dietary carbohydrate intake on the free testosterone: cortisol ratio responses to short-term intensive exercise training. *Eur J Appl Physiol* 2010;108:1125.

Li J, et al. Duration of exercise as a key determinant of improvement in insulin sensitivity in type 2 diabetes patients. *J Exp Med* 2012;227:289.

Iizuka K, et al. Skeletal muscle is an endocrine organ. *J Pharmacol Sci* 2014;125:125.

Maïmoun L, et al. Testosterone secretion in elite adolescent swimmers does not modify bone mass acquisition: a 1-year follow-up study. *Fertil Steril* 2013;99:270.

Märtins AS, et al. Hypertension and exercise training differentially affect oxytocin and oxytocin receptor expression in the brain. *Hypertension* 2005;46:1004.

Mäestu J, et al. Anabolic and catabolic hormones and energy balance of the male bodybuilders during the preparation for the competition. *J Strength Cond Res* 2010;24:1074.

Michelini LC. Oxytocin in the NTS. A new modulator of cardiovascular control during exercise . *Ann N Y Acad Sci* 2001;940:206.

McMurray RG, Hackney AC. Interactions of metabolic hormones, adipose tissue and exercise. *Sports Med* 2005;35:393.

Neville V, et al. Salivary IgA as a risk factor for upper respiratory infections in elite professional athletes. *Med Sci Sports Exerc* 2008;40:1228.

Nieman DC, et al. Influence of carbohydrate ingestion on immune changes after 2 h of intensive resistance training. *J Appl Physiol* 2004;96:1293.

Peake JM, et al. Metabolic and hormonal responses to isoenergetic high-intensity interval exercise and continuous moderate-intensity exercise. *Am J Physiol Endocrinol Metab* 2014;307:E539.

Pedersen BK, Febbraio MA. Muscle as an endocrine organ: focus on muscle-derived interleukin-6. *Physiol Rev* 2008;88:1379.

Pedersen BK, Edward F. Adolph distinguished lecture: muscle as an endocrine organ: IL-6 and other myokines. *J Appl Physiol* 2009;107:1006.

Pedersen BK, Febbraio MA. Muscles, exercise and obesity: skeletal muscle as a secretory organ. *Nat Rev Endocrinol* 2012;8:457.

Pedersen BK. Muscle as a secretory organ. *Compr Physiol* 2013;3:1337.

Peres SB, et al. Endurance exercise training increases insulin responsiveness in isolated adipocytes through IRS/PI3-kinase/Akt pathway. *J Appl Physiol* 2005;98:1037.

Ponjee GAE, et al. Androgen turnover during marathon running. *Med Sci Sports Exerc* 1994;26:1274.

Praet SE, van Loon LJ. Optimizing the therapeutic benefits of exercise in type 2 diabetes. *J Appl Physiol* 2007;103:1113.

Rahimi R, et al. Effects of very short rest periods on hormonal responses to resistance exercise in men. *J Strength Cond Res* 2010;24:1851.

Ratamess NA, et al. Androgen receptor content following heavy resistance exercise in men. *J Steroid Biochem Mol Biol* 2005;93:35.

Rosa C, et al. Order effects of combined strength and endurance training on testosterone, cortisol, growth hormone and IGFBP-3 in concurrent-trained men. *J Strength Cond Res* 2015;29:74.

Rubin MR, et al. High-affinity growth hormone binding protein and acute heavy resistance exercise. *Med Sci Sports Exerc* 2005;37:395.

Seo DI, et al. 12 weeks of combined exercise is better than aerobic exercise for increasing growth hormone in middle-aged women. *Int J Sport Nutr Exerc Metab* 2010;20:21.

Scharhag J, et al. Effects of graded carbohydrate supplementation on the immune response in cycling. *Med Sci Sports Exerc* 2006;38:286.

Schumann M, et al. Acute neuromuscular and endocrine responses and recovery to single-session combined endurance and strength loadings: "order effect" in untrained young men. *J Strength Cond Res* 2013;27:421.

Sillanpää E, et al. Serum basal hormone concentrations, nutrition and physical fitness during strength and/or endurance training in 39–64-year-old women. *Int J Sports Med* 2010;31:110.

Srikanthan P, Karlmangla AS. Relative muscle mass is inversely associated with insulin resistance and prediabetes. Findings from the third National Health and Nutrition Examination Survey. *J Clin Endocrinol Metab* 2011; 96:2898.

Teran-Garcia M, et al. Endurance training-induced changes in insulin sensitivity and gene expression. *Am J Physiol Endocrinol Metab* 2005;288:E1168.

Thomas GA, et al. Obesity, growth hormone and exercise. *Sports Med* 2013;168:797.

Trachta P, et al. Three months of regular aerobic exercise in patients with obesity improve systemic subclinical inflammation without major influence on blood pressure and endocrine production of subcutaneous fat. *Physiol Res* 2014;63:S299.

Tsai CL, et al. Executive function and endocrinological responses to acute resistance exercise. *Front Behav Neurosci* 2014;8:262.

Tremblay MS, et al. Effect of training status and exercise mode on endogenous steroid hormones in men. *J Appl Physiol* 2004;96:531.

Vaananen I, et al. Hormonal responses to 100 km cross-country skiing during 2 days. *J Sports Med Phys Fitness* 2004;44:309.

van der Heijden MM, et al. Effects of exercise training on quality of life, symptoms of depression, symptoms of anxiety and emotional well-being in type 2 diabetes mellitus: a systematic review. *Diabetologia* 2013;56:1210.

Váczi M, et al. Mechanical, hormonal, and hypertrophic adaptations to 10 weeks of eccentric and stretch-shortening cycle exercise training in old males. *Exp Gerontol* 2014;58C:69.

Vanheest JL, et al. Ovarian suppression impairs sport performance in junior elite female swimmers. *Med Sci Sports Exerc* 2014;46:156.

Wahl P, et al. Acute metabolic, hormonal, and psychological responses to different endurance training protocols. *Horm Metab Res* 2013;45:827.

Wahl P, et al. Active vs. passive recovery during high-intensity training influences hormonal response. *Int J Sports Med* 2014;35:583.

Walker S, et al. Effects of prolonged hypertrophic resistance training on acute endocrine responses in young and older men. *J Aging Phys Act* 2015; 23:230.

Walsh NP, et al. Position statement. Part one: immune function and exercise. *Exerc Immunol Rev* 2011;17:6. Review.

Weinstein AR, Sesso HD. Joint effects of physical activity and body weight on diabetes and cardiovascular disease. *Exerc Sport Sci Rev* 2006;34:10.

Weltman A, et al. Effects of continuous versus intermittent exercise, obesity, and gender on growth hormone secretion. *J Clin Endocrinol Metab* 2008; 93:4711.

Wesche MF, Wiersinga WM. Relation between lean body mass and thyroid volume in competition rowers before and during intensive physical training. *Horm Metab Res* 2001;33:423.

West DW, Phillips SM. Associations of exercise-induced hormone profiles and gains in strength and hypertrophy in a large cohort after weight training. *Eur J Appl Physiol* 2012;112:2693.

Wideman L, et al. The impact of sex and exercise duration on growth hormone secretion. *J Appl Physiol* 2006;101:1641.

Williams PT. Reduced diabetic, hypertensive, and cholesterol medication use with walking. *Med Sci Sports Exerc* 2008;40:433.

Witard OC, et al. High-intensity training reduces $CD8^+$ T-cell redistribution in response to exercise. *Med Sci Sports Exerc* 2012;44:1689.

Xu X, et al. Changes of cytokines during a spaceflight analog—a 45-day head-down bed rest. *PLoS One* 2013;8:e77401.

Yang X, et al. The longitudinal effects of physical activity history on metabolic syndrome. *Med Sci Sports Exerc* 2008;40:1424.

SECTION V

Exercise Training and Adaptations

Training for sports often entails more art than science. Individual achievements or win-loss records rather than scientific inquiry and discovery frequently gauge the success of physical conditioning. For example, in stop-and-go basketball, field hockey, lacrosse, and soccer, coaches often place considerable importance on developing aerobic capacity and fail to devote enough time to vigorous anaerobic training. These sports require a steady release of aerobic energy, yet crucial game situations frequently demand maximal glycolytic-anaerobic effort.

An overemphasis on training endurance athletes' glycolytic capacity would prove wasteful because of the minimal contribution of this energy system to successful performance. At the other extreme, one's aerobic metabolic capacity contributes little to overall success in sprint activities and power sports such as American football and discus, shot put, and hammer throw.

Developing a structured aerobic and anaerobic training regimen to achieve optimum performance requires a clear understanding of energy transfer and how specific training affects systems of energy delivery and utilization. *The basic approach to physiologic conditioning applies similarly to men and women within a broad age range; both respond and adapt to training in similar ways.*

Chapters 13 and 14 focus on training for aerobic and anaerobic power and muscular strength, the physiologic consequences of such training, and important factors that affect training success. Chapter 15 examines how different environmental conditions and special aids affect physiologic function and performance.

The test of a first-rate intelligence is the ability to hold two opposed ideas in mind at the same time and still retain the ability to function.

—F. Scott Fitzgerald

Training the Anaerobic and Aerobic Energy Systems

CHAPTER OBJECTIVES

- Define and provide two examples of each of the following four principles of training: *overload*, *specificity*, *individual differences*, and *reversibility*.
- Discuss the overload principle for training the intramuscular high-energy phosphate and glycolytic energy systems, and outline three specific adaptations in each system imposed by training.
- Describe how each of the following six factors affects an aerobic training program: initial fitness level, training specificity, genetics, training frequency, training duration, and training intensity.
- List five cardiovascular and pulmonary adaptations to aerobic training.
- For aerobic training, explain how heart rate can establish the appropriate intensity of effort.
- Define *training-sensitive zone*.
- Outline a typical training session for aerobic fitness improvement.
- Explain the need to adjust the training-sensitive zone for swimming and other modes of upper-body physical activity.
- Explain the influence of age on maximum heart rate and the training-sensitive zone.
- Contrast continuous versus intermittent aerobic training, including two advantages and disadvantages of each.
- Describe the most common form of overtraining syndrome and summarize two interacting factors contributing to overtraining among athletes.
- Outline five potential benefits and risks of physical activity during pregnancy.
- Summarize five recommendations for regular physical activity during pregnancy.

ANCILLARIES AT A GLANCE

Visit **http://thePoint.lww.com/MKKESS5e** to access the following resources.

- References: Chapter 13
- Interactive Question Bank

TRAINING MUST FOCUS ON ENERGY REQUIREMENTS

Different physical activities require rapid bursts of power during which energy requirements far exceed the body's oxygen delivery capacity. Even with available oxygen, cellular energy transfer from aerobic reactions progresses too slowly to match energy demands. This means that rapid anaerobic energy transfer capacity determines how fast a running back plows through the line in American football, a volleyball player leaps and smashes the ball over the net, and a softball player sprints to first base to beat out an infield hit. Even longer duration basketball, tennis, field hockey, lacrosse, ice hockey, and soccer involve sprinting, dashing, darting, and stop-and-go movements, during which the capacity to generate short bursts of anaerobic power plays an important role.

At the other extreme, success in sustained endurance activities necessitates a highly trained aerobic energy transfer system. This requires a cardiovascular system capable of delivering large quantities of blood to active tissues for an extended time and musculature with high capacity to process oxygen for the aerobic resynthesis of adenosine triphosphate (ATP).

ENERGY FOR MOVEMENT: KNOWING WHAT TO TRAIN FOR

A major ***training*** *objective stimulates structural and functional adaptations to improve performance in specific physical tasks.* Training for a particular sport or performance goal requires careful evaluation of the activity's energy components. This forms the basis for effectively managing the appropriate energy transfer system to match specific training objectives.

Recall that three energy systems operate concurrently: the ATP-phosphocreatine (PCr) system, lactic acid (glycolytic) system, and aerobic system. Their contributions to the total energy requirement differ markedly depending on activity duration and intensity, and the participant's fitness level.

A maximum burst of effort for a tennis serve, golf swing, gymnastics front flip, and even a 60- or 100-m sprint requires immediate energy transfer. This occurs anaerobically, almost exclusively from the intramuscular high-energy phosphates ATP and PCr. In performances lasting up to 90 seconds, anaerobic energy transfer reactions still predominate. In this case, the initial glycolytic phase of carbohydrate breakdown with subsequent lactate formation provides the primary energy source. One's capacity and tolerance for lactate accumulation determine the magnitude of energy generated from anaerobic sources. Effective training for anaerobic-type activities must achieve sufficient intensity and duration to enhance the glycolytic energy transfer system.

Wrestling, boxing, ice hockey, a 200-m swim, a 1500-m run, or a full-court press in basketball all require rapid anaerobic energy transfer, with important contributions from aerobic energy metabolism. As intensity of effort diminishes and duration extends between 2 and 4 minutes, reliance on energy from anaerobic metabolism decreases, while energy release from oxygen-consuming reactions predominates. Beyond 4 minutes, physical activity relies more on aerobic metabolism; energy from aerobic reactions almost exclusively powers a marathon run, long-distance swim, 25-mile continuous bicycle ride, and 4-hour nonstop hike to reach a mountain summit.

GENERAL TRAINING PRINCIPLES

Effective physiologic conditioning requires adherence to carefully planned and executed physical activity. Attention should focus on five interrelated components:

1. Appropriate competition
2. Workout frequency
3. Workout length
4. Type of training
5. Speed, intensity, duration, and repetition of the activity

These components displayed in **Figure 13.1** vary depending on the performance goal. Several general principles of physiologic conditioning underlie performance classifications based on intensity and duration of activity.

Overload Principle

The regular application of a specific **overload** enhances physiologic function to produce a positive training response. Exercising at intensities greater than normal induces a variety of highly specific adaptations so the body functions more efficiently. Achieving the appropriate overload requires judiciously manipulating combinations of training frequency, intensity, and duration, with focus on physical activity mode. We discuss these factors later in this chapter.

The concept of overload applies to the athlete, sedentary, disabled, and even cardiac patient. Physical rehabilitation for individuals in the latter group allows them to lead more normal and productive lives; through carefully crafted training regimens, many can eventually participate in marathons and almost every type of ultraendurance event.

Specificity Principle

Training specificity refers to adaptations in metabolic and physiologic systems that depend on the type of overload imposed and muscle mass activated. Just as strength-power training develops specific strength-power adaptations, regular aerobic activity elicits specific endurance training adaptations with essentially no effective transfer effects between strength-power training and aerobic training. The specificity principle also encompasses activities with *identical* metabolic components. For example, aerobic fitness for swimming, bicycling, running, or rowing improves most effectively when the exerciser aerobically trains the specific muscles required for the specific activity. In essence, specific training elicits specific training adaptations, creating specific **exercise training** effects referred to as the **SAID principle**—**S**pecific **A**daptations to **I**mposed **D**emands.

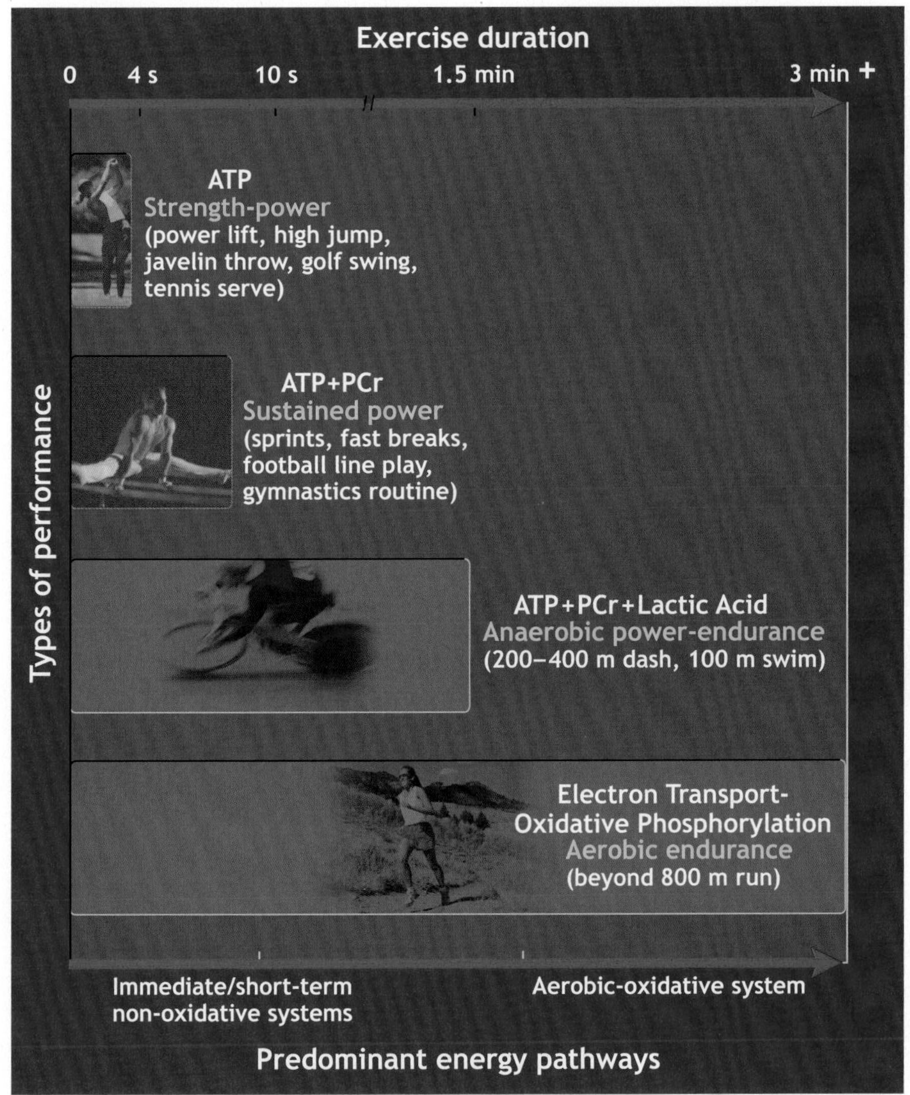

FIGURE 13.1 Classification of physical activity based on duration of all-out effort and the corresponding predominant intracellular energy pathways. (Reprinted with permission from McArdle WD, Katch FI, Katch VL. *Exercise Physiology: Nutrition, Energy, and Human Performance*. 8th Ed. Baltimore: Wolters Kluwer Health, 2015.)

Individual Differences Principle

A given training stimulus does not affect all individuals similarly. Many factors contribute to variations in training responses among individuals, including relative fitness level when training begins. People vary in initial fitness and training state prior to the start of a conditioning program and thus respond differently to the same training stimulus. Coaches and trainers should be mindful that all performers on a team or even those in the same event should not train the same way and at the same relative or absolute intensity. Such practices do not optimize specificity of training for a given individual. One also must be sensitive to recognize the importance of **individual differences** in training responsiveness. As such, training programs must strive to meet individual needs and capacities; individuals respond positively to an exercise stimulus when the physical activity prescription adjusts to their individual needs.

Reversibility Principle

The **reversibility of training effects**, referred to as **detraining**, occurs rapidly when a person ceases training. After only 1 to 2 weeks of detraining, measurable reductions occur in physiologic function and performance capacity, with a total loss of training improvements occurring within several months. **Figure 13.2** presents average percentage change reported from several studies that showed decreases in physiologic and metabolic variables with detraining, including bed rest.

In one experiment, $\dot{V}O_{2max}$ decreased 25% in five subjects confined to bed for 20 consecutive days; a similar decrease in maximal stroke volume and cardiac output accompanied the loss of aerobic capacity (~1% per day). Capillary number within trained muscle also decreased 14% to 25% over the detraining period. *These results highlight the transient and reversible nature of training improvements, even among high-performance athletes.* Thus, athletes typically begin a reconditioning program several months before the start of their competitive season or maintain some moderate level of off-season, sport-specific physical activity to minimize deconditioning.

EXERCISE TRAINING ADAPTATIONS

Individual differences in improvement generally represent the rule rather than the exception. Among individuals in the same physical activity training program, one person might show 10 times more improvement than another. Such variation in results is common; simply stated—some individuals respond more readily to an identical training stimulus than others.

The concept of **responders** and **nonresponders** emerged from training data collected on identical twins. In one study, 10 pairs of identical twins separated at birth and reared in different environments completed the same 20-week endurance training program. A strong genetic component occurred for improvements in cardiovascular and metabolic variables. Both members of the twin pair showed nearly the same training response; a large improvement in one twin mirrored similar improvement in the other and vice versa. In the mid-1960s, the renowned Swedish physiologist

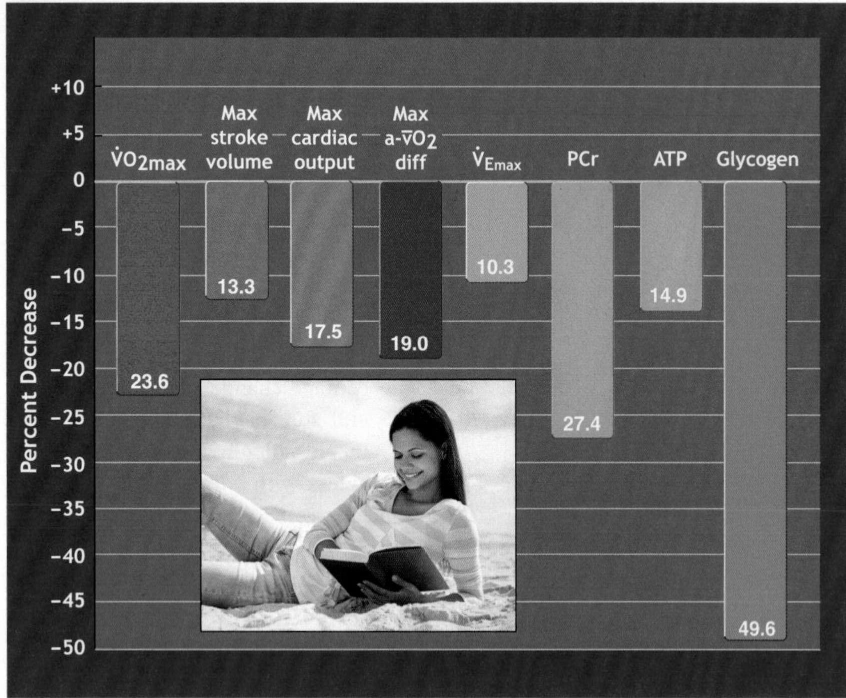

FIGURE 13.2 Average changes in physiologic and metabolic variables with different durations of detraining. Based on data from six studies. Values are as follows: $\dot{V}O_{2max}$ in L • min^{-1}; stroke volume in mL • b^{-1}; cardiac output in L • min^{-1}; a-$\bar{v}O_2$ diff = arteriovenous oxygen differences in mL • dL^{-1}; $\dot{V}_{Emax}$ = maximum minute ventilation in L • min^{-1}; PCr in mmol • g wet muscle^{-1}; ATP in mmol • g wet muscle^{-1}; and glycogen in mmol • g wet muscle^{-1}.

Dr. Per-Olof Åstrand (Chapter 1) prophetically commented concerning the role of genetics in physical performance: "To be an Olympic-caliber performer, you must choose your parents wisely."

Anaerobic System Changes

Figure 13.3 presents a generalized summary of the metabolic adaptations in anaerobic functions that accompany strenuous physical training that requires considerable overload of the anaerobic energy transfer systems. These changes occur *without* concomitant increases in aerobic functions. Three adaptations with sprint-power training include:

1. *Increased levels of anaerobic substrates.* Muscle biopsies taken before and after resistance training reveal an increase in trained muscle's resting levels of ATP, PCr, free creatine, and glycogen, including significant improvements in muscular strength (**Table 13.1**). Other studies show higher levels of ATP and total creatine content in the trained muscles of sprint runners and track speed cyclists compared with distance runners and road racers. Speed-power training also increases the PCr content of trained skeletal muscle.
2. *Increased quantity and activity of key enzymes that control glucose catabolism's anaerobic (glycolytic) phase.* The most dramatic increases in anaerobic enzyme function and fiber size occur in fast-twitch muscle fibers. These changes do not reach the magnitude observed for oxidative enzymes with aerobic training.
3. *Increased capacity to generate high levels of blood lactate during all-out physical activity.* Enhanced lactate-producing capacity probably results from training-induced increased levels of glycogen and glycolytic enzymes and improved motivation and "pain" tolerance to symptoms of fatiguing physical activity.

Aerobic System Changes

Table 13.2 summarizes important metabolic and physiologic differences when comparing typical values of healthy untrained individuals and endurance athletes. Aerobic training

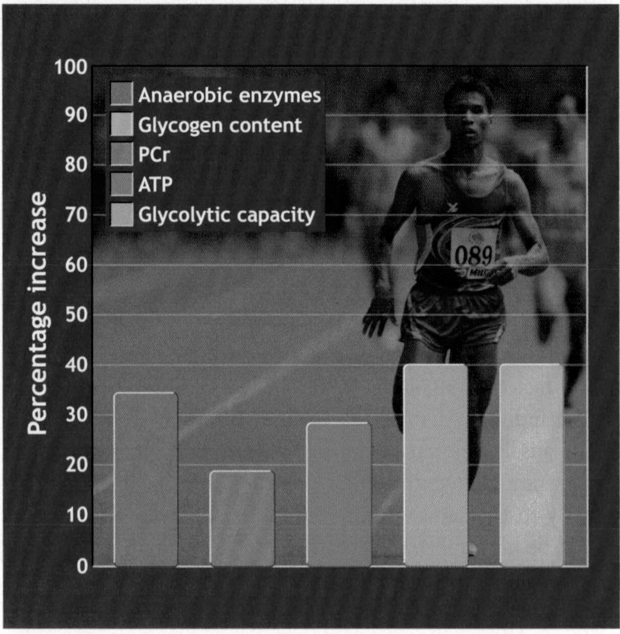

FIGURE 13.3 Generalized potential for increases in anaerobic energy metabolism of skeletal muscle with short-term sprint-power training. (Adapted with permission from McArdle WD, Katch FI, Katch VL. *Exercise Physiology: Nutrition, Energy, and Human Performance*. 8th Ed. Baltimore: Wolters Kluwer Health, 2015.)

TABLE 13.1 Changes in Resting Concentrations of PCr, Creatine, ATP, and Glycogen Following 5 Months of Heavy-Resistance Training in Nine Male Subjects

Variable[a]	Control	Posttraining	Percentage Difference[b]
PCr	17.07	17.94	+5.1
Creatine	14.52	10.74	+35.2
ATP	5.07	5.97	+17.8
Glycogen	113.90	86.28	+32.0

[a] All values are averages expressed in mM per gram of wet muscle.

[b] All percentage differences are statistically significant.

Source: Reprinted with permission from McArdle WD, Katch FI, Katch VL. *Exercise Physiology: Nutrition, Energy, and Human Performance.* 8th Ed. Baltimore: Wolters Kluwer Health, 2015; MacDougall JD, et al. Biochemical adaptation of human skeletal muscle to heavy resistance training and immobilization. *J Appl Physiol* 1977;43:700.

adaptations generally occur independent of gender and age. They also take place in medically cleared individuals with cancer, coronary heart disease, diabetes, hypertension, and chronic obstructive pulmonary disease (see Chapters 17 and 18).

Figure 13.4 displays four categories of diverse physiologic and metabolic factors related to oxygen transport and use: ventilation-aeration, central blood flow, active muscle metabolism, and peripheral blood flow.

TABLE 13.2 Typical Metabolic and Physiologic Values for Healthy, Endurance-Trained and Untrained Men[a]

Variable	Untrained	Trained	Percentage Difference[b]
Glycogen, mM · (g wet muscle)$^{-1}$	85.0	120	41
Number of mitochondria, mmol^{3}	0.59	1.20	103
Mitochondrial volume, % muscle cell	2.15	8.00	272
Resting ATP, mM · (g wet muscle)$^{-1}$	3.0	6.0	100
Resting PCr, mM · (g wet muscle)$^{-1}$	11.0	18.0	64
Resting creatine, mM · (g wet muscle)$^{-1}$	10.7	14.5	35
Glycolytic enzymes			
Phosphofructokinase, mM · (g wet muscle)$^{-1}$	50.0	50.0	0
Phosphorylase, mM · (g wet muscle)$^{-1}$	4–6	6–9	60
Aerobic enzymes			
Succinate dehydrogenase, mM · (kg wet muscle)$^{-1}$	5–10	15–20	133
Max lactate, mM · (kg wet muscle)$^{-1}$	110	150	36
Muscle fibers			
Fast twitch, %	50	20–30	−50
Slow twitch, %	50	60	20
Max stroke volume, mL	120	180	50
Max cardiac output, L · min^{-1}	20	30–40	75
Resting heart rate, b · min^{-1}	70	40	−43
Max heart rate, b · min^{-1}	190	180	−5
Max a-$\bar{v}O_2$ diff, mL · dL^{-1}	14.5	16.0	10
$\dot{V}O_{2max}$, mL · kg^{-1} · min^{-1}	30–40	65–80	107
Heart volume, L	7.5	9.5	27
Blood volume, L	4.7	6.0	28
$\dot{V}O_{2max}$, L · min^{-1}	110	190	73
Percentage body fat	15	11	−27

[a] In some cases, approximate values are used. In all cases, trained values represent data from endurance athletes. Caution is advised in assuming that percentage differences between trained and untrained necessarily result from training because genetic factors exert a strong influence on many of these factors.

[b] Percentage difference: trained versus untrained.

Source: Reprinted with permission from McArdle WD, Katch FI, Katch VL. *Exercise Physiology: Nutrition, Energy, and Human Performance.* 8th Ed. Baltimore: Wolters Kluwer Health, 2015.

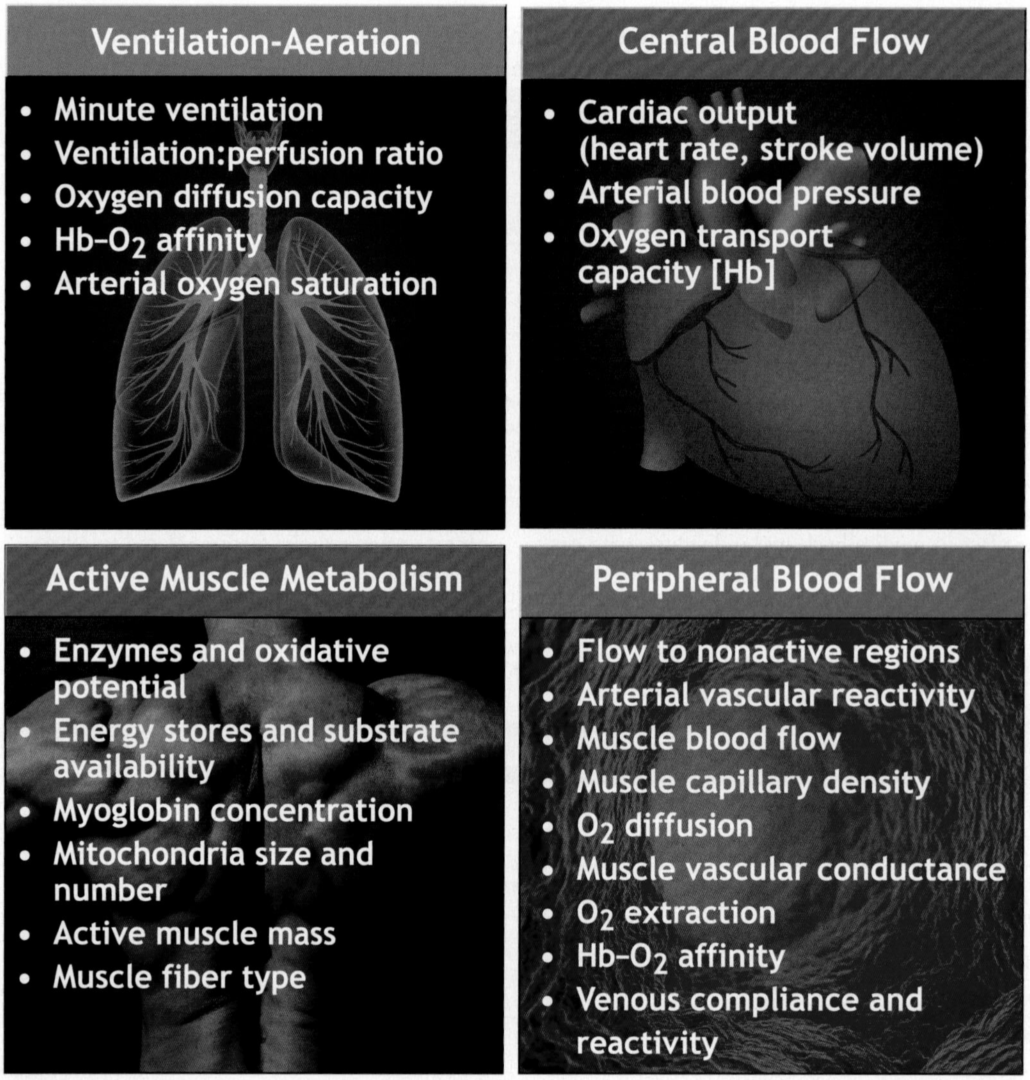

FIGURE 13.4 Physiologic factors that limit $\dot{V}O_{2max}$ and aerobic performance. *Hb*, hemoglobin. (Reprinted with permission from McArdle WD, Katch FI, Katch VL. *Exercise Physiology: Nutrition, Energy, and Human Performance*. 8th Ed. Baltimore: Wolters Kluwer Health, 2015.)

Metabolic Adaptations

Aerobic training induces intracellular changes that enhance a muscle fiber's capacity to aerobically generate ATP.

Metabolic Machinery

An increase in mitochondrial size and number in aerobically trained skeletal muscle improves its capacity to generate ATP by oxidative phosphorylation.

Enzymes

A twofold increase in **aerobic system enzymes** complements increases in mitochondrial size and number and coincides with increased mitochondrial capacity to generate ATP. These adaptations likely allow the trained person to sustain a high percentage of aerobic capacity during prolonged physical activity without accumulating blood lactate (i.e., achieve a higher blood lactate threshold [LT]).

Fat Catabolism

Regular aerobic physical activity profoundly improves ability to oxidize fatty acids, particularly triacylglycerols stored within active muscle during steady-rate physical activity (**Fig. 13.5**). Lipolysis increases from greater blood flow within trained muscle and a higher quantity of fat-mobilizing enzymes from adipocytes and fat-metabolizing enzymes within muscle fibers. This allows the endurance athlete to perform at a higher absolute level of submaximal physical activity than an untrained person before experiencing glycogen depletion's fatiguing effects.

Carbohydrate Catabolism

Aerobically trained muscle exhibits enhanced capacity to oxidize carbohydrate. This explains why during intense endurance activities, considerable pyruvate moves through aerobic energy pathways. A trained muscle's greater mitochondrial oxidative capacity and increased glycogen storage contribute to enhanced capacity for carbohydrate breakdown. An increased carbohydrate catabolism during intense aerobic physical activity serves two important functions:

1. Provides faster aerobic energy transfer compared to fat breakdown
2. Liberates about 6% more energy than fat per quantity of oxygen consumed

Muscle Fiber Type and Size

Endurance training produces aerobic metabolic adaptations in *both* muscle fiber types. This enhances each fiber's existing aerobic capacity and LT level without modifying the muscle fiber type. Selective hypertrophy also occurs in different muscle fiber types during specific overload training. In the same muscle, highly trained endurance athletes have larger slow-twitch than fast-twitch fibers. Conversely, for anaerobic power–trained athletes, fast-twitch fibers occupy more of their muscles' cross-sectional area. As might be expected, slow-twitch muscle fibers with high capacity to generate ATP aerobically contain large quantities of the iron-containing globular protein myoglobin, which facilitates oxygen transfer to mitochondria.

A CLOSER LOOK

An Example of Physical Activity Training Specificity

In an experiment in one of our laboratories on aerobic training specificity, 15 men swam 1 hour a day 3 days a week for 10 weeks at heart rates between 85% and 95% of maximum heart rate (HR_{max}). $\dot{V}O_{2max}$ was measured before and after training during treadmill running and tethered swimming (see Figure). Because vigorous swim training overloads the central circulation reflected by high activity heart rates, we anticipated at least some transfer in aerobic power improvements from swim training to running. This did not occur; an almost total specificity with swim training accompanied the $\dot{V}O_{2max}$ improvement.

Swim training improved $\dot{V}O_{2max}$ by 11% when measured during swimming but only 1.5% when measured during running. If only treadmill running had evaluated swim training effects, we would mistakenly have concluded *no training effect occurred.* For maximum performance during testing, subjects improved 34% in swim time to exhaustion but only 4.6% in treadmill test run time.

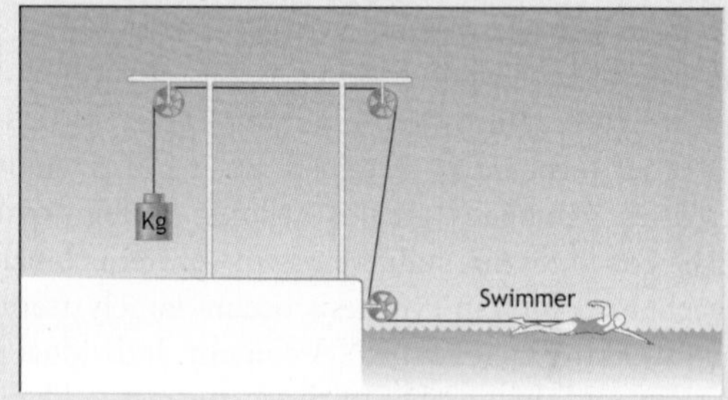

Measurement of energy expenditure during tethered swimming. (Adapted with permission from McArdle WD, Katch FI, Katch VL. *Exercise Physiology: Nutrition, Energy, and Human Performance.* 8th Ed. Baltimore: Wolters Kluwer Health, 2015.)

These findings and other research studies provide strong evidence that training for specific aerobic activities must provide an appropriate general level of cardiovascular stress and specific muscle overload required by the activity. Little improvement results when a dissimilar physical activity measures aerobic capacity or performance. In contrast, considerable improvements emerge when the training mode mimics aerobic adaptations.

Cardiovascular Adaptations

Figure 13.6 summarizes important adaptations in cardiovascular function with aerobic training. Such training produces structural and functional cardiovascular adaptations because of the intimate linkage between the cardiovascular system and aerobic metabolic processes.

Heart Size

Long-term aerobic training generally increases the heart's mass and volume with greater left ventricular end-diastolic volumes during rest and physical activity. This enlargement,

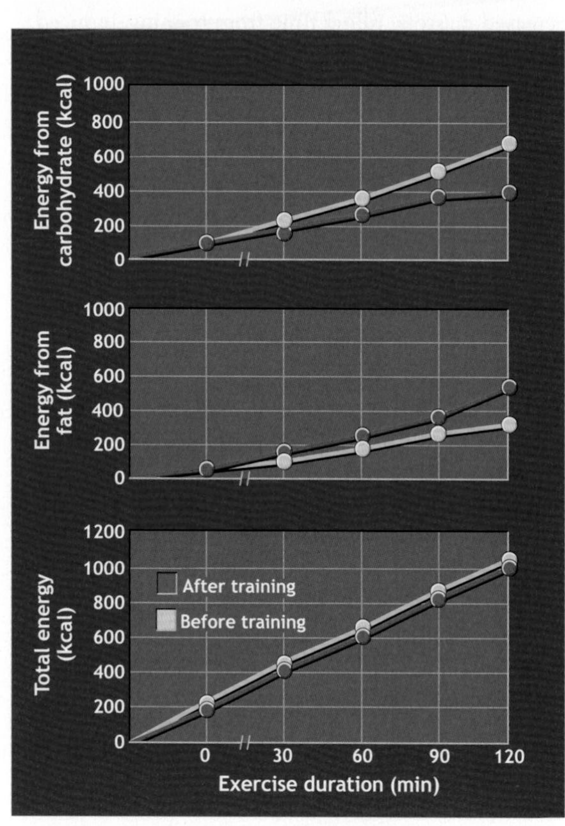

FIGURE 13.5 Aerobic training enhances fat catabolism in submaximal physical activity. During constant load, prolonged physical activity, total energy derived from fat oxidation increases considerably following training. The carbohydrate-sparing adaptation results from facilitated release of fatty acids from adipose tissue depots (augmented by a reduced blood lactate level) and an increased amount of triacylglycerol within the endurance-trained muscle fibers. (Reprinted with permission from Hurley BF, et al. Muscle triglyceride utilization during physical activity: effect of training. *J Appl Physiol* 1986;60:562.)

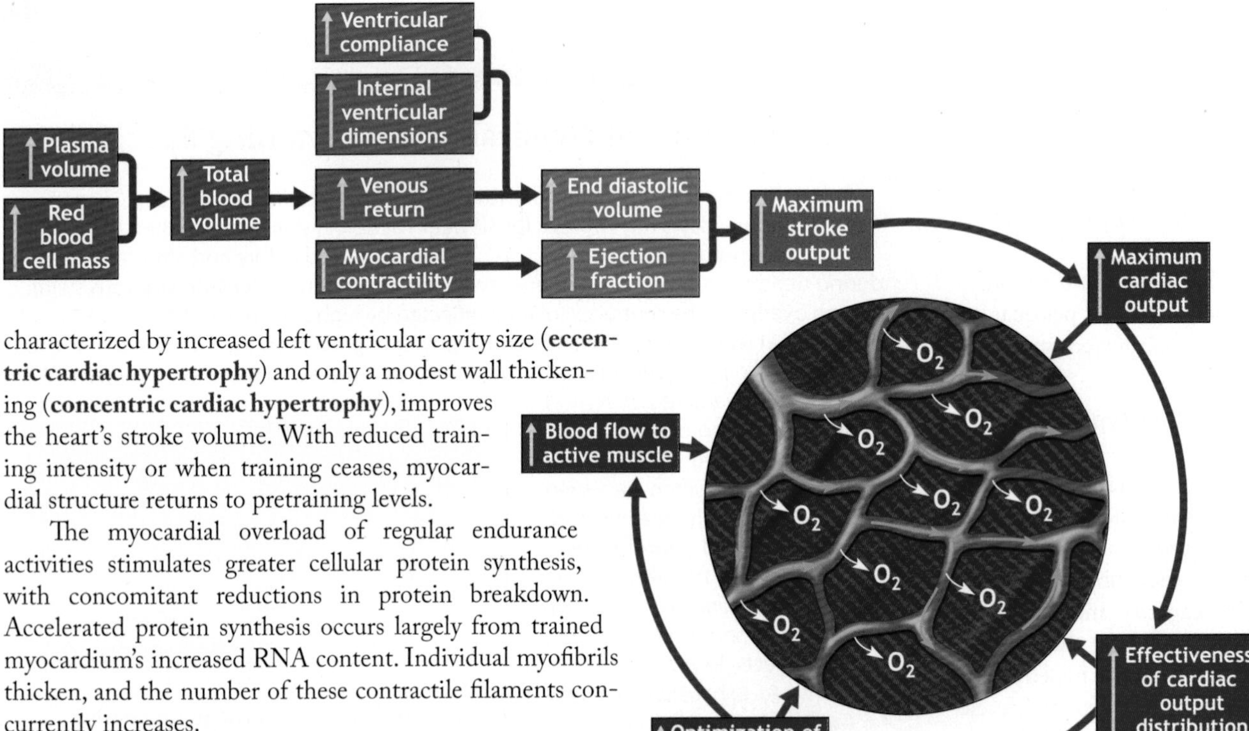

characterized by increased left ventricular cavity size (**eccentric cardiac hypertrophy**) and only a modest wall thickening (**concentric cardiac hypertrophy**), improves the heart's stroke volume. With reduced training intensity or when training ceases, myocardial structure returns to pretraining levels.

The myocardial overload of regular endurance activities stimulates greater cellular protein synthesis, with concomitant reductions in protein breakdown. Accelerated protein synthesis occurs largely from trained myocardium's increased RNA content. Individual myofibrils thicken, and the number of these contractile filaments concurrently increases.

FIGURE 13.6 Adaptations in cardiovascular function with aerobic training that increase oxygen delivery to active muscles. (Reprinted with permission from McArdle WD, Katch FI, Katch VL. *Exercise Physiology: Nutrition, Energy, and Human Performance*. 8th Ed. Baltimore: Wolters Kluwer Health, 2015.)

Important Contributors to Stroke Volume Increases

Four factors resulting from endurance training cause the heart's stroke volume to *increase* during rest and physical activity:

1. Increased internal left ventricular volume consequent to training-induced plasma volume expansion and mass
2. Reduced stiffness in coronary and other major arterial blood vessels
3. Increased diastolic filling time from training-induced bradycardia
4. Possibly improved intrinsic cardiac contractile function

Plasma Volume

Following four training sessions, plasma volume *increases* up to 20%. This adaptation enhances circulatory and thermoregulatory dynamics and facilitates oxygen delivery to muscle during physical activity. The rapid increase in plasma volume with aerobic training also contributes to training-induced eccentric hypertrophy with concomitant increases in stroke volume.

Stroke Volume

Figure 13.7 illustrates the typical stroke volume response for two groups of men during upright physical activity of increasing intensity. One group of endurance athletes trained for several years, while the other group included sedentary, healthy adults. Graded treadmill physical activity evaluated the sedentary adults' responses before and following a 2-month training program to improve aerobic fitness.

The data reveal five important and representative findings concerning aerobic training adaptations:

1. An endurance athlete's heart has a larger stroke volume at rest and during physical activity compared to an untrained person of similar age.
2. For trained and untrained individuals, the greatest stroke volume increase in upright physical activity occurs in the transition from rest to moderate physical activity, with only minimal further increases

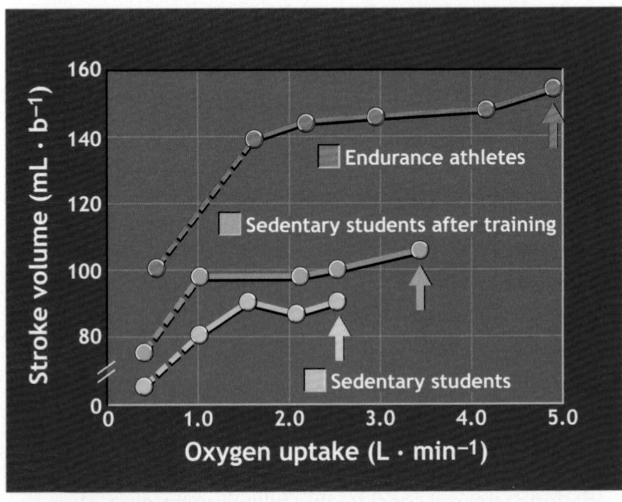

FIGURE 13.7 Stroke volume and oxygen uptake during upright physical activity in endurance athletes (■) and sedentary college students before (■) and after (■) 55 days of aerobic training (⬆ = maximal values). (Adapted with permission from McArdle WD, Katch FI, Katch VL. *Exercise Physiology: Nutrition, Energy, and Human Performance*. 8th Ed. Baltimore: Wolters Kluwer Health, 2015.)

in stroke volume with further increases in intensity

3. The heart's stroke volume achieves near-maximum values at 40% to 50% $\dot{V}O_{2max}$; in young adults, this usually represents a heart rate between 120 and 140 b · min^{-1}.
4. Only a small stroke volume increase occurs for untrained individuals in the transition from rest to physical activity.
5. Acceleration in heart rate produces the major increase in cardiac output.
6. For trained endurance athletes, *both* heart rate and stroke volume increases augment cardiac output, with stroke volume increasing 50% to 60% above resting values.
7. For previously sedentary subjects, 2 months of aerobic training increases stroke volume, but these values remain considerably below the average of elite athletes.

Heart Rate

A proportionate reduction in heart rate during submaximal physical activity accompanies the stroke volume increase with aerobic training. **Figure 13.8** illustrates this training effect for endurance athletes and sedentary adults for the heart rate versus oxygen uptake relationship.

A linear relationship between heart rate and oxygen uptake exists for both groups throughout the major portion of the activity range. As intensity increases, the athletes' heart rates accelerate to a lesser extent than in untrained adults; in contrast, the *slope* or rate of change in the lines differs considerably. This means the athlete or trained adult with an efficient cardiovascular response to physical activity achieves a higher oxygen uptake before reaching a particular submaximal heart rate than for sedentary adults. At an oxygen uptake of 2.0 L · min^{-1}, the athletes' heart rate averages 70 b · min^{-1} lower than sedentary counterparts. After sedentary adults trained for 2 months, the difference in submaximal heart rate decreases to 40 b · min^{-1}. In each case, cardiac output remains essentially unchanged, which means that larger stroke volumes explain the lower activity heart rates. If the heart pumps a large quantity of blood with each beat, then adequate oxygen delivery to active muscle requires only a small heart rate increase and vice versa for a heart with a smaller stroke volume.

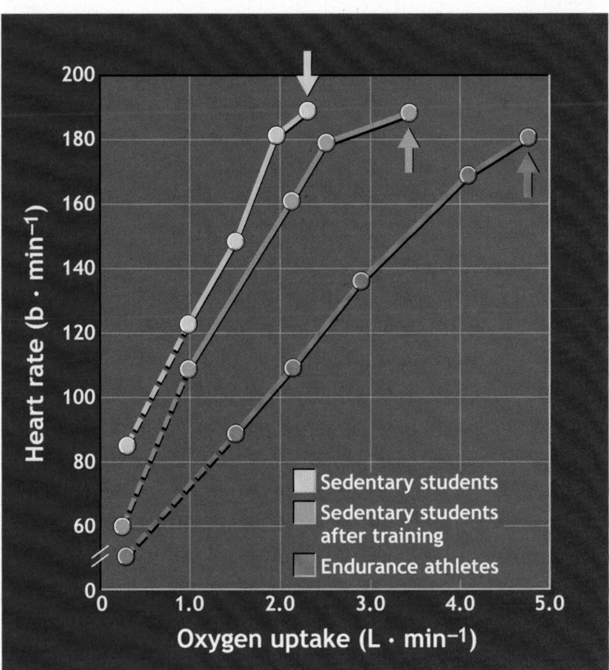

FIGURE 13.8 Heart rate and oxygen uptake during upright physical activity in endurance athletes (■) and sedentary college students before (■) and after (■) 55 days of aerobic training (⬆ = maximal values). (Adapted with permission from McArdle WD, Katch FI, Katch VL. *Exercise Physiology: Nutrition, Energy, and Human Performance*. 8th Ed. Baltimore: Wolters Kluwer Health, 2015.)

Cardiac Output

Increases in maximum cardiac output with aerobic training represent the most significant change in cardiovascular function (**Fig. 13.9**). Maximum heart rate decreases slightly with training, so the heart's increased outflow capacity results directly from the heart's improved stroke volume.

Aerobic training, while improving maximal cardiac output, reduces the heart's minute volume during moderate physical activity. In one study, average cardiac output of young men following 16 weeks of aerobic training decreased 1.1 and 1.5 L · min^{-1} at a specific submaximal oxygen uptake. As expected, maximal cardiac output increased 8% from 22.4 to 24.2 L · min^{-1}. With reduced submaximal cardiac output, a corresponding increase in oxygen extraction in the active muscles (i.e., increased a-$\bar{v}O_2$ difference) matched the exercise oxygen requirement.

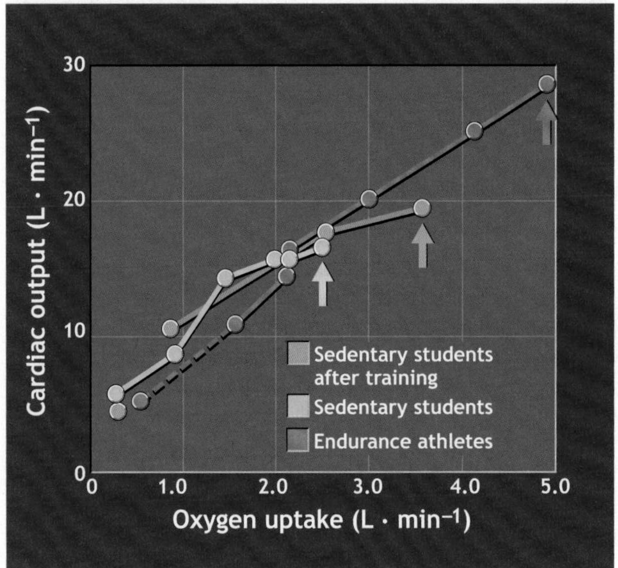

FIGURE 13.9 Cardiac output and oxygen uptake during upright physical activity in endurance athletes (■) and sedentary college students before (■) and after (■) 55 days of aerobic training (⬆ = maximal values). (Adapted with permission from McArdle WD, Katch FI, Katch VL. *Exercise Physiology: Nutrition, Energy, and Human Performance*. 8th Ed. Baltimore: Wolters Kluwer Health, 2015.)

A training-induced reduction in submaximal cardiac output reflects two factors:

1. More effective blood flow distribution
2. Trained muscles' increased capacity to generate ATP aerobically at a lower tissue Po_2

Oxygen Extraction—The a-$\bar{v}o_{2diff}$

Aerobic training increases the maximum quantity of oxygen extracted from arterial blood during intense physical activity. A more effective cardiac output distribution to working muscles and enhanced muscle fiber capacity to metabolize oxygen produce the increase in a-$\bar{v}o_2$ difference (a-$\bar{v}o_{2diff}$).

Figure 13.10 compares the relationship for trained athletes and untrained adults between oxygen extraction and physical activity intensity. For adults, the a-$\bar{v}o_{2diff}$ increases steadily during light and moderate physical activity to a maximum of 15 mL of oxygen per dL of blood. After 55 days of training, the adults' maximum a-$\bar{v}o_{2diff}$ increased 13% to 17 mL of oxygen per dL. This means that during intense physical activity, arterial blood released approximately 85% of its oxygen content. In fact, active muscle extracts even more oxygen because the a-$\bar{v}o_2$ difference reflects an average based on sampling of mixed venous blood. This sample contains blood returning from skin, kidneys, and nonactive musculature that requires much less oxygen during physical activity than active tissues. Posttraining values for maximal a-$\bar{v}o_{2diff}$ for the previously untrained adults equaled values for the endurance athletes. Obviously, the adults' lower cardiac output capacity explains the large difference in $\dot{V}O_{2max}$ that still differentiates athletes from lesser-trained counterparts (see **Fig. 13.9**).

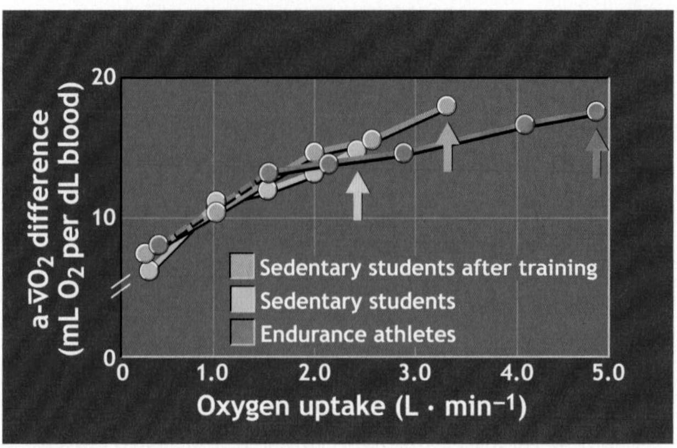

FIGURE 13.10 The a-$\bar{v}o_2$ difference and oxygen uptake during upright exercise in endurance athletes (■) and sedentary college students before (■) and after (■) 55 days of aerobic training (⬆ = maximal values). (Adapted with permission from McArdle WD, Katch FI, Katch VL. *Exercise Physiology: Nutrition, Energy, and Human Performance*. 8th Ed. Baltimore: Wolters Kluwer Health, 2015.)

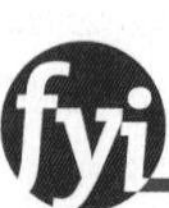

10,000 Steps a Day: A Practical Goal for Sedentary Americans

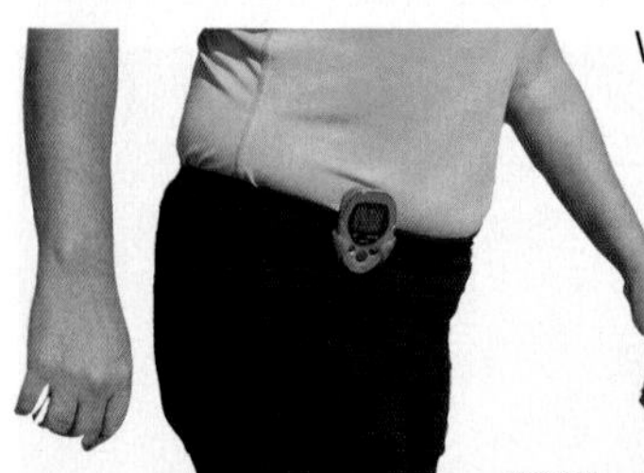

Walking represents "big muscle" low-impact physical activity performed with minimal equipment and little expense. The typical American achieves between 1000 and 3000 steps daily. A walking goal of 10,000 steps a day—the approximate equivalent of walking 5 miles—falls in line with most recommendations for optimal physical activity to reduce disease risk and capture the benefits of a healthier lifestyle. Smartphone "apps" and commercially available "trackers" (i.e., wristbands, watches, and buttons with microprocessor technology) easily monitor and log daily steps. The insert shows a waistband tracker to monitor daily activities; the results are expressed in kcal and steps. Positive feedback provides positive motivation to continue with the walking program.

For an added fitness bonus, individuals can intersperse their regular walking pace with 2- to 3-minute intervals of more brisk walking at a pace they rate as feeling "somewhat hard." For a walking program targeted toward weight loss, gradually increasing walking speed and number of daily steps to the 15,000-step range provides the necessary additional calorie-burning effects.

Blood Flow and Distribution

Three factors explain why aerobic training causes large increases in muscle blood flow during maximal physical effort:

1. Improved maximum cardiac output
2. Redistribution or shunting of blood from nonactive areas that temporarily compromise blood flow in all-out effort
3. Increased capillarization within trained muscle tissues

Blood Pressure

During rest and submaximal physical activity, aerobic training decreases systolic and diastolic blood pressures. The most apparent effect occurs for systolic pressure, particularly for hypertensive subjects. *Regular aerobic physical activity for previously sedentary adult men and women of all ages reduces systolic blood pressure approximately 6 to 10 mm Hg.*

A training-induced reduction in sympathetic nervous system catecholamines contributes to the lowering effect of physical activity on blood pressure, perhaps via reduced peripheral vascular resistance to blood flow. Regularly performed physical activity also facilitates the kidneys' elimination of sodium, which subsequently reduces fluid volume and thus blood pressure. *Regular physical activity represents a prudent first line of defense in most therapeutic programs to manage borderline hypertension.* More severe blood pressure elevations require combinations of diet, weight loss, physical activity, and ultimately pharmacologic intervention.

Pulmonary Adaptations

Aerobic training induces alterations in pulmonary dynamics. Such changes contribute to a more effective ventilatory response to the stress of physical activity.

Maximal Physical Activity

Training-induced improvements in $\dot{V}O_{2max}$ increase maximal minute ventilation $\dot{V}_{Emax}$. This adaptation makes sense physiologically because improved aerobic capacity reflects larger oxygen utilization and need to eliminate carbon dioxide by increased alveolar ventilation.

Submaximal Physical Activity

Regular training also improves ability to sustain high levels of submaximal ventilation. For example, 20 weeks of regular run training in healthy adult men and women increased ventilatory muscle endurance by 16%. Less lactate accumulated during submaximal breathing exercise, probably from increased aerobic enzyme levels in the ventilatory musculature. Enhanced ventilatory endurance reduces the feeling of breathlessness and pulmonary discomfort frequently experienced by untrained persons who perform prolonged submaximal exertion.

Only 4 weeks of submaximal physical activity training considerably *reduces* the ventilatory equivalent for oxygen ($\dot{V}_E/\dot{V}O_2$). Consequently, a particular level of submaximal oxygen uptake requires breathing less air; this reduces the percentage of the total oxygen cost of an activity attributable to breathing. Enhanced ventilatory economy contributes to overall endurance performance in two ways:

1. Reduces fatiguing effects of physical activity on ventilatory musculature
2. Frees oxygen from respiratory muscles by nonrespiratory active muscles

In general, tidal volume increases, breathing frequency decreases, and air remains in the lungs for a longer time interval between breaths. Slower breathing augments the amount of oxygen the alveoli extracts from the inspired air volume. For example, exhaled air of trained individuals contains only 14% to 15% oxygen during submaximal exertion, yet an untrained person's expired air contains about 17% oxygen at the same intensity. This means the untrained person must ventilate proportionately more air to achieve the same submaximal oxygen uptake.

Blood Lactate Concentration

Figure 13.11 illustrates the generalized endurance training effect in lowering blood lactate levels and extending duration of effort before onset of blood lactate accumulation or OBLA. The explanation underlying this effect centers on three possibilities related to central and peripheral adaptations to training:

1. Decreased rate of lactate formation during physical activity

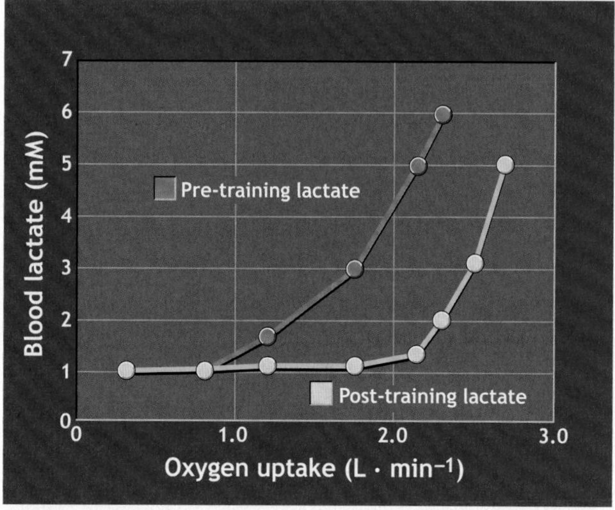

FIGURE 13.11 Generalized responses for pretraining and posttraining lactate accumulation during graded physical activity. (Adapted with permission from McArdle WD, Katch FI, Katch VL. *Exercise Physiology: Nutrition, Energy, and Human Performance*. 8th Ed. Baltimore: Wolters Kluwer Health, 2015; plots based on data from the Applied Physiology Laboratory, University of Michigan, Ann Arbor.)

2. Increased rate of lactate clearance during physical activity
3. Combined effects of increased lactate removal and decreased lactate formation

Body Composition Changes

For overly fat individuals, regular aerobic physical activity reduces body weight and body fat. Additionally, a regular program of resistance training typically increases fat-free body mass. Physical activity only, or activity combined with calorie restriction, reduces body fat more than fat lost with only dieting because enhanced physical activity conserves the body's lean tissue mass.

Temperature Regulation

Well-hydrated, aerobically trained individuals exercise more comfortably in hot environments because of a larger plasma volume and more-responsive thermoregulatory mechanisms. Trained men and women dissipate heat faster and more effectively than untrained persons. For trained individuals, the metabolic heat generated by physical activity poses less of a detriment to physical performance and overall safety.

Endurance Performance Changes

Enhanced endurance accompanies the physiologic adaptations of training. **Figure 13.12** depicts results for cycling performance after training performed 4 days weekly for 40 to 60 minutes for 10 weeks at an intensity of 85% $\dot{V}O_{2max}$. The performance test required subjects to maintain a constant work rate of 265 W for 8 minutes. Training produced less drop-off in power output during the prescribed 8-minute exercise test.

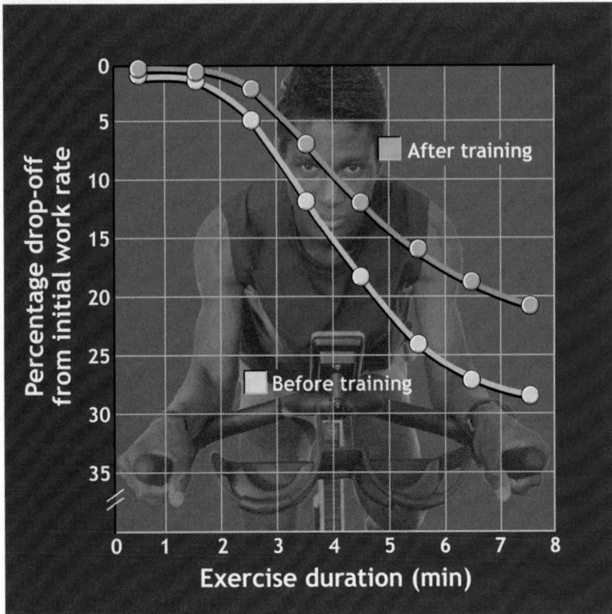

FIGURE 13.12 Percentage drop-off from initial intensity before and after 10 wk of endurance cycling training. (Reprinted with permission from the Applied Physiology Laboratory, University of Michigan, Ann Arbor.)

Psychological Benefits

Regular physical activity, either aerobic or resistance training, produces psychological benefits independent of age. Adaptations often occur to a degree equal to that achieved with other therapeutic interventions. Regular physical activity produces six potential psychological benefits:

1. Reduced anxiety state
2. Decreased mild to moderate depression
3. Reduced neuroticism as a long-term conditioning effect
4. Adjunct to professional treatment of severe depression
5. Improved mood, self-esteem, and self-concept
6. Reduced indices of stress

FACTORS AFFECTING THE AEROBIC TRAINING RESPONSE

Figure 13.13 indicates two important factors in formulating regimens of aerobic training:

1. Cardiovascular demands must reach an intensity to sufficiently increase or overload stroke volume and cardiac output.
2. Cardiovascular overload must activate sport-specific muscle groups to enhance local circulation and muscle's "metabolic machinery."

Proper endurance training overloads all components of oxygen transport and use. This consideration supports the specificity of training principle. *Simply stated—to improve—runners must run, cyclists must cycle, rowers must row, and swimmers must swim to achieve maximal performance benefits.*

The important factors that influence outcomes of aerobic training include initial level of cardiovascular fitness and training frequency, training duration, and training intensity. A Closer Look: "Quantity and Quality of Exercise for Developing and Maintaining Cardiorespiratory, Musculoskeletal, and Neuromotor Fitness in Apparently Healthy Adults: Guidance for Prescribing Exercise" provides guidelines on the types and amounts of physical activity for healthy adults ages 18 to 65.

Initial Aerobic Fitness Level

One's initial aerobic fitness level impacts the magnitude of training improvement. *Considerable improvement occurs when initial fitness remains low; conversely, an exceptionally high initial fitness level leaves little room for improvement.* For example, a 5% improvement in physiologic function for an elite athlete can be more significant than a 25% increase for a sedentary person. As a general guideline, aerobic fitness improvements range between 5% and 25% with endurance training. Some of this improvement occurs within the first training week.

Optimal Training Frequency

Exercising at least 3 days weekly generally initiates adaptive aerobic system changes. Several research studies report improvements when training only once weekly. Those subjects, however, had been sedentary; for them, any form of overload would have stimulated improvement. *In general, a training response occurs with physical activity performed at least three times weekly for at least 6 weeks.* Training four or five times a week generated only *slightly* greater physiologic improvements compared with thrice-weekly physical activity. For the average person, the small improvement in physiologic function assessed by $\dot{V}O_{2max}$ may not warrant the extra 1- or 2-day time investment in training. In contrast, the extra caloric expenditure needed for effective weight control with daily physical activity justifies more frequent and longer activity duration. To derive maximum health benefits, individuals should exercise most days of the week. Chapter 17 discusses health benefits of regular physical activity.

Optimal Training Duration

A common inquiry about physical activity participation concerns the optimal duration of daily workouts. For example, does 10 minutes of jogging provide twice the benefits of 5 minutes? Would a 2- or 3-minute run repeated 8 to 10 times provide greater training benefits than a continuous 20- to 30-minute run at similar intensity? Precise answers to these questions remain elusive because of an incomplete understanding of the mechanisms that underlie aerobic fitness improvements and proper criteria to evaluate such changes. Both continuous and more intense intermittent activity overload improve aerobic capacity. In general, performing less exhaustive, moderate-paced activity for the average person for at least 30 minutes a session establishes a realistic workout duration. In contrast, most competitive endurance athletes devote several hours each training session to enhance the aerobic system's functional capacity.

As for training volume, more does not necessarily produce greater results. In a study of collegiate swimmers, one group trained for 1.5 hours daily, and another group performed two 1.5-hour sessions each day. No differences emerged between groups in the improvement in swimming power, endurance, or performance time despite one group swimming twice the daily training volume. About 60 minutes of daily physical activity provides optimal health benefits and sets the lower limit for optimal duration to achieve weight loss.

Optimal Training Intensity

The most critical factor for successful aerobic training is properly managing intensity. Intensity generally reflects the activity's energy requirements per unit time, and specific energy systems activated relative to an individual's energy-generating capacity. One can express physical activity intensity in one of seven ways:

1. Energy expended per unit time (e.g., 9 kcal · min^{-1} or 37.8 kJ · min^{-1})
2. Absolute activity level or power output (e.g., cycle at 900 kg-m · min^{-1} or 147 W)
3. Relative metabolic level expressed as percentage of $\dot{V}O_{2max}$ (e.g., 85% $\dot{V}O_{2max}$)
4. Exercise below, at, or above the LT, or OBLA (e.g., 4 mM lactate)
5. Activity heart rate or percentage of maximum heart rate (e.g., 180 b · min^{-1} or 80% HR_{max})
6. Multiples of resting metabolic rate (e.g., 6 METs)
7. Rating of perceived exertion (e.g., RPE = 14)

By far, monitoring heart rate provides the most practical way to assess strenuousness of physical activity effort. Researchers frequently use heart rate to structure a training program and evaluate the effectiveness of different training intensities. For college-age men and women, a physical activity must attain a heart rate intensity at least 130 to 140 b · min^{-1}, which translates to about 50% to 55% of $\dot{V}O_{2max}$ or 70% HR_{max}. Generally, this intensity represents the *minimally optimal threshold stimulus* to improve cardiovascular function. More intense physical activity proves even more effective. Conversely, in untrained persons, extending duration induces fitness improvement if intensity does not achieve the threshold level.

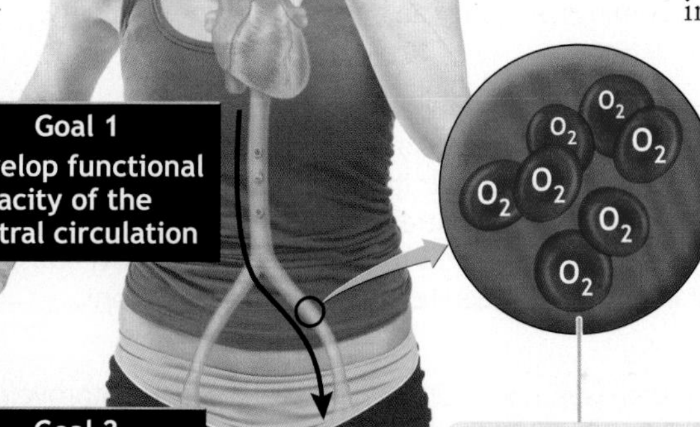

FIGURE 13.13 The two major goals of aerobic training: *Goal 1*, develop the functional capacity of the central circulation to deliver oxygen; *Goal 2*, enhance the aerobic capacity of the active musculature to supply and process oxygen. (Reprinted with permission from McArdle WD, Katch FI, Katch VL. *Exercise Physiology: Nutrition, Energy, and Human Performance*. 8th Ed. Baltimore: Wolters Kluwer Health, 2015.)

Overly Strenuous Physical Activity Not Required

A heart rate at 70% HR_{max} represents only moderate physical activity that can continue for a long duration with little or no physiologic discomfort. The term **conversational exercise** describes this training level. It refers to sufficiently intense activity to stimulate a training effect yet is not so strenuous to limit a person from talking during the workout.

Figure 13.14 shows that aerobic fitness improvements gradually decrease heart rate response at a given level of submaximal exertion or oxygen uptake. Consequently, the absolute activity level in running or swimming speed, or power output on a cycle ergometer, must increase accordingly to achieve the desired target heart rate. Consider a person who began training by slow walking but now walks more briskly; eventually, periods of the workout include jogging. Ultimately, activity at the training heart rate requires continuous movement.

A minimal threshold intensity exists below which no training effect occurs; a ceiling also can exist where a higher intensity workout produces little or no further gains. The lower and upper limits of the training-sensitive zone depend on the participant's age, initial fitness level, and training state. For people who begin with relatively poor aerobic fitness, including older men and women, the training threshold approaches 60% to 65% HR_{max}, which corresponds to about 45% $\dot{V}O_{2max}$; more fit individuals generally require a higher threshold level. The ceiling for training intensity remains unknown, although 90% HR_{max} probably represents the upper limit. Above this level, increases in intensity primarily overload the anaerobic energy transfer system. A Closer Look: "Predicting Maximum Heart Rate and the Training-Sensitive Zone" discusses common methods of

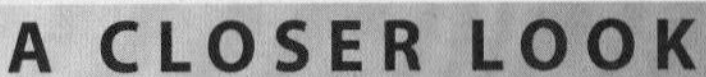

A CLOSER LOOK

Quantity and Quality of Physical Activity for Developing and Maintaining Cardiorespiratory, Musculoskeletal, and Neuromotor Fitness in Apparently Healthy Adults: Guidance for Prescribing Physical Activity

The American College of Sports Medicine (ACSM) provides guidance on physical activity prescription. Its basic recommendations are categorized by cardiorespiratory exercise, resistance exercise, flexibility exercise, and neuromotor exercise.

Cardiorespiratory Exercise

- Adults should complete at least 150 minutes of moderate-intensity physical activity weekly.
- Physical activity recommendations can be met through 30 to 60 minutes of moderate-intensity activity (5 days a week) or 20 to 60 minutes of vigorous-intensity physical activity (3 days weekly).
- One continuous session and multiple shorter sessions (of at least 10 min) are both acceptable to accumulate the desired amount of daily physical activity.
- Gradual progression of activity time, frequency, and intensity is recommended for best adherence and least injury risk.
- People unable to meet these minimums still can benefit from some activity.

Resistance Exercise

- Adults should train each major muscle group 2 or 3 days weekly using a variety of exercises and equipment.
- Very light or light intensity is best for older persons or previously sedentary adults starting exercise.
- Two to four sets of each activity will help adults improve strength and power.
- For each activity, 8 to 12 repetitions improve strength and power, 10 to 15 repetitions improve strength in middle-aged and older persons starting activity, and 15 to 20 repetitions improve muscular endurance.
- Adults should wait at least 48 hours between resistance-training sessions.

Flexibility Exercise

- Adults should do flexibility exercises at least 2 or 3 days each week to improve range of motion.
- Each stretch should be held for 10 to 30 seconds to the point of tightness or without pain.
- Repeat each stretch two to four times, accumulating 60 seconds per stretch.
- Static, dynamic, ballistic, and PNF stretches are all effective.
- Flexibility exercise is most effective when the muscle is "warm." Try light aerobic activity or a hot bath to warm the muscles before stretching.

Neuromotor Exercise

- Neuromotor exercise (sometimes called "functional fitness training") is recommended 2 or 3 days a week.
- Exercises should involve motor skills (balance, agility, coordination, and gait), proprioceptive exercise training, and multifaceted activities such as tai ji and yoga to improve physical function and prevent falls in the elderly.
- Twenty to 30 minutes a day is appropriate for neuromotor exercise.

In addition to outlining basic recommendations and their scientific reasoning, the ACSM position stand also clarifies these points of emphasis:

- Pedometers or step-counting devices used to measure physical activity are not an accurate measure of exercise quality and should not be used as the sole measure of physical activity.
- Though physical activity offers protective effects against heart disease, active adults can still develop heart problems. All adults must be able to recognize the warning signs of heart disease, and all healthcare providers should ask patients about these symptoms.
- Sedentary behavior—sitting for long periods of time—is distinct from physical activity and may pose a health risk in itself. Meeting the guidelines for physical activity does not make up for a sedentary lifestyle.

The ACSM position stand offers health-and-fitness professionals scientific, evidence-based recommendations to help them customize physical activity prescriptions for healthy adults.

Source: http://journals.lww.com/acsm-msse/Fulltext/2011/07000/Quantity_and_Quality_of_Exercise_for_Developing.26.aspx

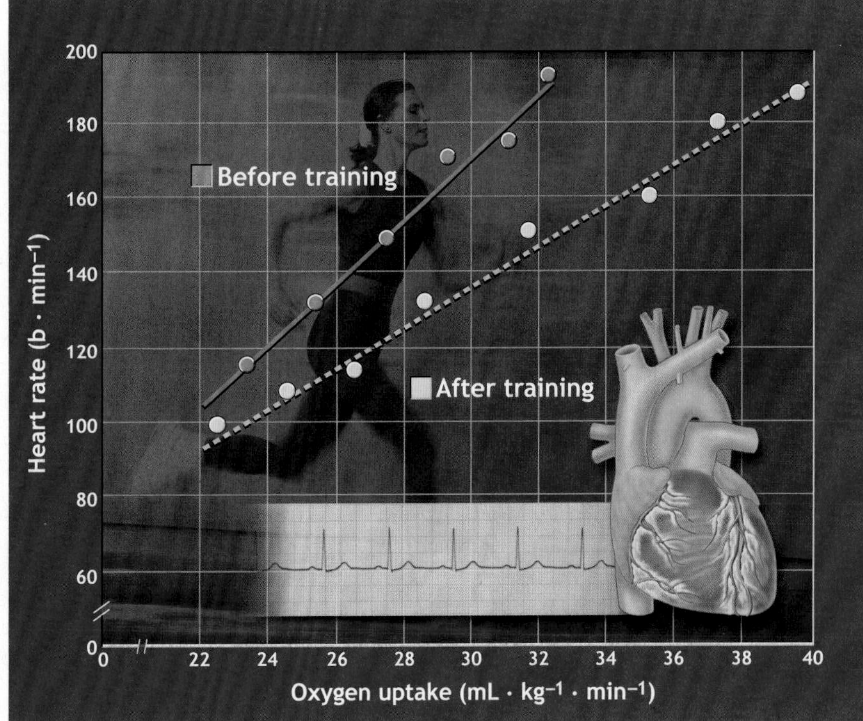

FIGURE 13.14 Improvements in heart rate response in relation to oxygen uptake with aerobic training. A reduction in heart rate with training usually reflects enhanced stroke volume. (Reprinted with permission from McArdle WD, Katch FI, Katch VL. *Exercise Physiology: Nutrition, Energy, and Human Performance*. 8th Ed. Baltimore: Wolters Kluwer Health, 2015.)

how heart rate can establish an appropriate aerobic training exertion level.

Optimal Window for Improvement

Positive adaptations with training in cardiorespiratory fitness and aerobic capacity generally occur within several weeks after beginning a conditioning program. **Figure 13.15** shows absolute and percentage improvements in $\dot{V}O_{2max}$ for men who trained 6 days weekly for 10 weeks. Training consisted of 30 minutes of bicycling 3 days a week combined with 40 minutes of running on alternate days. This produced continuous week-by-week aerobic capacity improvements. Adaptive responses to training eventually level off as a person reaches their genetically determined maximum. A Closer Look: "Cardiovascular Fitness Categories Using $\dot{V}O_{2max}$" presents fitness classification categories for typical adult men and women (excluding elite endurance-trained individuals) of different ages based on $\dot{V}O_{2max}$.

Trainability and Genes

The limits for developing fitness capacity link closely to natural endowment. For two individuals in the same physical conditioning program, one might show 10 times more improvement than the other. Genetic research indicates a genotype dependency for much of one's sensitivity in responding to maximal aerobic and anaerobic power training. This also includes muscle enzyme adaptations. Genetic makeup plays such a predominant role in training responsiveness that it makes it extremely difficult to predict a specific individual's response to a specific training stimulus.

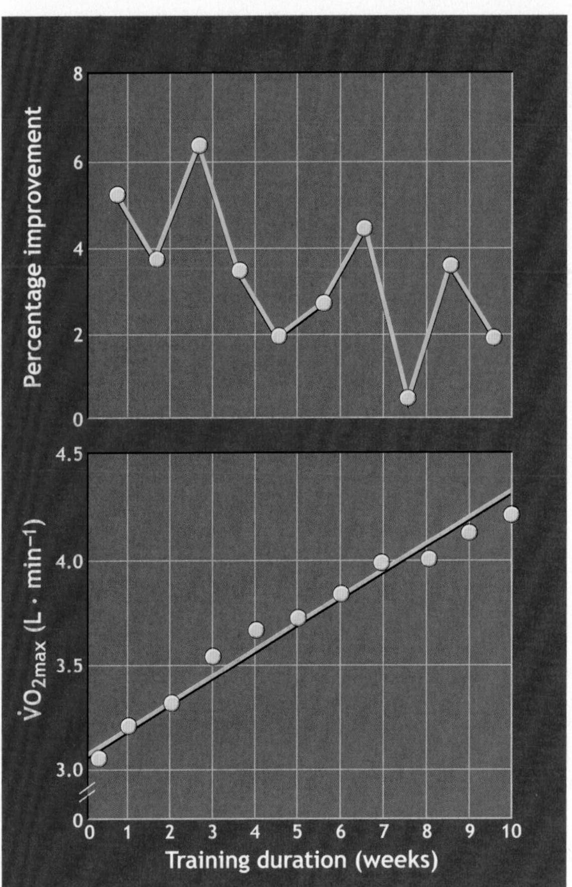

FIGURE 13.15 Continuous improvements in $\dot{V}O_{2max}$ during 10 wk of high-intensity aerobic training. (Reprinted with permission from Hickson RC, et al. Linear increases in aerobic power induced by a program of endurance exercise. *J Appl Physiol* 1977;42:373.)

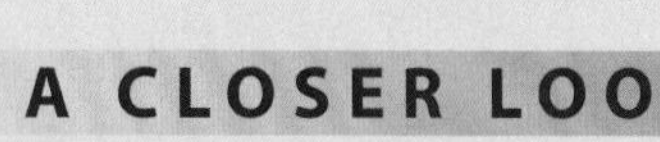

Predicting Maximum Heart Rate and the Training-Sensitive Zone

Predicting HR_{max}

Percentage of maximum HR predicts activity intensity (an activity's relative energy requirements). HR_{max} in beats per minute ($b \cdot min^{-1}$) can be predicted by age, independent of gender and physical activity status. For *average fat* men and women, HR_{max} predicts as:

$$\mathbf{HR_{max} = 208 - 0.7 \times (Age, y)}$$

Example

Calculate the HR_{max} for a 20-year-old man.

$$\mathbf{HR_{max} = 208 - 0.7 \times (Age, y) = 194\ bpm}$$

Predicting HR_{max} for Men and Women With ≥30% Body Fat

For *overfat* men and women with percentage body fat levels 30% or above, HR_{max} predicts as:

$$\mathbf{HR_{max} = 200 - 0.5 \times (Age, y)}$$

Example

Calculate the HR_{max} for a 25-year-old woman with a percentage body fat of 32%.

$$\mathbf{HR_{max} = 200 - 0.5 \times (Age, y) = 188\ bpm}$$

Computing Lower- and Upper-Limit Training Heart Rates

For men and women younger than age 60, the minimal- or lower-limit target threshold heart rate (LL_{THR}) stimulus for cardiovascular improvement ranges between 60% and 70% of HR_{max}, representing about 50% to 60% of $\dot{V}O_{2max}$. The upper-limit target heart rate (UL_{THR}) equals about 90% of HR_{max}, representing about 85% to 90% of $\dot{V}O_{2max}$. In individuals older than 60 years of age, LL_{THR} equals 60%, and UL_{THR} equals 75% of HR_{max}.

Method 1: Percentage Method

This method calculates the lower- and upper-limit target heart rates as a simple percentage of age-predicted HR_{max}.

1. Calculate LL_{THR} as:

$$\mathbf{LL_{THR} = Predicted\ HR_{max} \times Lower\text{-}limit\ percentage\ for\ age}$$

where lower-limit percentage = 70% for men and women 60 years and younger and 60% for men and women older than 60 years.

2. Calculate UL_{THR} as:

$$\mathbf{UL_{THR} = Predicted\ HR_{max} \times Upper\text{-}limit\ percentage\ for\ age}$$

where the upper-limit percentage = 90% for men and women 60 years and younger and 80% for men and women older than 60 years.

Example

Data: Male, age 55 years.

1. Calculate predicted HR_{max}:

$$\mathbf{HR_{max} = 208 - 0.7 \times (Age, y) = 170\ bpm}$$

$$\mathbf{LL_{THR} = 170 \times Lower\text{-}limit\ percentage\ for\ age = 170 \times 0.70 = 119\ bpm}$$

2. Calculate UL_{THR}

$$\mathbf{UL_{THR} = HR_{max} \times Upper\text{-}limit\ percentage\ for\ age = 170 \times 0.90 = 153\ bpm}$$

Method 2: Karvonen Method (Heart Rate Reserve)

An alternate, equally effective method calculates the lower- and upper-threshold HR levels at a percentage of the difference between resting and maximum HR, termed heart rate reserve (HRR; also referred to as the *Karvonen method* named after the Finnish physiologist who introduced this method; **www.briancalkins.com/HeartRate.htm**). The **Karvonen method** produces somewhat higher values compared with heart rate computed as percentage of HR_{max}. Karvonen's method requires about 50% of HRR as the LL_{THR} and 85% of HRR as UL_{THR}.

1. Calculate predicted HR_{max}:

$$\mathbf{HR_{max} = 208 - 0.7 \times Age, y}$$

2. Calculate LL_{THR}:

$$\mathbf{LL_{THR} = [(HR_{max} - HR_{rest}) \times 0.50] + HR_{rest}}$$

3. Calculate UL_{THR}:

$$\mathbf{UL_{THR} = [(HR_{max} - HR_{rest}) \times 0.85] + HR_{rest}}$$

Example

Data: Male, age 55 years, $HR_{rest} = 60\ b \cdot min^{-1}$.

1. Calculate predicted HR_{max}:

$$\mathbf{HR_{max} = 208 - 0.7 \times Age, y = 170\ bpm}$$

2. Calculate LL_{THR}:

$$\begin{aligned} LL_{THR} &= [(HR_{max} - HR_{rest}) \times 0.50] + HR_{rest} \\ &= [(170 - 60) \times 0.50] + 60 \\ &= 115 \text{ bpm} \end{aligned}$$

3. Calculate UL_{THR}:

$$\begin{aligned} UL_{THR} &= [(HR_{max} - HR_{rest}) \times 0.85] + HR_{rest} \\ &= [(170 - 60) \times 0.85] + 60 \\ &= 154 \text{ bpm} \end{aligned}$$

Adjust for Swimming and Other Upper-Body Activities

In trained and untrained subjects, swimming HR_{max} averages about 13 b · min^{-1} lower than in running. The smaller arm muscle mass activated during swimming probably causes this difference. Consequently, HR_{max} must be adjusted downward for swimming or other upper-body physical activity. Subtract 13 b · min^{-1} from the age-predicted HR_{max} values to calculate training heart rate during swimming. For example, a 25-year-old person wanting to swim at 80% of HR_{max} should select a swimming speed that produces an activity heart rate (percentage method) of about 142 b · min^{-1} (0.80 × [191 – 13]).

Method 3: Perhaps a Modification Required

Evidence from a longitudinal study of 132 persons, whose HR was measured an average of seven times over 9 years, indicates a bias in the widely used 220 – Age HR_{max} prediction. The bias *overestimates* this measure in men and women younger than age 40 and *underestimates* it in persons older than age 40 (see accompanying figure). This modified prediction equation (with a 5 to 8 b · min^{-1} standard deviation) is independent of gender, body mass index, and resting heart rate:

$$HR_{max} = 206.9 - 0.67 \times \text{Age (y)}$$

For example, use the above equation to estimate maximum heart rate for a 30-year-old man or woman:

$$\begin{aligned} HR_{max} &= 206.9 - (0.67 \times 30) \\ &= 206.9 - 20.1 \\ &= 187 \text{ b} \cdot \text{min}^{-1} \end{aligned}$$

These prediction formulas associate with a plus/minus error and should be used with caution. Each formula represents a convenient rule of thumb but should not determine a specific person's maximum heart rate. For example, within normal variation limits and using the 220 – Age formula, a maximum heart rate of 95% (±2 standard deviations) for 40-year-old men and women ranges between 160 and 200 b · min^{-1}.

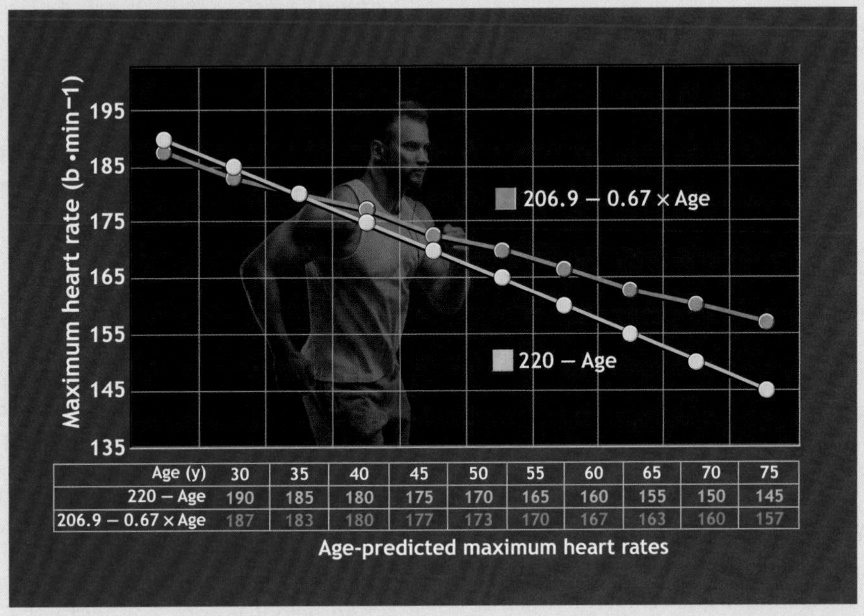

Age (y)	30	35	40	45	50	55	60	65	70	75
220 − Age	190	185	180	175	170	165	160	155	150	145
206.9 − 0.67 × Age	187	183	180	177	173	170	167	163	160	157

Age-predicted maximum heart rates

Sources: Davis JA, Convertino VA. A comparison of heart rate methods for predicting endurance training intensity. *Med Sci Sports Exerc* 1975;7:295.
Gellish RL, et al. Longitudinal modeling of the relationship between age and maximal heart rate. *Med Sci Sports Exerc* 2007;39:822.
Karvonen M, et al. The effects of training on heart rate. A longitudinal study. *Ann Med Exp Bio Fenn* 1957;35:307.
Miller WC, et al. Predicting max HR and the HR-V̇O_2 relationship for exercise prescription in obesity. *Med Sci Sports Exerc* 1993;25:1077.
Tanaka H, et al. Age-predicted maximal heart rate revisited. *J Am Coll Cardiol* 2001;37:153.

How to Maintain Aerobic Fitness Gains

An important question concerns optimal training frequency, duration, and intensity to *maintain* aerobic improvements. In one study, healthy young adults increased $\dot{V}O_{2max}$ 25% following 10 weeks of interval training by bicycling and running for 40 minutes, 6 days weekly. They then joined one of the two groups that continued to exercise for an additional 15 weeks at the same intensity and duration but at a reduced frequency of either 4 or 2 days weekly. Both groups maintained gains in aerobic capacity despite up to two-thirds reduced training frequency.

Improvement of aerobic capacity involves different training requirements than its maintenance. With intensity held constant, the required activity frequency and duration to maintain a certain aerobic fitness level remain considerably lower than required for its improvement. In contrast, a small decline in intensity reduces $\dot{V}O_{2max}$. *This means that intensity probably plays the principal role in maintaining training-induced* $\dot{V}O_{2max}$ improvement.

Fitness components other than $\dot{V}O_{2max}$ readily reflect adverse effects of reduced training volume. Well-trained endurance athletes who normally trained 6 to 10 hours a week reduced weekly training to one 35-minute session; this did not decrease their $\dot{V}O_{2max}$ over a 4-week interval. Endurance capacity at 75% $\dot{V}O_{2max}$ significantly decreased and related to depressed pre-exercise glycogen stores and diminished fat oxidation levels. *These findings indicate that a single* $\dot{V}O_{2max}$ *measure cannot adequately evaluate all of the important factors that impact the physiologic adaptations to training and detraining.*

A CLOSER LOOK

Cardiovascular Fitness Categories Using $\dot{V}O_{2max}$

The $\dot{V}O_{2max}$ test represents the most often cited criterion of cardiorespiratory fitness. Current practice evaluates the $\dot{V}O_{2max}$ score against criterion-referenced standards rather than norm-referenced standards. Criterion-referenced standards establish a *minimum* $\dot{V}O_{2max}$ consistent with good health similar to blood pressure and cholesterol standards, independent of the score's percentile ranking within a particular normative data set. The accompanying table presents a five-part classification for $\dot{V}O_{2max}$ for men and women of different ages. The poor category for each age group represents the lower limit of desirable cardiorespiratory fitness.

Individuals who regularly engage in distance running, swimming, bicycling, and cross-country skiing achieve the highest $\dot{V}O_{2max}$ values. These individuals have almost double the $\dot{V}O_{2max}$ of sedentary individuals.

Cardiovascular Fitness Classifications Based on $\dot{V}O_{2max}$ ($mL \cdot kg^{-1} \cdot min^{-1}$)

Gender	Age	Poor	Fair	Average	Good	Excellent
Men	≤29	≤24.9	25–33.9	34–43.9	44–52.9	≥53
	30–39	≤22.9	23–30.9	31–41.9	42–49.9	≥50
	40–49	≤19.9	20–26.9	27–38.9	39–44.9	≥45
	50–59	≤17.9	18–24.9	25–37.9	38–42.9	≥43
	60–69	≤15.9	16–22.9	23–35.9	36–40.9	≥41
Women	≤29	≤23.9	24–30.9	31–38.9	39–48.9	≥49
	30–39	≤19.9	20–27.9	28–36.9	37–44.9	≥45
	40–49	≤16:9	17–24.9	25–34.9	35–41.9	≥42
	50–59	≤14.9	15–21.9	22–33.9	34–39.9	≥40
	50–69	≤12.9	13–20.9	21–32.9	33–36.9	≥37

From a physiologic perspective, 4 to 7 days probably provides sufficient time to achieve maximum muscle and liver glycogen replenishment, optimal nutritional support and restoration, minimal residual muscle soreness, and quality healing of minor injuries.

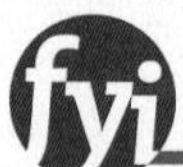

Determine Your "Fitness Age"

Data from Norwegian research at the K.G. Jebsen Center for Exercise in Medicine at the Norwegian University of Science and Technology, Trondheim, Norway, provide a low-tech method to estimate "fitness age (**www.ntnu.edu/cerg/fitness-numbers**)." Nearly 5000 men and women ages 20 to 90 were evaluated on a diverse set of variables including peak oxygen uptake to determine the best combination to predict aerobic capacity without maximal or near-maximal testing. These variables, entered into a simple formula, reliably predicted aerobic capacity to indicate "**fitness age**." For example, a 50-year-old with a peak oxygen uptake of a 70-year-old would have a fitness age of 70.

The following measures are required to estimate fitness age: resting heart rate measured after 10 minutes of quiet sitting, height, weight, waist girth, age, gender, estimated maximum heart rate, and frequency and intensity of physical activity. An online calculator is available at **www.worldfitnesslevel.org/determines fitness age.**

Source: Loe H, et al. Aerobic capacity reference data in 3816 healthy men and women 20–90 years. *PLoS ONE* 2013;8:5e64319 (**www.plosone.org/article/info%3Adoi%2F10.1371%2Fjournal.pone.0064319**).

Tapering for Peak Performance

During a competitive season, one should expect little improvement in the aerobic systems. At best, athletes must strive to prevent physiologic and performance deteriorations during this time. Before major competitions, athletes often reduce or **taper** training intensity, volume, or both, believing that such adjustments lead to peak performance. Unfortunately, generalizations about an optimal taper are not possible because each sport has its unique characteristics concerning the optimal taper interval. Thus, no clear answers exist about optimum taper duration or training modification.

FORMULATING AN AEROBIC TRAINING PROGRAM

This section presents guidelines for initiating aerobic training and describes a method to gauge and adjust training intensity. We also discuss advantages and possible limitations of intermittent and continuous aerobic training procedures.

General Guidelines

Regardless of present physiologic fitness, some basic research-based and commonsense guidelines provide the important element of structure when initiating an aerobic training program:

- **Start slowly.** Injuries often occur when initiating vigorous activity following years of sedentary living. Minor muscle aches and joint pain normally follow the start of a physical activity program, particularly with eccentric muscle actions (see Chapter 14). Severe muscular discomfort and excessive cardiovascular strain offer no additional training benefits; excessive fatigue frequently discourages beginners from continuing a regular physical conditioning program.
- **Allow a "warm-up" period.** Mild stretching and aerobic physical activity such as running in place, treadmill jogging, rope skipping, rowing, calisthenics, or stationary cycling for 5 to 10 minutes provide an adequate muscular and cardiovascular warm-up immediately before the aerobic workout phase. Rhythmic, moderate-intensity activity at a heart rate between 50% and 60% of maximum maintains optimal coronary blood flow for more favorable myocardial oxygenation.
- **Allow a "cool-down" recovery period.** Following the training phase, slow down gradually before stopping to allow metabolism to progress toward resting levels. A gradual cool down prevents blood from pooling in the large veins of the previously active muscles. Venous pooling could decrease blood pressure and reduce blood flow to the heart and brain, producing dizziness, nausea, and sometimes fainting. Reduced blood flow to the myocardium often precipitates a series of irregular heartbeats that could trigger a catastrophic cardiac episode.

Guidelines for Children

Children are not small adults. Children's physical activity programs should be general in nature compared with specific formulations used for adults. Guidelines from the National Association for Sport and Physical Education (**http://www.playgroundprofessionals.com/encyclopedia/n/national-association-sport-and-physical-education**) recommend the following:

1. Accumulate more than 60 minutes and up to several hours daily of age- and developmentally appropriate activities for elementary schoolchildren.
2. Some of the child's physical activity each day should be in blocks lasting 15 minutes or longer and include large muscle, rhythmic moderate to vigorous aerobic activity performed intermittently with brief rest and recovery periods.
3. Extended periods of inactivity (i.e., spending hours playing computer games and watching TV) are *not* appropriate for normal, healthy growing children.
4. Elementary schoolchildren should participate *regularly* in a variety of physical activities of various intensity levels.

Children's Cardiorespiratory Fitness Standards

A valid method to evaluate cardiorespiratory fitness in children uses time to complete a 1-mile walk-run. **Table 13.3** presents upper and lower end standards for the Healthy

TABLE 13.3 Standards for the Healthy Fitness Zone for 1-Mile Walk-Run Times and $\dot{V}O_{2max}$[a] for Children Ages 10 to 17 Years

Age	1-Mile Run Time (min:s)		$\dot{V}O_{2max}$ (mL · kg^{-1} · min^{-1})	
	Boys[b]	Girls[b]	Boys[b]	Girls[b]
10	11:30–9:00	12:30–9:30	42–52	39–47
11	11:00–8:30	12:00–9:00	42–52	38–46
12	10:30–8:00	12:00–9:00	42–52	37–45
13	10:00–7:30	11:30–9:00	42–52	36–44
14	9:30–7:00	11:00–8:30	42–52	35–43
15	9:00–7:00	10:30–8:00	42–52	35–43
16	8:30–7:00	10:00–8:00	42–52	35–43
17	8:30–7:00	10:00–8:00	42–52	35–43

[a] $\dot{V}O_{2max}$, maximal oxygen uptake.

[b] Number on left = lower end of Healthy Fitness Zone; number on right = upper end of Health Fitness Zone.

Source: From The Cooper Institute. *FITNESSGRAM/ACTIVITYGRAM Test Administration Manual*. 4th Ed. Champaign: Human Kinetics, 2007.

Fitness Zone consistent with good health for $\dot{V}O_{2max}$ and 1-mile times for different age children.

Setting fitness standards for children requires careful attention. The $\dot{V}O_{2max}$ expressed in $mL \cdot kg^{-1} \cdot min^{-1}$ remains relatively stable or decreases slightly between ages 5 and 19; walk-run performance almost doubles from growth and development and improved movement economy during this period; for example, a 12-year-old child completes a mile twice as fast as a 5-year-old. Also, $\dot{V}O_{2max}$ improves only slightly for children who undergo aerobic training, but performance considerably increases. This raises the question of whether aerobic capacity or performance represents the "best" expression of cardiorespiratory fitness in children and its improvement with training.

Applying a single mathematical equation to predict $\dot{V}O_{2max}$ based on a walk-run test in children poses problems because of continually increasing levels of running economy as children age. Variations in movement economy alter the relationship between aerobic fitness and running performance through all stages of growth and development.

ESTABLISHING TRAINING INTENSITY

What represents a considerable aerobic stress for a sedentary person falls below an elite athlete's threshold training intensity. Consequently, training intensity must be assessed relative to the stress it places on a person's aerobic system. Within this framework, one could justifiably maintain that three individuals performing their best marathon times of 2.5, 3.0, and 4.0 hours experience equivalent levels of physiologic stress despite large variations in running speed.

Train at a Percentage of $\dot{V}O_{2max}$

An individual can train at a percentage of $\dot{V}O_{2max}$ determined directly in the laboratory or estimated from intensity. For example, if an individual running at 5.5 mph requires an oxygen uptake of 33 $mL \cdot kg^{-1} \cdot min^{-1}$ and $\dot{V}O_{2max}$ equals 60 $mL \cdot kg^{-1} \cdot min^{-1}$, the exercise represents a stress of 55% of aerobic capacity. For another individual with a lower $\dot{V}O_{2max}$ of 40 $mL \cdot kg^{-1} \cdot min^{-1}$, the oxygen cost of running at 5.5 mph still requires 33 $mL \cdot kg^{-1} \cdot min^{-1}$, yet this person must exercise at 83% of maximum. To provide a similar overload intensity of 83% of $\dot{V}O_{2max}$ for the first jogger, the pace must increase to a speed requiring 48 mL O_2 $mL \cdot kg^{-1} \cdot min^{-1}$ or 8.6 mph.

Train at Percentage of Maximum Heart Rate

Assessing intensity accurately by direct measurement of oxygen uptake requires extensive laboratory measurements. A more practical alternative uses heart rate to classify intensity and individualizes aerobic training to keep pace as fitness improves. This approach applies the well-established relationship between percentage $\dot{V}O_{2max}$ and percentage HR_{max}.

The error averages about ±8% in estimating percentage $\dot{V}O_{2max}$ from percentage HR_{max}, or vice versa. Applying this intrinsic relationship, one needs only to monitor heart rate to estimate percentage $\dot{V}O_{2max}$. *Among healthy subjects, the relationship between percentage $\dot{V}O_{2max}$ and percentage HR_{max} remains the same for arm or leg activity in normal weight and overweight groups, cardiac patients, and those with spinal cord injuries.* Importantly, a lower HR_{max} occurs in upper-body arm compared with lower body leg activity; one must consider this difference in formulating the physical activity prescription for different modes (see A Closer Look: "Predicting Maximum Heart Rate and the Training-Sensitive Zone" earlier in this chapter).

To train at a percentage of HR_{max} requires knowledge of the heart rate during near-maximal effort. Three or 4 minutes of all-out running or swimming elicits HR_{max} values. Such intense activity requires considerable motivation and endangers those predisposed to coronary heart disease. For this reason, *predicting* HR_{max} has become standard practice. The following presents the most common formula (but not necessarily the most valid) to estimate maximum heart rate:

$$\mathbf{HR_{max} = 220 - age\ (y)}$$

Research suggests substantial individual differences using this method when applied to all individuals. Formulae

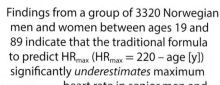

fyi A More Accurate Heart Rate Prediction Formula for Men and Women of Diverse Ages

Findings from a group of 3320 Norwegian men and women between ages 19 and 89 indicate that the traditional formula to predict HR_{max} (HR_{max} = 220 – age [y]) significantly *underestimates* maximum heart rate in senior men and women, with inaccuracies emerging at age 30 to 40 years. A more appropriate formula-tion for both sexes estimates maximum heart rate as 211 minus 64% of age. Thus, for a 70-year-old man or woman, the more appropriate estimate of maximum heart rate would = 166 beats a minute (211 – [0.64 × 70]) and not 150 beats a minute estimated by traditional formula. Although HR_{max} predicted by age alone regardless of formula may be practically convenient for various groups, its precision is limited and must be considered because the standard error of estimate approaches 10 beats a minute.

Source: Nes BM, et al. Age-predicted maximal heart rate in healthy subjects: the HUNT Fitness Study. *Scand J Med Sci Sports* 2013;23:697.

to predict HR_{max} results with less error are presented in A Closer Look: "Predicting Maximum Heart Rate and the Training-Sensitive Zone."

Effectiveness of Less-Intense Activity

Recommendation to train at 70% of HR_{max} for aerobic improvement represents a *general guideline* for a comfortable yet effective intensity. Twenty to 30 minutes of continuous activity at the 70% level stimulates a beneficial training effect; exercise at a lower intensity of 60% to 65% HR_{max} for 45 minutes also proves beneficial. *In general, longer duration offsets lower intensity, particularly for older and less fit individuals.* Regardless of activity level, more is not necessarily better because excessive activity increases the chance for sustaining bone, joint, and muscle injuries.

fyi Structured Physical Activity and High-Intensity Training Not Required for Health Benefits

The way you spend your free time profoundly affects the quality of life and the length of time lived. Research from Karolinska University Hospital in Stockholm followed 4232 men and women with an average age of 60. At the start of the study, nonexercise physical activity and exercise habits were assessed from a self-administrated questionnaire, and cardiovascular health established through physical examinations and laboratory tests. Over the next 12.5 years, 383 of the participants died from all causes and 476 suffered a fatal or nonfatal first-time cardiovascular event. As expected, those who engaged regularly in moderate- to high-intensity structured physical activity showed the highest survival level. However, those seniors involved in active leisure time had a greater survival rate than less active leisure time counterparts. Those involved in "active leisure" showed a 30% lower risk for all-cause mortality and 27% lower likelihood of suffering a cardiovascular event. Active leisure seniors also had smaller waist girths and more desirable blood lipid profiles. Men had better insulin and blood sugar levels than individuals who devoted their leisure time to sedentary pursuits. These findings support the wisdom of keeping physically active throughout life with either formal structured physical activity or varied leisure time pursuits, including popular gardening and hobby activities.

Source: Ekblom-Bak E, et al. The importance of non-exercise physical activity for cardiovascular health and longevity. *Br J Sports Med* 2014;48:233.

Train at a Perception of Effort

A psychophysiologic approach uses the **rating of perceived exertion (RPE)** as an indicator of intensity. With this approach, the exerciser rates on a numerical scale, sometimes called the Borg scale after Swedish researcher Gunnar Borg (**http://w3.psychology.su.se/staff/gbg/**) who developed the first of these scaling systems concerning perceived feelings relative to exertion level. Monitoring and adjusting RPE during physical activity provide an effective strategy to prescribe activities based on an individual's perception of effort that coincides with objective measures of physiologic or metabolic strain (%HR_{max}, %$\dot{V}O_{2max}$, blood lactate concentration). Activity levels corresponding to higher levels of energy expenditure and physiologic strain produce higher RPE ratings. For example, an RPE of 13 or 14 (activity that feels "somewhat hard"; **Fig. 13.16**) coincides with about 70% HR_{max} during cycle ergometer and treadmill activity; an RPE between 11 and 12 corresponds to physical activity at LT for trained and untrained individuals. Individuals learn quickly to exercise at a specific RPE. In this sense, the axiom "listen to your body" becomes apropos.

Lactate Threshold Training

Exercising at or slightly above the **lactate threshold (LT)**, particularly for more fit individuals, provides effective aerobic training with higher physical activity levels producing the greatest benefits. **Figure 13.17** illustrates how to determine the appropriate physical activity level by plotting intensity versus blood lactate level. In this example, the

RPE Scale	Equivalent % HR_{max}	Equivalent % $\dot{V}O_{2max}$
6		
7 Very, very light		
8		
9 Very light		
10		
11 Fairly light	52–66	31–50
12		
13 Somewhat hard	61–85	51–75
14		
15 Hard	86–91	76–85
16		
17 Very hard	92	85
18		
19 Very, very hard		

FIGURE 13.16 The Borg scale (and accompanying estimates of relative physical activity intensity) for obtaining the RPE during physical activity. (Adapted with permission from Borg GA. Psychological basis of physical exertion. *Med Sci Sports Exerc* 1982;14:377.)

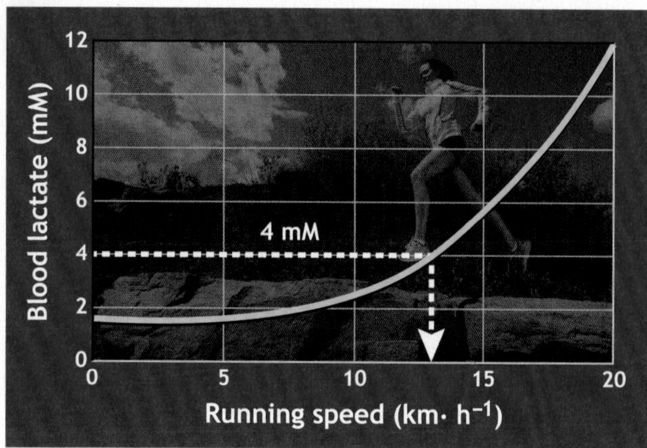

FIGURE 13.17 Blood lactate concentration in relation to running speed for one subject. At a lactate level of 4.0 mM, the corresponding running speed was approximately 13 km · h^{-1}. This speed establishes the subject's initial training intensity.

running speed that produced a blood lactate concentration at the 4-mM level or OBLA represented the recommended training intensity. Many coaches use the 4-mM blood lactate level as the optimal aerobic training intensity, yet no convincing evidence exists to justify this particular blood lactate level as most "ideal."

Regardless of the specific blood lactate level chosen for endurance training, the blood lactate–exercise intensity relationship should be evaluated periodically, with activity intensity adjusted to meet aerobic fitness improvements. If regular blood lactate measurement proves impractical, heart rate at the initial lactate determination remains a convenient and relatively stable marker for setting the appropriate predetermined intensity of effort. This notion is tenable because during incremental physical activity, no systematic training-induced change occurs in the heart rate–blood lactate relationship.

One important distinction between $\%HR_{max}$ and LT to establish training intensity rests with the physiologic dynamics each method reflects. The $\%HR_{max}$ method establishes a level of activity stress to overload the central circulation (e.g., stroke volume, cardiac output). The LT method places emphasis on peripheral vasculature and active muscles to sustain an aerobic metabolic steady-rate level.

TRAINING METHODS

Performance improvements occur each year in almost all athletic competitions. These advances generally relate to increased opportunities for participation; individuals with "natural endowment" more likely participate in particular sports. Also, improved nutrition and healthcare, better equipment, and more systematic and scientific approaches to athletic training contribute to superior performance. The following sections present general guidelines for anaerobic and aerobic training.

Anaerobic Training

The capacity to perform all-out physical activity for up to 60 seconds largely depends on ATP generated by the immediate and short-term anaerobic energy transfer systems (see **Fig. 13.1**).

Intramuscular High-Energy Phosphates

Football, weightlifting, and other brief, sprint-power sport activities rely exclusively on energy from ATP and PCr, the muscles' high-energy phosphates. Engaging performance-specific muscles in repeated 5- to 10-second maximum bursts of effort overloads this phosphagen pool. The intramuscular high-energy phosphates supply energy for intense but brief physical activity, so little lactate accumulates and recovery progresses rapidly. Thus, activity can begin again after about a 30-second rest. Brief, all-out physical activity interspersed with recovery represents a specific application of the interval training principle for anaerobic conditioning.

Activities selected to enhance ATP-PCr energy transfer capacity must engage the specific muscles at the movement speed and power output for which the athlete desires improved anaerobic power as dictated by the *specificity principle*. Not only does this enhance the metabolic capacity of the specifically trained muscle fibers, it also facilitates recruitment and modulation of the appropriate motor unit firing sequence activated in the movement.

Lactate-Generating Capacity

As the duration of maximal effort extends beyond 10 seconds, dependence on anaerobic energy from intramuscular high-energy phosphates decreases, with a proportionate increase in anaerobic energy transfer from anaerobic glycolysis. To improve energy transfer capacity by the short-term lactic acid energy system, training must overload this specific aspect of energy metabolism.

Anaerobic training to improve lactate-generating capacity requires extreme physiologic demands and considerable motivation. Repeated bouts of up to 1-minute maximum activity stopped 30 seconds before subjective feelings of exhaustion cause blood lactate to increase to their near-maximum levels. The individual repeats each bout following 3 to 5 minutes of recovery. Repetition of an activity causes **"lactate stacking,"** resulting in a higher blood lactate level than with just one exhaustive effort bout. As with all training regimens, exercise the specific muscle groups that require enhanced lactate-producing capacity. A backstroke swimmer should train by swimming the backstroke, a cyclist should bicycle, and basketball, hockey, or soccer players should perform movements and direction changes similar to those required by their sport.

Prolonged Recovery Following Anaerobic Physical Activity

Considerable recovery time occurs with intense physical activity that elevates core temperature, disrupts internal equilibrium, and elevates blood lactate. For this reason, intervals of anaerobic training should occur at the end of a workout. Otherwise, fatigue from training carries over and could hinder ability to perform subsequent aerobic training.

Aerobic Training: Continuous Versus Intermittent Methods

Relatively brief bouts of repeated activity, including continuous, long-duration efforts, enhance aerobic capacity provided the activity attains sufficient intensity to overload the aerobic system. **Continuous training, interval training,** and **fartlek training** represent three common methods to improve aerobic fitness.

Continuous Training

Continuous **long slow-distance (LSD) training** requires sustained, steady-rate aerobic activity. Because of its submaximal nature, physical activity continues for considerable time in relative comfort. This makes LSD training ideal for people just starting a conditioning program or wanting to enhance calorie output to reduce excess body fat. *The greatest health-related benefits of physical activity emerge when a person moves from a sedentary lifestyle to one that incorporates only a moderate level of continuous aerobic activity.* LSD training generally progresses at the relatively comfortable threshold intensity of 70% HR_{max}. It also can remain effective at the 85% or 90% level.

Endurance athletes overload the cardiovascular and energy transfer systems using continuous physical activity training at nearly the same intensity as competition. In sustained physical activity, this specifically activates slow-twitch muscle fibers. A champion middle-distance runner may run 5 miles continuously in 25 minutes during workouts at a heart rate of 180 $b \cdot min^{-1}$; this pace does not exhaust the athlete yet nearly duplicates race conditions. By finishing each session with several all-out sprints stopped 30 to 40 seconds before exhaustion, the athlete also trains the short-term glycolytic-anaerobic energy system that contributes to race performance, particularly at the finish. A marathon runner trains at a slightly slower pace than a middle-distance athlete to simulate the intensity, distance, and energy requirements of actual competition.

Interval Training

Periods of intense activity interspersed with moderate- to low-energy expenditure characterize many sport and life activities. Interval training simulates this variation in energy transfer intensity through regular spacing of activity and rest periods. With this approach, a person trains at an inordinately high intensity with minimal fatigue that would normally prove exhausting if done continuously. Rest-to-exercise intervals vary from a few seconds to several minutes depending on the energy system(s) overloaded. Four factors formulate the interval training prescription:

1. Intensity of interval
2. Duration of interval
3. Duration of recovery interval
4. Repetitions of recovery interval

One-Minute Bouts of Intense Physical Activity Improve Both Fitness and Health

Is the real question how much physical activity we need for improved health and fitness or rather how little is required?

To answer the question, Canadian researchers studied two groups of volunteers, one consisting of sedentary but healthy middle-aged men and women and the other consisting of middle-aged and older patients with diagnosed cardiovascular disease. Initial testing quantified HR_{max} and peak power output on a stationary bicycle with a relatively low starting resistance to pedaling. Participants then trained using repetitive short bursts of **high-intensity interval**

A CLOSER LOOK

A Typical Aerobic Physical Activity Session

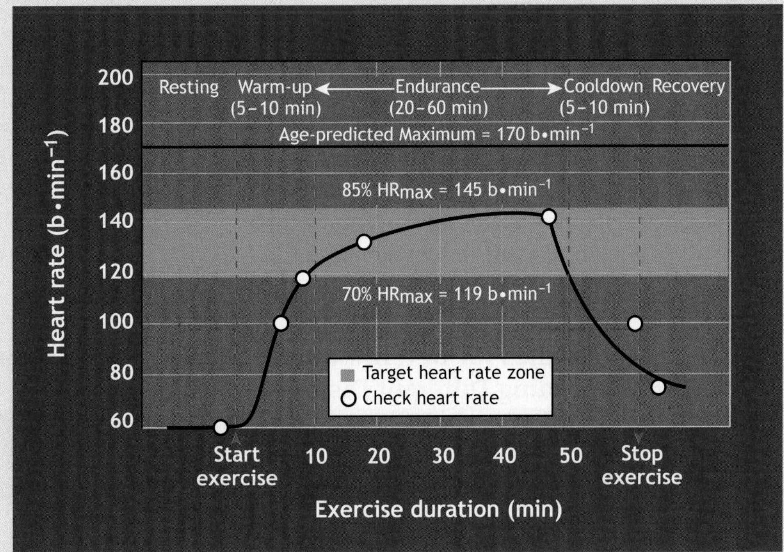

The figure above illustrates a typical aerobic training session for a 50-year-old woman. The session begins with a 5- to 10-minute warm-up period of light to moderate walking or jogging in place with a heart rate at about 120 $b \cdot min^{-1}$. This continues with the conditioning phase (30- to 60-min) with exercise heart rates within 70% to 85% of the age-predicted maximal heart rate. A 5- to 10-minute cool-down period follows as intensity exponentially declines toward the resting level.

training (HIIT). This routine involved 1-minute activity bouts at about 90% of HR_{max} followed by 1 minute of easy recovery with 10 total intervals of activity and recovery, for total workout time lasting only 20 minutes. Participants, particularly the cardiac patients, significantly improved overall health and cardiovascular fitness. The interesting finding was that all participants embraced the routine despite their ratings of perceived exertion during each activity bout at 7 or higher on a 10-point scale. Previous investigations with HIIT have demonstrated increases in the cellular proteins involved in energy transfer (i.e., mitochondrial biogenesis and increased glucose and fatty acid oxidation capacity) via aerobic processes, improved insulin sensitivity, and blood sugar regulation, which reduced type 2 diabetes risk.

Rationale for Interval Training

Running continuously at a 4-minute mile pace exhausts most people within a minute because of rapid lactate accumulation. Running at this speed for only 15 seconds followed by a 30-second rest period enables a person to accomplish 4 minutes of running at this near record pace. This does not equate to a 4-minute mile, but during 4 minutes of running, the person covers a 1-mile distance although the combined activity and rest intervals require 11 minutes and 30 seconds.

A sound rationale forms the basis for interval training. In the example of a continuous run by an average person at a 4-minute mile pace, the predominant energy comes from the short-term anaerobic energy pathway with rapid lactate accumulation. The individual becomes exhausted within 60 to 90 seconds. In contrast, running at this speed for 15-second intervals or less places significant demands on the immediate intramuscular ATP and PCr energy system without much lactate accumulation. Repetitively linking specific activity and rest intervals as part of interval training eventually places considerable demand on aerobic energy metabolism.

In interval training, as with other forms of physiologic conditioning, intensity must overload the specific energy system(s) desired for improvement through sport-specific muscle activation. **Table 13.4** outlines a practical method to determine intensity for interval training in running and swimming.

No one method has proved superior for either continuous or interval training to improve aerobic fitness. Both methods probably can be applied interchangeably. Importantly, continuous LSD training gives the endurance athlete a more "task-specific" cardiovascular and metabolic overload that more closely mimic the duration and intensity of race conditions. Likewise, sprint and middle-distance athletes benefit from the intense metabolic demands and specific neuromuscular and fiber-type activation provided by interval training.

Formulating the Exercise: Relief Interval

Exercise Interval

- Add 1.5 to 5 seconds to the exerciser's "best time" for training distances between 60 and 220 yards for running and 15 and 55 yards for swimming. If a person covers 60 yards from a running start in 8 seconds, the duration for each repeat equals 8 + 1.5 or 9.5 seconds. Add 3 seconds to the best running time for interval training distances of 110 yards and 5 seconds to a distance of 220 yards. This particular application of interval training most effectively trains the anaerobic energy system's intramuscular high-energy phosphate component.
- For training distances of 440 yards running or 110 yards swimming, determine the exercise rate by subtracting 1 to 4 seconds from the average 440-yard portion of a mile run or 110-yard portion of a 440-yard swim. If a person runs a 7-minute mile (averaging 105 s per 440 yd), the interval time for each 440-yard repeat ranges between 104 (105 − 1) and 101 seconds (105 − 4).
- For run training intervals beyond 440 yards and swim intervals beyond 110 yards, add 3 to 4 seconds to the average 440-yard portion of a mile run or 110-yard portion of a 440-yard swim. In running an 880-yard interval, the 7-minute miler runs each interval in about 216 seconds ([105 + 3] × 2 = 216).

TABLE 13.4 Guidelines for Determining Interval Training Intensities for Running and Swimming Different Distances

Interval Training Distances (Yards)		Work Rate for Each Activity Interval or Repeat	
Run	**Swim**		
55 110 220	15 25 55	1.5 3.0 5.0	Seconds *slower* than best times from running or swimming start for each distance
440	110	1–4 s *faster* than the average run or 110-yard swim time during 1-mile run or 440-yard swim	
660–1320	165–320	3–4 s *slower* than average 440-yard run or 100-yard swim time during 1-mile run or 440-yard swim	

Source: From Fox EL, Matthews DK. *Interval Training*. Philadelphia: W. B. Saunders, 1974.

Relief Interval

- The relief or recovery interval occurs either passively, called *rest to relief*, or actively, called *exercise to relief*. Recovery duration represents a multiple of the exercise interval. A 1:3 ratio overloads the immediate energy system. For a sprinter who runs 10-s intervals, the relief interval equals 30 seconds. For training the short-term glycolytic energy system, the relief interval doubles (ratio of 1:2). In this case, a 2-minute recovery follows a 1-minute run or swim. These specified ratios for the exercise-to-relief interval for training allow sufficient restoration of high-energy phosphates and lactate removal so subsequent activity proceeds with minimal fatigue.
- For training the long-term aerobic energy system, the exercise-to-relief interval usually equals 1:1 or 1:1.5. During a 60- to 90-second activity interval, for example, oxygen uptake increases rapidly to a relatively high level. Although some lactate accumulates during this relatively intense bout, the duration remains brief enough to prevent exhaustion. A 1- to 2-minute recovery allows activity to begin again before oxygen uptake returns to its pre-exercise level. Consecutive repeat exercise:relief intervals ensure that cardiovascular response and aerobic metabolism eventually maintain near-maximal levels throughout exercise and recovery. Performing continuously at this intensity exhausts the person within several minutes, causing training to cease.

Fartlek Training

Fartlek means "speed play" in Swedish. Fartlek training was developed in 1937 by Gösta Holmér (1891–1983). Holmér, the Swedish national track coach, based his training system after the incomparable and perhaps greatest runner of all time, Finnish world champion, and multiple Olympic gold medal winner, "The Flying Finn," Paavo Nurmi (1897–1973; **http://paavonurmi.fi/en/**). During his three Olympic Games from 1920 to 1928, Nurmi (5′9″ [1.74 m] and 143 lb [65 kg]) won nine gold and three silver medals. He also established 22 official world records at distances ranging between 1500 m and 20 km. In addition, at one point in his illustrious career, he held the world record in the mile, 5000 m, and 10,000 m races simultaneously. Nurmi was one of the first world-class athletes to apply systematic training regimens, particularly using a companion stopwatch during his runs to develop optimal pacing strategies combined with speed work. During the Nurmi era, many runners relied on self-developed methods to create a crudely blended mix of interval and continuous training introduced to the United States in the early 1940s. These methods were particularly suited to out-of-doors physical activity over natural terrain. The system used alternate running at fast and slow speeds over both level and hilly landscape.

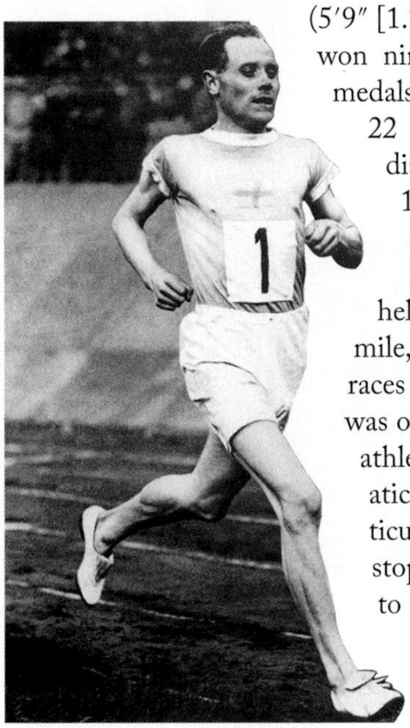

Fartlek training workouts do not require systematic manipulation of exercise and relief intervals, in contrast to the precise physical activity and rest sequences prescribed in interval training. In fartlek training, the performer determines the training schema based on "how it feels" at the time, in a way similar to gauging physical activity intensity based on one's rating of perceived exertion. If used properly, this method will overload one or all of the energy transfer systems. Fartlek training provides ideal general conditioning and off-season training methods but lacks the systematic, quantified approaches of interval and continuous training.

THE OVERTRAINING SYNDROME

Ten to 20% of athletes experience **overtraining syndrome** or "staleness." With this condition, an athlete can fail to endure and adapt to training so that normal performance deteriorates and the athlete encounters increasing difficulty fully recovering from a workout. This takes on added significance for elite athletes for whom performance decrements of less than 1% can cause a gold medalist to fail to qualify for competition. Stated somewhat differently, a 1% *improvement* in performance will make the difference between a gold and silver medal—or no medal at all.

Two clinical forms of overtraining exist:

1. The less common **sympathetic form** characterizes by increased sympathetic activity during rest and generally typified by hyperexcitability, restlessness, and impaired performance. This form reflects excessive psychological or emotional stress that accompanies the interaction among training, competition, and responsibilities of normal living.
2. The more common **parasympathetic form** characterizes by predominance of vagal activity during rest and exertion. More properly termed **overreaching** in the early stages within as few as 10 days, the syndrome is qualitatively similar in symptoms to the full-blown parasympathetic overtraining syndrome but of shorter duration. Excessive and protracted physical overload with inadequate recovery and rest causes overreaching. Initially, just to maintain performance requires greater effort, which eventually leads to performance deterioration in training and competition. A few days up to 2 weeks of rest usually eliminates overreaching and reestablishes full function. Untreated overreaching eventually progresses to the overtraining syndrome.

Symptoms of Overtraining and Staleness

Common overtraining characteristics include the following:

1. Unexplained and persistently poor athletic performance and substantial fatigue

2. Prolonged recovery from typical training sessions or competitive events
3. Disturbed mood states characterized by general fatigue, apathy, depression, irritability, and loss of competitive drive
4. Persistent muscle and joint soreness and stiffness
5. Elevated resting pulse and increased susceptibility to upper respiratory tract infections and gastrointestinal disturbances
6. Insomnia
7. Loss of appetite, weight loss, and inability to maintain ideal body weight for competition
8. Overuse injuries

No simple, reliable method can diagnose overtraining in its earliest stages. The best indications include deterioration in physical performance and alterations in mood rather than changes in immune function.

PHYSICAL ACTIVITY AND TRAINING DURING PREGNANCY

Forty percent or more of women in the United States participate in different forms of physical activity during pregnancy. **Figure 13.18** illustrates the prevalence and pattern of different activities during pregnancy between pregnant and nonpregnant women. Nonpregnant women were more likely to meet the moderate or vigorous physical activity recommendations than nonpregnant counterparts. For both groups, walking represented the most common activity (52% for pregnant and 45% for nonpregnant). Pregnant women who engaged in either moderate or vigorous physical activity were generally younger, non-Hispanic white, unmarried, more educated, and nonsmokers and had higher incomes than less physically active counterparts.

During pregnancy, walking, swimming, and aerobics are the most popular physical activities. Older mothers who delivered more than one child or had previous children, and unfavorable reproductive histories, are less likely to exercise during pregnancy.

Energy Cost and Physiologic Demands of Physical Activity

Cardiovascular responses during physical activity during pregnancy follow normal patterns. An uncomplicated pregnancy offers no greater physiologic strain to the mother during moderate exertion other than provided by the additional weight gain and the possible encumbrance of fetal tissue. Increases in maternal body mass add considerably to physical effort in weight-bearing walking, jogging, and stair climbing.

Fetal Blood Supply

Any factor that might compromise fetal blood supply raises medical concern regarding physical activity during pregnancy. Studies of uterine blood flow during physical exertion in various mammalian species indicate that healthy animals maintain adequate oxygen supply to the developing fetus during moderate to intense maternal physical activity.

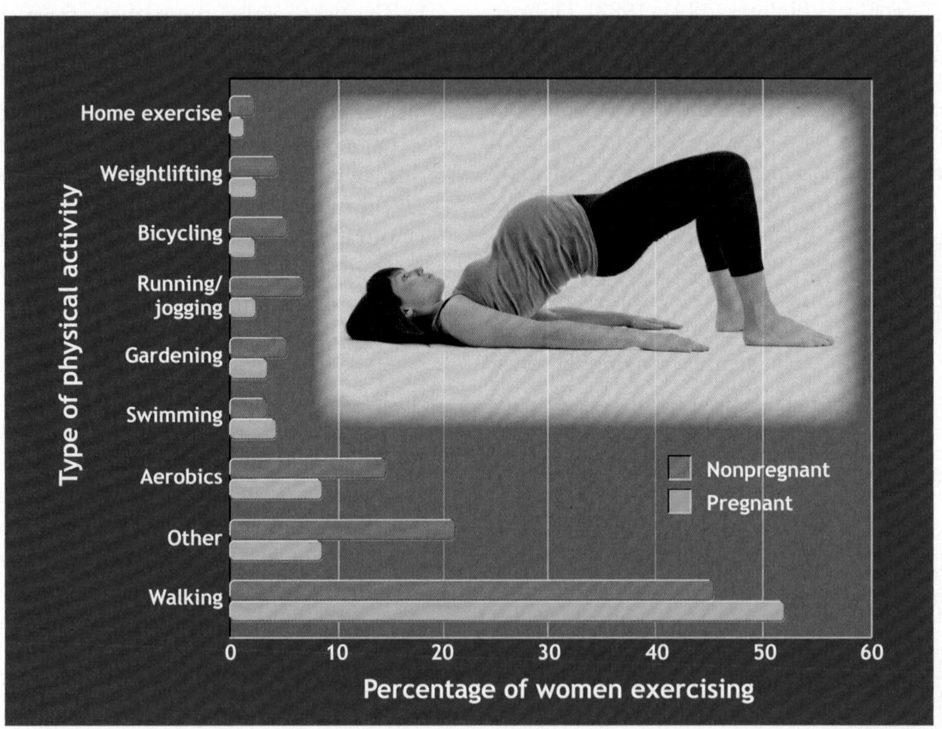

FIGURE 13.18 Common physical activities among pregnant and nonpregnant women (1994, 1996, 1998, and 2000 data combined). (Reprinted with permission from McArdle WD, Katch FI, Katch VL. *Exercise Physiology: Nutrition, Energy, and Human Performance*. 8th Ed. Baltimore: Wolters Kluwer Health, 2015; as reprinted with permission from Petersen AM, et al. Correlates of physical activity among pregnant women in the United States. *Med Sci Sports Exerc* 2005;37:1748.)

Physical activity participation probably diverts some blood from the uterus and visceral organs for preferential distribution to active muscles; as such, intense effort could pose a hazard to a fetus with restricted placental blood flow. In addition, elevated maternal core temperature hinders heat dissipation from the fetus through the placenta. Maternal hyperthermia negatively affects fetal development (e.g., increased risk for neural tube defect) early in pregnancy. During warmer weather in late spring, summer, and early fall, physical activity should take place in the cooler part of the day and for shorter intervals while the individual maintains regular fluid intake.

Current medical opinion maintains that 30 or 40 minutes of moderate aerobic activity by a previously active, healthy, low-risk woman during an uncomplicated pregnancy does not compromise fetal oxygen supply and acid-base status or produce other adverse effects to mother or fetus. Performed regularly, moderate physical activity maintains cardiovascular fitness with the added benefit of producing a beneficial training effect.

Fourteen Exercise Contraindications During Pregnancy

1. Pregnancy-induced hypertension
2. Preterm rupture of membranes
3. Preterm labor during the prior or current pregnancy
4. Incompetent cervix
5. Persistent second- to third-trimester bleeding
6. Intrauterine growth retardation
7. Type 1 diabetes
8. History of two or more spontaneous abortions
9. Multiple pregnancy
10. Smoking
11. Excessive alcohol intake
12. History of premature labor
13. Anemia
14. Excessive obesity

Pregnancy Course and Outcome

No overall consensus previously existed on whether regular physical activity enhanced the course of pregnancy, including labor, delivery, and outcome. Current data now support a recommendation for regular, moderate physical activity during pregnancy, even after the first trimester. In many ways, maternal physiologic responses and adaptations to activity beneficially interact with physiologic changes in pregnancy.

Regular aerobic physical activity throughout pregnancy accomplishes the following:

1. Reduces birth weight
2. Reduces birth weight percentile
3. Reduces the offspring's calculated percentage body fat and fat mass

Follow-up studies of children whose mothers remained regularly active during the second and third trimesters indicated these children maintained similar height and head girth. They also weighed less and had significantly lower sum of five skinfolds and lower upper-arm fat than children of sedentary women. The offspring of active mothers had higher scores on intelligence tests, including superior oral language skills. Benefits to fetal neurologic development and increased mental capacity have linked to one or more of the following five factors for providing the "stimulus" to create positive benefits associated with regular physical activity during pregnancy:

1. Intermittent stress
2. Vibration
3. Sound
4. Motion
5. Accelerated heartbeat

The offspring of physically active women did not show evidence of a comparative deficit in any area examined. These findings should reassure active women who chose to continue physical activity during an uncomplicated pregnancy.

SUMMARY

1. Activating a specific energy transfer system in exercise provides a way to classify different physical activities.
2. Effective training allocates time to overload the energy system(s) involved in the activity.
3. Intensity and duration largely determine anaerobic and aerobic energy transfer during physical activity.
4. During sprint-power activities, primary energy transfer involves the immediate and short-term energy systems.
5. The long-term aerobic system becomes progressively more important in activities longer than 2-minutes duration.
6. Proper training recognizes four principles for producing and maintaining optimum improvements: overload, specificity, individual differences, and reversibility.
7. Anaerobic training increases resting intramuscular anaerobic substrates and key glycolytic enzymes that typically increase all-out, sprint-power performance.
8. Aerobic training must overload both circulatory function and metabolic capacity of specific muscles.
9. Peripheral adaptations in active tissues exert substantial performance benefits.
10. Four major factors affecting aerobic training improvement include initial fitness level, frequency, duration, and intensity, the latter exerting the most profound influence.
11. Aerobic training adaptations to generate ATP aerobically include increased mitochondrial size and number, improved aerobic enzyme activity, greater trained muscle capillarization, and enhanced oxidation of fats during submaximal physical activity.
12. Functional and dimensional changes in the cardiovascular system induced by aerobic training include decreases in resting and submaximal heart rate, enlarged left ventricular cavity, enhanced stroke volume and cardiac output, and expanded $a\text{-}\bar{v}O_2$ difference.

13. Two ways to establish training intensity are (1) absolute basis and (2) relative basis geared to an individual's physiologic response.
14. Practical and effective methods to prescribe physical activity are based on percentage of HR_{max} (≥65% to 70% age-predicted HR_{max}), percentage of heart rate reserve, or rating of perceived exertion.
15. HR_{max} averages about 13 b · min^{-1} lower in upper-body arm cranking and swimming than in lower-body walking, running, cycling, and stair stepping.
16. At least 3 days a week represents optimal aerobic training frequency.
17. When intensity, duration, and frequency remain constant, similar training improvements occur regardless of training mode provided the evaluation test incorporates the training mode.
18. Prolonged and intense training can lead to overtraining or staleness with associated alterations in neuroendocrine and immune functions.
19. The overtraining syndrome includes chronic fatigue, poor performance, frequent infections, and general loss of interest in training.
20. Moderate aerobic physical activity by a previously active and healthy, low-risk woman during an uncomplicated pregnancy does not compromise fetal well-being and seldom produces adverse maternal effects.

THINK IT THROUGH

1. Discuss whether regular physical activity benefits a person, even if intensity of effort remains insufficient to stimulate a training effect.
2. Respond to the question, "How long must I train to 'get in shape'?"
3. What information is needed to develop an effective program to evaluate and improve aerobic capacity for firefighters, police officers, and oilfield workers?
4. A coach insists that a single activity mode improves aerobic capacity for all physical activities requiring a high level of aerobic fitness. Explain what you regard as the potential effectiveness of single-mode physical activity to produce generalized cross-training effects.

KEY TERMS

Aerobic system enzymes: Enzymes that catalyze the biochemical reactions in the aerobic synthesis of ATP (e.g., citric acid cycle and electron transport chain).

Concentric cardiac hypertrophy: Modest thickening of left ventricular walls when adding new sarcomeres without significant overall heart enlargement.

Continuous training: Physical training involving steady-paced prolonged activity; usually performed continuously for 30 to 90 minutes at moderate or high aerobic intensity.

Conversational exercise: Physical activity of moderate intensity performed without discomfort, allowing individual to achieve sufficient intensity to stimulate a training effect yet not produce discomfort to prevent talking during the activity.

Detraining: Also referred to as "reversibility of training effects"; loss of physiologic and performance adaptations, which rapidly occur upon terminating participation in regular physical activity.

Eccentric cardiac hypertrophy: Cardiac enlargement characterized by increased left ventricular cavity size and generally related to increased volume overload.

Exercise training: Structured physical activity program designed to stimulate structural and functional adaptations to improve components of good health, anatomy and physiology, and performance in specific physical tasks.

Fartlek training: Relatively unscientific blending of interval and continuous training; applicable to activity out of doors over natural terrain, without requiring systematic manipulation of exercise and relief intervals but a training schema based on "how it feels" at the time.

Fitness age: Comparison of physiologic or performance capacity to determine how well the body functions physically relative to how well it works for the typical person of a given age.

High-intensity interval training (HIIT): Also termed high-intensity intermittent exercise (HIIE) or sprint interval training (SIT). An enhanced form of interval training that alternates periods of short intense anaerobic exercise with less-intense recovery periods.

Individual differences: Exercise training principle that all individuals do not respond similarly to a given training stimulus but vary as influenced by age, genetics, and initial fitness level.

Interval training: Exercise training involving low- to high-intensity physical activity interspersed with rest or relief periods.

Karvonen method: Method to establish the training threshold, which requires individuals to exercise at a heart rate at least equal to 60% of the difference between resting and maximum and expressed as $HR_{threshold} = HR_{rest} + 0.60 (HR_{max} - HR_{rest})$.

Lactate stacking: Training that causes blood lactate to rise to near-peak levels with a 1-minute maximum exercise bout repeated multiple times following 3 to 5 minutes of recovery.

Lactate threshold (LT): Maximum steady-rate effort maintained without lactate increasing above 4 mM.

Long slow-distance (LSD) training: Continuous exercise training involving steady-paced, prolonged activity over extended distances or durations at moderate or high aerobic intensity between 60 and 80% $\dot{V}O_{2max}$.

Nonresponders: Individuals who show little or no response to a training stimulus.

Overload: Exercising at intensities greater than normal, or manipulating training frequency, intensity, and duration (or their combination), induces a variety of highly specific adaptations so the body functions more efficiently.

Overreaching: Describes the early stages of the parasympathetic form of the overtraining syndrome, which can occur within 10 days.

Overtraining syndrome: Excessive and protracted physical overload with inadequate recovery and rest, which produces chronic fatigue, sustained poor exercise performance, altered sleep patterns and appetite, frequent infections, altered immune and reproductive functions, mood disturbances and general malaise, and loss of interest in high-level training.

Parasympathetic form: Most common overtraining form characterized by predominance of vagal activity during rest and physical activity.

Rating of perceived exertion (RPE): Method to prescribe exercise from an individual's perception of effort, which coincides with objective measures of physiologic/metabolic strain that includes $\%HR_{max}$, $\%\dot{V}O_{2max}$, and blood lactate concentration.

Responders: Individuals who show a high responsiveness to a training stimulus.

Reversibility of training effects: Loss of physiologic and performance adaptations, which rapidly occur upon terminating participation in regular physical activity.

SAID principle: Specific Adaptations to Imposed Demands, which embodies the specificity of training principle.

Sympathetic form: Less common form of overtraining; characterized by increased sympathetic activity during rest, with symptoms of general hyperexcitability, restlessness, and impaired exercise performance.

Taper: One- to 3-week reduced training intensity and/or volume prior to competition to minimize physiologic and performance deteriorations.

Training specificity: Highly task-specific adaptations in metabolic and physiologic systems that depend on the type of overload imposed and muscle mass activated.

SELECTED REFERENCES

Ade CJ, et al. Effects of body posture and exercise training on cardiorespiratory responses to exercise. *Respir Physiol Neurobiol* 2013;188:39.

American College of Sports Medicine. *Guidelines for Exercise Testing and Prescription*. 8th Ed. Baltimore: Lippincott Williams & Wilkins, 2010.

American College of Sports Medicine. American College of Sports Medicine: Position stand on the recommended quantity and quality of exercise for developing and maintaining cardiorespiratory and muscular fitness, and flexibility in healthy adults. *Med Sci Sports Exerc* 1998;30:975.

Arbab-Zadeh A, et al. Cardiac remodeling in response to 1 year of intensive endurance training. *Circulation* 2014;130:2152.

Ashor AW, et al. Exercise modalities and endothelial function: a systematic review and dose-response meta-analysis of randomized controlled trials. *Sports Med* 2015;45:279.

Babaei P, et al. Effect of six weeks of endurance exercise and following detraining on serum brain derived neurotrophic factor and memory performance in middle aged males with metabolic syndrome. *J Sports Med Phys Fitness* 2013;53:437.

Bergouignan A, et al. Activity energy expenditure is a major determinant of dietary fat oxidation and trafficking, but the deleterious effect of detraining is more marked than the beneficial effect of training at current recommendations. *Am J Clin Nutr* 2013;98:648.

Binnie MJ, et al. Effect of surface-specific training on 20 m sprint performance on sand and grass surfaces. *J Strength Cond Res* 2013;27:3515.

Borg GA. Psychological basis of physical exertion. *Med Sci Sports Exerc* 1982;14:377.

Bosquet L, et al. Effects of tapering on performance: a meta-analysis. *Med Sci Sports Exerc* 2006;39:1358.

Bouchard C, et al. Genetics of aerobic and anaerobic performance. *Exerc Sport Sci Rev* 1992;20:27.

Bray SR, et al. Self-control training leads to enhanced cardiovascular exercise performance. *J Sports Sci* 2014;3:1.

Buchheit M, Laursen PB. High-intensity interval training, solutions to the programming puzzle. Part II: anaerobic energy, neuromuscular load and practical applications. *Sports Med* 2013;43:927.

Christensen B, et al. Whole body metabolic effects of prolonged endurance training in combination with erythropoietin treatment in humans: a randomized placebo controlled study. *Am J Physiol Endocrinol Metab* 2013;305:E879.

Church TS, et al. Effects of different doses of physical activity on cardiorespiratory fitness among sedentary, overweight or obese postmenopausal women with elevated blood pressure: a randomized controlled trial. *JAMA* 2007;297:2081.

Coggan AR. Plasma glucose metabolism during exercise: effect of endurance training in humans. *Med Sci Sports Exerc* 1997;29:620.

Coyle EF. Very intense exercise-training is extremely potent and time efficient: a reminder. *J Appl Physiol* 2005;98:1983.

Diffee GM. Adaptation of cardiac myocyte contractile properties to exercise training. *Exerc Sport Sci Rev* 2004;32:112.

Dishman RK, et al. Neurobiology of exercise. *Obesity (Silver Spring)* 2006; 14:345. Review.

El-Lithy A, et al. Effect of aerobic exercise on premenstrual symptoms, haematological and hormonal parameters in young women. *J Obstet Gynaecol* 2014;3:1.

Eston RG, et al. The validity of predicting maximal oxygen uptake from a perceptually-regulated graded exercise test. *Eur J Appl Physiol* 2005;94:221.

Friedlander AL, et al. Training-induced alterations of carbohydrate metabolism in women: women respond differently than men. *J Appl Physiol* 1998;85:1175.

García-Pallarés J, et al. Physiological effects of tapering and detraining in world-class kayakers. *Med Sci Sports Exerc* 2010;42:1209.

Gellish RL, et al. Longitudinal modeling of the relationship between age and maximal heart rate. *Med Sci Sports Exerc* 2007;39:822.

Gibala MJ, McGee SL. Metabolic adaptations to short-term high-intensity interval training: a little pain for a lot of gain? *Exerc Sport Sci Rev* 2008;36:58.

Gibala MJ, et al. Physiological adaptations to low-volume, high-intensity interval training in health and disease. *J Physiol* 2012;590:1077.

Gillen JB, et al. Acute high-intensity interval exercise reduces the postprandial glucose response and prevalence of hyperglycaemia in patients with type 2 diabetes. *Diabetes Obes Metab* 2012;14:575.

Gist NH, et al. Sprint interval training effects on aerobic capacity: a systematic review and meta-analysis. *Sports Med* 2014;44:269.

Glowacki SP, et al. Effects of resistance, endurance, and concurrent exercise on training outcomes in men. *Med Sci Sports Exerc* 2004;36:2119.

González-Alonso J. Point: Counterpoint: Stroke volume does/does not decline during exercise at maximal effort in healthy individuals. *J Appl Physiol* 2008;104:275.

Gormley SE, et al. Effect of intensity of aerobic training on VO_{2max}. *Med Sci Sports Exerc* 2008;40:1336.

Hafstad AD, et al. High intensity interval training alters substrate utilization and reduces oxygen consumption in the heart. *J Appl Physiol* 2011;111:1235.

Haskell WL, et al. Physical activity and public health: updated recommendation for adults from the American College of Sports Medicine and the American Heart Association. *Med Sci Sports Exerc* 2007;39:1423.

Helgerud J, et al. Aerobic high-intensity intervals improve VO_{2max} more than moderate training. *Med Sci Sports Exerc* 2007;39:665.

Holloszy JO, Coyle EF. Adaptations of skeletal muscle to endurance exercise and their metabolic consequences. *J Appl Physiol* 1984;56:831.

Jacobs RA, et al. Improvements in exercise performance with high-intensity interval training coincide with an increase in skeletal muscle mitochondrial content and function. *J Appl Physiol* 2013;115:785.

Jakeman J, et al. Extremely short duration high-intensity training substantially improves endurance performance in triathletes. *Appl Physiol Nutr Metab* 2012;37:976.

Konopka AR, et al. Myosin heavy chain plasticity in aging skeletal muscle with aerobic exercise training. *J Gerontol A Biol Sci Med Sci* 2011;66:835.

Lamina S, Agbanusi E. Effect of aerobic exercise training on maternal weight gain in pregnancy: a meta-analysis of randomized controlled trials. *Ethiop J Health Sci* 2013;23:59.

Laughlin MH, et al. Control of blood flow to cardiac and skeletal muscle during exercise. In: Rowell LB, Sheperd JT, eds. *Handbook of Physiology, Exercise: Regulation and Integration of Multiple Systems*. Bethesda: American Physiological Society, 1996.

Lazar JM, et al. Swimming and the heart. *Int J Cardiol* 2013;168:19.

Lee I-M, et al. Physical activity and coronary heart disease in women: is "no pain no gain" passé? *JAMA* 2001;285:1447.

Luden N, et al. Myocellular basis for tapering in competitive distance runners. *J Appl Physiol* 2010;108:1501.

Mann T, et al. Methods of prescribing relative exercise intensity: physiological and practical considerations. *Sports Med* 2013;43:613.

Manson JE, et al. Walking compared with vigorous exercise for the prevention of cardiovascular events in women. *N Engl J Med* 2002;347:716.

Martin WH III. Effect of endurance training on fatty acid metabolism during whole body exercise. *Med Sci Sports Exerc* 1997;29:635.

May LE, et al. Regular maternal exercise dose and fetal heart outcome. *Med Sci Sports Exerc* 2012;44:1252.

Menzies P, et al. Blood lactate clearance during active recovery after an intense running bout depends on the intensity of the active recovery. *J Sports Sci* 2010;28:975.

Moore RL, Palmer BM. Exercise training and cellular adaptations of normal and diseased hearts. *Exerc Sport Sci Rev* 1999;27:285.

Mudd LM, et al. Health benefits of physical activity during pregnancy: an international perspective. *Med Sci Sports Exerc* 2013;45:268.

Mujika I, Padilla S. Scientific basis for precompetition tapering strategies. *Med Sci Sports Exerc* 2003;34:1182.

Murtagh EM, et al. The effects of 60 minutes of brisk walking per week, accumulated in two different patterns, on cardiovascular risk. *Prev Med* 2005;41:92.

Nelson ME, et al. Physical activity and public health in older adults: recommendation from the American College of Sports Medicine and the American Heart Association. *Med Sci Sports Exerc* 2006;39:1435.

Owe KM, et al. Exercise during pregnancy and the gestational age distribution: a cohort study. *Med Sci Sports Exerc* 2012;44:1067.

Ozkaya O, et al. An elliptical trainer may render the Wingate all-out test more anaerobic. *J Strength Cond Res* 2014;28:643.

Padua DA, et al. Seven steps for developing and implementing a preventive training program: lessons learned from JUMP-ACL and beyond. *Clin Sports Med* 2014;33:615.

Parfitt G, et al. Perceptually regulated training at RPE13 is pleasant and improves physical health. *Med Sci Sports Exerc* 2012;44:1613.

Persinger RC, et al. Consistency of the talk test for exercise prescription. *Med Sci Sports Exerc* 2004;36:1632.

Price BP, et al. Exercise in pregnancy: effect on fitness and obstetric outcomes—a randomized trial. *Med Sci Sports Exerc* 2012;44:2263.

Raglin J, Bardukas A. Overtraining in athletes: the challenge of prevention. A consensus statement. *ACSM's Health Fitness J* 1999;3:27.

Robertson RJ, Noble BJ. Perception of physical exertion: methods, mediators, and applications. *Exerc Sport Sci Rev* 1997;25:407.

Rønnestad BR, Mujika I. Optimizing strength training for running and cycling endurance performance: a review. *Scand J Med Sci Sports* 2014;24:603.

Ruchat SM, et al. Nutrition and exercise reduce excessive weight gain in normal-weight pregnant women. *Med Sci Sports Exerc* 2012;44:1419.

Rudra CB, et al. A prospective analysis of recreational physical activity and pre-eclampsia risk. *Med Sci Sports Exerc* 2008;40:1581.

Sakamoto A, et al. Hyperventilation as a strategy for improved repeated sprint performance. *J Strength Cond Res* 2014;28:1119.

Santos-Concejero J, et al. OBLA is a better predictor of performance than Dmax in long and middle-distance well-trained runners. *J Sports Med Phys Fitness* 2014;54:553.

Sarzynski MA, et al. Measured maximal heart rates compared to commonly used age-based prediction equations in the heritage family study. *Am J Hum Biol* 2013;25:695.

Slettaløkken G, Rønnestad BR. High intensity interval training every second week maintains VO_{2max} in soccer players during off-season. *J Strength Cond Res* 2014;28:1946.

Special communications: roundtable consensus statement. Impact of physical activity during pregnancy and postpartum on chronic disease risk. *Med Sci Sports Exerc* 2006;38:989.

Stanley J, et al. Cardiac parasympathetic reactivation following exercise: implications for training prescription. *Sports Med* 2013;47:9424.

Stoudemire NM, et al. The validity of regulating blood lactate concentration during running by rating perceived exertion. *Med Sci Sports Exerc* 1996;28:490.

Talanian JL, et al. Two weeks of high-intensity aerobic interval training increases the capacity for fat oxidation during exercise in women. *J Appl Physiol* 2007;102:1439.

Tanaka H, et al. Age predicted maximal heart rate revisited. *J Am Coll Cardiol* 2001;37:153.

Trinity JD, et al. Maximal mechanical power during a taper in elite swimmers. *Med Sci Sports Exerc* 2006;38:1643.

Treuth MS, et al. Pregnancy-related changes in physical activity, fitness, and strength. *Med Sci Sports Exerc* 2005;36:832.

Unnithan VB, et al. Oxygen uptake kinetics in trained adolescent females. *Eur J Appl Physiol* 2015;115:213.

Urhausen A, et al. Impaired pituitary hormonal response to exhaustive exercise in overtrained endurance athletes. *Med Sci Sports Exerc* 1998;30:407.

Uusitalo AL, et al. Overtraining: making a difficult diagnosis and implementing targeted treatment. *Phys Sportsmed* 2001;29:35.

Venables MC, Jeukendrup AE. Endurance training and obesity: effect on substrate metabolism and insulin sensitivity. *Med Sci Sports Exerc* 2008;40:495.

Vollaard NB, et al. Exercise-induced oxidative stress in overload training and tapering. *Med Sci Sports Exerc* 2006;38:1335.

Walther C, et al. The effect of exercise training on endothelial function in cardiovascular disease in humans. *Exerc Sport Sci Rev* 2004;32:129.

Wang Z, et al. Adapted low intensity ergometer aerobic training for early and severely impaired stroke survivors: a pilot randomized controlled trial to explore its feasibility and efficacy. *J Phys Ther Sci* 2014;26:1449.

Warburton DER, Gledhill N. Counterpoint: Stroke volume does not decline during exercise at maximal effort in healthy individuals. *J Appl Physiol* 2008;104:276.

Warner SO, et al. The effects of resistance training on metabolic health with weight regain. *J Clin Hypertens* 2010;12:64.

Weltman A, et al. Exercise training at and above lactate threshold in previously untrained women. *Int J Sports Med* 1992;13:257.

Weltman A, et al. Repeated bouts of exercise alter the blood lactate-RPE relation. *Med Sci Sports Exerc* 1998;30:1113.

White E, et al. Resistance training during pregnancy and birth outcomes. *J Phys Act Health* 2013;11(6):1141.

Wilmore JH, et al. Cardiac output and stroke volume changes with endurance training: the HERITAGE family Study. *Med Sci Sports Exerc* 2001;33:99.

Yan Z, et al. Exercise training-induced regulation of mitochondrial quality. *Exer Sport Sci Rev* 2012;40:159.

Zhang J, Savitz DA. Exercise during pregnancy among U.S. women. *Ann Epidemiol* 1996;6:53.

Training Muscles to Become Stronger

CHAPTER OBJECTIVES

- Describe the following four methods to assess muscular strength: cable tensiometry, dynamometry, one-repetition maximum (1-RM), and computer-assisted isokinetic dynamometry.
- Outline the general procedure to assess 1-RM for bench press and leg press.
- Explain five ways to ensure test standardization and fairness when evaluating muscular strength.
- Compare absolute and relative upper- and lower-body muscular strength in men and women.
- Define *concentric*, *eccentric*, and *isometric* muscle actions, and provide two examples of each action.
- Recommend the appropriate frequency, overload, and sets and repetitions for dynamic resistance training.
- Explain the specificity of training response for muscular strength related to enhanced performance in sports and occupational tasks.
- Compare isokinetic resistance training with conventional dynamic and static resistance training.
- Describe the rationale for plyometric training to improve muscular strength and power, and give two examples of exercises for these purposes.
- Indicate how psychological and muscular factors interact to influence maximum strength capacity.
- Outline six major physiologic adaptations to resistance training.
- Describe how to develop a circuit resistance-training program to improve muscular strength and aerobic fitness simultaneously.
- Describe two tests to assess muscular endurance for the abdominals and chest-shoulder areas.
- Describe the proposed six phases for delayed onset muscle soreness (DOMS) following unaccustomed exercise.

ANCILLARIES AT A GLANCE

Visit **http://thePoint.lww.com/MKKESS5e** to access the following resources:

- References: Chapter 14
- Interactive Question Bank

PART 1 Muscular Strength: Measurement and Improvement

Lifting weights began as a spectator sport in the United States and Europe in the early 1840s as "strongmen" showcased their prowess in traveling carnivals and sideshows. Much of the "science" of strength development at that time is attributed to **Pehr Henrik Ling** (see Chapter 1). Ling is remembered as the father of Swedish gymnastics; in 1813, he founded the current Swedish School of Sport and Health Sciences under the name of the Royal Central Institute of Gymnastics, Stockholm. Both he and his son **Hjalmar Ling** (1820–1886; see photo) were influential writers and practitioners during the genesis of early "movement science" education and methodology. Their many disciples became experts in physical education in Sweden and Europe, and their influential techniques of strength development migrated to the British Isles and eventually the United States. Other notable achievements in "strength" activities or gymnastics occurred during this same time frame, mainly from German and European educators.

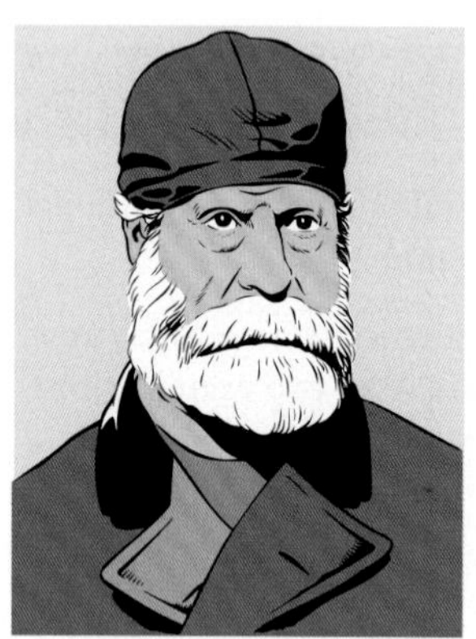

Hjalmar Ling

Figure 14.1 shows examples of late 19th century "strength and exercise machines" popularized by Swedish physician **Gustav Zander** (1835–1920), the development of which was strongly influenced by the Lings' Swedish Gymnastic movement. Zander's methods for treating patients and the common person included standard gymnastic exercise regimens, mostly calisthenics, balance, and core trunk and limb strengthening routines. Included were workouts on his mechanical exercise machines that served double duty for general strength development and "mechanical gymnastic treatments" for morbid disorders and diseases of the heart, nerves, respiratory and abdominal organs, obesity, gout, and rheumatism of the bony articulations including scoliosis. Zander's many successful treatment clinics in the 1890s featured his machines and opened up a new vista and attitudes toward self-enhancement through exercise for fitness and health. During this period in the United States, measuring muscular strength became popular to evaluate physical fitness and body development, particularly in schools, colleges, physiotherapy centers, and local gymnasia and exercise training centers.

In 1897 at a meeting of the American College Gymnasium Directors, strength contests were established to determine overall body strength based on measures of back, leg, arm, and chest strength. The first six colleges to participate were Amherst College, Columbia University, Harvard University, the University of Minnesota, Dickinson College, and Wesleyan College. Harvard University was the overall winner, followed closely by Columbia University. By the mid-1900s, physical culture specialists, bodybuilders, competitive weightlifters, field-event athletes, and some wrestlers were using traditional weightlifting exercises rather than the passive methods of massage and electrical vibration that also flourished during this time. Research in the late 1950s and early 1960s dispelled the myth that traditional muscle-strengthening exercise

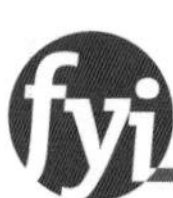

Contributions to the Early Science of "Strength" Activities

The following individuals and events are remembered for their contributions to the early science of "strength" activities:

- Johann Basedow (1723–1790), German educator, founded the Philanthropinum and Education of the Mind and Body (**www.academia.edu/931788/The_History_of_Physical_Education_Book_Chapter**).
- Johann Christoph Friedrich "Guts" Muth (1759–1839), German educator and writer, described workout routines for balance on swinging beams, poles, ropes, and other apparatus (Goodbody J. *The Illustrated History of Gymnastics.* London: Stanley Paul & Co., 1982. ISBN 0-09-143350-9).
- Francis Amoros (1770–1848), Spanish educator, helped to establish gymnastics in France, emphasizing upper body strength routines on the trapeze, rings, and ropes.
- Franz Nachtegall (1777–1847) operated a private gymnastic club in Denmark, emphasizing mass calisthenics incorporating vaulting and specific routines with dumbbells and small, weighted balls.
- Gerhard Vieth (1759–1839), German author, devised specific exercise routines emphasizing "strength/power movements" on ropes, beams, and horizontal pole vaulting.
- Friedrich Ludwig Jahn (1778–1852) promoted gymnastic exercise to develop muscular strength and endurance and influenced other education leaders, including Francis Lieber (1800–1872) who emigrated to the United States in 1824, along with Charles Follen (1796–1840; started the first college gymnasium in America) and Charles Beck (1798–1866); this trio formally introduced and promoted gymnastics to America; subsequently, strongmen and circus performers incorporated it into their strength-training regimens.

Teachers were trained not only as physical education instructors in the schools and YMCAs (first American YMCA founded in Boston at the Old South Church in 1851; **www.ymca.net/history/founding.html**) but also for government work as military gymnastics instructors and physiotherapists. In 1887, the YMCA founded a college in Springfield, Massachusetts (formerly International Young Men's Christian Association Training School and now Springfield College), also emphasizing teaching and organizing gymnastic activities and other individual and dual sports. Both football, introduced in 1890 by student-instructor Amos Alonzo Stagg (1862–1965), and basketball, developed in 1891 by James Naismith (1861–1938), who also led classes in indoor exercise routines and "strengthening" calisthenics, had their start at the Springfield YMCA Training School.

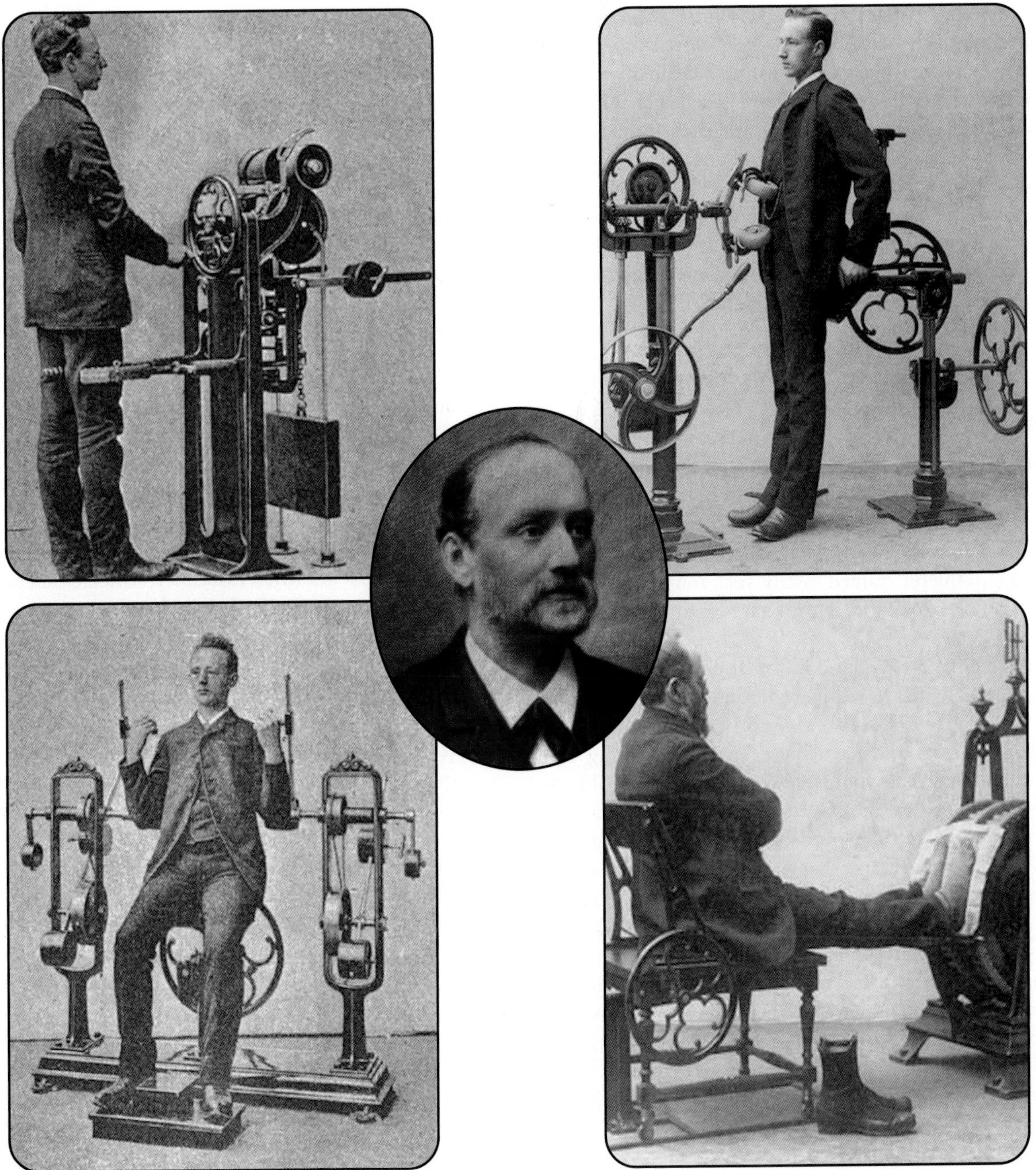

FIGURE 14.1 Four examples of late 19th century "strength machines" popularized by Swedish physician Gustav Zander, MD (1835–1920), who produced 27 mechanical apparatuses that became prototypes of common equipment now ubiquitous in physical fitness gymnasiums and training centers worldwide. The successful Nautilus line of exercise equipment was remarkably similar in design to many of Zander's machines (**www.nps.gov/hosp/historyculture/upload/zander.pdf**). Zander and his followers believed that their complex mechanized machines using pulleys and counterbalances that emphasized "progressive exertion" to control the body's muscles to build strength could play a decisive role to create more positive health outcomes than bloodletting, purging, or strenuous acrobatics and nonphysician-approved allopathic "cures" of the time. Zander marketed his steam-powered machines as a "preventative against the evils engendered by a sedentary life and the seclusion of the office." At the turn of the 20th century, Zander's machines were showcased at elite East Coast health spas including the Fordyce Bathhouse in Little Rock, AK (**www.nps.gov/hosp/historyculture/fordyce-bathhouse.htm**), at the Massachusetts General Hospital outpatient department beginning in 1904, and at private clinics near Central Park in New York City. While strapped into the apparatus, the motor provided the power to passively exercise the joints and muscles throughout their range of motion. Each machine was designed to exercise a different body region. Zander's mechanized machines disappeared after the Great Depression, replaced by smaller, more compact equipment that evolved over the next 75 years into modern strength and fitness training "active machines." (Photos from Levertin A. *Dr. G. Zanders Medico-Mechanical Gymnastics. Its Method, Importance and Application*. Stockholm: Norstead & Sonner, 1893.)

reduced movement speed or range of joint motion. Instead, the opposite usually occurred: elite weightlifters, bodybuilders, and "muscle men" had exceptional joint flexibility without limitations in general limb movement speed. For untrained healthy individuals, heavy-resistance exercises increased the speed and power of muscular effort without impairing subsequent sports performance.

The sections that follow explore the underlying rationale for strength training, including acute and chronic physiologic adjustments as muscles become stronger with training.

FOUNDATIONS FOR STUDYING MUSCULAR STRENGTH

The inclusion of strength development programs as part of athletic training regimens is not new; strength development prepared men for warfare in ancient China, Japan, India, Greece, and Rome. When the Olympic games first began in 776 B.C., athletes trained nearly year-round and incorporated muscle-strengthening exercises into their arduous regimens.

The scientific foundations for strength training for athletes began with the Chinese in 3600 B.C. During the Chou dynasty (1122–249 B.C.), conscripts had to pass weightlifting tests and participate in chariot racing and running and jumping contests before becoming soldiers. Weight training also took place in ancient Egypt and India; sculptures and illustrations depict athletes training with heavy stone weights. Women practiced weight training; wall mosaics recovered from Roman villas showed young women exercising with handheld weights. During the *"Age of Strength"* in the sixth century, weightlifting competitions often took place between soldiers and athletes. The Greek physician Galen (see Chapter 1), in his insightful treatise *The Preservation of Health*, referred to exercising with dumbbell-type weighted objects called halteres made of stone or metal and weighing between 12 and 35 kg (26 and 77 lb).

OBJECTIVES OF RESISTANCE TRAINING

Resistance training and strength development are used for multiple purposes:

1. Weightlifting and powerlifting competition (who is the strongest?)
2. Bodybuilding (maximize muscular development for aesthetic goals)
3. General strength training (fitness and health enhancement)
4. Physical therapy (rehabilitation from injury or disease)
5. Maximizing sport performance (sport-specific resistance training)
6. Muscle physiology (understanding structure and function)

RESISTANCE-TRAINING VOCABULARY

Many terms and much jargon abound in the area of resistance training, yet certain terms consistently appear in the research literature and popular writings about resistance-training methods and outcomes. **Table 14.1** defines common resistance-training terms.

MUSCLE ACTION TYPES

The three types of muscle action are:

1. **Concentric action**, the most common form of muscle action, occurs in dynamic activities where muscles shorten and produce tension through the range of motion. **Figure 14.2A** illustrates the concentric muscle action that occurs when raising a dumbbell from the extended to the flexed elbow position.
2. **Eccentric action** (also called lengthening or plyometrics) occurs when external resistance exceeds muscle force and muscle lengthens as tension develops. In **Figure 14.2A**, the dumbbell is slowly lowered as it resists gravity's force. The sarcomeres in the activated muscle fibers of the upper arm muscles lengthen eccentrically to prevent the dumbbell from crashing to the surface. In weightlifting, muscles frequently act eccentrically as the weight slowly returns to the starting position to begin the next concentric (shortening) muscle action. Eccentric action during this "recovery" phase adds to the total work and effectiveness of the exercise repetition.
   a. The term isotonic, derived from the Greek word isotonos (*iso* meaning the same or equal, *tonos* meaning tension or strain), commonly refers to concentric and eccentric muscle actions because movement occurs with a constant (the same) resistance. However, *isotonic* necessarily lacks precision when applied to muscle actions that involve movement because the muscle's effective force-generating capacity continually varies as the joint angle changes throughout the ROM.
3. **Isometric action** (also called static or stationary) **(Fig. 14.2B)** occurs when a muscle generates force and attempts to shorten but cannot overcome the external resistance during muscular action against an immovable bar in an isometric rack.

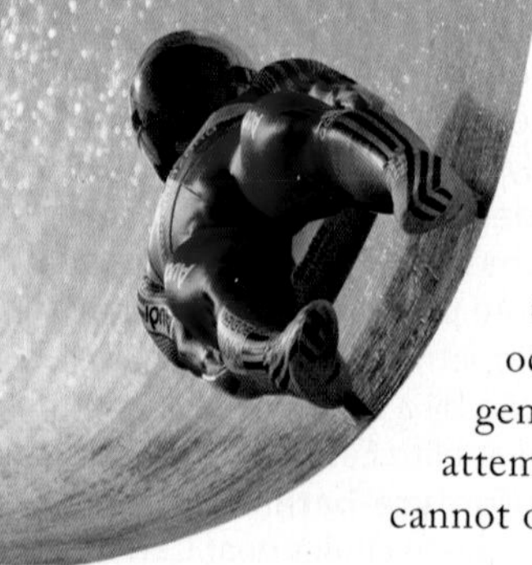

The winter sliding sport *Skeleton* involves racing a small sled at nearly 80 mph (130 km · h^{-1}) down an ice track lying face down and facing forward without steering or braking mechanisms.

Other near-sustained isometric-type muscle

TABLE 14.1 Definition of Selected Terms Appearing in the Resistance-Training Literature

Term	Definition
Cheating	Breaking from strict form when performing an exercise to increase the resistance moved when performing the movement (e.g., rather than maintaining an erect upper body when performing a standing arm curl, a slight body swing at the start of the movement allows the person to lift a heavier weight or the same weight more times with potentially harmful consequences)
Circuit resistance training	Series of resistance exercises performed in sequence from one exercise "station" to the next with minimal rest, usually 20 to 30 seconds, between exercises
Concentric action	Muscle shortening occurs during force application
Dynamic constant external resistance training	Resistance training in which external resistance or weight does not change, yet joint flexion and extension occurs with each movement repetition
Eccentric action	Muscle lengthening occurs during force application
Exercise intensity	Muscle force expressed as a percentage of a muscle's maximum force-generating capacity or some level of maximum
Isokinetic action	Muscle action performed at constant angular limb velocity where constant torque or tension is maintained as muscle shortens or lengthens
Isometric action	Muscle action without noticeable outward change in muscle length
Maximal voluntary muscle action (MVMA)	Maximal force generated in one repetition (1-RM), or performing a series of submaximal actions to momentary failure
Muscular endurance	Sustaining maximum or submaximum force, often determined by assessing the maximum number of exercise repetitions at a percentage of maximum strength
Overload	A muscle acting against a resistance greater than normally encountered
Periodization	Variation in training volume and intensity over a specified time period, with the goal to prevent staleness while peaking physiologically for competition
Plyometrics	Exercise that repeatedly stretches and loads a muscle suddenly and then immediately contracts it (e.g., repeated standing long jumps, hops, vertical jumps, and box jumps)
Power	Rate of performing work (force × distance ÷ time or force × velocity)
Progressive overload	Incrementally increasing the stress placed on a muscle to produce greater force or greater endurance in subsequent workouts
Range of motion (ROM)	Maximum ROM through a joint's arc
Repetition	One complete exercise movement, usually consisting of concentric and eccentric muscle action or one complete isometric muscle action
Repetition maximum (RM)	Maximum force generated for one repetition of a movement (1-RM) or predetermined number of repetitions (e.g., 5- or 10-RM)
Set	Preset number of repetitions performed in resistance training
Sticking point	Region in an exercise ROM against a set resistance that provides the greatest difficulty to complete the movement with good form
Strength	Maximum force-generating capacity of a muscle or group of muscles
Suspension training	Leveraging a person's body weight during exercise without reliance on externally fixed weights, pulleys, or cams by increasing or decreasing the suspension coordinates—the height of ropes, pulleys, slings, or bungee cords—relative to the suspension point
Torque	Force that produces a turning, twisting, or rotary movement in any plane about an axis; commonly expressed in Newton meters (Nm)
Training volume	Total work performed in a single training session
Variable resistance training	Training with equipment that either uses a lever arm, cam, hydraulic system, or pulley to alter the resistance to match the increases and decreases in a muscle's capacity throughout a joint's ROM

actions occur in surfing, sailing, and wind boarding and in most snow and ice sports, including alpine ski racing, snowmobiling, bobsleigh, luge, and skeleton, which require prolonged, static posture during the activity. The approximately 1-minute duration of the skeleton race requires intense, near-maximum isometric muscle actions to the finish following the push-off (**www.topendsports.com/videos/category/sports/winter/skeleton/**). From a physics standpoint, an isometric muscle action does not produce external work, yet this action can generate considerable force despite the lack of noticeable lengthening or shortening of muscle with joint movement.

Dynamic constant external resistance (DCER) refers to resistance training where external resistance or weight does not change throughout each repetition of both raising (concentric) and lowering (eccentric) phases. DCER implies that the external weight or resistance remains constant throughout the movement.

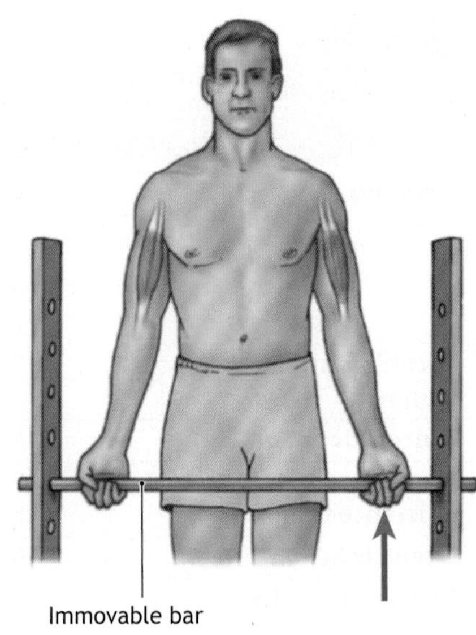

FIGURE 14.2 Muscular force during (**A**) concentric (shortening) and eccentric (lengthening) and (**B**) isometric (static) muscle actions. (Reprinted with permission from McArdle WD, Katch FI, Katch VL. *Exercise Physiology: Nutrition, Energy, and Human Performance*. 8th Ed. Baltimore: Wolters Kluwer Health, 2015.)

MUSCULAR STRENGTH MEASUREMENT AND TESTING

Different methods commonly assess isometric and concentric/eccentric **muscular strength**. Strength refers to the maximum force, tension, or torque generated by a muscle or muscle groups.

Isometric Muscle Testing

Isometric testing measures muscle force at a specific joint angle. **Figure 14.3** shows three different isometric testing devices. In **Figure 14.3A**, a cable tensiometer assesses

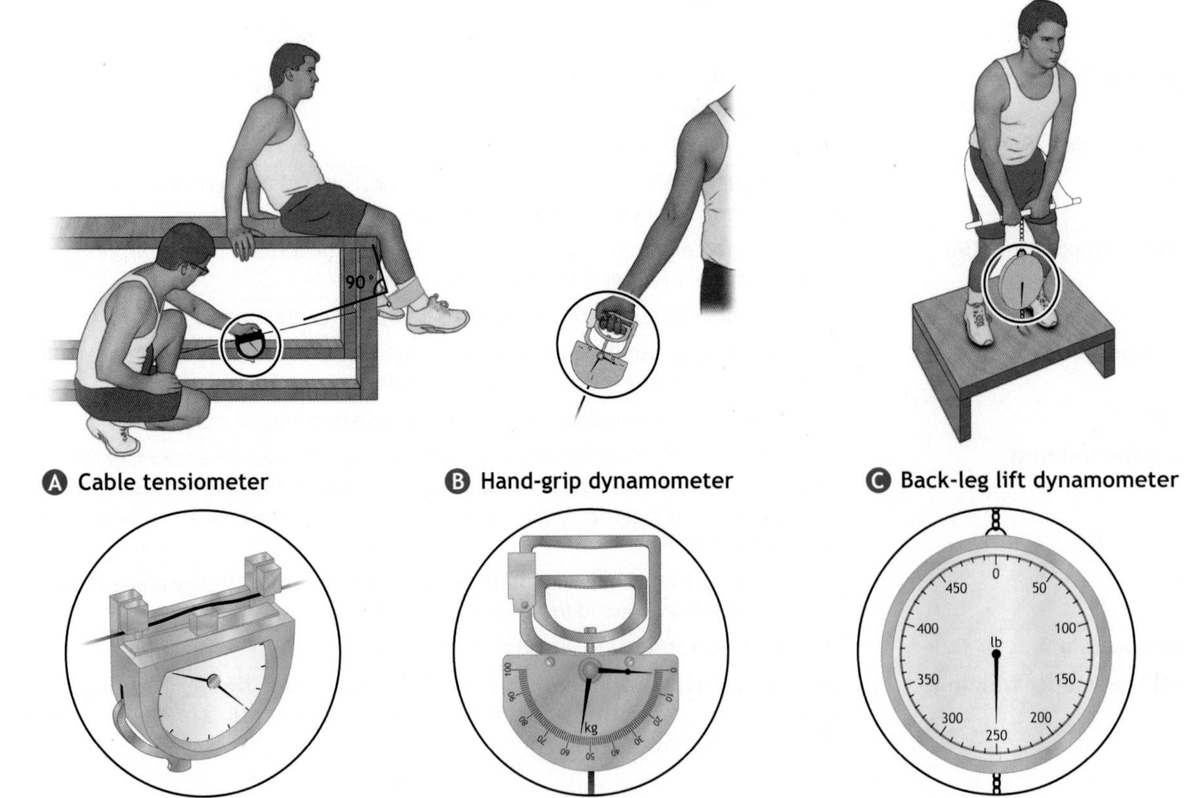

FIGURE 14.3 Measurement of static strength by (**A**) cable tensiometer, (**B**) handgrip dynamometer, and (**C**) back-leg lift dynamometer.

static muscular force during knee extension. Increased force on the cable depresses a riser over which the cable passes; this deflects the pointer and indicates the amount of force applied. The application of the tensiometer for strength measurements differs considerably from its original use for measuring tension on steel cables linking various parts of an airplane's tail and wing assemblies.

Figure 14.3B and C displays handgrip and backlift **dynamometers** to assess static strength. Both devices operate on the principle of compression. Application of external force to the dynamometer compresses a steel spring and moves a pointer. Knowing how much force must move the pointer, a given distance determines how much external "static" force the dynamometer absorbs.

Computer-assisted devices also can assess isometric muscle force.

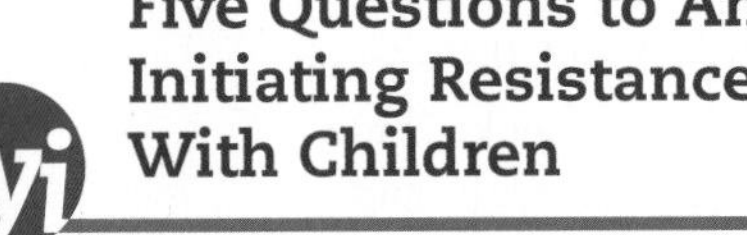

Five Questions to Answer Before Initiating Resistance Training With Children

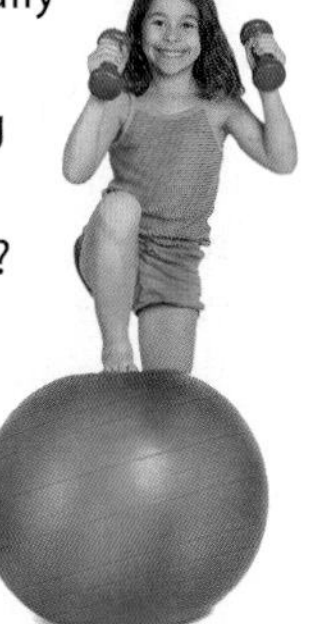

1. Is the child psychologically and physically ready to participate?
2. Does the child understand proper lifting techniques for each exercise?
3. Does the child understand safety concerns?
4. Does the equipment fit the child?
5. Does the child have a balanced overall physical activity program?

Eccentric/Concentric Muscle Strength Testing

One-Repetition Maximum

The **one-repetition maximum (1-RM)** technique refers to a dynamic method to assess eccentric/concentric muscle actions. To assess 1-RM for single or multiple muscle groups, choose the initial weight close to but below maximum lifting capacity (see A Closer Look: "How to Assess and Evaluate One-Repetition Maximum for Bench Press and Leg Press"). Weight is incrementally added on successive lifts until the person achieves maximum lift capacity. The weight increments range between 1 and 5 kg depending on the muscle group evaluated. Rest intervals of 1 to 5 minutes provide sufficient recuperation before attempting a lift at the next heavier weight.

Figure 14.4 illustrates two submaximal methods (5-RM and 10-RM) used as alternatives to the 1-RM method, and the percentage of maximum each represents to evaluate a muscle's force- and power-generating capacity. In these tests (shown for the bench press), the greatest amount of weight lifted five or 10 times becomes the repetition maximum to assess strength. The measurement procedure in these cases assesses 5-RM (generally 90% of maximum) or 10-RM (~78% of maximum). The 5- and 10-RM methods provide appropriate markers to assess muscular strength in children and older adults in whom maximal lifting may be contraindicated.

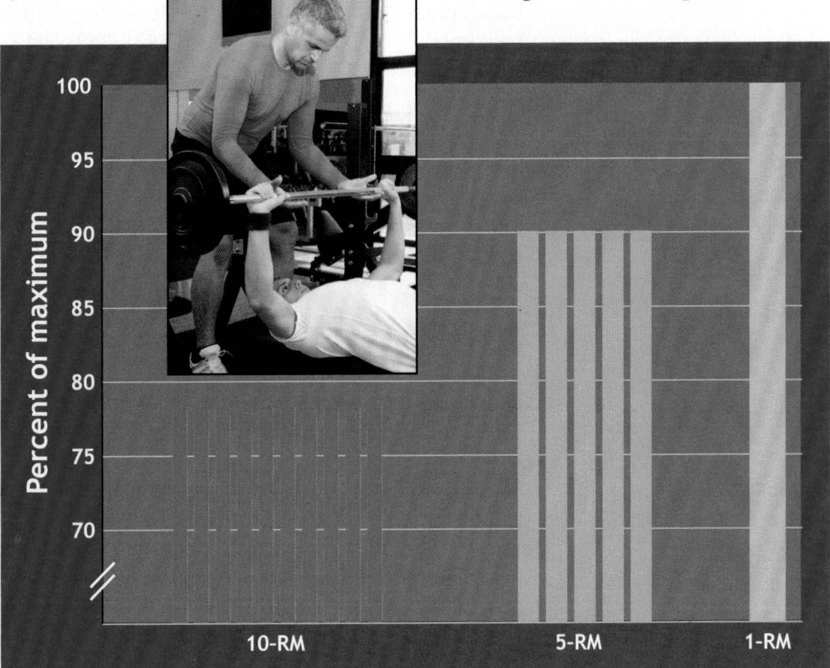

FIGURE 14.4 Three methods, 1-RM, 5-RM, and 10-RM, to assess force-generating capacity in the bench-press dynamic movement.

Estimating 1-RM Strength Using Submaximum Repetitions-to-Fatigue Test Scores

A strong inverse relationship exists between muscular endurance (e.g., number of repetitions to fatigue using a submaximum resistance) and percentage of 1-RM lifted. Stated differently, lifting a heavier load produces a fewer number of repetitions (see Load-Repetition Relationship in A Closer Look: "How to Assign Load [Resistance] and Repetition Number to Achieve Different Training Goals"). When 1-RM testing is unwarranted or ill advised (i.e., in preadolescents, the elderly, poorly conditioned individuals, or those with cardiovascular disease or physical limitations), repetitions to fatigue with a submaximum weight can predict 1-RM strength. The two equations shown below for trained and untrained differ because previous resistance training alters the relationship between a submaximal performance (7- to 10-RM) and maximal lift capacity (1-RM). Generally, a weight one can lift for 7- to 10-RM represents about 68% of the 1-RM score for the untrained person and 79% of the new 1-RM after training.

Untrained: 1-RM (kg) = 1.554 × 7- to 10-RM weight (kg) − 5.181

Trained: 1-RM (kg) = 1.172 × 7- to 10-RM weight (kg) + 7.704

For example, estimate 1-RM bench press score for a trained person whose 10-RM bench press equals 70 kg as follows:

1-RM (kg) = 1.172 × 70 kg + 7.704 = 89.7 kg

Testing Protocol

Determine the maximum number of repetitions to fatigue a person can achieve at a given weight lifted. Use this number to predict the 1-RM. (Refer to A Closer Look: "How To Assign Load [Resistance] and Repetition Number to Achieve Different Training Goals" for procedures

A CLOSER LOOK

How to Assess and Evaluate One-Repetition Maximum for Bench Press and Leg Press

The maximum weight or resistance for 1-RM for a particular muscle action with proper form measures maximum eccentric/concentric muscle strength. A trial-and-error approach determines the 1-RM strength value. After each successful single lift (rest 2 to 3 min between attempts), increase the weight by 5 to 10 lb until achieving the maximum weight lifted.

The 1-RM bench press (illustrated on the facing page) assesses maximum muscular strength of the major muscle groups of the upper body, and the leg press assesses maximum strength of major portions of the lower-body musculature. Dividing the 1-RM score by body weight (1-RM [lb or kg] ÷ body weight [lb or kg]) assesses relative muscular strength and provides a frame of reference to evaluate different body weight comparisons (see Table below).

Reference Values for 1-RM Bench Press and Leg Press Expressed Relative to Body Weight[a]

	Age, y			
Rating	**20–29**	**30–39**	**40–49**	**50–59**
Men				
Excellent				
Bench press	>1.26	>1.08	>0.97	>0.86
Leg press	>2.08	>1.88	>1.76	>1.66
Good				
Bench press	1.17–1.25	1.01–1.07	0.91–0.96	0.81–0.85
Leg press	2.00–2.07	1.80–1.87	1.70–1.75	1.60–1.65
Average				
Bench press	0.97–1.16	0.86–1.00	0.78–0.90	0.70–0.80
Leg press	1.83–1.99	1.63–1.79	1.56–1.69	1.46–1.59
Fair				
Bench press	0.88–0.96	0.79–0.85	0.72–0.77	0.65–0.69
Leg press	1.65–1.82	1.55–1.62	1.50–1.55	1.40–1.45
Poor				
Bench press	<0.87	<0.78	<0.71	<0.60
Leg press	<1.64	<1.54	<1.49	<1.39
Women				
Excellent				
Bench press	>0.78	>0.66	>0.61	>0.54
Leg press	>1.63	>1.42	>1.32	>1.26
Good				
Bench press	0.72–0.77	0.62–0.65	0.57–0.60	0.51–0.53
Leg press	1.54–1.62	1.35–1.41	1.26–1.31	1.13–1.25
Average				
Bench press	0.59–0.71	0.53–0.61	0.48–0.56	0.43–0.50
Leg press	1.35–1.53	1.20–1.34	1.12–1.25	0.99–1.12
Fair				
Bench press	0.53–0.58	0.49–0.52	0.44–0.47	0.40–0.42
Leg press	1.25–1.34	1.13–1.19	1.06–1.11	0.86–0.98
Poor				
Bench press	<0.52	<0.48	<0.43	<0.39
Leg press	<1.25	<1.12	<1.05	<0.85

Adapted from Cooper Institute for Aerobics Research, 1997.
[a]Score = 1-RM (lb) ÷ body weight (lb).

Procedures for Bench Press Test

Muscle Groups	Equipment	Starting Position	Movement
Shoulder flexors and adductors; elbow extensors	Barbell or bench press station on a single- or multistation resistance machine	1. Overhand (pronated) grip, slightly wider than shoulder width apart. 2. Lay supine on a bench with the feet on the floor straddling the bench. 3. Signal a spotter to position the bar at arms' length above the chest with arms extended.	1. Downward movement: lower the bar until it touches the chest. 2. Upward movement: push the bar up to full elbow extension while maintaining body position without arching the back. The spotter maintains grip on the bar throughout the movement without offering assistance; also helps to place the bar on the supports.

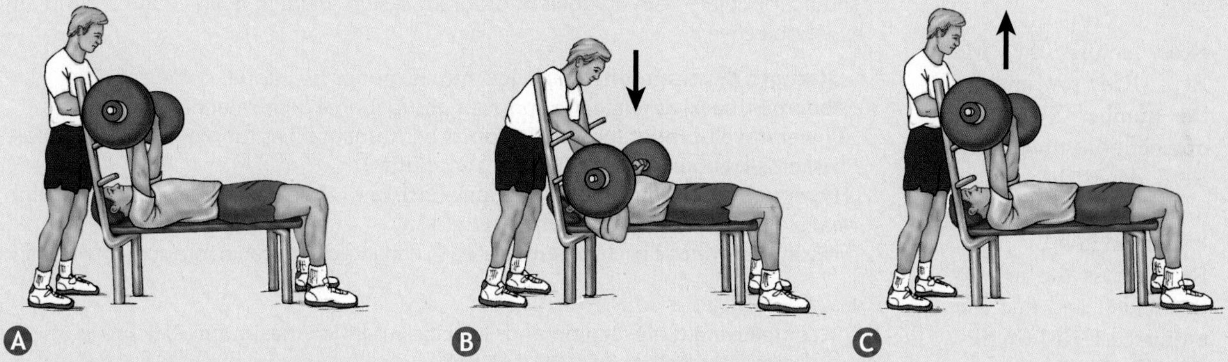

A B C

Procedures for Leg Press Test

Muscle Groups	Equipment	Starting Position	Movement
Knee extensors and hip extensors	Leg press on a single- or multistation resistance machine	1. Sit with the legs parallel and feet on the machine's foot rests. 2. Grasp the seat or the side handle.	1. Forward movement: push the foot rests steadily forward; do not forcefully lock out the knees during extension. 2. Backward movement: move the footrests slowly back to the starting position.

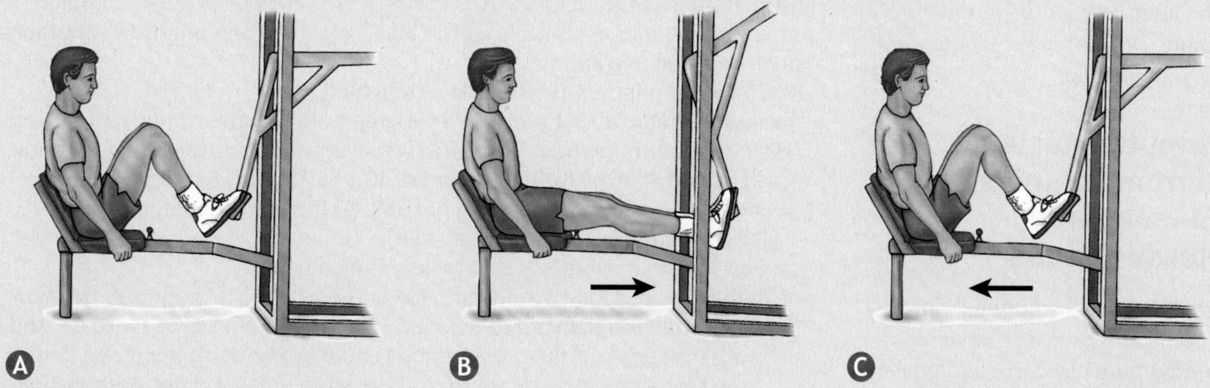

A B C

A = beginning; B = forward; C = return.

to determine the maximum number of repetitions.) Use the data in **Table 14.2** and these three steps to determine 1-RM:

1. Read across the Max Reps (RM) row and find the number of repetitions completed.
2. Read down the column to the load lifted (weight completed, in lb).
3. Read across the row to the far left to find the estimated 1-RM.

For example, if individual performs a 5-RM test and lifts 174 lb:

1. Read across the Max Reps (RM) row and find the number 5 (number of repetitions to fatigue).
2. Read down the column to the number 174 (the load lifted in lb).
3. Read across the row to the far left and find the estimated 1-RM (in this example, 200 lb).

The data in **Table 14.2** also estimate the load (weight in lb) at a given percentage of 1-RM. For example, find the 1-RM load in column 1 (e.g., 120 lb); go across to the desired percentage in row 2 (%1-RM; 80%) and find the weight (in lb) corresponding to that percentage in the intersecting cell (in this example, 96 lb; see *yellow highlights* in table).

Computer-Assisted Electromechanical and Isokinetic Determinations

Microprocessor technology integrated with exercise equipment quantifies muscular force and power during a variety of movements. Modern instrumentation measures force, acceleration, and velocity of body segments in various movement patterns. For example, force platforms measure external application of muscular

A CLOSER LOOK

How to Assign Load (Resistance) and Repetition Number to Achieve Different Training Goals

Assigning combinations of load (resistance) and repetition number (repetitions) constitutes the most important aspects of establishing a resistance-training program. Research and practical experience indicate that performing a maximum of 6 or fewer repetitions elicits the greatest increase in strength and maximal power output. Resistances that produce 10 to 15 or even 20 and above repetitions greatly impact muscular endurance development. This knowledge makes it possible to specifically train for a desired muscular performance.

Identify Training Goals

Age, physical maturity, training history, and psychological and physical tolerance should formulate training goals or program design. Training goals center around four major objectives:

1. **Strength development** of specific muscle groups (i.e., upper or lower body, abdomen, back) as related to sports or occupational performance
2. **Power development** for specific sports performance (i.e., running back in football, basketball rebounder, high jumper, shot-putter)
3. **Hypertrophic development** for appearance or to alter body size (i.e., weight gain) and to improve overall muscular strength
4. **Muscle endurance development** related to enhanced occupation or sports performance

Assigning Load and Repetition

The accompanying table recommends specific repetition maximum (RM) and load expressed as a percentage of 1-RM (%1-RM).

The following five-step sequence to determine loads and repetition number for individualized training makes use of data from **Table 14.2**:

1. Determine the 1-RM in kg or lb as follows:
   a. Warmup using five to seven repetitions with light resistance.
   b. Rest for 1 to 2 minutes; perform slow stretching.
   c. Increase the load by 10 to 20 lb (4 to 9 kg) or 8% to 10% for upper-body exercise and by 30 to 40 lb (14 to 18 kg) or 10% to 20% for lower-body exercise. Complete 3 to 10 repetitions; stop at 10 repetitions.
   d. Rest for 1 to 2 minutes; perform slow stretching.
   e. Increase load above previous level (step c above), attempting to approach "near" maximum; increase 10 to 20 lb (4 to 9 kg) or 8% to 10% for upper-body exercise and 30 to 40 lb (14 to 18 kg) or 10% to 20% for lower-body exercise; complete as many repetitions as possible (at this load, maximum repetitions will probably range between two and six).
   f. Rest for 2 to 3 minutes; perform slow stretching.
   g. Increase the load above previous level (step e above), attempting to approach "near" maximum; increase 10 to 20 lb (4 to 9 kg) or 8% to 10% for upper-body exercise and 30 to 40 lb (14 to 18 kg) or 10% to 20% for lower-body exercise. Complete as many repetitions as possible (at this load, repetitions will probably range between one and four).
   h. Rest for 2 to 3 minutes; perform slow stretching.
   i. If the previous load produced 1-RM or more, rest 2 to 3 minutes (perform slow stretching). Increase the load 5 to 10 lb (2 to 4 kg) or 1% to 5% and attempt again. If the previous load could not be completed one time, rest for 2 to 3 minutes (perform slow stretching) and decrease the load by 5 to 10 lb (2 to 4 kg) or 1% to 5% for upper-body exercise and by 10 to 20 lb (4 to 9 kg) for lower-body exercise; attempt the lift again, trying to achieve the 1-RM.
2. Determine training goal(s) (e.g., strength, power, hypertrophy, endurance).
3. Determine the appropriate *repetition number* for the specific training goal (see **Table 14.2**).

Load: Repetition Continuum for Specific Training Goals

Training Goal	Load (%1-RM)	Goal Repetitions
Strength	≥85	≤6
High power	80–90	1–2
Low power	75–85	3–5
Hypertrophy	67–85	6–12
Endurance	≤67	≥12

From Baechle TR, et al. Resistance training. In: Baechle TR, Earle RW, eds. *Essentials of Strength Training and Conditioning*. 2nd Ed. Champaign: Human Kinetics Press, 2000.

4. Determine the specific %1-RM based on the repetition number (see **Table 14.2**).
5. Determine the training load (weight).
   a. Multiply the 1-RM load by the %1-RM (expressed as a decimal) selected for training.

Examples

With a training goal to achieve muscle hypertrophy, and 1-RM of 200 lb, follow the five-step procedure outlined previously to determine load and repetition number:

1. Determine the 1-RM.

$$1\text{-}RM = 200\ lb$$

2. Determine the training goal.

Muscle hypertrophy

3. Determine the appropriate repetition number for the specific training goal (see Table).

The repetition number is 6 to 12; use 8.

4. Determine the specific %1-RM based on the repetition number (see **Table 14.2**).

For goal repetitions 6 to 12,
the %1-RM is 67% to 85%; use 75%.

5. Determine the training load or weight; multiply the 1-RM load by the %1-RM (expressed as a decimal) selected for training.

$$Training\ load = 200 \times 0.75 = 150\ lb$$

This person would train using eight repetitions with a weight of 150 lb. Retest the 1-RM as improvement progresses about every 2 weeks to adjust the training load.

Sources: Baechle TR, Earle RW, eds. *Essentials of Strength Training and Conditioning*. 3rd Ed. Champaign: Human Kinetics Press, 2008.
Fleck SJ, Kraemer WJ. *Designing Resistance Training Programs*. 3rd Ed. Champaign: Human Kinetics Press, 2004.
Kraemer WJ, Koziris LP. Muscle strength training: techniques and considerations. *Phys Ther Pract* 1992;2:54.

force by limbs during jumping. Other electromechanical devices measure forces generated during all movement phases of cycling, rowing, supine bench press, seated and upright leg press, and exercises for other trunk, arm, and leg movements.

An **isokinetic dynamometer** (**Fig. 14.5**), an electromechanical accommodating resistance instrument with a speed-controlling mechanism, accelerates to a preset, constant velocity with applied force regardless of the force exerted on the device movement arm. At the attained velocity, the isokinetic loading mechanism adjusts automatically to provide a counterforce to variations in force generated by muscle as movement continues throughout the "strength curve." Thus, maximum force or any percentage of maximum effort generates throughout the full ROM at a pre-established velocity of limb movement. This allows training and measurement along a continuum from high-velocity (low-force) to low-velocity (high-force) conditions. A multifunction microprocessor within the dynamometer continuously monitors the immediate level of applied force. An electronic integrator in series with a monitor displays the average or peak force generated during any interval for almost instantaneous feedback about performance (e.g., force, torque, work).

The interface of microprocessor technology with mechanical devices provides the sport and exercise scientist, physical therapist, sports physician, and coach with valuable data to evaluate, test, train, and rehabilitate individuals. The argument in support of isokinetic strength measurement maintains that muscle strength dynamics involve considerably more than just the final outcome of 1-RM, 5-RM, or 10-RM testing. For example, two individuals with identical 1-RM bench press scores could exhibit dissimilar force curves throughout the movement ROM. Individual differences in force dynamics (e.g., time to peak tension) throughout the full ROM may reflect an entirely different underlying neuromuscular physiology unavailable with standard 1-RM free weight or mechanical device testing.

STRENGTH-TESTING CONSIDERATIONS

Seven important considerations exist for muscle strength testing regardless of the measurement method:

1. Provide standardized instructions before testing.
2. Ensure uniformity for warm-up duration and intensity.
3. Provide adequate practice before testing to minimize "learning" that could compromise initial results and unfairly bias final test results.
4. On the test device, ensure consistency among subjects in the angle of limb measurement or body position.

TABLE 14.2 **Estimating 1-RM From Submaximum Load (Weight) and Number of Repetitions**

To Use the Table, (1) Read Across the Max Reps (RM) Row and Find the Number of Repetitions Completed, (2) Read Down the Column to the Load (Weight Completed, lb) Lifted, and (3) Read Across the Row to the Far Left to Find the Estimated 1-RM

Max Reps (RM)	1	2	3	4	5	6	7	8	9	10	12	15
%1-RM	*100*	*95*	*93*	*90*	*87*	*85*	*83*	*80*	*77*	*75*	*67*	*65*
Load lifted (weight completed, lb)	10	10	9	9	9	9	8	8	8	8	7	7
	20	9	19	18	17	17	17	16	15	15	13	13
	30	9	28	27	26	26	25	24	23	23	20	20
	40	38	37	36	35	34	33	32	31	30	27	26
	50	48	47	45	44	43	42	40	39	38	34	33
	60	57	56	54	52	51	50	48	46	45	40	39
	70	67	65	63	61	60	58	56	54	53	47	46
	80	76	74	72	70	68	66	64	62	60	54	52
	90	86	84	81	78	77	75	72	69	68	60	59
	100	95	93	90	87	85	83	80	77	75	67	65
	110	105	102	99	96	94	91	88	85	83	74	72
	120	114	112	108	104	102	100	96	92	90	80	78
	130	124	121	117	113	111	108	104	100	98	87	85
	140	133	130	126	122	119	116	112	108	105	94	91
	150	143	140	135	131	128	125	120	116	113	101	98
	160	152	149	144	139	136	133	128	123	120	107	104
	170	162	158	153	148	145	141	136	131	128	114	111
	180	171	167	162	157	153	149	144	139	135	121	117
	190	181	177	171	165	162	158	152	146	143	127	124
	200	190	186	180	174	170	166	160	154	150	134	130
	210	200	195	189	183	179	174	168	162	158	141	137
	220	209	205	198	191	187	183	176	169	165	147	143
	230	219	214	207	200	196	191	184	177	173	154	150
	240	228	223	216	209	204	199	192	185	180	161	156
	250	238	233	225	218	213	208	200	193	188	168	163
	260	247	242	234	226	221	206	208	200	195	174	169
	270	257	251	243	235	230	224	216	208	203	181	176
	280	266	260	252	244	238	232	224	216	210	188	182
	290	276	270	261	252	247	241	232	223	218	194	189
	300	285	279	270	261	255	249	240	231	225	201	195
	310	295	288	279	270	264	257	248	239	233	208	202
	320	304	298	288	278	272	266	256	246	240	214	208
	330	314	307	297	287	281	274	264	254	248	221	215
	340	323	316	306	296	289	282	272	262	255	228	221
	350	333	326	315	305	298	291	280	270	263	235	228
	360	342	335	324	313	306	299	288	277	270	241	234
	370	352	344	333	322	315	307	296	285	278	248	241
	380	361	353	342	331	323	315	304	293	285	255	247
	390	371	363	351	339	332	324	312	300	293	261	254
	400	380	372	360	348	340	332	320	308	300	268	260

Note: *Yellow* highlighted numbers are used in the example on the prior pages.

From Baechle TR, et al. Resistance training. In: Baechle TR, Earle RW, eds. *Essentials of Strength Training and Conditioning*. 2nd Ed. Champaign: Human Kinetics Press, 2000.

5. Predetermine a minimum number of trials (repetitions) to establish a criterion strength score. For example, if administering five repetitions of a test, what score represents the individual's strength score? Is the highest score best, or should one use the average? In most cases, an average of the last of several trials provides a more representative (reliable) strength or power score than a single measure, even if that measure was obtained on the first attempt.
6. Select test measures with high test score reproducibility. This crucial but often overlooked aspect

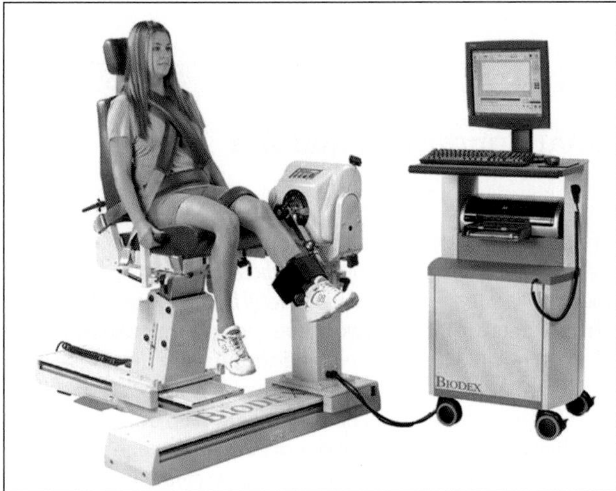

FIGURE 14.5 Biodex advanced isokinetic electromechanical dynamometer. (Photo from Biodex; **www.biodex.com/physical-medicine/products/dynamometers/system-4-quick-set.**)

of testing evaluates the variability of the subject's responses on repeated efforts. A lack of test score consistency or unreliability can mask an individual's representative performance on the measure or change in performance when evaluating strength improvement.

7. Account for individual differences in body weight and lean body mass and body composition (total and regional body fat) using appropriate statistical models when evaluating strength scores among diverse individuals and groups.

Minimally Invasive Microtechniques for Lower Back Surgery

Approximately 500,000 people in the United States and hundreds of thousands worldwide have surgery annually to gain relief from lower back and leg pain.

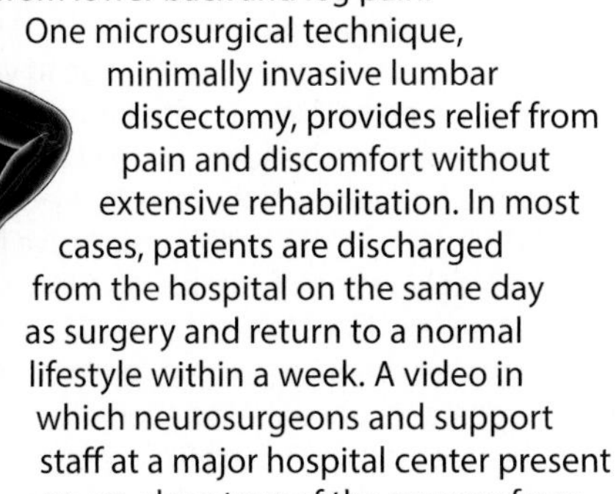

One microsurgical technique, minimally invasive lumbar discectomy, provides relief from pain and discomfort without extensive rehabilitation. In most cases, patients are discharged from the hospital on the same day as surgery and return to a normal lifestyle within a week. A video in which neurosurgeons and support staff at a major hospital center present an up-close tour of the surgery from the first incision to the operation's completion is available online at **www.orlive.com/baptisthealth/videos/minimally-invasive-lumbar-discectomy?view=displayPageNLM.**

Weightlifting Belts Help Reduce Injurious Compressive Forces on Spinal Disks

Wearing a relatively stiff weightlifting belt during heavy lifts (squats, dead lifts, clean-and-jerk maneuvers) reduces intra-abdominal pressure compared with lifting without a belt. The belt reduces potentially injurious compressive forces on spinal disks during near-maximal lifting, including most Olympic and powerlifting events and associated training. In one study, nine experienced weightlifters lifted barbells up to 75% of body weight under three conditions: (1) while inhaling and wearing a belt, (2) while inhaling and not wearing a belt, and (3) while exhaling and wearing a belt. Measurements included intra-abdominal pressure, trunk muscle electromyography (EMG), ground reaction forces, and kinematics. The belt reduced compression forces by about 10% but only when the weightlifter inhaled before lifting. The authors concluded that wearing a tight and stiff back belt while inhaling before lifting reduces spinal loading during the lift.

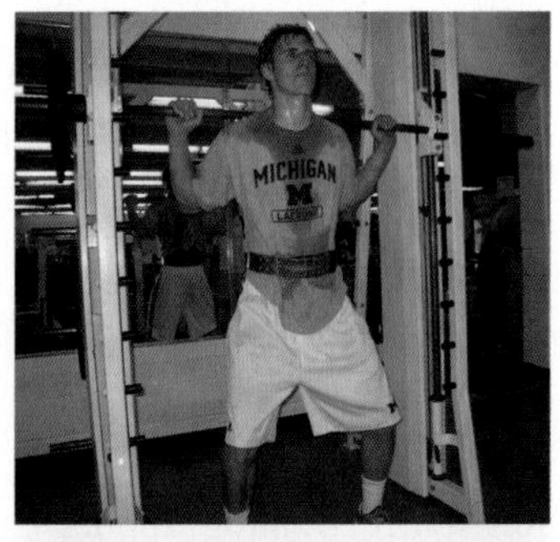

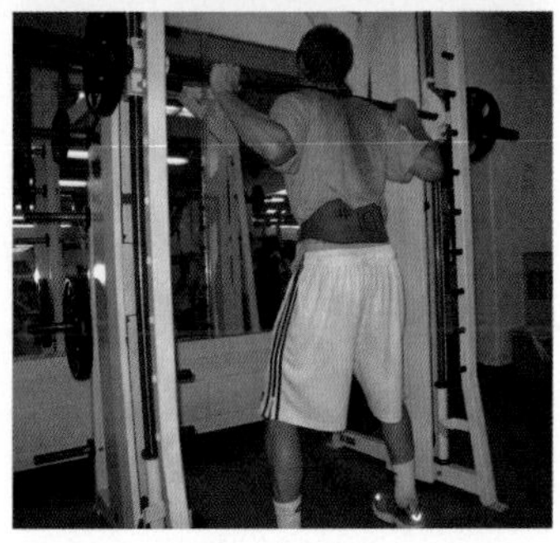

A person who normally trains wearing a belt should generally refrain from lifting without one. Further recommendations include performing at least some submaximal resistance training without a belt to strengthen the deep abdominal and pelvic-stabilizing muscles. This also develops the proper pattern of muscle recruitment to generate high intra-abdominal pressures when not wearing a belt. Wearing a back belt to ameliorate low back injuries in the workplace does not provide a clear-cut biomechanical advantage. A 2-year prospective study of nearly 14,000 material-handling employees in 30 states evaluated the effectiveness of using back belts to reduce back injury worker's compensation claims and reports of low back pain. Neither frequent back belt use (usually once a day and once or twice a week) nor a store policy that required the use of these belts reduced injury or reports of low back pain. Researchers worldwide continue to probe for answers about the cause of low back pain syndrome and how to minimize its severity and reduce its occurrence.

TRAINING MUSCLES TO BECOME STRONGER

A muscle strengthens when trained near its current maximal force-generating capacity. Standard weightlifting equipment, pulleys, slings, springs, immovable bars, resistance bands, and a variety of isokinetic, pneumatic, and hydraulic devices provide effective muscle overload. Certain exercise methods lend themselves to precise and systematic overload applications. **Progressive resistance weight training, isometric training**, and **isokinetic training** represent three common exercise systems to train muscles to become stronger. Strengthening muscles requires adherence to basic exercise training principles and specific guidelines.

Overload (Intensity)

Resistance training applies the **overload principle** regardless of the device used to produce the overload. In each case, the muscle responds to the level of tension placed on muscle (intensity of the overload) rather than the form of overload. The amount of overload reflects a percentage of the maximum strength (1-RM) of a nonfatigued muscle or muscle group. Performing a **voluntary maximal muscle action** means a muscle must exert as much force as its present capacity allows. A partially fatigued muscle cannot generate the same force as a nonfatigued muscle. The last repetition to momentary failure in a set denotes a voluntary maximal muscle action. Muscular overload in resistance training usually requires such voluntary maximal muscle actions.

Three approaches, either singularly or in combination apply the principles of muscular overload in resistance training:

1. Increase load or resistance
2. Increase repetition number
3. Increase speed of muscle action

A CLOSER LOOK

Musculoskeletal Conditions and the Lower Back

According to the National Center for Health Statistics and other data sources, including the *Healthcare Cost and Utilization Project, Medical Expenditures Panel Survey*, and the 2014 edition of *"The Burden of Musculoskeletal Diseases in the United States"* (**www.boneandjointburden.org**), one in two adults report a musculoskeletal condition requiring medical attention. Musculoskeletal disorders and diseases include approximately 150 different diseases and syndromes typically associated with pain or inflammation and most economically advanced countries remain the leading cause of disability in more than half of all chronic conditions in people over age 50. The incidence and burden of musculoskeletal conditions are likely to escalate in the next 10 to 20 years due to an aging population and sedentary lifestyles.

In particular, back injuries account for one-fourth of all work-related injuries and one-third of all compensation costs, which, according to the Bureau of Labor Statistics (**www.bls.gov**), cost about $90 billion yearly in related health costs. Most cases result from on-the-job injuries, particularly in men in lumber and building retailing (highest risk) and construction (most cases); major risk industries for women include nursing and work in personal care centers (highest risk) and hospitals (most cases). Work in grocery stores and agricultural crop production rank among the top 10 occupations for lower back injury for men and women.

Muscular weakness, particularly in the abdominal and lower lumbar back regions, lumbar spine instability, and poor joint flexibility in the back and legs represent primary external factors related to lower back pain syndrome.

Prevention of and rehabilitation from chronic lower back strain commonly use muscle-strengthening and joint flexibility exercises. Continuing normal activities of daily living within limits dictated by pain tolerance yields more rapid recovery from acute back pain than bed rest. Maintaining normal physical activity facilitates greater recovery than specific back-mobilizing exercises performed following pain onset. Prudent resistance-training isolates and strengthens the abdomen and lower lumbar extensor muscles that support and protect the spine through its full ROM. Patients with low back pain who strengthen these muscle groups experience fewer acute and chronic symptoms, improved muscular strength and endurance, and increased ROM.

Resistance-Training Exercises: Potential Risks to the Lower Back

Resistance-training exercise poses a dilemma for those with lower back syndrome. Improper performance of a typical resistance exercise movement with a relatively heavy load with hips thrust forward and arched back creates considerable lower spine compressive forces. For example, pressing and curling exercises with back hyperextension creates unusually high shearing stress on lumbar vertebrae, often triggering lower back pain accompanied by regional muscle instability.

Compressive forces with heavy lifting also can hasten damage to vertebral disks that cushion and protect vertebrae. Performing half squats with barbell loads from 0.8 to 1.6 times body mass produces huge compressive loads on the L3 to L4 spine segment, often the equivalent of 6 to 10 times body mass. For example, a person who weighs 90 kg and squats with 144 kg (318 lb) can create peak compressive forces in excess of 1367 kg (13,334 N)! A sudden amplification of compressive force can precipitate anterior disk prolapse or herniation (see Fig. 11.4 in Chapter 11). A lower-intensity but sustained compressive force that produces fatigue can increase posterior bulging of the lamellas in the posterior annulus. In national-level male and female powerlifters, average compressive loads on L4 to L5 reached 1757 kg (17,192 N).

At the practical level during sports training with resistance methods (i.e., functional training with free weights), one must not sacrifice meticulous execution of an exercise just to lift a heavier load or "squeeze out" additional repetitions. The extra weight lifted through improper technique (*cheating*) does not facilitate muscle strengthening; rather, improper body alignment or unwarranted muscle substitution during the lift can trigger debilitating injury and result in the need for surgery.

This unnerving fact should encourage proper strengthening of "core" abdominal and lower back muscles.

General Back Exercises

The figure illustrates 12 exercises that provide general strengthening of the abdomen, pelvic region, and lower back. They improve hamstring and lower back flexibility for individuals with no apparent lower back and spinal injuries, while symptomatic individuals including athletes require targeted exercises to minimize symptoms yet provide incremental steps as they return to normal function.

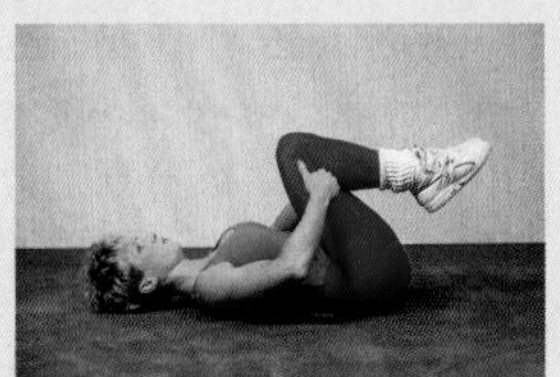

(A) ***Knees-to-chest stretch:*** Lie supine and pull knees into chest while keeping lower back flat on the surface.

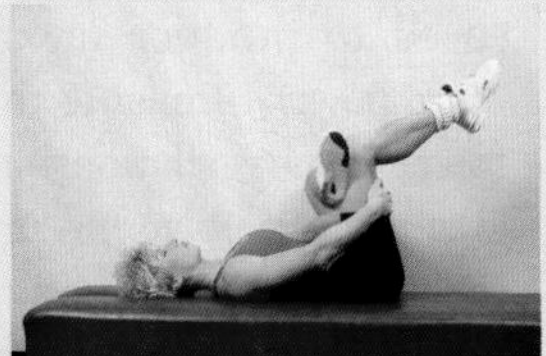

(B) ***Cross-leg stretch:*** Cross legs like sitting male. Cross legs and pull 90°-flexed knee toward chest.

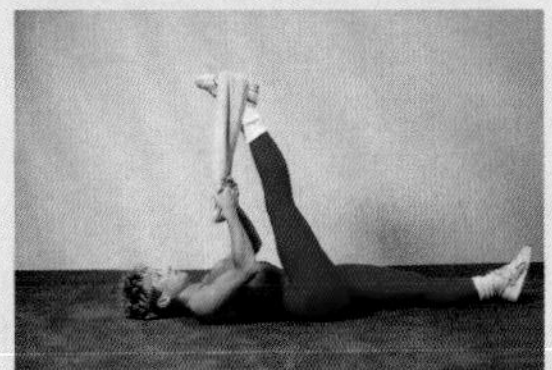

(C) ***Hamstring stretch:*** Wrap strap over foot, keeping lower back flat; pull leg upward toward head.

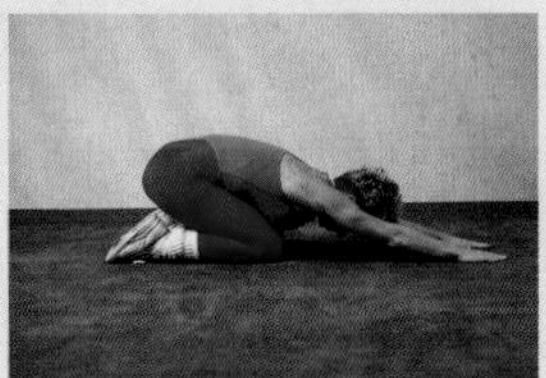

(D) ***Snail stretch:*** Sit with buttocks on bilateral heels; move hands as far forward along the surface as possible.

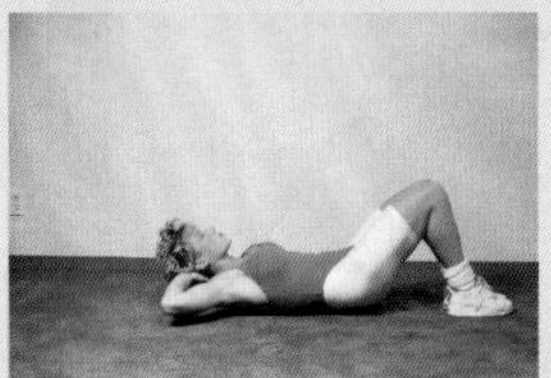

(E) ***Bent-knee sit-up:*** Keep hands low on neck (or across chest) with head positioned over the shoulders. Roll up slowly, engaging one row of abdominals at a time. Raise the shoulders 4 to 6 inches off the surface.

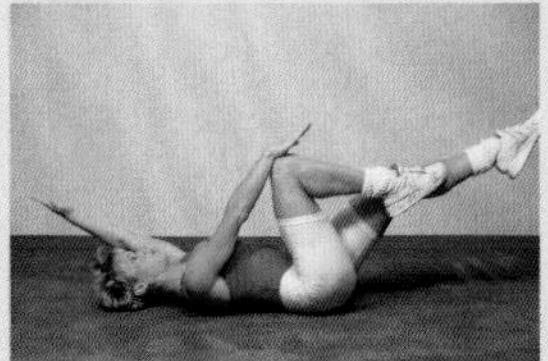

(F) ***Dying bug:*** Flex the pelvis to flatten the lower back against the surface. Over one side, bring an extended arm and flexed knee together. The opposing side should extend a straight arm overhead and straight leg backward. Maintain pelvic flexion while exchanging opposing arms and legs in this position.

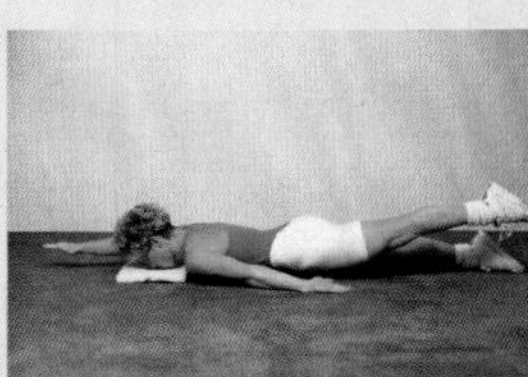

(G) ***Dry-land swimming:*** Lying prone with pelvic flexion, alternate lifting opposite arm and legs.

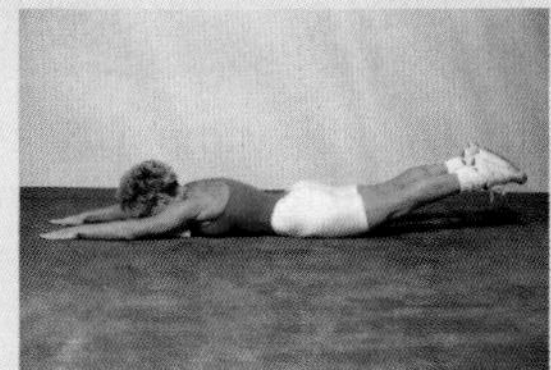

(H) ***Both legs up:*** Lying prone with pelvic flexion, lift both legs simultaneously while keeping the head on the floor.

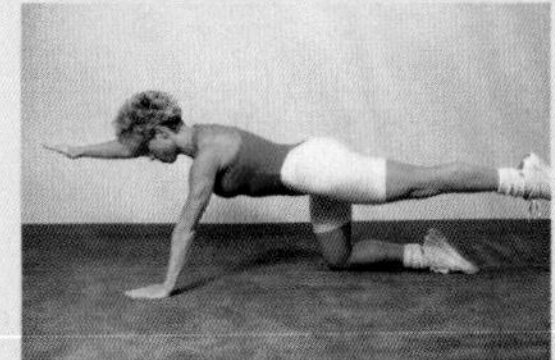

(I) ***Pointer (bird dog):*** Start with hands and knees on the floor. Flex pelvis into counter position. Exchange pointing opposite arm and leg while keeping the torso level.

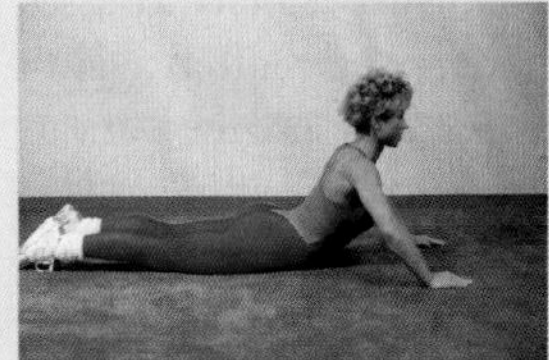

(J) ***Upper body up:*** Lying prone with pelvic flexion and arms outstretched or behind the back, lift the upper torso while keeping the legs on the floor.

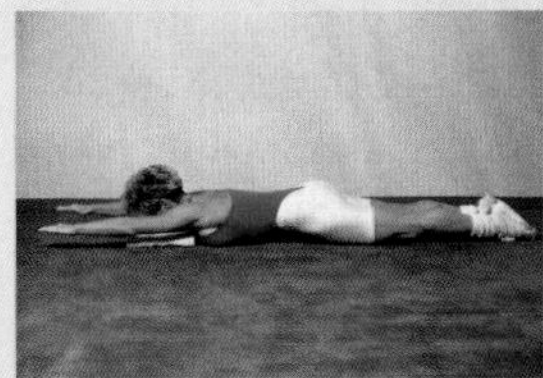

(K) ***Prone cobra push-up:*** Keep the pelvis on the floor while pressing up with the arms, causing lower back extension.

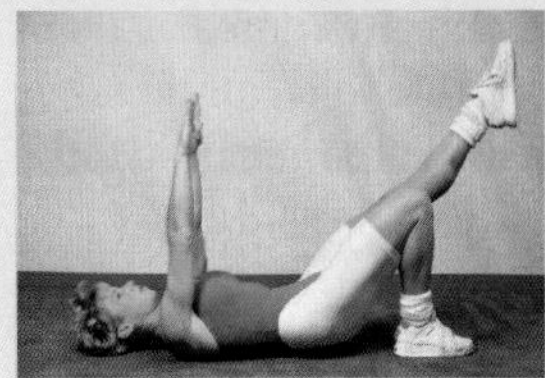

(L) ***Leg pointer:*** Lie supine on the floor and flex the pelvis with the lower abdominals to flatten the lower back into the surface. Extend one arm upward and one leg outward while keeping the quadriceps level.

Twelve examples of general exercises to strengthen the abdomen and lower back and increase hamstring and lower back flexibility. (Photos courtesy of Dr. Robert S. Swanson, DC. Robert Swanson Chiropractic Clinic. Santa Barbara, CA.).

The degree of muscular overload, often called training intensity, represents the most important factor in strength development; it requires training above a minimum threshold level to induce a training response. Minimal intensity for muscular overload occurs between 60% and 70% of 1-RM. This means that performing a large number of repetitions with light resistance at a low percentage of 1-RM produces only minimal, if any, real strength improvements.

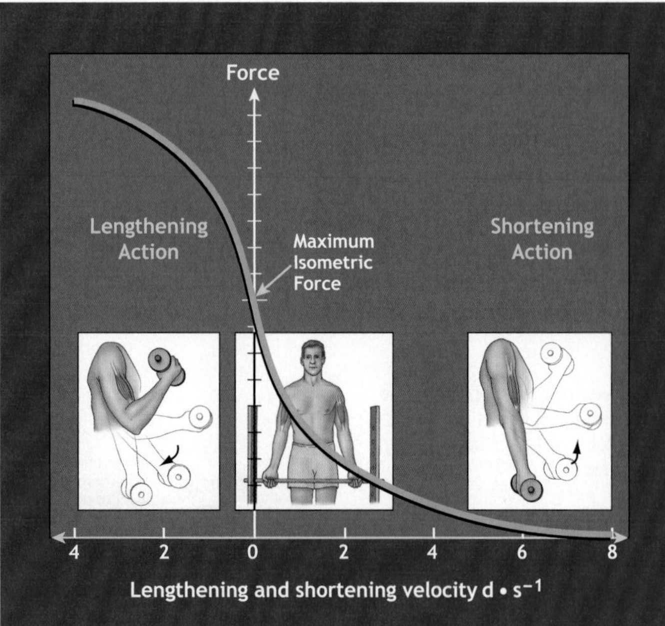

FIGURE 14.6 Maximum force-velocity relationship for shortening and lengthening muscle actions. Rapid shortening velocities (degrees per second, d · s^{-1}) generate the least maximum force. Shortening velocity becomes zero (maximum isometric force) when the curve crosses the *y* axis. Force-generating capacity increases to its highest as the muscle lengthens at rapid velocities.

Force-Velocity Relationship

Different physical activities require different amounts of strength (force) and power. Absolute or peak force generated in a movement depends on the speed of muscle lengthening and shortening. **Figure 14.6** shows the **force-velocity relationship** for concentric and eccentric muscle actions. The force-velocity relationship, denoted by a curve, represents an intrinsic relationship when a muscle shortens (or lengthens) against a constant load, with velocity assessed during muscle shortening or lengthening and plotted against the resistive force. Muscles both shorten and lengthen at different maximum velocities depending on the load placed on them (horizontal axis of graph). Shortening velocity becomes zero at maximum isometric force when the curve crosses the *y* axis. Force-generating capacity increases to its highest as the muscle lengthens at rapid velocities. As the load increases, maximum shortening velocity decreases. Conversely, a muscle's force-generating capacity rapidly declines with increased shortening velocity. This helps to explain difficulty attempting to rapidly move a heavy weight.

A shortening (concentric) action becomes a lengthening or (eccentric) action when the external load exceeds a muscle's maximum isometric force capacity (noted as point *0* on the horizontal axis). In contrast to a concentric muscle action, rapid eccentric actions generate the greatest force. This may explain the relatively greater muscle damage and delayed muscle soreness that accompanies an eccentric exercise bout. Muscle fiber type also influences the force-velocity relationships; fast-twitch muscle fibers produce greater muscle force at fast movement speeds than slow-twitch fibers because they possess higher ATPase activity, which accelerates adenosine triphosphate breakdown. Athletes who possess a high percentage of fast-twitch fibers have a distinct performance advantage in power-type physical activities.

Power-Velocity Relationship

Figure 14.7 illustrates the inverted-U relationship between a muscle's maximal power output and limb movement speed during a concentric muscle action. Peak power rapidly increases with increasing velocity to a region of peak velocity. Thereafter, maximal power output decreases because of reduced maximum force at faster movement speeds. Each muscle group has an optimum movement speed to produce maximum power. Similar to the force-velocity relationship, greater peak power at any movement velocity occurs in fast-twitch muscle fibers than in slow-twitch fibers.

Load-Repetition Relationship

The total work accomplished by muscle action depends on the load or resistance placed on the muscle. One can perform high repetitions with light loads but only few repetitions with near-maximal loads. **Figure 14.8A** shows this relationship for the full range of percentages of 1-RM. The area from 60%

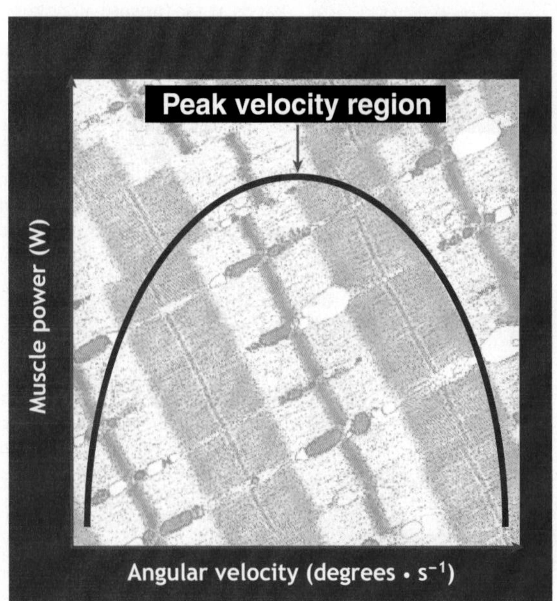

FIGURE 14.7 Inverted-U relationship between muscle's maximal power output and limb movement speed during concentric muscle actions. Power (work per unit time) increases as a function of movement velocity up to a peak velocity region. Thereafter, power decreases with further increases in angular velocity.

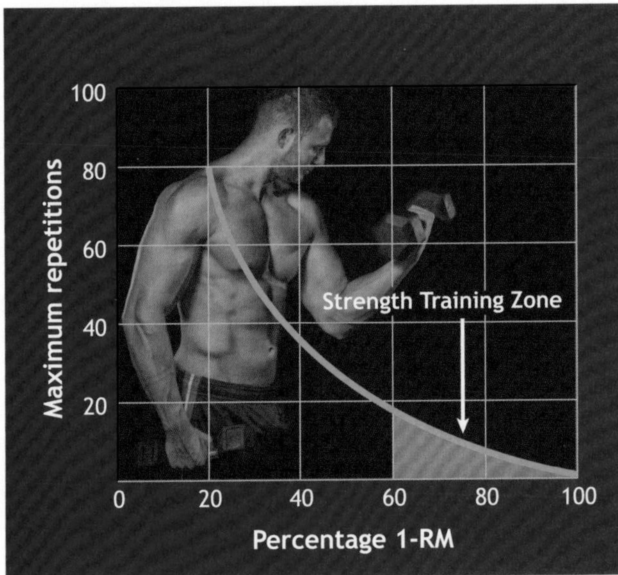

FIGURE 14.8 Relationship between maximum number of repetitions to failure and load at 20% to 100% 1-RM. (From Siff MC, Verkhoshansky YV. *Supertraining: Special Strength Training for Sporting Excellence*. Perry: Strength Coach, Inc., 1997.)

to 100% 1-RM represents the **strength-training zone**, the overload stimulus that optimizes strength improvement.

GENDER DIFFERENCES IN MUSCULAR STRENGTH

Two strength-testing approaches determine whether true gender differences exist in muscular strength:

1. Assessment of absolute strength (total force exerted)
2. Assessment of relative strength (force exerted related to body mass, fat-free body mass [FFM], or muscle cross-sectional area [MCSA])

Absolute Muscle Strength

Comparisons of muscular strength on an absolute score basis (i.e., total force in lb or kg) reveal that men possess considerably greater strength than women for all muscle groups tested. Women score about 50% lower than men for upper-body strength and about 30% lower for lower-body leg strength. This gender disparity exists independent of the measuring device and generally coincides with gender-related difference in muscle mass distribution. Exceptions usually emerge for strength-trained female track-and-field athletes and bodybuilders who have strength trained for many years for national and international competitions.

Table 14.3 provides the strength ratios for different muscle groups (female strength score ÷ male strength score). These data represent averages from the research literature based on strength scores of men and women for concentric and eccentric muscle actions. Overall, the typical woman's total body strength represents 64% of the typical man's strength; for upper-body strength, women average 56% of the men's score, and lower-body strength averages 72% of values achieved by men.

TABLE 14.3 Ratio of Female Strength to Male Strength for Different Muscle Groups[a]

Muscle Group	Strength Ratio (Female Score ÷ Male Score)
Elbow flexors	0.55
Elbow extensors	0.48
Knee flexors	0.69
Knee extensors	0.68
Shoulder flexors	0.55
Trunk extensors and flexors	0.60
Hip extensors and flexors	0.80
Finger flexors	0.60

[a]Data represent an average of values in the literature that reported female-to-male data. The ratios were obtained by dividing the female mean strength for a given muscle(s) by the mean male strength score. These data can be used to (1) evaluate performance of women relative to men, (2) select first approximations of suitable loads for women based on data for men, or (3) approximate data for men if only data for women are available.

Relative Muscle Strength

Human skeletal muscle fibers *in vitro* (outside of the body) generate 16 to 30 Newtons (N) maximal force per square centimeter of **muscle cross-sectional area (MCSA)** (MCSA refers to a cross-section of the largest diameter in an intact, contracted muscle regardless of gender). In the body (*in vivo*), force-output capacity varies depending on the bony lever's arrangement and muscle architecture.

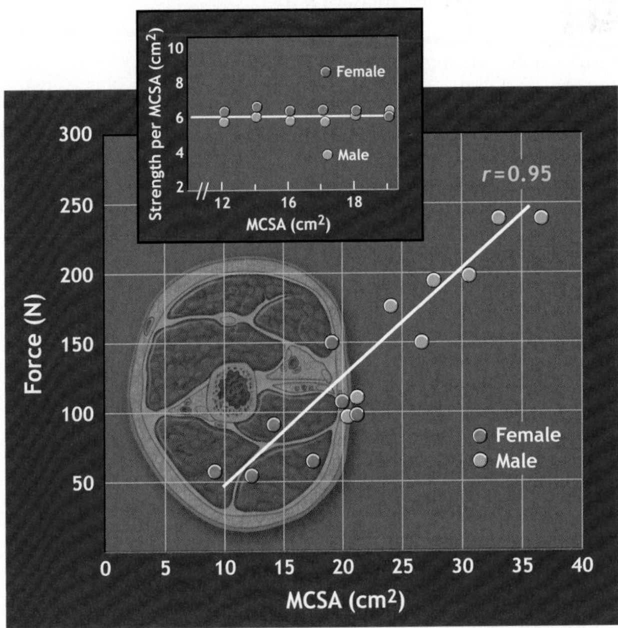

FIGURE 14.9 Plot of force (Newtons, N) versus muscle cross-sectional area (MCSA, cm^2). Data represent elbow flexion. The inset figure shows the strength per unit MCSA. (Data from Miller JD, et al. Gender differences in strength and muscle fiber characteristics. *Eur J Appl Physiol* 1992;66:254, and Ikai M, Fukunaga R. Calculation of muscle strength per unit cross-sectional area of human muscle by means of ultrasonic measurements. *Arbeitsphysiologie* 1968;26:26.)

Figure 14.9 depicts the results of a classic study that compared arm flexor strength of men and women related to MCSA. The strong linear, positive relationship of $r = 0.95$ indicates that individuals with larger MCSA generate the greatest muscular force, and those with smaller MCSA generate the lowest force. This is true for the entire range of force outputs from the lowest to highest scores. The inset graph shows equality in strength between genders when expressing arm flexor strength per unit MCSA. See A Closer Look: "Determining Upper Arm Muscle and Fat," for how to determine MCSA.

Relative strength computes by relating strength to one of three variables:

1. Body mass (strength score in lb or kg ÷ body mass in lb or kg)
2. Segmental or total FFM (strength score in lb or kg ÷ FFM in lb or kg)
3. MCSA (strength score in lb or kg ÷ MCSA)

A relative score increases the "fairness" when comparing two individuals' strength performances (or the same person assessed before, during, and after a training regimen or weight loss program).

A CLOSER LOOK

Determining Upper Arm Muscle and Fat

Girth measurements include bone surrounded by a mass of muscle tissue ringed by a subcutaneous fat layer (Fig. 1). Muscle represents the largest component of the girth except in obese and elderly individuals, so girth indicates one's relative muscularity. Estimating limb muscle area assumes similarity between a limb and a cylinder, with subcutaneous fat evenly distributed around the cylinder (Fig. 1).

Measurements

Determine the following:

1. Upper-arm girth (relaxed triceps; G_{arm}): With a cloth tape, measure with arm extended relaxed at the side (or parallel to the ground in an abducted position). Measure girth (cm) midway between the acromial and olecranon process (Fig. 2).

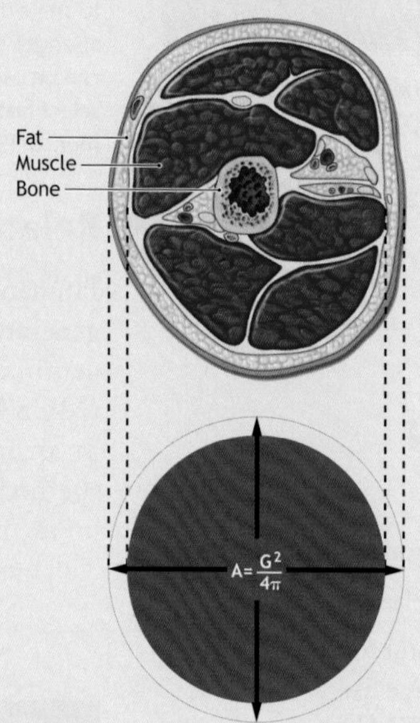

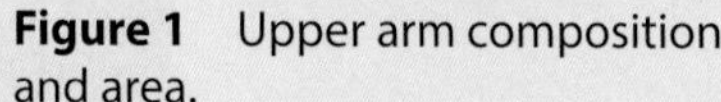

Figure 1 Upper arm composition and area.

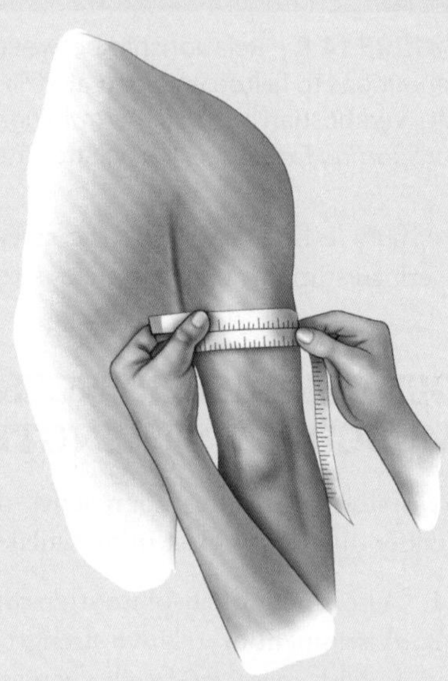

Figure 2 Relaxed triceps arm girth, cm.

RESISTANCE TRAINING FOR CHILDREN

Resistance training for children has gained popularity over the past two decades, yet its benefits and possible risks remain fertile ground for further research. Incomplete skeletal development in young children and adolescents raises concern about the potential for bone and joint injury with heavy muscular overload. One might question whether resistance training improves strength at a relatively young age because the hormonal profile continues to develop, particularly for the tissue-building hormones testosterone and growth hormone. *Closely supervised resistance-training programs using concentric-only muscle actions with high repetitions and low resistance improve children's muscular strength without adverse effect on bone or muscle.* Consensus exists among health care and fitness professional organizations—American Academy of Pediatrics (**www.aap.org/en-us/Pages/Default.aspx**), American College of Sports Medicine (**www.acsm.org/**), American Orthopaedic Society for Sports (**www.sportsmed.org**), and National Strength and Conditioning Association (**www.nsca.com**)—that child and adolescent supervised strength training programs that adhere to established training guidelines and precautions are both safe and effective. **Table 14.4** provides basic guidelines for resistance exercise progressions for children at different ages.

RESISTANCE-TRAINING SYSTEMS

Many systems of "strength training" have been developed over the past several centuries. When we think of modern methods to develop muscular strength, we usually think of some variation of free weights or barbells. For historical perspective, the Ling system referenced earlier in this chapter devised routines of progressive exercises to strengthen total body musculature. The method of progressive sling suspension training shown in **Figure 14.10 (top)** was pioneered in

2. Triceps skinfold (Sf_{tri}): With a skinfold caliper, measure in millimeters and convert to decimeters (dm; mm ÷ 10) on the back of the arm, over the triceps muscle, as a vertical fold at the same level as the relaxed arm girth (Fig. 3).

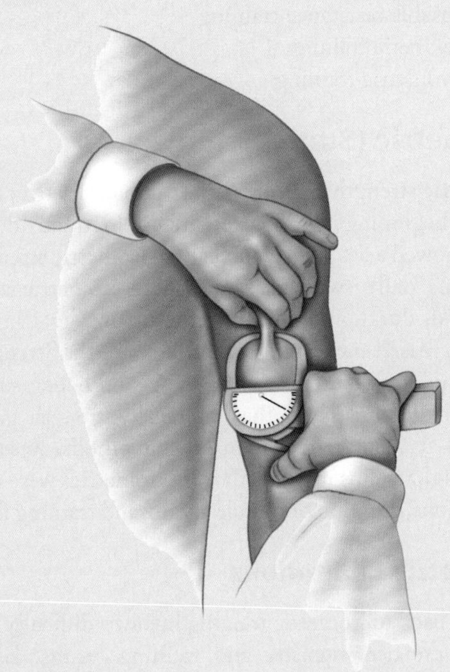

Figure 3 Triceps skinfold, mm.

Example

Data

Upper arm girth (G_{arm}) in cm (30.0 cm); triceps skinfold (Sf_{tri}) in dm (2.5 dm).

Computations

1. **Arm muscle girth, cm** $= G_{arm} - (\pi Sf_{tri})$
   $= 30.0\text{ cm} - (\pi 2.5\text{ dm})$
   $= 30.0 - 7.854$
   $= 22.1\text{ cm}$

2. **Arm muscle area, cm²** $= [G_{arm} - (\pi Sf_{tri})] \div 4\pi$
   $= (30.0\text{ cm}) - (\pi 2.5\text{ dm})^2 \div 4\pi$
   $= 488.4 \div 12.566$
   $= 38.9\text{ cm}^2$

3. **Arm area (A), cm²** $= (G_{arm})^2 \div 4\pi$
   $= (30.0\text{ cm})^2 \div 4\pi$
   $= 900 \div 12.566$
   $= 71.6\text{ cm}^2$

4. **Arm fat area, cm² = Arm area − Arm muscle area**
   $= 71.6\text{ cm}^2 - 38.9\text{ cm}^2$
   $= 32.7\text{ cm}^2$

5. **Arm fat index, % fat area**
   $= (\text{Arm fat area} \div \text{Arm area}) \times 100$
   $= (32.7\text{ cm}^2 \div 71.6\text{ cm}^2) \times 100$
   $= 45.7\%$

TABLE 14.4 Guidelines for Resistance Exercise for Children[a]

Age, y	Guideline
5–7	Introduce child to basic exercises with little or no weight; develop the concept of a training session; teach exercise techniques; progress from body weight calisthenics, partner exercises, and lightly resisted exercises; keep volume low.
8–10	Gradually increase the exercise number; practice exercise techniques for all lifts; start gradual progressive loading of exercises; keep exercises simple; increase volume slowly; carefully monitor tolerance to exercise stress.
11–13	Teach all basic exercise techniques; continue progressive loading of each exercise; emphasize exercise technique; introduce more advanced exercises with little or no resistance.
14–15	Progress to more advanced resistance exercise programs; add sport-specific components; emphasize exercise techniques; increase volume.
16+	Entry level into adult programs after the person masters all background experience

[a]Note: If a child at a particular age level has no previous experience, progression must start at previous levels and move to more advanced levels as exercise tolerance, skill, and understanding permit.

From Kraemer WJ, Fleck SJ. *Designing Resistance Training Programs*. Champaign: Human Kinetics, 2014.

Sweden beginning in the 1840s. Between 1914 and 1918, more advanced suspension and sling exercise and training methods (**Fig. 14.10, middle**) were developed by physiotherapists working in English hospitals and rehabilitation facilities during and after World War I. Norwegian sling suspension training methods developed in the early 1990s (**Fig. 14.10, bottom**) also complemented physical therapy applications and general and specific fitness training. Sling suspension methodologies leverage the person's body weight as resistance increases or decreases by altering the suspension coordinates, sling height, or body position relative to the suspension point.

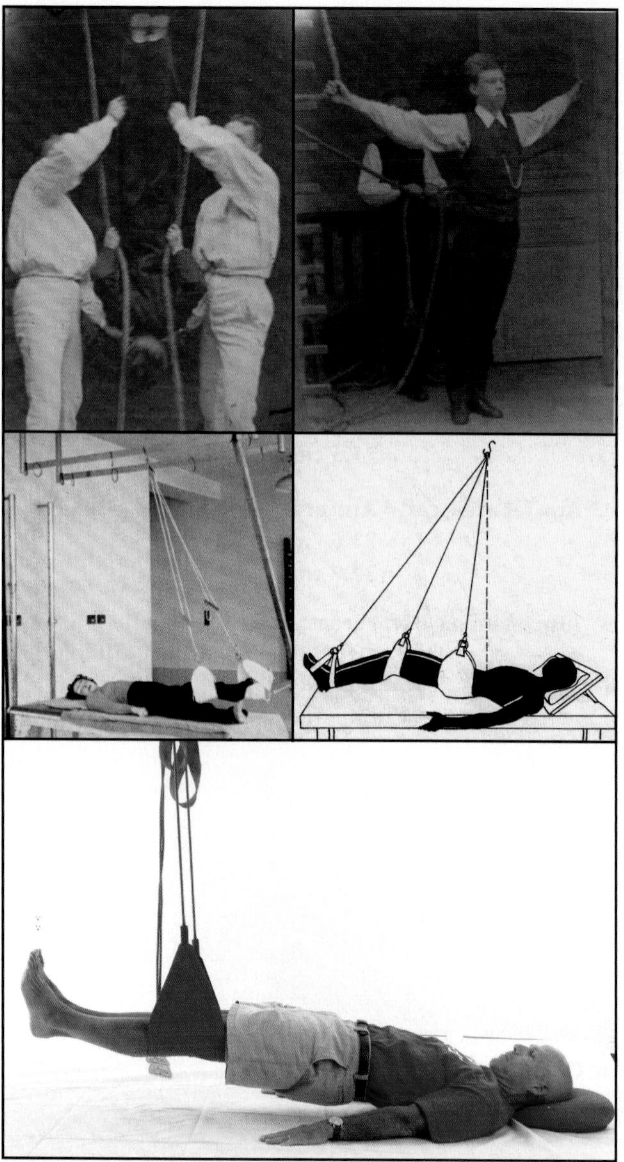

FIGURE 14.10 Different systems of sling suspension progressive exercise to strengthen total body musculature. **Top**. Progressive rope and sling suspension remedial exercise regimens pioneered in Sweden beginning in the 1840s. **Middle**. Sling suspension and reciprocal weight and pulley exercise training methods pioneered in the British Isles in the 1920s to 1950s by Olive Frances Guthrie Smith (1883–1956) with A.E. Porritt in 1931. (From Smith OFGS, Porritt AE. A method of exciting incipient movement in weakened and paralyzed muscles. *Br Med J* 1931;1:54.) **Bottom**. Suspension training techniques developed in the 1990s emphasize unstable, closed kinetic chain exercise for physical therapy applications, strength development, and general and specific fitness training. (Photo copyright Victor Katch. Ann Arbor.)

Muscular strength can be developed by five different but interrelated popular training systems:

1. Isometric training
2. DCER training
3. Variable resistance training
4. Isokinetic training
5. Plyometric training

Isometric (Static) Training

Isometric strength training gained popularity over a 10-year period beginning in 1955. Research in Germany during this time showed a 5% weekly increase in isometric strength from only one daily, two-thirds maximum isometric action for 6 seconds duration. Repeating this action 5 to 10 times further increased measured isometric strength. Strength gains from this simple exercise seemed beyond belief; subsequent research demonstrated that isometric strength gains progressed at a slower rate than other methods. Research also showed that gains in strength from isometrics were related to repetitions, duration of muscle action, and training frequency.

Isometric Limitations

A drawback to isometric training involves difficulty in monitoring exercise intensity and training results. Essentially, no external movement occurs during the muscle action, so it becomes difficult to determine objectively if the person's strength actually improves and whether the person applies an appropriate overload force during training.

Isometric Benefits

Isometric exercise effectively improves the strength of a particular muscle or group of muscles when the applied isometric force covers four or five joint angles through the ROM. Isometric training works well in orthopedic and physical therapy applications that isolate strengthening movements during rehabilitation. Isometric measurement pinpoints an area of muscle weakness, and isometric training strengthens muscles at the appropriate joint angle in the ROM.

Dynamic Constant External Resistance Training

This popular system of resistance training involves both lifting (concentric) and lowering (eccentric) phases, with each repetition using weight plates (barbells and dumbbells) or exercise machines that feature different muscular overload strategies.

Progressive Resistance Exercise

Following World War II, rehabilitation medicine researchers devised a resistance-training method to improve the force-generating capacity of previously injured muscles and limbs. Their method involved three sets of resistance exercise, each consisting of 10 repetitions done consecutively without rest. The first set involved one-half the maximum weight lifted 10 times or one-half 10-RM; the second set used three-quarters 10-RM; the final set required maximum weight for 10 repetitions or 10-RM. As patients increased their strength, the resistance increased periodically to match strength improvements. This technique of **progressive resistance exercise (PRE)**, a practical application of the overload principle, forms the basis for most current resistance-training programs.

Variations of Progressive Resistance Exercise

Research has altered PRE regimens to determine an optimal number of sets, repetitions, frequency, and relative intensity of training to improve strength. The list that follows summarizes 13 general research findings on the ideal number of sets and repetitions, including frequency and relative intensity of PRE training for optimal strength improvement:

1. Eight- to 12-RM proves effective loading for novice trainers, and 1- to 12-RM for intermediate training. The 1- to 12-RM protocol can then increase to heavy loading using 1- to 6-RM.
2. Rest for 3 minutes between sets of an exercise at moderate movement velocity (1 to 2 s of concentric; 1 to 2 s of eccentric).
3. For PRE at a specific RM load, increase the load from 2% to 10% when performing 1 to 2 repetitions above the current workload.
4. Performing one exercise set induces only slightly less strength improvement in recreational weightlifters than performing two or three sets. For those wishing to maximize muscle strength and size gains, higher volume, multiple-set paradigms emphasizing 6- to 12-RM at moderate velocity with 1- to 2-minute rests between sets prove most effective.
5. Single-set programs generally produce most of the health and fitness benefits of multiple-set programs. These "lower-volume" programs also produce greater compliance and reduce the time commitment.
6. Novices and intermediates train 2 to 3 days a week, whereas advanced exercisers typically train 3 to 4 days a week and sometimes more. Such a generalization is not without a potential downside. High training frequency extends the transient activation of inflammatory signaling cascades, concomitant with persistent suppression of key mediators of anabolic responses, which could blunt the training response.
7. Training twice every second day produces overall superior results compared with daily training. This may occur from the effects of low muscle glycogen content (with training twice every second day) on enhanced gene transcription involved in training adaptations.
8. If training includes multiple exercises, 4 or 5 days a week may produce less improvement than training 2 or 3 days a week because near-daily training of the same muscles impairs muscle recuperation between training sessions. Inadequate recovery retards progress in neuromuscular and structural adaptations and strength development.
9. A fast rate of moving a given resistance generates more strength improvement than moving at a slower rate. Neither free weights (barbells, weight plates, dumbbells, kettlebells) nor an array of exercise machines show inherent superiority for developing overall muscle strength.
10. Exercise should sequence to optimize workout quality by engaging large before small muscle groups, multiple-joint exercises before single-joint exercises, and higher-intensity exercise before lower-intensity exercise.
11. Combined resistance-training concentric and eccentric muscle actions augment effectiveness and include both single- and multiple-joint exercises to potentiate a muscle's strength and fiber size.
12. Overload training with concentric-eccentric muscle actions preserves strength gains better during a maintenance phase than concentric-only training.
13. Power training should apply the strategy to improve muscular strength plus include lighter loads (30% to 60% 1-RM) performed at fast contraction velocity. Use 2- to 3-minute rest periods between sets. Emphasize multiple-joint exercises that activate large muscle groups.

The American College of Sports Medicine (ACSM) position stand on progression models in resistance training for healthy adults can be downloaded free as a PDF (**http://journals.lww.com/acsm-msse/Fulltext/2009/03000/Progression_Models_in_Resistance_Training_for.26.aspx**).

Responses of Men and Women to Dynamic Constant External Resistance Training (DCER)

Figure 14.11 depicts strength changes for men and women with DCER training based on an average from 12 experiments. Women achieved a higher percentage strength improvement than men, although considerable overlap existed in between sex comparisons. These findings indicate a relative equality

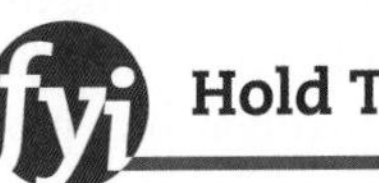

Hold That Stretch!

Stretching with fast, bouncing, jerky movements that use the body's momentum can strain or tear muscles and create a reflex action that resists the muscle stretch. Go into the stretch slowly with good form, hold the stretch position for 10 to 15 seconds, then try to increase the ROM as you continue to hold the stretch for another 10 seconds.

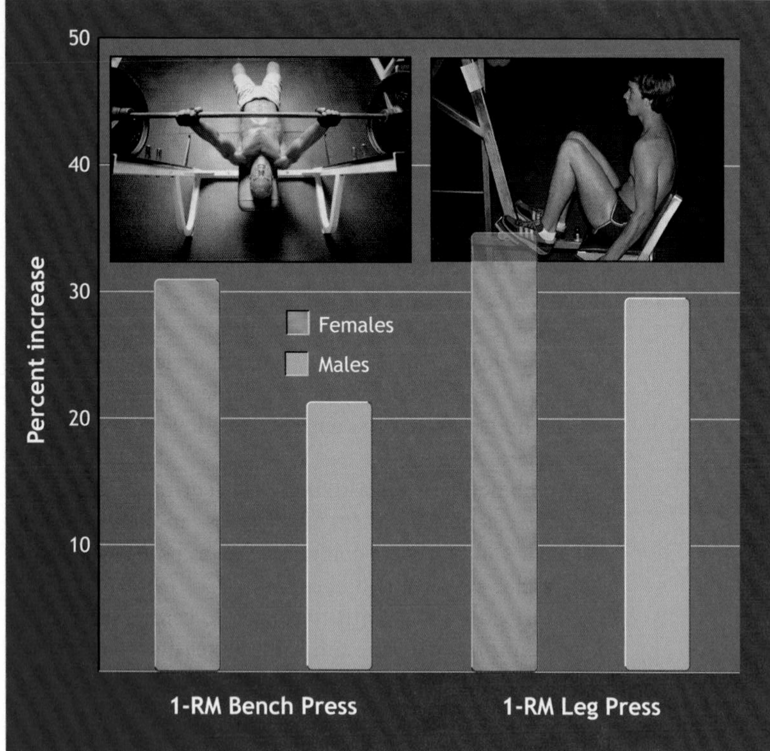

FIGURE 14.11 Percentage increase in one-repetition maximum (1-RM) bench press and leg press of women and men in response to resistance training. Values represent an average of 12 studies using dynamic constant external resistance (DCER) training for a minimum of 9 weeks duration 3 days per week with two or more sets per session.

in trainability between women and men, at least with short-duration resistance training.

Variable Resistance Training

A limitation of typical DCER weightlifting exercise involves failure of muscles to generate maximum force through all movement phases. **Variable resistance-training equipment** alters external resistance to movement by use of a lever arm, irregularly shaped metal cam, air, hydraulics, or a pulley to match increases and decreases in force capacity related to joint angle and hence lever characteristics throughout an ROM. This adjustment, based on average physical dimensions of a population, supposedly should facilitate strength gains because it theoretically allows near-maximal force production throughout the full ROM.

Biomechanical research shows that a single cam-based device cannot possibly compensate fully for individual differences in mechanics in force applications during all phases of a particular movement. Variations in limb length, point of attachment of muscle tendons to bone, body size, and muscle force output at different joint angles all affect maximum force generated throughout an ROM. Variable resistance devices do, however, provide improvements in strength comparable to improvements seen with other weightlifting and resistance equipment.

Isokinetic Training

Isokinetic resistance training differs markedly from isometrics, DCER, and variable resistance methods. Isokinetic training uses a muscle action performed at constant angular limb velocity. Unlike dynamic resistance exercise, isokinetic exercise does not require a specified initial resistance; rather, the isokinetic device controls movement velocity. The muscles exert maximal forces as they shorten (a concentric action) throughout the ROM at a specific velocity. Advocates of isokinetic training argue that exerting maximal force throughout the full ROM optimizes strength development. Also, concentric-only actions minimize the potential for muscle and joint injury and pain frequently noted from the high force generated with the movement's eccentric component.

Experiments With Isokinetic Exercise and Training

Experiments using isokinetic exercise explored the force-velocity relationship in various exercises and related this to the muscle's fiber-type composition. **Figure 14.12** displays the progressive decline in concentric peak torque output with increasing angular velocity of knee extensor muscles in two groups that differed in sports training and muscle fiber composition. For movement at $180° \cdot s^{-1}$, elite Swedish track-and-field sprinters and jumper power athletes achieved higher torque per kilogram of body mass than

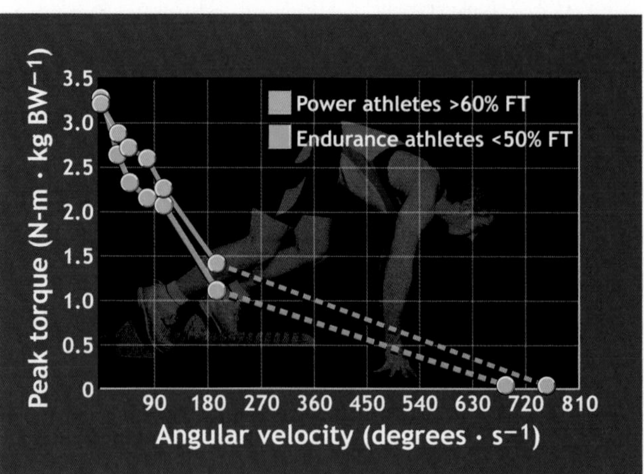

FIGURE 14.12 Peak torque per unit body mass related to angular velocity in two groups of athletes with different muscle fiber compositions. The torque-velocity curves were extrapolated (*dashed line*) to an estimated maximal velocity for knee extension. (Reprinted with permission from McArdle WD, Katch FI, Katch VL. *Exercise Physiology: Nutrition, Energy, and Human Performance*. 8th Ed. Baltimore: Wolters Kluwer Health, 2015; data from Throstensson A. Muscle strength, fiber types, and enzyme activities in man. *Acta Physiol Scand* 1976;(Suppl):443.)

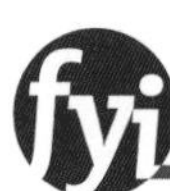

ACSM Top Ten Fitness Trends in 2013

The American College of Sports Medicine (ACSM) conducts an annual survey of fitness leaders to reveal needs and trends and to focus in various fitness environments. In essence, ACSM determines "what's hot and what's not" in the health and fitness industry. The seventh survey, released in November 2014, was completed by 3346 health and fitness professionals worldwide who are certified by ACSM or other organizations.

Body weight–loaded training made the list for the first time in 7 years. Pilates and balance and stability ball training had been trending higher in prior surveys, but did not reappear on the current list. The top ten trends in the field of fitness include:

1. Educated, certified, and experienced fitness professionals
2. Strength training
3. Body weight–loaded training
4. Children and obesity
5. Exercise and weight loss
6. Fitness programs for older adults
7. Personal training
8. Functional fitness
9. Core training
10. Group personal training

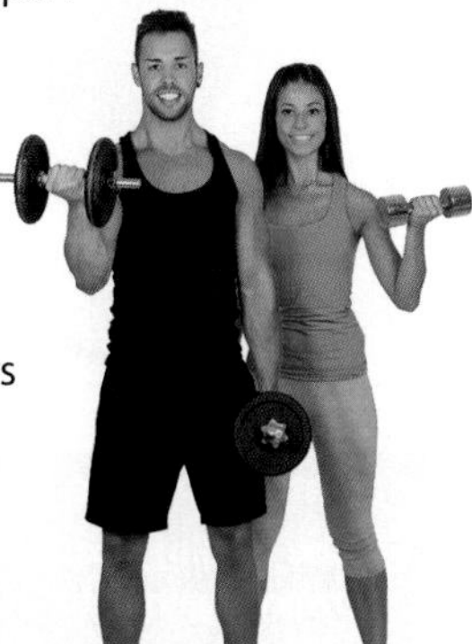

competition walkers and cross-country endurance runners. At this angular velocity, maximal torque equaled about 55% of maximal isometric force ($0° \cdot s^{-1}$). The athletes' muscle fiber composition distinguishes the two curves in **Figure 14.12**. At zero velocity shortening, an isometric action, the same peak force per unit body mass occurred for athletes with relatively high (power athletes) or low (endurance athletes) percentages of fast-twitch muscle fibers; this indicated that maximal isometric knee extension activated both fast- and slow-twitch motor units. Increasing movement velocity produced greater torque by individuals with a higher percentage of fast-twitch fibers. More than likely, fast-twitch muscle fibers favor performance in power activities where torque generation at rapid movement velocities often dictates success.

Plyometric Training

For sports that require powerful, propulsive movements—football, volleyball, sprinting, high jump, long jump, and basketball—athletes apply a special form of exercise training termed **plyometrics** or explosive jump training. These exercises repeatedly stretch and load muscles suddenly and then immediately activate them. Plyometric exercise usually requires jumps in place or rebound jumping, or drop jumping from a preset height, to mobilize the inherent stretch-recoil characteristics of skeletal muscle and its modulation via the stretch or myotatic reflex.

Stated somewhat differently, plyometric exercise involves rapid stretching followed by shortening of a muscle group during a dynamic movement. Prior stretching produces a stretch reflex and elastic recoil within muscle. When combined with a vigorous muscle contraction, plyometric actions greatly increase the force that overloads the muscles, thereby facilitating increases in strength and power. Plyometric exercises range in difficulty from calf jumps off the ground with a rebound jump to multiple one-leg jumps to and from boxes ranging in height from 1 to 6 feet. **Figure 14.13** illustrates four examples of plyometric exercise drills. The basic principle for all jumping and plyometric exercises is to absorb the shock with the arms or legs and then immediately contract the muscles. For example, when doing a series of squat jumps, the person should jump again as quickly into the air as possible after landing while at the same time, if possible, thrusting both heels up toward the buttocks. Quicker jumps provide greater overload to the muscles. In essence, "fast" plyometric exercise "trains" the neural pathways to respond quickly to activate muscles rapidly.

Plyometric maneuvers avoid the disadvantage of having to decelerate a mass in the latter part of the joint ROM during a fast movement; this provides for maximal power production. **Figure 14.14** compares a traditional bench press movement to achieve maximal power output versus a ballistic bench "throw" to maximize power output by simulating an attempt to project the barbell from the hands. The results were unequivocal. During a standard bench press, deceleration begins at about 60% of the bar position relative to the total concentric movement distance (*orange line*). In contrast, velocity during the bench throw (*yellow line*) continues to increase throughout the ROM and remains higher at all bar positions following movement. This translates into greater average force, average power, and peak power outputs. Achieving a faster average and peak velocity throughout the ROM produces greater power output and muscle activation assessed by EMG than the traditional weightlifting exercise movement. The throw condition produced greater muscle activity for the pectoralis major (+19%), anterior deltoid (+34%), triceps brachii (+44%), and biceps brachii (+27%).

Allowing the athlete to develop greater power at the end of the movement more closely simulates the projection phase of throwing a ball or implement, maximal effort jumping movements, or impact in striking movements. In this form of training, called **ballistic resistance training**, the person moves the weight or projectile as fast as possible with good form while trying to generate maximal force before releasing it. Sports performance examples include the shot put, overhead soccer throw, and javelin and discus throws; the push away from the pole vigorously in the pole vault; the takeoff jump for a volleyball spike; positioning and jumping for a basketball rebound; multiple punches in boxing, and takeoff in the high jump.

Plyometric exercise overloads a muscle to provide forcible and rapid stretch (eccentric or stretch phase) immediately

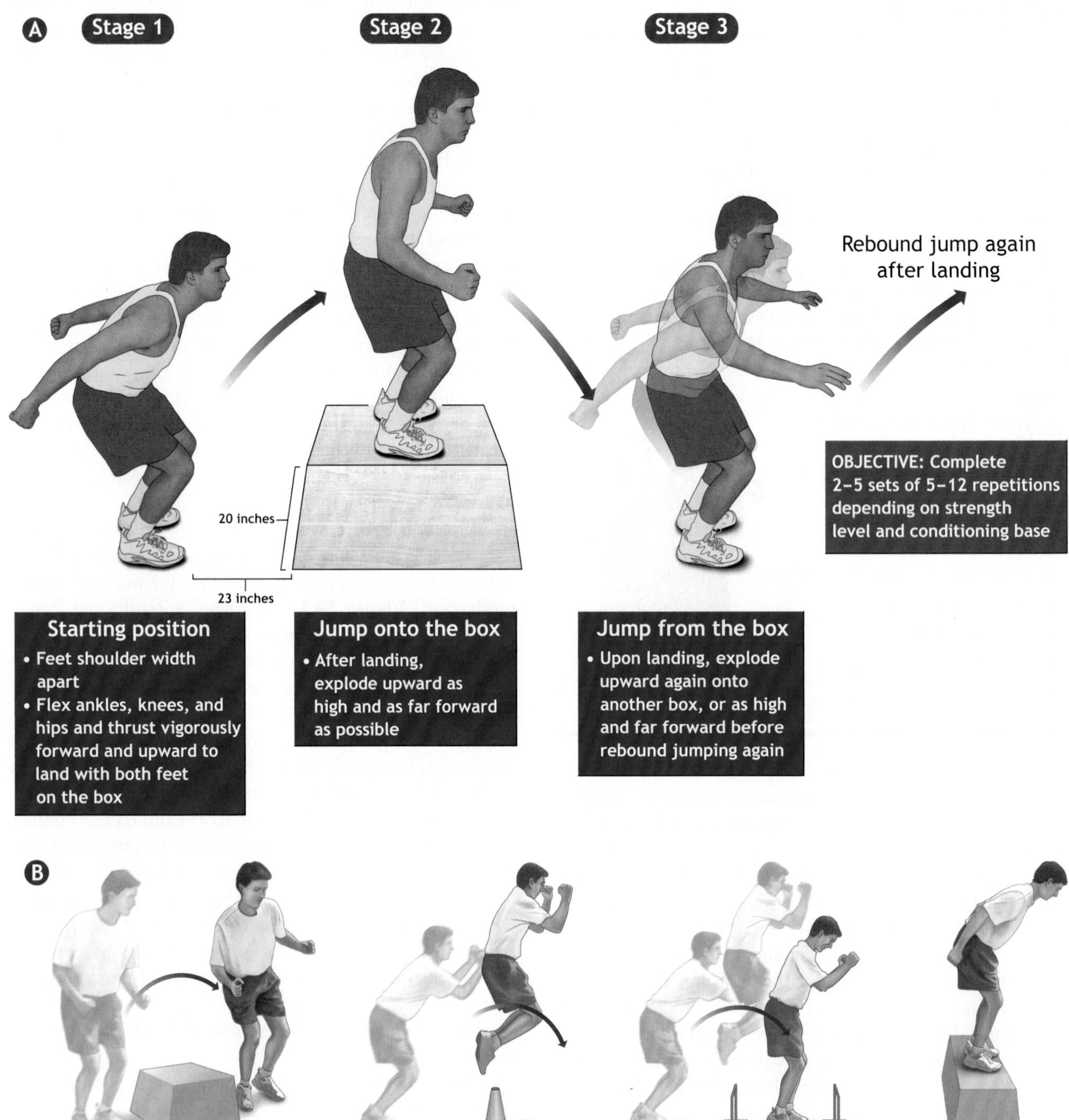

Rebound Jumping Technique in Polymetric Training
A
Stage 1
Stage 2
Stage 3
Rebound jump again after landing
OBJECTIVE: Complete 2–5 sets of 5–12 repetitions depending on strength level and conditioning base
20 inches
23 inches
Starting position
• Feet shoulder width apart
• Flex ankles, knees, and hips and thrust vigorously forward and upward to land with both feet on the box
Jump onto the box
• After landing, explode upward as high and as far forward as possible
Jump from the box
• Upon landing, explode upward again onto another box, or as high and far forward before rebound jumping again
B

FIGURE 14.13 **A.** Rebound jumping technique in plyometric training. **B.** Four examples of plyometric exercise drills: (1) box jump, (2) cone hop, (3) hurdle hop, and (4) long jump from a box. (Reprinted with permission from McArdle WD, Katch FI, Katch VL. *Exercise Physiology: Nutrition, Energy, and Human Performance*. 8th Ed. Baltimore: Wolters Kluwer Health, 2015; examples courtesy of Dr. Thomas D. Fahey, California State University at Chico, Chico.)

before the concentric or shortening phase of action. The **stretch-shortening cycle (SSC)** represents an important concept that describes how skeletal muscles function efficiently in unrestricted human locomotor activities. When gastrocnemius muscle spindles suddenly stretch, their sensory receptors fire with the impulses traveling through the dorsal root into the spinal cord to activate the anterior motor neuron to the muscle and trigger the stretch reflex (see Chapter 11), the timing of which relies on the speed of movement. The sequence of stretching and shortening muscle fibers as in the contact phase of running serves a fundamental purpose—to enhance the final push-off phase. In many sports situations, the rapid lengthening phase in the SSC produces a more powerful subsequent movement.

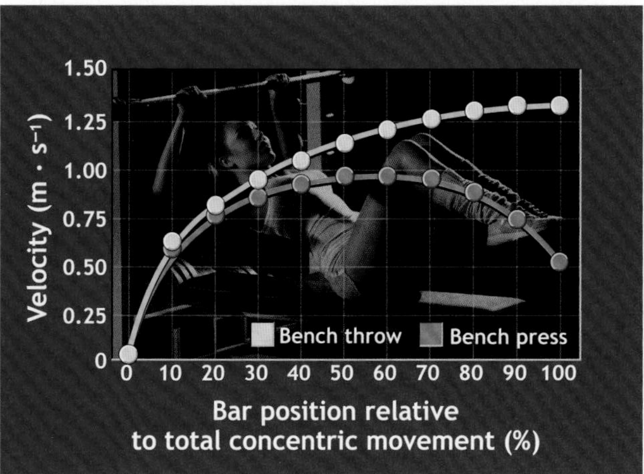

FIGURE 14.14 Mean bar velocity related to total concentric bar movement for bench throw and traditional bench press performed rapidly. (Reprinted with permission from McArdle WD, Katch FI, Katch VL. *Exercise Physiology: Nutrition, Energy, and Human Performance*. 8th Ed. Baltimore: Wolters Kluwer Health, 2015; data from Newton RU, et al. Kinematics, kinetics, and muscle activation during explosive upper body movements. *J Appl Biomech* 1996;12:31.)

From a practical standpoint, a plyometric drill uses body mass and gravity for the important SCC rapid prestretch or "cocking" phase to activate the muscles' natural elastic recoil elements. Prior stretch augments subsequent concentric muscle action in the opposite direction. Forcibly dropping the arms to the side before vertical jumping produces quadriceps muscle eccentric prestretch and exemplifies a natural plyometric movement. Lower body plyometric drills include a standing jump, multiple jumps, repetitive jumping in place, depth jumps or drop jumping from a height of about 1 m, single- and double-leg jumps, and various modifications. Proponents believe that repetitive plyometric actions provide neuromuscular training to enhance specific muscles' power output and sport-specific power performances as in jumping.

fyi Body Weight–Loaded Training

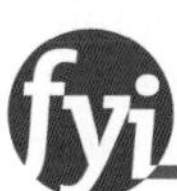

Body weight–loaded training has gained popularity as another modality to strengthen muscles and activate neural control mechanisms to support such training. In the example of body weight–supported push-up exercise (see image), the arms in the slings and not the contact surface of the floor bear the person's body weight. This activates both agonists and antagonist muscles about a joint, including additional muscle groups along the kinetic chain. While an individual performs this maneuver, the added component of instability further challenges trunk and back muscle neuromuscular control mechanisms. Individuals accustomed to doing regular push-ups on a flat surface can find this way of supporting the body during the push-up maneuver a difficult task. The hands may begin to wobble in trying to maintain balance during the movement. Some individuals may not be able to even hold the starting position, let alone complete the full range of muscle actions. For them, starting the push-up with the knees on the ground often serves as a lead-up to eventually completing the exercise without knee support.

The role of adding perturbation during relatively simple or complex movements may play a key role in "training" the intricate signaling patterns that control the basics of human movement.

Core Training

Core training—also referred to as lumbar stabilization, core strengthening, dynamic stabilization, neutral spine control, trunk stabilization, abdominal strength, core "pillar" training, and core functional strength training—has become an important part of many athletes training regimen.

The concept considers the core as a four-sided muscular frame with abdominal muscles in front, the paraspinals and gluteals in back, the diaphragm at the top, and the pelvic floor and hip girdle musculature framing the bottom. The "core" does not simply refer to muscles that cross the midsection of the body to form the "six-pack" abdominals commonly portrayed in magazine advertisements. The core region includes 29 pairs of muscles that hold the trunk steady, in addition to balancing and stabilizing the bony structures of the spine, pelvis, thorax, and other areas activated during most movements. Without adequate "strength and balance," the totality of these spine-frame structures would become mechanically unstable. A properly functioning core provides appropriate distribution of forces along the muscle-joint-bone axis for optimal movement control and efficiency; adequate absorption of ground-impact forces; and absence of excessive compressive, translational, and shearing forces on joints along the kinetic chain that must support the body weight.

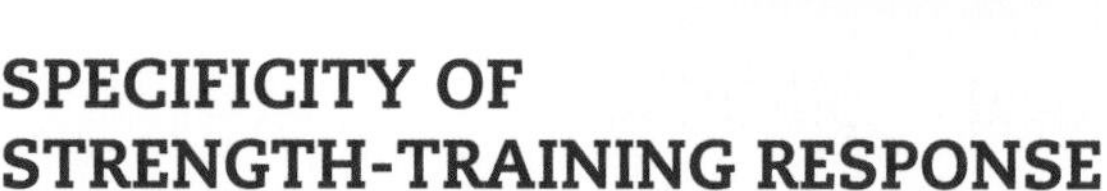

SPECIFICITY OF STRENGTH-TRAINING RESPONSE

An isometrically trained muscle shows greatest strength improvement when measured isometrically; similarly, a dynamically trained muscle tests best when evaluated in resistance activities that require movement. Isometric strength developed at or near one joint angle does not readily transfer to other angles or body positions that use the same muscles. In contrast, muscles trained dynamically through movement over a limited ROM show the greatest strength improvement when measured in that ROM. Even body position specificity exists; muscular strength of ankle plantar and dorsiflexors developed in the standing position with concentric and eccentric muscle actions showed little transfer with the same muscles evaluated in the supine position. Resistance-training specificity makes sense because strength improvement blends adaptations in two areas:

1. Muscle fiber and connective tissue harness of the specific muscle or muscles
2. Neural organization and excitability of motor units that power discrete voluntary movement patterns

A muscle's maximal force output depends on neural factors that effectively recruit and synchronize firing of motor units, not just the intrinsic factors of muscle fiber type and cross-sectional area.

A 3-month study of young adult men and women emphasized the highly specific nature of resistance-training adaptations. One group trained the hand's adductor pollicis muscle isometrically with 10 daily actions of 5 seconds duration at a frequency of 1 per minute. The other group trained the same muscle dynamically with 10 daily 10-repetition bouts of weight movement at one-third maximal strength. The untrained muscle served as the control. To eliminate any training influence from psychological factors and central nervous system adaptations, a supermaximal electrical stimulation applied to the motor nerve evaluated the trained muscles' force capacity. The results were clear—both training groups improved maximal force capacity and peak rate of force development. The improvement in maximal force for the isometrically trained group nearly doubled the improvement for the dynamically trained group. Conversely, improvement in the speed of force development averaged about 70% greater in the group trained with dynamic muscle actions. Such findings provide strong evidence that resistance training *per se* does not induce all-inclusive "general" adaptations in muscle structure and function. Rather, a muscle's contractile properties—maximal force, velocity of shortening, and rate of tension development—improve in a highly specific way that relates directly to the muscle action in training. Both static and dynamic training methods produce strength increases, yet no one system rates consistently superior to the other in how best to train and assess muscle function. The crucial consideration before making decisions about the most effective training strategy requires resolving the intended purpose of the newly acquired "strength."

Practical Implications

The complex interaction between nervous and muscular systems helps to explain why leg muscles strengthened in squats or deep knee bends fail to show equivalent improved force capability in other leg movements as in jumping or leg extension. Low relationships emerge between dynamic measures of leg extension force at any speed and vertical jumping height. This means individuals who exhibit superior leg extension force do not necessarily have the best vertical jump and vice versa for individuals with low leg extension force. A muscle group strengthened and enlarged by dynamic resistance training does not demonstrate equal improvement in force capacity when measured isometrically or isokinetically. Consequently, strengthening muscles for a specific athletic or occupational activity (e.g., golf, tennis, rowing, swimming, football, firefighting, package handling) demands more than just identifying and overloading the muscles in the movement; it also requires neuromuscular training specifically in the important movements that require improved strength. A more appropriate name for this type of training is **functional strength training** or functional resistance movement training.

To improve a specific physical performance through resistance training, it is crucial to train the muscle(s) in movements that mimic the movement requiring force-capacity improvement, with a focus on force, velocity, and power requirements rather than simply an isolated joint or muscle action. To train a specific muscle or group of muscles, the coach and athlete must carefully assess the muscle group(s) involved in a particular movement. Performing triceps extensions with weights would not seem appropriate to train the specific upper arm musculature involved in the skilled movements required in the shot put or rapid downswing in the golf swing, even though both skills require triceps activation.

Training should develop maximum force-generating capacity for those muscle groups throughout the ROM at a movement pattern and speed that closely mimics actual sports performance. Isometric training cannot accomplish this goal because no limb movement occurs; isokinetic actions provide maximal overload potential at diverse movement velocities because movement speed with electromechanical dynamometers can approach $400° \cdot s^{-1}$.

Even moving at this relatively "fast" speed does not mimic movement velocity during some sports in which limb velocity approaches $2000° \cdot s^{-1}$. For example, arm velocity measured about the elbow joint during a baseball pitch by major league pitchers routinely exceeds 600 to $700° \cdot s^{-1}$, and leg velocity during a football, rugby, or soccer kick nearly doubles the speed of the fastest electromechanical measuring device and "strength"-training equipment.

PERIODIZATION

In the early 1960s, Russian sports scientist **Leonid Matveyev** introduced the concept of strength-training **periodization** or training planning. This concept has since become incorporated into the training regimens of novice and champion athletes. Conceptually, periodization varies training intensity and volume to ensure optimal conditions so that peak performance coincides with major competitions. Periodization for resistance training subdivides a specific resistance-training period for 1 year (macrocycle) into smaller periods or phases (mesocycles), with each mesocycle again separated into weekly microcycles. In essence, the training model progressively decreases training volume and increases intensity as program duration progresses to maximize newly acquired improvements in muscular strength and power. Fractionating the macrocycle into components allows manipulation of training intensity, volume, frequency, sets, repetitions, and rest periods to prevent overtraining. It also provides workout variety. Periodization variation can reduce negative overtraining or "staleness" effects so athletes achieve peak performance at competition. **Figure 14.15A** depicts the generalized design for periodization and a typical macrocycle's four distinct phases. As competition approaches, training volume gradually decreases, and training intensity concurrently increases. The four phases of periodization are as follows:

1. Preparation phase emphasizes modest strength development with high-volume (3 to 5 sets; 8 to12 reps), low-intensity workouts (50% to 80% 1-RM plus flexibility and aerobic and anaerobic training).
2. First transition phase emphasizes strength development with workouts of moderate volume (3 to 5 sets; 5 to 6 reps) and moderate intensity (80% to 90% 1-RM plus flexibility and interval aerobic training).
3. Competition phase lets the participant peak for competition. Selective strength development emphasized with low-volume, high-intensity workouts (3 to 5 sets; 2 to 4 reps at 90% to 95% 1-RM) plus short periods of interval training that emphasize sport-specific exercises.

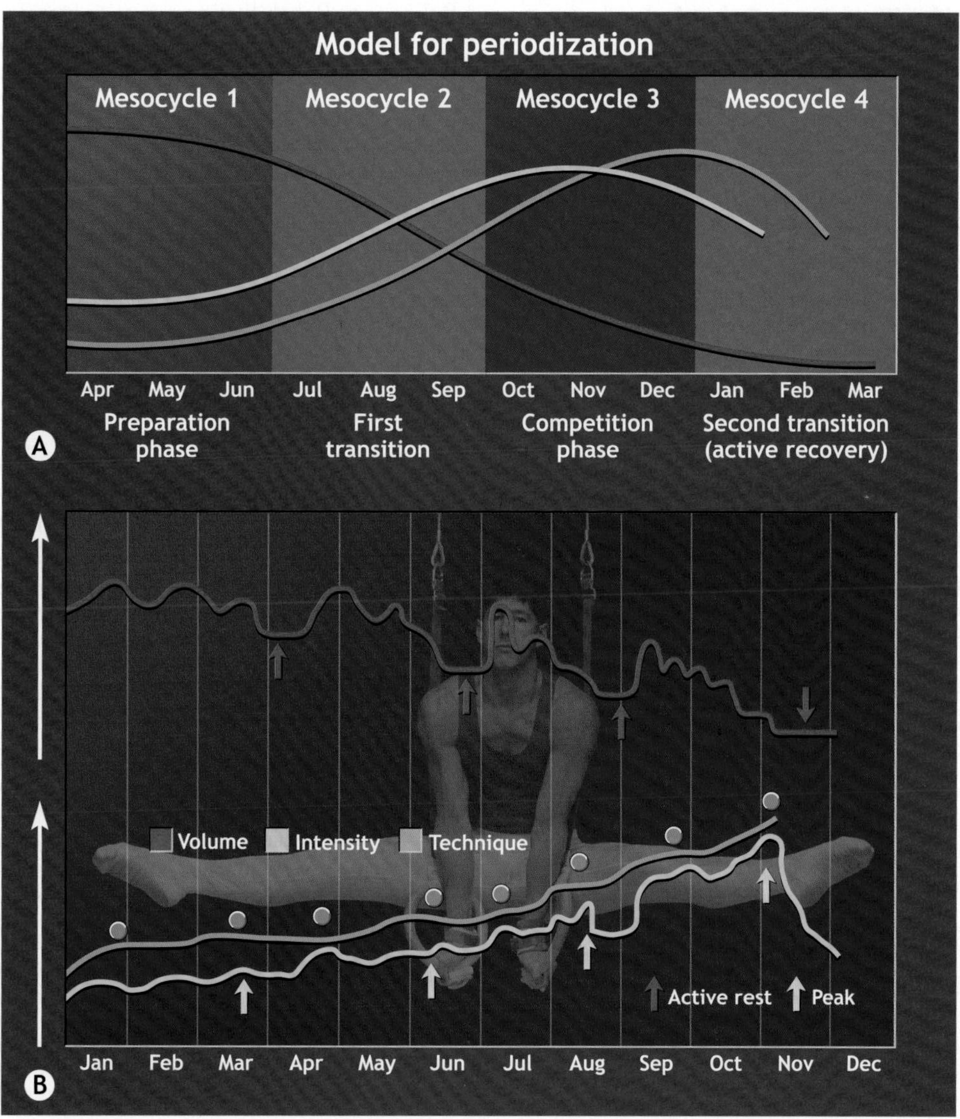

FIGURE 14.15 **A.** Periodization subdivides a macrocycle into distinct phases or mesocycles. These in turn separate into weekly microcycles. The general plan provides modifications, but mesocycles typically include four parts: (1) preparation phase, (2) first transition phase, (3) competition phase, and (4) a second transition or active recovery phase. **B.** Example of periodization for an elite gymnast preparing for competition. Competitions took place throughout the yearly training program, so periodization focused on achieving peak performance at the end of each macrocycle. Periodization places training into context for intensity, duration, and frequency of strength/power workouts. The major purpose of this focus attempts to avoid overtraining (staleness), minimize injury potential, and reduce training monotony while progressing toward peak competition performance (*filled green circles*). (Reprinted with permission from McArdle WD, Katch FI, Katch VL. *Exercise Physiology: Nutrition, Energy, and Human Performance*. 8th Ed. Baltimore: Wolters Kluwer Health, 2015.)

4. Second transition phase (active recovery) emphasizes recreational activities and low-intensity workouts that incorporate different exercise modes. The athlete repeats the periodization cycle in planning for the next competition.

Periodization structures an inverse relation between training volume and training intensity through the competition phase; it then decreases both aspects during the second transition or recuperation period. Note the increase in time devoted to technique training as competition approaches, with training volume at the periodization cycle's lowest point. **Figure 14.15B** illustrates how training volume and intensity interact within a mesocycle for an athlete in a specific sport.

Sport-Specific Training Principles

Sport-specific training principles usually apply in periodization when designing a training regimen based on a sport's distinct strength, power, and endurance requirements. A detailed analysis of the sport's metabolic and technical requirements frames the training paradigm. The concept of periodization makes intuitive sense, yet few studies present conclusive evidence for the superiority of this training approach. Confounding factors include difficulty controlling for differences in training intensity, training volume, and the participants' fitness capacities. One critical review of periodized strength training concluded that it produced greater improvements in muscular strength, body mass, lean body mass, and percentage body fat than nonperiodized multiple- and single-set training programs.

PRACTICAL RECOMMENDATIONS FOR INITIATING A RESISTANCE-TRAINING PROGRAM

1. Avoid maximum lifts in the beginning stages of resistance training. Excessive resistance contributes little to strength development and greatly increases risk of muscle or joint injury. A load equal to 60% to 80% of a muscle's force-generating capacity sufficiently stimulates increases in muscular strength. This load generally allows completion of about 10 repetitions of a particular movement.
2. Use lighter resistance to perform more repetitions at the start of training. Novices should initially attempt 12 to 15 repetitions. This regimen does not place excessive strain on the musculoskeletal system during the program's early phase. Use a heavier load if 12 repetitions feel too easy. The resistance is too heavy if the exerciser cannot complete 12 repetitions. This trial-and-error process may take several exercise sessions to establish the proper starting resistance.
3. After several weeks of training, decrease the repetitions to between 6 and 8 when muscles adapt and the exerciser becomes proficient in executing correct movements.
4. Add more resistance after achieving the target repetition number. This regimen represents progressive resistance training; as muscles become stronger, resistance increases with the lifting of a heavier load.
5. The exercise sequence should proceed from larger to smaller muscle groups to avoid premature fatigue of the smaller group.

RESISTANCE-TRAINING GUIDELINES FOR SEDENTARY ADULTS, ELDERLY INDIVIDUALS, AND CARDIAC PATIENTS

Currently, the American College of Sports Medicine (**www.acsm.org**), the American Heart Association (**www.aha.org**), the Centers for Disease Control and Prevention (**www.cdc.gov**), the American Association of Cardiovascular and Pulmonary Rehabilitation (**www.aacvpr.org**), and the U.S. Surgeon General's Office (**www.surgeongeneral.gov**) consider regular resistance exercise an important component of a comprehensive, health-related physical fitness program. Resistance-training goals for competitive athletes focus on optimizing muscular strength, power, and muscular hypertrophy "with high-intensity" 1- to 6-RM training loads. In contrast, goals for most middle-aged and older adults focus on maintenance and possible increase of muscle and bone mass and muscular strength and endurance to enhance the overall health and physical fitness profile. Adequate muscular strength in midlife maintains a margin of safety above the necessary threshold required to minimize musculoskeletal injuries in later life.

The resistance-training program recommended for middle-aged and older men and women is classified as "moderate intensity." In contrast to the multiple-set, heavy-resistance approach used by younger athletes, the program uses single sets of different exercises performed between 8- and 15-RM a minimum of twice weekly.

Resistance Training Plus Aerobic Training Equals Less Strength Improvement

Concurrent resistance and aerobic training programs produce less muscular strength and power improvement than training for strength only. This partly explains why power athletes and bodybuilders refrain from endurance activities while participating in resistance training. More than likely, the added energy and perhaps protein demands of intense endurance training impose a limit on a muscle's growth and metabolic responsiveness to resistance training. Also, an acute, short-term bout of intense endurance exercise inhibits performance in subsequent muscular strength activities.

SUMMARY

1. Resistance training and strength development serve multiple purposes including strength and physique competitions, fitness and health enhancement, physical rehabilitation, enhanced sports performance, and means for increased knowledge of muscle structure and function.

2. Common methods to measure muscular strength include tensiometry, dynamometry, 1-RM testing with weights, and computer-assisted force and work-output determinations, including isokinetic assessment.
3. Resistance training performed incorrectly with excessive hyperextension or back arch create shearing forces that produce undesirable muscle strain or spinal pressure that can trigger low back pain.
4. Substantial physiologic and performance specificity in response to training cast doubt on the appropriateness of general fitness measures, including strength tests to determine success in specific physical tasks or occupations.
5. Regardless of gender, human skeletal muscle theoretically generates a maximum of 16 to 30 N of maximum force per cm^2 of muscle cross-section.
6. On an absolute basis, men outperform women on strength tests because of men's larger muscle mass.
7. Muscles become stronger with overload training that increases the load or speed of muscle action or that combines increases in load and speed.
8. Strength gains occur when overload represents at least 60% to 80% of a muscle's maximum force-generating capacity.
9. Closely supervised resistance training for children using moderate levels of concentric exercise improves muscular strength without adverse effects on bone or muscle.
10. Three major exercise systems that develop muscular strength spotlight DCER training, isometric training, and isokinetic training.
11. Isokinetic training generates maximum force throughout the full ROM at different limb movement velocities.
12. Plyometric training incorporates the inherent stretch-recoil characteristics of the neuromuscular system to develop specific muscular power. These exercises repeatedly stretch and load muscles suddenly and then immediately contract them (e.g., repeated standing long jumps, hops, vertical jumps, and box jumps).
13. Body weight loading with suspension training activates agonists and antagonist muscles about a joint, including additional muscle groups along the kinetic chain.
14. Periodization divides a distinct period or macrocycle of resistance training into smaller training mesocycles; these subdivide into weekly microcycles.
15. Compartmentalization of training minimizes staleness and overtraining effects to maximize peak performance that coincides with competition.
16. Resistance training for competitive athletes optimizes muscular strength, power, and hypertrophy.
17. Resistance-training goals for middle-aged and older adults aim to modestly improve muscular strength and endurance, maintain muscle and bone mass, and enhance overall health and fitness.
18. Resistance training for specific sports should develop maximum force-generating capacity throughout a muscle's ROM at a speed that closely mimics the actual performance.
19. Concurrent training to improve muscular strength and aerobic capacity inhibits the magnitude of strength improvement compared with training only for muscular strength.

THINK IT THROUGH

1. Explain why athletes have spotters apply external force to the bar in the early phase of a bench press with weight to increase difficulty and then provide assistance toward its completion.
2. Based on your knowledge of gender-related differences in muscular strength, devise a physical test that (1) minimizes and (2) maximizes performance differences between men and women.
3. If a man and a woman of the same age, body weight, and training status could be matched for muscle cross-sectional area of the upper arms and shoulders and they both performed a 1-RM seated press, who would achieve the higher press score, the man or the woman?
4. Discuss the statement: "There is no one best system of resistance training."

PART 2 Adaptations to Resistance Training

Both acute responses and chronic adaptations occur with resistance training. An **acute response** refers to immediate changes in muscle or other cells, tissues, or systems during or immediately following a single exercise bout. For example, energy stores and cardiovascular dynamics change in response to specific muscle actions. Repeated exposure to a stimulus produces a longer-lasting change that influences the acute response over time (e.g., less disruption in cellular integrity [muscle damage] with a given level of exercise). **Adaptation** refers to how the body adjusts to a repeated, chronic stimulus.

Knowing the acute and chronic responses to resistance training facilitates exercise prescription and program design. Adaptations to repeated muscular overload ultimately determine a training program's effectiveness. The time course of adaptations varies among individuals and depends on the nature and magnitude of prior adaptations. Also, a resistance-training program must consider the expression of individual differences in adaptation or training responsiveness.

Adaptations to resistance training occur from the cellular to systemic levels. **Figure 14.16** displays six factors that impact muscle mass development and maintenance. More than likely, genetic factors strongly influence the effect of each factor on the ultimate training outcome. Resistance training contributes little to tissue growth without appropriate nutrition. Similarly, training outcomes depend on

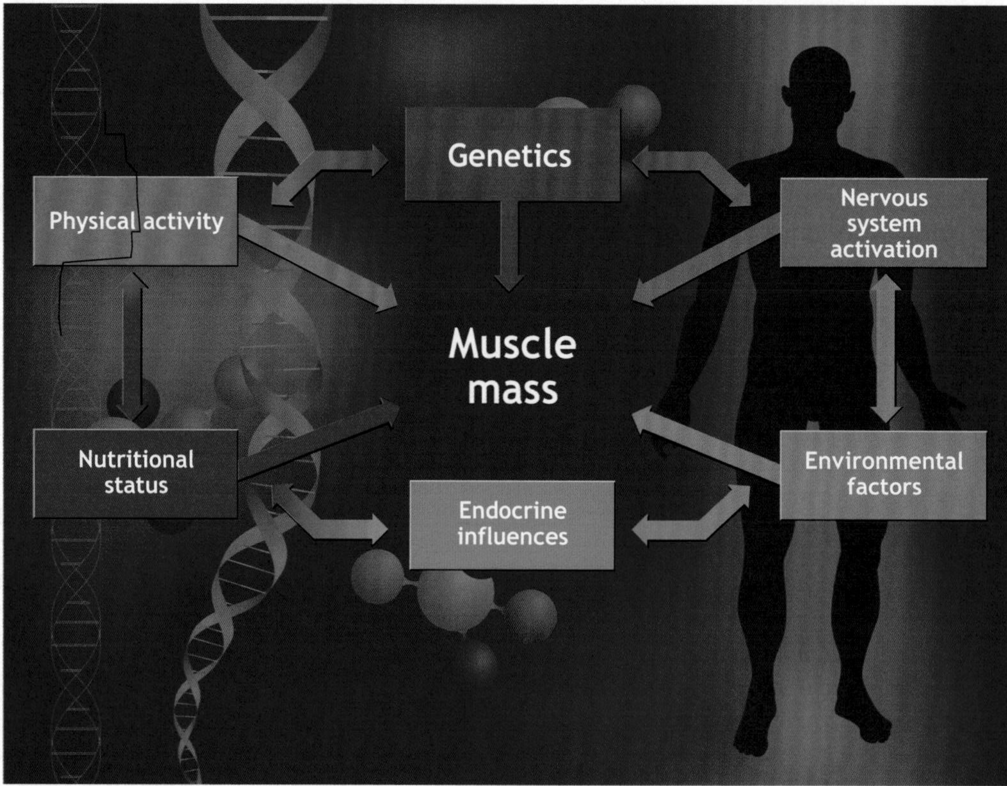

FIGURE 14.16 Interaction of six factors that develop and maintain muscle mass. (Reprinted with permission from McArdle WD, Katch FI, Katch VL. *Exercise Physiology: Nutrition, Energy, and Human Performance*. 8th Ed. Baltimore: Wolters Kluwer Health, 2015.)

targeted hormones and patterns of nervous system activation. Without muscular overload, these six factors cannot work synergistically to increase muscle mass and muscle strength.

NEURAL AND MUSCULAR ADAPTATIONS WITH RESISTANCE TRAINING

Well-documented changes from overload training occur in the gross structural and microscopic architecture within muscle tissue. **Figure 14.17** showcases the relative roles of neural and muscular adaptations in strength improvement with resistance training. Neural adaptations predominate in the early phase of training; this phase encompasses the duration of most research studies. Hypertrophy-induced adaptations create an upper limit on longer-term training improvements. This tempts many athletes to use anabolic steroids and/or human growth hormone (dashed line) to induce continual hypertrophy if training alone fails.

NEURAL ADAPTATIONS

A classic series of experiments illustrates the importance of psychological factors in expressing human muscular strength. The researchers measured arm strength in college-age men under five scenarios: (1) normal conditions, (2) immediately following a loud noise, (3) while the subject screamed loudly

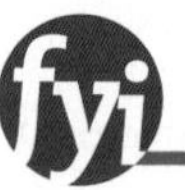

Knee Pain and Fear Avoidance: A Real-Life Experience

In some cases, fear avoidance turns into a chronic problem with negative consequences for recovery in rehabilitation from prior musculoskeletal issues. For example, one of the authors (FK) had knee pain (the medial side of the left knee joint marked by blue tape in the image) that made it nearly impossible to step down from a 6-inch stair out of "fear" of experiencing pain. Degeneration of articular surfaces and trauma from jumping off a rock while climbing had precipitated the injury, which persisted for over a year. "Fear avoidance was so real FK couldn't overcome it. When attempting to just step down from a stair during a physical therapy session, FK stood on the bench unable to perform the simple step down! The physical therapist would not offer physical support, and it took 5 more therapy sessions before FK would try the step down. The "fear effect" was real as if there was a huge "brain stop" mechanism at work. Once the threshold for experiencing pain diminished, the fear disappeared and stepping down was no longer a problem—but it did take some time."

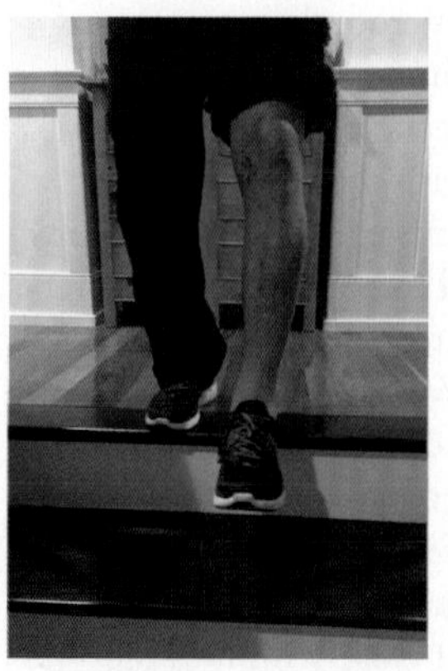

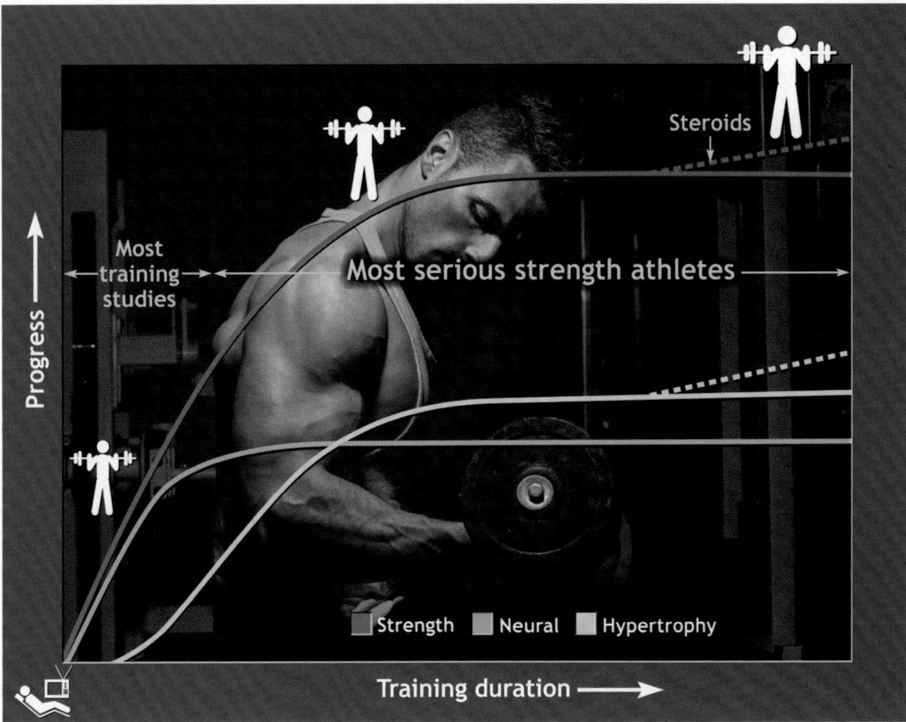

FIGURE 14.17 Relative roles of neural and muscular adaptations in strength improvement with resistance training. Note that neural adaptations predominate in the early phase of training (this phase encompasses the duration of most research studies). Hypertrophy-induced adaptations place the upper limit on longer-term training improvements. This tempts many athletes to use anabolic steroids and/or human growth hormone (*dashed line*) to induce continual hypertrophy if training alone fails. (Adapted with permission from McArdle WD, Katch FI, Katch VL. *Exercise Physiology: Nutrition, Energy, and Human Performance.* 8th Ed. Baltimore: Wolters Kluwer Health, 2015; from Sale DG. Neural adaptation to resistance training. *Med Sci Sports Exerc* 1988;20:135.)

at the time of exertion, (4) under the influence of alcohol and amphetamines ("pep pills"), (5) and under hypnosis when told they possessed considerable strength and should not fear injury. Each of the alterations generally increased strength above normal levels; hypnosis, the most "mental" of all treatments, produced the greatest increments.

The investigators theorized that temporary modifications in central nervous system function accounted for strength improvements under the various conditions. They contended that most persons normally operate at a level of neural inhibition, perhaps via protective reflex mechanisms that constrain the expression of strength capacity. Neuromuscular inhibition can occur from unpleasant past experiences with exercise, an overly protective home environment, or exaggerated fear of musculoskeletal pain or injury referred to as *fear avoidance*.

Regardless of the reason, such individuals typically cannot express maximum strength capacity as long as the psychological "thoughts" persist. In contrast, increased neurologic arousal may account for "unexplainable" feats of strength and power during highly charged emergency and rescue situations. An example would be a relatively small person lifting an extremely heavy object off an injured person. In athletics, the excitement of intense competition or influence of disinhibitory drugs or hypnotic suggestion can induce a "supermaximal" performance from greatly muted neural inhibition and optimal motor neuron recruitment. Rapid improvements in muscular strength during the first few weeks of resistance training largely result from a "learning" phenomenon, or lessening of fear and psychological inhibition, as the novice becomes more practiced with the specific strength activity (e.g., proper form in bench press or squat exercise).

Highly trained athletes often create an almost self-hypnotic state by intensely concentrating, or "psyching," before competition. It sometimes takes years of training to perfect the "block out" of extraneous stimuli such as crowd noise so the muscle action ties in directly to the performance. This practice has been perfected in powerlifting competition where success depends on precise, coordinated movements combined with maximal muscle tension output. Enhanced arousal level and accompanying neural disinhibition or facilitation can fully activate muscle groups.

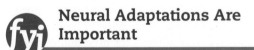

Neural Adaptations Are Important

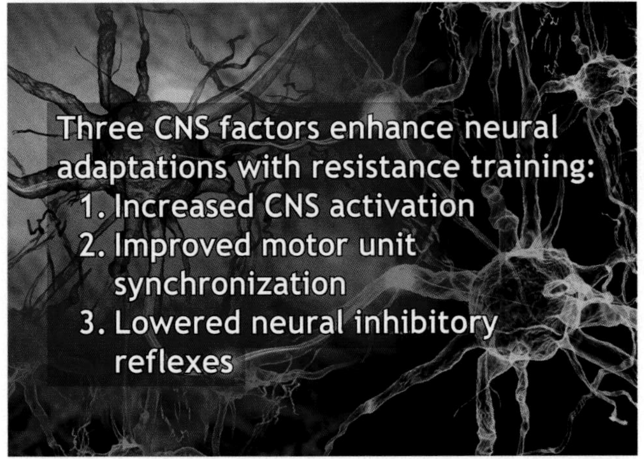

Three CNS factors enhance neural adaptations with resistance training:
1. Increased CNS activation
2. Improved motor unit synchronization
3. Lowered neural inhibitory reflexes

Motor Unit Activation: Size Principle

Motor unit recruitment occurs in sequence from low to high thresholds and from low to high muscle force output. An increased rate of motor unit firing also increases a muscle's

Muscular Strength and Puberty

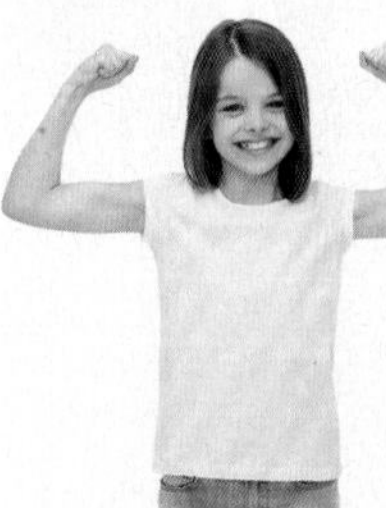

Until puberty, boys maintain about 10% greater muscle strength than girls. After age 12, boys continue to increase in strength, while strength plateaus in girls. Gender-related changes in body composition account for much of these strength difference.

Adapted with permission from Kraemer WJ, Newton RU. Training for muscular power. *Phys Med Rehabil Clin* 2000;11:341.

force output. These two factors—recruitment of motor units and increase in their firing rate—produce a continuum of a muscle's voluntary force output.

Type II motor units have a high twitch force; they become activated in activities requiring significant force. In contrast, type I motor units that generate less force activate under lower force requirements. Individuals unaccustomed to high physical demands probably cannot voluntarily recruit all higher threshold type II motor units, so they cannot maximally tap their muscle's true strength potential. An adaptation to resistance training allows an untrained person to recruit more motor units to achieve a maximal muscle action. Increased motor unit firing synchronization provides another neural adjustment to increase force production with training. Greater synchronization causes more motor units to fire simultaneously.

In experienced weightlifters, neural components also contribute to strength improvement. In one study, minimal changes took place in muscle fiber size, yet 2 years of training increased absolute strength and power. Electromyography (EMG) analyses revealed enhanced voluntary muscle activation over the training period. This supports the contention that the neural component contributes significantly to strength improvements with training.

MUSCLE ADAPTATIONS

Three factors explain strength capacity: (1) muscle cross section, (2) fiber type, and (3) mechanical arrangement of muscle and bone. As emphasized previously, psychological inhibitions and learning factors greatly modify muscular strength, yet the anatomic and intrinsic physiologic factors within the muscle determine both strength capacity and the ultimate limit of strength development. Gross and ultrastructural changes in muscle with chronic resistance training generally produce adaptations in the contractile apparatus accompanied by substantial gains in muscular strength and power. An increase in a muscle's external size, reflecting an increase in its internal volume, represents the most visible adaptation to resistance training. The training response of the biceps and triceps muscle regions often serves as the "criterion" anatomical sites for changes in a muscle's architecture from overload training. **Muscle fiber hypertrophy** (increased size of individual fibers) usually explains increases in gross muscle size, although increased fiber number (**fiber hyperplasia**) provides a controversial complementary hypothesis.

Muscle Fiber Hypertrophy

An increase in muscular tension (force) with exercise training provides the primary stimulus to initiate the process of skeletal muscle growth or hypertrophy. True changes in muscle size become detectable after only 3 weeks of training, and the remodeling of muscle architecture precedes gains in MCSA. In essence, muscle hypertrophy with resistance training represents a fundamental biologic adaptation. The extraordinarily large muscle size and well-defined "ripped" musculature of fitness enthusiasts, gymnasts, and bodybuilders results from enlargement of individual muscle cells, mainly the fast-twitch fibers. Growth takes place from one or more of the following four adaptations:

1. Increased actin, myosin, and other contractile proteins
2. Increased number and size of myofibrils per muscle fiber
3. Increased connective, tendinous, and ligamentous tissues
4. Increased quantity of enzymes and stored nutrients

Not all muscle fibers undergo the same degree of enlargement with resistance training. Muscle growth depends on the muscle fiber type activated and their recruitment pattern. As discussed previously, improving muscular strength and power does not necessarily require muscle fiber hypertrophy because important neurologic factors initially affect the expression of human strength. Thereafter, slower occurring strength improvements generally coincide with noticeable alterations in a muscle's subcellular molecular architecture.

As training continues, contractile proteins increase in conjunction with enlarged muscle fiber cross-sectional area. *Overload training enlarges individual muscle fibers with subsequent muscle growth.* Weightlifters' fast-twitch fibers average about 45% larger than corresponding fibers of healthy sedentary persons and endurance athletes. The hypertrophic process synchronizes directly to increased mononuclear number and synthesis of cellular components, particularly the contractile myosin heavy-chain and actin protein filaments. Skeletal muscle remodels its internal architecture, potentially reconfiguring external orientation and hence its shape. **Table 14.5** lists important resistance-training effects on muscle's cellular adaptations.

Significant Metabolic Adaptations Occur

Success at elite levels of sport performance requires a particular muscle fiber distribution. The relatively fixed nature of muscle fiber type suggests a genetic predisposition for exceptional, world-class level performance. Considerable plasticity exists for metabolic potential, however, as specific training enhances the anaerobic and aerobic energy transfer capacity of both fiber types. The heightened oxidative capacity of fast-twitch fibers with endurance training brings them to a

TABLE 14.5 Physiologic Adaptations to Resistance Training

System/Variable	Response
Muscle Fibers	
Number	Equivocal
Size	Increase
Type	Unknown
Capillary Density	
In bodybuilders	No change
In powerlifters	Decrease
Mitochondria	
Volume	Decrease
Density	Decrease
Twitch Contraction Time	
Enzymes	Decrease
Creatine phosphokinase	Increase
Myokinase	Increase
Enzymes of Glycolysis	
Phosphofructokinase	Increase
Lactate dehydrogenase	No change
Aerobic Metabolism Enzymes	
Carbohydrate	Increase
Triacylglycerol	Not known
Intramuscular Fuel Stores	
Adenosine triphosphate	Increase
Phosphocreatine	Increase
Glycogen	Increase
Triacylglycerols	Not known
$\dot{V}O_{2max}$	
Circuit resistance training	Increase
Heavy-resistance training	No change
Connective Tissue	
Ligament strength	Increase
Tendon strength	Increase
Collagen content of muscle	No change
Bone	
Mineral content	Increase
Cross-sectional area	No change
Resistance to fracture	Increase

Modified from Fleck SJ, Kramer WJ. Resistance training: physiological responses and adaptations (Part 2 of 4). *Phys Sports Med* 1988;16:108.

fyi Neural and Muscular Factors Determine Strength

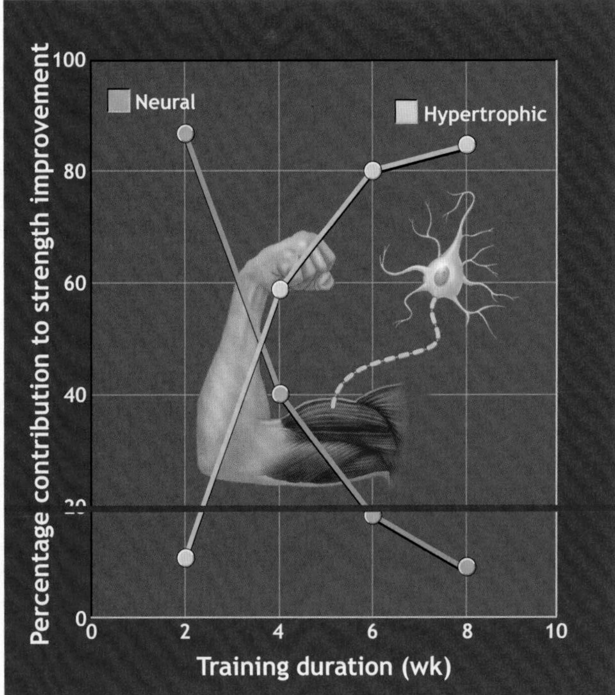

A generalized response curve for gains in muscle strength with resistance training occurs from neural (*orange*) and/or muscular (*yellow*) factors. During a typical 8-week training period, neural factors account for approximately 90% of the strength gained over the first 2 weeks. In the subsequent 2 weeks, between 40% and 50% of the strength improvement still relates to nervous system adaptation. Thereafter, muscle fiber adaptations become progressively more important to strength improvement. Experiments of this type generally evaluate neural factors from integrated EMG recordings of the muscle groups trained.

Image reprinted with permission from McArdle WD, Katch FI, Katch VL. *Exercise Physiology: Nutrition, Energy, and Human Performance.* 8th Ed. Baltimore: Wolters Kluwer Health, 2015.

level nearly equal to the aerobic potential of the slow-twitch fibers of untrained counterparts. Advancing age generally presents no barrier to training adaptations of muscle fibers. With an adequate training stimulus, skeletal muscle fiber size, capillarization, and glycolytic and respiratory enzymes of older men and women adapt to both endurance and resistance training similar to younger persons.

Endurance training induces some intraconversion of type IIb fibers to the more aerobic type IIa fibers. The well-documented increase in mitochondrial size and number and corresponding increase in total quantity of citric acid cycle and electron transport enzymes accompany these fiber subdivision changes. Within a particular muscle group, only the specifically trained muscle fibers adapt to regular exercise; this explains why well-trained athletes who change to a sport demanding use of primarily different muscle groups (or different portions of the same muscle) often feel untrained for the new activity. Within this framework, swimmers or canoeists (with well-trained upper body musculature) do not necessarily transfer their upper body fitness to a running sport that relies predominantly on a highly conditioned lower body musculature.

Muscle Remodeling: Can Fiber Type Be Changed?

Skeletal muscle represents dynamic tissue whose cell populations do not remain fixed throughout life. Rather, muscle fibers undergo regeneration and remodeling and alter their phenotypic profile to meet diverse functional demands from resistance or endurance training. Muscle activation via specific types and intensities of long-term use stimulates otherwise dormant myogenic stem cells called **satellite cells** beneath a muscle fiber's basement membrane to proliferate and differentiate to form new fibers. Fusion of satellite cell nuclei and incorporation into existing muscle fibers allow the fiber to synthesize more proteins to form additional myofibril contractile elements. Chronic overload most likely contributes directly to muscular hypertrophy and may stimulate transformation of existing fibers from one type to another.

Many extracellular signal molecules, primarily insulinlike growth factor (IGF), fibroblast growth factors, transforming growth factors, and hepatocyte growth factor, govern satellite cell activity and possibly muscle fiber proliferation and differentiation resulting from specific exercise training. **Figure 14.18** proposes a model for muscle cell remodeling involving satellite cell incorporation into an existing muscle fiber. A specific set of genes (gene A in the figure within the pre-existing nucleus) is expressed within the fiber. Chronic activation from physical activity stimulates satellite cell proliferation, with some cells differentiating and fusing with pre-existing muscle fibers. The new muscle nuclei alter gene expression in the adapting muscle depicted by gene B within the myofibril.

Muscle fiber-type transformation occurs with specific training. In one study, four athletes trained anaerobically for 11 weeks followed by 18 weeks of aerobic training. Anaerobic training increased the percentage of type IIc fibers (a previous subclassification) and decreased the percentage of type I fibers; the opposite occurred during the aerobic training phase. Similarly, 4 to 6 weeks of sprint training increased the percentage of fast-twitch fibers, with a commensurate decrease in slow-twitch fiber

A CLOSER LOOK

How to Assess Muscular Endurance

Muscular endurance refers to how well a muscle or group of muscles exerts submaximum force repeatedly in a given time period, or the duration a given muscle action can sustain a percentage of its 1-RM either dynamically or isometrically. The number of total repetitions of a muscle action in a given time (e.g., number of curl-ups, sit-ups, or push-ups within 1 min or while maintaining a given cadence) provides a common yardstick for expressing muscular endurance. Muscular endurance depends somewhat on a muscle's maximum strength but little on cardiorespiratory fitness because components of aerobic fitness represent separate physiological and fitness entities. To test muscular endurance using weights, the weight lifted should coincide with either a percentage of body weight (**Table 1**) or a percentage of 1-RM. An arbitrary goal would be to achieve between 15 and 20 total repetitions.

Two of the more popular muscular endurance tests do not require weights to assess endurance of the abdominal (curl-up) and upper body (push-up) musculatures.

Curl-Up Muscular Endurance Test

Initial Position

The individual lies supine with knees flexed and feet about one foot from the buttocks. The arms extend forward with fingers palm-down on the thighs pointing toward the knees (**Fig. 1A**). The tester kneels behind the person with hands cupped under the individual's head (about 2 in off the floor).

TABLE 1 Recommended Percentage of Body Weight Lifted in Different Resistance Exercise Movements to Assess Muscular Endurance

	Percentage of Body Weight	
Exercise	**Men**	**Women**
Arm curl	0.33	0.25
Bench press	0.66	0.50
Lateral pull down	0.66	0.50
Triceps extension	0.33	0.33
Leg extension	0.50	0.50
Leg curl	0.33	0.33

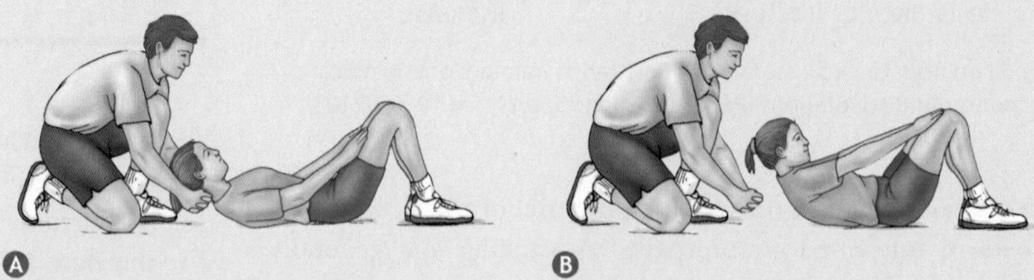

Figure 1 Start (**A**) and finish (**B**) positions for the curl-up test.

Movement

The person curls up slowly, sliding the fingers up the legs until the fingertips touch the patellae (knee caps; **Fig. 1B**), followed by slowly returning to the starting position with the back of the head touching the tester's hands. To reduce lower back strain, minimize rectus femoris involvement and emphasize abdominal muscle action; no assistance should anchor or support the feet.

The Test and Standards

Required curl-up rate equals 20 repetitions per minute (3 s per curl-up; metronome set at 40 b · min^{-1}, or 2 beats per curl-up and recovery).

Individuals perform as many curl-ups as possible at a cadence (which must be maintained) to a maximum of 75. **Table 2** presents standards for evaluating scores on the curl-up test.

Push-Up Muscular Endurance Test

The push-up muscular endurance test can be performed in one of two ways: (1) full-body push-up and (2) modified push-up that reduces the body mass move to areas of the arms, chest, and shoulders. The modified push-up serves as an alternative to assess individual differences in upper-body strength for females because they possess considerably less relative strength in upper body musculature compared with males.

TABLE 2 Test Standards to Assess Curl-Up Performance

	Number of Curl-Ups Completed		
	Age, y		
Rating	**<35**	**35–44**	**>45**
Excellent			
Men	60	50	40
Women	50	40	30
Good			
Men	45	40	25
Women	40	25	15
Fair			
Men	30	25	15
Women	25	15	10
Poor			
Men	15	10	5
Women	10	6	4

From Faulkner RA, et al. A partial curl-up protocol for adults based on an analysis of two procedures. *Can Sport Sci* 1989;14:135; Sparling PB, et al. Development of a cadence curl-up for college students. *Res Q Exerc Sport* 1997;68:309.

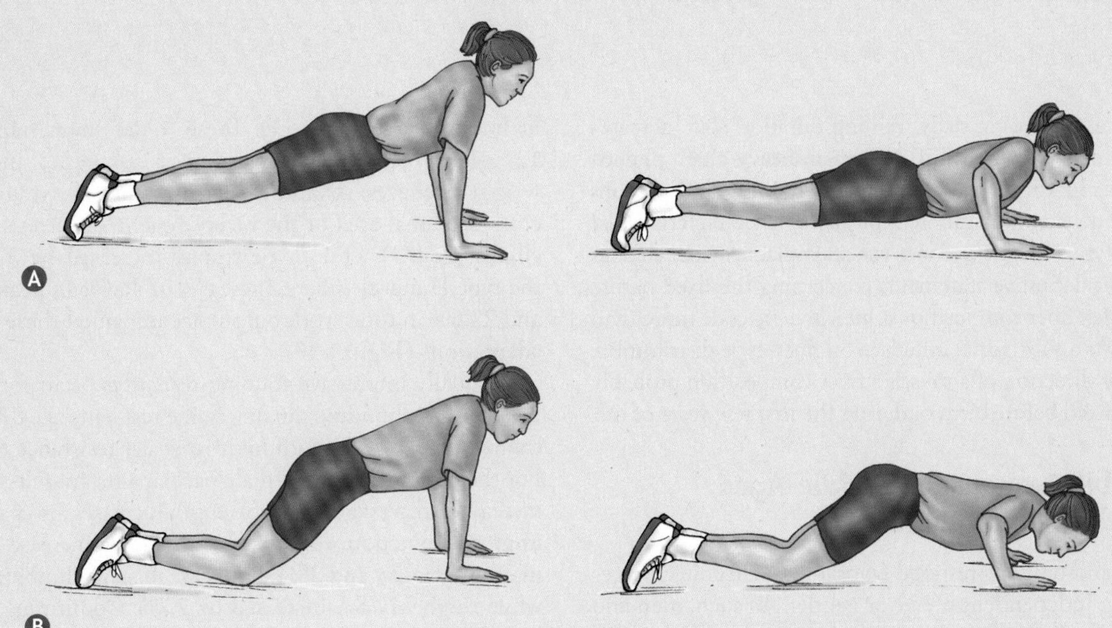

Figure 2 Start and finish positions for (**A**) full-body push-up and (**B**) modified push-up.

(*Continues on next page*)

A CLOSER LOOK (Continued)

Initial Position

Full-Body Push-Up: The person assumes a relatively stiff prone position from head to ankles, keeping the hands shoulder width apart and arms fully extended **(Fig. 2A)**.

Modified Push-Up: The person assumes the bent-knee position with hips and buttocks pressing downward in line with the neck and shoulders **(Fig. 2B)**.

Movement

Full-Body Push-Up and Modified Push-Up: Lower the body until elbows reach 90-degree of flexion; the return action requires pushing up until the arms fully extend. The push-up action should proceed in a continuous motion without rest pauses between flexion-extension movements.

Standards

Table 3 presents standards for scoring the full-body push-up (men) and modified push-up (women) tests.

TABLE 3 Test Standards to Assess Push-Up Performance of Men (Full-Body Push-Up) and Women (Modified Push-Up)

	Number of Push-Ups Completed				
	Age, y				
Rating	**20–29**	**30–39**	**40–49**	**50–59**	**60+**
Full-body push-up					
Excellent	>54	>44	>39	>34	>29
Good	45–54	35–44	30–39	25–34	20–29
Average	35–44	25–34	20–29	15–24	10–19
Fair	20–34	15–24	12–19	8–14	5–9
Poor	<20	<15	<12	<8	<5
Modified push-up					
Excellent	>48	>39	>34	>29	>19
Good	34–48	25–39	20–34	15–29	5–19
Average	17–33	12–24	8–19	6–14	3–4
Fair	6–16	4–11	3–7	2–5	1–2
Poor	<6	<4	<3	<2	<1

From Pollock ML, et al. *Health and Fitness Through Physical Activity*. New York: John Wiley & Sons, 1984.

percentage. Increasing daily training duration also increases the fast- to slow-twitch shift in myosin heavy-chain phenotype in rat hindlimb muscles. Specific training and perhaps inactivity may convert different physiologic characteristics of type I to type II fibers and vice versa. Available evidence does not permit definitive statements concerning the fixed nature of a muscle's fiber composition. One's genetic code more than likely exerts a substantial influence on fiber-type distribution. The major direction of a muscle's fiber composition probably becomes fixed before birth or during the first few years of life.

Favorable Response of Middle-Aged and Elderly Individuals

Muscles and tendons respond favorably to chronic changes in loading independent of age or gender. As such, men and women experience considerable physiologic and performance adaptations with resistance training, uninfluenced by aging effects. A study of five older healthy men age 68 years clearly demonstrated the remarkable plasticity of human skeletal muscle. These "older" men trained for 12 weeks using heavy-resistance, isokinetic, and free-weight exercises. Training increased muscle volume and cross-sectional area of the biceps brachii (13.9%) and brachialis (26.0%) while hypertrophy increased by 37.2% in the type II muscle fibers. Increases of 46.0% in peak torque and 28.6% in total work output accompanied these cellular adaptations (**Fig. 14.19**).

Equally impressive training responses occur for elderly persons. One hundred nursing home residents age 87.1 years trained for 10 weeks with high-intensity resistance training. For the 63 female and 37 male participants, muscle strength increased an average 113%. Strength increases also paralleled improved function, reflected by an 11.8% increase in normal gait velocity and 28.4% increase in stair-climbing speed, while thigh MCSA increased by 2.7%. Confirming studies have verified the benefits of functional strength training to improve activities of daily living (ADL) in the older elderly, including countering the devastating medical consequences of slip and fall mishaps.

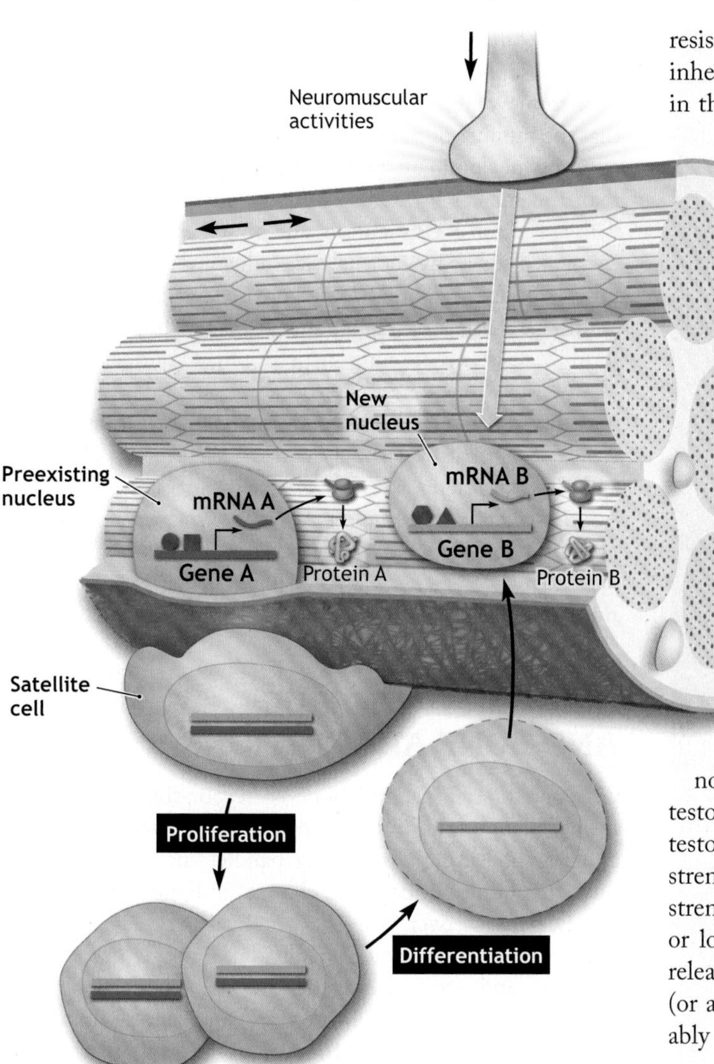

FIGURE 14.18 Model for skeletal muscle adaptation involving satellite cells. A specific set of genes (*gene A*) is expressed in the pre-existing myonuclei. Upon stimulation from increased neuromuscular activity, the satellite cells proliferate, with some differentiating and fusing with pre-existing myofibers. These myonuclei may alter gene expression (*gene B*) in the adapting muscle because they undergo altered differentiation from increased neuromuscular activities. (Reprinted with permission from McArdle WD, Katch FI, Katch VL. *Exercise Physiology: Nutrition, Energy, and Human Performance.* 8th Ed. Baltimore: Wolters Kluwer Health, 2015; as adapted with permission from Yan Z. Skeletal muscle adaptation and cell cycle regulation. *Exerc Sport Sci Rev* 2000;1:24.)

Changes in Muscle Fiber–Type Composition With Resistance Training

Research has evaluated the effects of resistance exercise training on leg extensor muscle fiber size and fiber composition. Biopsy specimens from the vastus lateralis muscle before and following resistance training revealed no change in percentage distribution of fast- and slow-twitch muscle fibers indicated by changes in myofibrillar ATPase.

Metabolic characteristics of specific fibers and fiber subdivisions undergo modification within 4 to 8 weeks of resistance training. This occurs despite dramatic changes in inherent muscle fiber types with chronic exercise. A decrease in the percentage of type IIb and corresponding increase in type IIa fibers denote one of the more prominent and rapid resistance-training adaptations.

Muscle Fiber Hypertrophy and Testosterone Levels

Popular dogma maintains that testosterone (the chief male sex hormone) facilitates muscle hypertrophy with resistance training. Testosterone binds with special receptor sites on muscle and other tissues to contribute to male secondary sex characteristics. These include gender differences in muscle mass and strength that develop at puberty's onset. Variation in testosterone levels would then explain individual differences in muscular enlargement with resistance training and the smaller hypertrophic response of women to muscular overload. Research to date does not support such notions about female's response to overload training and testosterone. Essentially no correlation exists between plasma testosterone levels and body composition and muscular strength in men and women. Individuals with high muscle strength and/or FFM can either have high, intermediate, or low testosterone levels. Acute increases in sex hormone release following a single bout of maximal resistance training (or any maximal effort exercise) remain transient and probably of little consequence to training responsiveness.

Muscle Fiber Hypertrophy: Male Versus Female

Computed tomography scans to evaluate MCSA show that men and women experience similar hypertrophic responses to resistance training. Men achieve a greater absolute increase in muscle size because of a larger initial total muscle mass but without a difference in muscle enlargement on a percentage basis compared with women of similar training status.

Other comparisons between elite male and female bodybuilders verify these observations. Women who train with conventional resistance methods gain strength and size on a similar percentage basis as men.

Muscle Fiber Hyperplasia

A common question concerns whether resistance training produces hyperplasia, defined as an increased number of muscle cells. If this does occur, to what extent does it contribute to muscle enlargement? Chronic skeletal muscle overload in various animal species develops new muscle fibers from normally dormant satellite cells between the basement layer and plasma membrane or by longitudinal splitting. With longitudinal splitting, a relatively large muscle fiber splits into two or more smaller individual daughter cells through lateral budding. These fibers function more efficiently than the large single fiber from where they originated.

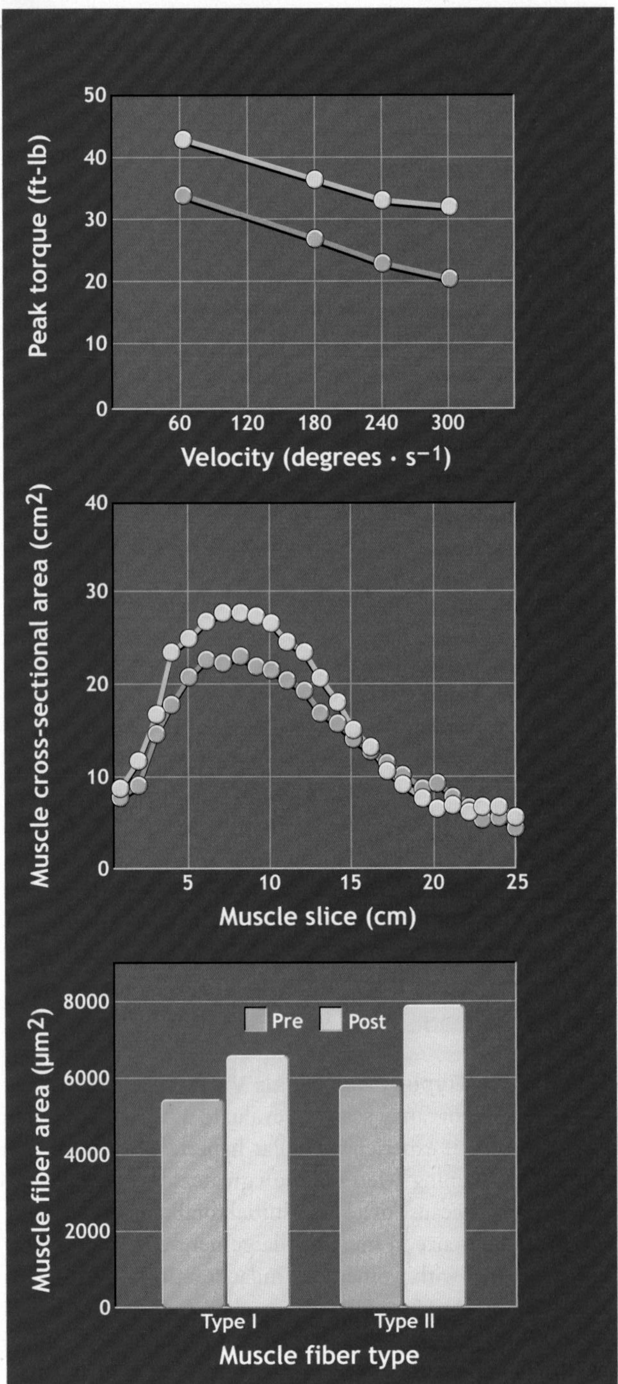

FIGURE 14.19 Plasticity of aging muscle. Data from five older men before (*orange*) and after (*yellow*) 12 weeks of heavy-resistance training. **Top.** Peak torque of elbow flexors. **Middle.** Plot of flexor cross-sectional area computed from MRI scans from proximal (*right*) to distal (*left*) end of muscle. **Bottom.** Average for type I and type II fiber areas. (Reprinted with permission from McArdle WD, Katch FI, Katch VL. *Exercise Physiology: Nutrition, Energy, and Human Performance*. 8th Ed. Baltimore: Wolters Kluwer Health, 2015; from Roman WJ, et al. Adaptations in the elbow flexors of elderly males after heavy-resistance training. *J Appl Physiol* 1993;74:750.)

Generalizing findings from research on animals to humans poses a problem. The massive cellular hypertrophy in humans with resistance training does not occur in many animal species. In cats, for example, muscle fiber hyperplasia reflects the primary compensatory adjustment to muscular overload. Some evidence supporting hyperplasia in humans does exist. Autopsy data from young, healthy men who died accidentally show that the number of muscle fibers of the larger and stronger leg opposite the dominant hand contained 10% more muscle fibers than the smaller leg. Cross-sectional studies of bodybuilders with large limb circumferences and muscle mass failed to show they possessed above–normal-size individual muscle fibers. The possibility does exist that some bodybuilders inherited an initially large number of small muscle fibers that then with certain forms of resistance training "hypertrophy" to normal size.

Muscle fibers may adapt differently to high-volume, high-intensity training used by bodybuilders than to the typical low-repetition, heavy-load system favored by strength and power athletes. *Even if other human studies replicate a training-induced hyperplasia, and even if the response reflects a positive adjustment, hypertrophy of existing individual muscle fibers represents the most important contribution from overload training to increased muscle size.*

CONNECTIVE TISSUE AND BONE ADAPTATIONS

Ligaments, tendons, and bone correspondingly strengthen as muscle strength and size increase. Increases in ligament and tendon strength generally parallel the rate of muscle fiber adaptation. In contrast, changes in bone improve more slowly, perhaps over a 6- to 12-month period. Connective tissue proliferates around individual muscle fibers; this thickens and strengthens the muscle's connective tissue structures. Such adaptations from resistance training help to protect joints and muscles from injury and also justify resistance exercise for preventive and rehabilitative strategies. Resistance training also positively affects bone dynamics in young individuals. Elite 14- to 17-year-old junior Olympic weightlifters, for example, have higher bone densities in the hip and femur regions than age-matched controls or adults.

CARDIOVASCULAR ADAPTATIONS

Training volume and intensity influence the effect of resistance training on cardiovascular system adaptations (**Table 14.6**).

Subtle yet important differences exist between myocardial enlargement from resistance training (physiologic hypertrophy) and enlargement from chronic hypertension (pathologic hypertrophy). In pathologic conditions, ventricular wall thickness increases beyond age and gender normal limits independent of assessment method and evaluative criteria. Left ventricle dilation and weakening, a frequent response to chronic hypertension and subsequent congestive heart failure, do not accompany the compensatory increase in myocardial wall thickness that occurs with resistance training. The hearts of champion resistance-trained athletes usually exceed the size of the hearts of their untrained counterparts, but heart size generally falls within the upper range of normal limits related to body size or cardiac function variables.

Resistance exercise more acutely increases blood pressure than lower-intensity dynamic movements, yet does

TABLE 14.6 Cardiovascular Adaptations to Resistance Training

Variable	Adaptation
Rest	
Heart rate	No change
Blood pressure	
Diastolic	Decrease or no change
Systolic	Decrease or no change
Rate-pressure product (HR × SBP)	Decrease or no change
Stroke volume	Increase or no change
Cardiac function	Increase or no change
Left ventricular wall thickness	Increase
Right ventricular wall thickness	No change
Left ventricular chamber volume	No change
Right ventricular chamber volume	No change
Left ventricular mass	Increase
Lipid profile	
Total cholesterol	Decrease
HDL-C	Increase or no change
LDL-C	Decrease or no change
During Exercise	
Heart rate	No change
Blood pressure	
Diastolic	Decrease
Systolic	Decrease
Rate-pressure product	Decrease
Stroke volume	Increase or no change
Cardiac output	Increase or no change
$\dot{V}O_{2peak}$	Increase or no change

not produce any long-term increase in resting blood pressure. Weightlifters and bodybuilders with hypertension can exhibit these four characteristics:

1. Probably essential hypertension with no identifiable cause
2. Experience chronic overtraining syndrome
3. Use anabolic steroids or other performance-enhancing substances
4. Possess an undesirable level of body fat or other hypertension risks established for the general population.

Metabolic Stress of Resistance Training

Metabolic and cardiovascular evaluations indicate that traditional resistance-training methods offer little benefit for aerobic fitness or as a calorie burner for weight control and do not significantly modify risk factors related to cardiovascular disease. Oxygen uptake for both isometric and typical weightlifting exercises would classify as "light to moderate" along the energy expenditure continuum, even though subjects report considerable muscular stress. A person can perform 15 or 20 different resistance exercises during a 1-hour training session, yet the net total time to perform exercise usually lasts no longer than 6 or 7 minutes. This relatively brief activity period with only moderate-energy expenditure reinforces the notion that traditional resistance-training programs would not improve endurance capacity in sports such as soccer, field hockey, or basketball that rely on a large aerobic component. Resistance-training exercises provide only limited utility as the primary activities in a weight-loss program because of the relatively low total energy expenditure during "typical" training sessions. In contrast, resistance training incorporated into a "circuit" routine as explained below will produce a substantial caloric expenditure if the participant rotates through 8 to 15 different exercise stations with minimal rest intervals and continues essentially nonstop for approximately 60 minutes at a moderate- to high-intensity effort.

Circuit Resistance Training: Increased Energy Expenditure

Modifying standard resistance training by de-emphasizing heavy overload increases exercise caloric expenditure and workout volume, thus improving more than one aspect of physical fitness. Research has focused on the energy cost and cardiorespiratory demands of **circuit resistance training (CRT)**. In CRT, a pre-established exercise-to-rest sequence usually consists of 8 to 15 different exercise stations, with 15 to 20 repetitions performed for each exercise. Exercise resistance requires between 40% and 50% of 1-RM. After a 15- to 30-second rest interval, participants move to succeeding exercise stations to complete the circuit. **Figure 14.20** outlines the sequence of progression through a multilevel, 5- to 12-station circuit. In this example, the person exercises at a particular station before moving on to the next

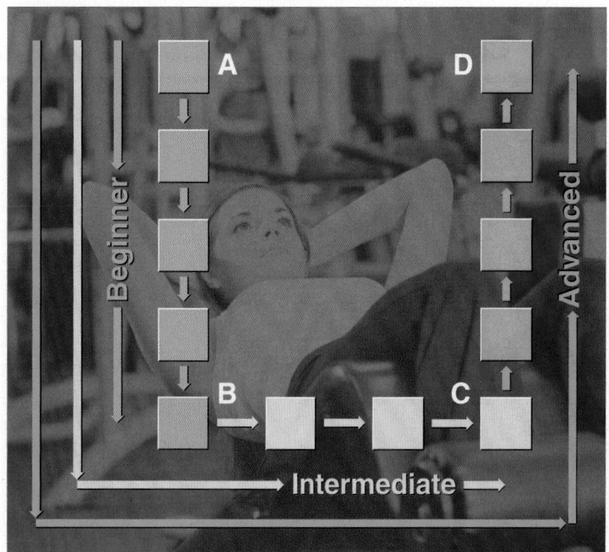

FIGURE 14.20 A basic multilevel exercise circuit. Beginners can work twice through the circuit from A to B; after several weeks, they progress three times through this portion of the circuit; finally, they increase the number of circuit revolutions up to six, depending on the number of stations. At the intermediate level, add several stations; participants proceed three to six times through circuit A to C. Build progression into each circuit by increasing the number of stations (A to D) and/or exercise load, repetitions, and duration.

TABLE 14.7 Energy Expenditure for Different Modes of Resistance Exercise Compared With Walking[a]

Mode	Gender	kJ · min⁻¹	kcal · min⁻¹
Nautilus, circuit	M F	29.7 24.3	7.1 5.8
Nautilus, circuit	M	22.6	5.4
Universal, circuit	M F	33.1 28.5	7.9 6.8
Isokinetic, slow	M	40.2	9.6
Isokinetic, fast	M	41.4	9.9
Isometric and free weight	M	25.1	6.0
Hydra-Fitness, circuit	M	37.7	9.0
Walking on level	M	22.6	5.4

[a]Based on a body weight of 68 kg.

Data from Katch FI, et al. Evaluation of acute cardiorespiratory responses to hydraulic resistance exercise. *Med Sci Sports Exerc* 1985;17:168.

station in sequence. Successful programs have incorporated music into the workout—upbeat music tempo during the exercise, with the music lowered to signify the individual should move to the next exercise station. The basic idea is to accomplish as many repetitions with good form during each exercise interval.

In one experiment, net energy expended (excluding resting metabolism) equaled 129 kcal for men and 95 kcal for women over the total exercise period. Heart rate averaged 142 $b \cdot min^{-1}$ (72% HR_{max}; 40% $\dot{V}O_{2max}$) for men and 158 $b \cdot min^{-1}$ (82% HR_{max}; 45% $\dot{V}O_{2max}$) for women.

CRT provides an alternative for fitness enthusiasts who desire a general conditioning program that improves both muscular strength and aerobic capacity. It also can supplement an off-season fitness program for sports that require a high level of muscular strength, power, and endurance.

Table 14.7 presents energy expenditure data for different types of resistance-type exercises compared to walking on the level. Isokinetic CRT procedures produced the highest energy expenditures.

BODY COMPOSITION ADAPTATIONS

Table 14.8 lists changes in body composition with DCER training from different experiments. For the most part, small decreases occur in body fat, with minimal increases in total body mass and FFM. The largest FFM increases amount to about 3 kg (6.6 lb) over 10 weeks, or about 0.3 kg weekly, with results about the same for men and women. Adherence to stringent, daily dietary intake potentially can accelerate the weight loss. Body composition data for other dynamic strength-training systems show similar results. No one resistance-training system proves superior for changing body composition.

MUSCLE SORENESS AND STIFFNESS

Most people experience soreness and stiffness in newly exercised joints and muscles following an extended exercise layoff. Temporary soreness may persist for several

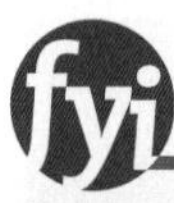

Components of Explosive Power Development

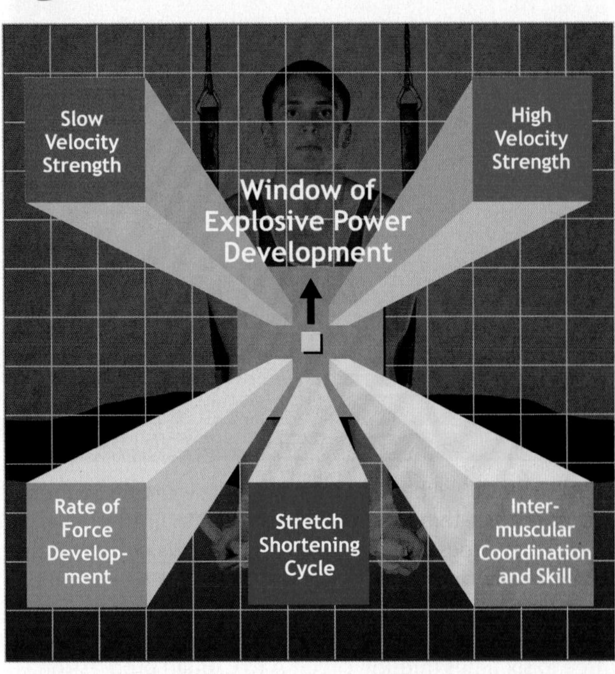

Each of the five components in the proposed model shown at the left makes important neuromuscular contributions to maximal power training. The window of adaptation opportunity shrinks for an athlete with already well-developed components but expands for components in need of considerable improvement. As an athlete approaches their high-velocity strength potential, that component's contribution to overall maximal power development diminishes. It may seem counterintuitive, but athletes must focus on training their least-developed components. Stated somewhat differently, maximal power performance improves more readily when targeting specific training routines to improve the weakest links because these have the largest adaptation opportunity window to develop superior explosive power.

Image reprinted with permission from McArdle WD, Katch FI, Katch VL. *Exercise Physiology: Nutrition, Energy, and Human Performance.* 8th Ed. Baltimore: Wolters Kluwer Health, 2015; as adapted with permission from Dr. William J. Kraemer, Human Performance Laboratory, University of Connecticut, Storrs; Adapted with permission from Kraemer WJ, Newton RU. Training for muscular power. *Phys Med Rehabil Clin* 2000;11:341.

TABLE 14.8 Body Composition Changes With Resistance Training[a]

Gender	Training Duration, wk	# of Exercises	Body Composition Changes		
			Body Mass, kg	FFM, kg	% Body Fat
F	10	10	0.1	1.3	−1.8
M	20	10	0.7	1.7	−1.5
M	9	5	0.5	1.4	−1.0
F	24	4	−0.04	1.0	−2.1
F	9	11	0.4	1.5	−1.3
M	8	10	1.0	3.1	−2.9
M	10	11	1.7	2.4	−9.1
F	10	8	−0.1	1.1	−1.9
M	10	8	0.3	1.2	−1.3
M	20	10	0.5	1.8	−1.7

[a]Data from different studies in the literature.

F = female; M = male; FFM = fat-free mass.

hours immediately following unaccustomed exercise, whereas a residual **delayed-onset muscle soreness (DOMS)** appears later and can last for 3 or 7 days. Any of the following 6 factors or a combination of them can produce DOMS:

1. Minute tears in muscle tissue or damage to its contractile components with accompanying release of creatine kinase, myoglobin, and troponin I—the muscle-specific marker of muscle fiber damage
2. Osmotic pressure changes that cause fluid retention in the surrounding tissues
3. Muscle spasms
4. Overstretching and perhaps tearing of portions of the muscle's connective tissue harness
5. Acute inflammation
6. Alteration in the cell's mechanism for calcium regulation

Eccentric Actions Produce Muscle Soreness

The precise cause of muscle soreness remains unknown. The degree of discomfort and muscle disturbance depends largely on the intensity and duration of effort and type of exercise performed. The magnitude of active strain imposed on a muscle fiber, rather than absolute force, precipitates muscle damage and soreness. Eccentric and to some extent isometric muscle actions generally trigger the greatest postexercise discomfort, especially among older individuals. Existing muscle damage or soreness from previous exercise does not exacerbate subsequent muscle damage or impair the regenerative process.

Cell Damage

The first bout of repetitive, unaccustomed physical activity disrupts the integrity of the cells' internal environment. This can produce microlesions and temporary ultrastructural damage in a pool of stress-susceptible or degenerating muscle fibers. Damage becomes more extensive several days following exercise than in the immediate postexercise period. A single bout of moderate concentric exercise provides a prophylactic effect on muscle soreness from subsequent high-force eccentric exercise, with the beneficial effect lasting up to 6 weeks. Such results support the wisdom of initiating a training program with repetitive, moderate concentric exercise to protect against muscle soreness following exercise with an eccentric component.

Altered Sarcoplasmic Reticulum

Four factors produce major alterations in sarcoplasmic reticulum structure and function with unaccustomed exercise:

1. Changes in pH
2. Changes in intramuscular high-energy phosphates
3. Changes in ionic balance
4. Changes in temperature

These four effects depress the rates of Ca^{2+} uptake and release and increase free Ca^{2+} concentration as the mineral rapidly moves into the damaged fibers' cytosol. Intracellular Ca^{2+} overload contributes to the autolytic process within damaged muscle fibers that degrades contractile and noncontractile structures.

Vitamin E supplementation (and perhaps supplementation with vitamin C and the mineral selenium) protects against cellular membrane disruption and enzyme loss following muscle damage from resistance exercise. Postexercise protein supplementation also may protect against muscle soreness in severely exercise-stressed individuals. In contrast, supplementing daily with either fish oil high in omega-3 and omega-6 fatty acids, or with soy isolate isoflavones for 30 days prior to and during the week of testing to reduce the inflammatory response produced no benefit to DOMS compared with placebo treatment. This included strength measures, pain ratings, limb girth, and blood measures related to muscle damage, inflammation, and lipid peroxidation. Supplementation with 750 mg a day of phosphatidylserine for 10 days did not afford additional protection against DOMS and markers of muscle damage, inflammation, and oxidative stress following prolonged downhill running. Similarly, taking a protease supplement did not affect pain perception associated with DOMS or blood markers of muscle damage.

Delayed-Onset Muscle Soreness Model

Figure 14.21 diagrams the probable six phases in DOMS development that ultimately lead to an inflammatory process and subsequent recuperation. Cellular adaptations to short-term exercise provide enhanced resistance to subsequent damage and pain.

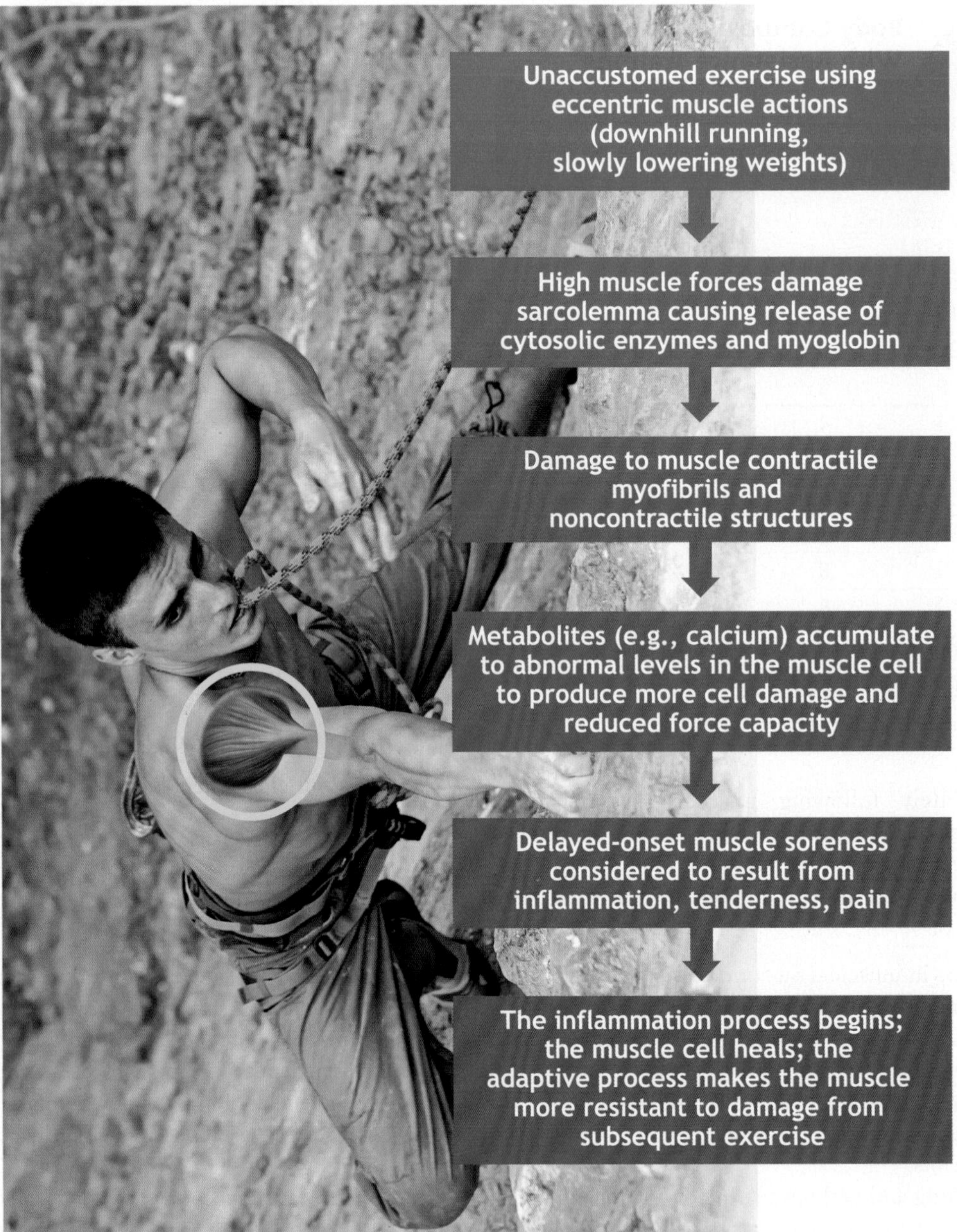
Unaccustomed exercise using eccentric muscle actions (downhill running, slowly lowering weights)
High muscle forces damage sarcolemma causing release of cytosolic enzymes and myoglobin
Damage to muscle contractile myofibrils and noncontractile structures
Metabolites (e.g., calcium) accumulate to abnormal levels in the muscle cell to produce more cell damage and reduced force capacity
Delayed-onset muscle soreness considered to result from inflammation, tenderness, pain
The inflammation process begins; the muscle cell heals; the adaptive process makes the muscle more resistant to damage from subsequent exercise

FIGURE 14.21 Proposed six-phase sequence for delayed-onset muscle soreness following unaccustomed exercise.

SUMMARY

1. Six factors—genetics, exercise, nutritional, hormonal, environmental, and neural—interact to regulate skeletal muscle mass and corresponding strength development.
2. Muscle fiber size, fiber type, and anatomic-lever arrangement of bone and muscle determine an individual's muscular strength.
3. CNS neural influences that activate prime movers in a specific movement greatly affect one's ability to express muscular strength.
4. Muscular strength with resistance training occurs from improved capacity for neuromuscular activation and significant alterations in a muscle fiber's contractile elements.
5. As muscle overload progessively increases, individual muscle fibers normally grow larger, a process termed muscle hypertrophy.
6. Total muscle enlargement involves increased protein synthesis within the fiber's contractile elements and proliferation of cells that thicken and strengthen the muscle's connective tissue harness.
7. Muscle fiber hypertrophy involves structural changes within the contractile mechanism, particularly for fast-twitch fibers, and increases in intramuscular anaerobic energy stores.
8. Intense resistance training does not induce cellular component adaptations that enhance aerobic energy transfer.

9. Women and men improve strength and muscle size with resistance training at about the same relative percentage.
10. Conventional resistance-training exercises contribute little to enhanced cardiovascular-aerobic fitness.
11. Most resistance-training programs without dietary constraint do not significantly reduce body fat because of their relatively low-energy cost.
12. Circuit resistance training using lower resistance (load) and higher repetitions combines the muscle-training benefits of resistance exercise with the cardiovascular, calorie-burning benefits of continuous, more intense physical activity.
13. Eccentric muscle actions produce significantly more delayed-onset muscle soreness or DOMS compared with concentric-only and isometric exercise.
14. DOMS includes muscle tears and connective tissue damage as part of the inflammatory response.

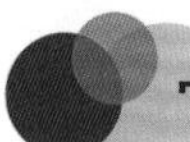

THINK IT THROUGH

1. For a football lineman, how would you apply the principle of specificity to evaluate current muscular strength and power and improve specific sport muscular performance?
2. Outline a sequence of steps in designing a resistance-training program for sedentary, middle-age men and women.
3. Outline two tests to evaluate muscular performance to best reflect the force-power requirements for firefighters.
4. Respond to a friend who comments: "I run and workout with free weights regularly, yet every spring my muscles are sore a day or two after a few hours of yard work."

KEY TERMS

Acute response: Immediate changes in muscle or other cells, tissues, or systems during or immediately following a single exercise bout.

Adaptation: How the body adjusts to a repeated, chronic stimulus.

Ballistic resistance training: Mode of training where a person moves a weight or projectile as rapidly as possible through the full range of motion with good form while trying to generate maximal force before releasing it.

Circuit resistance training (CRT): Resistance training with a pre-established exercise-to-rest sequence, usually consisting of 8 to 15 different exercise stations, with 15 to 20 repetitions performed for each exercise.

Concentric action: Muscle shortening during force application.

Core training: Exercise training of abdominal muscles, paraspinals and gluteals, diaphragm, and pelvic floor and hip girdle musculature.

Delayed-onset muscle soreness (DOMS): Soreness and stiffness in exercised joints and muscles that can persist for up to 7 days following a bout of unaccustomed exercise.

Dynamic constant external resistance (DCER): Resistance training in which external resistance or weight does not change, yet joint flexion and extension occurs with each repetition.

Dynamometers: Force-measuring instruments to assess a mechanically derived output—force, power, torque, speed, and velocity—during diverse muscle actions.

Eccentric action: Muscle lengthening that occurs during force application.

Fiber hyperplasia: Increase in muscle fiber number.

Force-velocity relationship: Intrinsic relationship when a muscle shortens against a constant load, with velocity assessed during shortening and plotted against the resistive force.

Functional strength training: Type of training that requires neuromuscular adaptations in the important movements that necessitate improved strength.

Hypertrophic development: Increase in muscle fiber size from strength development techniques.

Isokinetic dynamometer: Electromechanical accommodating resistance instrument with a speed-controlling mechanism, which accelerates to a preset, constant velocity with applied force regardless of the force exerted on the device movement arm, and where resistance increases or decreases with a muscle's capacity that varies throughout a joint's ROM.

Isokinetic resistance training: Training that uses a muscle action performed at constant angular limb velocity and where resistance increases or decreases with a muscle's capacity that varies throughout a joint's ROM.

Isokinetic training: Common exercise strategy to train muscles to become stronger via muscle action performed at constant angular limb velocity.

Isometric action: Muscle action performed at constant limb position where no noticeable movement occurs.

Isometric testing: Assessing muscle action at a specific joint angle without noticeable outward change in muscle length.

Isometric training: Common exercise strategy to train muscles to become stronger in performing static muscle actions.

Ling, Hjalmar: Swedish educator; helped to found early movement science education and methodology in the mid-1850s in Europe.

Ling, Pehr Henrik: Father of Swedish gymnastics; in 1813, founded the current Swedish School of Sport and Health Sciences under the name of the Royal Central Institute of Gymnastics, Stockholm.

Matveyev, Leonid: Russian sports scientist; in 1962, he introduced the concept of strength-training periodization or sequential training planning.

Muscle cross-sectional area (MCSA): Measured cross-section of the largest diameter in an intact, contracted muscle.

Muscle endurance development: Developing sustained maximum or submaximum force, often determined by assessing maximum number of exercise repetitions at a percentage of maximum strength.

Muscle fiber hypertrophy: Increased size of individual muscle fibers.

Muscular strength: Maximum force, tension, or torque generated by a muscle or muscle groups.

One-repetition maximum (1-RM): Maximum force generated for one repetition of a movement.

Overload principle: Basic tenant of training strategy whereby a muscle makes physiological adaptations to the progressive level of tension placed on it.

Periodization: Training planning that varies training intensity and volume to ensure optimal conditions so that peak performance coincides with major competitions.

Plyometrics: Special form of training to develop powerful, propulsive movements—requiring jumping in place or rebound jumping or drop jumping from a preset height—to mobilize the inherent stretch-recoil characteristics of skeletal muscle and its modulation via the stretch or myotatic reflex.

Power development: Procedures that determine and/or enhance the rate of performing work (force × distance ÷ time or force × velocity).

Progressive resistance exercise (PRE): Practical application of the overload principle, which forms the basis for most resistance-training programs; influenced by number of sets, repetitions, frequency, and relative intensity of training to improve strength.

Progressive resistance weight training: Common exercise strategy to train muscles to become stronger using standard weightlifting equipment, pulleys, slings, springs, immovable bars, resistance bands, and a variety of isokinetic, pneumatic, and hydraulic devices.

Relative strength: Computed relative to either body mass, segmental or total FFM, or MCSA to help introduce "fairness" when comparing men and women of widely different strength and body composition profiles.

Satellite cells: Dormant myogenic stem cells that activate and replicate under certain conditions.

Strength development: Using a variety of methods to enhance maximum force-generating capacity of a muscle or group of muscles.

Strength-training zone: Intensity of effort from 60% to 100% of 1-RM during resistance training to increase muscular strength.

Stretch-shortening cycle (SSC): Concept that describes how skeletal muscles function efficiently in unrestricted human locomotor activities; sequence of stretching and shortening muscle fibers to reflexly enhance subsequent movement performance.

Variable resistance-training equipment: Training with equipment that either uses a lever arm, cam, hydraulic system, or pulley to alter the resistance to match the increases and decreases in a muscle's force capacity that varies throughout a joint's ROM.

Voluntary maximal muscle action: Highest force a muscle produces under voluntary control.

Zander, Gustav: Swedish physician (1835–1920) devised methods to treat patients and common persons with standard gymnastic exercise emphasizing mechanical machines, calisthenics, balance, and core trunk and limb strength.

SELECTED REFERENCES

Adamson M, et al. Unilateral arm strength training improves contralateral peak force and rate of force development. *Eur J Appl Physiol* 2008;103:553.

Alcaraz PE, et al. Physical performance and cardiovascular responses to an acute bout of heavy resistance circuit training versus traditional strength training. *J Strength Cond Res* 2008;22:667.

Allison GT, et al. Feedforward responses of transversus abdominis are directionally specific and act asymmetrically: implications for core stability theories. *J Orthop Sports Phys Ther* 2008;38:228.

Andersen LL, et al. Neuromuscular adaptations to detraining following resistance training in previously untrained subjects. *Eur J Appl Physiol* 2005;93:511.

Andersen LL, et al. The effect of resistance training combined with timed ingestion of protein on muscle fiber size and muscle strength. *Metabolism* 2005;54:151.

Areta JL, et al. Reduced resting skeletal muscle protein synthesis is rescued by resistance exercise and protein ingestion following short-term energy deficit. *Am J Physiol Endocrinol Metab* 2014;306:E989.

Arts MP, et al.; The Hague Spine Intervention Prognostic Study (SIPS) Group. Management of sciatica due to lumbar disc herniation in the Netherlands: a survey among spine surgeons. *J Neurosurg Spine* 2008;9:32.

Azegami M, et al. Effect of single and multi-joint lower extremity muscle strength on the functional capacity and ADL/IADL status in Japanese community-dwelling older adults. *Nurs Health Sci* 2007;9:168.

Baker D, Newton RU. Acute effect on power output of alternating an agonist and antagonist muscle exercise during complex training. *J Strength Cond Res* 2005;19:202.

Bartolomei S, et al. Block versus weekly undulating periodized resistance training programs in women. *J Strength Cond Res* 2015. In press as of March 29, 2015.

Beck TW, et al. Effects of a protease supplement on eccentric exercise-induced markers of delayed-onset muscle soreness and muscle damage. *J Strength Cond Res* 2007;21:661.

Bgeginski R, et al. Cardiorespiratory responses of pregnant and nonpregnant women during resistance exercise. *J Strength Cond Res* 2015;29:596.

Black CD, et al. High specific torque is related to lengthening contraction-induced skeletal muscle injury. *J Appl Physiol* 2008;104:639.

Bodine SC. mTOR signaling and the molecular adaptation to resistance exercise. *Med Sci Sports Exerc* 2007;38:1950.

Bohannon RW. Hand-grip dynamometry predicts future outcomes in aging adults. *J Geriatr Phys Ther* 2008;31:3.

Brocherie F, et al. Electrostimulation training effects on the physical performance of ice hockey players. *Med Sci Sports Exerc* 2005;37:455.

Buford TW, et al. A comparison of periodization models during nine weeks with equated volume and intensity for strength. *J Strength Cond Res* 2007;21:1245.

Caserotti P, et al. Changes in power and force generation during coupled eccentric-concentric versus concentric muscle contraction with training and aging. *Eur J Appl Physiol* 2008;103:151.

Castagna C, et al. Aerobic and explosive power performance of elite Italian regional-level basketball players. *J Strength Cond Res* 2009;23:1982.

Chapman MA, et al. Disruption of both nesprin 1 and desmin results in nuclear anchorage defects and fibrosis in skeletal muscle. *Hum Mol Genet* 2014;23:5879.

Cholewicki J, et al. Lumbar spine stability can be augmented with an abdominal belt and/or increased intra-abdominal pressure. *Eur Spine J* 1999;8:388.

Choo A, et al. Muscle gene expression patterns in human rotator cuff pathology. *J Bone Joint Surg Am* 2014;96:1558.

Coeffey VG, et al. Effect of high-frequency resistance exercise on adaptive responses in skeletal muscle. *Med Sci Sports Exerc* 2007;39:2135.

Coffey VG, Hawley JA. The molecular basis of training adaptation. *Sports Med* 2007;37:737.

Colado JC, Triplett NT. Effects of a short-term resistance program using elastic bands versus weight machines for sedentary middle-aged women. *J Strength Cond Res* 2008;22:1441.

Cronin J, Crewther B. Training volume and strength and power development. *J Sci Med Sport* 2004;7:144.

Cronin JB, Hansen KT. Strength and power predictors of sports speed. *J Strength Cond Res* 2005;19:349.

Cronin NJ, et al. Effects of contraction intensity on muscle fascicle and stretch reflex behavior in the human triceps surae. *J Appl Physiol* 2008;105:226.

Crowther RG, et al. Kinematic responses to plyometric exercises conducted on compliant and noncompliant surfaces. *J Strength Cond Res* 2007;21:460.

Daly RM, et al. Muscle determinants of bone mass, geometry and strength in prepubertal girls. *Med Sci Sports Exerc* 2008;40:1135.

Dayanidhi S, Lieber RL. Skeletal muscle satellite cells: mediators of muscle growth during development and implications for developmental disorders. *Muscle Nerve* 2014;50:723.

de Villarreal ES, et al. Determining variables of plyometric training for improving vertical jump height performance: a meta-analysis. *J Strength Cond Res* 2009;23:495.

de Vos NJ, et al. Optimal load for increasing muscle power during explosive resistance training in older adults. *J Gerontol A Biol Sci Med Sci* 2005;60:638.

DeLorme TL, Watkins AL. *Progressive Resistance Exercise*. New York: Appleton-Century-Crofts, 1951.

Egan B, Zierath JR. Exercise metabolism and the molecular regulation of skeletal muscle adaptation. *Cell Metab* 2012;17:162.

Elvested P, et al. The effects of a worksite neuromuscular activation program on sick leave: a pilot study. *Med Sci Sports Exerc* 2008;40:S434.

Enoka RM, Stuart DG. Neurobiology of muscle fatigue. *J Appl Physiol* 1992; 72:1631.

Falla D, Farina D. Neural and muscular factors associated with motor impairment in neck pain. *Curr Rheumatol Rep* 2007;9:497.

Farina D, et al. The extraction of neural strategies from the surface EMG. *J Appl Physiol* 2004;96:1486.

Flanagan EP, et al. Reliability of the reactive strength index and time to stabilization during depth jumps. *J Strength Cond Res* 2008;5:1677.

Frost DM, et al. A proposed method to detect kinematic differences between and within individuals. *J Electromyogr Kinesiol* 2015;25:479.

Gillies AR, et al. Three-dimensional reconstruction of skeletal muscle extracellular matrix ultrastructure. *Microsc Microanal* 2014;2:1.

Goodpaster BH, et al. Attenuation of skeletal muscle and strength in the elderly: The Health ABC Study. *J Appl Physiol* 2001;90:2157.

Goto K, et al. The impact of metabolic stress on hormonal responses and muscular adaptations. *Med Sci Sports Exerc* 2005;37:955.

Gotshalk LA, et al. Cardiovascular responses to a high-volume continuous circuit resistance training protocol. *J Strength Cond Res* 2004;18:760.

Graves JE, et al. Specificity of limited range of motion variable resistance training. *Med Sci Sports Exerc* 1989;21:84.

Hackney KJ, et al. Resting energy expenditure and delayed-onset muscle soreness after full-body resistance training with an eccentric concentration. *J Strength Cond Res* 2008;22:1602.

Hakkinen A, et al. Effects of home strength training and stretching versus stretching alone after lumbar disk surgery: a randomized study with a 1-year follow-up. *Arch Phys Med Rehabil* 2005;86:865.

Harber MP, et al. Single muscle fiber contractile properties during a competitive season in male runners. *Am J Physiol Regul Integr Comp Physiol* 2004;287: R1124.

Hartmann H, et al. Effects of different periodization models on rate of force development and power ability of the upper extremity. *J Strength Cond Res* 2009;23:1921.

Haswell K, et al. Clinical decision rules for identification of low back pain patients with neurologic involvement in primary care. *Spine* 2008;33:68.

Hawkins SB, et al. The effect of different training programs on eccentric energy utilization in college-aged males. *J Strength Cond Res* 2009;23:1996.

Hedayatpour N, et al. Sensory and electromyographic mapping during delayed-onset muscle soreness. *Med Sci Sports Exerc* 2008;40:326.

Henwood TR, Taaffe DR. Improved physical performance in older adults undertaking a short-term programme of high-velocity resistance training. *Gerontology* 2005;51:108.

Hubal MJ, et al. Mechanisms of variability in strength loss after muscle-lengthening actions. *Med Sci Sports Exerc* 2007;39:461.

Ikai M, Steinhaus AH. Some factors modifying the expression of human strength. *J Appl Physiol* 1961;16:157.

Impellizzeri FM, et al. Effect of plyometric training on sand versus grass on muscle soreness and jumping and sprinting ability in soccer players. *Br J Sports Med* 2008;42:42.

Ishikawa M, Komi PV. Muscle fascicle and tendon behavior during human locomotion revisited. *Exerc Sport Sci Rev* 2008;36:193.

Ishikawa M, Komi PV. The role of the stretch reflex in the gastrocnemius muscle during human locomotion at various speeds. *J Appl Physiol* 2007;103:1030.

Ispirlidis I, et al. Time-course of changes in inflammatory and performance responses following a soccer game. *Clin J Sport Med* 2008;18:423.

Issurin V. Block periodization versus traditional training theory: a review. *J Sports Med Phys Fitness* 2008;48:65.

Jensen I, Harms-Ringdahl K. Strategies for prevention and management of musculoskeletal conditions. Neck pain. *Best Pract Res Clin Rheumatol* 2007;21:93.

Katch VL. The Lumbopelvic system: anatomy, physiology, motor control, instability and description of a unique treatment modality. In: Donatell RA, Wooden MJ, eds. *Orthopaedic Physical Therapy*. 4th Ed. St. Louis: Churchill Livingstone: Elsevier, 2010.

Kemmler WK, et al. Effects of single- vs. multiple-set resistance training on maximum strength and body composition in trained postmenopausal women. *J Strength Cond Res* 2004;18:689.

Kubo K, et al. Effects of plyometric and weight training on muscle-tendon complex and jump performance. *Med Sci Sports Exerc* 2007;39:1801.

Lamon S, et al. Regulation of STARS and its downstream targets suggest a novel pathway involved in human skeletal muscle hypertrophy and atrophy. *J Physiol* 2009;587:1795.

Larsson L, et al. Muscle strength and speed of movement in relation to age and muscle morphology. *J Appl Physiol* 1979;46:451.

Leukel C, et al. Influence of falling height on the excitability of the soleus H-reflex during drop-jumps. *Acta Physiol (Oxf)* 2008;192:569.

Lieber RL, Ward SR. Cellular mechanisms of tissue fibrosis. 4. Structural and functional consequences of skeletal muscle fibrosis. *Am J Physiol Cell Physiol* 2013;305:C241.

Lieber RL. *Skeletal Muscle Structure, Function, and Plasticity: The Physiological Basis of Rehabilitation*. 3rd Ed. Baltimore: Lippincott, Williams & Wilkins, 2010.

Lin JD, et al. The effects of different stretch amplitudes on electromyographic activity during drop jumps. *J Strength Cond Res* 2008;22:32.

Lund H, et al. Learning effect of isokinetic measurements in healthy subjects, and reliability and comparability of Biodex and Lido dynamometers. *Clin Physiol Funct Imaging* 2005;25:75.

McCaulley GO, et al. Mechanical efficiency during repetitive vertical jumping. *Eur J Appl Physiol* 2007;101:115.

McCurdy KW, et al. The effects of short-term unilateral and bilateral lower-body resistance training on measures of strength and power. *J Strength Cond Res* 2005;19:9.

McGill S. *Low Back Disorders: Evidence-Based Prevention and Rehabilitation*. 2nd Ed. Champaign: Human Kinetics, Inc., 2007.

McGill S, et al. Passive stiffness of the lumbar torso in flexion, extension, lateral bending, and axial rotation. Effect of belt wearing and breath holding. *Spine (Phila Pa 1976)* 1994;19:696.

McGill SM, et al. The effect of an abdominal belt on trunk muscle activity and intra-abdominal pressure during squat lifts. *Ergonomics* 1990;33:147.

Meyer GA, et al. Role of the cytoskeleton in muscle transcriptional responses to altered use. *Physiol Genomics* 2013;45:321.

Miyaguchi K, Demura S. Relationships between stretch-shortening cycle performance and maximum muscle strength. *J Strength Cond Res* 2008;22:19.

Mjolsnes R, et al. A 10-week randomized trial comparing eccentric vs. concentric hamstring strength training in well-trained soccer players. *Scand J Med Sci Sports* 2004;14:311.

Molski M. Two-wave model of the muscle contraction. *Biosystems* 2009;96:136.

Myers NL, et al. Increasing ball velocity in the overhead athlete: a meta-analysis of randomized controlled trials. *J Strength Cond Res* 2015. In Press as of 25.06.2015.

Narici MV, Maganaris CN. Plasticity of the muscle-tendon complex with disuse and aging. *Exerc Sport Sci Rev* 2007;35:126.

Nosaka K, et al. Partial protection against muscle damage by eccentric actions at short muscle lengths. *Med Sci Sports Exerc* 2005;37:746.

Palmisano MG, et al. Muscle intermediate filaments form a stress-transmitting and stress-signaling network in muscle. *J Cell Sci* 2015;128:219.

Petrella JK, et al. Age differences in knee extension power, contractile velocity, and fatigability. *J Appl Physiol* 2005;98:21.

Prestes J, et al. Comparison between linear and daily undulating periodized resistance training to increase strength. *J Strength Cond Res* 2009;23:2437.

Prokopy M, et al. Closed-kinetic chain upper-body training improves throwing performance of NCAA Division I softball players. *J Strength Cond Res* 2009;22:1790.

Reeves ND, et al. Plasticity of dynamic muscle performance with strength training in elderly humans. *Muscle Nerve* 2005;31:355.

Regueme SC, et al. Delayed influence of stretch-shortening cycle fatigue on large ankle joint position coded with static positional signals. *Scand J Med Sci Sports* 2008;18:373.

Sangnier S, Tourny-Chollet C. Study of the fatigue curve in quadriceps and hamstrings of soccer players during isokinetic endurance testing. *J Strength Cond Res* 2008;22:1458.

Santana JC, et al. A kinetic and electromyographic comparison of the standing cable press and bench press. *J Strength Cond Res* 2007;21:1271.

Seeman E. Structural basis of growth-related gain and age-related loss of bone strength. *Rheumatology (Oxford)* 2008;47:iv2.

Seger JY, Thorstensson A. Effects of eccentric versus concentric training on thigh muscle strength and EMG. *Int J Sports Med* 2005;26:45.

Seiler S, Sæterbakken A. A unique core stability training program improves throwing velocity in female high school athletes. *Med Sci Sports Exerc* 2008; 40:S248.

Seyennes OR, et al. Early skeletal muscle hypertrophy and architectural changes in response to high-intensity resistance training. *J Appl Physiol* 2007;102:373.

Shaw WS, et al. Patient clusters in acute, work-related back pain based on patterns of disability risk factors. *J Occup Environ Med* 2007;49:185.

Shepstone TN, et al. Short-term high- vs low-velocity isokinetic lengthening training results in greater hypertrophy of the elbow flexors in young men. *Scand J Med Sci Sports* 2005;15:135.

Shimano T, et al. Relationship between the number of repetitions and selected percentages of one repetition maximum in free weight exercises in trained and untrained men. *J Strength Cond Res* 2006;20:819.

Sidorkewicz N, et al. Examining the effects of altering hip orientation on gluteus medius and tensor fascae latae interplay during common non-weight-bearing hip rehabilitation exercises. *Clin Biomech (Bristol, Avon)* 2014;29:971.

Signorile JF, et al. Early plateaus of power and torque gains during high- and low-speed resistance training of older women. *J Appl Physiol* 2005 ;98:1213.

Smith LR, Meyer G, Lieber RL. Systems analysis of biological networks in skeletal muscle function. *Wiley Interdiscip Rev Syst Biol Med* 2013;5:55.

Spiering BA, et al. Resistance exercise biology: manipulation of resistance exercise programme variables determines the responses of cellular and molecular signaling pathways. *Sports Med* 2008;38:527.

Storch EK, Kruszynski DM. From rehabilitation to optimal function: role of clinical exercise therapy. *Curr Opin Crit Care* 2008;14:451.

Symons TB, et al. Effects of maximal isometric and isokinetic resistance training on strength and functional mobility in older adults. *J Gerontol A Biol Sci Med Sci* 2005;60:777.

Takahashi M, et al. Muscle excursion does not correlate with increased serial sarcomere number after muscle adaptation to stretched tendon transfer. *J Orthop Res* 2012;30:1774.

Thomas GA, et al. Maximal power at different percentages of one repetition maximum: influence of resistance and gender. *J Strength Cond Res* 2007; 21:336.

Thomas K, et al. The effect of two plyometric training techniques on muscular power and agility in youth soccer players. *J Strength Cond Res* 2009;23:332.

Tirrell TF, et al. Human skeletal muscle biochemical diversity. *J Exp Biol* 2012;215:2551.

Tuttle LJ, et al. Post-mortem timing of skeletal muscle biochemical and mechanical degradation. *J Biomech* 2014;47:1506.

Tuttle LJ, et al. Sample size considerations in human muscle architecture studies. *Muscle Nerve* 2012;45:742.

Twist C, et al. The effects of plyometric exercise on unilateral balance performance. *J Sports Sci* 2008;10:1073.

Ullrich B, et al. Neuromuscular responses to 14 weeks of traditional and daily undulating resistance training. *Int J Sports Med* 2015;36:554.

Veqar Z, Imtiyaz S. Vibration Therapy in Management of Delayed Onset Muscle Soreness (DOMS). *J Clin Diagn Res* 2014;8:1.

Verghese J, et al. Self-reported difficulty in climbing up or down stairs in nondisabled elderly. *Arch Phys Med Rehabil* 2008;89:100.

Vikne J, et al. A randomized study of new sling exercise treatment vs traditional physiotherapy for patients with chronic whiplash-associated disorders with unsettled compensation claims. *J Rehabil Med* 2007;39:252.

Walts CT, et al. Do sex or race differences influence strength training effects on muscle or fat? *Med Sci Sports Exerc* 2008;40:229.

Wilson JM, Flanagan EP. The role of elastic energy in activities with high force and power requirements: a brief review. *J Strength Cond Res* 2008;5:1705.

Winter EM, Fowler N. Exercise defined and quantified according to the Système International d'Unités'. *J Sports Sci* 2009;27:447.

Wood LE, et al. Elbow flexion and extension strength relative to body or muscle size in children. *Med Sci Sports Exerc* 2004;36:1977.

Zammit PS. All muscle satellite cells are equal, but are some more equal than others? *J Cell Sci* 2008;121:2975.

Factors Affecting Physiologic Function: The Environment and Special Aids to Performance

CHAPTER OBJECTIVES

- Explain the statement: The hypothalamus plays the most important role in regulating thermal balance.
- Name four physical factors that contribute to heat exchange during rest and physical activity.
- Describe how the circulatory system serves as a "workhorse" for thermoregulation.
- List three desirable clothing characteristics during physical effort in cold and warm weather.
- Describe how cardiac output, heart rate, and stroke volume respond during submaximal and maximal physical activity during environmental heat stress.
- Describe circulatory adjustments that maintain blood pressure during hot weather physical activity.
- Quantify fluid loss during physical activity in hot weather.
- Identify three physiologic consequences of dehydration.
- Explain how acclimatization, training, age, gender, and body fat modify heat tolerance during physical activity.
- Identify three factors that comprise the heat-stress index.
- Explain the purpose of the windchill index.
- Describe four physiologic adjustments to cold stress.
- Outline the effects of increasingly higher altitudes on oxygen's partial pressure in ambient air, hemoglobin saturation with oxygen in pulmonary capillaries, and maximal oxygen uptake ($\dot{V}O_{2max}$).
- Describe three immediate and three long-term physiologic adjustments to altitude exposure.
- Describe the typical time course for red blood cell reinfusion and mechanism for its ergogenic effect on endurance performance and aerobic capacity.
- Explain the major medical use of erythropoietin and its potential dangers for healthy athletes.
- Contrast "general warm-up" with "specific warm-up."
- Identify two potential cardiovascular benefits of moderate warm-up immediately before extreme physical effort.
- Provide a rationale for breathing a hyperoxic gas mixture to enhance physical activity performance and quantify its potential to increase tissue oxygen availability.

ANCILLARIES AT A GLANCE

Visit **http://thePoint.lww.com/MKKESS5e** to access the following resources:

- References: Chapter 15
- Interactive Question Bank
- Appendix SR-6: Additional Video Links
- Animation: Thermal Regulation
- Animation: Water Balance

This chapter discusses specific problems encountered during physical activity in hot and cold environments and at high altitude. We present this information within the framework of the immediate physiologic adjustments and longer-term adaptations as the body strives to maintain internal consistency despite severe environmental challenges. We also explore three common ergogenic interventions—blood doping, warm-up, and hyperoxic gas—strategies proported to improve physiologic function, physical activity capacity, and athletic performance.

PART 1 Mechanisms of Thermoregulation

THERMOREGULATION

Normal body **temperature** fluctuates several degrees during the day in response to physical activity, emotions, and ambient temperature variations; oral temperature averages about 1.0°F (0.56°C) less than rectal temperature. Body temperature also exhibits diurnal fluctuations—the lowest temperatures occur during sleep, and slightly higher temperatures persist when awake even when the person relaxes in bed.

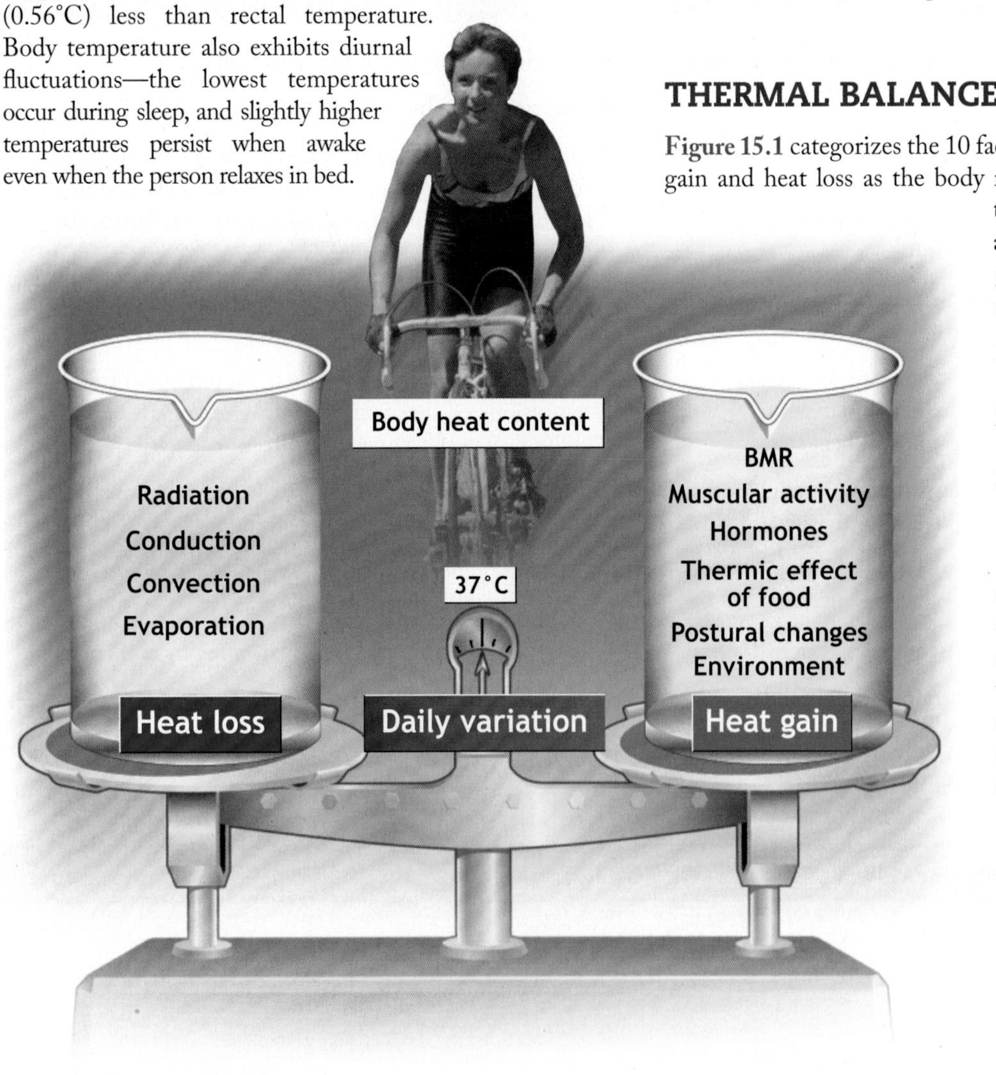

Thermoregulation plays such an important role in the body's homeostatic balance mechanisms that the price of failure can be death. A person can tolerate a drop in core temperature of 18°F (10°C) but an increase of only 9°F (5°C). Over the past 35 years, more than 100 football players and collegiate wrestlers have died from excessive heat stress during practice or competition. Heat injury also often occurs during military training and operations, during longer duration athletic events, and in industry (miners) and farming (migrant farmworkers).

Understanding thermoregulation and the most effective line of attack to support temperature control mechanisms dramatically reduces heat-related tragedies. Coaches, athletes, and race and event organizers must reduce factors that promote heat gain and dehydration. Concern should also focus on the most effective behavioral approaches, including prudent scheduling of events, acclimatization, proper clothing, and fluid and electrolyte replacement before, during, and following physical activity to blunt any negative thermal effects on performance and safety.

See the animation "Thermal Regulation" on **http://thePoint.lww.com/MKKESS5e** for a demonstration of this process.

THERMAL BALANCE

Figure 15.1 categorizes the 10 factors that contribute to heat gain and heat loss as the body rapidly adjusts to maintain thermal neutrality. This balance results from three integrative mechanisms that accomplish the following:

1. Alter heat transfer to the periphery (**shell**)
2. Regulate evaporative cooling
3. Vary the rate of heat production

The temperature of the deeper tissues or **core** rises quickly when heat gain exceeds heat loss during vigorous exertion in a warm environment. In the cold, in contrast, heat loss begins to exceed heat production and core temperature plummets.

Body heat content
Radiation
Conduction
Convection
Evaporation
Heat loss
37°C
Daily variation
BMR
Muscular activity
Hormones
Thermic effect of food
Postural changes
Environment
Heat gain

FIGURE 15.1 Ten contributing factors to heat gain and heat loss to regulate core temperature at about 98.6°F (37°C).

Body Temperature Measurement

A thermal gradient exists within the body, with core body temperature (T_{core}) the highest and shell temperature (T_{skin}) the lowest. Mean body temperature

($\bar{T}_{body}$) represents an average of skin and internal temperatures. Common sites to estimate average core temperature ($\bar{T}_{core}$) include the rectum (rectal temperature), eardrum (tympanic temperature), and esophagus (esophageal temperature). Temperature sensors placed at various skin locations estimate T_{skin}. Mean skin temperature ($\bar{T}_{skin}$) represents the weighted average of different skin temperatures that reflect the portion of the body's surface that each site represents (e.g., arm, trunk, leg, head). $\bar{T}_{body}$ computes as follows:

$$\bar{T}_{body} = (0.6 \times \bar{T}_{core}) + (0.4 \times \bar{T}_{skin})$$

The relative proportion of the body's average temperature represented by the core equals 0.6 (60%) and 0.4 (40%) for the skin.

HYPOTHALAMIC REGULATION OF BODY TEMPERATURE

The brain's hypothalamus contains the central coordinating center for temperature regulation. This group of specialized neurons at the floor of the brain serves as an extremely sensitive thermostat to carefully regulate temperature within a narrow range of 98.6°F ± 1.8°F (37°C ± 1°C). Unlike a home thermostat, the hypothalamus cannot turn the heat on or off; it only initiates responses to protect the body when core temperature changes from its "norm" due to heat gain and heat loss. Temperature-regulating mechanisms become activated in two ways:

1. Thermal skin receptors provide peripheral input to the hypothalamic central control center.
2. Temperature changes in blood that perfuses the hypothalamus directly stimulate the hypothalamic control center.

The hypothalamic regulatory center plays the most important role in maintaining thermal balance. Cells in the anterior hypothalamus directly detect changes in blood temperature in addition to receiving peripheral input. Cells then activate either the posterior hypothalamus to initiate coordinated responses for heat conservation or the anterior hypothalamus to initiate responses to heat loss. Peripheral skin receptors primarily detect cold; the hypothalamus monitors body warmth by the temperature of the blood that perfuses this area. **Table 15.1** summarizes the mechanisms that regulate body temperature; each responds in a graded manner, increasing or decreasing as required to preserve thermoregulation within narrow limits.

Oral Temperature Does Not Always Measure Core Temperature

Oral temperature does not accurately measure deep body or core temperature following strenuous physical activity. Large and consistent differences occurred between oral and rectal temperatures after a 14-mile race in a tropical climate; whereas rectal temperature averaged 103.5°F (39.7°C), oral temperature remained normal at 98.6°F (37°C). This discrepancy partly results from evaporative cooling of the mouth and airways from relatively high ventilatory volumes during and immediately following intense exertion.

REGULATING BODY TEMPERATURE DURING COLD AND HEAT EXPOSURE

Cold Stress

Excessive heat loss occurs in extreme cold at rest. This increases the body's heat production and slows heat loss as physiologic adjustments combat a decrease in core temperature.

Three integrated factors regulate body temperature during cold exposure:

1. **Vascular adjustments:** Circulatory adjustments "fine tune" temperature regulation. Stimulation of cutaneous cold receptors constricts peripheral blood vessels. Vasoconstriction immediately reduces the flow of warm blood to the body's cooler surface and redirects it to the warmer core that includes cranial, thoracic, and abdominal cavities and portions of the muscle mass. Consequently, skin temperature decreases toward ambient temperature to optimize the insulatory benefits of skin and subcutaneous fat.
2. **Muscular activity:** Shivering generates metabolic heat (maximum of three to five times resting metabolism), but physical activity provides the greatest contribution in defending against cold. Energy metabolism during physical activity sustains a constant core temperature when air temperatures decrease to −22°F (−30°C) without need for insulating clothing.
3. **Hormonal output:** Increased release of the adrenal medulla's "calorigenic" hormones epinephrine and norepinephrine partially accounts for increased basal heat production during cold exposure. Prolonged cold stress also increases the thyroid gland's release of thyroxine to elevate resting metabolism.

TABLE 15.1 Mechanisms for Temperature Regulation

Stimulated by Cold	Mechanism
Decreases heat loss	Vasoconstriction of skin vessels; postural reduction of surface area (curling up)
Increases heat production	Shivering and increased voluntary activity; increased thyroxine and epinephrine secretion
Stimulated by Heat	
Increases heat loss	Vasodilation of subcutaneous skin vessels; sweating
Decreases heat production	Decreased muscle tone and voluntary activity; decreased thyroxine and epinephrine secretion

Heat Stress

Thermoregulatory mechanisms primarily protect against overheating. Thwarting excessive body heat buildup becomes important during sustained intense effort when metabolic rate increases 20 to 25 times resting levels—heat production that could increase core temperature by 1.8°F (1°C) every 5 minutes. Here, physiologic competition exists between mechanisms that maintain a large muscle blood flow and mechanisms that regulate body temperature. **Figure 15.2** illustrates the following four potential avenues for heat exchange during physical activity:

1. **Radiation:** Objects continually emit electromagnetic heat waves. The body is usually warmer than the environment, so the net exchange of radiant heat energy occurs from the body through air to solid, cooler objects in the environment. Despite subfreezing temperatures, a person can remain warm by absorbing sufficient radiant heat energy directly from direct sunlight or from sunlight reflected from snow, sand, or water. The body absorbs radiant heat energy when an object's temperature in the environment exceeds skin temperature, making evaporative cooling the only avenue for heat loss.
2. **Conduction:** Heat loss by conduction directly transfers heat from one molecule to another through a liquid, solid, or gas. The circulatory system transports most of the body heat to the outer shell, but a small amount continually moves by conduction directly through warmer deep tissues to cooler outer surfaces. Conductive heat loss then warms air molecules and cooler surfaces that contact skin. The rate of conductive heat loss depends on two factors—the temperature gradient between skin and surrounding surfaces and their thermal qualities. For example, when hiking outdoors in the heat, some relief comes from lying on a cool rock shielded from the sun. Conductance between the rock's colder surface and the hiker's warmer surface enhances body heat loss until the rock warms to body temperature.
3. **Convection:** Heat loss by conduction depends on how rapidly air near the body exchanges after warming. With little or no air movement (convection), air next to the skin warms and acts as an insulation zone to minimize further conductive heat loss. Conversely, if cooler air continuously replaces warmer air surrounding the body, as it does on a breezy day, in a room with a fan, or during running, heat loss increases because convective currents carry the heat away. For example, air currents at 4 mph cool twice as effectively as air moving at 1 mph.
4. **Evaporation:** *Evaporative cooling provides the major physiologic defense against overheating.* Water vaporization from the respiratory passages and skin surface continually transfers heat to the environment. In response to heat stress, the body's 2 to 4 million sweat or eccrine glands secrete large quantities of hypotonic

A CLOSER LOOK

Assessing Heat Quality of the Environment: How Hot Is Too Hot?

Seven factors determine the physiologic strain imposed by environmental heat:

1. Air temperature and relative humidity
2. Individual differences in body size and fatness
3. State of training
4. Degree of acclimatization
5. Environmental influences—convective air currents and radiant heat gain
6. Physical activity intensity
7. Clothing amount, type, and color

Football deaths from heat injury have occurred with air temperature below 75°F (23.9°C) but with relative humidity above 95%. *Prevention remains the most effective way to control heat-stress injuries.* Most importantly, acclimatization minimizes the likelihood of heat injury. Another consideration requires evaluating the environment for its potential thermal challenge using the wet bulb-globe temperature (WB-GT) index. This index of environmental heat stress developed by the military provides important information to the National Collegiate Athletic Association to establish thresholds for increased risk of heat injury and physical performance decrements. The WB-GT index depends on ambient temperature, relative humidity, and radiant heat as related in the following equation:

$$\text{WB-GT} = (0.1 \times \text{DBT}) + (0.7 \times \text{WBT}) + (0.2 \times \text{GT})$$

where DBT represents the dry bulb temperature

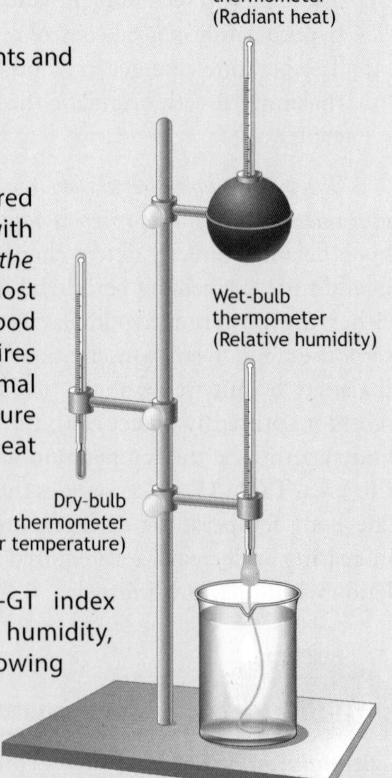

Figure 1 • Apparatus to measure wet bulb-globe temperature (WB-GT).

saline solution (0.2% to 0.4% NaCl). Cooling occurs when sweat reaches the skin and fluid evaporates. The cooled skin then cools the blood shunted from the interior to the surface. Along with heat loss through sweat evaporation, approximately 350 mL of water known as insensible perspiration seeps through the skin each day and evaporates to the environment. Also, 300 mL of water vaporizes daily from respiratory passages' moist mucous membranes. In cold weather, respiratory tract evaporation appears as "foggy breath."

Evaporative Heat Loss at High Ambient Temperatures

Increased ambient temperature reduces the effectiveness of heat loss by conduction, convection, and radiation. As ambient temperature exceeds body temperature, these three mechanisms of thermal transfer actually contribute to heat gain. When this occurs, or when conduction, convection, and radiation cannot adequately dissipate a large metabolic heat load, sweat evaporation and water vaporization from the respiratory tract provide the *only* avenue for heat dissipation. For someone relaxing in a hot, humid environment, the normal 2-L daily fluid requirement doubles or even triples from evaporative fluid loss.

Heat Loss in High Humidity

Three factors impact sweat evaporation from skin:

1. Surface exposed to the environment
2. Temperature and relative humidity of ambient air
3. Convective air currents around the body

(air temperature) recorded by an ordinary mercury thermometer, and WBT equals the wet bulb temperature recorded by a similar thermometer except that a wet wick surrounds the mercury bulb (**Fig. 1**). With high relative humidity, little evaporative cooling occurs from the wetted bulb, so this thermometer's temperature remains similar to the dry bulb. On a dry day, considerable evaporation occurs from the wetted bulb to maximize the difference between the two thermometer readings. A small difference between thermometer readings indicates high relative humidity, whereas a large difference indicates little air moisture and rapid evaporation. GT represents the globe temperature recorded by a thermometer with a black metal sphere enclosing its bulb. The black globe absorbs radiant energy from the surroundings to measure this source of heat gain. Most industrial supply companies sell this relatively inexpensive thermometer. One can also assess ambient heat load from wet bulb thermometer (WBT) because this reading reflects both air temperature and relative humidity.

The American College of Sports Medicine proposes the following recommendations concerning risk for heat injury with continuous physical activity such as endurance running and cycling based on the WB-GT:

- *Very high risk*: Above 82°F (28°C)—postpone race.
- *High risk*: 73°F to 82°F (23°C to 28°C)—heat-sensitive individuals (e.g., obese, low physical fitness, unacclimatized, dehydrated, previous history of heat injury) should not compete.
- *Moderate risk*: 65°F to 73°F (18°C to 23°C)
- *Low risk*: Below 65°F (18°C)

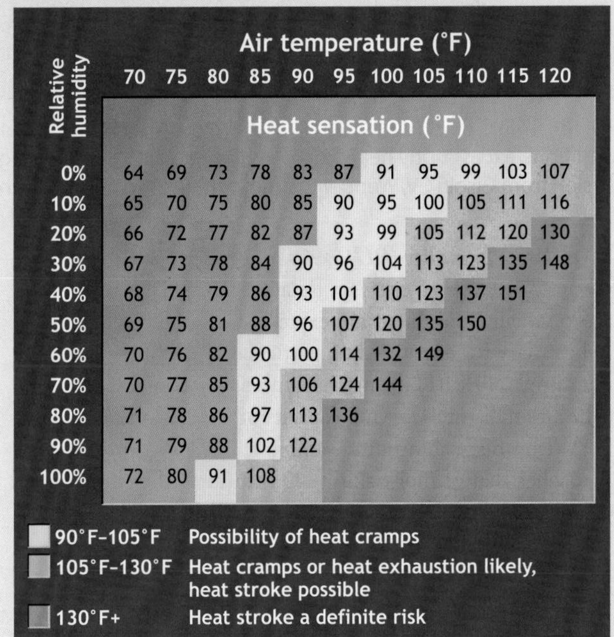

Air temperature (°F) / Heat sensation (°F)

Relative humidity	70	75	80	85	90	95	100	105	110	115	120
0%	64	69	73	78	83	87	91	95	99	103	107
10%	65	70	75	80	85	90	95	100	105	111	116
20%	66	72	77	82	87	93	99	105	112	120	130
30%	67	73	78	84	90	96	104	113	123	135	148
40%	68	74	79	86	93	101	110	123	137	151	
50%	69	75	81	88	96	107	120	135	150		
60%	70	76	82	90	100	114	132	149			
70%	70	77	85	93	106	124	144				
80%	71	78	86	97	113	136					
90%	71	79	88	102	122						
100%	72	80	91	108							

90°F–105°F Possibility of heat cramps
105°F–130°F Heat cramps or heat exhaustion likely, heat stroke possible
130°F+ Heat stroke a definite risk

Figure 2 • The heat-stress index.

Without the WBT, but knowing relative humidity (local meteorologic stations or media reports), the heat-stress index (**Fig. 2**) evaluates the relative heat stress. The index should rely on data close to the actual sport site to eliminate potential error from meteorologic data some distance from the event.

Source: Reproduced with permission from McArdle WD, Katch FI, Katch VL. *Exercise Physiology: Nutrition, Energy, and Human Performance*. 8th Ed. Baltimore: Wolters Kluwer Health, 2015.

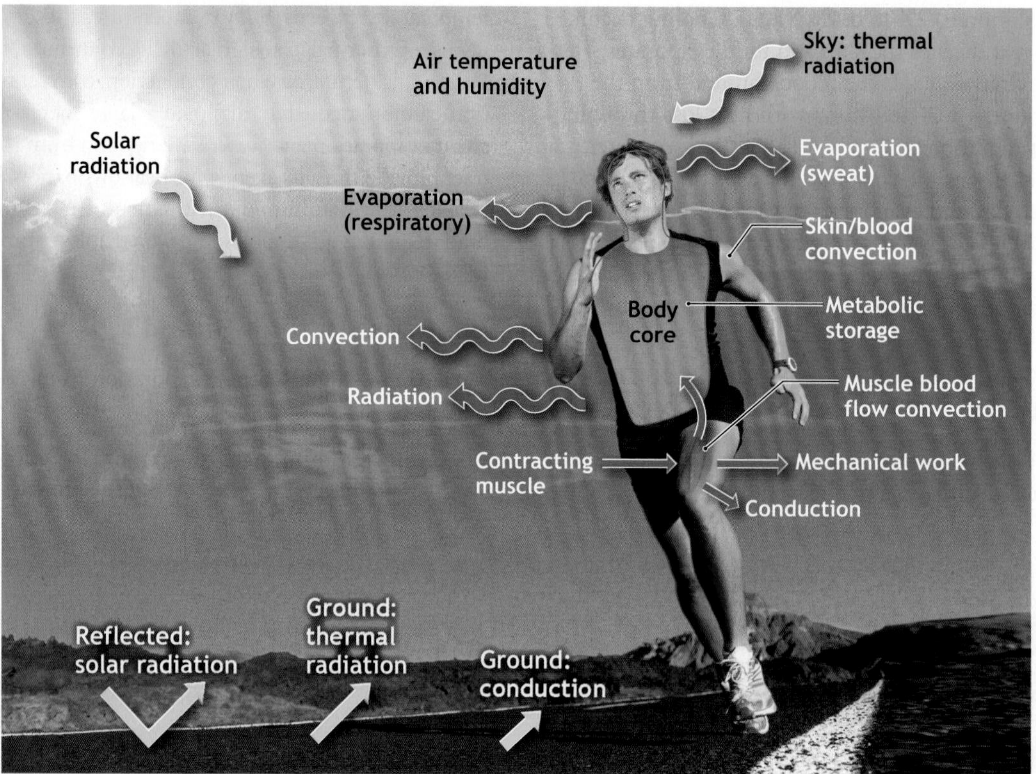

FIGURE 15.2 Heat production within active muscle and its transfer from the core to the skin. Under appropriate environmental conditions, excess body heat dissipates to the environment to regulate core temperature within a narrow range. (Adapted with permission from Gisolfi CV, Wenger CB. Temperature regulation during exercise: old concepts, new ideas. *Exerc Sport Sci Rev* 1984;12:339.)

***Relative humidity (RH)** exerts the greatest effect on the effectiveness of evaporative heat loss.* Relative humidity describes the ratio of water in ambient air, expressed as a percentage, to its total capacity for moisture at a particular ambient temperature. For example, 40% RH means that ambient air contains only 40% of the air's moisture-carrying capacity at a specific temperature.

With high humidity, ambient air's vapor pressure approaches that of moist skin (~40 mm Hg). When this happens, evaporation decreases even though large quantities of sweat bead on the skin and eventually roll off. This response represents a useless water loss that can precipitate dehydration and heat-related disorders. Continually drying the skin with a towel before sweat evaporates also hinders evaporative cooling. *Sweat does not cool the skin; rather, skin cooling occurs when sweat evaporates from the skin surface.* Individuals can tolerate relatively high environmental temperatures when humidity remains low. For this reason, hot, dry desert climates are more thermally "comforting" than cooler but more humid tropical climates.

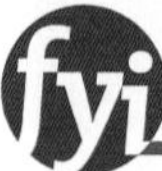

Different Liquids Evaporate at Different Rates

Why does alcohol evaporate from the skin rapidly while water takes a longer time? Evaporation or vaporization continually occurs at a liquid's surface, but the rate of evaporation varies depending largely on five factors:

1. Temperature or average kinetic energy of its molecules, with higher temperature directly increasing molecular movement and evaporation rate.
2. Magnitude of cohesion or intermolecular force of attraction between the liquid's molecular bonds.
3. Heavier-weight molecules evaporate more slowly than lower-weight molecules.
4. Molecules escape from the liquid's surface; the larger the exposed surface, the greater the molecular escape.
5. The evaporation rate of liquids increases with the flow of air currents above its surface.

Ethyl alcohol, known commonly as rubbing alcohol, evaporates nearly five times more rapidly than water because the molecular force of attraction is less than exists between the atoms of water molecules. When molecules with higher kinetic heat energy evaporate from a liquid, lower-kinetic energy, lower-temperature molecules remain, which accounts for the cooling effect on the skin of rapidly evaporating alcohol. Oils, in contrast, evaporate at a more "sluggish" rate than either alcohol or water.

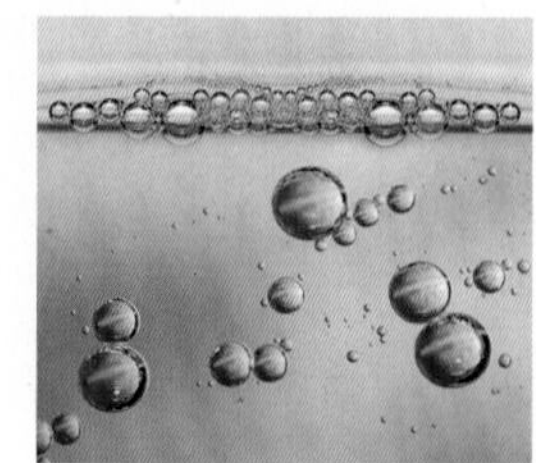

INTEGRATION OF HEAT-DISSIPATING MECHANISMS

Heat dissipation involves integration of three physiologic mechanisms:

1. Circulation
2. Evaporation
3. Hormonal adjustments

Circulation

The circulatory system serves as the "workhorse" for thermal balance. When an individual is at rest in hot weather, heart rate and cardiac output increase, and superficial arterial and venous blood vessels dilate to divert warm blood to the body's cooler outer shell. Peripheral vasodilation causes a flushed or reddened face on a hot day or during vigorous physical activity. With extreme heat stress, 15% to 25% of cardiac output passes through the skin, greatly increasing the peripheral tissues' thermal conductance. This favors radiative heat loss to the environment, mostly from the hands, forehead, forearms, ears, and tibial region.

Evaporation

Sweating begins several seconds after initiation of vigorous activity. After about 30 minutes, it reaches equilibrium directly related to exercise load. A large cutaneous blood flow coupled with evaporative cooling usually produces an effective thermal defense. Cooled peripheral blood then returns to deeper tissues to acquire additional heat on its return to the heart.

Hormonal Adjustments

Heat stress initiates hormonal adjustments to conserve electrolytes and fluid lost in sweat. In response to a thermal challenge, the pituitary gland releases vasopressin (**antidiuretic hormone [ADH]**). *ADH stimulates water resorption from the kidney tubules to form concentrated urine during heat stress.* Concurrently, with even a single bout of physical activity or repeated days of physical activity in hot weather, the adrenal cortex releases the sodium-conserving hormone **aldosterone** to increase the renal tubules' resorption of sodium. Aldosterone also acts on sweat glands to reduce sweat's osmolality to further conserve electrolytes.

EFFECTS OF CLOTHING ON THERMOREGULATION

Clothing insulates the body from its surroundings. It reduces radiant heat gain in a hot environment and retards conductive and convective heat loss in the cold.

Cold Weather Clothing

The mesh of clothing's fibers traps air and warms it to insulate from the cold. This establishes a barrier to heat loss because cloth and air both conduct heat poorly. A thicker zone of trapped air next to the skin provides more effective insulation. Several layers of light clothing or garments lined with animal fur, feathers, or synthetic (man-made) fabrics with numerous layers of trapped air insulate better than a single bulky layer of winter clothing.

The ideal winter garment in cold, dry weather blocks air movement but also allows water vapor from sweating to escape through clothing for subsequent evaporation. Wool or synthetics like polypropylene and such derivative "moisture-wicking" fabrics have excellent insulating and quick-dry properties. Wicking-engineered fabrics rely on capillary action to draw moisture off the skin to the outside of the fabric where it evaporates more readily. When clothing becomes wet, through either external moisture or condensation from sweating, it loses nearly 90% of its insulating properties. *Wet clothing speeds heat transfer from the body because water conducts heat faster than air.*

When working or exercising in cold air, the adequacy of insulation does not usually present a problem; rather, the key factor involves metabolic heat and sweat dissipation through a thick air-clothing barrier. Cross-country skiers alleviate this dilemma by removing layers of clothing as the body warms to maintain core temperature without reliance on evaporative cooling.

Warm Weather Clothing

Dry clothing, no matter how lightweight, *retards* heat exchange more than the same clothing fully wet. Switching from a soaked garment to a dry tennis, basketball, or football uniform in hot weather makes little sense for temperature regulation because evaporative heat loss occurs only when clothing becomes thoroughly wet. A dry uniform simply prolongs the time between evaporative heat loss from sweating and its cooling effects.

Different materials absorb water at different rates. Cottons and linens, for example, readily absorb moisture. In contrast, heavy sweatshirts and rubber or plastic garments produce high relative humidity close to the skin, retarding sweat evaporation and cooling. Wearing loose-fitting clothing permits free convection of air between the skin and environment to promote evaporation from the skin. Moisture-wicking fabrics adhere closely to the skin to optimally transfer heat and moisture from the skin to the environment, particularly during intense hot weather exertion. These fabrics wick moisture away from the skin. They also offer benefits during physical activity in cold environments because dry clothing, in contrast to sweat-drenched clothing, greatly reduces hypothermia risk. Clothing color also plays an important role; dark colors absorb light rays and add to radiant heat gain, whereas lighter color clothing reflects heat rays.

Football Uniforms

Of all athletic uniforms and equipment, football clothing plus pads plus helmet present the greatest barrier to heat dissipation. The 6 or 7 kg of equipment carried over a relatively hot artificial playing surface adds considerably to the body's total metabolic load.

Wearing football gear while exercising produces higher rectal and skin temperatures during physical activity and recovery than similar acivity without equipment. The skin temperature directly beneath the padding averages only 1°C less than rectal temperature. This indicates that subcutaneous blood in these areas cooled only about one fifth as much as blood near the skin surface directly exposed to the environment. Rectal temperature remains elevated in recovery with uniforms, making a rest period of limited value in normalizing thermal status unless the athlete removes the uniform.

SUMMARY

1. Humans tolerate only relatively small variations in internal core temperature.
2. Exposure to heat or cold stress initiates thermoregulatory responses that either generate or conserve heat at low ambient temperatures and dissipate heat at high temperatures.
3. The hypothalamus serves as the "thermostat" to regulate adjustments from skin's peripheral thermal receptors and changes in hypothalamic blood temperature.
4. Heat conservation in cold stress occurs by vascular adjustments that shunt blood from the cooler periphery to the warmer deep tissues of the body's core. If this proves ineffective, shivering increases metabolic heat.
5. Heat stress causes warm blood to divert from the body's core to the shell.
6. Heat loss occurs by radiation, conduction, convection, and evaporation.
7. Evaporation provides the major physiologic defense against overheating at high ambient temperatures and during physical activity.
8. Humid environments dramatically decrease evaporative heat loss effectiveness.
9. Physically active persons are particularly vulnerable to a dangerous state of dehydration and spiraling core temperature.
10. Ideal warm weather clothing includes lightweight, loose-fitting, and light-colored clothes.
11. Even when wearing ideal clothing, heat loss slows until evaporative cooling achieves optimal levels.
12. Several layers of light clothing provide a thick zone of trapped air near the skin for more effective insulation than a single thick layer of clothing.
13. Wearing wet clothing decreases insulation so heat readily escapes from the body.

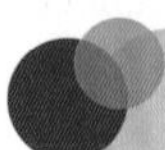

THINK IT THROUGH

1. What mechanism might explain how improved aerobic fitness increases physical activity tolerance in a warm, humid environment?
2. From the standpoint of survival, discuss why the body's physiology is better geared to regulate temperature in heat stress than in cold stress.
3. Describe the ideal personal physical and physiologic characteristics to minimize heat injury risk during physical activity during environmental heat stress.
4. How should a person dress who wishes to play 90 minutes of outdoor paddle tennis at 20°F (26.7°C)?
5. A person walks along a beach on a cloudy day at a constant speed of 4 mph. The wind blows from the west at a steady 12 mph. The westerly portion of the walk feels cooler than the return walk to the east, which feels warmer. Give a possible reason for this discrepancy based on the physical principles of heat gain-heat loss.

PART 2 Physical Activity, the Environment, and Thermoregulation

PHYSICAL ACTIVITY IN THE HEAT

Cardiovascular adjustments and evaporative cooling facilitate metabolic heat dissipation during physical activity, particularly in hot weather. A trade-off occurs because fluid loss in thermoregulation with sweating often creates a relative state of dehydration. Excessive sweating leads to more serious fluid loss that reduces plasma volume. The extreme result ends in circulatory failure, with core temperature increasing to lethal levels.

Circulatory Adjustments

Two competitive cardiovascular demands exist when exercising in hot weather:

1. Oxygen delivery to active muscles must increase to sustain energy metabolism.
2. Peripheral blood flow to skin must increase to transport metabolic heat generated during physical activity for dissipation at the body's surface, with this blood no longer available to active muscles.

Cardiac output remains similar during submaximal effort in hot and cold environments, but the heart's stroke volume becomes smaller when exercising in the heat. In fact, stroke volume decreases in proportion to fluid deficit created during the activity. This produces *higher* heart rates at all submaximal activity levels. Maximal cardiac output and aerobic capacity decrease during exertion in the heat because the compensatory increase in heart rate does not offset the stroke volume decrease.

Vascular Constriction and Dilation

Adequate skin and muscle blood flow during heat stress occurs at the expense of other tissues, which temporarily compromise their blood supply. For example, compensatory constriction of splanchnic vascular bed and renal tissues rapidly counters vasodilation of subcutaneous vessels. Prolonged blood flow reduction to visceral tissues contributes to liver and renal complications often noted with exertional heat stress.

Maintaining Blood Pressure

Arterial blood pressure remains stable during physical activity in heat because visceral vasoconstriction increases total vascular resistance as blood redirects to areas in need. During near-maximal exertion with accompanying dehydration, less blood diverts to peripheral areas for heat dissipation. This reflects the body's attempt to maintain cardiac output despite sweat-induced decreases in plasma volume. *Circulatory regulation and maintenance of muscle blood flow take precedence over temperature regulation, often at the expense of a spiraling core temperature and compromised health risk.*

Core Temperature During Physical Activity

Heat generated by active muscles can increase core temperature to fever levels that would incapacitate a person if they were caused by external heat stress alone. Champion distance runners show no ill effects from rectal temperatures as high as 105.8°F (41°C) recorded at the end of a 3-mile race or other similar endurance events.

Within limits, increased core temperature with physical activity does not reflect heat dissipation failure. To the contrary, this well-regulated response occurs even during cold weather. **Figure 15.3** illustrates the relationship between esophageal (core) temperature and oxygen uptake expressed as a percentage of $\dot{V}O_{2max}$ during physical activity of increasing severity for men and women of varying fitness levels. Core temperature increases in proportion to intensity of effort. *More than likely, a modest core temperature increase reflects favorable internal adjustments that create an optimal thermal environment for physiologic and metabolic functions.*

A CLOSER LOOK

Recognizing and Treating Signs and Symptoms of Heat-Related Disorders

Human heat dissipation occurs by one of two mechanisms:

1. Redistribution of blood from deeper tissues to the periphery
2. Activation of the cooling mechanism from evaporation of sweat from the skin's surface and respiratory passages

What Happens During Heat Stress?

During heat stress at rest, cardiac output increases, vasoconstriction and vasodilation move central blood volume toward the skin, and thousands of previously dormant capillaries threading through the upper skin layer open to accommodate blood flow. Conduction of heat away from warm blood at the skin's cooled surface occurs without undue strain on the body's heat-dissipating functions. In contrast, heat production during physical activity often strains heat-dissipating mechanisms, especially in high ambient temperature and high humidity.

Signs and Symptoms of Heat-Related Disorders

Each year in the United States, extreme heat causes on average 658 deaths—more than tornadoes (**http://cdc.gov/media/releases/2013/p0606-extreme-heat.html**). About half of the fatalities are men and women age 65 years and older. If the normal signs of heat stress—thirst, tiredness, grogginess, and visual disturbances—go unheeded, cardiovascular compensation begins to fail. This initiates a cascade of disabling complications collectively termed **heat illness**.

Heat cramps, **heat syncope**, **heat exhaustion**, and **heat stroke** constitute the major heat illnesses in order of increasing severity. No clear-cut demarcation exists among these maladies because symptoms often overlap. When symptoms of serious heat illness occur, immediate action must include reducing heat stress and rehydrating the person until medical help arrives. The table lists the causes, signs, and symptoms and preventive methods for the four categories of heat illness.

Heat Illness: Causes, Signs and Symptoms, and Prevention

Condition	Causes	Signs and Symptoms	Prevention
Heat cramps	Intense, prolonged activity in the heat	Tightening, cramps, involuntary spasms of active muscles; low serum Na^+	Cease activity; rehydrate
Heat syncope	Peripheral vasodilatation and pooling of venous blood; hypotension; hypohydration	Light-headedness; syncope, mostly in upright position during rest or activity; pallor; high rectal temperature	Ensure acclimatization and fluid replenishment; reduce exertion on hot days; avoid standing
Heat exhaustion	Cumulative negative water balance	Exhaustion; hypohydration, flushed skin; reduced sweating in extreme dehydration syncope, high rectal temperature	Proper hydration before activity and adequate replenishment during activity ensure acclimatization
Heat stroke	Extreme hyperthermia leads to thermoregulatory failure; aggravated by dehydration	Acute medical emergency; includes hyperpyrexia (rectal temperature >105.8°F, 41°C); lack of sweating and neurologic deficit (disorientation, twitching, seizures, coma)	Ensure acclimatization; identify and exclude individuals at risk; adapt activities to climatic constraints

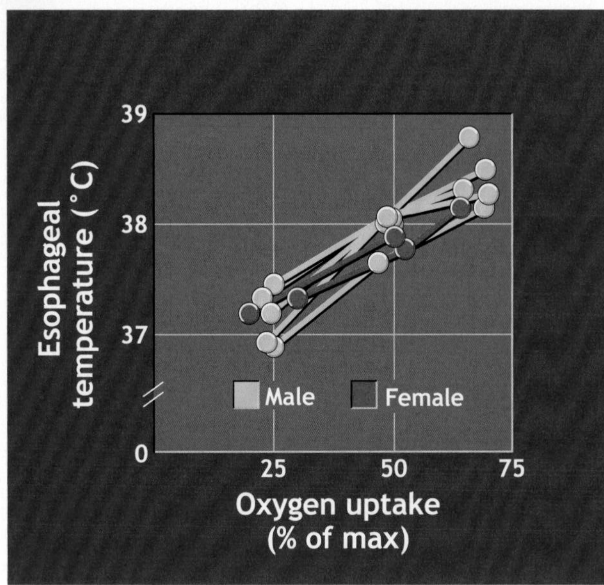

FIGURE 15.3 Relationship between esophageal temperature and oxygen uptake as a percentage of $\dot{V}O_{2max}$. (Adapted with permission from McArdle WD, Katch FI, Katch VL. *Exercise Physiology: Nutrition, Energy, and Human Performance*. 8th Ed. Baltimore: Wolters Kluwer Health, 2015; data from Saltin B, Hermansen L. Esophageal, rectal, and muscle temperature during exercise. *J Appl Physiol* 1966;21:1757.)

Water Loss in the Heat: Dehydration

Dehydration induced by 2 to 3 hours of intense physical effort in the heat often reaches levels that impede heat dissipation and severely compromise cardiovascular function and performance capacity. **Figure 15.4** shows average water loss per hour from sweating at various air temperatures for a typical adult during rest and light and moderate physical activity.

 See the animation "Water Balance" on **http://thePoint.lww.com/MKKESS5e** for an overview.

Magnitude of Fluid Loss in Physical Activity

For an acclimatized person, sweat loss peaks at about 3 L · h^{-1} during intense physical effort in the heat and averages nearly 12 L (26.4 lb) on a daily basis. Intense sweating for several hours can induce sweat gland fatigue and impair core temperature regulation. Elite marathon runners frequently sweat in excess of 5 L of fluid during competition; this represents 6% to 10% of body mass. For slower paced marathons or ultramarathons, the average fluid loss rarely exceeds 500 mL · h^{-1}. For more intense effort even in a temperate climate, soccer players lose approximately 2 L of sweat during a 90-minute game played at about 50°F (10°C).

Hot, humid environments impede the effectiveness of evaporative cooling from high ambient air vapor pressure, with such environments promoting large fluid losses. **Figure 15.5** illustrates the linear relationship between sweat rate during rest and physical activity and the air's moisture content expressed as wet bulb temperature (see A Closer Look: "Assessing Heat Quality of the Environment: How Hot is Too Hot?")

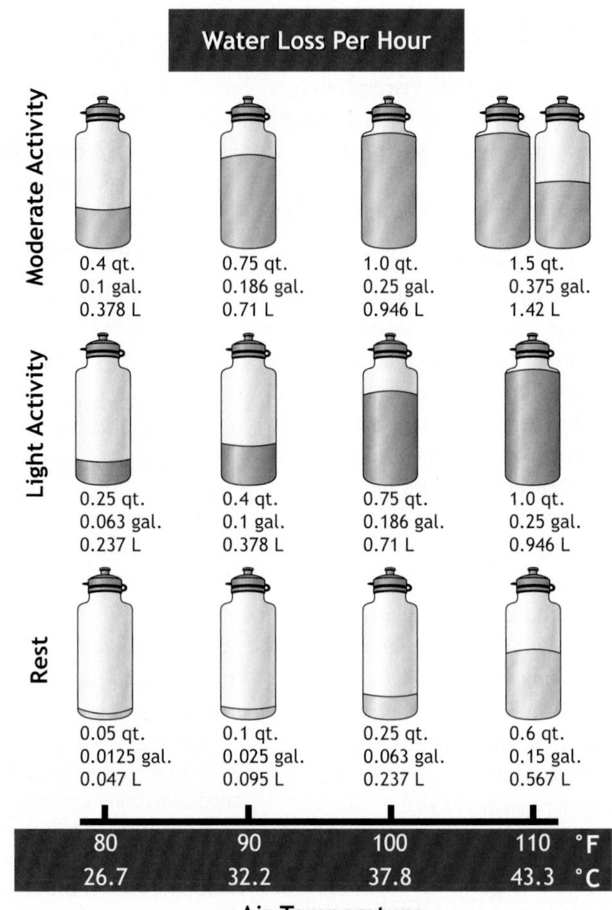

FIGURE 15.4 Average water loss per hour for a typical adult caused by sweating at various air temperatures during rest and light and moderate physical activity.

Ironically, excessive sweat output in high humidity contributes little to cooling because minimal evaporation takes place. In this regard, clothing that retards rapid evaporation of sweat creates an extremely humid microclimate at the skin's surface that promotes dehydration and overheating.

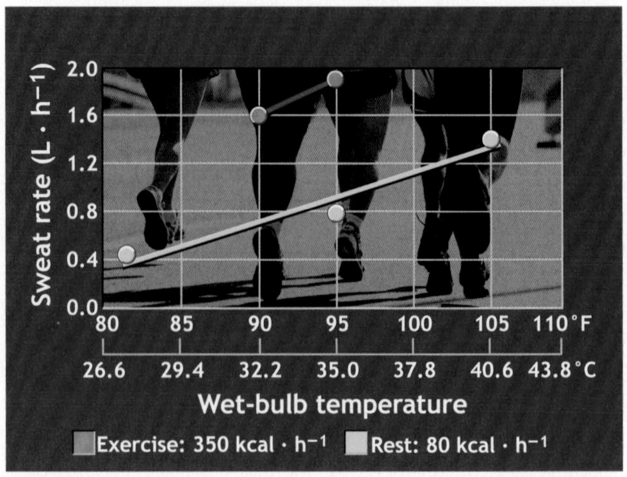

FIGURE 15.5 Effect of humidity (wet bulb temperature) on sweat rate during rest and exercise in the heat. Ambient temperature (dry bulb) equaled 110°F (43.3°C). (Data from Iampietro PF. Exercise in hot environments. In: Shephard RJ, ed. *Frontiers of Fitness*. Springfield: Charles C. Thomas, 1971.)

Consequences of Dehydration

Any degree of dehydration can impair physiologic function and thermoregulation. When plasma volume decreases as dehydration progresses, peripheral blood flow and sweating rate also decrease to make the body's control of thermoregulation progressively more difficult. Compared with normal hydration, premature performance fatigue can occur from reduced plasma volume that increases heart rate, perception of effort, and core temperature. A fluid loss equivalent to only 1% of body mass increases rectal temperature compared with the same physical activity performed fully hydrated. Dehydration equivalent to 5% of body mass increases rectal temperature and heart rate while decreasing sweating rate, $\dot{V}O_{2max}$, and physical activity capacity compared with a normal hydrated condition.

Blood plasma supplies most of the water lost through sweating; thus, maintaining cardiac output becomes problematic as sweat loss progresses. Loss of plasma volume produces two effects:

1. Initiates increases in systemic vascular resistance to maintain blood pressure
2. Reduces skin blood flow, which thwarts a major avenue for heat dissipation

Dehydration reduces circulatory and temperature-regulating capacity to meet the metabolic and thermoregulatory demands of physical activity.

Seven factors affect sweat-loss dehydration:

1. Activity intensity
2. Activity duration
3. Environmental temperature
4. Solar load
5. Wind speed
6. Relative humidity
7. Clothing ensemble

Table 15.2 shows theoretical water requirements at different ambient temperatures and relative humidities with and without a solar load. A 100°F (37.8°C) ambient air temperature increases the resting water requirement by 50% to 60%. Adding physical activity and radiant heat increases the requirement even more. Eight hours of strenuous outdoor physical effort at temperatures of 96°F (35°C) or higher at a relative humidity ≥20% could increase total fluid requirements to 15 L. Replacing this much fluid requires drinking water at regular intervals throughout the day.

fyi Impact of Weather on Running Performance

Marathon performance decreases progressively as wet bulb–globe temperature (WB-GT) increases. The accompanying figure illustrates the slowing of marathon running performance of men and women as the WB-GT increased from 50°F to 77°F (10°C to 25°C), with performance more negatively affected for slower runners.

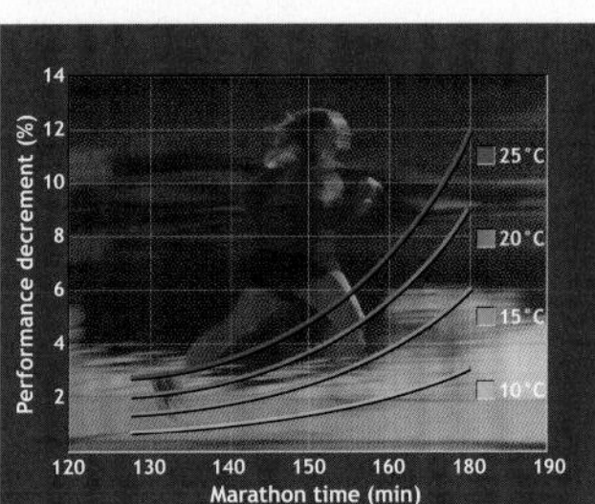

Source: From Ely MR, et al. Impact of weather on marathon running performance. *Med Sci Sports Exerc* 2007;39:487.

Fluid Loss in Winter Environments

Dehydration becomes a serious risk during cold weather physical activity. For example, colder air contains less moisture than air at a warmer temperature, particularly at higher altitudes. Fluid volume loss increases from the respiratory passages as incoming cold, dry air fully humidifies and warms to body temperature, with about 1 L of fluid lost daily. In addition, cold stress increases urine production, which also adds to body fluid loss. Ironically, many people overdress for outdoor winter activities. Sweating begins as activity continues because body heat production exceeds heat loss. This discrepancy can magnify if individuals consider it unimportant to consume fluids before, during, and following strenuous cold weather physical activity.

Diuretic Use

Athletes who take diuretics to rapidly lose body water and body weight reduce their plasma volume, negatively impacting

TABLE 15.2 Water Requirements ($L \cdot H^{-1}$) for Rest and Varying Intensities of Work in the Heat: Indoors and Outdoors at Diverse Temperatures and Relative Humidity

Air Temp (°F) and RH	Indoors (No Solar Load)				Outdoors (Clear Sky)			
	Rest	Light	Medium	Heavy	Rest	Light	Medium	Heavy
85 @ 50%	0.2	0.5	1.0	1.5	0.5	0.9	1.3	1.8
96 @ 30%	0.3	0.9	1.3	1.9	0.8	1.2	1.7	2.0
105 @ 30%	0.6	1.0	1.5	2.0	0.9	1.3	1.9	2.0
115 @ 20%	0.8	1.2	1.7	2.0	1.1	1.5	2.0	2.0
120 @ 20%	0.9	1.3	1.9	2.0	1.3	1.7	2.0	2.0

RH, relative humidity.

Source: From Askew EC. Nutrition and performance in hot, cold, and high altitude environments. In: Wolinsky I, ed. *Nutrition in Exercise and Sport.* 3rd Ed. Boca Raton: CRC Press, 1997.

thermoregulation and cardiovascular function. Diuretic drugs also can impair neuromuscular function when comparable fluid loss occurs through physical activity. Individuals who vomit and take laxatives to reduce body mass not only become dehydrated but also lose minerals, which weakens muscles and can impair motor function. Dehydration also can disrupt normal sodium and potassium ion balance across electrochemical gradients, and in the heart, can trigger fatal arrhythmias.

Water Replacement and Rehydration

Adequate fluid replacement in acclimatized humans sustains evaporative cooling. Properly scheduling fluid replacement maintains plasma volume so that circulation and sweating progress optimally. This may be "easier said than done" because some coaches and athletes cling to the misguided notion that water consumption hinders physical performance. When left on their own, athletes often voluntarily replace only about half of the water they lose during vigorous physical activity (<500 mL · h^{-1}).

Chronic dehydration to lose weight becomes a "way of life" for many athletes, from high performance dance specialists who strive to maintain a thin appearance to power athletes who try to "make weight" to compete in a lighter weight category. Coaches and exercise specialists must remain vigilant about each athlete's hydration status and its potential impact on physical performance and safety. *All participants in sports and recreation activities from novice to champion must replenish fluids regularly!*

Periodic application of cold towels to the forehead and abdomen during exertion or taking a cold shower before exercising in a hot environment at best provide only minimal benefits to facilitate heat transfer at the body's surface compared with the same activity without skin wetting. Adequate hydration—and not the often used pouring water over the head or body—affords the most effective defense against heat stress by balancing water loss with water intake. *A well-hydrated athlete always functions at a higher physiologic and performance level than a dehydrated one.*

A CLOSER LOOK

ACSM's Optimal Goals for Fluid Intake When Exercising

How to Optimally Rehydrate for Physical Activity

Pre-activity Hyperhydration

Start the activity euhydrated and with normal plasma electrolyte levels. Ingesting "extra" water (**hyperhydration**) before physical activity in the heat offers some protection because it delays hypohydration, increases sweating during physical activity, and brings about a smaller increase in core temperature.

Acute hyperhydration results from consuming (1) at least 500 mL of water before sleeping the night before exercising in the heat, (2) another 500 mL upon awakening, and (3) 400 to 600 mL (13 to 20 oz) of cold water about 20 minutes before physical activity. This final pre-activity intake provides fluid and increases stomach volume to optimize gastric emptying.

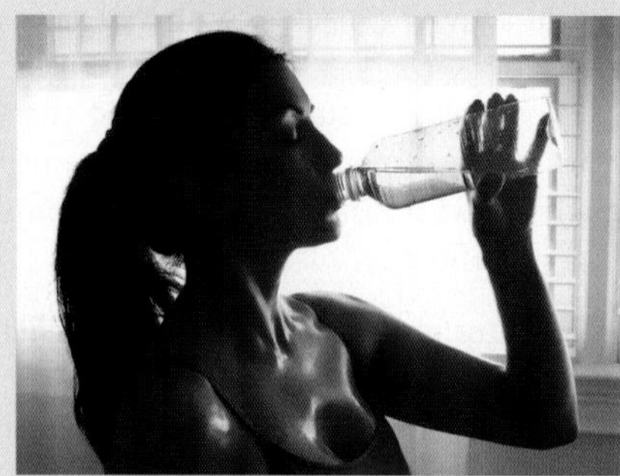

During intense physical activity in the heat, matching fluid loss with fluid intake becomes virtually impossible because only 800 to 1000 mL of fluid empty from the stomach each hour. This rate of stomach emptying does not match a water loss that may average nearly 2000 mL per hour. Consuming beverages containing electrolytes and carbohydrates generally provide benefits over water alone.

Adequacy of Rehydration

Changes in body weight indicate water loss and rehydration adequacy. Voiding small volumes of dark yellow urine with a strong odor also provides a qualitative indication of inadequate hydration. Well-hydrated individuals typically produce copious amounts of urine without a strong smell.

Each pound of weight lost represents 450 mL (15 fluid oz) of dehydration. Periodic water breaks during activity can deter fluid depletion (see American College of Sports Medicine Clarifies Indicators for Fluid Replacement at **www.acsm-msse.org/**). Alcohol-containing beverages generally impede fluid balance restoration, particularly if the rehydration fluid contains 4% or more alcohol content.

Determining the Rate and Quantity of Rehydration

Table 15.3 shows sample computations for determining the quantity and rate of fluid loss during physical activity. The data under headings A to H show the calculations of sweat rate (column H) for a person who exercises for 90 minutes (column G), with a urine volume (in milliliters; column E) measured before postexercise body weight measurement (rows A, B, and C). With a sweat rate of 1152 mL · h^{-1}, this person needs to consume about 1000 mL (32 oz) during each hour at a rate of 250 mL (8.5 oz) at 15-minute intervals to match total fluid loss during activity.

Partitioning rehydration periods into 10- to 15-minute intervals allows one to maintain optimal stomach volume and properly match fluid loss with fluid intake. This dictum applies: provide for unrestricted access to water during

Optimizing Hydration

Before Physical Activity

- Drink approximately 17–20 oz 2–3 h before activity.
- Consume another 7–10 oz after the warm-up (10–15 min before physical activity).

During Physical Activity

- Drink approximately 28–40 oz every hour of physical activity (7–10 oz every 10–15 min).
- Rapidly replace lost fluids (sweat and urine) within 2 h after activity to enhance recovery by drinking 20–24 oz for every pound of body weight lost through sweating.

Electrolyte Replacement

The volume of ingested fluid after physical activity must exceed by 25% to 50% of the activity sweat loss to restore fluid balance because the kidneys continually form urine regardless of hydration status. Unless the beverage contains sufficiently high sodium content, excess fluid intake merely increases urine output without benefit to rehydration. Maintaining a relatively high plasma concentration of sodium by adding sodium to ingested fluid sustains the thirst drive, promotes retention of ingested fluids (less urine output), and more rapidly restores lost plasma volume. The American College of Sports Medicine recommends that sports drinks contain 0.5 to 0.7 g of sodium per liter of fluid consumed during activities lasting more than 1 hour. A beverage that tastes good to the individual also contributes to voluntary rehydration during physical activity and recovery.

With prolonged physical activity in the heat, sweat loss can deplete the body of 13 to 17 g of salt (2.3 to 3.4 g per L of sweat) daily, about 8 g more than typically consumed. With heavy sweating, increasing the intake of potassium-rich citrus fruits and bananas replaces potassium losses. A glass of orange juice or tomato juice replaces almost all the potassium, calcium, and magnesium excreted in 3 L of sweat.

practice and competition. *Athletes in most sports should rehydrate on a regular schedule because the thirst mechanism imprecisely gauges the body's water needs.*

FACTORS AFFECTING HEAT TOLERANCE

Factors that interact with and affect physiologic adjustments and physical activity tolerance during environmental heat stress include acclimatization, training, age, gender, and body composition.

Acclimatization

Light physical activity performed easily in cool weather becomes taxing when attempted on a hot day. The early stages of spring training often prove hazardous for heat injury because thermoregulatory mechanisms have not adjusted to the dual

TABLE 15.3 Computing Magnitude of Sweat Loss and Rate of Sweating During Physical Activity

A: BW before activity	61.7 kg
B: BW after activity	60.3 kg
C: BW difference (A − B)	1400 g
D: Drink volume	420 mL
E: Urine volume output	90 mL[a]
F: Sweat loss (C + D − E)	1730 mL
G: Activity time	90 min (1.5 h)
H: Sweat rate (F ÷ G)	19.2 mL · min^{-1} (1152 ml · h^{-1})[b]

[a]Weight of urine should be subtracted if urine was excreted before postexercise body weight measurement.

[b]1152 mL · h^{-1}; in this example, a person should drink about 1000 mL (32 oz) of fluid during each hour of activity (250 mL [8.5 oz] every 15 min) to remain well hydrated.

Source: Modified from Gatorade Sports Science Institute, Vol. 9, No. 4, 1996.

BW, body weight in kg. Calculations of sweat rate (row H) for a person who exercises for 90 min (row G) and who consumes 420 mL of fluid (row D); BM, body mass; DBM, difference in body mass before and after exercise (row C); urine volume (in milliliter; row E) measured before postexercise body mass measurement.

challenge of physical activity and environmental heat. *Repeated exposure to hot environments combined with physical activity improves physical capacity with less discomfort during heat stress.*

***Heat acclimatization** refers to the physiologic adaptive changes that improve heat tolerance.* **Figure 15.6** illustrates findings from a classic study in the 1960s of thermoregulatory adjustments over a 9-day heat acclimatization period. Two to four hours daily of heat with physical activity produce essentially complete acclimatization after 10 days. In practical terms, the first several activity sessions in a hot environment should be light in intensity and last about 15 to 20 minutes. Thereafter, activity sessions can increase systematically to achieve normal training duration and intensity.

Table 15.4 summarizes the main physiologic adjustments during heat acclimatization. *Optimal acclimatization necessitates adequate hydration.* Proportionately larger quantities of blood transfer to cutaneous vessels as acclimatization progresses, which facilitates heat exchange from the core to the shell. More effective cardiac output distribution maintains blood pressure during physical activity; a lowered threshold or earlier sweating onset complements the circulatory acclimatization. These responses initiate cooling before internal temperature increases substantially. Following 10 days of heat exposure, sweating capacity nearly doubles, and sweat dilutes with fewer electrolytes lost and more even distribution on the skin surface to facilitate greater cooling. For an acclimatized individual, increased sweat loss increases the need to rehydrate during and following physical activity. A heat-acclimatized person performs physical activity with a lower skin and core temperature and heart rate than an unacclimatized individual from adjustments in circulatory function and evaporative cooling. Unfortunately, major benefits of acclimatization to hot environments dissipate within 2 to 3 weeks following return to more temperate climates.

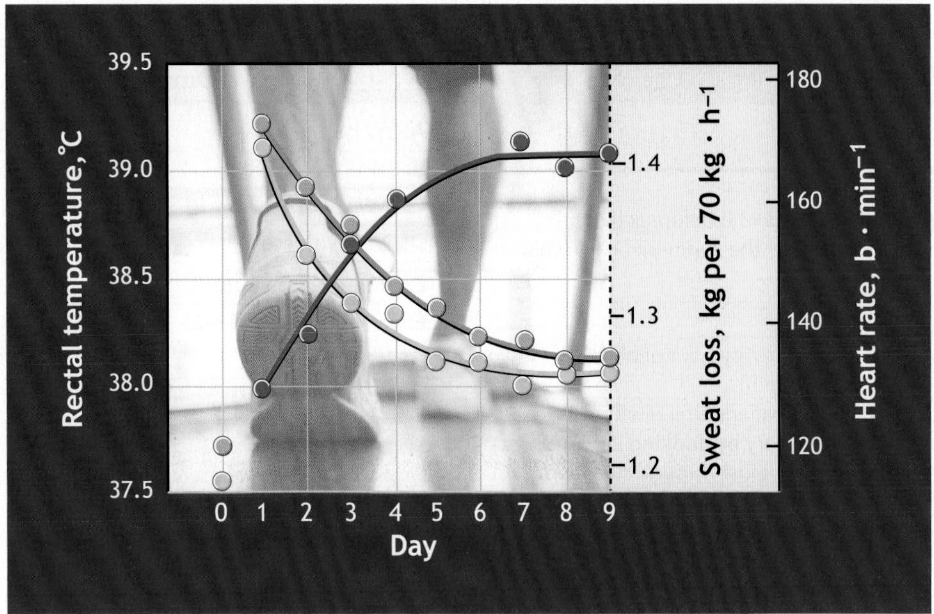

FIGURE 15.6 Average rectal temperature (●), heart rate (●), and sweat loss (●) during 100 minutes of daily heat-exercise exposure for 9 consecutive days. On day 0, the men walked on a treadmill at an intensity of 300 kcal • h^{-1} in a cool climate. Thereafter, they performed the same daily activity in the heat at 48.9°C (26.7°C wet bulb). (Data from Lind AR, Bass DE. Optimal exposure time for development of acclimatization to heat. *Fed Proc* 1963;22:704.)

Exercise Training

The normal exercise-induced "internal" heat stress from strenuous physical activity in a cool environment adjusts peripheral circulation and evaporative cooling in a manner *qualitatively* similar to hot ambient temperature acclimatization. This enables well-conditioned individuals to respond more effectively to severe heat stress than their sedentary counterparts.

Training alone increases sweating response sensitivity and capacity so sweating begins at a lower core temperature. It also produces larger volumes of more dilute sweat. These beneficial responses relate to the increase in plasma volume early in endurance training. Increased plasma volume aids sweat gland function during heat stress and maintains adequate plasma volume to support the demands of physical activity on skin and muscle blood flow. A trained person stores less heat early during exercise training and reaches a thermal steady state and a lower core temperature sooner than an untrained person. The training advantage for thermoregulation occurs *only* if the individual fully hydrates during the activity.

Exercise "heat conditioning" in cool weather proves less effective than acclimatization from similar training in the heat. *Full heat acclimatization does not occur without exposure to environmental heat stress.* Athletes who train and compete in hot weather have a distinct thermoregulatory advantage over those who train in cooler climates but periodically compete in hot weather.

Age

Studies that have considered four factors—body size and composition, aerobic fitness level, hydration status, and degree of acclimatization—show little age-related effects on

TABLE 15.4 Physiologic Adjustments During Heat Acclimatization

Acclimatization Response	Effect
Improved cutaneous blood flow	Transports metabolic heat from deep tissues to the body's shell
Effective distribution of cardiac output	Appropriate circulation to skin and muscles to meet demands of metabolism and thermoregulation; greater stability in blood pressure during physical activity
Lowered threshold for start of sweating	Evaporative cooling begins early in physical activity
More effective distribution of sweat over skin surface	Optimum use of effective surface for evaporative cooling
Increased sweat output	Maximizes evaporative cooling
Lowered salt concentration in sweat	Dilute sweat preserves electrolytes in extracellular fluid.

Source: Reprinted with permission from McArdle WD, Katch FI, Katch VL. *Exercise Physiology: Nutrition, Energy, and Human Performance*. 8th Ed. Baltimore: Wolters Kluwer Health, 2015.

thermoregulatory capacity or acclimatization to heat stress. For example, in comparing young and middle-aged competitive runners, no age-related decrements emerged in thermoregulatory ability during marathon running. Likewise, temperature regulation was not impaired in physically trained 50-year-old men compared with younger men during physical activity in the heat.

On the negative side, older adults do not recover from dehydration as readily as younger counterparts owing to a reduced thirst drive. This places elderly individuals in a chronic state of hypohydration with less than optimal plasma volume that would impede thermoregulatory dynamics. An altered thirst mechanism and shift in the operating point for control of body fluid volume and composition also decrease total blood volume in older individuals.

Existing Age-Related Thermoregulatory Differences

Several age-related factors affect thermoregulatory dynamics despite equivalence between young and older adults in capacity to regulate core temperature during heat stress. Aging delays the onset of sweating and blunts the magnitude of the sweating response due to three factors:

1. Modified sensitivity of thermoreceptors
2. Limited sweat gland output
3. Dehydration-limited sweat output with insufficient fluid replacement

Aging also alters the intrinsic structure and function of the skin and its vasculature to impair mechanisms that mediate cutaneous vasodilation, which attenuates the vasodilation response.

Age-related vascular changes include depressed peripheral sensitivity that impairs cutaneous vasodilation from two factors:

1. Smaller release of vasomotor tone
2. Less active vasodilation when sweating begins

Children

Despite their larger number of heat-activated sweat glands per unit of skin area, prepubescent children show a lower sweating rate and higher core temperature during heat stress than adolescents and adults. Thermoregulatory differences probably persist through puberty without limiting exercise capacity except during extreme environmental heat stress. Sweat composition also differs between children and adults; children show higher sweat concentrations of sodium and chlorine but lower lactate, H^+, and potassium concentrations. Children also take longer to acclimatize to heat than adolescents and young adults. *From a practical and health standpoint, children exposed to environmental heat stress should exercise at a reduced intensity and receive additional time to acclimatize than more mature competitors.*

Gender

Women and men equally tolerate the physiologic and thermal stress of physical activity when matched for fitness and acclimatization levels. Gender differences occur in four thermoregulatory mechanisms:

1. **Sweating**: Women possess more heat-activated sweat glands per unit of skin area than men. Women begin sweating at higher skin and core temperatures; they produce less sweat for a similar heat-exercise load, even when acclimatized comparably to men.
2. **Evaporative versus circulatory cooling:** Women exhibit heat tolerance similar to men of equal aerobic fitness at the same physical activity level despite their lower sweat output. Women rely more on circulatory mechanisms for heat dissipation, whereas men exhibit greater evaporative cooling. Women who sweat less to maintain thermal balance have less chance of experiencing dehydration during physical activity at high ambient temperatures.
3. **Body surface area-to-mass ratio:** Women possess a larger body surface area-to-mass ratio, a favorable dimensional characteristic to dissipate heat. Under identical conditions of heat exposure, women cool at a rate faster than men through a smaller body mass across a relatively large surface area. Compared with adults, children also possess a "geometric" advantage during heat stress because boys and girls have larger surface areas per unit of body mass.
4. **Menstruation:** Initiation of sweating requires a higher core temperature threshold during the menstrual cycle's luteal phase. This change in thermoregulatory sensitivity does not affect physical activity ability or ability perform strenuous physical work in a hot environment.

Body Fat Level

Excess body fat negatively impacts physical performance in hot environments. Fat's specific heat exceeds that of muscle tissue and subsequently insulates the body's shell to retard peripheral heat conduction. Larger overfat persons also possess a smaller body surface area-to-mass ratio for sweat evaporation compared with leaner smaller persons. Excess body fat also directly adds to energy expended in weight-bearing activities. Additional compounding factors include the added weight of sports equipment and intense competition. Fatal heat stroke occurs 3.5 times more frequently in obese young adults than in nonobese counterparts.

COLD WEATHER ACTIVITY

Human exposure to extreme cold produces considerable physiologic and psychological challenges. Cold ranks high among the differing terrestrial environmental stressors for its potentially lethal consequences. Core temperature regulation during cold stress becomes further compromised during these five circumstances:

1. Chronic exertional fatigue
2. Sleep loss
3. Inadequate nourishment
4. Reduced tissue insulation
5. Depressed shivering heat production

Table 15.5 presents the physiologic changes associated with hypothermia that range from mild to severe.

TABLE 15.5 Core Temperature and Associated Psychological Changes That Occur as Core Temperature Falls; Individuals Respond Differently at Each Level of Core Temperature

Stage	Core Temperature		Physiological Changes
	°F	°C	
Normothermia	98.6	37.0	
Mild hypothermia	95.0	35.0	Maximal shivering, increased blood pressure
	93.2	34.0	Amnesia; dysarthria; poor judgment; behavior change
	91.4	33.0	Ataxia; apathy
Moderate hypothermia	89.6	32.0	Stupor
	87.8	31.0	Shivering ceases; pupils dilate
	85.2	30.0	Cardiac arrhythmias; decreased cardiac output
	85.2	29.0	Unconsciousness
Severe hypothermia	82.4	28.0	Ventricular fibrillation likely; hypoventilation
	80.6	27.0	Loss of reflexes and voluntary motion
	78.8	26.0	Acid-base disturbances; no response to pain
	77.0	25.0	Reduced cerebral blood flow
	75.2	24.0	Hypotension; bradycardia; pulmonary edema
	73.4	23.0	No corneal reflexes; areflexia
	66.2	19.0	Electroencephalographic silence
	64.4	18.0	Asystole
	59.2	15.2	Lowest infant survival from accidental hypothermia
	56.7	13.7	Lowest adult survival from accidental hypothermia

Source: From American College of Sports Medicine Position Stand. Prevention of cold injuries during exercise. *Med Sci Sports Exerc* 2007;38:2012.

Water represents an excellent medium to study physiologic adjustment to cold. The body loses heat about two to four times faster in cool water compared with air at the same temperature. Metabolic heat generated by muscular activity contributes to thermoregulation during cold stress. Shivering frequently occurs when people remain inactive in a pool or ocean environment because of the large conductive heat loss. Swimming at a relatively slow submaximal pace in 64°F (18°C) water requires about 500 mL more oxygen each minute than similar swimming in 79°F (26°C) water. The extra oxygen directly relates to the added energy cost of shivering as the body attempts to combat heat loss. At this point, core temperature declines because additional metabolic heat from shivering and physical activity cannot counter the large thermal drain.

In 1998, in one of the most amazing solo Transatlantic endurance ocean swimming feats without a kickboard, French-born ultraendurance swimmer Benoit Lecomte swam 6 to 8 hours a day for 2-hour intervals in 40°F to 50°F water and relentless waves for 3736 nautical miles, crossing the Atlantic ocean from Hyannis (Cape Cod), MA, to Quiberon, France, 73 days later (**http://news.bbc.co.uk/2/hi/europe/180273.stm**)!

Individual differences in body fat content exert a considerable effect on physiologic function in a cold environment during rest and exertion. Successful ocean swimmers have more subcutaneous fat than other endurance athletes. When these individuals swim in cold water, their additional fat greatly increases insulations' effectiveness because peripheral blood moves centrally to the body's core in cold water. They can swim for many hours in cold ocean waters with almost no decrease in core temperature compared with leaner swimmers who cannot counter the heat drain to the water.

Acclimatization to Cold

Humans adapt more successfully to chronic heat exposure than regular cold exposure. Avoiding the cold or minimizing its effects represents the basic response of Eskimos and those who inhabit Siberia and Greenland. The clothing of these cold-weather inhabitants provides a near-tropical microclimate.

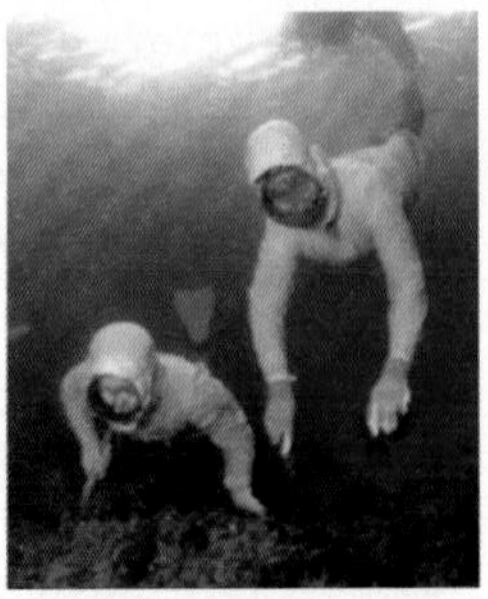

Some indication of cold adaptation comes from studies of the Ama (*AmaSan*), the women breathhold divers of Korea and southern Japan who tolerate daily prolonged cold exposure while diving for shellfish, seaweed, and other food in 50°F (10°C) water. In addition to an apparent psychological toughness (they dive throughout pregnancy), a 25% increase in resting metabolism contributes to their cold tolerance. Interestingly, Ama divers possess body fat levels similar to nondiving counterparts.

thePoint® Appendix SR-6: Additional Video Links, provides a source for a video of the Ama.

A type of general cold adaptation occurs after prolonged cold air exposure. Increased heat production does not accompany body heat loss, and individuals regulate at a lower core temperature in the cold, including improved ability to sleep in the cold. Some peripheral adaptations also reflect a form of acclimation with severe localized cold stress. Repeated cold exposure of the hands or feet brings about blood flow increases through these areas, as occurs in individuals who handle nets and fish in the cold. Such local adaptations facilitate regional heat loss because they provide a form of self-defense. Vigorous circulation in exposed areas defends against tissue damage from localized hypothermia known as *congelation* or injury or destruction of skin and underlying tissues, of which **frostbite** serves as an excellent example. This serious tissue injury occurs in body parts farthest from the heart (fingers, toes, nose, ears) and areas with larger exposed areas.

EVALUATING ENVIRONMENTAL COLD STRESS

Heightened participation in outdoor winter activities increases cold injuries from overexposure. Pronounced peripheral vasoconstriction during severe cold exposure causes skin temperature in the extremities to decline to dangerous levels. *Early warning signs of cold injury include tingling and numbness in the fingers and toes or a burning sensation in the nose and ears.* Disregarding signs of overexposure leads to frostbite (see next page).

Windchill Temperature Index

The **windchill temperature index** presented in **Figure 15.7** has been used by the National Weather Service (**www.nws.noaa.gov**) since 1973; it was modified in 2001. Based on

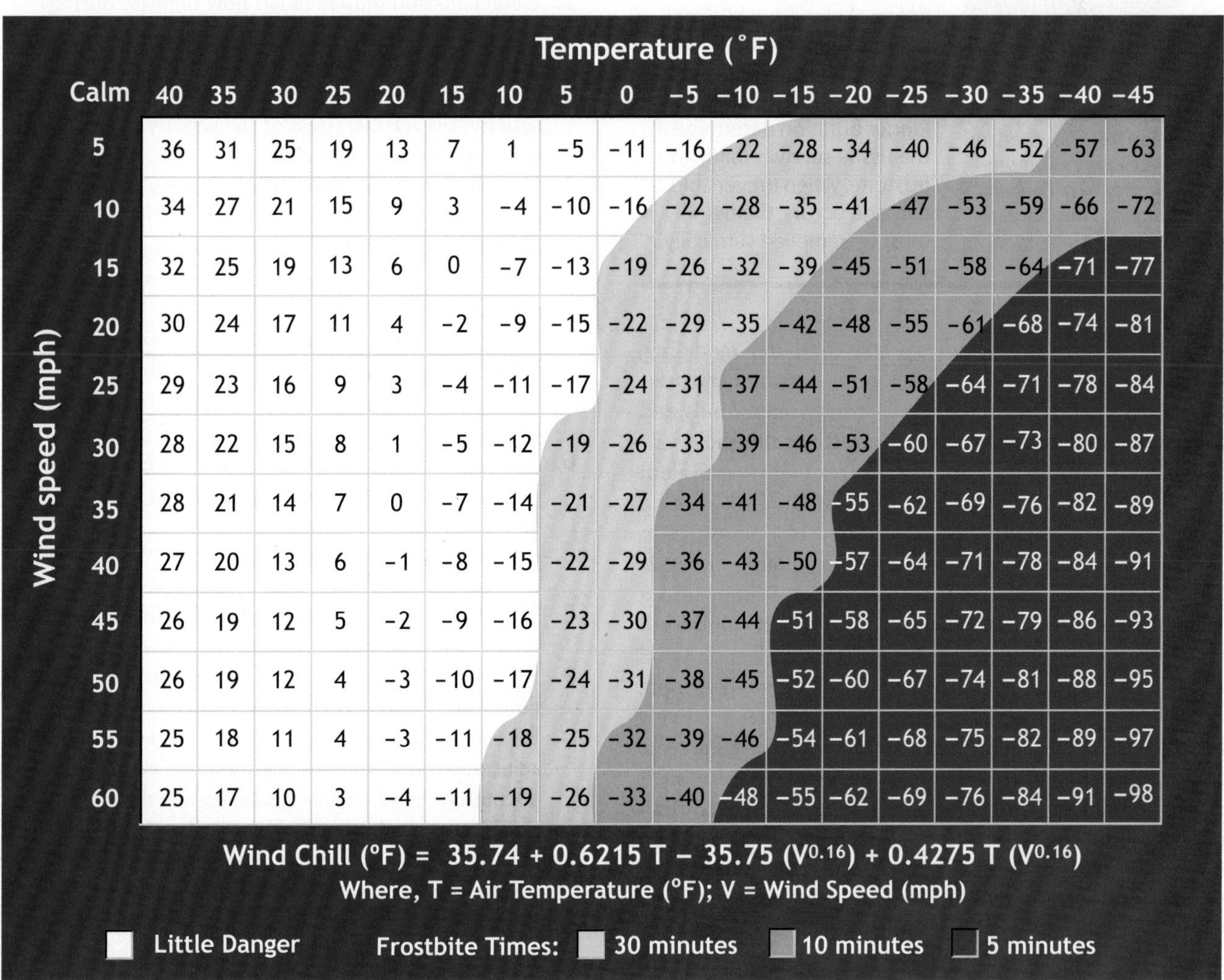

Temperature (°F)

Wind speed (mph) / Calm	40	35	30	25	20	15	10	5	0	−5	−10	−15	−20	−25	−30	−35	−40	−45
5	36	31	25	19	13	7	1	−5	−11	−16	−22	−28	−34	−40	−46	−52	−57	−63
10	34	27	21	15	9	3	−4	−10	−16	−22	−28	−35	−41	−47	−53	−59	−66	−72
15	32	25	19	13	6	0	−7	−13	−19	−26	−32	−39	−45	−51	−58	−64	−71	−77
20	30	24	17	11	4	−2	−9	−15	−22	−29	−35	−42	−48	−55	−61	−68	−74	−81
25	29	23	16	9	3	−4	−11	−17	−24	−31	−37	−44	−51	−58	−64	−71	−78	−84
30	28	22	15	8	1	−5	−12	−19	−26	−33	−39	−46	−53	−60	−67	−73	−80	−87
35	28	21	14	7	0	−7	−14	−21	−27	−34	−41	−48	−55	−62	−69	−76	−82	−89
40	27	20	13	6	−1	−8	−15	−22	−29	−36	−43	−50	−57	−64	−71	−78	−84	−91
45	26	19	12	5	−2	−9	−16	−23	−30	−37	−44	−51	−58	−65	−72	−79	−86	−93
50	26	19	12	4	−3	−10	−17	−24	−31	−38	−45	−52	−60	−67	−74	−81	−88	−95
55	25	18	11	4	−3	−11	−18	−25	−32	−39	−46	−54	−61	−68	−75	−82	−89	−97
60	25	17	10	3	−4	−11	−19	−26	−33	−40	−48	−55	−62	−69	−76	−84	−91	−98

Wind Chill (°F) = $35.74 + 0.6215\,T - 35.75\,(V^{0.16}) + 0.4275\,T\,(V^{0.16})$

Where, T = Air Temperature (°F); V = Wind Speed (mph)

Little Danger Frostbite Times: 30 minutes 10 minutes 5 minutes

FIGURE 15.7 The windchill temperature index—the proper way to evaluate the "coldness" of an environment. The figure shows the windchill temperatures for the relative risk of frostbite and the predicted times to freezing of exposed facial skin. Wet skin exposed to wind cools even faster: if the skin is wet and exposed to wind, the ambient temperature used for the windchill table should be 50°F (10°C) lower than the actual ambient temperature. (Reprinted with permission from American College of Sports Medicine Position Stand. Prevention of cold injuries during exercise. *Med Sci Sports Exerc* 2006;38:2012.)

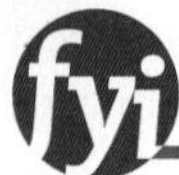

Three Stages of Frostbite

Stage 1: Skin appears yellow or white, often with slight burning sensations. This relatively mild stage can be reversed by gradually warming the affected area.
Stage 2: Disappearance of pain with skin reddening and swelling. Treatment may produce blisters and skin peeling.
Stage 3: Skin becomes waxy and hard, skin dies, and edema can occur from impaired blood flow at stage 3, damage usually becomes permanent, with nerve loss from oxygen deprivation. Frostbitten areas turn discolored—purplish at first and then black. Nerve damage produces a loss of feeling in the frostbitten areas. Without feeling in the damaged area, checking it for cuts and breaks in the skin is vital. Infected open skin can lead to gangrene (tissue necrosis) and need for amputation.

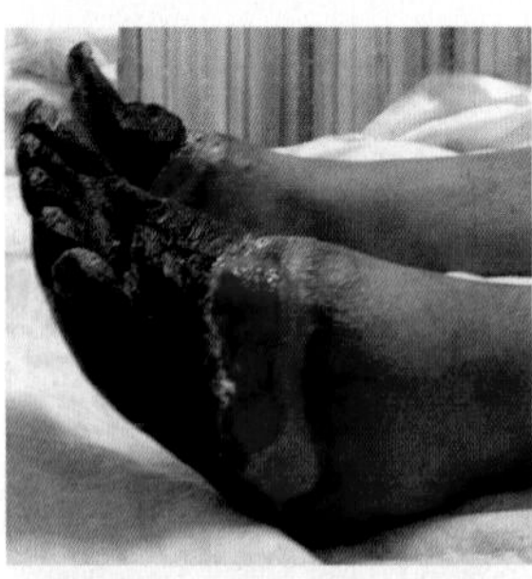

Image reprinted with permission from Southerland J, et al. *McGlamry's Comprehensive Textbook of Foot and Ankle Surgery*. Philadelphia: Wolters Kluwer Health, 2012.

The accompanying image shows deep bilateral frostbite injury to both feet. Rewarming and preventing infection over a 6-week or longer duration determine if the tissue survives following frostbite. When irreversible damage occurs, the tissue must be removed surgically.

advances in science, technology, and computer modeling, the 2001 revised formula offers a more accurate and useful way to understand the dangers from winter winds and freezing temperatures and provides frostbite threshold values. For example, a 30°F ambient air reading is equivalent to 9°F with a wind speed of 25 mph, and a 10°F reading equals −11°F at the same wind velocity. If a person runs, skis, or skates into the wind, the effective cooling increases directly with forward velocity. Running at 8 mph into a 12-mph headwind creates the equivalent of a 20-mph wind speed. Conversely, running at 8 mph with a 12-mph wind at one's back creates a relative wind speed of only 4 mph. The *white zone* in the left of the figure denotes relatively little danger from cold injury for a properly clothed person. In contrast, the *yellow-, orange-, and red-shaded zones* indicate frostbite threshold values; the danger to exposed flesh increases, especially for the ears, nose, and fingers, when moving to the right of the chart. In the *red-shaded zone,* the equivalent windchill temperatures pose serious risk of exposed flesh freezing within minutes.

Respiratory Tract During Cold Weather Activity

Cold ambient air does not damage respiratory passages. Even in extreme cold, incoming air warms to between 80°F (27°C) and 90°F (32°C) as it enters the bronchi. Warming an incoming breath of cold air greatly increases its capacity to hold moisture. Thus, humidification of inspired cold air produces water and heat loss from the respiratory tract, particularly with large ventilatory volumes during intense physical activity. This contributes to dryness of the mouth, a burning sensation in the throat, respiratory passage irritation, and general dehydration. Wearing a scarf or mask-type "baklava" that covers the nose and mouth and traps the water in exhaled air (and warms and moistens the next incoming breath) helps minimize uncomfortable respiratory symptoms.

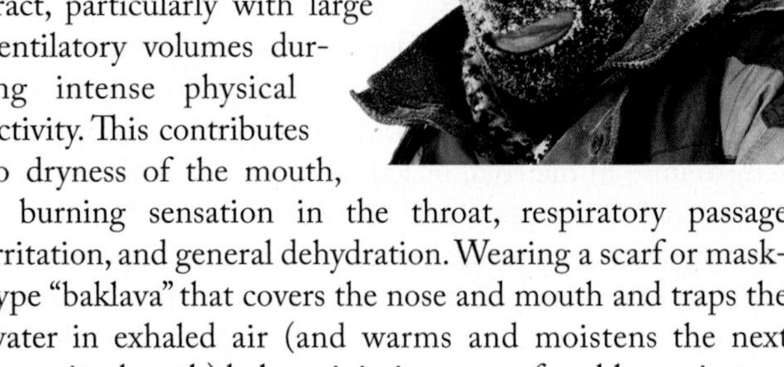

SUMMARY

1. Cutaneous and muscle blood flow increase during physical activity in the heat; other tissues temporally compromise their blood supply.
2. Core temperature normally increases during physical activity; the relative stress of the activity determines the magnitude of increase.
3. Excessive sweating strains fluid reserves and creates a relative state of dehydration.
4. Sweating without fluid replacement decreases plasma volume and causes a precipitous, dangerous increase in core temperature.
5. Physical activity in a hot, humid environment poses a thermoregulatory challenge because the large sweat loss in high humidity contributes little to evaporative cooling.
6. A small degree of dehydration thwarts heat dissipation, compromises cardiovascular function, and diminishes physical capacity.
7. Adequate fluid replacement preserves plasma volume to maintain circulation and sweating at optimal levels.
8. The ideal fluid replacement schedule during physical activity matches fluid intake to fluid loss.
9. Electrolytes added to a rehydration beverage replenish fluid more effectively than plain water.
10. Repeated heat stress initiates thermoregulatory adjustments that improve physical capacity and reduce discomfort on subsequent heat exposure; this redistributes cardiac output while increasing sweating capacity.
11. Full acclimatization generally requires about 10 days of heat exposure.
12. Body size and composition, aerobic fitness, level of hydration, and degree of acclimatization show little age-related decrement in thermoregulatory capacity during moderate heat-exercise stress or ability to acclimatize to heat stress.
13. Women and men show equivalent efficiency in thermoregulation during physical activity, but women sweat less than men at the same core temperature.

14. The heat-stress index uses ambient temperature and relative humidity to evaluate the environment's potential heat challenge to a physically active person.
15. Water conducts heat about 25 times greater than air; thus, immersion in water of only 28°C to 30°C provides considerable cold stress.
16. Subcutaneous fat provides excellent insulation against cold stress; it enhances vasomotor effectiveness to help the body maintain a large percentage of metabolic heat.
17. Fatter individuals exhibit less thermal and cardiovascular strain and greater exercise tolerance during cold exposure than leaner counterparts.
18. The windchill temperature index determines the interacting effects of ambient temperature and wind speed on exposed flesh.
19. Inspired ambient air temperature does not pose a danger to the respiratory tract, and water evaporation from the respiratory passages during cold weather activity magnifies fluid loss.

THINK IT THROUGH

1. What information contributes to predicting an individual's survival time during extreme cold exposure?
2. In deciding on the starting time for an upcoming July marathon in Florida, indicate what past meteorologic information would be most valuable and why.
3. Explain whether significant thermoregulatory benefits result for a marathoner who splashes water over her body during the run.
4. Suppose you have to jog across a desert for 8 hours (sea level, 115°F [46.1°C], 20% relative humidity) while carrying only a backpack. What items would you take and why?

PART 3 Physical Activity at Altitude

Native populations live in permanent settlements in the Andes and Himalayan mountains at altitudes as high as 5486 m (18,000 ft). Prolonged exposure of an unacclimatized person to this altitude can precipitate death from ambient air's subnormal oxygen pressure, termed **hypoxia**, even if the person remains sedentary. The physiologic challenge of even medium altitude becomes apparent during physical activity for newcomers unacclimatized to oxygen's decreased partial pressure.

ALTITUDE STRESS

Figure 15.8 illustrates the barometric pressure, respired gas pressures, and percentage saturation of hemoglobin at various terrestrial elevations. The density of air decreases progressively with ascents above sea level. For example, whereas the barometric pressure at sea level averages 760 mm Hg, at 3048 m, the barometer reads 510 mm Hg; at an elevation of 5486 m, the pressure of a column of air at the earth's surface represents about half of its pressure at sea level. Dry ambient air, whether at sea level or altitude, contains 20.9% oxygen. The Po_2 (density of oxygen molecules) decreases proportionately to the decrease in barometric pressure upon ascending to higher elevations ($Po_2 = 0.209 \times$ barometric pressure). Ambient Po_2 at sea level averages 150 mm Hg but averages only 107 mm Hg at 3048 m. *Reduced Po_2 and accompanying arterial hypoxia precipitate the immediate physiologic adjustments to altitude and longer-term process of acclimatization.*

Figure 15.9 shows changes that occur in oxygen availability reflected by Po_2 in ambient air, alveolar air, and arterial and mixed-venous blood as one ascends from sea level to an altitude of Pikes Peak. The **oxygen transport cascade** refers to the progressive change in the environment's oxygen pressure and in various body tissues.

Oxygen Loading at Altitude

The inherent nature of the oxyhemoglobin dissociation curve discussed in Chapter 9 dictates only a small change in hemoglobin's percentage saturation with decreasing Po_2 until about 3048 m (10,000 ft). At 1981 m (6500 ft), alveolar Po_2 lowers from its sea-level value of 100 to 78 mm Hg, yet hemoglobin still remains 90% saturated with oxygen. This relatively small decrease in oxygen carried by blood has little effect on a resting or mildly active individual but exerts a major effect during more intense endurance performance.

In transitioning from moderate to higher elevations, values for alveolar (arterial) oxygen partial pressure exist on the steep part of the oxyhemoglobin dissociation curve. This reduces hemoglobin oxygenation dramatically and negatively impacts even moderate aerobic activities. An acute exposure to 4300 m (14,107 ft), for example, reduces aerobic capacity 32% compared with the value at sea level. Above 5182 m (17,000 ft), permanent living becomes nearly impossible, and mountain climbing usually relies on using supplemental oxygen equipment. However, acclimatized mountaineers have lived for weeks at 6706 m (22,002 ft) breathing only ambient air. Members of two Swiss expeditions to Mt. Everest remained at the summit for 2 hours without using oxygen equipment; quite an impressive feat considering arterial Po_2 equals 28 mm Hg with a corresponding 58% arterial blood oxygen saturation. An unacclimatized person traversing under these conditions would become unconscious within 30 seconds. Such performances clearly represent an exception, but they do demonstrate the enormous adaptive capability of humans to play, work, and survive without external support at extreme terrestrial elevations.

Not Much Oxygen at the Top

At the summit of Mt. Everest (8848 m; 28,028 ft), ambient air pressure averages 250 mm Hg with a concomitant alveolar oxygen pressure of 25 mm Hg or about 30% of sea-level

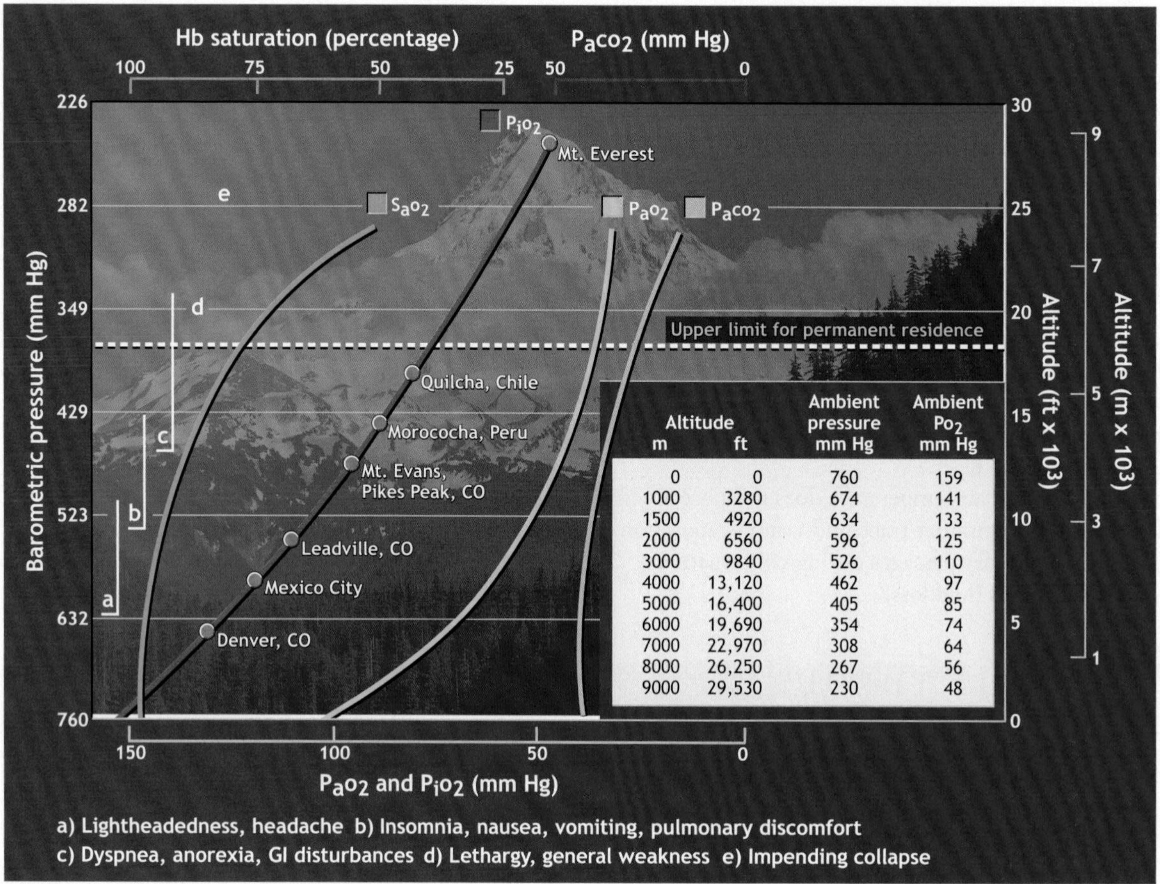

Altitude m	Altitude ft	Ambient pressure mm Hg	Ambient PO_2 mm Hg
0	0	760	159
1000	3280	674	141
1500	4920	634	133
2000	6560	596	125
3000	9840	526	110
4000	13,120	462	97
5000	16,400	405	85
6000	19,690	354	74
7000	22,970	308	64
8000	26,250	267	56
9000	29,530	230	48

FIGURE 15.8 Changes in environmental and physiologic variables with progressive elevations in altitude (P_aO_2, partial pressure of arterial oxygen; P_aCO_2, partial pressure of arterial carbon dioxide; P_iO_2, partial pressure of oxygen in inspired air; S_aO_2, oxygen saturation of hemoglobin).

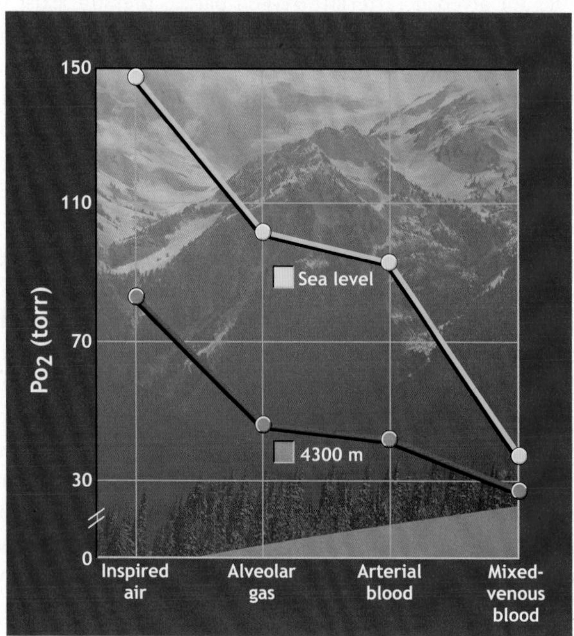

FIGURE 15.9 Oxygen transport cascade from sea level to 4300 m (14,108 ft). (Reprinted with permission from McArdle WD, Katch FI, Katch VL. *Exercise Physiology: Nutrition, Energy, and Human Performance*. 8th Ed. Baltimore: Wolters Kluwer Health, 2015.)

oxygen availability. At this altitude, $\dot{V}O_{2max}$ decreases to the sea-level value of an average 80-year-old man. Concerning the importance of conserving oxygen during a Mt. Everest climb, one experienced mountaineer commented: *"This is a place where people will cut their toothbrush in half to reduce weight carried."*

ACCLIMATIZATION

***Altitude acclimatization** broadly describes the adaptive responses in physiology and metabolism that improve tolerance to altitude hypoxia.* Acclimatization adjustments occur progressively to each higher elevation, and full acclimatization requires time. As a general guideline, it takes about 2 weeks to adapt to 2300 m (7545 ft). Thereafter, each 610-m (2000 ft) altitude increase requires an additional week for full adaptation up to 4572 m (15,000 ft). As summarized in **Table 15.6**, some compensatory responses to altitude occur almost immediately, but others take weeks or even months.

Immediate Adjustments to Altitude Exposure

At elevations above 2300 m (7546 ft), rapid physiologic adjustments compensate for thinner air and reduced alveolar

TABLE 15.6 Immediate and Longer-Term Adjustments to Altitude Hypoxia

System	Immediate	Longer Term
Pulmonary acid-base	Hyperventilation	Hyperventilation
	Body fluids become more alkaline due to reduced CO_2 (H_2CO_3) with hyperventilation	Excretion of base (HCO_3^-) via kidneys with reduced alkaline reserve
Cardiovascular	Increased submaximal heart rate	Submaximal heart rate remains elevated.
	Increased submaximal cardiac output	Submaximal cardiac output falls to or below sea-level values.
	Stroke volume remains the same or lowers slightly	Stroke volume lowers
	Maximum cardiac output remains the same or lowers slightly	Maximum cardiac output lowers
Hematologic		Decreased plasma volume
		Increased hematocrit
		Increased hemoglobin concentration
		Increased total number of RBCs
		Possible increased capillarization of skeletal muscle
Local		Increased RBC 2,3-DPG
		Increased mitochondria
		Increased aerobic enzymes

Source: Reprinted with permission from McArdle WD, Katch FI, Katch VL. *Exercise Physiology: Nutrition, Energy, and Human Performance*. 8th Ed. Baltimore: Wolters Kluwer Health, 2015.

oxygen pressure. The two most important of these responses include:

1. **Hyperventilation triggered by increased respiratory drive:** *Hyperventilation represents the immediate first line of defense to altitude exposure.* Chemoreceptors located in the aortic arch and branching of the carotid arteries in the neck detect reduced arterial Po_2. Chemoreceptor stimulation increases ventilation, raising alveolar oxygen concentration toward the ambient air level. Any increase in alveolar Po_2 with hyperventilation facilitates oxygen loading in the lungs.
2. **Increased cardiac output (blood flow) during rest and submaximal physical activity:** Submaximal cardiac output and heart rate increase 50% above sea-level values in the early stages of altitude acclimatization, but the heart's stroke volume remains essentially unchanged. Sea level and altitude-exercise oxygen uptake remain similar, but increased *submaximal exercise* blood flow at altitude compensates for the reduced arterial oxygen content. In contrast, circulatory adjustments to acute altitude exposure with *maximal exercise* cannot compensate for the lower oxygen content of arterial blood, dramatically decreasing $\dot{V}O_{2max}$ and physical capacity.

Fluid Loss

A depressed thirst sensation at altitude negatively impacts body fluid balance. The cool, dry air in mountainous regions also causes considerable body water to evaporate as air warms and moistens the respiratory passages. Respiratory fluid loss often leads to moderate dehydration and accompanying symptoms of dryness of the lips, mouth, and throat, particularly for physically active people with relatively large daily pulmonary ventilations and exercise-related sweat loss. For such active people, body weight should be monitored frequently. Unlimited fluids should be available to ensure against dehydration.

Longer-Term Adjustments to Altitude Exposure

Hyperventilation and increased submaximal cardiac output provide a rapid, effective countermeasure to an acute altitude challenge. Other *slower-acting* physiologic adjustments commence during a prolonged altitude stay. The three most important longer-term adjustments include:

1. **Acid-base adjustment:** Hyperventilation at altitude favorably increases alveolar oxygen concentration, while carbon dioxide concentration decreases. Ambient air contains essentially no carbon dioxide, so the increased alveolar ventilation at altitude washes out or dilutes carbon dioxide temporarily in transit through the alveoli. This creates a larger than normal gradient for carbon dioxide diffusion from blood into the lungs, reducing arterial carbon dioxide considerably. During prolonged high-altitude exposure, alveolar carbon dioxide pressure can decrease to 10 mm Hg compared with the typical sea-level value of 40 mm Hg. Carbon dioxide loss from

body fluids causes pH to increase as the blood becomes more alkaline. Control of respiratory alkalosis produced by hyperventilation occurs in the kidneys, which slowly excrete base or HCO_3^- through the renal tubules. The establishment of acid-base equilibrium with acclimatization occurs with a loss of alkaline reserve. Altitude does not affect anaerobic metabolic pathways per se; instead, blood's buffering capacity for acids gradually decreases, thereby reducing the critical level for accumulation of the acid metabolite lactic acid.

2. **Hematologic changes:** *An increase in the blood's oxygen-carrying capacity provides the most important long-term altitude adaptation.* Two factors account for this adaptation:
   a. Initial plasma volume decrease
   b. Increase in erythrocytes and hemoglobin synthesis

A rapid decrease in plasma volume increases red blood cell (RBC) concentration during the first few days at altitude. This response causes arterial blood's oxygen *concentration* to increase above values observed on immediate altitude ascent. The reduced arterial Po_2 stimulates a concurrent increase in RBC mass, a response termed **polycythemia**, that directly increases the blood's *capacity* to transport oxygen. Within 15 hours after an individual reaches moderate altitude, the kidneys release the erythrocyte-stimulating hormone **erythropoietin (EPO)**. In the following weeks, RBC production in the marrow of long bones increases and remains elevated. For well-acclimatized mountaineers, oxygen transport capacity for each dL or 100 mL of blood ranges between 25 and 30 mL compared with about 20 mL for lowland residents. For example, the

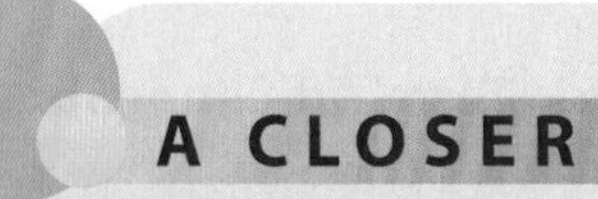

A CLOSER LOOK

Identification and Treatment of Altitude-Related Medical Problems

Newcomers to high altitudes risk various medical problems associated with reduced arterial Po_2. These problems usually remain mild and dissipate within several days, depending on the speed of ascent and degree of exposure. Other medical complications, however, can compromise overall health and safety. Three medical conditions threaten those who ascend to high altitude:

1. *Acute mountain sickness (AMS)*, the most common malady
2. *High-altitude pulmonary edema (HAPE)*, which reverses if the person returns quickly to a lower altitude
3. *High-altitude cerebral edema (HACE)*, a potentially fatal condition if not diagnosed and treated immediately

Acute Mountain Sickness

Most people experience AMS discomfort during the first few days at altitudes of 2500 m (8202 ft) and above. Factors that predispose to AMS include individual susceptibility, rapid rate of ascent, and lack of prealtitude exposure. Nonspecific symptoms include headache, nausea, dizziness, fatigue, insomnia, and peripheral edema. This relatively benign condition, which becomes exacerbated by physical activity in the first few hours of exposure, possibly results from acute reduction in cerebral oxygen saturation. Maintenance of hydration and adequate sleep allowance may be critical performance requirements at altitude. AMS occurs most frequently in those who ascend rapidly to a high altitude without benefiting from gradual and progressive acclimatization to lower altitudes. Symptoms described in **Table 1** usually begin within 4 to 12 hours and dissipate within the first week. Exertion does not exacerbate these symptoms. Headache, the most frequent symptom, probably results from increased cerebral hemodynamics from short-term hyperventilation. Most symptoms become prevalent above 3000 m. Rapid ascent to 4200 m almost guarantees some AMS maladies.

TABLE 1 Altitude-Related Medical Conditions and Symptoms

Condition	Symptoms
Acute mountain sickness (AMS)	Severe headache, fatigue, irritability, nausea, vomiting, loss of appetite, indigestion, flatulence, generalized weakness, constipation, decreased urine output with normal hydration, sleep disturbance
High-altitude pulmonary edema (HAPE)	Debilitating headache and severe fatigue; excessively rapid breathing and heart rate; rales[a]; cough producing pink frothy sputum; bluish skin color (from low blood Po_2); disruption of vision, bladder, and bowel functions; poor reflexes; loss of coordination of trunk muscles; paralysis on one side of the body
High-altitude cerebral edema (HACE)	Staggered gait, dyspnea upon exertion, severe weakness/fatigue, persistent cough with pulmonary infection, pain or pressure in substernal area, confusion, impaired mental processing, drowsiness, ashen skin color, loss of consciousness

For current information about physical/medical problems at altitude: **www.uptodate.com/contents/high-altitude-illness-including-mountain-sickness-beyond-the-basics**.
[a]Excess mucus in the lungs, diagnosed as clicking sounds heard through a stethoscope.

Decreased thirst sensation and severe appetite suppression occur during the early stages, often resulting in a 40% reduction in energy intake and consequent body mass loss. Diets low in salt and high in carbohydrates are well tolerated during the early stay at high altitude. A potential benefit of maintaining carbohydrate reserves through dietary intake lies in the liberation of more energy per unit oxygen with carbohydrate oxidation than with fat (5.0 kcal vs. 4.7 kcal per L of oxygen). Also, high blood lipid levels following a high-fat meal may reduce arterial oxygen saturation. Three other benefits of maintaining a high-carbohydrate diet include:

1. Enhanced altitude tolerance
2. Reduced mountain sickness severity
3. Lessened physical performance decrements during the early stages of altitude exposure

Even moderate physical activity becomes intolerable for persons who suffer AMS effects, although symptoms subside and often disappear as acclimatization progresses. Acclimatizing slowly to moderate altitudes below 3048 m (10,000 ft), followed by a gradual progression to higher elevations (termed *staged ascent*), usually prevents AMS. Climbers should spend several nights at 2500 to 3000 m (8200 to 9800 ft) before going higher, and an extra night should be added for each additional 600 to 900 m (1968 to 2952 ft) climbed. Abrupt increases of more than 600 m in the altitude for sleeping should be avoided at 2500 m (8202 ft) or above ("climb high-sleep low"). If acclimatization proves ineffective, a 300-m (984-ft) descent usually alleviates symptoms; supplemental oxygen and the drug acetazolamide (Diamox) facilitate recovery.

High-Altitude Pulmonary Edema

For unknown reasons, about 2% of sojourners to altitudes above 3000 m (9842 ft) experience HAPE. The symptoms shown in Table 1 usually manifest within 12 to 96 hours following rapid ascent. Major predisposing factors for HAPE include level of altitude, rate of ascent, and individual susceptibility. Changes in pulmonary function test variables after rapid ascent to high altitude fail to predict susceptibility to HAPE.

Fluid accumulates in the brain and lungs in HAPE, a life-threatening condition. At first, symptoms do not seem severe, but the syndrome progresses to pulmonary edema and fluid retention by the kidneys. Chest examination reveals wheezy, raspy sounds known as rales. Even in well-acclimatized individuals, HAPE can develop with severe exertion at elevations above 5486 m (18,000 ft), probably the result of increased pulmonary artery pressure with damage to the blood-gas barrier.

Table 2 lists appropriate methods to avoid and treat HAPE. Treatment to prevent severe disability or even death requires immediate descent to lower altitude on a stretcher or being flown to safety, as physical activity from walking potentiates complications. With proper treatment, symptoms subside within hours, with complete clinical recovery within days. HAPE poses no problem for healthy individuals who journey to and recreate without acclimatization at altitudes below 1676 m (5499 ft).

TABLE 2 Prevention and Treatment of High-Altitude Pulmonary Edema

Prevention

1. Slow ascent for susceptible individuals (average increase in sleeping altitude of 300 to 350 m · d^{-1} [984 to 1148 ft · d^{-1}] above 2500 m [8200 ft])
2. No ascent to higher altitude with symptoms of AMS
3. Descent when AMS symptoms do not improve after a day of rest
4. Under circumstances of high risk: Avoid vigorous activity when not acclimatized
5. Nifedipine: 20 mg slow-release formulation every 6 hours (or 30 to 60 mg sustained-release formulation once daily) for susceptible individuals when slow ascent is impossible

Treatment

1. Descent by at least 1000 m (3280 ft) (primary choice in mountaineering)
2. Supplemental oxygen: 2 to 4 L · min^{-1} (primary choice in areas with medical facilities)
3. When #1 and/or #2 are not possible:
   - Administer 20 mg nifedipine slow-release formulation every 6 h.
   - Use a portable hyperbaric chamber.
   - Descend to low altitude immediately.

High-Altitude Cerebral Edema

HACE, a potentially fatal neurologic syndrome, develops within hours or days in individuals with AMS. HACE occurs in about 1% of persons exposed to altitudes above 2700 m (8858 ft); it involves increased intracranial pressure and if left untreated causes coma and death. The early symptoms, similar to those of AMS and HAPE, progressively worsen as the altitude stay progresses (Table 1). Cerebral edema probably results from cerebral vasodilation and elevations in capillary hydrostatic pressure that moves fluid and protein from the vascular compartment across the blood-brain barrier. An enlarged cerebral fluid volume eventually distorts brain structures, particularly the white matter, which exacerbates symptoms and increases sympathetic nervous system activity. Tissue hypoxia caused by high-altitude exposure also initiates a series of local events that stimulate angiogenesis in brain tissue (new capillary vessel growth). Immediate descent to a lower elevation is mandatory because of the difficulty in adequately diagnosing HACE at high altitude.

Other Conditions

Chronic mountain sickness (CMS), prevalent in a small number of altitude natives, can develop after months and years at altitude. CMS relates to excessive polycythemia, perhaps from a genetically linked variation in the EPO response to hypoxic stress. CMS symptoms include lethargy, weakness, sleep disturbance, bluish skin coloring (cyanosis), and change in mental status. **High-altitude retinal hemorrhage (HARH)** affects virtually all climbers at altitudes above 6700 m (21,982 ft). HARH usually progresses unnoticed, with no specific treatment or means for prevention. Hemorrhage in the macula of the eye—the oval "yellow spot" region in the back of the eyeball close to the optic disc—produces irreversible visual defects. Retinal bleeding probably results from surges in blood pressure with exercise that cause blood vessels in the eye to dilate and rupture from increased cerebral blood flow.

oxygen-carrying capacity of blood for high-altitude residents of Peru averages 28% above sea-level natives. Even with hemoglobin's reduced oxygen saturation at altitude, the actual *quantity* of oxygen in arterial blood of elite mountaineers at altitude nearly equals values of counterparts living at sea-level.

Figure 15.10A illustrates the general trend for increased hemoglobin and hematocrit during altitude acclimatization for eight young women at the University of Missouri in Columbia, MO (altitude 213 m), who lived and worked for 10 weeks at the 4267-m summit of Pikes Peak, CO. Upon reaching Pikes Peak, their RBC concentrations increased rapidly from reduced plasma volume during the first 24 hours. Over the following month, hemoglobin concentration and hematocrit continued to increase and then stabilized thereafter. Two weeks after the women returned to the university, their hemoglobin and hematocrit levels returned to prealtitude values.

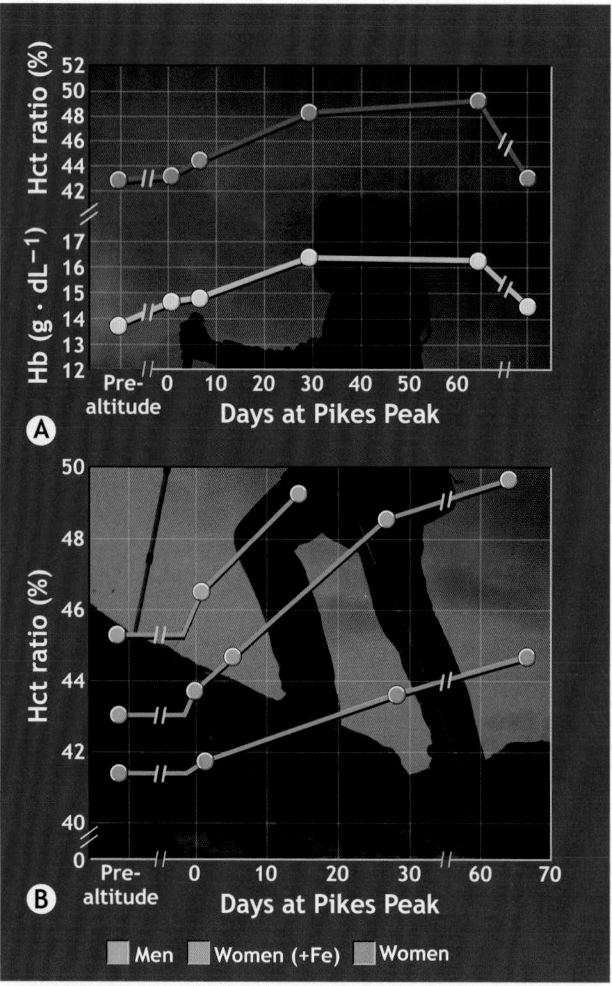

FIGURE 15.10 **A.** Effects of altitude on hemoglobin (Hb; *yellow line*) and hematocrit (Hct; *red line*) levels of eight young women from the University of Missouri (213 m [699 ft]) prior to, during, and 2 weeks after exposure to 4267 m (13,999 ft) at Pikes Peak, Colorado. (Adapted with permission from Hannon JP, et al. Effects of altitude acclimatization on blood composition of women. *J Appl Physiol* 1968;26:540.) **B.** Hematocrit response of young women receiving supplemental iron [+Fe] prior to and during altitude exposure compared with male and female subjects receiving no supplemental iron. (Courtesy of Dr. J. P. Hannon.) (**A** and **B**, reprinted with permission from McArdle WD, Katch FI, Katch VL. *Exercise Physiology: Nutrition, Energy, and Human Performance.* 8th Ed. Baltimore: Wolters Kluwer Health, 2015.)

Figure 15.10B shows that iron supplementation progressively increased prealtitude hematocrit and hemoglobin values. One might anticipate this finding because young women frequently suffer from mild dietary iron insufficiency with depressed iron reserves (see Chapter 2). Comparison of the acclimatization curves for the iron-supplemented women and another group of women not given additional iron showed greater hematocrit increase in the supplemented group. Iron supplementation enhanced hematocrit increases at altitude to a level equivalent to men at the same location. Athletes with borderline iron stores may not respond to acclimatization as effectively as individuals who arrive at altitude with iron reserves adequate to sustain increased erythrocyte production.

3. **Cellular adaptations:** Long-term altitude acclimatization initiates peripheral changes that facilitate aerobic metabolism. Three important adaptive changes occur:
   a. Increased capillary concentration in skeletal muscle, which reduces the distance for oxygen diffusion between blood and tissues
   b. Formation of additional mitochondria and increase in aerobic enzyme concentration to facilitate aerobic energy transfer
   c. Expanded oxygen storage within specific muscle fibers via increased myoglobin, which facilitates intracellular oxygen delivery and utilization, particularly at low tissue Po_2

METABOLIC, PHYSIOLOGIC, AND EXERCISE CAPACITIES AT ALTITUDE

The stress of high altitudes imposes meaningful limitations on exercise capacity and physiologic functions. Even at lower altitudes, the body's acclimation adjustments do not fully compensate for reduced oxygen pressure and diminishing physical performance.

Aerobic Capacity

Figure 15.11A depicts the relationship between $\dot{V}O_{2max}$ decreases (percent of sea-level value) and increasing altitude or simulated exposures reported in civilian and military studies. Small declines in $\dot{V}O_{2max}$ become noticeable at an altitude of 589 m. *Thereafter, arterial desaturation decreases $\dot{V}O_{2max}$ by 7% to 9% per 1000-m altitude increase to 6300 m, where aerobic capacity declines at a more rapid, nonlinear rate.* For example, aerobic capacity at 4000 m averages 75% of the sea-level value. At 7000 m, $\dot{V}O_{2max}$ averages half that at sea level. The $\dot{V}O_{2max}$ of fit men at the summit of Mt. Everest averages the low value of about 1000 mL · min^{-1} (4 METs or about four times the value for oxygen uptake at rest); this corresponds to a maximal power output of only 50 watts on a bicycle ergometer.

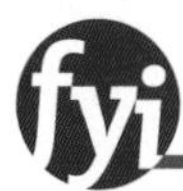

Same Oxygen Cost But a Greater Stress at Altitude

The oxygen cost of submaximal exercise at 100 watts on a bicycle ergometer at sea level and high altitude remains unchanged at about 2.0 L · min^{-1} (roughly 5 kcal · min^{-1}), but the relative strenuousness of effort increases dramatically at altitude. In this example, submaximal exercise representing 50% of sea-level $\dot{V}O_{2max}$ equals 70% of $\dot{V}O_{2max}$ at 4300 m.

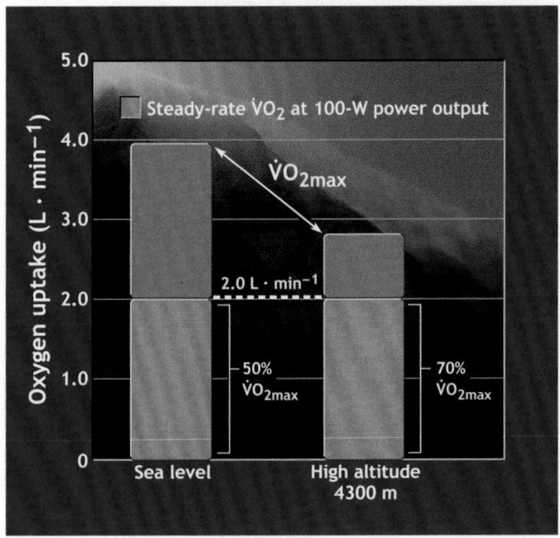

Comparison of oxygen cost and relative strenuousness of submaximal exercise at sea level and high altitude.

Circulatory Factors

Aerobic capacity remains below sea-level values despite several months of acclimatization. Reduced circulatory efficiency in moderate and strenuous activity generally offsets any acclimatization benefits. The immediate altitude response increases submaximal physical activity blood flow; cardiac output decreases in the days that follow and does not improve with longer altitude exposure. A decrease in stroke volume as the altitude stay progresses accounts for diminished cardiac output. At maximal effort, a decrease in maximum cardiac output occurs after about 1 week above 3048 m (10,000 ft) and persists throughout the altitude stay. *The combined effect of decreased maximum heart rate and maximum stroke volume explains the reduced maximum exercise blood flow.*

Difficult to Maintain Body Weight at High Altitude

Prolonged high-altitude exposure reduces lean body mass (muscle fibers atrophy by 20%) and body fat, with the magnitude of weight loss directly related to terrestrial elevation. This loss results from a reduced energy intake at altitude. In addition to depressed appetite and food intake during high-altitude exposure, intestinal absorption efficiency decreases, compounding the difficulty to sustain prealtitude body weight.

Exercise Performance

Figure 15.11B illustrates the generalized trend in performance decrements, primarily for athletes who compete at different altitude exposures. *Altitude exerts no adverse effect on events lasting less than 2 minutes.* The threshold for decrements in longer duration events appears at about 1600 m for events of 2- to 5-minute duration, but only a 600- to 700-m (2000- to 2300-ft) altitude induces poorer performance in events longer than 20 minutes. For the 1- and 3-mile runs, medium altitude (2300 m; 7500 ft) decreases performance by 2% to 13%. This coincides with the 7.2% increase in 2-mile run-times for highly trained middle-distance runners. After 29 days of acclimatization, high-altitude exposure still increases 3-mile runtime compared with sea-level runs. The small improvements in endurance at high altitude during acclimatization probably relate to three factors:

1. Increases in minute pulmonary ventilation (ventilatory acclimatization)
2. Increases in arterial oxygen saturation
3. Blunted lactate response

The Lactate Paradox

On immediate high-altitude ascent, a given submaximal activity load increases blood lactate concentration compared with sea-level values. Greater reliance on anaerobic glycolysis with altitude hypoxia presumably increases lactate accumulation. Surprisingly, after several weeks of hypoxic exposure, the same submaximal and maximal effort with large muscle groups produces *lower* lactate levels. This occurs despite no increases in either $\dot{V}O_{2max}$ or active tissue regional blood flow. A general depression in maximum lactate concentrations becomes apparent in maximal exertion above 4000 m (13,123 ft). A question arises concerning this apparent physiologic contradiction, termed the **lactate paradox**: How is lactate accumulation reduced without a corresponding increase in tissue oxygenation, which does not occur with altitude exposure? In fact, the hypoxemia associated with high altitude should instead promote lactate accumulation and not reduced blood lactate.

Research to resolve the lactate paradox points to reduced epinephrine output during chronic high-altitude exposure. A reduced epinephrine output lowers glucose mobilization from the liver, thus diminishing capacity for lactate formation. Suboptimal intracellular ADP during long-term altitude exposure can inhibit glycolytic pathway activation. Depressed lactate formation during maximal effort may partly reflect an overall diminished central nervous system drive, which would reduce one's capacity for all-out physical effort. Interestingly, lower blood lactate accumulation at high altitude does not relate to decreased buffering capacity with high-altitude acclimatization.

HIGH-ALTITUDE TRAINING AND SEA-LEVEL PERFORMANCE

Altitude acclimatization improves one's capacity to exercise at high altitudes, yet the effect of high-altitude exposure and altitude training on $\dot{V}O_{2max}$ and endurance performance immediately on return to sea level remains equivocal.

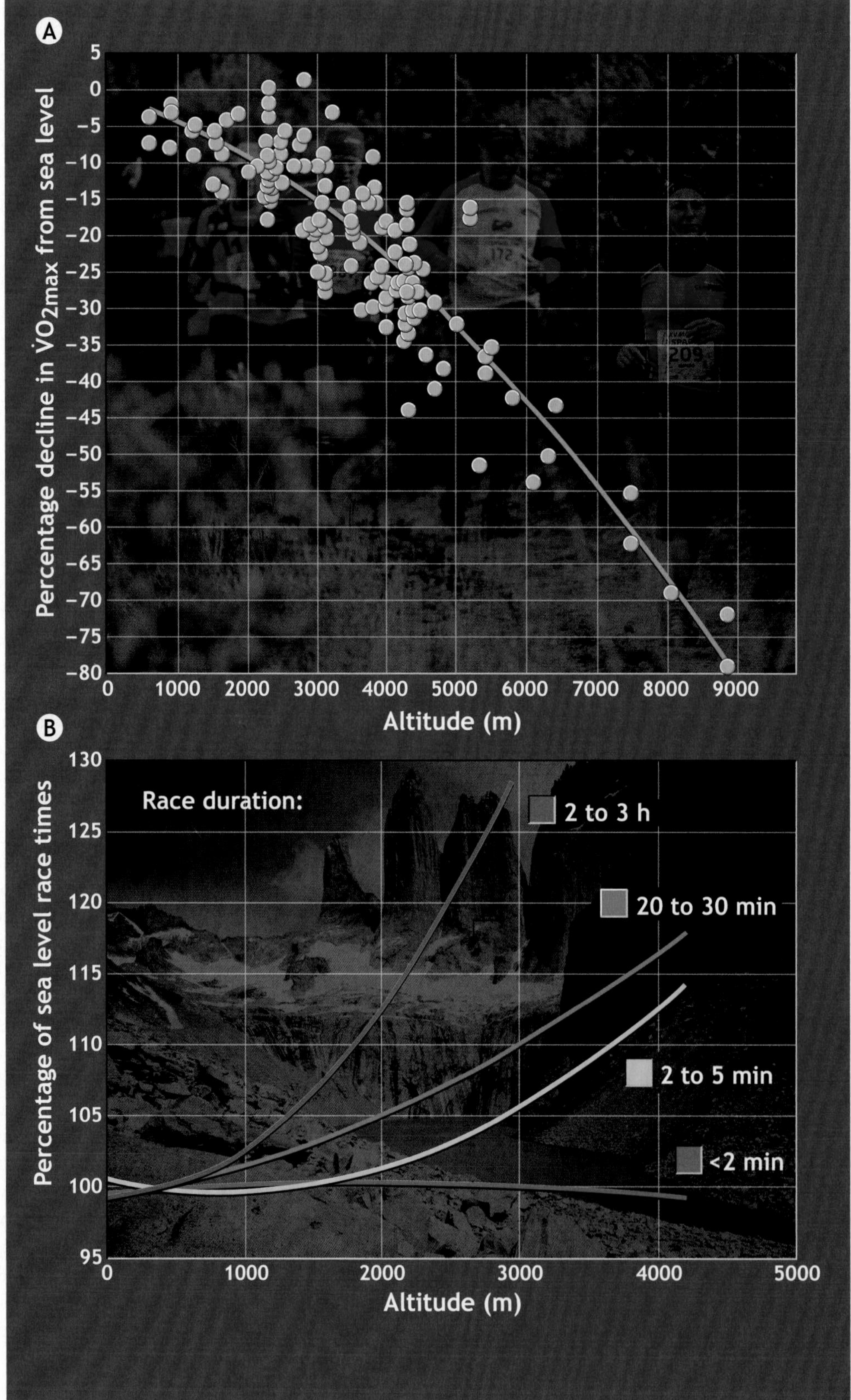

FIGURE 15.11 **A.** Reduction in $\dot{V}O_{2max}$ as a percentage of the sea-level value related to altitude exposure derived from 146 average data points from 67 different civilian and military investigations conducted at altitudes from 580 m (1902 ft) to 8848 m (29,021 ft). "Altitude" represents data from actual terrestrial elevations or simulated elevations with hypoxic chambers or hypoxic gas breathing. The *orange curvilinear line* is a database regression line drawn using the 146 points. **B.** Generalized trend in performance decrements related to altitude exposure for runners and swimmers, primarily during competition. (Adapted with permission from Fulco CS, et al. Maximal and submaximal exercise performance at altitude. *Aviat Space Environ Med* 1998;69:793.)

Altitude adaptations in local circulation and cellular function and compensatory increases in the blood's oxygen-carrying capacity theoretically should enhance sea-level physical performance. Unfortunately, altitude exercise–related research has not adequately evaluated this possibility. Often, poor control exists over subjects' physical activity level, making it difficult to determine whether any improved sea-level $\dot{V}O_{2max}$ or performance score on return from altitude represents a training effect, an altitude effect, or synergism between altitude and training.

$\dot{V}O_{2max}$ on Return to Sea Level

Sea-level aerobic capacity generally does *not* improve after living at high altitude. Compared with prealtitude measures, no change in $\dot{V}O_{2max}$ occurred for young runners on return to sea level after 18 days at 3100 m (10,170 ft). Training in chambers designed to simulate high altitude provided no additional benefit to sea-level performance compared with similar training at sea level. As expected, the high-altitude–trained group showed superior physical performance in the altitude experiments compared with sea-level counterparts.

Some physiologic changes produced during prolonged altitude exposure actually *negate* adaptations that could improve performance upon return to sea level. The residual effects of muscle mass loss and reduced maximum heart rate and stroke volume observed with prolonged high-altitude exposure would not enhance immediate physical performance on return to sea level. Any reduction in maximum cardiac output during a stay at a high altitude offsets benefits derived from the blood's greater oxygen-carrying capacity.

Can Sea-Level Training Be Maintained at High Altitude?

Exposure to 2300 m (7500 ft) and higher makes it nearly impossible for athletes to train at the same intensity as sea level. At 4000 m (13,123 ft), runners only can train at 40% of sea-level $\dot{V}O_{2max}$ compared with 80% of this value when at sea level. This high-altitude–related reduction in absolute training intensity makes it nearly impossible for athletes to maintain peak condition for sea-level competition.

High-Altitude Training Versus Sea-Level Training

To evaluate the effectiveness of training at high altitude, middle-distance runners trained at sea level for 3 weeks at 75% of sea-level $\dot{V}O_{2max}$. Another group of six runners trained an equivalent distance at the same percentage $\dot{V}O_{2max}$ measured at 2300 m. The groups then exchanged training sites and continued 3 weeks of similar training. Initially, 2-mile run times decreased by 7.2% at altitude compared with sea-level times. The times improved about 2.0% for both groups following altitude training, but postaltitude performance on return to sea level remained unchanged compared to prealtitude sea-level runs. The $\dot{V}O_{2max}$ for both groups at altitude decreased initially by about 17% and improved only slightly after 20 training days at high altitude. When the runners returned to sea level, aerobic capacity averaged 2.8% *below* prealtitude sea-level values! Clearly, for these highly conditioned runners, no synergistic effect occurred with relatively intense aerobic training at medium altitude compared with equally severe sea-level training.

Altitude Natives May Respond Differently

For endurance athletes native to moderate altitude, total hemoglobin and blood volume synergistically increase by training and altitude exposure compared to endurance athletes native to sea level. This adaptive response, unique to athletes born and living at altitude (e.g., Kenyan runners, Colombian cyclists, Mexican walkers), may contribute to their extraordinary endurance performance. Longer-term altitude-acclimatized cyclists also show improved aerobic capacity and peak power output during sea-level exercise simulations.

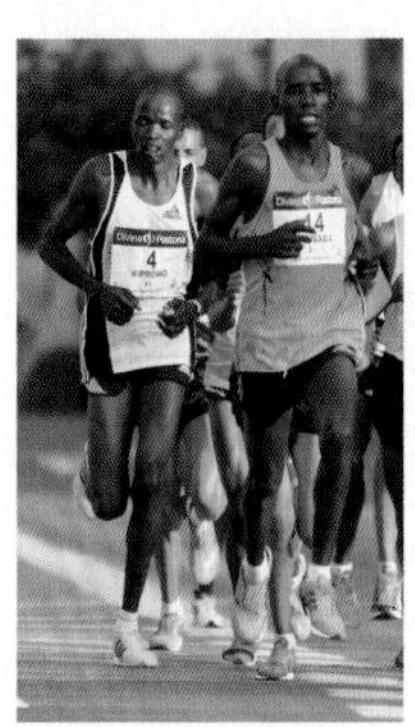

Sources: Brothers MD, et al. GXT responses to altitude-acclimatized cyclists during sea-level simulation. *Med Sci Sports Exerc* 2007;39:1727.

Schmidt W, et al. Blood volume and hemoglobin mass in endurance athletes from moderate altitude. *Med Sci Sports Exerc* 2002;34:1934.

"Live High, Train Low"

Failure to maintain absolute power outputs of sea-level training at high altitude may initiate a detraining effect. For these reasons, elite endurance athletes have resorted to the banned and dangerous practices of blood doping or EPO injections to increase hematocrit and hemoglobin concentration. They undertake these undesirable practices to achieve the benefits of physiologic changes without the inconvenience and negative effects of sojourning to higher altitudes.

Strategies that combine altitude acclimatization and maintenance of sea-level training intensity provide *synergistic benefits* to sea-level endurance performance. Regular training exposure to a near–sea-level environment prevents the reduced maximum stroke volume and cardiac output (i.e., impaired systolic function) typically observed during altitude training. Athletes who lived at 2500 m (8200 ft) but returned regularly to 1250 m (4100 ft) to a **"live high, train low"** strategy showed greater performance increases in the 5000-m (16,400-ft) run than athletes who lived and trained at 2500 m or athletes who lived and trained at sea level. Altitude acclimatization and maintaining sea-level training intensity provide important additive endurance sea-level benefits.

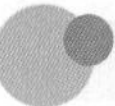

SUMMARY

1. Reduced ambient Po_2 upon high-altitude ascent causes inadequate oxygenation of hemoglobin and produces noticeable performance decrements in aerobic physical activities at 2000 m and higher.
2. Reduced arterial Po_2 and accompanying tissue hypoxia stimulate immediate physiologic responses that improve high-altitude tolerance during rest and physical activity.
3. Longer-term acclimatization involves physiologic adjustments that mitigate intolerance to altitude hypoxia.
4. The three main longest-term acclimatization adjustments involve re-establishing the acid-base balance of body fluids, increased hemoglobin and RBC synthesis, and enhanced local circulation and cellular metabolic functions.
5. Gradations in high-altitude dictates the rate and magnitude of acclimatization. Noticeable improvements occur within several days, but major adjustments require about 2 weeks. Near-full acclimatization to high altitude takes 4 to 6 weeks.
6. For individuals at a simulated altitude that approaches the summit of Mt. Everest, alveolar Po_2 equals 25 mm Hg, reducing $\dot{V}O_{2max}$ by 70%.
7. Acclimatization does not fully compensate for altitude stress. Even after acclimatization, $\dot{V}O_{2max}$ decreases about 2% for every 300 m above 1500 m, with impaired endurance performance paralleling the reduced aerobic capacity.
8. Altitude-related decrements in maximum heart rate and stroke volume offset the beneficial effects of acclimatization and partially explain an inability to achieve sea-level $\dot{V}O_{2max}$.
9. Sea-level $\dot{V}O_{2max}$ and endurance performance do not improve following altitude acclimatization.
10. High-altitude training provides no additional benefit to sea-level physical performance compared with equivalent training only at sea level.

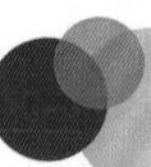

THINK IT THROUGH

1. To climb Mt. Everest, elite mountaineers take 3 months to establish 5 base camps at 16,600 ft (4216 m), 19,500 ft (4953 m), 21,300 ft (5410 m), 24,000 ft (6096 m), and 26,000 ft (6604 m) before the final ascent. Explain the physiologic rationale for this "stage ascent" approach to mountaineering.
2. If altitude acclimatization improves endurance performance at high altitude, why does it not improve similar performance immediately upon return to sea level?
3. Explain whether periodic breath-holding while exercising at sea level brings about similar physiologic adaptations as training at a high altitude.
4. What advice would you give to an athlete who plans to train for an endurance race at high altitude in 2 months?
5. Respond to this question: If altitude has such negative effects on the body, why are some track-and-field records broken during competition at higher elevations?
6. From a physiologic perspective, what represents a safe altitude for flight in an airplane with a nonpressurized cabin?

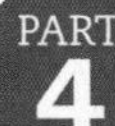

PART 4 Physiologic Agents to Enhance Performance

Four common nonnutritional, nonpharmacologic procedures attempt to enhance physiologic response to physical activity and physical performance:

1. RBC reinfusion
2. Exogenous use of the hormone EPO
3. Pre-exercise warm-up
4. Breathing hyperoxic gas mixtures

RED BLOOD CELL REINFUSION

Red blood cell (RBC) reinfusion, often called *induced erythrocythemia, blood boosting,* or *blood doping*, came into public prominence as a possible ergogenic technique during the 1972 Munich and 1976 Montreal Olympics—when Finnish quadruple gold medalist Lasse Virin (**www.olympic.org/videos/lasse-viren-wins-the-distance-double-double-montreal-1976-olympic-games**) reportedly used the procedure (legal at that time) to prepare for his 5000- and 10,000-m endurance runs (**http://news.google.com/newspapers?nid=1310&dat=19760730&id=2qtVAAAAIBAJ&sjid=3uADAAAAIBAJ&pg=3194,7526139**).

How It Works

RBC reinfusion requires withdrawal of between 1 and 4 units of a person's blood (1 unit = 450 mL). The plasma is removed and immediately reinfused, and the packed RBCs are frozen for storage. To prevent dramatic reductions in blood cell concentration, removal of each unit of blood occurs over 3 to 8 weeks, the time needed to re-establish normal RBC levels. Reinfusion of an individual's own stored RBCs (referred to as **autologous transfusion**) occurs up to 7 days before endurance competition. **Homologous transfusion** infuses type-matched donor's blood. Infusion by either method increases hematocrit and hemoglobin levels by 8% to 20% and increases average hemoglobin concentration for men from a normal of 15 g per dL of blood to about 19 g per dL. Theoretically, the added blood volume increases maximal cardiac output, and increased hematocrit augments blood's oxygen-carrying capacity to increase available oxygen to working muscles. This effect benefits endurance athletes, especially long-distance runners for whom oxygen transport often limits maximal physical capacity.

Infusing 900 to 1800 mL of preserved autologous blood usually provides ergogenic benefits. Each 500-mL infusion of whole blood, or its equivalent of 275 mL of RBCs, adds about 100 mL of oxygen to the blood's total oxygen-carrying capacity. This occurs because each deciliter of whole blood normally carries approximately 20 mL of oxygen. An endurance athlete's total blood volume circulates five times each minute in intense physical activity. The potential "extra" available oxygen to tissues from each unit of reinfused blood, or its RBC component, equals 500 mL (5 × 100 mL extra O_2).

Blood doping can create effects opposite to those intended. A large infusion of RBCs and resulting inordinately large increase in cellular concentration could theoretically increase blood viscosity or thickness and subsequently decrease cardiac output, thus *reducing* aerobic capacity. Any large increase in blood viscosity also would compromise blood flow through diseased, narrowed coronary vessels.

Does It Work?

Research generally confirms physiologic and performance improvements with RBC reinfusion. Differences in results among various studies originate largely from blood storage methods. Frozen RBCs store in excess of 6 weeks without loss of cells compared with those at conventional storage at 4°C employed in earlier studies; substantial hemolysis or cell destruction occurs at 4°C after only 3 weeks. This is important because it usually takes a person about 6 weeks to replenish RBCs after withdrawal of 2 units of whole blood (**Fig. 15.12**).

RBC reinfusion elevates hematologic characteristics in both men and women. This effect translates to a 5% to 13% increase in aerobic capacity, reduced submaximal heart rate and blood lactate for a standard exercise task, and improved endurance at sea level and high altitude.

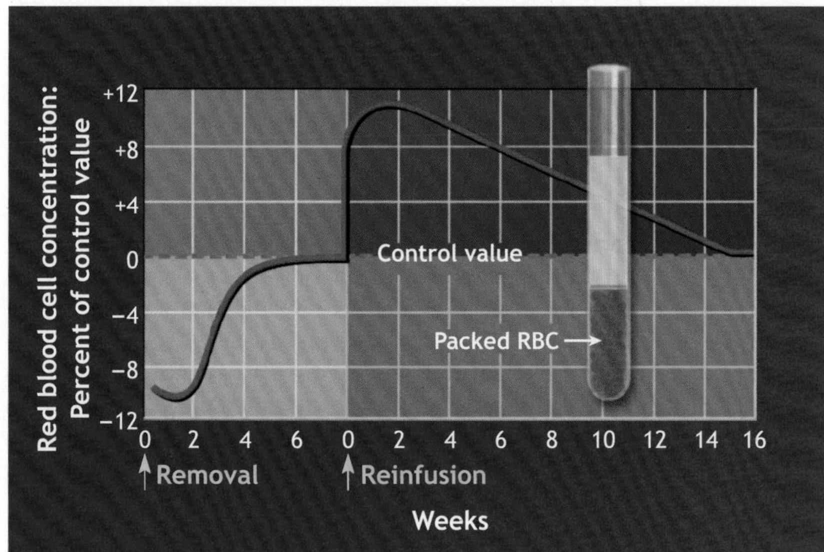

FIGURE 15.12 Time course of hematologic changes after removal and reinfusion of 900 mL of freeze-preserved blood. (Data from Gledhill N. Blood doping and related issues: a brief review. *Med Sci Sports Exerc* 1982;14:183.)

Table 15.7 illustrates hematologic, physiologic, and performance responses for adult men during submaximal and maximal physical activity before and 24 hours after a comparatively large 750-mL RBC infusion.

Hormonal Blood Boosting

To eliminate the cumbersome and lengthy process of blood doping, some endurance athletes use erythropoietin (EPO), a kidney hormone that stimulates bone marrow to increase RBC production. Medically, EPO combats anemia in patients with severe kidney disease. Normally, with low hematocrit or when arterial oxygen pressure decreases, as in severe lung disease or ascent to a high altitude, EPO release stimulates RBC synthesis.

Simply injecting the hormone requires much less sophistication than blood-doping procedures; unfortunately, hematocrit can dangerously exceed levels in excess of 60% if EPO is administered exogenously in an unregulated and unmonitored fashion. Excessive hemoconcentration increases blood viscosity and augments exercise-induced increases in systolic blood pressure. This potentiates the likelihood for stroke, heart attack, heart failure, pulmonary embolism, and even death.

The International Cycling Union (**www.uci.ch**) established a hematocrit threshold for disqualification of 50% for men and 47% for women; the International Skiing Federation (**www.fis-ski.com**) uses a hemoglobin concentration of 18.5 $g \cdot dL^{-1}$ as the threshold for disqualification. Hematocrit cutoff values of 52% for men and 48% for women, approximately 3 standard deviations above the mean, represent "abnormally high" or extreme values.

The enhancement of oxygen availability to muscles by EPO analog and mimetics constitutes one of the main challenges to doping control. The concern of sports-governing bodies has now shifted from simple RBC reinfusion to concern about transfection to athletes' genes (transfer to an athlete's body of genes that code for erythropoietin) and the subsequent impact on performance. Sports authorities now categorize "gene doping" as a prohibited practice.

Iron Anomaly Among Cyclists

Current concern centers on an anomaly in iron metabolism frequently observed among high-level international cyclists. Many riders have serum iron levels that exceed 500 $ng \cdot L^{-1}$ (normal: 100 $ng \cdot L^{-1}$), with some values exceeding 1000 $ng \cdot L^{-1}$. The elevated iron level comes from regular injections of supplemental iron to support increased RBC synthesis induced by repeated EPO use. Chronic iron overload in vital organs increases risk for liver dysfunction, including cirrhosis and liver cancer. Excess iron deposition, considered iron "toxicity," can

TABLE 15.7 Physiologic, Performance, and Hematologic Characteristics Before and 24 Hours After the Reinfusion of 750 mL of Packed Red Blood Cells

Variable	Preinfusion	Postinfusion	Difference	Difference, %
Hemoglobin, g · 100 mL blood^{-1}	13.8	17.6	3.8[b]	+27.5[b]
Hematocrit, %[a]	43.3	54.8	11.5[b]	+26.5[b]
Submaximal $\dot{V}O_2$, L · min^{-1}	1.6	1.5	−0.01	−0.6
Submaximal HR, b · min^{-1}	127.4	109.2	18.2	−14.3[b]
$\dot{V}O_2$, L · min^{-1}	3.3	3.7	0.4[b]	+12.8[b]
HR_{max}, b · min^{-1}	181.6	180.0	−1.6	−0.9
Treadmill runtime, s	793.0	918.0	125.0[b]	+15.8

[a]Hematocrit presented as the percent (%) of 100 mL of whole blood occupied by RBCs.

[b]Statistically significant difference.

Source: From Robertson RJ, et al. Effect of induced erythrocythemia on hypoxia tolerance during physical exercise. *J Appl Physiol* 1982;53:490.

negatively affect the heart's bundle of His and Purkinje fibers, which increase chances of irregular heart dysfunction when the iron lodges in those structures. Other medical complications of iron overload include chronic fatigue, diabetes, hair loss, heart attack or heart failure, hypopituitarism, hypothyroidism, hypogonadism, infertility, impotence, metabolic syndrome, osteoarthritis, osteoporosis, and persistent physical symptoms including premature death. According to the Iron Disorders Institute (**www.irondisorders.org/iron-overload**), iron mismanagement resulting in overload can accelerate neurodegenerative diseases such as Alzheimer, early-onset Parkinson, Huntington, epilepsy, and multiple sclerosis. The treatment for iron overload can include physician-prescribed iron reduction therapy, including blood removal (phlebotomy), blood donation, and iron chelation with prescription drugs. These procedures are not without risk, and most times the best strategy is "watchful waiting" until higher iron levels return to normal.

WARM-UP

Coaches, trainers, and athletes at all levels of competition believe in the benefit of some type of mild physical activity or **warm-up** preceding vigorous exertion. Preliminary physical activity enables the performer to:

1. Prepare either physiologically or psychologically for an upcoming event
2. Reduce likelihood of joint and muscle injury

In animals, greater forces and increases in muscle length are required to injure a "warmed-up" muscle compared with a muscle in a "cold" condition. The explanation maintains that warming up stretches the muscle-tendon unit to allow for greater length and less tension at any given load.

Warm-up is classifies into two categories, although overlap exists:

1. **Category 1. General warm-up** involves calisthenics, stretching, and general body movements or "loosening-up" activities usually *unrelated* to the specific neuromuscular actions of the anticipated performance.
2. **Category 2. Specific warm-up** provides *skill rehearsal* for the activity. Typical examples include swinging a golf club before the "real" attempt; throwing a baseball or football; practicing tennis volleys and baseline shots, or basketball layups and jump shots; and preliminary lead-up in the high jump or pole vault.

Psychological Considerations

Competitors at all levels believe that some prior activity prepares them mentally for their event so they can concentrate on the upcoming performance. *Evidence supports that a specific warm-up related to the activity improves required skill and coordination patterns.* Athletes participating in sports requiring accuracy, timing, and precise movements benefit from specific or formal preliminary practice.

Competitors also believe that prior physical activity, particularly before strenuous effort, gradually prepares them to go "all out" with less fear of injury. The ritual warm-up of baseball pitchers provides a case in point. Would a starting or relief pitcher enter a game throwing at competitive speeds without previously warming up? Would any elite athlete begin competition without first engaging in a particular form, intensity, or duration of warm-up? Because topflight athletes believe in warming up, it becomes nearly impossible to design an experiment with individuals to factually resolve whether or not warm-up actually improves subsequent performance and reduces injury potential.

In certain situations, peak performance occurs when play begins, without time for warming up. When a reserve player enters a game in the last few minutes, no time exists for preliminary stretching, vigorous calisthenics, or taking practice shots. The player must go all out with no warm-up except for that done before the game or at intermission.

Physiological and Performance Effects

Little evidence exists that warm-ups per se directly improve subsequent physical performance. Lack of scientific justification does not mean that warm-ups should be disregarded.

Warm-Up: Physiologic Considerations

The following five physiologic mechanisms suggest how warm-up might improve subsequent performance:

1. Increased speed of contraction and relaxation of warmed muscles.
2. Greater economy of movement because of lowered viscous resistance within warmed muscles.
3. Facilitated oxygen utilization by warmed muscles because hemoglobin releases oxygen more readily at higher muscle temperatures.
4. Facilitated nerve transmission and muscle metabolism at higher temperatures; a specific warm-up facilitates motor unit recruitment required in subsequent all-out physical activity.
5. Increased blood flow through active tissues as local vascular beds dilate in response to increases in metabolism and muscle temperatures.

Source: O'Leary JD, et al. Improving clinical performance using rehearsal or warm-up: an advanced literature review of randomized and observational studies. *Acad Med* 2014;89:1416.

We advocate, although without strong conviction, that such procedures continue because of the strong psychological component and "possible" physical benefits of warming up, whether passive (massage, heat applications, and diathermy), general (calisthenics and jogging), or specific (practice of actual movements). Until substantial evidence justifies elimination, a brief warm-up provides a comfortable way to lead into more vigorous activity.

A gradual warm-up to moderate intensity can increase muscle and core temperature 1°C to 3°C without inducing fatigue or reducing immediate energy stores. This consideration makes the warm-up highly individualized. For example, the duration and intensity of an Olympic swimmer's warm-up might exhaust a recreational swimmer.

In accordance with the principle of exercise specificity, muscles should be engaged in a way that mimics the anticipated activity and brings about a full range of joint motion. Optimally, a competitive event or activity should begin within several minutes from the end of the warm-up. Ironically, some coaches advocate that swimmers continue the traditional practice of repeatedly swimming laps at the start of a meet, even if their events do not occur for upward of an hour or more before their swim.

Warm-Up and Sudden Strenuous Physical Activity: Clinical Considerations

Several studies have evaluated the effects of preliminary activity on cardiovascular responses to sudden, strenuous exercise. The findings provide a different physiologic framework for justifying warm-up for individuals in adult fitness and cardiac rehabilitation programs and in occupations and sports requiring a sudden burst of intense physical effort.

In one study, 44 men free from overt symptoms of coronary heart disease performed intense, uphill running on a treadmill for 10 to 15 seconds without prior warm-up. Evaluation of postexercise electrocardiographic (ECG) tracings revealed that 70% of the subjects displayed abnormal ECG changes attributed to inadequate myocardial oxygen supply. These changes did not relate to age or fitness level. To evaluate the effects of warming up, 22 of the men jogged in place at moderate intensity with a heart rate of 145 $b \cdot min^{-1}$ for 2 minutes before the treadmill run. With warm-ups, 10 men with previously abnormal ECG responses to the treadmill run showed normal tracings, and 10 men improved their ECG results; only two subjects showed ischemic changes or poor oxygen supply following the warm-up. Warm-ups also improved the blood pressure response. For seven subjects with no warm-up, systolic blood pressure averaged 168 mm Hg immediately after the treadmill run. This decreased to 140 mm Hg with the 2-minute warm-up.

Coronary blood flow adjustments to sudden, intense exertion do not occur instantaneously, and transient myocardial ischemia can occur in apparently healthy and fit individuals. *The positive effect of prior warm-up ($\geq$2 min of easy jogging) on ECG and blood pressure indicates a more favorable relationship between myocardial oxygen supply and demand in the warmed-up condition.*

Warm-up preceding strenuous physical activity probably benefits all people, yet the greatest effect occurs for those with compromised myocardial oxygen supply. A brief activity warm-up optimizes blood pressure and hormonal adjustments at the onset of subsequent strenuous exertion and serves two important purposes:

1. Reduces myocardial work load and thus myocardial oxygen requirements
2. Enhances coronary blood flow to augment myocardial oxygen supply

BREATHING HYPEROXIC GAS

Athletes often breathe oxygen-enriched or **hyperoxic gas mixtures** during time out, at half time, or following strenuous exertion at sea level. They believe that this procedure enhances the blood's oxygen-carrying capacity to facilitate exercise recovery. When healthy people breathe ambient air at sea level, hemoglobin in arterial blood leaving the lungs contains nearly 98% of its full oxygen complement. In physiologic terms, this indicates one of two things:

1. Breathing higher than normal sea-level concentrations of oxygen (hyperoxic mixtures) increases hemoglobin's oxygen transport by only 10 mL of extra oxygen for every 1000 mL of blood.
2. Oxygen dissolved in plasma when breathing a hyperoxic mixture at sea level increases only slightly from its normal quantity of 3 mL to about 7 mL per 1000 mL of blood.

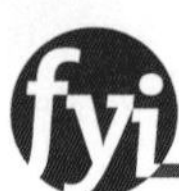

A Warmed-Up Muscle Enhances Sprint Cycling Performance

A study shed light on the effects on thigh muscle temperature and subsequent maximal sprint performance of passive insulation versus external heating during recovery after a sprint-specific warm-up. Eleven male cyclists on three different occasions completed a 15-minute intermittent warm-up on a cycle ergometer followed by a 30-minute passive recovery before attempting a 30-second maximal "all-out" sprint test. Indwelling microelectrodes to assess average muscle temperature ($\overline{T}m$) were inserted into the vastus lateralis at 1-, 2-, and 3-cm depth before and following the warm-up and prior to the sprint test. Absolute and relative peak power output gauged performance on the sprint test, including measurement of blood lactate concentration immediately following physical activity. During recovery from warming up, cyclists wore a tracksuit top and standard tracksuit pants (SUIT), insulated athletic pants (IPANTS), or insulated athletic pants infused with an electric heating elements (HEAT).

Warm-up increased $\overline{T}m$ by approximately 2.5°C at all depths, with no differences between the three warmed-up conditions. During recovery, $\overline{T}m$ remained elevated in HEAT compared with IPANTS and SUIT at all microelectrode depths ($P < 0.001$). Both peak and relative power output were significantly elevated by 9.6% in HEAT and 9.1% compared with IPANTS. The increase in blood lactate concentration was significantly enhanced following the sprint in SUIT but not IHEAT versus IPANTS. The authors concluded that passive thigh heating between warm-up completion and performance execution using pants incorporating electrically heated pads reduces the decline in thigh muscle temperature and therefore improves sprint cycling performance.

Source: Faulkner SH, et al. Reducing muscle temperature drop after warm-up improves sprint cycling performance. *Med Sci Sports Exerc* 2013;45:359.

Breathing hyperoxic gas at sea level increases oxygen-carrying capacity by 14 mL of oxygen for every 1000 mL of blood; 10-mL extra attaches to hemoglobin and 4-mL extra dissolves in plasma.

Before Physical Activity

The blood volume of a 70-kg person equals approximately 5000 mL. A hyperoxic breathing mixture potentially adds about 70 mL of oxygen in the total blood volume (5000 mL blood × 14.0 mL extra O_2 per 1000 mL blood = 70 mL O_2). Despite any potential psychological benefit to the athlete who believes that pre-exercise oxygen breathing helps performance, only a slight performance advantage exists from the small 70 mL of extra oxygen. Further, any advantage occurs only if subsequent physical activity takes place *immediately* after hyperoxic breathing. This means that the athlete cannot breathe ambient air in the interval between hyperoxic breathing and physical activity. Breathing ambient air, with considerably lower Po_2 than the previously inspired hyperoxic mixture, facilitates oxygen's movement from the body to the environment. A halfback who breathes oxygen on the sideline before returning to the game or a swimmer who takes a few deep breaths of oxygen before moving to the blocks for starting instructions gains *no* competitive edge from physiologic benefits if they still breathe ambient air. This is particularly ironic in American football because the energy to power each play generates almost completely from metabolic reactions that do *not* require oxygen!

During Physical Activity

Breathing hyperoxic gas during submaximal and maximal aerobic activity enhances endurance performance. Oxygen breathing *during* submaximal activity reduces blood lactate, heart rate, and ventilation volume and increases maximal oxygen uptake.

In one study, subjects performed a 6.5-minute endurance ride on a bicycle ergometer at an activity level equivalent to 115% of $\dot{V}O_{2max}$ while breathing either room air or 100% oxygen. Subjects breathed both air and oxygen from identical tanks of compressed gas to mask knowledge of the breathing mixture.

Figure 15.13A gives the details of the ride, showing superiority in endurance with less drop-off in pedal revolutions during the hyperoxic trials. **Figure 15.13B** shows oxygen uptake curves while participants cycled while breathing either oxygen or room air. A higher oxygen uptake occurred when participants breathed 100% oxygen, with a correspondingly faster increase in oxygen uptake early in physical activity. The small increase in hemoglobin saturation with hyperoxic breathing and additional oxygen dissolved in plasma increase oxygen availability during maximal physical activity. During this time, total blood volume circulates up to seven times each minute in an elite endurance athlete. Quantitatively, the 70 mL of extra oxygen in the total blood volume with hyperoxic breathing circulated seven times each minute provides an additional 490 mL of oxygen each minute during intense aerobic activity. Also, increased partial pressure of oxygen in solution while breathing hyperoxic gas facilitates oxygen diffusion across the capillary-tissue membrane to the mitochondria. This accounts for more rapid oxygen utilization early in physical activity.

Breathing hyperoxic mixtures provides physiologic benefits during some forms of physical activity, but the sports application of mixtures seems limited. The added weight of an appropriate breathing system would negate any ergogenic benefit. Also, the legality of the system's use during competition seems highly unlikely.

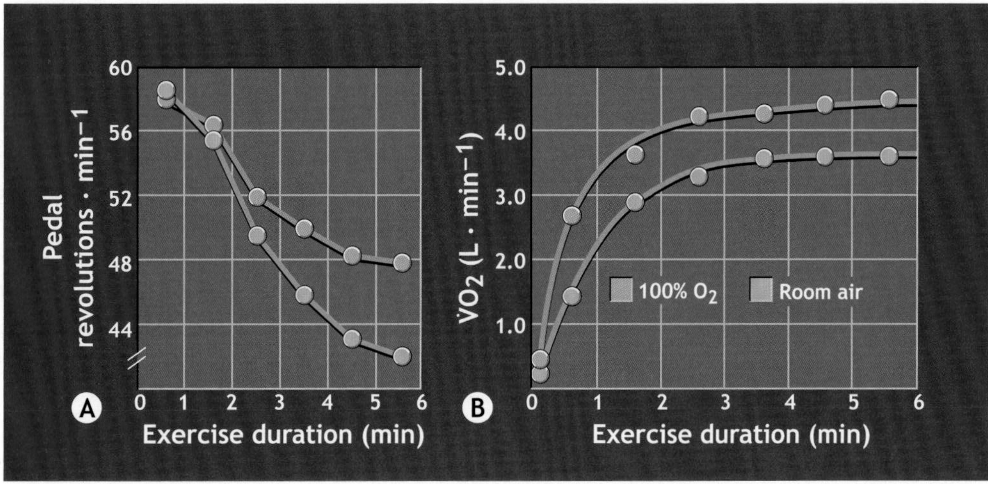

FIGURE 15.13 **A.** Superiority of endurance (measured by pedal revolutions each minute) breathing pure oxygen versus breathing ambient air at sea level. **B.** Oxygen uptake curves during the endurance rides show enhanced oxygen uptake while breathing pure oxygen. (Data from Weltman A, et al. Effects of increasing oxygen availability on bicycle ergometer endurance performance. *Ergonomics* 1978;21:427.)

In Recovery

Figure 15.14 illustrates the effects of breathing hyperoxic gas during recovery from strenuous physical activity on subsequent cycle performance. After 1 minute of all-out bicycle ergometer exercise, subjects recovered either passively by sitting quietly or actively by pedaling lightly while breathing room air or 100% oxygen for either 10 or 20 minutes. They then repeated the all-out bicycle ride. No differences emerged in cumulative revolutions (**Fig. 15.14A**) or the 6-second × 6-second revolutions (**Fig. 15.14B**) for the 1-minute ride after breathing either room air or pure oxygen in recovery. Also, no difference resulted between trials when comparing blood lactate levels at 10 and 20 minutes of recovery. This indicated that oxygen inhalation did not preferentially alter lactate removal. Subsequent research supports these findings; breathing hyperoxic mixtures following short intervals of submaximal or maximal activity does not alter the kinetics for minute ventilation, heart rate, or serum lactate, or the level of subsequent performance.

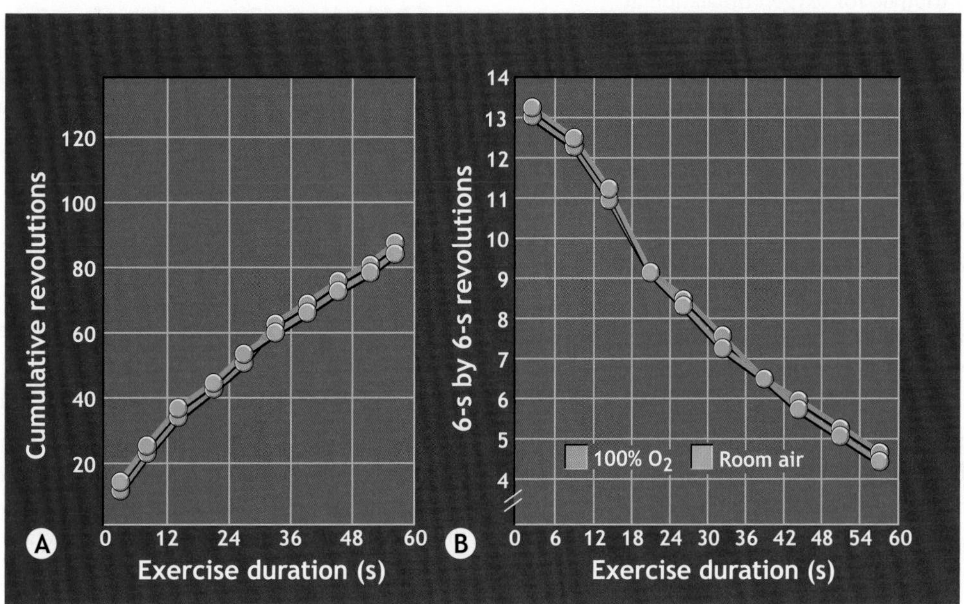

FIGURE 15.14 Cumulative **(A)** and absolute **(B)** pedal revolutions on a bicycle ergometer during 1 minute of maximal exercise subsequent to breathing either oxygen or ambient air during recovery from a previous maximal exercise bout. (Adapted with permission from Weltman A, et al. Exercise recovery, lactate removal, and subsequent high intensity exercise performance. *Res Q* 1977;48:786.)

SUMMARY

1. RBC reinfusion (blood doping) involves drawing, storing, and reinfusing concentrated RBCs for use several weeks later.
2. Added blood volume and RBC concentration theoretically create a larger maximum cardiac output and increase the blood's oxygen-carrying capacity to increase $\dot{V}O_{2max}$.
3. Research supports the ergogenic benefits of RBC reinfusion for aerobic exercise performance and thermoregulation.
4. Diverse physiologic rationales justify warm-up for ergogenic purposes and injury prevention.
5. Limited research supports the performance benefits of warm-up other than its potentially positive psychological effects.
6. A moderate cardiovascular warm-up before sudden strenuous exertion reduces cardiac work load and enhances coronary blood flow by depressing transient myocardial ischemia at intense physical activity onset.
7. Breathing 100% oxygen during exercise at sea level extends endurance by increasing oxygen uptake, reducing blood lactate, and lowering pulmonary ventilation.
8. Breathing hyperoxic mixtures before or after sea-level exercise provides no ergogenic benefit.

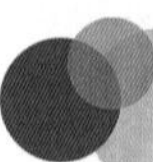

THINK IT THROUGH

1. As a basketball coach, what warm-up procedures would you recommend before a game?
2. Explain the rationale for oxygen inhalation at the sidelines during a football game played at the moderately high altitude of Denver, CO.

KEY TERMS

Aldosterone: Adrenal cortex sodium-conserving hormone, which acts on the renal tubules to increase sodium resorption and reduce sweat's osmolality.

Altitude acclimatization: Broadly describes adaptive responses in physiology and metabolism to improve tolerance to hypoxia.

Antidiuretic hormone (ADH): Hormone from the neurohypophysis of the hypothalamus; increases the permeability of the kidney's collecting tubules to facilitate fluid retention.

Autologous transfusion: Infusion of an individual's own blood.

Chronic mountain sickness (CMS): Prevalent in a small number of altitude natives; relates to excessive polycythemia, perhaps from a genetically linked variation in the EPO response to hypoxic stress. Symptoms include lethargy, weakness, sleep disturbance, bluish skin coloring (cyanosis), and change in mental status.

Core: Body's central tissues including the deep cranial, thoracic, and abdominal cavities.

Dehydration: Body water loss from states of hyperhydration to euhydration or from euhydration to hypohydration.

Erythropoietin (EPO): Kidney-produced hormone in response to reduced oxygen pressure in arterial plasma; regulates RBC production, synthesis and functioning of erythrocyte membrane proteins.

Frostbite: Localized damage caused by freezing to skin and other tissues; most likely occurs in body parts farthest from the heart and those with relatively large exposed surface areas.

Heat acclimatization: Describes the improved heat tolerance from collective physiologic adaptive changes.

Heat cramps: Severe involuntary, sustained, and spreading muscle spasms in the specifically active muscles during or following intense physical activity in the heat.

Heat exhaustion: Excessive sweating produces ineffective circulatory adjustments compounded by extracellular fluid depletion, principally in plasma volume.

Heat illness: Cascade of disabling complications when the normal signs of heat stress—thirst, fatigue, grogginess, and visual disturbances—go unheeded.

Heat stroke: Most serious of the heat-stress maladies reflecting failure of heat-regulating mechanisms from excessively high core temperature.

Heat syncope: Mild form of heat illness, also known as orthostatic dizziness. Refers to a fainting episode experienced in high environmental temperatures.

High-altitude retinal hemorrhage (HARH): Hemorrhage in the macula of the eye that affects virtually all climbers at altitudes above 6700 m and produces irreversible visual defects. Retinal bleeding probably results from surges in blood pressure with exercise that cause blood vessels in the eye to dilate and rupture from increased cerebral blood flow.

Homologous transfusion: Infusion of a type-matched donor's blood.

Hyperhydration: Ingesting "extra" water prior, during, or following physical activity.

Hyperoxic gas mixtures: Oxygen-enriched gas mixtures often breathed during time-outs, at half time, or following strenuous activity.

Hypoxia: Subnormal oxygen pressure in ambient air.

Lactate paradox: Addresses the question about why lactate accumulation reduces without a corresponding increase in tissue oxygenation when the hypoxemia associated with high altitude should instead promote lactate accumulation.

Live high, train low: Training strategy that combines altitude acclimatization and maintenance of sea-level training intensity to provide synergistic benefits to sea-level endurance performance.

Oxygen transport cascade: Changes in oxygen partial pressure as oxygen moves from ambient air at sea level to the mitochondria of maximally active muscle tissue.

Polycythemia: Abnormally high concentration of red blood cells.

Red blood cell (RBC) reinfusion: Withdrawing 1 to 4 units of blood, immediately reinfusing its plasma, and placing the packed red blood cells in frozen storage for later reinfusion.

Relative humidity (RH): Ratio of water in ambient air at a particular temperature compared to the total quantity of moisture that air could contain expressed as a percentage.

Shell: Peripheral tissues of the body including skin and subcutaneous fat.

Temperature: Mean kinetic energy of a substance's atoms as they move.

Warm-up: Preparatory physical activity performed in the belief that prior, preliminary physical activity, either mimicking the activity or more general in nature, prepares a person to perform "all out" without fear of injury.

Windchill temperature index: National Weather Service data that provides an accurate and understandable way to recognize dangers from winter winds and freezing temperatures, including frostbite threshold values.

SELECTED REFERENCES

Alderman BL, et al. Factors related to rapid weight loss practices among international-style wrestlers. *Med Sci Sports Exerc* 2004;36:249.

Amann M, et al. Altitudeomics: on the consequences of high altitude acclimatization for the development of fatigue during locomotor exercise in humans. *J Appl Physiol* 2013;115:634.

American College of Sports Medicine. American College of Sports Medicine position stand on heat and cold illnesses during distance running. *Med Sci Sports Exerc* 1996;28:1.

American College of Sports Medicine. American College of Sports Medicine position stand. Exertional heat illness during training and competition. *Med Sci Sports Exerc* 2007;39:556.

Anholmm JD, et al. Radiographic evidence of interstitial pulmonary edema after exercise at altitude. *J Appl Physiol* 1999;86:503.

Armstrong LE, et al. Limitations to the use of plasma osmolality as a hydration biomarker. *Am J Clin Nutr* 2013;98:503.

Arnaud MJ, Noakes TD. Should humans be encouraged to drink water to excess? *Eur J Clin Nutr* 2011;65:875; author reply 877.

Audran M, et al. Effects of erythropoietin administration in training athletes and possible indirect detection in doping control. *Med Sci Sports Exerc* 1999;31:639.

Baker LB, et al. Progressive dehydration causes a progressive decline in basketball skill performance. *Med Sci Sports Exerc* 2007;39:1114.

Barnard RJ, et al. Cardiovascular responses to sudden strenuous exercise: heart rate, blood pressure, and ECG. *J Appl Physiol* 1973;34:883.

Barnard RJ, et al. Ischemic response to sudden strenuous exercise in healthy men. *Circulation* 1973;48:936.

Bärtsch P, Swenson ER. Clinical practice: acute high-altitude illnesses. *N Engl J Med* 2013;368:2294.

Beidleman BA, et al. Seven intermittent exposures to altitude improves exercise performance at 4300 m. *Med Sci Sports Exerc* 2008;40:141.

Bender PR, et al. Decreased exercise muscle lactate release after high altitude acclimatization. *J Appl Physiol* 1989;67:1456.

Bergeron MF. Reducing sports heat illness risk. *Pediatr Rev* 2013;34:270.

Bergeron MF, et al. International Olympic Committee consensus statement on thermoregulatory and altitude challenges for high-level athletes. *Br J Sports Med* 2012;46:770.

Berglund B, et al. The Swedish Blood Pass project. *Scand J Med Sci Sports* 2007;17:292.

Bonne TC, et al. "Live High-Train High" increases hemoglobin mass in Olympic swimmers. *Eur J Appl Physiol* 2014;114:1439.

Booth J, et al. Improved running performance in hot humid conditions following whole body precooling. *Med Sci Sports Exerc* 1997;29:943.

Brajkovic D, et al. Influence of localized auxiliary heating on hand comfort during cold exposure. *J Appl Physiol* 1998;85:2054.

Braun B. Effects of high altitude on substrate use and metabolic economy: cause and effect? *Med Sci Sports Exerc* 2008;40:1495.

Brothers MD, et al. GXT responses to altitude-acclimatized cyclists during sea-level simulation. *Med Sci Sports Exerc* 2007;39:1727.

Browne A, et al. The ethics of blood testing as an element of doping control in sport. *Med Sci Sports Exerc* 1999;31:497.

Butterfield GE. Nutrient requirements at high altitude. *Clin Sports Med* 1999;18:607.

Buyrnley M, et al. Effects of prior warm-up regime on severe-intensity cycling performance. *Med Sci Sports Exerc* 2005;36:838.

Carter R III. Exertional heat illness and hyponatremia: an epidemiological prospective. *Curr Sports Med Rep* 2008;7:S20.

Casa DJ, et al. Cold water immersion: the gold standard for exertional heatstroke treatment. *Exerc Sport Sci Rev* 2007;35:141.

Ceretelli P, Samaja M. Acid-base balance at exercise in normoxia and in chronic hypoxia. Revisiting the "lactate paradox." *Eur J Appl Physiol* 2003;90:431.

Chapman RF, et al. Timing of return from altitude training for optimal sea level performance. *J Appl Physiol* 2014;116:837.

Chen SM, et al. Altitude training improves glycemic control. *Chin J Physiol* 2013;56:4.

Cheung SS, McLellan TM. Heat acclimation, aerobic fitness, and hydration effects on tolerance during uncompensable heat stress. *J Appl Physiol* 1998;84:1731.

Cheung SS, Sleivert GG. Multiple triggers for hyperthermic fatigue and exhaustion. *Exerc Sport Sci Rev* 2004;32:100.

Cheuvront SN, et al. No effect of moderate hypohydration or hyperthermia on anaerobic exercise performance. *Med Sci Sports Exerc* 2006;38:1093.

Chinevere TD, et al. Effect of heat acclimation on sweat minerals. *Med Sci Sports Exerc* 2008;40:886.

Cleary MA, et al. Thermoregulatory, cardiovascular, and perceptual responses to intermittent cooling during exercise in a hot, humid outdoor environment. *J Strength Cond Res* 2013;28:792.

Cotter JD, Tipton MJ. Moving in extreme environments: what's extreme and who decides? *Extrem Physiol Med* 2014;3:11.

Coyle EF, Montain SJ. Benefits of fluid replacement with carbohydrate during exercise. *Med Sci Sports Exerc* 1992;24:S324.

Cymerman A, et al. Operation Everest II: maximal oxygen uptake at extreme altitude. *J Appl Physiol* 1989;66:2446.

DeLorey DS, et al. Prior exercise speeds pulmonary O_2 uptake kinetics by increases in both local muscle O_2 availability and O_2 utilization. *J Appl Physiol* 2007;103:771.

Dematte JE, et al. Near-fatal heat stroke during the 1995 heat wave in Chicago. *Arch Intern Med* 1998;129:173.

Distefano LJ, et al. Hypohydration and hyperthermia impair neuromuscular control after exercise. *Med Sci Sports Exerc* 2013;45:1166.

Eastwood A, et al. Within-subject variation in hemoglobin mass in elite athletes. *Med Sci Sports Exerc* 2012;44:725.

Eichner ER. Heat cramps in sports. *Curr Sports Med Rep* 2008;7:178.

Ekblom B, et al. Central circulation during exercise after venesection and reinfusion of red blood cells. *J Appl Physiol* 1976;40:379.

Evans RK, et al. Effects of warm-up before eccentric exercise on indirect markers on muscle damage. *Med Sci Sports Exerc* 2002;34:1892.

Faiss R, et al. Responses to exercise in normobaric hypoxia: comparison between elite and recreational ski-mountaineers. *Int J Sports Physiol Perform* 2014;9:978.

Falk B, et al. Response to rest and exercise in the cold: effects of age and aerobic fitness. *J Appl Physiol* 1994;76:72.

Faulkner SH, et al. Reducing muscle temperature drop after warm-up improves sprint cycling performance. *Med Sci Sports Exerc* 2013;45:359.

Fulco CS, et al. Maximal and submaximal exercise performance at altitude. *Aviat Space Environ Med* 1998;69:793.

Gagnon D, et al. Mean arterial pressure following prolonged exercise in the heat: influence of training status and fluid replacement. *Scand J Med Sci Sports* 2012;22:e99.

Giesbrecht GG. Cold stress, near drowning and accidental hypothermia: a review. *Aviat Space Environ Med* 2000;71:733.

Gonzalez-Alonso J, et al. Stroke volume during exercise: interaction of environment and hydration. *Am J Physiol Heart Circ Physiol* 2000;278:H321.

Gore CJ, et al. Nonhematological mechanisms of improved sea-level performance after hypoxic exposure. *Med Sci Sports Exerc* 2007;39:1600.

Gray SC, et al. Effect of active warm-up on metabolism prior to and during intense dynamic exercise. *Med Sci Sports Exerc* 2002;34:2091.

Green HJ, et al. Human skeletal muscle exercise metabolism following an expedition to Mount Denali. *Am J Physiol Regul Integr Comp Physiol* 2000;279:R1872.

Hajoglou A, et al. Effect of warm-up on cycle time trial performance. *Med Sci Sports Exerc* 2005;37:1608.

Hales JRS. Hyperthermia and heat illness: pathological implications for avoidance and treatment. *Ann N Y Acad Sci* 1997;813:534.

Hamouti N, et al. Ingestion of sodium plus water improves cardiovascular function and performance during dehydrating cycling in the heat. *Scand J Med Sci Sports* 2014;24:507.

Hamouti N, et al. Sweat sodium concentration during exercise in the heat in aerobically trained and untrained humans. *Eur J Appl Physiol* 2011;111:2873.

Hew-Butler T, et al. Consensus Statement of the 1st International Exercise-Associated Hyponatremia Consensus Development Conference, Cape Town, South Africa 2005. *Clin J Sport Med* 2005;15:208.

Holliss BA, et al. Influence of intermittent hypoxic training on muscle energetics and exercise tolerance. *J Appl Physiol* 2013;114:611.

Holowatz LA, et al. Altered mechanisms of vasodilation in aged human skin. *Exerc Sport Sci Rev* 2007;35:119.

Honigman B, et al. Acute mountain sickness in a general tourist population at moderate altitude. *Ann Intern Med* 1993;118:587.

Inoue Y, et al. Mechanisms underlying the age-related decrement in the human sweating response. *Eur J Appl Physiol* 1999;79:121.

Jacobs RA. Live high-train low does not improve sea-level performance beyond that achieved with the equivalent living and training at sea level. *High Alt Med Biol* 2013;14:328.

Janse de Jonge XA, et al. Exercise performance over the menstrual cycle in temperate and hot, humid conditions. *Med Sci Sports Exerc* 2012;44:2190.

Johnson JM. Physical training and the control of skin blood flow. *Med Sci Sports Exerc* 1998;30:382.

Judelson DA, et al. Effect of hydration state on strength, power, and resistance exercise performance. *Med Sci Sports Exerc* 2007;39:1817.

Junglee NA, et al. Exercising in a hot environment with muscle damage: effects on acute kidney injury biomarkers and kidney function. *Am J Physiol Renal Physiol* 2013;305:F813.

Katayama K, et al. Effect of intermittent hypoxia on oxygen uptake during submaximal exercise in endurance athletes. *Eur J Appl Physiol* 2004;92:75.

Kenefick RW, et al. Impact of skin temperature and hydration on plasma volume responses during exercise. *J Appl Physiol (1985)* 2014;117:413.

Kenney WL, Chiu P. Influence of age on thirst and fluid intake. *Med Sci Sports Exerc* 2001;332:1524.

Kenney WL, et al. Decreased active vasodilator sensitivity in aged skin. *Am J Physiol* 1997;272:H1605.

Knight DR, et al. Hyperoxia increases lung maximal oxygen uptake. *J Appl Physiol* 1993;75:2586.

Lambert GP. Role of gastrointestinal permeability in exertional heatstroke. *Exerc Sport Sci Rev* 2004;32:185.

LeBlanc J. Factors affecting cold acclimation and thermogenesis in man. *Med Sci Sports Exerc* 1988;20:S193.

Levine BD, Stray-Gunderson J. "Living high—training low": effect of moderate-altitude acclimatization with low-altitude training on performance. *J Appl Physiol* 1997;83:102.

Lippi G, Banfi G. Blood transfusions in athletes: old dogmas, new tricks. *Clin Chem Lab Med* 2006;44:1395.

Lönnberg M, Lundby C. Detection of EPO injections using a rapid lateral flow isoform test. *Anal Bioanal Chem* 2013;405:9885.

Luetkemeier MJ, Thomas EL. Hypervolemia and cycling time trial performance. *Med Sci Sports Exerc* 1994;26:503.

Lundby C, Robach P. Assessment of total haemoglobin mass: can it detect erythropoietin-induced blood manipulations? *Eur J Appl Physiol* 2010;108:197.

Lundby C, et al. Does altitude training increase exercise performance in elite athletes? *Br J Sports Med* 2012;46:822.

MacDonald M, et al. Acceleration of VO_2 kinetics in heavy submaximal exercise by hyperoxia and prior high-intensity exercise. *J Appl Physiol* 1997;83:1318.

Masschelein E, et al. High twin resemblance for sensitivity to hypoxia. *Med Sci Sports Exerc* 2015;47:74.

Maughan RJ, et al. Restoration of fluid balance after exercise-induced dehydration: effect of food and fluid intake. *Eur J Appl Physiol* 1996;73:317.

Maughan RJ, Meyer NL. Hydration during intense exercise training. *Nestle Nutr Inst Workshop Ser* 2013;76:25.

McAllister RM. Adaptations in control of blood flow with training: splanchnic and renal blood flows. *Med Sci Sports Exerc* 1998;30:375.

McArdle WD, et al. Thermal adjustment to cold-water exposure in exercising men and women. *J Appl Physiol* 1984;56:1572.

McArdle WD, et al. Thermal responses of men and women during cold-water immersion: influence of exercise intensity. *Eur J Appl Physiol* 1992;65:265.

McCullough EA, Kenney WL. Thermal insulation and evaporative resistance of football uniforms. *Med Sci Sports Exerc* 2003;35:832.

McDermott BP, et al. The influence of rehydration mode following exercise dehydration on cardiovascular function. *J Strength Cond Res* 2013;27:2086.

McLean BD, et al. Application of 'live low-train high' for enhancing normoxic exercise performance in team Sport athletes. *Sports Med* 2014;44:1275.

McLean BD, et al. Physiological and performance responses to a pre-season altitude training camp in elite team sports athletes. *Int J Sports Physiol Perform* 2013;8:391.

Montain SJ, et al. Aldosterone and vasopressin responses in the heat: hydration level and exercise intensity effects. *Med Sci Sports Exerc* 1997;29:661.

Montain SJ. Hydration recommendations for sport 2008. *Curr Sports Med Rep* 2008;7:187.

Mora-Rodriguez R. Influence of aerobic fitness on thermoregulation during exercise in the heat. *Exerc Sport Sci Rev* 2012;40:79.

Moran DS, et al. Evaluating physiological strain during cold exposure using a new cold strain index. *Am J Physiol* 1999;277:R556.

Noakes TD, Speedy DB. Case proven: exercise associated hyponatremia is due to overdrinking. *Br J Sports Med* 2006;40:567.

Noakes TD. Commentary: role of hydration in health and exercise. *BMJ* 2012;345:e4171.

Noakes TD. *Waterlogged: The Serious Problem of Overhydration in Endurance Sports*. Champaign: Human Kinetics, 2012.

Nolte HW, et al. Ad libitum vs. restricted fluid replacement on hydration and performance of military tasks. *Aviat Space Environ Med* 2013;84:97.

Nolte HW, et al. Protection of total body water content and absence of hyperthermia despite 2% body mass loss ('voluntary dehydration') in soldiers drinking ad libitum during prolonged exercise in cool environmental conditions. *Br J Sports Med* 2011;45:1106.

Nolte HW, et al. Trained humans can exercise safely in extreme dry heat when drinking water ad libitum. *J Sports Sci* 2011;29:1233.

Nordsborg NB, et al. Four weeks of normobaric "live high-train low" do not alter muscular or systemic capacity for maintaining pH and K^+ homeostasis during intense exercise. *J Appl Physiol* 2012;112:2027.

Norris JN, et al. High altitude headache and acute mountain sickness at moderate elevations in a military population during battalion-level training exercises. *Mil Med* 2012;177:917.

O'Toole ML, et al. Hematocrits of triathletes: is monitoring useful? *Med Sci Sports Exerc* 1999;31:372.

Periard JD, Racinais S. Self-paced exercise in hot and cool conditions is associated with the maintenance of $\%VO_2$peak within a narrow range. *J Appl Physiol (1985)* 2015. In press as of 04.01.15.

Perry CGR, et al. Effects of hyperoxic training on performance and cardiorespiratory response to exercise. *Med Sci Sports Exerc* 2005;37:1175.

Pope RP, et al. A randomized trial of preexercise stretching for prevention of lower-limb injury. *Med Sci Sports Exerc* 2000;32:271.

Poppendieck W, et al. Cooling and performance recovery of trained athletes: a meta-analytical review. *Int J Sports Physiol Perform* 2013;8:227.

Richard NA, et al. Acute mountain sickness, chemosensitivity and cardiorespiratory responses in humans exposed o hypobaric and normobaric hypoxia. *J Appl Physiol* 2013;116:945.

Rivera-Brown AM, et al. Drink composition, voluntary drinking and fluid balance in exercising, trained, heat-acclimatized boys. *J Appl Physiol* 1999;86:78.

Robach P, et al. Serum hepcidin levels and muscle iron proteins in humans injected with low- or high-dose erythropoietin. *Eur J Haematol* 2013;91:74.

Robach P, et al. The role of haemoglobin mass on VO_{2max} following normobaric 'live high-train low' in endurance trained athletes. *Br J Sports Med* 2012;46:822.

Robbins MK, et al. Effect of oxygen breathing following submaximal and maximal exercise on recovery and performance. *Med Sci Sports Exerc* 1992;24:270.

Robergs RA, et al. Effects of warm-up on muscle glycogenolysis during intense exercise. *Med Sci Sports Exerc* 1991;23:7.

Roberts WO. Exertional heat stroke during a cool weather marathon: a case study. *Med Sci Sports Exerc* 2006;38:1197.

Roberts WO. Fractured fairy tales: hyponatraemia and the American College of Sports Medicine fluid recommendations. *Br J Sports Med* 2007;41:109; author reply.

Rodriguez R, et al. Aerobically trained individuals have a greater increase in rectal temperature than untrained ones during exercise in the heat a similar relative intensities. *Eur J Appl Physiol* 2010;109:973.

Roy ML, et al. Effect of sodium in a rehydration beverage when consumed as a fluid or meal. *J Appl Physiol* 1998;85:1329.

Rozycki TJ. Oral and rectal temperatures in runners. *Phys Sportsmed* 1984;12:105.

Rupp T, et al. The effect of hypoxemia and exercise on acute mountain sickness symptoms. *J Appl Physiol* 2013;1144:180.

Russell G, et al. Effects of prolonged low dosage of recombinant human erythropoietin during submaximal and maximal exercise. *Eur J Appl Physiol* 2002;86:442.

Saltin B, et al. Morphology, enzyme activities and buffer capacity in leg muscles of Kenyan and Scandinavian runners. *Scand J Med Sci Sports* 1995;5:209.

Sawka MN, Coyle EF. Influence of body water and blood volume on thermoregulation and exercise performance in the heat. *Exerc Sport Sci Rev* 1999;27:167.

Sawka MN, et al. American College of Sports Medicine position stand. Exercise and fluid replacement. *Med Sci Sports Exerc* 2008;39:377.

Sawka MN, et al. Integrated physiological mechanisms of exercise performance, adaptation, and maladaptation to heat stress. *Compr Physiol* 2011;1:1883.

Sawka MN, Noakes TD. Does dehydration impair exercise performance? *Med Sci Sports Exerc* 2006;37:1209.

Sheffield-Moore M, et al. Thermoregulatory responses to cycling with and without a helmet. *Med Sci Sports Exerc* 1997;29:755.

Shirreffs SM, Maughan RJ. Rehydration and recovery of fluid balance after exercise. *Exerc Sport Sci Rev* 2000;1:27.

Shirreffs SM, Maughan RJ. Restoration of fluid balance after exercise-induced dehydration: effects of alcohol consumption. *J Appl Physiol* 1997;83:1152.

Sims ST, et al. Sodium loading aids fluid balance and reduces physiological strain of trained men exercising in the heat. *Med Sci Sports Exerc* 2007;39:123.

Stapleton JM., et al. At what level of heat load are age-related impairments in the ability to dissipate heat evident in females? *PLoS One* 2015. In press as of 04.01.15.

Subudhi AW, et al. AltitudeOmics: the integrative physiology of human acclimatization to hypobaric hypoxia and its retention upon reascent. *PLoS One* 2014;9:e92191.

Tam N, Noakes TD. The quantification of body fluid allostasis during exercise. *Sports Med* 2013;43:1289. Review.

Thomsen JJ, et al. Prolonged administration of recombinant erythropoietin increases the submaximal performance more than maximal aerobic capacity. *Eur J Appl Physiol* 2007;101:481.

Toner MM, McArdle WD. Human thermoregulatory responses to acute cold stress with special reference to water immersion. In: Fregly MJ, Blatteis CM, eds. *Handbook of Physiology. Sect. 4: Environmental Physiology, Vol. 1.* New York: Oxford University Press, 1996.

Truijens MJ, et al. The effect of intermittent hypobaric hypoxic exposure and sea level training on submaximal economy in well-trained swimmers and runners. *J Appl Physiol* 2008;104:328.

Tyler CJ, et al. The effect of cooling prior to and during exercise on exercise performance and capacity in the heat: a meta-analysis. *Br J Sports Med* 2015;49:7.

U.S. Department of Health and Human Services. Hyperthermia and dehydration-related deaths associated with intentional weight loss in three collegiate wrestlers—North Carolina, Wisconsin, and Michigan, November–December, 1997. *MMWR Morb Mortal Wkly Rep* 1998;47:105.

von Duvillard SP, et al. Sports drinks, exercise training, and competition. *Curr Sports Med Rep* 2008;7:202.

Wagner PD, Lundby C. The lactate paradox: does acclimatization to high altitude affect blood lactate during exercise? *Med Sci Sports Exerc* 2007;39:747.

Watson G, et al. Influence of diuretic-induced dehydration on competitive sprint and power performance. *Med Sci Sports Exerc* 2005;37:1168.

Weavil JC, et al. Endurance exercise performance in acute hypoxia is influenced by expiratory flow limitation. *Eur J Appl Physiol* 2015 In press as of 04.01.15.

Wehrlin JP, et al. Live high–train low for 24 days increases hemoglobin mass and red cell volume in elite endurance athletes. *J Appl Physiol* 2006;101:1938.

Weltman AL, et al. Effects of increasing oxygen availability on bicycle ergometer endurance performance. *Ergonomics* 1978;21:427.

West JB. Barometric pressure on Mt. Everest: new data and physiological significance. *J Appl Physiol* 1999;86:1062.

West JB. *High Life: A History of High Altitude Physiology and Medicine.* New York: Oxford University Press, 1998.

West JB. Point:counterpoint: the lactate paradox does/does not occur during exercise at high altitude. *J Appl Physiol* 2007;102:2398.

Wilber RL. Live high+train low does improve sea level performance beyond that achieved with the equivalent living and training at sea level. *High Alt Med Biol* 2013;14:325.

Wilhite DP, et al. Increases in $\dot{V}O_{2max}$ with "live high-train low" altitude training: role of ventilatory acclimatization. *Eur J Appl Physiol* 2013;113:419.

Willie CK, et al. Regional cerebral blood flow in humans at high altitude: gradual ascent and two weeks at 5050m. *J Appl Physiol* 2013;116:905.

Winter FD, et al. Effects of 100% oxygen on performance of professional soccer players. *JAMA* 1989;262:227.

SECTION VI

Optimizing Body Composition and Weight Control, Successful Aging, and Health-Related Physical Activity Benefits

Approximately one third of all deaths globally occur from ailments linked to four factors—excess body fat, diminished physical activity, suboptimal dietary intake, and smoking—and this trend knows no economic, racial, or cultural borders.

Forty years ago, age 65 represented the onset of "old" age. Gerontologists now consider 85 as a demarcation of "oldest old" and age 75 as "young old." The Office of the Chief Actuary of the Social Security Administration (**www.socialsecurity.gov**) estimates that a male born on April 3, 2015 will live to age 83.1 while his female counterpart will achieve age 86.8. These evolving demographics call for a new gerontologic viewpoint that addresses areas beyond age-related diseases and recognizes that *successful, healthy aging* requires enhanced physiologic function through optimal dietary strategies and increased physical activity.

The physiologic and physical activity capacities of older people generally rate below those of younger counterparts, yet one can question whether such differences reflect true biologic aging or simply the effects of disuse that usually accompany aging.

From the glaciers of the Arctic to the palm-fringed beaches of the South Pacific, there are now more overfat people in the world than hungry people! It should occasion little surprise that obesity has become one of the world's leading causes of morbidity and mortality.

— *Anonymous*

A meaningful upswing has occurred in participation of older individuals in a broad range of physical activities. A physically active lifestyle contributes to the ability of these individuals to retain a relatively high level of functional capacity, thus enabling them to safely engage in leisure recreational pursuits and **activities of daily living (ADL)** (e.g., eating, bathing, dressing, and movement; **http://aspe.hhs.gov/daltcp/reports/meacmpes.htm**). Moreover, maintaining an active lifestyle helps to counter obesity and other diseases related to sedentary living (e.g., degenerative musculoskeletal and cardiovascular disorders).

Clinical exercise physiologists have become part of a team approach to individual healthcare. Where physical dysfunction exists, these professionals primarily focus on restoring an individual's mobility and functional capacity in concert with physical therapists, occupational therapists, and physicians. Clinical exercise physiologists assume an increasingly important clinical role in sports medicine as they assist in evaluating and reconditioning individuals with diverse diseases and physical limitations and may also provide significant input in preventive aspects related to disability and disease.

Chapter 16 focuses on body composition and its components and assessment, the differences between men and women and trained and untrained individuals, and topics relevant to the staggering revelations about the obesity epidemic. We also include basic information about obesity and the role of optimal nutrient intake and increased physical activity to reverse the energy balance equation in favor of weight loss. In Chapters 17 and 18, we explore aspects of the aging process and the exercise physiologist role as a healthcare professional in the clinical setting.

CHAPTER 16

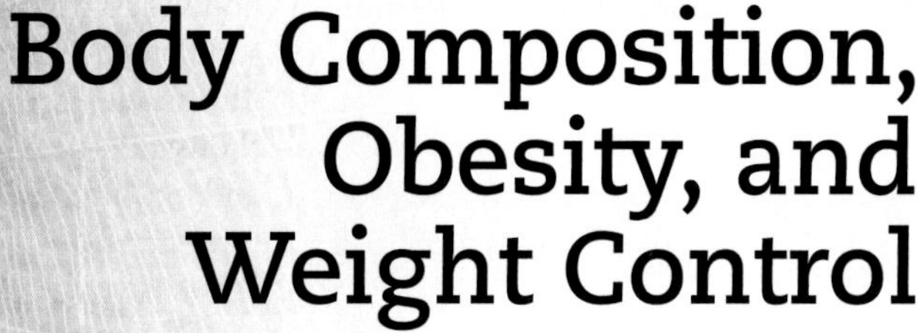

Body Composition, Obesity, and Weight Control

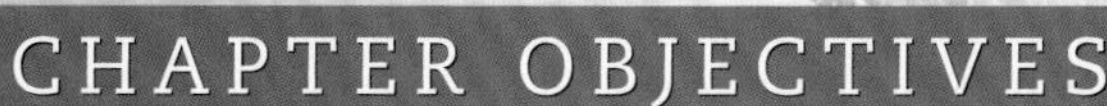

CHAPTER OBJECTIVES

- Outline five body composition characteristics of the "reference man" and "reference woman."
- Define *lean body mass*, *fat-free body mass*, and *minimal body mass*.
- Describe Archimedes' principle and its application to human body volume measurement.
- List two assumptions for computing percentage body fat from body density.
- Explain how population-specific skinfold and girth equations predict body fat.
- Give three weaknesses of the use of body mass index to assess excess weight, excess fat, and disease risk.
- Describe the current status of overweight and obesity among American adults and children.
- List eight significant health risks of obesity.
- Provide two criteria that define obesity in adult men and women.
- Explain how fat cell hypertrophy and hyperplasia each contributes to obesity and whether changes in body weight can modify these factors.
- Outline how "unbalancing" the energy balance equation can impact body weight.
- Explain the rationale for including regular physical activity in a prudent weight-loss program.
- Explain how a moderate increase in regular physical activity for a previously sedentary, overweight person affects daily food intake and overall energy expenditure.
- Explain the rationale for and effectiveness of specific physical activity for localized fat loss.
- Give two diet and physical activity recommendations for gaining weight to enhance sports performance.

ANCILLARIES AT A GLANCE

Visit **http://thePoint.lww.com/MKKESS5e** to access the following resources:

- References: Chapter 16
- Interactive Question Bank
- Appendix D: Evaluation of Body Composition—Girth Method
- Appendix SR-6: Additional Video Links

This chapter describes the gross composition of the human body, including direct and indirect methods to partition the body into two basic compartments—fat mass (FM) and fat-free body mass (FFM). We also present simple, noninvasive methods to analyze an individual's body composition and discuss the important role increased physical activity and dietary restraint play in achieving optimal body composition and improving overall health status.

PART 1 Human Body Composition

In the last 80 years, numerous studies have evaluated body composition and how best to measure its various components. Most methodologies partition the body into two distinct compartments: **fat mass (FM)** and **fat-free body mass (FFM)**. The density of homogenized snippets of fat-free body tissues in small mammals averages 1.100 $g \cdot cm^{-3}$ at 37°C. Fat stored in adipose tissue has an average density of 0.900 $g \cdot cm^{-3}$ at 37°C.

Subsequent body composition studies have expanded the two-component model to three (water, protein, and fat) or four components (water, protein, bone minerals, and fat) to account for biologic variability. Not surprisingly, men and women differ in relative quantities of specific body components. Consequently, gender-specific reference standards provide a framework to evaluate "normal" body composition.

MULTICOMPONENT MODEL OF BODY COMPOSITION

Figure 16.1 illustrates a five-level model to examine the human body's components. Each level of the model becomes more elaborate (atoms, molecules, cells, tissue systems, and whole body) as the body's complexity of biologic organization increases. Note that subdivisions exist within each of the five levels. The model primarily attempts to identify and then quantify each level's various components. An essential feature of the model provides separate and distinct levels, each with directly or indirectly measurable characteristics.

Due to practical limitations, body composition analyses mostly centers on the tissue and whole-body level. Gender differences in several body composition components provide a convenient foundation to understand body composition from the framework of a **reference man and reference woman**, a concept developed in the 1960s by Dr. **Albert Behnke** (1898–1993; American College of Sports Medicine [ACSM] Honor Award; Navy physician and pioneer body composition research scientist).

BEHNKE'S REFERENCE MAN AND REFERENCE WOMAN MODELS

Figure 16.2 illustrates the body composition models representing Behnke's reference man and reference woman. The different color schema partitions body mass into lean body mass (LBM), muscle, and bone, with total body fat subdivided into **storage fat** and **essential fat** components. This model integrates the average physical dimensions from thousands of individuals measured in large-scale civilian and military anthropometric surveys and separate laboratory cadaver studies of detailed tissue composition and structure.

The reference man is taller and heavier, his skeleton weighs more, and he possesses a larger muscle weight and lower body fat content than does the reference woman. These differences exist even when one expresses fat, muscle, and bone as a percentage of body weight. Just how much of the gender difference in body fat relates to biologic, behavioral, or lifestyle factors remains unclear. More than likely, hormonal differences play an important role.

The concept of reference standards does not mean that men and women should strive to achieve this "ideal" body composition, nor should the reference man and woman reflect the desirable standard for optimal health status. Rather, the reference model proves useful for statistical comparisons and data interpretations based on population studies of elite athletes, individuals involved in exercise training and physical activity, different racial and ethnic groups, those at the extremes of underweight and obesity, and individuals intent on improving physique status.

Storage and Essential Fat

In the reference model, total body fat exists in two sites or depots—storage fat and essential fat. The storage fat depot includes fat or triacylglycerol packed primarily in adipose tissue. The adipose tissue energy reserve contains approximately 83% pure fat, 2% protein, and 15% water within its supporting structures. Storage fat includes the visceral fatty tissues that protect thoracic and abdominal cavity internal organs from trauma. Essential fat consists of fat in the heart, lungs, liver, spleen, kidneys, intestines, muscles, and lipid-rich tissues of the central nervous system and bone marrow. *Normal physiologic functioning requires this fat.* In the heart, for example, dissectible cadaver fat represents approximately 18.4 g or 5.3% of an average 349 g male heart and 22.7 g or 8.6% of a 256 g female heart. In women, essential fat also includes **sex-specific essential fat**.

A larger adipose tissue volume called **subcutaneous fat** exists beneath the skin's surface. A similar proportional distribution of storage fat exists in men and women (12% of body weight in men and 15% in women), but the total percentage of essential fat in women, which includes sex-specific fat, averages four times that in men. *A woman's additional essential fat likely serves biologically important functions related*

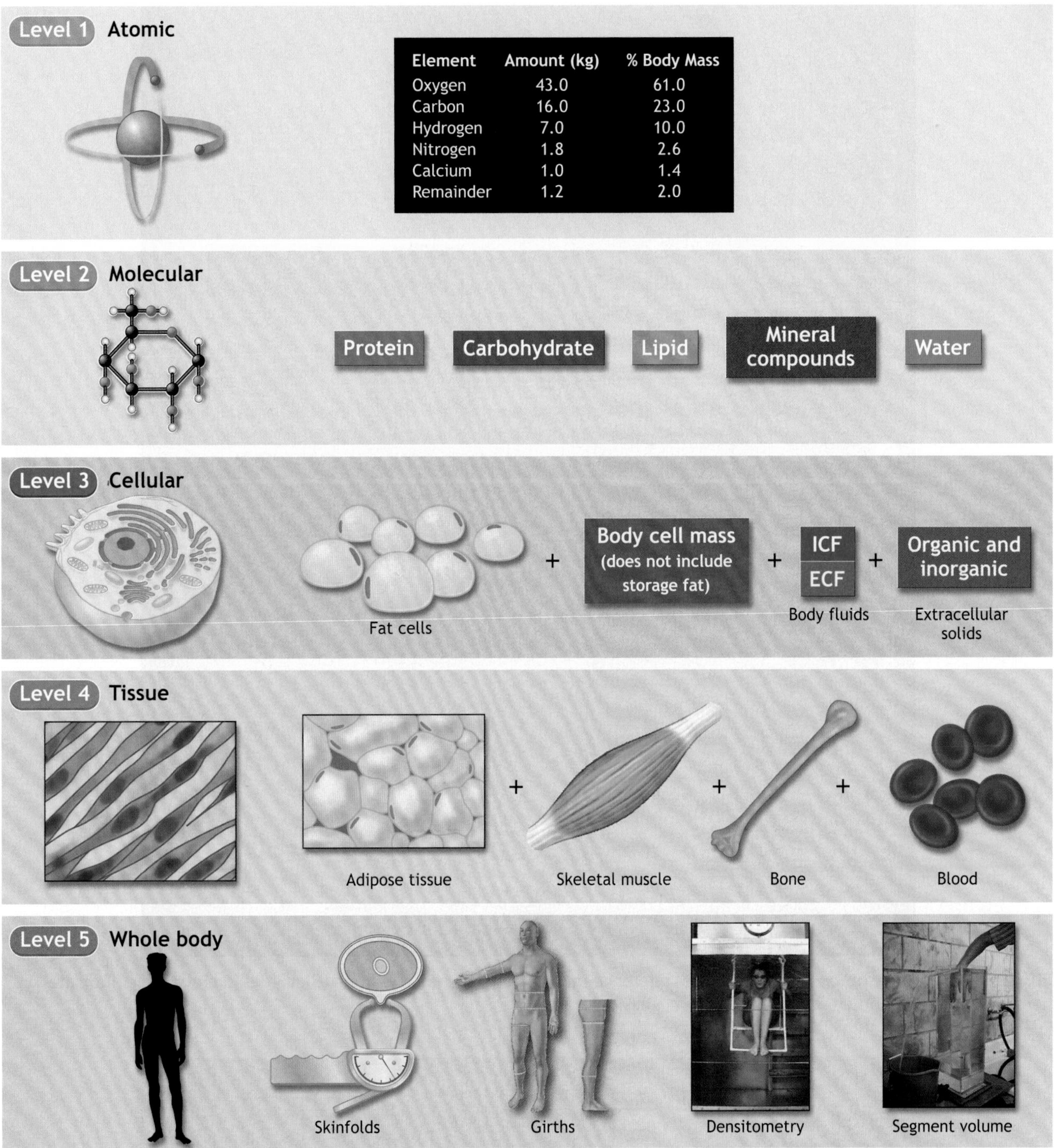

FIGURE 16.1 Five-level, multicomponent model to assess and interpret body composition. Each level progresses in complexity of biologic organization. ECF, extracellular fluid; ICF, intracellular fluid. (Adapted with permission from Wang ZM, et al. The five-component model. A new approach to organizing body composition research. *Am J Clin Nutr* 1992;56:19.)

to childbearing and other hormonal functions. Considering the reference body's total quantity of about 8.5 kg (18.7 lb) of storage fat, this depot theoretically represents 63,500 kcal of available energy, or the energy equivalent of playing pickup basketball nonstop for 107 hours, golfing without a cart/walking at a normal pace on a track for 176 to 180 continuous hours, or treading water in a swimming pool without a break for 10 days straight. In terms of running, this quantity of fat represents the equivalent of performing nonstop at a 9-minute-per-mile pace for 114 hours to complete about 29 consecutive marathons!

Figure 16.3 partitions the distribution of body fat for the reference woman. As part of the 5% to 9% sex-specific fat reserves, breast fat probably contributes no more than 4% of body weight for women; total fat content as a percentage of body weight in women ranges between 14% and 35%. We

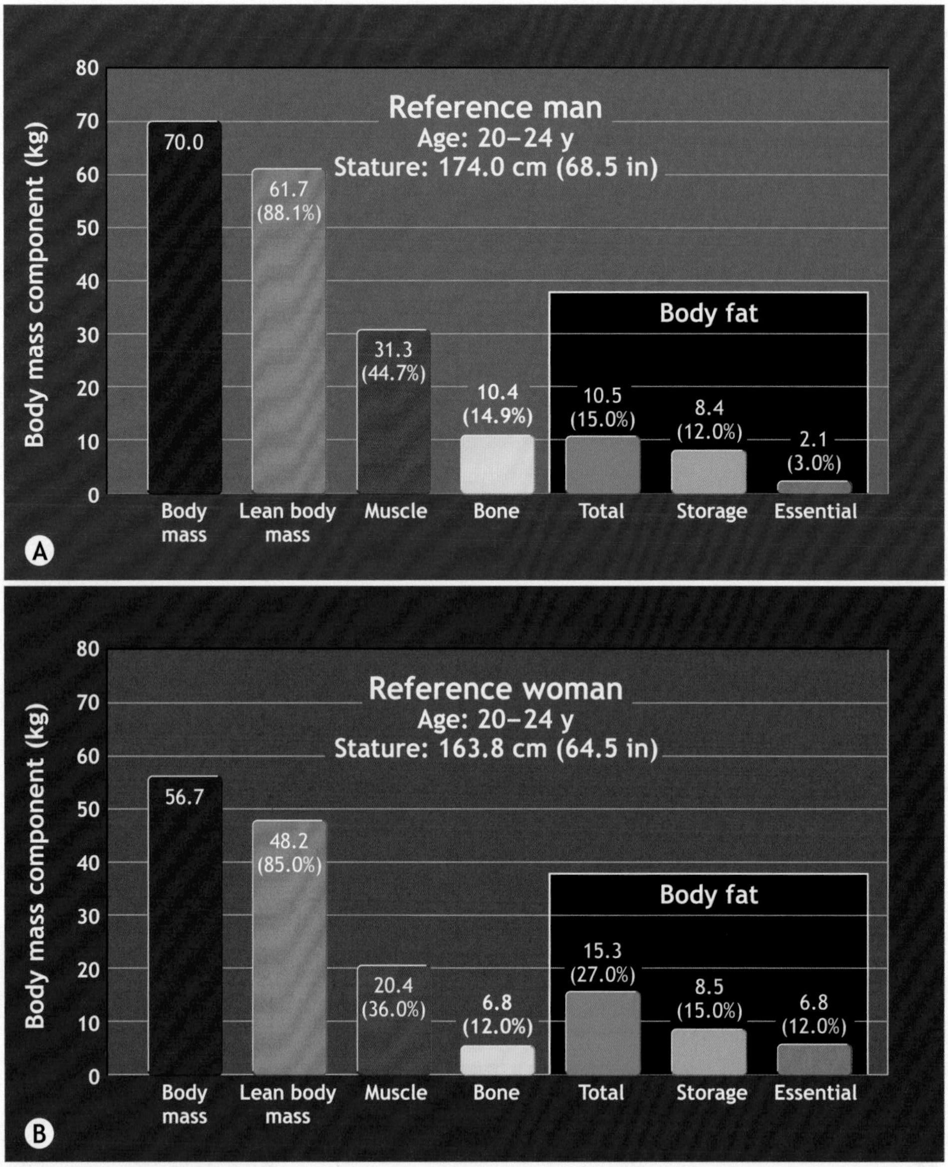

FIGURE 16.2 Body composition of Behnke's reference man **(A)** and reference woman **(B)**. Values in *parentheses* indicate percentage of total body mass.

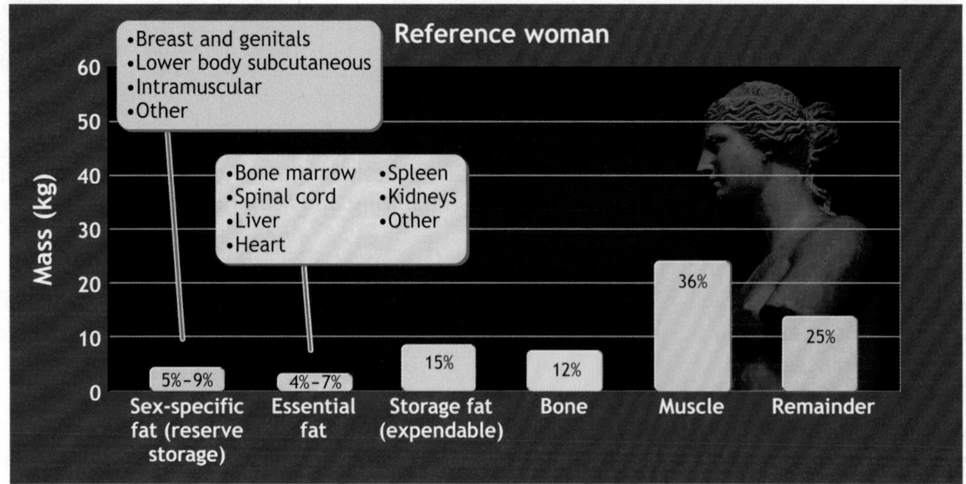

FIGURE 16.3 Theoretical model for body fat distribution for the reference woman with body mass of 56.7 kg, stature of 163.8 cm, and 27% body fat. (From Katch VL, et al. Contribution of breast volume and weight to body fat distribution in females. *Am J Phys Anthropol* 1980;53:93.)

interpret this to mean that other substantial sex-specific fat depots exist in pelvic, buttock, and thigh regions that contribute to the female's total body fat stores.

Fat-Free Body Mass and Lean Body Mass

The terms FFM and LBM refer to specific body components. These terms often are used interchangeably, and the differences are subtle but real. **Lean body mass (LBM)**, a theoretical entity, contains the small percentage of non–sex-specific essential fat (equivalent to ~4% to 7% of body weight) located chiefly within the central nervous system, bone marrow, and internal organs. In contrast, fat-free mass (FFM) represents body mass devoid of all extractable fat (FFM = Body mass − Fat mass). Behnke emphasized that FFM refers to an *in vitro* entity appropriate to carcass analysis. He considered the LBM an *in vivo* entity relatively constant in water, organic matter, and mineral content throughout an active adult's life span. *In normally hydrated, healthy adults, FFM and LBM differ only in the essential fat component.*

LBM in men and **minimal body mass** in women consist chiefly of essential fat (plus sex-specific fat for women), muscle, water, and bone (see Fig. 16.2). If the reference man's total body fat percentage equals 15.0% (storage fat plus essential fat), the density of a hypothetical fat-free body attains the upper limit of 1.100 $g \cdot cm^{-3}$. In the reference woman, the average whole-body density of 1.040 $g \cdot cm^{-3}$ represents a body fat percentage of 27%; of this, approximately 12% consists of essential body fat. A density of 1.072 $g \cdot cm^{-3}$ represents the minimal body weight of 48.5 kg. In practical terms, density values exceeding 1.068 for women (14.8% body fat) and 1.088 $g \cdot cm^{-3}$ for men (5% body fat) rarely occur except in young, exceptionally lean athletes.

Table 16.1 presents data for percentage body fat for selected groups of male and female athletes. Striking differences exist among these groups, including variability within each athletic category.

TABLE 16.1 Percentage Body Fat for Male and Female Athletes

Sport[a]	Percentage Body Fat	
	Male	Female
Ballet dancing	8–14	13–20
Baseball/softball	12–15	12–18
Basketball	6–12	20–27
Bodybuilding	5–8	10–15
Canoe/kayak	6–12	10–16
Cycling	5–15	15–20
Football		
Backs	9–12	
Linebackers	13–14	
Lineman	15–19	
Quarterbacks	12–14	
Gymnastics	5–12	10–16
Horse racing	8–12	10–16
Ice/field hockey	8–15	12–18
Orienteering	5–12	12–24
Racquetball	8–13	15–22
Rock climbing	5–10	13–18
Rowing	6–14	12–18
Rugby		10–17
Skiing		
Alpine	7–14	18–24
Cross-country	7–12	16–22
Jumping	10–15	12–18
Speed skating	10–14	15–24
Synchronized swimming		12–24
Swimming	9–12	14–24
Tennis	12–16	16–24
Track and field		
Discus throwing	14–18	22–27
Jumping	7–12	10–18
Long distance running	6–13	12–20
Shot put	16–20	20–28
Sprinting	8–10	12–20
Decathlon	8–10	
Triathlon	5–12	10–15
Volleyball	11–14	16–25
Weightlifting	9–16	
Wrestling	5–16	

[a]Data for specific sports compiled from the research literature.

Minimal Leanness Standards

A biologic lower limit exists beyond which a person's body weight cannot decrease without presumably impairing health status or altering normal physiologic functions. Malnutrition in men and women falls into this category, notably the complex eating disorder anorexia nervosa and body dysmorphic disorder (BDD; **www.adaa.org/understanding-anxiety/related-illnesses/other-related-conditions/body-dysmorphic-disorder-bdd**).

Men

To estimate the lower body fat limit in men or LBM, subtract storage fat from body weight. For the reference man, the LBM (61.7 kg; 135.7 lb) includes approximately 3% (2.1 kg; 4.6 lb) essential body fat. Encroachment into this reserve may impair optimal health and capacity for vigorous physical activity.

Minnesota Semistarvation Experiments

Low body fat values exist for male world-class endurance athletes and also for conscientious objectors or pacifists to military service who voluntarily reduced their body fat stores with semistarvation during a year-long nutritional experiment near the end of World War II. From November 1944 through October 1945, University of Minnesota physiologist Ancel Keys (1904–2004; **www.nytimes.com/2004/11/23/obituaries/23keys.html?_r=0**) conducted one of the classic

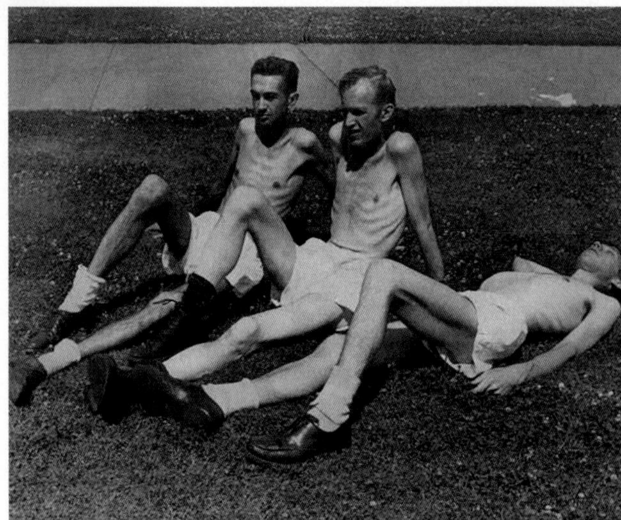

FIGURE 16.4 Three of the 36 volunteers resting during their daily routines in the Minnesota Semistarvation experiments. (Image reprinted with permission from Minnesota Historical Society, **http://www.mnopedia.org/event/starvation-experiment-dr-ancel-keys-1944-1945**.)

nutrition experiments on body wasting and physiologic functioning sponsored by the US Army (**www.mnopedia.org/event/starvation-experiment-dr-ancel-keys-1944-1945**) (**Fig. 16.4**).

In 1941, Keys created the famous "K rations," compact nutritional packets used by the military in World War II. A subsequent experiment at the opposite end of the spectrum studied how to "refeed" the millions of war victims, prisoners, and refugees worldwide. The government had speculated that starvation during the war could pose serious refeeding challenges when the war ended. A two-volume report of the experiment, *The Biology of Human Starvation*, can be accessed at **www.ncbi.nlm.nih.gov/pmc/articles/PMC1526048/** and is recommend reading about food consumption, dietary practices, and psychological ramifications including physiological effects of wasting disease with suboptimal dietary intake.

Women

In contrast to the lower limit of body weight for the reference man with 3% essential fat, the lower limit for the reference woman equals approximately 12% essential fat. This theoretical limit, called minimal body weight, represents 48.5 kg (107.3 lb) for the reference woman. Generally, the leanest women in the population do not fall below 10% to 12% body fat, which represents a narrow range that is probably at the lower limit for most women in good health. As a point of interest, remain skeptical if skinfold assessment of body fat yields values below this lower body fat range. We are unaware of skinfold conversion formulae validated on "ultrathin" females (e.g., those with anorexia nervosa or "apparently thin" female marathoners). *Behnke's theoretical concept of minimal body weight in women, incorporating approximately 12% essential fat, corresponds to the LBM in men that includes 3% essential fat.*

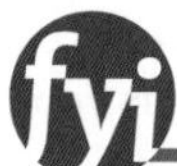

Low Body Fat in Marathoners

The low body fat levels of marathon runners, ranging from 1% to 8% of body weight, probably reflect both self-selection and a combination of an adaptation to long-term training for distance running and a reduced energy intake relative to energy output from intense training. A relatively low body fat reduces the energy cost of weight-bearing physical activity; it also provides an effective gradient to dissipate metabolic heat generated during prolonged physical activity. Top-level marathoners must adhere to careful dietary practices to maintain sufficient body weight to support the typical 80 to 120 miles a week of arduous training. Over the past 60 years, the body size of competitive marathoners has diminished—they remain mostly thin with low body fat levels. The male winner of the 2014 New York City Marathon, Kenyan Wilson Kipsang Kiprotich, weighed 62 kg (137 lb) with a height of 1.82 m (5′11″). The female winner (below), Kenyan Mary Jepkosgei Keitany, weighed 42 kg (93 lb).

Source: Stellingwerff T. Contemporary nutrition approaches to optimize elite marathon performance. *Int J Sports Physiol Perform* 2013;8:573.

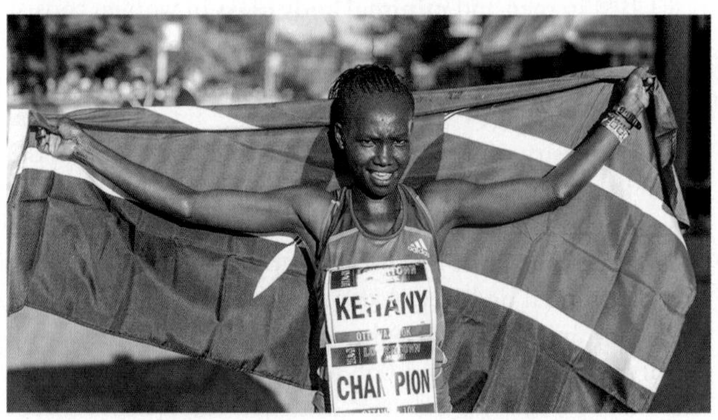

Underweight and Thin

The terms *underweight* and *thin* describe considerably different physical conditions. Measurements in our laboratories have focused on the structural characteristics of "apparently" thin women. We initially screened subjects subjectively as thin or "skinny." Twenty-six women were measured for skinfolds, circumferences, bone diameters, and percentage body fat and FFM by **densitometry** (one of the gold standards of measurement explained later in this chapter).

Unexpectedly, the "skinny" women's percentage of body fat averaged 18.2%, only 7 to 9 percentage points below the values of 25% to 27% body fat typically reported for young adult women. Another striking finding included equivalence in four trunk and four extremity bone diameter measurements for the thin-appearing women compared with 174 women who averaged 25.6% fat and 31 women who averaged 31.4% body fat. Thus, appearing thin or skinny did not necessarily correspond to a diminutive frame size or critically low body fat percentage as proposed in Behnke's model for minimal body weight and essential body fat.

Three criteria identify an underweight female:

1. Body weight lower than minimal body weight calculated from skeletal measurements
2. Body weight lower than the 20th percentile by **stature**
3. Percentage body fat lower than 17% assessed by a criterion method (e.g., hydrodensitometry or DXA)

LEANNESS, REGULAR PHYSICAL ACTIVITY, AND MENSTRUAL IRREGULARITY

Physically active women, particularly participants in the "low-weight" or "body appearance" sports (e.g., distance running, bodybuilding, figure skating, diving, ballet, and gymnastics), increase their likelihood for one of three medical maladies:

1. Delayed menstruation onset
2. Irregular menstrual cycle (oligomenorrhea)
3. Complete menses cessation (amenorrhea)

In the general population, amenorrhea occurs in 2% to 5% of women of reproductive age, but it reaches 40% in some athletic groups. As a group, ballet dancers remain lean, with a greater incidence of menstrual dysfunction and eating disorders and a higher mean age at menarche than age-matched, nondance counterparts. Nearly one third to one half of female endurance athletes exhibit some menstrual irregularity. In premenopausal women, menstrual function irregularity or absence accelerates bone loss and increases musculoskeletal injury risk during physical activity.

The **exercise stress hypothesis** posits that prolonged levels of chronic physical stress can disrupt the hypothalamic-pituitary-adrenal axis and gonadotropin-releasing hormone output (see Chapter 12), which results in irregular menstruation. A concurrent hypothesis maintains that an inadequate energy reserve to sustain pregnancy induces cessation of ovulation (**energy availability hypothesis**).

Some researchers argue that 17% body fat represents a *critical level* for menstruation onset, with 22% fat needed to sustain a normal cycle. They reason that body fat below these levels triggers hormonal and metabolic disturbances that impact the menses. Research with animals has identified **leptin** (see Part 3 of this chapter), a hormone intimately linked to body fat levels and appetite control, as a principal puberty-imitating chemical. Thus, a link exists between hormonal regulation of sexual maturity onset (and perhaps continued optimal sexual function) and level of stored energy reflected by accumulated body fat.

LBM-to-Body Fat Ratio

The LBM-to-body fat ratio may play a key role in normal menstrual function. This could occur through peripheral fat's role in converting androgens to estrogens or through leptin production in adipose tissue. Other factors also may be operative as many physically active women below the supposedly critical 17% body fat level have normal menstrual cycles without sacrificing a high level of physiologic and performance capacity. Conversely, some amenorrheic athletes maintain body fat levels considered average for the population. Potential causes of menstrual dysfunction include the complex interplay of physical, nutritional, genetic, hormonal, psychological, and environmental factors, and an individual's regional fat distribution.

Intense bouts of physical activity trigger the release of an array of hormones, some of which disrupt normal reproductive function. Intense and/or prolonged exertion that releases cortisol and other stress-related hormones also can alter ovarian function via the hypothalamic-pituitary-adrenal axis.

In all likelihood, 13% to 17% body fat probably represents a minimum range associated with regular menstrual function. The effects and risks of sustained amenorrhea on the reproductive system remain unknown. A gynecologist or endocrinologist should evaluate failure to menstruate or cessation of the normal cycle. Such disrupted function may signal a significant medical condition—pituitary or thyroid gland malfunction or premature menopause.

Consuming well-balanced, nutritious meals on a regular basis helps to prevent or reverse athletic amenorrhea without

When a Model Is Not Ideal

Forty years ago, only an 8% difference existed in body weight between professional fashion models and the average American woman. In 2014, a model's body weight averaged approximately 20% to 25% lower than the national average weight of females of similar age. Tremendous commercial pressure dominates the top modeling agencies worldwide to recruit models in the lower body weight range of what most would consider "thin." At a trending Web site for those considering a position as a top fashion model (**www.modelingadvice.com/fashionModelSize.html**), the following tips were given for the "ideal model look":

> For body size, ... tall and very thin —5'9" to 5'10", size 2 to 4 but I think they would love size 0. If you are USA average of 5'6" size 10/12 forget about any hope of being a high fashion model this season. ... The industry looks for someone who is small to medium boned, fit but not buff. With a long graceful swan like neck, a square jaw and high strong cheek bones. ... Shoulder should be broad and squared and you should have a long legged look (more leg than torso).

Twenty years ago, gymnasts weighed about 20 lb more than today. Thus, it should come as little surprise that disordered eating patterns and unrealistic weight goals, and general dissatisfaction with one's body, remain common among girls and women of *all* ages.

requiring a reduction in training volume or intensity. The approach may take up to 1 year of nonpharmacologic intervention of weight gain with continuation of physical activity. When injuries to young amenorrheic ballet dancers prevent them from exercising regularly, normal menstruation resumes even though body weight remains low.

SUMMARY

1. Total body fat consists of essential fat and storage fat. Essential fat contains fat in bone marrow, nerve tissue, and organs; it does not represent an energy reserve but an important component for normal biologic function.
2. Storage fat, the energy reserve, accumulates mainly as adipose tissue beneath the skin and deeper visceral depots.
3. Storage fat averages 12% of body weight for young adult men and 15% of body weight for women.
4. True gender differences exist for essential fat. It averages 3% body weight for men and 12% body weight for women.
5. The greater percentage of essential fat for women most likely relates to childbearing and hormonal functions (i.e., sex-specific essential fat).
6. A person probably cannot reduce body fat below the essential fat level and still maintain good health and optimal physiologic capacity.
7. Menstrual dysfunction occurs among female athletes who train hard, incur an energy deficit, and maintain low levels of body fat.
8. Potential causes of menstrual dysfunction include a complex interplay of factors including the psychological stress of consistent training and competition, hormonal balance, energy and nutrient intake, and body composition.

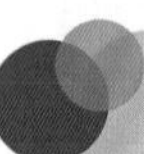

THINK IT THROUGH

1. What arguments counter the position that no true sex difference exists in body fat, but only a difference caused by gender-related patterns of regular physical activity and caloric intake?

PART 2 Assessing Body Size and Composition

Two general approaches can determine the fat and fat-free components of the human body:

1. Direct measurement by chemical analysis or dissection
2. Indirect estimation by hydrostatic weighing, simple anthropometric measurements, and other clinical and laboratory procedures, including body stature and body weight

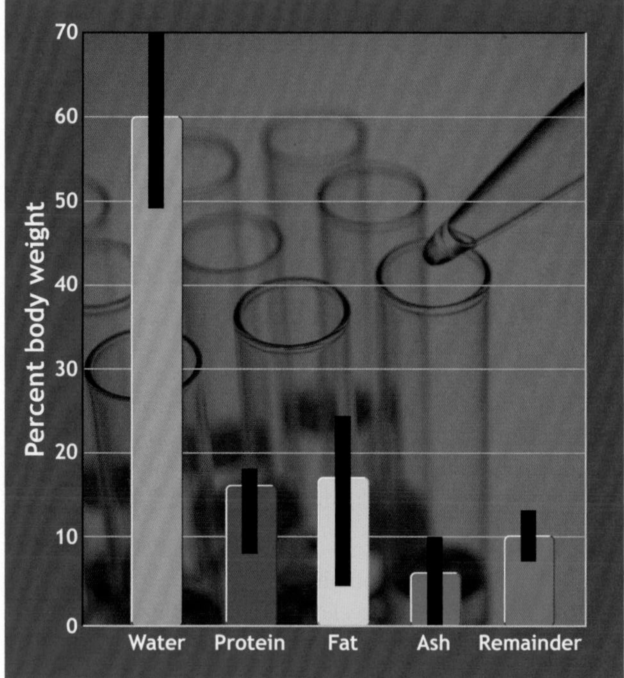

FIGURE 16.5 Various tissues in the adult male and female body based on cadaver analysis expressed as a percentage of total body mass (in kilogram). (Adapted with permission from Clarys JP, et al. Gross tissue weights in the human body by cadaver dissection. *Hum Biol* 1984;56:459.)

DIRECT ASSESSMENT

Two methods directly assess body composition. One technique dissolves a cadaver in a chemical solution to determine its mixture of fat and fat-free components. The other technique involves physical dissection of fat, fat-free adipose tissue, muscle, and bone. Such analyses require extensive time, meticulous attention to detail, and specialized laboratory equipment and pose ethical questions and legal problems in obtaining cadavers for research purposes.

The most complete physical dissection study was published in 1984. Analyses for each cadaver included removing skeletal muscle and the brain, heart, lungs, liver, kidneys, and spleen. Bones were then separated at their articulations and scraped to leave surfaces free of muscle and adipose tissue. Muscle included the ligaments, and bone retained the cartilage of any articular surface. Airtight plastic buckets stored all dissected tissues, including scrapings. The tissues were weighed to within 0.1 g and their densities determined as the ratio of weight to volume. Complete dissection took approximately 15 hours and required a team of 10 to 12 anatomists and kinesiologists.

Figure 16.5 presents the combined results from 25 male and female embalmed cadavers ranging in age from 55 to 94. The height of each bar indicates the arithmetic mean for the cadaver components expressed as a percentage of body weight, and the black vertical bars represent the range.

A separate analyses of the males and females revealed that the average adipose tissue weight in women equated to 40.5% of total body weight and 28.1% in men. The researchers introduced the concept of **adipose tissue–free weight (ATFW)**—the whole-body weight minus the weight of all dissectible adipose tissue that contains about 83% pure fat. Muscle accounted for 52% of the ATFW in men and 48.1% in women, and bone constituted 19.9% of ATFW in men and 21.3% in women. For the combined men and women data, the average proportion of the ATFW included 8.5% skin, 50.0% muscle, and 20.6% bone.

Direct body composition assessment suggests that while considerable individual differences exist in total body fatness, the compositions of skeletal weight and the fat-free and fat tissues remain relatively stable. The assumed constancy of these tissues allows researchers to develop mathematical equations to indirectly predict the body's fat percentage.

INDIRECT ASSESSMENT

Many indirect procedures assess body composition. One involves **Archimedes' principle** applied to hydrostatic weighing (also referred to as *hydrodensitometry* or *underwater weighing*). This method computes percentage body fat from **body density (Db)**; ratio of body weight to body volume). Other procedures predict body fat from skinfold thickness and girth measurements (**anthropometry**), x-ray, total body electrical conductivity (TOBEC) or bioelectrical impedance analysis (BIA) (including segmental impedance), near-infrared interactance (NIR), ultrasound, computed tomography (CT), **air plethysmography (BOD POD)**, and magnetic resonance imaging (MRI).

Hydrostatic Weighing (Archimedes' Principle)

The Greek mathematician, engineer, researcher, and inventor Archimedes (287–212 B.C.) discovered a fundamental principle currently applied to evaluate human body composition (**Fig. 16.6**) (**http://ed.ted.com/lessons/mark-salata-how-taking-a-bath-led-to-archimedes-principle**). Legend has it that an itinerant scholar of that time described the circumstances surrounding the event as follows:

> King Hieron of Syracuse suspected that his pure gold crown had been altered by substitution of silver for gold. The King directed Archimedes to devise a method for testing the crown for its gold content without dismantling it. Archimedes pondered over this problem for many weeks without succeeding, until one day, he stepped into a bath filled to the top with water and observed the overflow. He thought about this for a moment, and then, wild with joy, jumped from the bath and ran naked through the streets of Syracuse shouting, "Eureka, Eureka! I have discovered a way to solve the mystery of the king's crown."

Archimedes reasoned that a substance such as gold must have a volume proportional to its weight; measuring the volume of an irregularly shaped object would require submersion in water with collection of the overflow. Essentially,

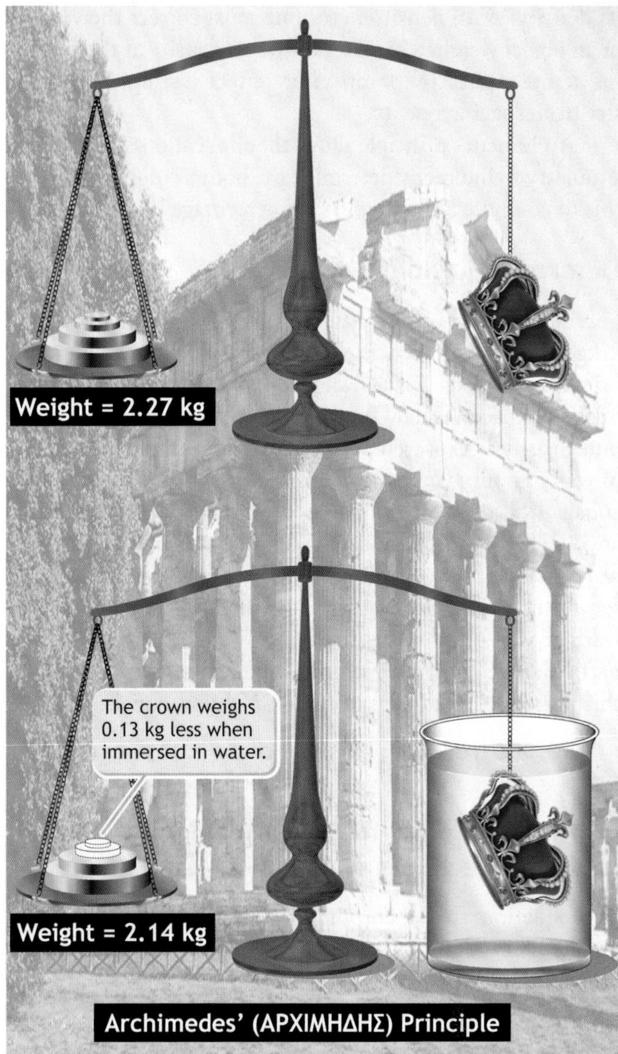

FIGURE 16.6 Archimedes' principle for determining the volume and specific gravity of the king's crown.

Archimedes compared the **specific gravity** of the crown with the specific gravities for gold and silver. He also reasoned that an object submerged or floating in water becomes buoyed up by a counterforce that equals the weight of the volume of water it displaces. This buoyant force supports an immersed object against gravity's downward pull so an object loses weight in water. *The object's loss of weight in water equals the weight of the volume of water it displaces, so its specific gravity refers to the weight of an object in air divided by its loss of weight in water.* The loss equals the weight in air minus the weight in water.

$$\text{Specific gravity} = \text{Weight in air} \div \text{Loss of weight in water}$$

One can think of specific gravity as an object's "heaviness" related to its volume. Objects of the same volume may vary considerably in density (defined as weight per unit volume). One gram of water occupies exactly 1 cm^3 at a temperature of 39.2°F (4°C); the density equals 1 $g \cdot cm^{-3}$. Water achieves its greatest density at 4°C; increasing water temperature increases the volume of 1 g of water and decreases its density. With densitometry, one must correct the volume of an object weighed in water for water density at the weighing temperature. The temperature effect distinguishes density from specific gravity.

Archimedes' principle allows the application of hydrodensitometry to indirectly determine the body's volume and from this to compute body density and percentage body fat.

Determining Body Density

For illustrative purposes, suppose a 50-kg woman weighs 2 kg when submerged in water. According to Archimedes' principle, a 48-kg *loss* of weight in water equals the weight of the displaced water. The volume of water displaced computes easily because chemists have determined the density of water at any temperature. In this example, 48 kg of water equals 48 L or 48,000 cm^3 (1 g of water = 1 cm^3 by volume at 39.2°F [4°C]). If the woman were measured at the cold water temperature of 39.2°F (4°C), no density correction for water would be necessary. In practice, researchers use warmer water and apply the density value for water at the particular weighing temperature. The whole-body density of this person, computed as Weight ÷ Volume, equals:

$$\mathbf{50{,}000\ g\ or\ 50\ kg \div 48{,}000\ cm^3 = 1.0417\ g \cdot cm^3}$$

Computing Percentage Body Fat, Fat Mass, and Fat-Free Body Mass

The equation that incorporates whole-body density from underwater weighing to estimate the body's fat percentage is derived from the following three premises:

1. Densities of the FM (all extractable lipid from adipose and other body tissues) and FFM (remaining lipid-free tissues and chemicals, including water) remain relatively constant (fat tissue = 0.90 $g \cdot cm^{-3}$; fat-free tissue = 1.10 $g \cdot cm^{-3}$), even with variations in total body fat and FFM components of bone and muscle.
2. Densities for the components of the FFM at a body temperature of 98.6°F (37°C) remain constant within and among individuals: water, 0.9937 $g \cdot cm^{-3}$ (73.8% of FFM); mineral, 3.038 $g \cdot cm^{-3}$ (6.8% of FFM); and protein, 1.340 $g \cdot cm^{-3}$ (19.4% of FFM).
3. The person measured differs from the reference body only in fat content (reference body assumed to possess 73.8% water, 19.4% protein, and 6.8% mineral).

Siri Equation to Predict Percentage Body Fat

Berkeley biophysicist Dr. **William Siri** (1926–2004) collaborated with Dr. Albert Behnke, then working at Berkeley's School of Public Health on a way to convert body density measurements to body fat, which led to his formulation of the "Siri equation" to compute percentage body fat from whole-body density.

Siri's simplified equation substitutes 0.90 $g \cdot cm^{-3}$ for the density of fat and 1.10 $g \cdot cm^{-3}$ for the density of the fat-free tissues:

$$\mathbf{Percentage\ body\ fat = 495 \div Body\ density - 450}$$

Based on the previous three assumptions, the following example incorporates the body density value of

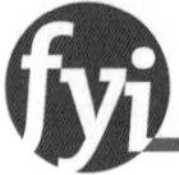

William Siri: Another Side of an Extraordinary Scientist

William "Will" Siri, a leading biophysics researcher at the Lawrence Berkeley National Laboratory, CA (**www.lbl.gov**), a past president of the Sierra Club, and a longtime environmental activist, climbed some of the world's tallest mountains in the name of science and in 1963 was deputy leader and scientific coordinator of the first American expedition to successfully climb Mt. Everest. Regarded as one of the world's foremost mountain-climbing scientists, Siri participated in or led scientific climbing expeditions around the world to study the effects of altitude and oxygen deprivation on the human body, including his own.

Siri led a 1954 effort to reach the top of 27,765-foot Makalu in the Himalayas, the fifth highest peak in the world. The 10-man party made it as high as 23,000 feet before bad weather forced abandonment of the effort. While on the same venture, Siri helped rescue a member of Sir Edmund Hillary's climbing team from an icy crevasse. Hillary and his Nepalese Sherpa guide, Tenzing Norgay, had made history a year earlier when they became the first men to reach the summit of Everest, the world's tallest mountain.

Ten years after Hillary and Norgay's feat, Siri made news himself as deputy leader and scientific coordinator of the 1963 expedition that succeeded in putting five Americans atop the 29,035-foot Everest. Siri, who did not attempt to reach the summit, spent most of his time at the 22,000-foot base camp but was at the 24,000-foot level for several days. Before the Everest climb, Siri spent 4 days in a decompression chamber at Donner Laboratory (**www2.lbl.gov/Publications/75th/files/04-lab-history-pt-3.html**) on the UC Berkeley campus in an experiment to measure physiological response to high altitudes. His experiment and the Everest climb were part of his ongoing research on the stress induced by hypoxia (lack of oxygen) and high-altitude fatigue and the resulting effects on the production of red blood cells.

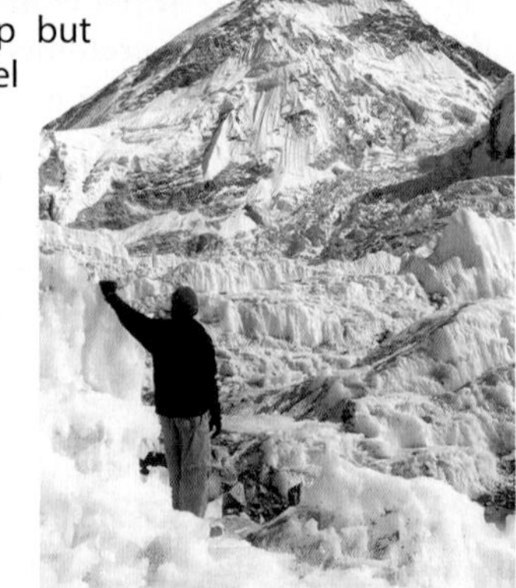

"If nothing else," Siri told a San Francisco newspaper after the successful Everest climb, and before he was honored by President Kennedy at the White House for the accomplishment, "we proved to the world that not all Americans are soft and flabby."

1.0417 g · cm^{-3} (determined for the woman in the previous example):

$$\text{Percentage body fat} = 495 \div \text{Body density} - 450 = 495 \div 1.0417 - 450 = 25.2\%$$

The weight of body fat is calculated by multiplying body weight by percentage fat:

$$\text{Fat mass (kg)} = \text{Body mass (kg)} \times (\text{Percentage fat} \div 100) = 50\ \text{kg} \times 0.252 = 12.6\ \text{kg}$$

Subtracting mass of fat from body mass yields FFM:

$$\text{FFM (kg)} = \text{Body mass (kg)} - \text{Fat mass (kg)} = 50\ \text{kg} - 12.6\ \text{kg} = 37.4\ \text{kg}$$

In this example, 25.2% or 12.6 kg (27.8 lb) of the 50-kg body mass consists of fat, with the remaining 37.4 kg (82.5 lb) representing the FFM component.

Several other equations also estimate percentage body fat from body density. The basic difference among the formulae to calculate body fat generally averages less than 1% body fat units for body fat levels between 4% and 30%.

Limitations of Density Assumptions

The generalized density values for fat-free tissue (1.10 g · cm^{-3}) and fat tissue (0.90 g · cm^{-3}) represent averages for young and middle-aged white adults. These "constants" vary among individuals and demographic groups, particularly the density and FFM chemical composition. Such variation places some limitation in partitioning body mass into fat and fat-free components and predicting percentage body fat from whole-body density. Specifically, average density of the FFM is higher for blacks and Hispanics than for whites (1.113 g · cm^{-3} blacks, 1.105 g · cm^{-3} Hispanics, and 1.100 g · cm^{-3} whites). Racial differences also exist among adolescents. Consequently, existing equations formulated from assumptions for whites to calculate body composition from body density in blacks or Hispanics *overestimate* FFM and *underestimate* percentage body fat. The following modification of Siri's equation computes percentage body fat from body density for blacks:

$$\text{Percentage body fat} = 437.4 \div \text{Body density} - 392.8$$

Applying constant density values for different tissues in growing children or aging adults also introduces errors in predicting body composition. For example, the water and mineral contents of the FFM continually change during growth; at the other end of the age spectrum, the demineralization of osteoporosis occurs with aging. Reduced bone density makes the density of the fat-free tissue of young children and older adults lower than the assumed 1.10 g · cm^{-3} constant. This invalidates assumptions of constant densities of fat and FFMs in the two-compartment model and *overestimates* **relative body fat (%BF)** calculated from densitometry. For this reason, many researchers do not convert body density to percentage body fat in children and aging adults. Others apply a multicompartment model to adjust for such factors to compute percentage body fat from body density in prepubertal children. **Table 16.2** provides equations adjusted to maturation level to predict percentage body fat from whole-body density of boys and girls ages 7 to 17.

Table 16.3 presents density estimates of FFM for different adult male and female population subgroups and equations to predict percentage body fat. These were derived from whole-body density based on assumptions regarding the densities and proportions of the body's protein, mineral, and water content. Obviously, different equations to convert body density to percentage body fat yield different values depending on their underlying assumptions. This variation does not reflect an inherent error in the underwater weighing method; rather, hydrostatic weighing to assess body volume generates a relatively small technical error for this variable of less than 1%.

Body Volume Measurement

Figure 16.7 illustrates three examples of body volume measurements by hydrostatic weighing. First, the subject's body mass in air is assessed to the nearest ±50 g (1.76 oz). A diver's belt secured around the waist prevents less dense (more fat) subjects from floating to the surface during submersion. Seated with the head out of water, the subject then makes a forced maximal exhalation while lowering the head just beneath the water. The breath is held for several seconds while the underwater weight is recorded.

TABLE 16.2 Percentage Body Fat Estimated From Body Density (Db) Using Age- and Gender-Specific Conversion Constants to Account for Changes in the Density of the Fat-Free Body Mass as a Child Matures

Age, y	Boys	Girls
7–9	%Fat = (5.38/Db – 4.97) × 100	%Fat = (5.43/Db – 5.03) × 100
9–11	%Fat = (5.30/Db – 4.86) × 100	%Fat = (5.35/Db – 4.95) × 100
11–13	%Fat = (5.23/Db – 4.81) × 100	%Fat = (5.25/Db – 4.84) × 100
13–15	%Fat = (5.08/Db – 4.64) × 100	%Fat = (5.12/Db – 4.69) × 100
15–17	%Fat = (5.03/Db – 4.59) × 100	%Fat = (5.07/Db – 4.64) × 100

From Lohman T. Applicability of body composition techniques and constants for children and youth. *Exerc Sports Sci Rev* 1986;14:325.

TABLE 16.3 Equations to Predict Percentage Body Fat From Body Density (Db) Based on Different Estimates of the Fat-Free Body Density (FFDb)

Age, y	Equation	FFDb[a]
Male		
White		
7–12	%Fat = 5.08/Db – 4.89	1.084
13–16	%Fat = 5.07/Db – 4.64	1.094
17–19	%Fat = 4.99/Db – 4.55	1.098
20–80	%Fat = 4.95/Db – 4.50	1.100
African American		
18–22	%Fat = 4.37/Db – 3.93	1.113
Japanese		
18–48	%Fat = 4.97/Db – 4.52	1.099
61–78	%Fat = 4.87/Db – 4.41	1.105
Female		
White		
7–12	%Fat = 5.35/Db – 4.95	1.082
13–16	%Fat = 5.10/Db – 4.66	1.093
17–19	%Fat = 5.05/Db – 4.62	1.095
20–80	%Fat = 5.01/Db – 4.57	1.097
Native American		
18–60	%Fat = 4.81/Db – 4.34	1.108
African American		
24–79	%Fat = 4.85/Db – 4.39	1.106
Hispanic		
20–40	%Fat = 4.87/Db – 4.41	1.105
Japanese		
18–48	%Fat = 4.76/Db – 4.28	1.111
61–78	%Fat = 4.95/Db – 4.50	1.100
Anorexic		
15–30	%Fat = 5.26/Db – 4.83	1.087
Obese		
17-62	%Fat = 5.00/Db – 4.56	1.098

Equations from the research literature.

[a]Each estimate of the fat-free body density (FFDB) uses slightly different values for the proportions of the body's protein, mineral, and water content.

The subject repeats this procedure 8 to 12 times to obtain a dependable or "true" underwater weight score. Even when achieving a full exhalation, a small volume of air, the **residual lung volume (RLV)**, remains in the lungs. Thus, the calculation of body volume requires subtraction of this buoyant effect of the RLV. This can be measured immediately before, during, or shortly following underwater weighing.

Rationale for Measuring Residual Volume

The largest source of error in calculating body volume by hydrostatic weighing results from errors in measuring RLV. Failure to account for RLV *underestimates* whole-body density because the lungs' air volume contributes to buoyancy. This omission creates a "fatter" person when converting body density to percentage body fat. Even under field conditions (i.e., at a sports training site; **Fig. 16.7A, C**), assessment of residual volume cannot be neglected. Its measurement requires specialized equipment and trained personnel. In situations that do not demand research-level accuracy (general screening, fitness assessments, teaching laboratories), RLV prediction equations based on age, stature, body mass, or vital capacity provide an appropriate estimate (see A Closer Look: "Predicting Residual Lung Volume").

Menstrual Cycle Effects on Body Fat Computations

Normal fluctuations in body mass, chiefly body water, during the menstrual cycle generally do not affect body density and body fat assessed by hydrostatic weighing. Some females, however, experience noticeable increases in body water exceeding 1.0 kg (2.2 lb) just preceding and during menstruation. Water retention of this magnitude affects body density slightly and introduces a small error in computing percentage body fat.

Body Volume Measurement by Air Displacement

Techniques other than hydrodensitometry can reliably assess body volume. **Figure 16.8** illustrates the BOD POD, a plethysmographic device used to assess body volume and its changes for groups that range from infants to older adults to collegiate wrestlers and exceptionally large NFL professional football and NBA basketball players. Essentially, body volume equals the chamber's reduced air volume when the subject enters the 750-L volume, dual-chamber fiberglass shell. The molded front seat separates the unit into front and rear chambers. The electronics housed in the rear chamber contain the pressure

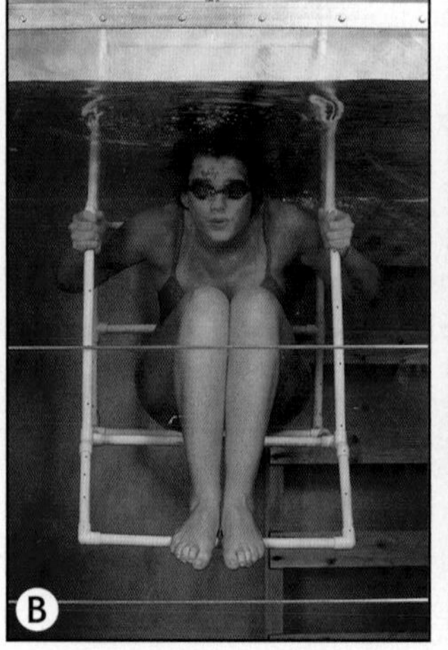

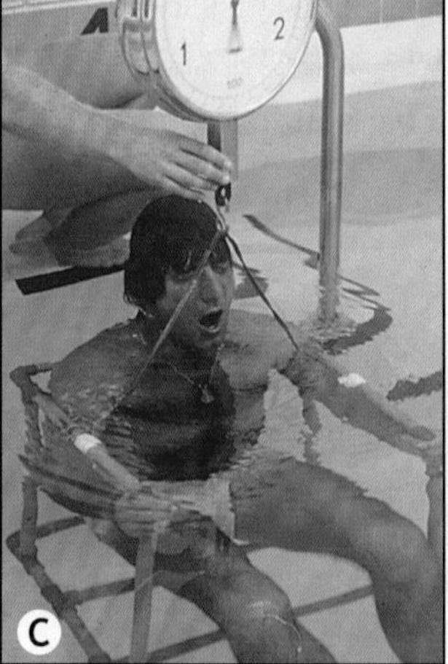

FIGURE 16.7 Measuring body volume using underwater weighing in **(A)** swimming pool, **(B)** stainless steel tank in the laboratory, **(C)** therapy pool at a pro football training facility.

transducers, breathing circuit, and air circulation system. Changes in pressure between the two chambers oscillate the diaphragm, which directly reflects any change in chamber volume. The subject makes several breaths into an air circuit to assess thoracic gas volume (which when subtracted from measured body volume yields true body volume). Body density computes as body mass (measured in air) ÷ body volume (measured by BOD POD), including a correction for a small negative volume caused by isothermal effects related to skin surface area. The Siri equation converts body density to percentage body fat. Numerous studies have assessed reliability and validity of BOD POD compared with other criterion body composition methods in children; young, middle-aged, and older adults; diverse ethnic groups; obese individuals; persons with disabilities and diseases including diabetes and obesity; and different categories of male and female athletes.

A CLOSER LOOK

Predicting Residual Lung Volume

The RLV represents a large and variable gas volume that must be subtracted to accurately determine body volume. Laboratory techniques such as helium dilution (**http://nutrition.uvm.edu/bodycomp/uww/helium.html**) and nitrogen washout routinely measure RLV. Each procedure requires complicated and expensive laboratory equipment. An alternate, although less valid, approach estimates RLV with gender-specific prediction equations based on age, stature, and body mass. The standard error of estimate to predict RLV ranges between ±325 and 500 mL; this can correspond to errors in predicting percentage body fat of up to ±2.5% or more body fat units.

Residual Lung Volume Prediction Equations

Variables: Age, years; stature (St), cm; body mass (BM), kg

Normal-weight men:

$$\text{RLV, L} = (0.022 \times \text{Age}) + (0.0198 \times \text{St}) - (0.015 \times \text{BM}) - 1.54$$

Normal-weight women (uses only age and stature):

$$\text{RLV, L} = (0.007 \times \text{Age}) + (0.0268 \times \text{St}) - 3.42$$

Overfat men (%Fat ≥25) and women (%Fat ≥30):

$$\text{RLV, L} = (0.0167 \times \text{Age}) + (0.0130 \times \text{BM}) \times (0.0185 \times \text{St}) - 3.3413$$

Examples

1. Man: Age, 21 years; body mass, 80 kg (176.4 lb); stature, 182.9 cm (72 in.)

$$\begin{aligned}\text{RLV (L)} &= (0.022 \times 21) + (0.0198 \times 182.9) - (0.015 \times 80) - 1.54\\ &= 0.462 + 3.621 - 1.2 - 1.54\\ &= 1.34\ \text{L}\end{aligned}$$

2. Woman: Age, 19 years; stature, 160.0 cm (63 in.)

$$\begin{aligned}\text{RLV (L)} &= (0.007 \times 19) + (0.0268 \times 160.0) - 3.42\\ &= 0.133 + 4.288 - 3.42\\ &= 1.00\ \text{L}\end{aligned}$$

3. Overfat man: Age, 35 years; body mass, 104 kg (229.3 lb); stature, 179.5 cm (70.7 in.)

$$\begin{aligned}\text{RLV (L)} &= (0.0167 \times 35) + (0.0130 \times 104) + (0.0185 \times 179.5) - 3.3413\\ &= 0.5845 + 1.352 + 3.321 - 3.3413\\ &= 1.39\ \text{L}\end{aligned}$$

Sources: Grimby G, Söderholm B. Spirometric studies in normal subjects III: static lung volumes and maximum ventilatory ventilation in adults with a note on physical fitness. *Acta Med Scand* 1963;173:199.

Miller WCT, et al. Derivation of prediction equations for RV in overweight men and women. *Med Sci Sports Exerc* 1998;30:322.

Morrow JR Jr, et al. Accuracy of measured and predicted residual lung volume on body density measurement. *Med Sci Sports Exerc* 1986;18:647.

Skinfold Measurements

Simple anthropometric procedures can successfully predict body fatness. The most common of these procedures uses **skinfolds**. The rationale for using skinfolds to estimate the body's fat composition results from the close interrelationships among three factors:

1. Subcutaneous fat in adipose tissue deposits directly beneath the skin
2. Body's internal fat stores
3. Density of the intact human body

The Caliper

As early as 1930, a special pincer-type caliper was in use to accurately measure subcutaneous fat at selected body sites. **Skinfold calipers** work on the same principle as a micrometer to measure the distance between two points. The pincer jaws exert a constant tension of 10 g · mm^{-2} at the point of contact with the double layer of skin plus subcutaneous tissue. The caliper dial indicates skinfold thickness in millimeters.

Figure 16.9 illustrates three different types of skinfold calipers. Compared with the most costly calipers (Harpenden and Lange), the less expensive plastic models are less precise,

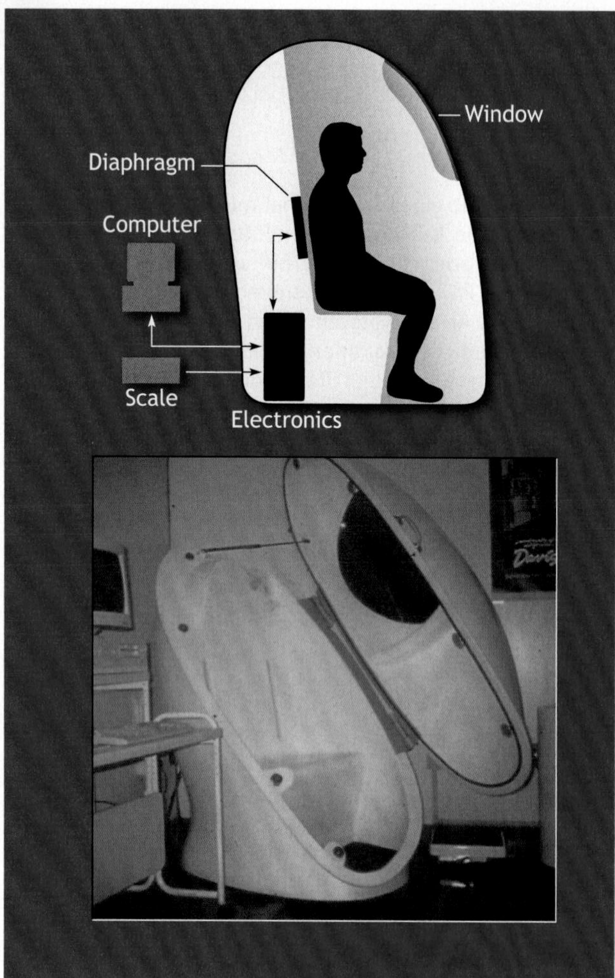

FIGURE 16.8 **(Top)** Major system components of the BOD POD (**bottom image**), the air displacement chamber used to measure total body volume by air displacement. (Photo courtesy of Life Sciences Instruments, Concord, CA.)

exert nonconstant jaw tension throughout the range of measurement, usually have a smaller measurement scale (<60 mm), and produce less consistent scores at the same skinfold site when used by inexperienced testers.

Measuring skinfold thickness requires grasping a fold of skin and subcutaneous fat firmly with the thumb and forefingers and pulling it away from the underlying muscle tissue following the skinfold's natural contour. The skinfold is recorded within 2 seconds after applying the full force of the caliper. This time limitation avoids skinfold compression (see A Closer Look: "When Should Skinfold Readings Be Taken"). For research purposes, the investigator should attain considerable experience in taking measurements and demonstrate consistency in duplicating skinfold values at multiple sites for the same subject made on the same day, consecutive days, or even weeks apart. A good rule of thumb to achieve consistency requires taking duplicate or triplicate practice measurements at all skinfold sites on approximately 50 males and females who range in body fat from "thin" to "obese," including athletes of various body configurations (e.g., diminutive gymnasts, lightweight wrestlers, tall rowers, volleyball and basketball players). Careful attention to details before making "real" measurements helps to ensure greater measurement reproducibility.

Skinfold Sites

Common anatomic sites for skinfold measurement include triceps, subscapular, suprailiac, abdominal, and upper thigh sites. The investigator should take a minimum of two or three measurements in rotational order at each site on the right side of the body with the subject standing. The average value represents the skinfold score. Except for the subscapular and suprailiac sites, which should be measured diagonally, all measurements should be taken in the vertical plane. The *lower right schematic* in **Figure 16.10** shows a skinfold caliper and compression of a double layer of skin and underlying tissue during the measurement along with the anatomic location for five of the most frequently measured skinfold sites:

1. *Triceps*: Vertical fold at the posterior midline of the upper arm, halfway between the tip of the shoulder and tip of the elbow; elbow remains in an extended, relaxed position
2. *Subscapular*: Oblique fold just below the bottom tip of the scapula
3. *Suprailiac* (iliac crest): Slightly oblique fold just above the hip bone (crest of ileum); the fold follows the natural diagonal line
4. *Abdomen*: Vertical fold 1 inch to the right of the umbilicus
5. *Thigh*: Vertical fold at the midline of the thigh, two thirds of the distance from the middle of the patella (knee cap) to the hip

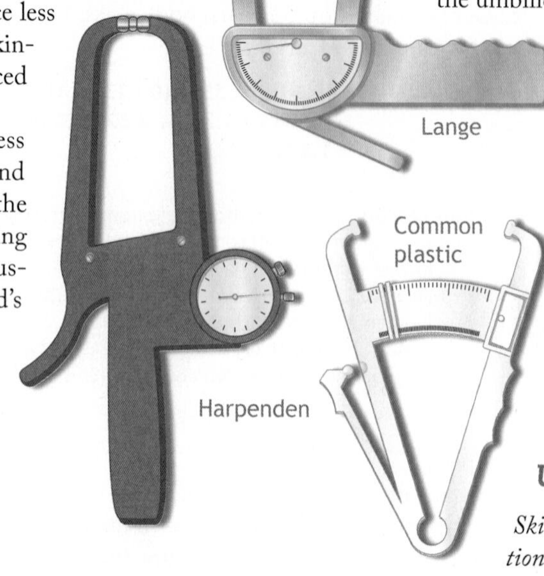

FIGURE 16.9 Common calipers to measure subcutaneous fat.

Additional measurement sites include *chest* (diagonal fold with long axis directed toward the right nipple; on the anterior axillary fold as high as possible) and *biceps* (vertical fold at the posterior midline of the right upper arm).

Usefulness of Skinfolds

Skinfolds provide meaningful information about body fat and its distribution. We recommend two practical ways to use skinfolds:

1. Sum individual skinfold values; this "sum of skinfolds" (ΣSkf) indicates relative fatness among individuals; it also reflects either absolute or percentage skinfold changes before and after an intervention program.
2. Apply mathematical equations to predict body density or percentage body fat from the individual skinfold values or the ΣSkf. The equations prove accurate for subjects similar in age, gender, training status, fatness, and race to the group from which they were derived.

When meeting these two criteria, predicted body fat for an individual usually ranges between 3% and 5% body fat units computed from body density with hydrostatic weighing.

A CLOSER LOOK

When Should Skinfold Readings Be Taken?

A frequently asked question about taking skinfold measurements concerns when to read the caliper value. Should the caliper be left on the site for 1, 3, or 5 seconds or until the pointer stops moving?

Research-quality skinfold calipers exert an average compression force of 10 g per mm^2 at all jaw openings. This means that the caliper always exerts the same pressure regardless of skin-plus-fat thickness. After it is applied to the skinfold site, the caliper continues to displace subcutaneous interstitial water, connective tissue, and fat throughout the measurement period until the skinfold's rebound force counteracts the caliper pressure.

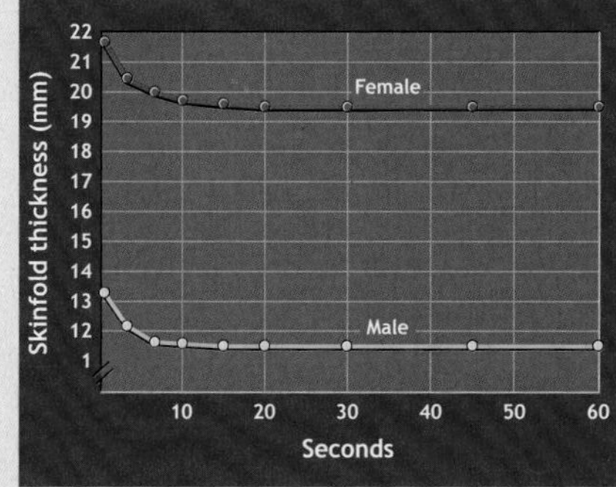

The *inset* chart shows the compression data for triceps skinfold for 18 men and 18 women. Modification of the caliper provided for an instantaneous record of skinfold thickness throughout the measurement period. More than 70% of the total compression of skin and underlying fat takes place within the first 4 seconds after applying the caliper. Thus, to record the uncompressed skin-plus-fat measurement, the reading should be made when applying the caliper to the skin as it exerts its full pressure and certainly within 1 or 2 seconds. Any prolonged delay in reading the caliper *underestimates* the actual skinfold value.

The absolute change in skinfold thickness among subjects over 60 seconds ranged between 0.3 and 4.5 mm. Although not a dramatic absolute change, this error can affect the accuracy of percentage body fat when using skinfold prediction equations. For example, using the initial uncompressed versus the final compressed skinfold value (after 60 s) produced differences in predicted percentage body fat that ranged between 2 and 8 fat percentage units (a 10% to 50% error). This large error cannot be ignored. Almost all of the research studies using skinfolds have not specified when they recorded their readings. One can only surmise that it occurred immediately after placing the calipers on the skin to obtain an uncompressed value.

Source: Becque DM, et al. Time course of skin-plus-fat compression in males and females. *Hum Biol* 1986;58:33.

Skinfolds, Body Fat, and Age

In young adults, approximately half of the body's total fat consists of subcutaneous fat, with the remainder stored as visceral and organ fat. With advancing age, a proportionately greater quantity of fat deposits internally compared with subcutaneous fat. Thus, the same skinfold score reflects a *greater* percentage body fat as one ages. *For this reason, age-adjusted, generalized equations should be used to predict body fat from skinfolds that apply to a broad age range of adult men and women* (see A Closer Look: "Choosing the Appropriate Skinfold Equation to Predict Body Fat in Diverse Populations"). We recommend ΣSkf and specific equations as the best alternative to accurately estimate the body's amount and distribution of fat. Researchers also have cautioned that acceleration of the "obesity epidemic" may require adjustment of generalized equations to predict body fat in subjects whose sum of seven skinfolds (chest, axilla, triceps, subscapular, abdominal, iliac, thigh) exceeds 120 mm.

A person can become a skilled skinfold technician by adhering to the following nine guidelines:

1. Precisely locate and mark anatomical landmarks for each site before taking any measurement.
2. Read caliper dial to nearest half marking (e.g., 0.5 mm) within 1 to 2 seconds of application of caliper to the skin.
3. Take a minimum of two measurements at each site and use the average as the skinfold score.
4. Take duplicate or triplicate measurements in rotational order rather than consecutive readings at each site to avoid a compression of the skin plus subcutaneous fat.
5. Do not take measurements for at least 15 minutes after the individual stops physical activity; the shift in body fluid to the skin spuriously increases the reading.
6. Practice on at least 50 males and females who vary in body size from "thin" to "obese" including athletes in different sports. As part of that practice, make multiple measurements at the different skinfold sites to gain experience before using the scores as "real" skinfold values.
7. Obtain training from previously skilled technicians in how to take skinfolds; this allows you to compare your results with the results of an "expert."
8. Take measurements on dry, lotion-free skin.

9. If possible, enroll in a course that deals with body composition assessment; some continuing education providers offer courses that award certifications of completion in body composition assessment procedures.

User Beware

Assessing skinfolds requires expertise with the proper measurement techniques. The particular caliper style, whether metal, spring-loaded, plastic, electronic, or wide and thin pincer pads, can contribute to measurement errors. Another error source occurs when assessing extremely overfat people; in such nonathletic individuals (usually weighing more than 300 lb), skinfold thickness often exceeds the width of the caliper's jaws. For these reasons, we advocate using girths as the anthropometric technique of choice for these individuals.

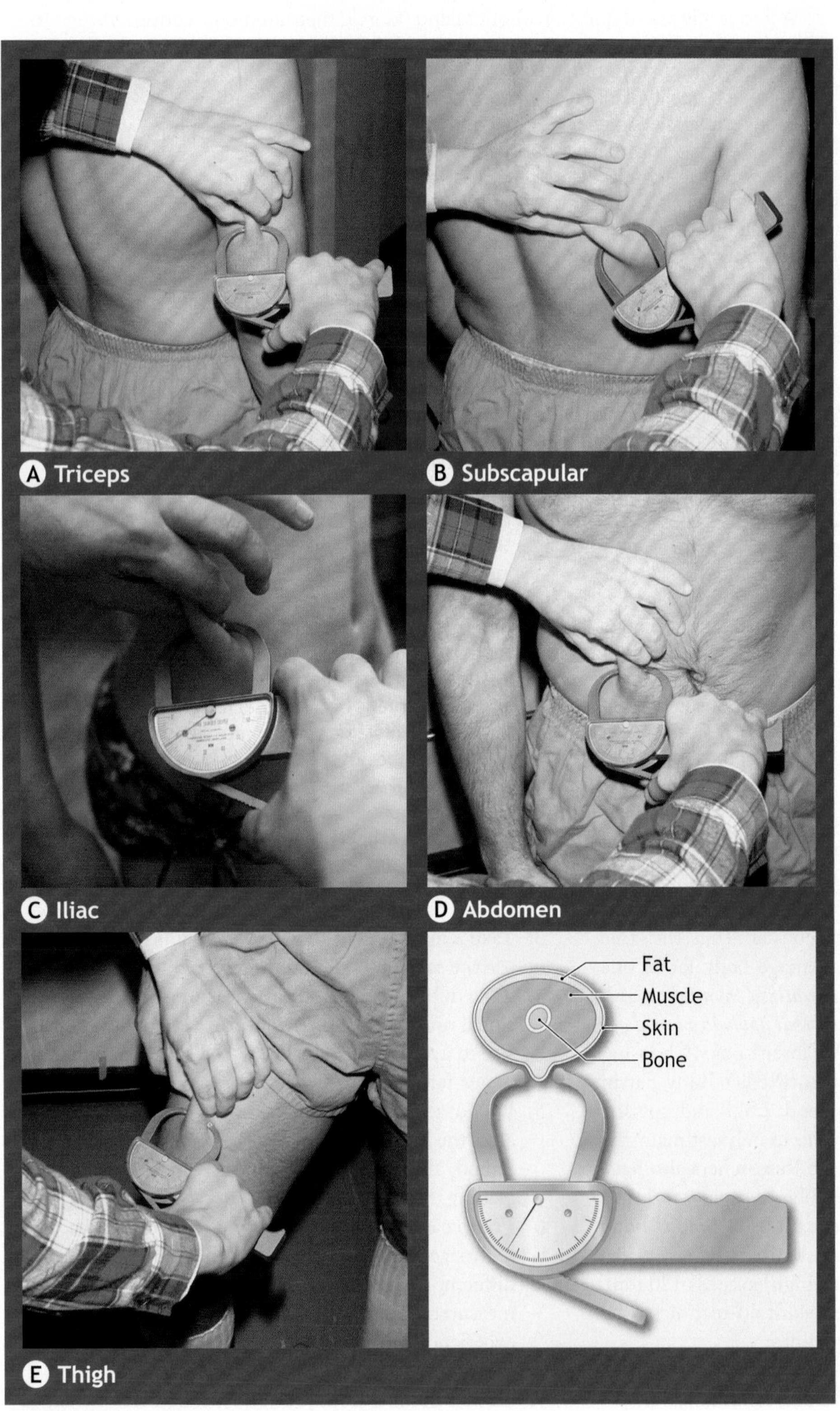

FIGURE 16.10 Anatomic location of five common skinfold sites: triceps **(A)**, subscapular **(B)**, suprailiac **(C)**, abdomen **(D)**, and thigh **(E)**.

Girth Measurements

Figure 16.11 shows the six most common sites for girth measurements. These include *abdomen, buttocks, thigh, right upper arm, right forearm,* and *calf.* Girths offer an easily administered and valid alternative to skinfolds. To avoid skin compression, apply a linen or plastic measuring tape lightly to the skin surface at the measurement site so the tape remains taut but not tight. Take duplicate measurements at each site and average the scores.

Usefulness of Girth Measurements

Girths prove most useful in ranking individuals within a group according to relative fatness. As with skinfolds, girth-based equations predict body density and/or percentage body fat with a certain amount of error, albeit relatively small. On average, for about 70 of every 100 people measured, the equations will predict body fat within the 2.5% to 4.0% body fat compared to predictions assessed by the more valid criteria hydrostatic weighing, DXA, or BOD POD. The extent of prediction error or measurement uncertainty depends largely on whether individuals have similar physical characteristics to the original validation group. In a

A CLOSER LOOK

Choosing the Appropriate Skinfold Equation to Predict Body Fat in Diverse Populations

More than 100 different equations exist to predict body density and percentage body fat from skinfolds. The equations, often formulated from homogeneous groups, incorporate between two and seven measurement sites to predict body density. The density value then converts to percentage body fat using an appropriate equation for the specific population. The different equations yield predicted values that at best usually fall within ±3% to 5% body fat units assessed by hydrostatic weighing.

Different Equations

The table presents examples of skinfold equations for different populations. The following abbreviations apply (all skinfolds in mm): ΣSkf = sum of skinfolds; tri = tricep; calf = calf; scap = subscapular; midax = midaxillary; iliac = suprailiac; abdo = abdomen; thigh = thigh; Db = whole-body density, g · cm^{-3}; BF = body fat; age in years (y).

Equations to Predict Percentage Body Fat From Skinfolds

Population	Age, y	Variables	Equation	Comments
Children				
Boys	6–10	tri + calf	%BF = 0.735 (Σ2Skf) + 1.0	
		tri + scap	%BF = 0.783 (Σ2Skf) + 1.6	Use when ΣSkf >35 mm
Girls	6–10	tri + calf	%BF = 0.610 (Σ2Skf) + 5.1	
		tri + scap	%BF = 0.546 (Σ2Skf) + 9.7	Use when ΣSkf >35 mm
Native Americans				
Women	18–60	tri + midax + iliac	Db = 1.061 – 0.000385 (Σ3Skf) – 0.000204 (age)	%BF = [(4.81 ÷ Db) – 4.34]100
African Americans				
Women	18–55	chest + abdo + thigh + tri + scap + iliac + midax	Db = 1.0970 – 0.00046971 (Σ7Skf) + 0.00000056 $(Σ7Skf)^2$ – 0.00012828 (age)	%BF = [(4.85 ÷ Db) – 4.39]100
Men	8–61	chest + abdo + thigh + tri + scap + iliac + midax	Db = 1.1120 – 0.00043499 (Σ7Skf) + 0.00000055 $(Σ7Skf)^2$ – 0.00028826 (age)	%BF = [(4.37 ÷ Db) – 3.93]100
Hispanics				
Women	20–40	chest + abdo + thigh + tri + scap + iliac + midax	Db = 1.10970 – 0.00046971 (Σ7Skf) + 0.00000056 $(Σ7Skf)^2$ – 0.00012828 (age)	%BF = [(4.87 ÷ Db) – 4.41]100
Native Japanese				
Women	18–23	tri + scap	Db = 1.0897 – 0.00133 (Σ2Skf)	%BF = [(4.76 ÷ Db) – 4.28]100
Men	18–27	tri + scap	Db = 1.0913 – 0.00116 (Σ2Skf)	%BF = [(4.97 ÷ Db) – 4.52]100
White Americans				
Women	18–55	tri + iliac + thigh	Db = 1.0994921 – 0.0009929 (Σ3Skf) + 0.00000023 $(Σ3Skf)^2$ – 0.0001392 (age)	%BF = [(5.01 ÷ Db) – 4.57]100
Men	18–55	chest + abdo + thigh	Db = 1.109380 – 0.0008267 (Σ3Skf) + 0.00000016 $(Σ3Skf)^2$ – 0.0002574 (age)	%BF = [(4.95 ÷ Db) – 4.50]100
Athletes (all sports)				
Men	18–29	tri + iliac + abdo + thigh	Db = 1.112 – 0.00043499 (Σ7Skf) + 0.00000055 $(Σ7Skf)^2$ – 0.00028826 (age)	%BF = [(5.01 ÷ Db) – 4.57]100
Women	18–29	chest + midax + tri + scap + abdo + iliac + thigh	Db = 1.096095 – 0.0006952 (Σ4Skf) + 0.0000011 $(Σ4Skf)^2$ – 0.0000714 (age)	%BF = [(4.95 ÷ Db) – 4.50]100

practical sense, such relatively small prediction errors make girth estimations of body fat useful to those without access to laboratory facilities, as in fitness and sports centers, and hospital and physical therapy facilities. Stated in another way, the most desirable situation occurs when the magnitude of measurement uncertainty remains as low as possible.

These equations should *not* be used to predict fatness in individuals who appear excessively thin or who participate regularly in strenuous sports or resistance training that can increase girth without altering subcutaneous fat. Specific equations based on girths are required to estimate body composition for clinically obese adult men and women (see A Closer Look: "How to Predict Percentage Body Fat from Girths for Overly Fat Men and Women"). Girths also can be used to analyze patterns of body fat distribution (**fat patterning**), including changes in fat distribution during weight loss and weight gain.

Predicting Body Fat From Girths

From the appropriate tables in Appendix D: Evaluation of Body Composition—Girth Method, substitute the corresponding constants A, B, and C in the formula shown at the bottom of each table. This requires one addition and two subtraction steps. The following five-step example shows how to compute percentage fat, FM, and FFM for a 21-year-old man who weighs 79.1 kg:

Step 1. Measure the upper arm, abdomen, and right forearm girths with a cloth tape to the nearest 0.25 inches (0.6 cm): upper arm = 11.5 inches (29.21 cm), abdomen = 31.0 inches (78.74 cm), right forearm = 10.75 inches (27.30 cm).

Step 2. Determine the three constants A, B, and C corresponding to the three girths from Appendix D: constant A corresponding to 11.5 inches = 42.56, constant B corresponding to 31.0 inches = 40.68, and constant C corresponding to 10.75 inches = 58.37.

Step 3. Compute percentage body fat by substituting the appropriate constants in the formula for young men shown at the bottom of Chart 1 in Appendix D as:

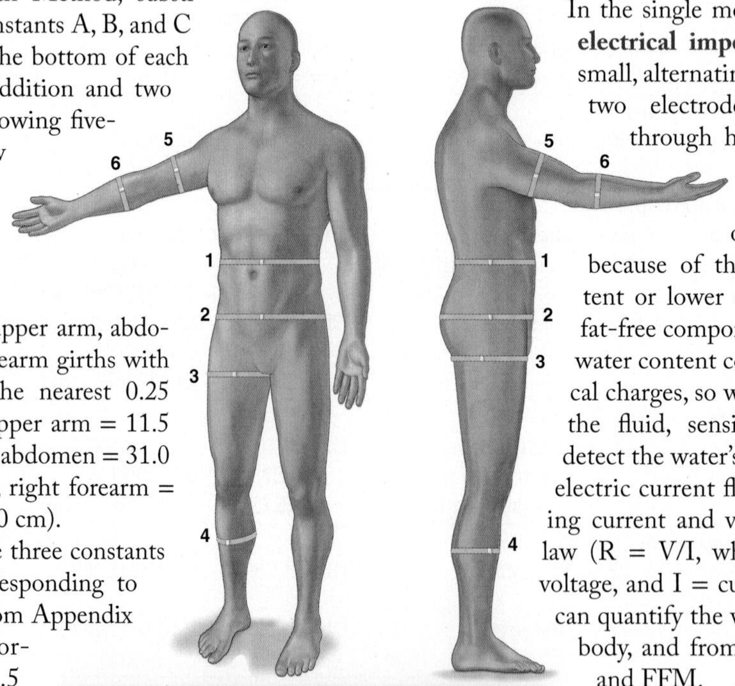

$$\begin{aligned}\textbf{Percentage Fat} &= \textbf{Constant A} + \textbf{Constant B} - \textbf{Constant C} - \textbf{10.2}\\ &= 42.56 + 40.68 - 58.37 - 10.2\\ &= 83.24 - 58.37 - 10.2\\ &= 24.87 - 10.2\\ &= 14.7\%\end{aligned}$$

Step 4. Calculate the mass of body fat as:

$$\begin{aligned}\textbf{Fat mass} &= \textbf{Body mass} \times (\%\textbf{Fat} \div 100)\\ &= 79.1\text{ kg} \times (14.7 \div 100)\\ &= 79.1\text{ kg} \times 0.147\\ &= 11.6\text{ kg}\end{aligned}$$

Step 5. Determine FFM as:

$$\begin{aligned}\textbf{FFM} &= \textbf{Body mass} - \textbf{Fat mass}\\ &= 79.1\text{ kg} - 11.63\text{ kg}\\ &= 67.5\text{ kg}\end{aligned}$$

1. **Abdomen:** 1 in above the umbilicus
2. **Buttocks:** Maximum protrusion of buttocks with the heels together
3. **Right thigh:** Upper thigh, just below the buttocks
4. **Right calf:** Widest girth midway between the ankle and knee
5. **Right upper arm (biceps):** Palm up, arm straight and extended in front of the body; taken at the midpoint between the shoulder and the elbow
6. **Right forearm:** Maximum girth with the arm extended in front of the body

FIGURE 16.11 Landmarks for measuring various girths at six common anatomic sites (see text for description). (Reproduced with permission from McArdle WD, Katch FI, Katch VL. *Exercise Physiology: Nutrition, Energy, and Human Performance*. 8th Ed. Baltimore: Wolters Kluwer Health, 2015.)

Bioelectrical Impedance Analysis

In the single mode of low-frequency **bioelectrical impedance analysis (BIA)**, a small, alternating current flowing between two electrodes passes more rapidly through hydrated fat-free body tissues and extracellular water compared with fat or bone tissue. This occurs because of the greater electrolyte content or lower electrical resistance of the fat-free component. In essence, the body's water content conducts the flow of electrical charges, so when current flows through the fluid, sensitive instrumentation can detect the water's impedance. Impedance to electric current flow, calculated by measuring current and voltage, is based on Ohm's law (R = V/I, where R = resistance, V = voltage, and I = current). These relationships can quantify the volume of water within the body, and from this, percentage body fat and FFM.

Bioelectrical impedance analysis requires measurement by trained personnel under strictly standardized conditions, particularly electrode placement and the subject's body position, hydration status, previous food and beverage intake, skin temperature, and recent physical activity. As **Figure 16.12** illustrates, the person lies on a flat nonconducting surface. Injector or source electrodes attach on the dorsal surfaces of the foot and wrist, and detector or sink electrodes attach between the radius and ulna (styloid process) and at the ankle between the medial and lateral malleoli.

Figure 16.12C illustrates the segmental measurement approach including electrode configuration to assess electric current (I) and voltage (V) for the right arm, trunk, and right leg. The person receives a painless, localized electrical current, and the impedance or resistance to current flow between the source and detector electrodes determined. Conversion of the impedance value to body density—adding body mass and stature, gender, age, and sometimes race, level of fatness, and several girths to the equation—computes percentage body fat from the Siri equation or other similar density conversion equation.

Hydration Level Affects Bioelectrical Impedance Analysis Accuracy

Hydration level negatively impacts BIA accuracy in determining body fat content. Hypohydration and hyperhydration alter the body's normal electrolyte concentrations; this in turn affects current flow independent of a real body composition change. For example, voluntary fluid restriction decreases impedance. This lowers percentage body fat estimate; hyperhydration produces the opposite effect and produces a higher body fat estimate. Skin temperature, influenced by ambient conditions, also affects whole-body resistance and BIA body fat prediction. Predicted body fat is lower in a warm environment than a cold one because moist skin produces less impedance to electrical flow

Even with normal hydration and environmental temperature, body fat predictions may be less valid compared with the criterion hydrostatic weighing method. BIA tends to overpredict body fat in lean and athletic subjects and underpredict body fat in fatter subjects. BIA often

A CLOSER LOOK

How to Predict Percentage Body Fat From Girths for Overly Fat Men and Women

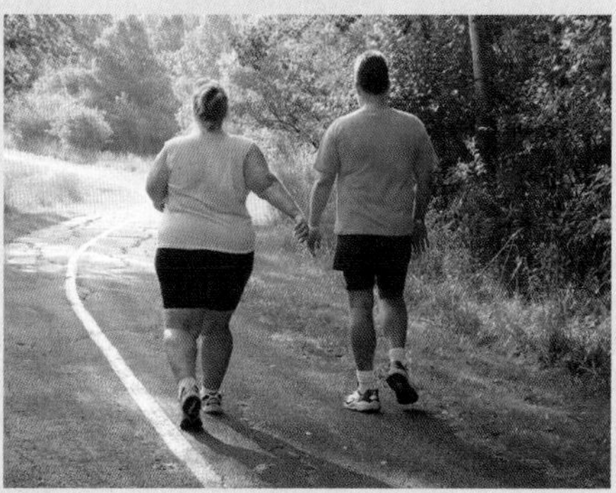

Estimating percentage body fat (%BF) in overly fat individuals by skinfold prediction becomes problematic from difficulty securing accurate and repeatable measurements owing to an extensive, unevenly distributed mass of subcutaneous fat. In addition, with increasing levels of body fatness, the proportion of subcutaneous fat to total body fat changes, thereby affecting the relationship between skinfolds and body density (Db). The following four factors limit skinfold use with overly fat individuals:

1. Difficulty of site selection and palpation of body landmarks
2. Skinfold thickness may exceed caliper jaw aperture
3. Variability in adipose tissue composition affects skinfold compressibility
4. Poorer objectivity in skinfold measures as body fat increases

Predicting Percentage Body Fat

Use the following equations to predict %BF in obese (>30%BF) women (age 20 to 60 y) and obese (>20%BF) men (age 24 to 68 y).

Women

$$\%BF = 0.11077(ABDO) - 0.17666(HT) + 0.14354(BW) + 51.03301$$

Men

$$\%BF = 0.31457(ABDO) - 0.10969(BW) + 10.8336$$

where ABDO = the average of (1) waist girth (taken horizontally at the level of the natural waist—narrowest part of the torso, as seen from the anterior) and (2) abdomen girth (taken horizontally at the level of the greatest anterior extension of the abdomen, usually, but not always, at the level of the umbilicus). Duplicate measurements are taken and averaged. BW = body weight in kilograms; HT = stature in centimeters.

Examples

1. Overly Fat Woman

Waist girth = 115 cm
Abdomen girth = 121 cm; HT = 165.1 cm; BW = 97.5 kg

$$\begin{aligned}\%BF &= 0.11077(ABDO) - 0.17666(HT) + 0.14354(BW) + 51.03301\\ &= 0.11077[(115+121)/2] - 0.17666(165.1)\\ &\quad + 0.14354(97.5) + 51.03301\\ &= 13.07 - 29.17 + 13.995 + 51.03301\\ &= 48.9\%\end{aligned}$$

2. Overly Fat Man

Waist girth = 131 cm
Abdomen girth = 136 cm; BW = 135.6 kg

$$\begin{aligned}\%BF &= 0.31457(ABDO) - 0.10969(BW) + 10.8336\\ &= 0.31457[(131.0+136.0)/2] - 0.10969(135.6) + 10.8336\\ &= 41.995 - 14.873 + 10.8336\\ &= 37.9\%\end{aligned}$$

Sources: Tran ZV, Weltman A. Predicting body composition of men from girth measurements. *Hum Biol* 1988;60:167.
Weltman A, et al. Accurate assessment of body composition in obese females. *Am J Clin Nutr* 1988;48:1178.

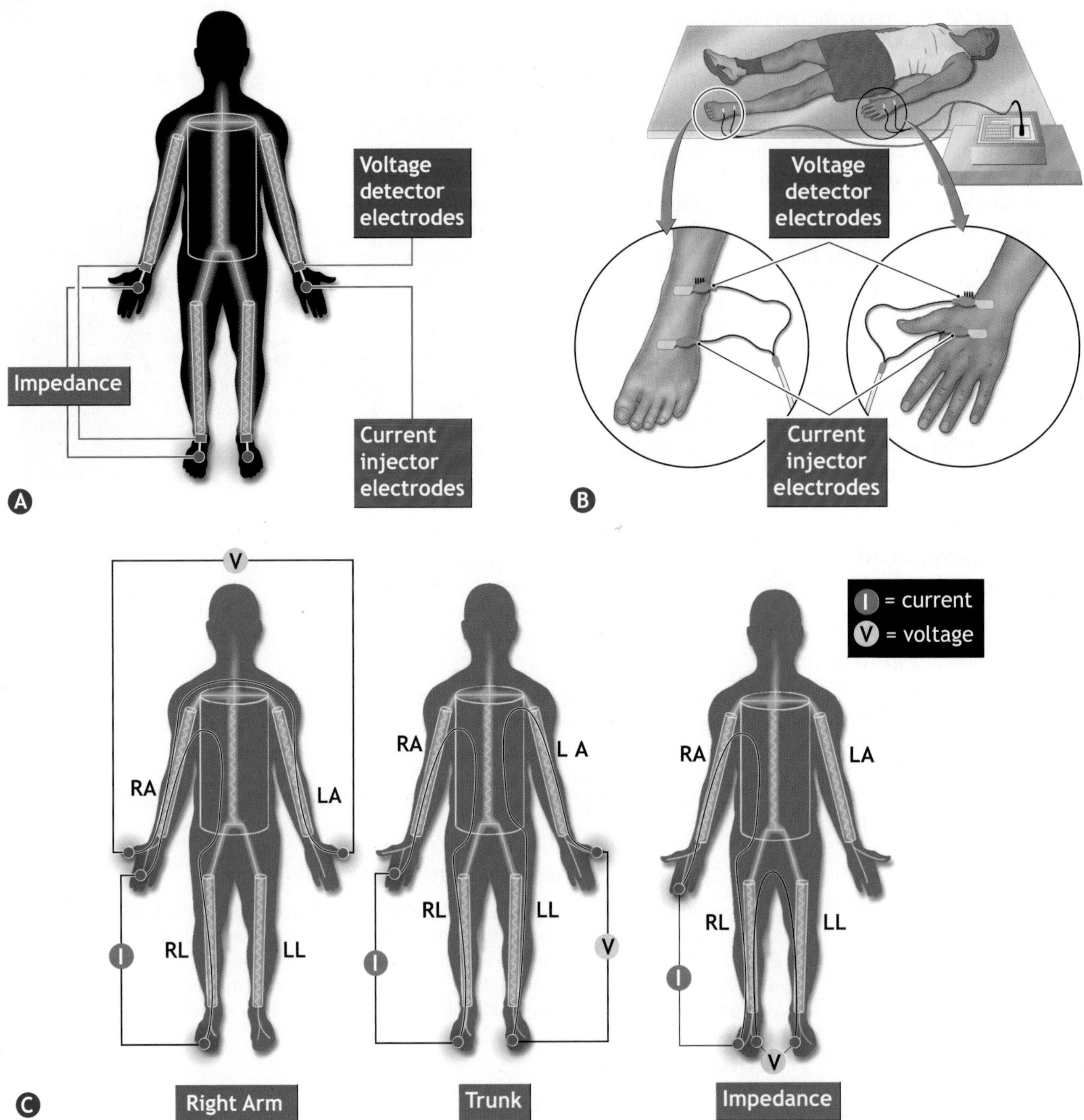

FIGURE 16.12 Method to assess body composition by bioelectrical impedance analysis. **A.** Whereas the four-surface electrode technique (whole-body impedance) applies current via one pair of distal (injector) electrodes, the proximal (detector) electrode pair measures electrical potential across the conducting segment. **B.** Standard placement of electrodes and body position during whole-body impedance measurement. **C.** Segmental measurement illustrating assessment of current (I) and voltage (V) for the right arm, trunk, and right leg.

predicts body fat less accurately than do girths and skinfolds. Whether BIA detects small changes in body composition during weight loss remains unclear. At best, BIA represents a noninvasive, safe, relatively easy, and generally reliable way to assess total body water. The tendency to overestimate percentage body fat increases when BIA is used for black athletes and lean subjects. Fatness-specific BIA equations exist that predict body fat for overfat and nonoverfat American Indian, Hispanic, white men and women, and diverse population groups. With proper measurement standardization, the menstrual cycle does not appear to affect body composition assessment by BIA. This area of research continues to remain active; a PubMed search from February 1975 through June, 2015 returned over 3428 articles (search terms "bioelectrical impedance body composition"), and 424 articles when the search terms added "exercise."

A Word of Caution When Using BIA for Athletes

Coaches and athletes require a safe, easily administered, and valid tool to assess body composition and detect *changes* with caloric restriction or physical conditioning in their athletes. A major limitation in achieving these goals concerns BIA's ack of instrument sensitivity to detect small body-compositional changes, particularly without appropriate control over factors that impact measurement accuracy and reliability. For example, sweat loss dehydration in endurance runners from prior physical activity or reduced glycogen reserves, and associated loss of glycogen-bound water from an intense training session, reduces body resistance or impedance to electrical current flow. This results in overestimates of FFM and underestimates of percentage body fat.

Dual-Energy X-Ray Absorptiometry

Dual-energy x-ray absorptiometry (DXA) (**Fig. 16.13**) accurately quantifies fat and nonbone regional LBM, including the mineral content of the body's deeper bony structures. DXA has become the accepted clinical tool to assess spinal osteoporosis for bone mineral density in osteoporosis screening. DXA also can quantify fat and muscle around bony areas of the body, including regions without bone present. When used for body composition assessment, DXA does not require assumptions about the biologic constancy of the fat and fat-free components as does hydrostatic weighing.

With DXA, two distinct low-energy x-ray beams with short exposure and low radiation dosage penetrate bone and soft tissue areas to a depth of approximately 30 cm. The subject lies supine on a table as the source and detector probes slowly pass across the body over a short time period (~12 min). Computer software reconstructs the attenuated x-ray beams to produce an image of underlying tissues and quantifies bone mineral content, total FM, and FFM. Analyses can include selected trunk and limb regions for detailed study of tissue composition in relation to disease risk and effects of training and detraining.

DXA estimates show excellent agreement with other independent estimates of bone mineral content. Strong relationships exist between DXA-determined total body fat and body fat by densitometry, segmental upper and lower extremity mass, total body potassium, or total body nitrogen and abdominal adiposity. The DXA error is usually less than 2% body fat units when compared with densitometry-determined body fat in a heterogeneous age group of male and female adults.

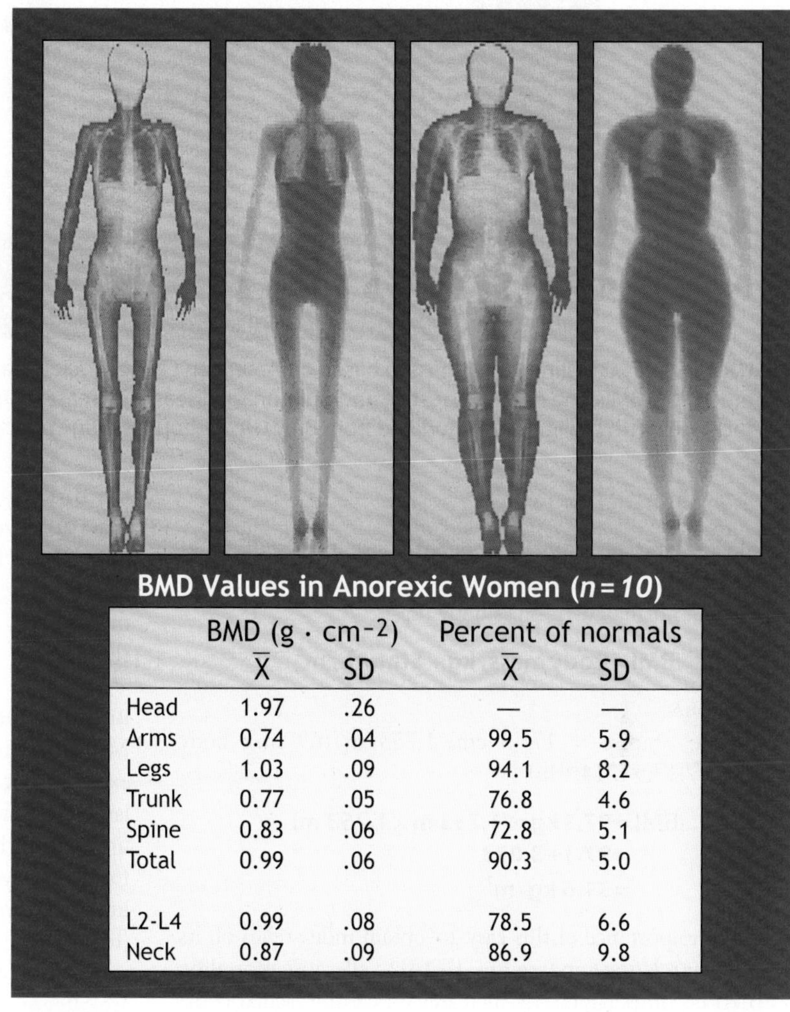

BMD Values in Anorexic Women ($n = 10$)

	BMD ($g \cdot cm^{-2}$) $\bar{X}$	BMD SD	Percent of normals $\bar{X}$	Percent of normals SD
Head	1.97	.26	—	—
Arms	0.74	.04	99.5	5.9
Legs	1.03	.09	94.1	8.2
Trunk	0.77	.05	76.8	4.6
Spine	0.83	.06	72.8	5.1
Total	0.99	.06	90.3	5.0
L2-L4	0.99	.08	78.5	6.6
Neck	0.87	.09	86.9	9.8

FIGURE 16.13 Dual-energy x-ray absorptiometry (DXA). Example of an anorexic woman **(two left images)** and a typical woman **(two right images)** whose body fat percentage averages 25% of her total body mass of 56.7 kg (125 lb). The average anorexic subject weighed 44.4 kg (97.9 lb) with DXA-estimated 7.5% body fat from the fat percentages at the arms, legs, and trunk regions. The values in the *inset table* present the average percentage values for bone mineral density (BMD) for different regional body areas in the anorexic group compared with a group of 287 normal-weight women ages 20 to 40 years. (Photo courtesy of R.B. Mazess, Department of Medical Physics, University of Wisconsin, Madison, WI, and the Lunar Radiation Corporation, Madison, WI. Data from Mazess RB, et al. *Skeletal and Body Composition Effects of Anorexia Nervosa*. Paper presented at the International Symposium on In Vivo Body Composition Studies, June 20–23, 1989, Toronto, Ontario, Canada.)

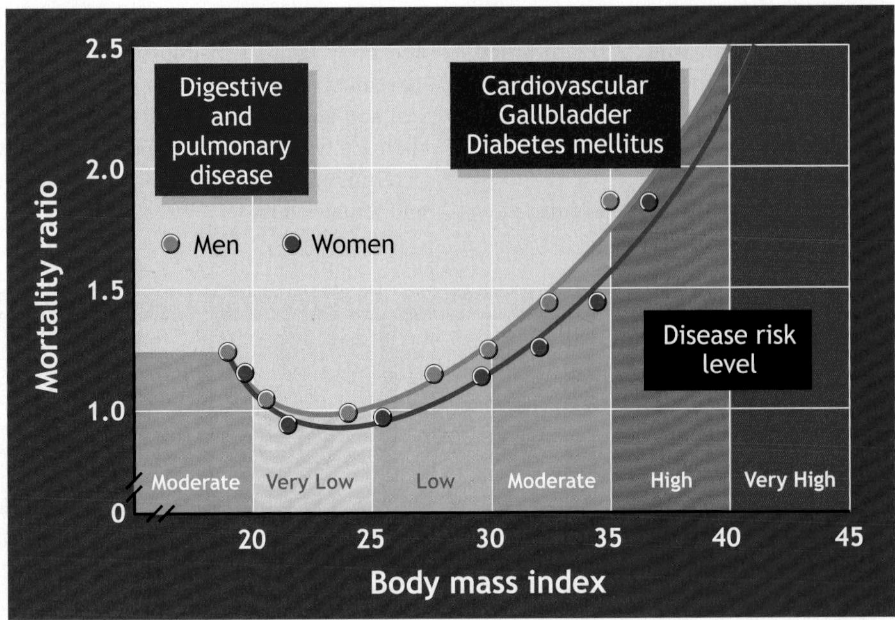

FIGURE 16.14 Curvilinear relationship based on American Cancer Society data between all-cause mortality and BMI. At extremely low BMIs, the risk for digestive and pulmonary diseases increases; cardiovascular, gallbladder, and type 2 diabetes risk increases with higher BMIs. (Modified from Bray GA. Pathophysiology of obesity. *Am J Clin Nutr* 1992;55:488S).

Body Mass Index

Clinicians and researchers frequently use the **body mass index (BMI)**, derived from body mass related to stature, to assess the "normalcy" of one's body mass:

$$\mathbf{BMI = Body\ mass,\ kg \div Stature,\ m^2}$$

Example

Man: Stature = 175.3 cm, 1.753 m (69 in.); body mass = 97.1 kg (214.1 lb)

$$\begin{aligned}\mathbf{BMI} &= \mathbf{97.1\ kg \div (1.753\ m \times 1.753\ m)}\\ &= \mathbf{97.1 \div 3.073}\\ &= \mathbf{31.6\ kg \cdot m^2}\end{aligned}$$

The importance of this easy-to-obtain index relies on its curvilinear relationship (see **Fig. 16.14**) to all-cause mortality; as BMI becomes larger, risk increases for cardiovascular complications including hypertension, diabetes, certain cancers, and renal disease. The level of disease risk along the bottom of the figure represents the degree of risk with each 5-unit change in BMI. The lowest health risk category occurs for those with BMIs in the range of 20 to 25, with the highest risk for those with BMIs that exceed 40. For women, 21.3 to 22.1 represents the desirable BMI range; the corresponding range for men equals 21.9 to 22.4. An increased disease incidence occurs when BMI exceeds 27.8 for men and 27.3 for women.

Classifications established by the National Heart, Lung, and Blood Institute (NHLBI) define "**overweight**" as a BMI of 25 to 29.9 and "**obesity**" as a BMI of 30 or above (see Part 3 of this chapter).

Limitations of Body Mass Index for Athletes

As with height and weight tables, BMI does not consider the body's fat and nonfat components. Specifically, factors other than excess body fat affect the numerator of the BMI equation. These factors include bone and muscle mass and even increased plasma volume induced by training. A high BMI can lead to an incorrect interpretation of excess body fat in lean individuals with excessive muscle mass when genetic makeup or training actually elevates the BMI.

BMI Misclassifies Athletes as Overweight or Obese

Misclassifying athletes as overweight with implications of excessive fat using a BMI standard applies particularly to large-size, field-event athletes, bodybuilders, weightlifters, upper–weight class wrestlers, and American professional football players. For example, the BMI for seven defensive linemen from a former NFL Super Bowl team averaged 31.9 (team BMI averaged 28.7), clearly signaling these professional athletes as overweight and placing them in the moderate category for mortality risk. Their body fat content, 18.0% for lineman and 12.1% for the team, misclassified them for fatness using BMI as the overweight standard.

In contrast to the professional football players, the average player in the National Basketball Association (NBA) for the 1993 to 1994 season had a BMI of below 25. This relatively low BMI placed them at low risk and keeps them out of the overweight category, although they would be classified as overweight by height-weight standards. Consider two contemporary NBA superstars—Kobe Bryant of the Los Angeles Lakers and LeBron James of the Cleveland Cavaliers. Bryant weighs 220 lb (99.8 kg) at 76.75 inches (195 cm) and James weighs 250 lb (113 kg) at 78 inches (203.2 cm).

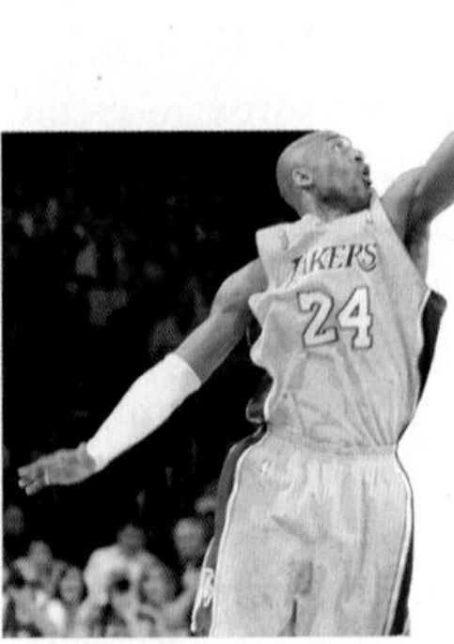

Kobe Bryant

Both players, by BMI standards (**www.nhlbi.nih.gov/health/educational/lose_wt/BMI/bmicalc.htm**), would classify as "overweight" with a BMI for Bryant at 26.3 and James at 27.4! Clearly, both players are fit, not overweight, and possess a large lean tissue component.

OTHER INDIRECT PROCEDURES TO ESTIMATE BODY COMPOSITION

Near-Infrared Interactance

Near-infrared interactance (NIR) applies technology developed by the U.S. Department of Agriculture to assess the body composition of livestock and the lipid content of various grains (**http://naldc.nal.usda.gov/download/12493/PDF**). The commercial versions to assess body composition in humans use a safe, portable, lightweight monitor; require minimal training; and necessitate little physical contact with the subject during measurement. These test administration aspects make NIR popular for body composition assessment in health clubs, hospitals, and weight-loss centers. Unfortunately, research with humans has not confirmed NIR's validity compared with hydrostatic weighing and skinfold measurement. In general, research does not support NIR as a robust, valid method to assess human body composition across a broad range of ages, sexes, and racial and athletic categories.

Ultrasound Assessment of Body Fat

Ultrasound technology can assess thickness of fat and muscle and image deeper tissues such as a muscle's cross-sectional area, including the abdominal region for fetal monitoring during pregnancy. The method converts electrical energy through a probe into high-frequency pulsed sound waves that penetrate the skin surface into the underlying tissues. The sound waves pass through adipose tissue and penetrate the muscle layer. The waves then reflect against the bone to the fat-muscle interface to produce an echo, which returns to a receiver within the probe. The simplest A-mode type of ultrasound does not produce an image of the underlying tissues. Rather, the time required for sound wave transmission through the tissues and back to the transducer converts to a distance score that indicates fat or muscle thickness. Color and multiple-frequency imaging allows clinicians to trace blood flow through organs and tissues or, with the use of miniaturized probes, identify internal tissues, vessels, and organs. In consumer-oriented research, ultrasonic imaging of thigh fat depth provided evidence that treatments using two topical cream applications to the thighs and buttocks to reduce "cellulite" (so-called dimpled fat) failed to reduce local fat thickness compared with control conditions.

Ultrasonography to map muscle and fat thickness at different body regions quantifies changes in the topographic fat pattern and serves as a valuable adjunct to whole-body composition assessment. In hospitalized patients, ultrasonic fat and muscle thickness determinations aid in nutritional assessment during weight loss and gain.

Computed Tomography and Magnetic Resonance Imaging

Computed Tomography

Computed tomography (CT) scanning revolutionized medicine when first introduced in the mid-1970s; it made organs and bones visible with the clarity of anatomy textbooks. Using an array of x-ray emitters and detectors, CT generates detailed cross-sectional, two-dimensional radiographic images of body segments when an x-ray beam of ionizing radiation passes through tissues of different densities. CT produces pictorial and quantitative information about total tissue area, total fat and muscle area, and thickness and volume of tissues within an organ.

Figure 16.15A and B shows CT scans of the upper legs and a cross section at the midthigh of a professional walker who walked 11,200 miles through the 50 United States in 50 weeks. Total cross section and muscle cross section increased, and subcutaneous fat decreased correspondingly in the midthigh region in the "after" scans (not shown). CT has established the relationship between simple skinfolds and girths at the abdomen and total adipose tissue volume measured from single or multiple pictorial "slices" through this region. The single cut through the L4–L5 region minimizes the radiation dose and provides the best view of visceral and subcutaneous fat. A high association exists between **visceral adipose tissue (VAT)** and waist girth—people with larger waist girth possess greater VAT. An increased amount of deep abdominal adipose tissue (VAT) relates to increased risk for type 2 diabetes, blood lipid profile disorders, lung disease, and hypertension, including cardiometabolic factors and cardiovascular disease.

Magnetic Resonance Imaging

Magnetic resonance imaging (MRI) offers a valuable, noninvasive assessment of the body's tissue compartments. Physician and research scientist Raymond Vahan Damadian (1936) first proposed the idea for MRI in 1969 dealing with soft tissue imaging of cancer tissue. The first published article on the topic appeared in 1971. MRI, patented in 1974 and first constructed in 1976 at the Downstate Medical Center in Brooklyn, New York, provides a noninvasive assessment of detailed, high-resolution contrasts of the body's tissue compartments without the potential risks of damaging ionizing radiation common with x-ray and CT scanning. The schematic drawing in **Figure 16.16A** shows the arrangement of the different muscular structures. The *yellow areas* that surround the thigh correspond to both subcutaneous and internal fat, with minimal fat intrusion located among and within the different muscles. The femur bone appears at the center of the cross section. **Figure 16.16B** shows a transaxial image of the midthigh of a 30-year-old male middle-distance runner. Computer

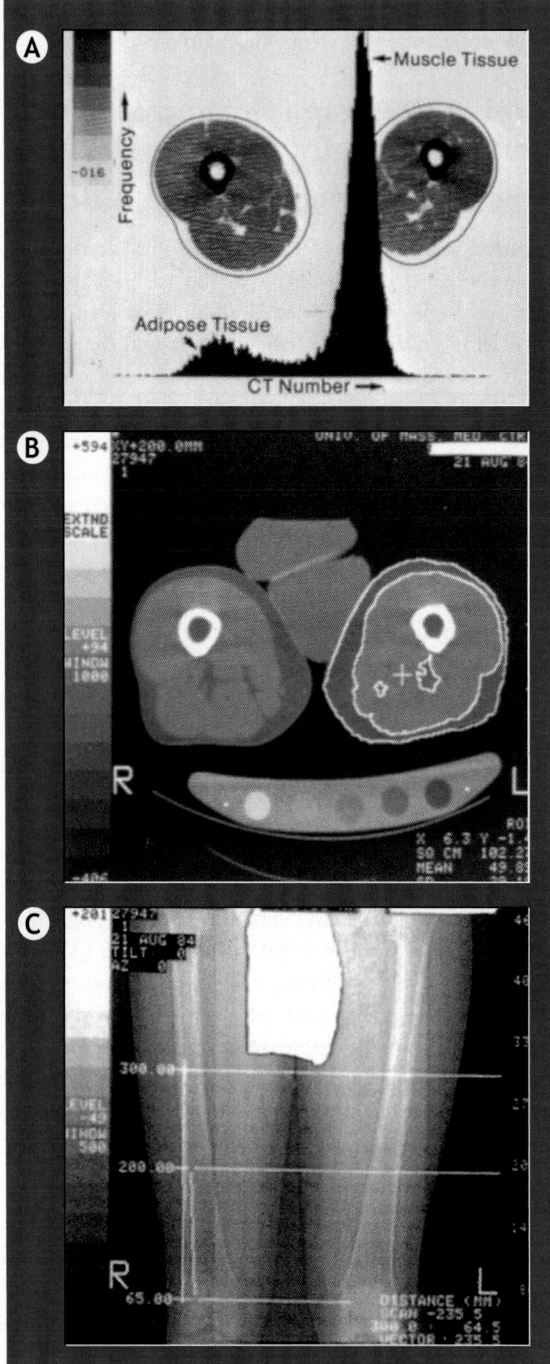

FIGURE 16.15 CT scans. **(A)** Plot of pixel elements (CT scan) illustrating the extent of adipose and muscle tissue in a cross section of the thigh. The two other views show **(B)** a cross section of the midthigh and **(C)** an anterior view of the upper legs prior to a 1-year walk across the United States by a champion walker. (CT scans courtesy of Dr. Steven Heymsfeld, George A. Bray, Jr., Endowed Chair in Nutrition, Pennington Biomedical Research Center, Louisiana State University, Baton Rouge, LA.)

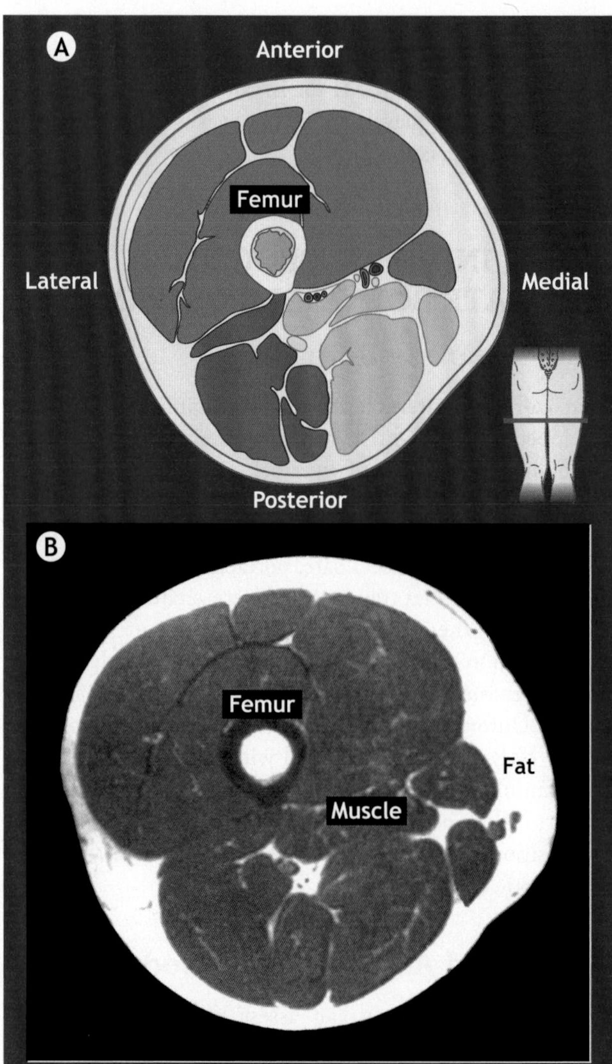

FIGURE 16.16 **A.** Arrangement of muscular structures at the midthigh region as shown at the top of the cross-sectional drawing. The *yellow* areas that surround the thigh correspond to subcutaneous and internal fat, with minimal fat located among the different muscles. The femur bone appears at the center of the cross section. **B.** Transverse MRI scan of the right thigh that corresponds to the structures in **(A)**. (Adapted with permission from Moore KL, et al. *Clinically Oriented Anatomy*. 7th Ed. Baltimore: Wolters Kluwer Health, 2013.)

software subtracts fat and bony tissues (*white areas*) to compute thigh muscle cross-sectional area. With MRI, electromagnetic radiation in a strong magnetic field excites the hydrogen nuclei of the body's water and lipid molecules. These molecules vary in concentration depending on the tissue source; they are more concentrated in fat, less so in water and blood, and least in bone. The nuclei then project a detectable signal that rearranges under computer software to visually represent various body tissues. MRI can quantify total and subcutaneous adipose tissue in individuals of varying body fatness.

AVERAGE VALUES FOR BODY FAT

Table 16.4 presents average values for percentage body fat for men and women from different US regions. The column headed "68% Variation Limits" indicates the range for percentage body fat that includes ±1 standard deviation or

TABLE 16.4 Average Percentage Body Fat for Younger and Older Women and Men From Selected Studies

Study	Age Range, y	Stature, cm	Body Mass, kg	%Fat	68% Variation Limits
Younger Women					
North Carolina, 1962	17–25	165.0	55.5	22.9	17.5–28.5
New York, 1962	16–30	167.5	59.0	28.7	24.6–32.9
California, 1968	19–23	165.9	58.4	21.9	17.0–26.9
California, 1970	17–29	164.9	58.6	25.5	21.0–30.1
Air Force, 1972	17–22	164.1	55.8	28.7	22.3–35.3
New York, 1973	17–26	160.4	59.0	26.2	23.4–33.3
North Carolina, 1975		166.1	57.5	24.6	—
Army recruits, 1986	17–25	162.0	58.6	28.4	23.9–32.9
Massachusetts, 1994	17–30	165.3	57.7	21.8	16.7–27.8
Older Women					
Minnesota, 1953	31–45	163.3	60.7	28.9	25.1–32.8
	43–68	160.0	60.9	34.2	28.0–40.5
New York, 1963	30–40	164.9	59.6	28.6	22.1–35.3
	40–50	163.1	56.4	34.4	29.5–39.5
North Carolina, 1975	33–50	—	—	29.7	23.1–36.5
Massachusetts, 1993	31–50	165.2	58.9	25.2	19.2–31.2
Younger Men					
Minnesota, 1951	17–26	177.8	69.1	11.8	5.9–11.8
Colorado, 1956	17–25	172.4	68.3	13.5	8.2–18.8
Indiana, 1966	18–23	180.1	75.5	12.6	8.7–16.5
California, 1968	16–31	175.7	74.1	15.2	6.3–24.2
New York, 1973	17–26	176.4	71.4	15.0	8.9–21.1
Texas, 1977	18–24	179.9	74.6	13.4	7.4–19.4
Army recruits, 1986	17–25	174.7	70.5	15.6	10.0–21.2
Massachusetts, 1994	17–30	178.2	76.3	12.9	7.8–18.9
Older Men					
Indiana, 1966	24–38	179.0	76.6	17.8	11.3–24.3
	40–48	177.0	80.5	22.3	16.3–28.3
North Carolina, 1976	27–50	—	—	23.7	17.9–30.1
Texas, 1977	27–59	180.0	85.3	27.1	23.7–30.5
Massachusetts, 1993	31–50	177.1	77.5	19.9	13.2–26.5

about 68 of every 100 persons measured. As an example, the average percentage body fat of 15.0% for young men from the New York sample includes the ±68% variation limits from 8.9% to 21.1% body fat. Interpreting this statistically, for 68 of every 100 young men measured, percentage fat ranges between 8.9% and 21.1%. Of the remaining 32 young men, 16 possess more than 21.1% body fat, and the 16 other men have a body fat percentage of less than 8.9%. *In general, percentage body fat for young adult men averages between 12% and 15%; the average fat value for women ranges between 25% and 28%.*

The trend of available body composition data of men and women of different ages indicates a distinct tendency for percentage body fat to steadily increase with advancing age. The mechanisms that lead to increased body fat with age are not clearly understood. The trend does not necessarily imply a desirable or normal aging process because participation in vigorous physical activity throughout life frequently blunts body fat accretion with age. Regular physical activity maintains or increases bone mass while preserving muscle mass. In contrast, a sedentary lifestyle results in increased storage fat, particularly in the abdominal region, and definitively reduces muscle mass. This occurs even if daily caloric intake remains unchanged.

DETERMINING GOAL BODY WEIGHT

No one really knows the optimum body fat or body weight for a particular individual. Inherited genetic factors greatly influence body fat distribution and play an important role in programming body size and its link to disease risk with aging. Values for percentage body fat for young adults average approximately 15% for men and 25% for women. Women and men who exercise regularly or train for athletic competition typically have lower body fat levels than do their age-matched sedentary counterparts. In contact sports and activities requiring muscular power (e.g., American football, rugby, sprint swimming, and running), successful performance usually requires a large body mass with average to low body fat. In contrast, successful athletes in weight-bearing endurance activities generally possess a relatively light body mass with low body fat. *Proper assessment of body composition, not body weight, determines a person's ideal body weight. For athletes,* ***goal body weight*** *must coincide with optimizing sport-specific measures of physiologic functional capacity and performance.*

To compute a "goal" body weight target that uses a desired (and healthy) percentage of body fat, employ this equation:

Goal body weight = FFM ÷ (1.00 – %fat desired)

Suppose a 23-year-old, 120-kg (265-lb) large man currently with 24% body fat wants to know how much fat weight to lose to attain a body fat composition of 15% (average value for young men). The following computations provide this information:

Fat mass = Body mass, kg × Decimal % body fat
= 120 kg × 0.24
= 28.8 kg

FFM = Body mass, kg – Fat mass, kg
= 120 kg – 28.8 kg
= 91.2 kg

Goal body weight = FFM, kg ÷ (1.00 – Decimal % fat desired)
= 91.2 kg ÷ (1.00 – 0.15)
= 91.2 kg ÷ 0.85
= 107.3 kg (236.6 lb)

Desirable fat loss = Present body weight, kg – Goal body weight, kg
= 120 kg – 107.3 kg
= 12.7 kg (28.0 lb)

A Desirable Range for Goal Body Weight

For practical purposes, recommend a "desirable body weight range" rather than a single goal weight. This should range within ±2 lb of the computed "goal body weight." For example, if goal body weight equals 135 lb, the person should strive for a weight between 133 and 137 lb.

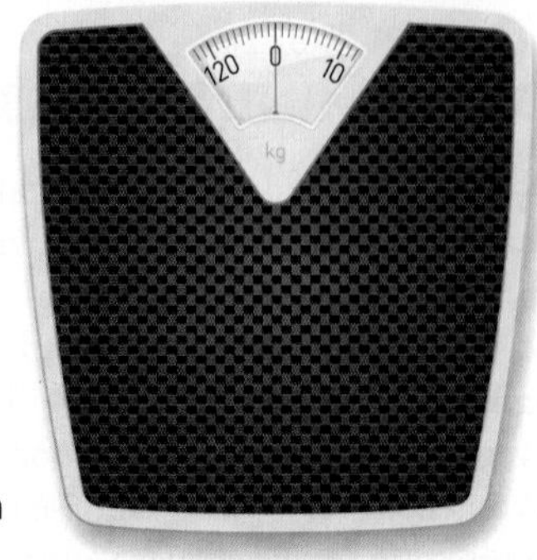

If this person lost 12.7 kg (26.5 lb) of body fat, his new body mass of 91.2 kg (210.1 lb) would have a fat content equal to 15% of body mass. These calculations assume no change in FFM during weight loss. Moderate caloric restriction plus increased daily energy expenditure reduces body fat and can conserves lean tissue. Part 4 of this chapter discusses prudent yet effective approaches to reduce body fat and maintain and/or increase the FFM component.

SUMMARY

1. Two approaches directly assess body composition. In one technique, a chemical solution literally dissolves the body into its fat and nonfat (fat-free) components. The other approach involves physical dissection of fat, fat-free adipose tissue, muscle, and bone.
2. Hydrostatic weighing determines body volume with subsequent calculation of body density and percentage body fat.
3. Subtracting fat mass from body mass yields fat-free body mass (FFM).
4. Air displacement technology (BOD POD) offers an alternative means to quantify body composition because of ease of administration, high reproducibility of body volume scores, and generally high validity using hydrostatic weighing as the criterion method to estimate body fat.
5. Common field methods to assess body composition use population-specific prediction equations from relationships among selected skinfolds and girths and body density and percentage body fat.
6. Skinfold and girth equations predict most accurately with subjects similar to those who participated in the equations' original derivation.
7. BMI relates more closely to body fat and health risk than simply body mass and stature; as with height–weight tables, BMI does not consider the body's proportional composition.
8. The concept of BIA states that hydrated, fat-free body tissues and extracellular water facilitate electrical flow better compared with fat tissue because of the greater electrolyte content of the fat-free component.
9. Impedance to electric current flow relates directly to the body's fat content.
10. NIR should be used with caution when assessing body composition; this methodology currently lacks verification of adequate validity.
11. Ultrasonography, CT, MRI, and DXA indirectly assess body composition.
12. The average healthy young man possesses 15% body fat, and the average woman possesses 25% body fat.
13. Average body fat values for average-size men and women can serve as a common yardstick to evaluate

deviations from the "average" for the body fat of individual athletes and specific athletic groups.

14. Goal body weight computes as FFM ÷ 1.00 – Desired %fat.
15. Top male and female endurance runners represent the lower end of the fat-to-lean continuum.

THINK IT THROUGH

1. How would you use anthropometric data to estimate optimal body composition?
2. Discuss whether the established differences in body composition between men and women justify gender-specific normative standards to evaluate different components of physical fitness and motor performance.
3. A friend complains that three fitness centers determined her percentage body fat from skinfolds as 19%, 25%, and 31%. How can you reconcile these discrepancies?

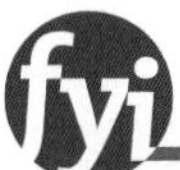

The Supersizing of America

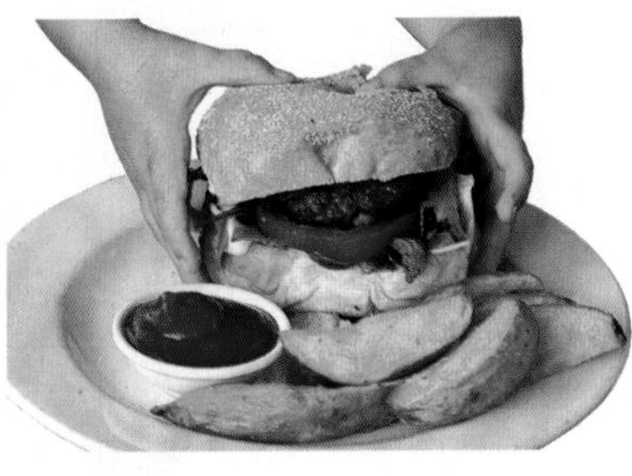

Substantial changes in genetic makeup cannot account for the rapid increase in obesity among Americans over the past 20 years. More than 69% of the US population now classify as either overweight or obese. More than likely, the culprits in the fattening of America are a sedentary lifestyle and ready availability of tasty, lipid- and calorie-rich foods currently served in increasingly larger portions.

PART 3 Overweight, Overfat, and Obesity

Shockingly, the American Medical Association (**AMA**) now classifies one third of all American as ill! At its annual 2013 meeting, the AMA (**www.ama-assn.org**) formally recognized obesity as a disease, a decision that will now make physicians pay more attention to this condition that affects one in three Americans and causes insurance companies to cover prevention and treatment strategies that include drugs, surgery, and counseling. Those opposing this decision argue that the popular way for classification of desirable and undesirable body weight—the body mass index—is simplistic and flawed. For example, some individuals classified as obese are healthy with no specific disease symptoms or treatment requirements, whereas others below this classification have excess body fat and other comorbidities that represents a "multimetabolic and hormonal disease state" leading to undesirable medical outcomes such as type 2 diabetes and cardiovascular disease.

To gain insights into the magnitude of the obesity epidemic, a random-digit telephone survey of nearly 110,000 adults in the United States found that nearly 70% struggle to lose weight or just maintain their current body weight. Fifty-eight percent of Americans would like to lose weight and 36% are following a particular diet plan, yet less than 19% of those following such plans closely track their intake of fats, carbohydrates, proteins, and calories. Only 20% of the 50 to 65 million Americans trying to lose weight use the recommended combination of eating fewer calories and engaging in at least 150 minutes of weekly increased physical activity over and above the common activities of daily living. Those attempting to lose weight spend nearly $60 billion annually on weight-reduction products and services, often using potentially harmful dietary practices and drugs while ignoring sensible weight-loss programs. Approximately 2 million Americans spend more than $140 million on appetite-suppressing, over-the-counter diet pills that line the shelves of drugstores, health food and fitness centers, and supermarkets, and products marketed through TV, radio, direct mail, and the Internet.

Despite the upswing in attempts to lose weight, Americans are considerably more overweight than a generation ago, and the trend is for further increases in all regions of the United States. Data from the **Centers for Disease Control and Prevention** (**CDC**; **www.cdc.org**) Behavioral Risk Factor Surveillance Survey (BRFSS 2013; **www.cdc.gov/obesity/data/prevalence-maps.html**) provide state-by-state prevalence rates for obesity in the United States (**Fig. 16.17**). The data were collected through the CDC's Behavioral Risk Factor Surveillance System (BRFSS). Each year, state health departments use a series of monthly telephone interviews with US adults to collect data, including height and weight to calculate BMI. In 2011 to 2012, the prevalence of obesity was higher among middle-aged adults (39.5%) than among younger (30.3%) or older (35.4%) adults.

Figure 16.17 displays the data for 2013, including the state-by-state obesity prevalence ranked from highest prevalence to lowest, with Guam and Puerto Rico included at the bottom of the insert. The first 20 states in the listing had an obesity prevalence rating at 30% or higher. The prevalence rates for Mississippi and West Virginia exceeded 35%, while Arkansas, Tennessee, Kentucky, and Louisiana ranked in the five top "fattest" states. The South had the highest obesity prevalence of 30.2%, followed by the Midwest (30.1%), Northeast (26.5%), and West (24.9%). The states with the highest adult obesity rates also have the highest prevalence of type 2 diabetes. Combining data from

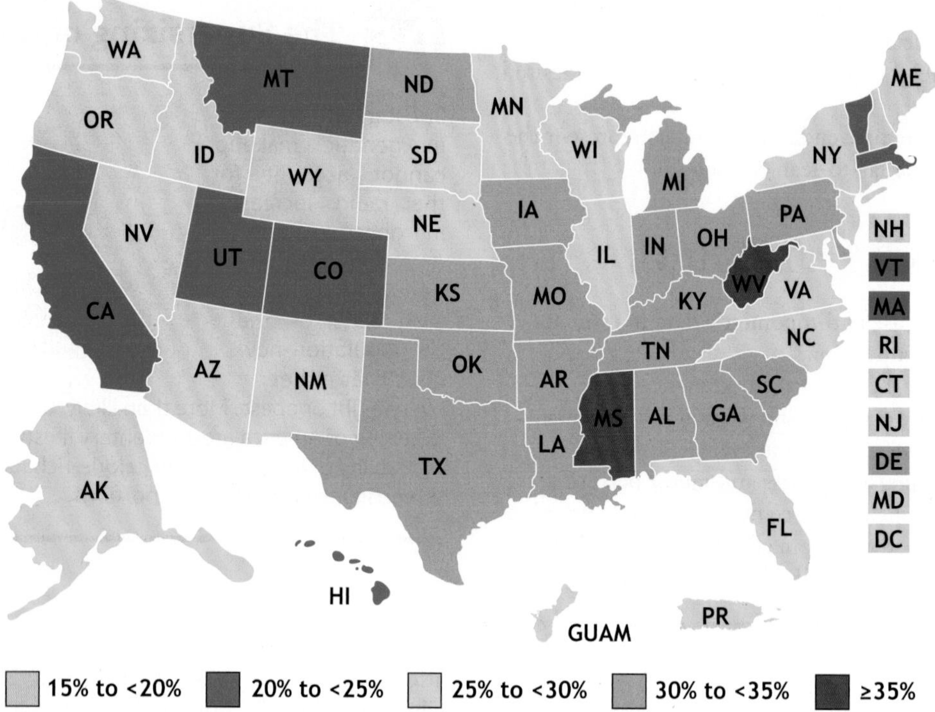

FIGURE 16.17 Prevalence of Self-Reported Obesity Among U.S. Adults by State and Territory, BRFSS, 2013. Prevalence estimates reflect BRFSS methodological changes started in 2011. These estimates should not be compared to prevalence estimates before 2011. Guam and Puerto Rico were the only US territories with obesity data available on the 2013 BRFSS. (Reprinted from Behavioral Risk Factor Surveillance Systems [BRFSS], Centers for Disease Control. *Overweight and Obesity: Obesity Prevalence Maps*, **www.cdc.gov/obesity/data/prevalence-maps.html**.)

2011 through 2013, non-Hispanic blacks had the highest prevalence of self-reported obesity (37.6%), followed by Hispanics (30.6%) and non-Hispanic whites (26.6%). Unfortunately, no state had a prevalence of obesity less than 20%. This contrasts markedly with similar data from 2006, where the obesity rate was only above 30% in four states (currently 20 states for 2013). To say the least, from 2007 to 2013, the obesity rates for US adults have skyrocketed. Even Colorado, which had the lowest obesity prevalence (below 20% in 2006), now has inched above 21% for the first time (21.3%), and Hawaii's obesity prevalence crept up to 21.8%. The next three states with the lowest obesity prevalence include Massachusetts (23.6%), Utah (24.2%), and Montana (24.6%).

A 2009 report, *"How Obesity Policies Are Failing in America"* from the Trust for America's Health (**healthyamericans.org/reports/obesity2009/**), provided further alarming data and trends about current strategies, including school nutrition and physical activity policies regarding the obesity epidemic. The report predicts that by the year 2018, 108 million American adults will classify as obese, and weight gain not only in adults but in children as well could drive up healthcare costs by $344 billion. At a minimum in 2016, the percentage of obese and overweight children in 30 states will exceed 30%! Obesity also disproportionately affects those from minority populations (see the FYI box).

fyi One in Five American Children Is Obese

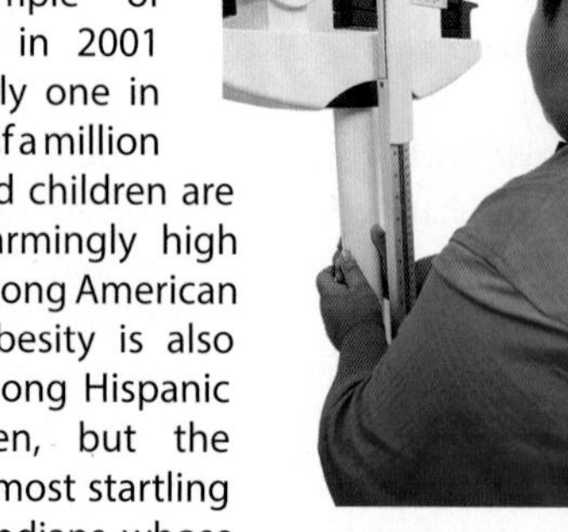

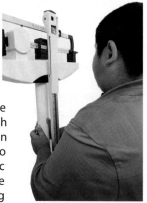

Research appearing in the *Archives of Pediatrics & Adolescent Medicine* on a nationally representative sample of preschoolers born in 2001 indicates that nearly one in five or more than half a million American 4-year-old children are obese with an alarmingly high one in three rate among American Indian children. Obesity is also more prevalent among Hispanic and black children, but the disparity becomes most startling among American Indians whose obesity doubles that of whites.The alarming statistics are that 13% of Asian children, 16% of whites, 21% of blacks, 22% of Hispanics, and 31% of American Indians are obese.

DEFINITIONS: OVERWEIGHT, OVERFAT, AND OBESE

Confusion surrounds the precise meaning of the terms *overweight*, ***overfat***, and *obesity* as applied to body composition. Each term often takes on a different meaning depending on the situation and contextual use. The medical literature generally defines *overweight* as an overfat condition relative to other individuals of the same age or height despite the absence of accompanying body fat measures. Within this context, *obesity* refers to individuals at the extreme of the overfat continuum. This frame of reference delineates the body fat range by BMI (discussed earlier in this chapter).

Research and debate among diverse disciplines reinforce the need to distinguish between overweight, overfat, and obese to ensure consistency in use and interpretation. In proper context, the overweight condition refers to a body weight that exceeds some average for stature, and perhaps age, usually by some standard deviation unit or percentage. The overweight condition frequently accompanies an increase in body fat, but not always (as prevalent in male power athletes), and it may or may not coincide with the comorbidities glucose intolerance, insulin resistance, dyslipidemia, and hypertension.

When measures of body fat are available, researchers can accurately place an individual's body fat level on a continuum from low to high, independent of body weight. Overfatness then would refer to a condition in which body fat exceeds an age- or gender-appropriate average by a predetermined amount. In most situations, *overfatness* represents the correct term to assess individual and group body fat levels.

Obese refers to the overfat condition that accompanies a constellation of disease comorbidities that include one or all of the following nine components of the "**obese syndrome**:"

1. Glucose intolerance
2. Insulin resistance
3. Dyslipidemia
4. Type 2 diabetes
5. Hypertension
6. Elevated plasma leptin concentrations
7. Increased VAT
8. Increased risk of coronary heart disease
9. Presence of certain cancers

Men and women may classify as overweight or overfat and yet not exhibit "obese syndrome" components. We urge caution in using the term *obese* in all cases of excessive body weight. In the medical and lay press, the terms overweight, overfat, and obese are often but mistakenly used interchangeably to designate the same condition.

OBESITY: A GLOBAL EPIDEMIC

According to the **World Health Organization** (**WHO**; **www.who.int**) and data from several National Health and Nutrition Examination Surveys (**www.cdc.gov/nchs/nhanes.htm**), obesity represents a complex condition with serious social and psychological dimensions that impact all age and socioeconomic groups. It threatens to overwhelm both developed and developing countries.

Highlights from WHO's 2014 global data include the following grim statistics:

1. Approximately 1.6 billion adults age 15+ years were overweight.
2. At least 500 million adults were obese (200 million men; 300 million women).
3. By 2016, over 2 billion adults will be overweight, and more than 700 million obese.
4. At least 42 million children younger than 5 years of age were overweight; contrast this with "only" 20 million overweight children in 2008.
5. Sixty-five percent of the world's population lives in countries where overweight and obesity kill more people than does the underweight condition. This is equivalent to 2.5 times the proportion of adults and children who are undernourished!
6. The prevalence of obesity among adults did not change between 2009 and 2010 and 2011 and 2012.
7. In 2011 to 2012, the prevalence of obesity was higher among middle-aged adults (39.5%) than among younger (30.3%) or older (35.4%) adults.

WHO posits that increased consumption of more energy-dense, nutrient-poor foods with high levels of sugar and saturated fats, combined with reduced physical activity, has led to obesity rates that have risen threefold or more since 1980. This phenomenon is not limited to the United States but includes the United Kingdom, Eastern Europe, the Middle East, the Pacific Islands, Australia, and especially China (about one fifth of the 1 billion overweight or obese people in the world are Chinese). In 2014, the skyrocketing obesity rate in China tallied 46 million obese and 300 million overweight adults, or more than one in four Chinese adult men and women.

Despite hunger in many parts of the world, there are more overfat than underweight individuals. On a global basis, about every fourth person on the planet has the distinction of being overfat!

Compared to the rest of the world, the United States accounts for the greatest percentage of the world's obese (13%), while India and China combined account for about 15% of the total. Ten countries worldwide account for 671 million obese adults—about 50% of the world's obese. More disturbingly, and in line with statistics about childhood obesity in the United States, 23% of boys and 14% of girls under age 20 are either obese or overweight.

The prevalence of overweight and adult obesity in the United States represents about 134 million Americans (66% of adults age 20 years or older and 35% of college students). Currently, more than 4 million individuals exceed 136.4 kg (300 lb), and more than 500,000 people, mostly men, exceed 181.8 kg (400 lb). The average woman now weighs an unprecedented 75.4 kg (166.2 lb) with a waist girth of 37.5 inches (95.3 cm; **www.cdc.gov/nchs/fastats/body-measurements.htm**)! Some researchers maintain that if this trend continues, 70% to 75% of the US adult population may reach overweight or obesity status by the year 2020, with essentially the entire adult population becoming overweight within three generations!

TABLE 16.5 **Classification of Overweight and Obesity by BMI, Waist Circumference, and Associated Disease Risk**

Category	BMI (kg · m^{-2})	Obesity Class	Disease Risk[a] (Relative to Normal Weight and Waist Circumference[b])	
			Men: ≤40 in. (102 cm) Women: ≤35 in. (88 cm)	Men: >40 in. (102 cm) Women: >35 in. (88 cm)
Underweight	<18.5			
Normal[c]	18.5–24.9			
Overweight	25.0–29.9		Increased	High
Obesity	30.0–34.9 35.0–39.9 ≥40.0	I II III	High Very high Extremely high	Very high Very high Extremely high

[a]Disease risk for type 2 diabetes, hypertension, and coronary heart disease.

[b]Waist girth measured at the level of the top of the right iliac crest; the tape should be snug but not compressing the skin and held parallel to the floor; make at normal ventilation.

[c]Increased waist circumference can also be a marker for increased risk even in persons of normal weight.

From Aronne LJ. Classification of obesity and assessment of obesity-related health risks. *Obesity Res* 2002;10:105.

Obesity and Minorities

The obesity rate for Mexican American adults exceeds 40%, about 5 to 6 percentage points greater than the average rate of about 35% for adult Americans. Second- and third-generation Mexican Americans are more than twice as likely to become excessively fat due to "societal switching" from a more customary Mexican diet featuring fresh corn, beans, and vegetables to a more American-style diet that relies on processed foods (**www.timigustafson.com/2012/minorities-are-hit-the-hardest-by-the-obesity-crisis/#sthash.QzcAFGbI.dpuf**).

Hispanics in general are approaching a 25% obesity prevalence. Hispanics represent the fastest-growing ethnic group in the United States; in about 35 years in 2050, the Hispanic population will swell to over 130 million individuals. Currently, over 20% of this ethnic group exhibits weight-related high blood pressure and high cholesterol.

The obesity rate for African Americans averages almost 50%, with values greater for women than men as four out of five African American women are either overweight or obese (**http://minorityhealth.hhs.gov**).

In its 2008 CDC report, "Differences in Prevalence of Obesity," (**www.cdc.gov/nchs/data/databriefs/db131.htm**), the US government set a specific goal to level the playing field by eliminating health disparities among racial and ethnic populations:

> Given the overall high prevalence of obesity and the significant differences among non-Hispanic blacks, non-Hispanic whites and Hispanics, effective policies and environmental strategies that promote healthy eating and physical activity are needed for all populations and geographic areas, but particularly for those populations and areas disproportionally affected by obesity.

Table 16.5 presents a classification schema of overweight and obesity by BMI, waist circumference, and associated disease risk. The WHO Obesity Task Force initially developed this BMI classification system, which has been adopted by the NIH's National Heart, Lung, and Blood Institute (**www.nhlbi.nih.gov**).

CAUSES OF OVERFATNESS

Overfatness frequently begins during childhood. Overfat children have a threefold risk of becoming overfat adults compared with children of normal body weight. Simply stated, a child usually does not grow out of obesity. Tracking body weight through generations indicates that overfat parents likely give birth to children who become overfat and whose offspring also often become overfat. This pattern continues from generation to generation.

Excessive fatness also develops slowly through adulthood, with most of the weight gain occurring between ages 25 and 44 years. Beginning at age 30 for the typical American male and at age 27 for the typical American female, individuals gain between 0.2 and 0.8 kg (0.5 to 1.8 lb) of body weight each year until age 60. Thus, the average 20-year-old college students will weigh an additional 40 lb (18.1 kg) at age 60. The degree to which this creeping obesity during adulthood reflects a "normal biologic pattern" of aging remains unclear.

Overeating and Other Causative Factors

Human obesity results from a complex interaction among at least 11 specific factors that predispose humans to excessive weight gain. They include the following 11 factors:

1. Eating patterns
2. Eating environment
3. Body image
4. Resting metabolic rate
5. Diet-induced thermogenesis
6. Level of spontaneous activity or "fidgeting"

7. Body temperature
8. Susceptibility to specific viral infections
9. Levels of cellular adenosine triphosphatase
10. Lipoprotein lipase and other enzymes
11. Levels of metabolically active **brown adipose tissue (BAT)**

Regardless of specific obesity causes and their interactions, five common treatment procedures—diets, drugs, physical activity, psychological methods, and surgery, either alone or in combination—often fail when tracked on a long-term basis. Researchers continue to devise strategies to try to prevent and treat this health catastrophe.

Effect of Global Changing of Dietary Patterns

Changes in diet and reduced energy expenditure via patterns of work and leisure, often referred to as the *nutrition transition*, contribute greatly to the increase in obesity worldwide. Moreover, the pace of these changes continues to accelerate, especially in low- and middle-income countries. Dietary changes that characterize the nutrition transition are both quantitative and qualitative: shifts in dietary structure toward higher energy density foods with greater fat and added sugars, greater saturated fat (mostly from animal sources), reduced intake of complex carbohydrates and dietary fiber, and reduced intake of fruits and vegetables. These trends in food consumption suggest a causal link to increasing obesity rates.

Worldwide Food Consumption Patterns

Food consumption, expressed in kcal per capita per day, provides a key variable to measure and evaluate energy storage. Analysis of worldwide data shows steadily increasing daily kcal per capita from the mid-1960s to 2009, increasing globally by approximately 450 kcal and by more than 600 kcal in developing countries (**Table 16.6**). These data, coupled with decreased energy expenditure for all populations of the world, help to explain the worldwide creeping obesity epidemic. Viewing the data in an interactive graphic plots the daily caloric intake per capita in European countries (Belgium, England, Finland, France, Germany, Iceland, Italy, Netherlands, Norway) and the United States from 1700 to 2010 (**www.ourworldindata.org/data/food-agriculture/food-per-person/**). For most countries, the clear upward trend shows little evidence of abating, although the daily peak 3804 kcal in the United States in the early 2000s declined by about 100 kcal in 2010. For some countries, the changes have been nothing short of breathtaking; the salient example is the energy value of the typical diet in France at the start of the 18th century, where energy intake was as low as that of Rwanda in 1965, the most malnourished nation in the world for that year! Since about 1850, however, the French, Belgian, and English trends parallel US trends.

Fast Food and Obesity Link in Adolescents

An estimated 75% of all US adolescents ages 12 to 18 eat fast food one or more times weekly. This increase in fast-food consumption parallels the escalating obesity epidemic, increasing the possibility of a causal relationship. Six fast-food characteristics link to excess energy intake and subsequent adiposity:

1. Enormous portion sizes
2. High-energy density
3. Palatability
4. Excessive amounts of refined starch and added sugars
5. High fat content
6. Low dietary fiber levels

TABLE 16.6 Global and Regional Per Capita Food Consumption (kcal Per Capita Per Day)

Region	1964–1966	1974–1976	1984–1986	1997–1999	2015	2030
World	2358	2435	2655	2803	2940	3050
Developing countries	2054	2152	2450	2681	2850	2980
Near East and North Africa	2290	2591	2953	3006	3090	3170
Sub-Saharan Africa (excluding South Africa)	2058	2079	2057	2195	2360	2540
Latin America + Caribbean	2393	2546	2689	2824	2980	3140
East Asia	1957	2105	2559	2992	3060	3190
South Asia	2017	1986	2205	2403	2700	2900
Industrialized countries	2947	3065	3206	3380	3440	3500

From Diet, Nutrition and The Prevention of Chronic Diseases. *WHO Technical Report Series #916. Report of a Joint WHO/FAO Expert Consultation.* Geneva, Switzerland: World Health Organization, 2003.

Enormous Portion Sizes

The enormity of popular food portions has increased dramatically over the last decade. Consider the choices for specialty hamburgers at McDonald's, Burger King, Carl's Jr., and Wendy's and their select nutrient composition values for calories, total fat, protein, carbohydrate, and sodium, shown in **Figure 16.18**. These four fast-food restaurants are not the only ones that supersize their selections. *Hardee's* 2/3-lb Monster Thickburger (**www.hardees.com**) packs in a whopping 1290 kcal with 92 g fat and 2840 mg sodium, the latter representing 118% of the daily recommended intake. But the winner goes to the *Red Robin Gourmet Burger* topped with hardwood-smoked bacon, melted Pepper Jack cheese, peppercorn spread, tomatoes, and crispy onion straws—3540 kcal (**www.redrobin.com/menu**)! The calories in this supersized burger represent the equivalent of the *2-day* total calorie requirement for a 5′6″ college-age female.

The total number of calories in a particular food item, although high, tells only part of the story. Adding other food items to the meal easily can propel the total calories well above the recommended daily requirement. For example, adding one large 5.4 oz order of French fries (500 kcal) and a chocolate *McCafe* shake (510 kcal) to a *McDonald's* Bacon Clubhouse Burger (1470 kcal) adds up to a whopping 2480 kcal! If you substitute a vanilla cone (170 kcal) for the shake, substitute a Premium Southwest Salad (450 kcal) for the fries, and a Southern Style Crispy Chicken Sandwich (430 kcal) for the Bacon Clubhouse Burger, you reduce the number of calories consumed by about 1500 kcal. This "calorie savings" still amounts to more than half of the recommended daily calorie consumption for a young woman of average body build. An important point worth considering is even when one selects supposedly more healthful food choices, the end result for total calories consumed probably will exceed the calories required for weight maintenance.

Research demonstrates, and as evident from **Figure 16.18**, fast-food consumption for one of the most popular categories of food entrees—the hamburger sandwich—relates directly to total energy intake and inversely to diet quality. Moreover, a positive association exists between fast-food consumption and body weight in adolescents and primarily overweight and obese individuals.

McDonald's	Big Mac	Bacon Clubhouse Burger	Bacon Habanero Ranch Quarter Pounder	Bacon & Cheese Quarter Pounder	Double Quarter Pounder w Cheese
Calories	530	720	610	600	740
Fat (g)	27	40	31	29	42
Carbohydrate (g)	47	52	47	48	43
Protein (g)	24	38	36	36	47
Sodium (mg)	960	1470	1190	1380	1300

Burger King	Whopper Sandwich	Double Whopper Sandwich	Double Whopper w Cheese w/o Mayo	Triple Whopper Sandwich	Four Cheese Whopper
Calories	650	900	1070	1160	850
Fat (g)	37	56	70	75	57
Carbohydrate (g)	50	50	52	50	47
Protein (g)	22	35	44	49	32
Sodium (mg)	910	980	1780	1050	1160

Carl's Jr.	Famous Star w Cheese	Super Star w Cheese	Double Western Bacon Cheeseburger	Guacamole Bacon Six Dollar Burger	Western Bacon Six Dollar Burger
Calories	680	940	1000	1030	1030
Fat (g)	39	59	54	69	55
Carbohydrate (g)	57	59	75	56	81
Protein (g)	28	48	53	48	53
Sodium (mg)	1220	1560	1840	2130	2440

Wendy's	Hot 'N Juicy w Cheese	Bacon Portabella	Hot 'N Juicy 1/2 lb	Baconator	Hot 'N Juicy 3/4 lb
Calories	580	610	820	940	1090
Fat (g)	35	31	46	57	66
Carbohydrate (g)	43	41	42	41	43
Protein (g)	39	34	48	57	69
Sodium (mg)	1220	1220	1510	1850	1960

McDonald's. 2014. (www.mcdonalds.com/us/en/food/full_menu/full_menu_explorer.html)
Burger King USA Nutritionals. 2014 (www.bk.com/pdfs/nutrition.pdf)
Carl's Jr. 2014 (www.carlsjr.com/)
Wendy's. 2014 (www.wendys.com/en-us/hamburgers)

FIGURE 16.18 Nutritional values of popular fast-food choices.

Genetics Play a Role

In our modern scientific era, molecular geneticists are committed to unraveling the intimate secrets of subcellular function related to obesity,

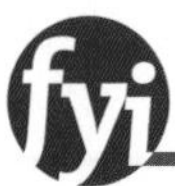

The Good and Bad of Body Fat

Three studies from researchers in Boston, Finland, and the Netherlands published in the *New England Journal of Medicine* show that some brown fat—the "good fat," which spurs the body to burn calories to generate body heat without ATP production (via uncoupled metabolism)—remains in adults. This energy-generating fat form stores mostly around the neck and under the collarbone; its energy-storing white (yellow) fat counterpart concentrates around the waistline to store energy and release chemicals that control metabolism and insulin use. The research indicates:

1. Lean individuals have more brown fat than do overweight counterparts.
2. Brown fat accelerates its energy release in cooler environments.
3. Women tend to have more brown fat than do men, with larger and more active deposits.

Devising a means to fully activate the body's brown fat might serve as the Holy Grail in treating the obese condition.

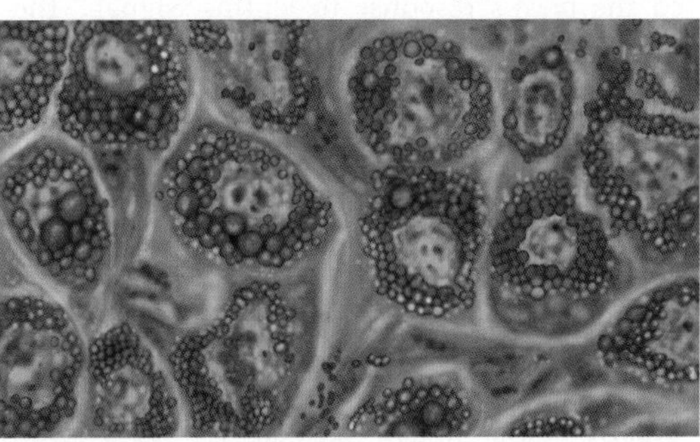

trying to answer a seemingly simple question: "Why have so many people become so fat, and what can be done to ameliorate the problem?" British researchers in December 2009 provided clear evidence of a biological mechanism that helps to explain why some people are more susceptible to gaining weight in a world dominated by high-calorie food and a sedentary lifestyle. The experiment turned the spotlight on the protein-coding **FTO gene**, which affects a person's risk of becoming obese or overweight. The FTO gene exists in two varieties, and all individuals inherit two copies of the gene. Children who inherit two copies of one variant were 70% more likely to be obese than those who inherited two copies of the other variant. Fifty percent of the children who inherited one copy of each FTO variant had a 30% higher obesity risk. The groundbreaking part of the study involved a subgroup of 76 children whose metabolism was monitored for 10 days and who consumed test meals at the school. The available food was measured before and after consumption to determine how much food the children consumed. Those tests showed the FTO variant did not depress metabolism but instead increased the tendency to eat more high-calorie foods in the test meals. In each case, the extra weight was explained entirely by more body fat, not increased muscle mass or structural differences such as being taller.

Genetic makeup does not necessarily cause obesity, but it does lower the threshold for its development and contributes to differences in weight gain for individuals fed identical daily caloric excess. **Figure 16.19** summarizes findings from a large number of individuals representing nine different background types. Genetic factors determined about 25% of transmissible variation in percentage body fat and total FM and largest transmissible variation related to a cultural effect. *In an obesity-producing environment characterized as sedentary and stressful with easy access to calorie-dense food, the genetically susceptible individuals gain weight.*

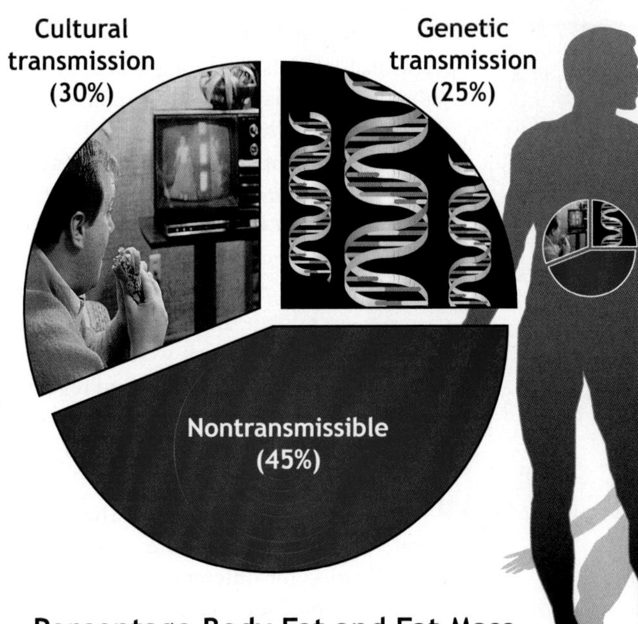

FIGURE 16.19 Total transmissible variance for body fat. Total body fat and percentage body fat determined by hydrostatic weighing. (Data from Bouchard C, et al. Inheritance of the amount and distribution of human body fat. *Int J Obes* 1988;12:205.)

A Mutant Gene and Leptin

In 2013, researchers linked human obesity to a **mutant gene**. Studies at the University of Cambridge in England identified a specific defect in two body weight–controlling genes. Two cousins from a Pakistani family in England inherited a defect in the gene that synthesizes leptin, a crucial hormonal body weight–regulating substance produced by fat and released into the bloodstream, where it acts on the hypothalamus. Congenital absence of leptin produced continual hunger and marked obesity in these children. The second genetic defect observed in an English patient affected the body's response to leptins "signal." The triggering signal largely determines how much one eats, how much energy one expends, and ultimately how much one weighs.

The genetic model in **Figure 16.20** proposes that the *ob* gene normally becomes activated in adipose tissue and perhaps muscle tissue, where it encodes and stimulates production of a body fat–signaling hormonelike protein called *ob* protein (or leptin), which then enters the bloodstream. This satiety signal molecule travels to the arcuate nucleus, a collection of specialized neurons in the mediobasal hypothalamus that controls appetite and metabolism and develops soon after birth. Normally, leptin blunts the urge to eat when caloric intake maintains ideal fat stores. Leptin may affect specific hypothalamic region neurons that stimulate production of chemicals that suppress appetite or reduce the levels of neurochemicals that stimulate appetite. Such mechanisms would explain how body fat remains intimately "connected" via a physiologic pathway to the brain to regulate energy balance. In essence, leptin availability or its lack affects the neurochemistry of appetite and the brain's dynamic "wiring" to possibly impact appetite and obesity in adulthood.

Gender, hormones, pharmacologic agents, and the body's current energy requirements also affect leptin production. Neither short- nor long-term physical activity meaningfully affects leptin, independent of the effects of activity on total adipose tissue mass.

The linkage of genetic and molecular abnormalities to obesity allows researchers to view overfatness as a disease instead of a psychological flaw.

fyi Obesity-Related Illness

Obesity causes more than 100,000 deaths in the United States each year, according to the latest statistics released by the American Institute of Cancer Research (**www.aich.org**). Excessive body fat causes nearly one half of endometrial cancers and one third of esophageal cancers. If Americans maintained normal body weights (BMI ≤25.0), endometrial cancer would decrease by 49%, esophageal cancer by 35%, pancreatic cancer by 28%, kidney cancer by 24%, gallbladder cancer by 21%, breast cancer by 17%, and colon cancer by 9%. Obesity-related illness accounts for nearly 10% of all medical costs in the United States—estimated at greater than $147 billion yearly.

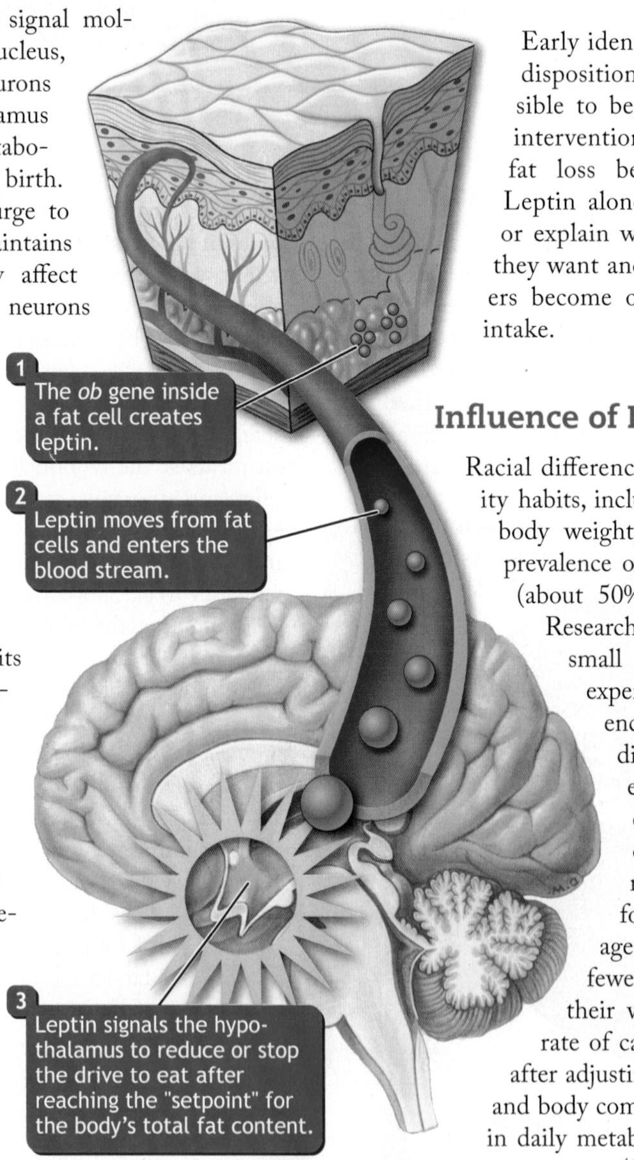

Early identification of one's genetic predisposition toward obesity makes it possible to begin diet and physical activity interventions before obesity sets in and fat loss becomes exceedingly difficult. Leptin alone does not determine obesity or explain why some people eat whatever they want and gain little weight while others become overfat with the same caloric intake.

1 The *ob* gene inside a fat cell creates leptin.
2 Leptin moves from fat cells and enters the blood stream.
3 Leptin signals the hypothalamus to reduce or stop the drive to eat after reaching the "setpoint" for the body's total fat content.

FIGURE 16.20 Genetic model of obesity. A malfunction of the satiety gene affects production of the satiety hormone leptin. Underproduction of leptin disrupts proper function of the hypothalamus (*step 3*), the center that regulates the body's fat level. (Model based on research conducted at Rockefeller University, New York.)

Influence of Racial Factors

Racial differences in food and physical activity habits, including cultural attitudes toward body weight, help to explain the greater prevalence of obesity among black women (about 50%) than white women (33%). Research with overfat women shows small differences in resting energy expenditure (REE) related to differences in LBM contribute to racial differences in obesity. A "racial" effect, which also exists among children and adolescents, predisposes black women to more readily gain weight and regain it following weight loss. On average, black women burn nearly 100 fewer kcal daily during rest than do their white counterparts. The slower rate of caloric expenditure persists even after adjusting for differences in body mass and body composition. A 100-kcal reduction in daily metabolism translates to nearly 1 lb (0.45 kg) of body fat gained each month. Total daily energy expenditure (TDEE) of black women averages 10% lower than whites, owing to a 5% lower REE and 19% lower physical activity energy expenditure. Additionally, overfat black women showed greater decreases in REE than did overfat white women after energy restriction and weight loss. The combination of a lower initial REE and more profound depression of REE with weight loss suggests that black women, including athletes, experience greater difficulty achieving and maintaining goal body weight than do overweight white women.

When evaluating purported racial differences in body composition characteristics and their implications for health and physical performance, one must carefully evaluate methods to explore such differences. Interethnic and interracial differences in body size, structure, and total body fat and its distribution can mask true differences in body fat at a given BMI. On the downside, single race-neutral, ethnicity-neutral generalized BMI health risk models obscure the potential to document actual chronic disease risks among different population groups. Perhaps, future research will determine a racially and ethnically based BMI model.

Physical Inactivity: An Important Component for Fat Accumulation

Regular physical activity, through either recreation or occupation, helps impede weight gain and adverse changes in body composition. Individuals who maintained weight loss over time showed greater muscle strength and engage in more physical activity than do their counterparts who regained lost weight. Variations in physical activity alone accounted for more than 75% of regained body weight. Such findings point to the need to identify and promote strategies that increase regular physical activity. In 2008, the U.S. Department of Health and Human Services (**www.health.gov/paguidelines/guidelines/default.aspx**) published national guidelines that recommended 60 or more minutes of daily moderate physical activity. We strongly endorse an increase to about 90 minutes of daily activity, 6 to 7 days a week over and above regular routines, to help to combat the obesity epidemic in the US population.

Physically active lifestyles lessen the "normal" pattern of fat gain in adulthood. For young and middle-aged men who exercise regularly, time spent in physical activity relates inversely to body fat level. Middle-aged long-distance runners remain leaner than their sedentary counterparts. Surprisingly, no relationship emerges between the runners' body fat level and caloric intake. Perhaps, the relatively greater body fat among middle-aged runners results from less-vigorous training, *not* greater food intake.

From age 3 months to 1 year, the total energy expenditure of infants who later became overweight averaged 21% less than infants with normal weight gain. For children ages 6 to 9 years, percentage body fat inversely related to physical activity level in boys but not girls. Overfat preadolescent and adolescent children generally spent less time engaging in physical activity or engaged in lower intensity physical activity than did normal-weight peers. The most discouraging news is that by the time young girls attain adolescence, many do not engage in regular physical activity. Specifically for girls, the decline in time spent in physical activity averaged nearly 100% among blacks and 64% among whites between ages 9 or 10 and ages 15 or 16. By age 16, 56% of the black girls and 31% of the white girls reported no leisure time physical activity.

Benefits of Increased Energy Output With Aging

Maintaining a lifestyle that includes a regular, consistent level of endurance physical activity attenuates but does not fully forestall the tendency to add extra weight through middle age. Sedentary men and women who begin a physical activity regimen lose weight and body fat compared with those who remain sedentary. Those who stop exercising gain body weight relative to those who remain active. Moreover, the amount of weight change relates proportionally to the change in physical activity dose. **Figure 16.21**

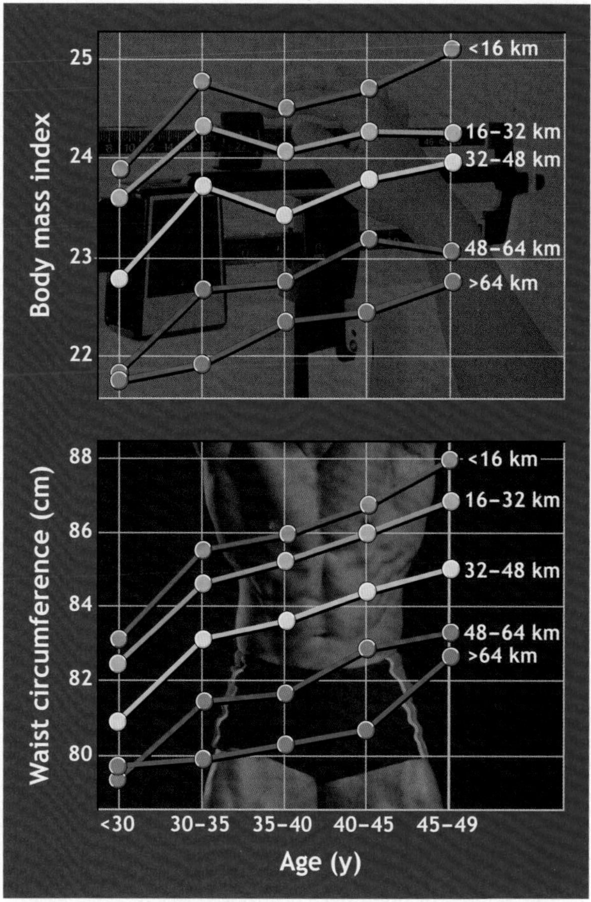

FIGURE 16.21 Relationship among average body mass index **(top)** and waist circumference **(bottom)** and age for men who maintained constant weekly running for varying distances (<16 to >64 km • wk^{-1}). Men who annually increase their running distance by 1.39 miles (2.24 km) per week compensate for the anticipated weight gain during middle age. (From Williams PT. Evidence for the incompatibility of age-neutral overweight and age-neutral physical activity standards from runners. *Am J Clin Nutr* 1997;65:1391.)

displays the inverse association among distance run and BMI and waist circumference in all age categories. Active men typically remained leaner than sedentary counterparts for each age group; men who ran longer distances weekly weighed less than did those who ran shorter distances. The typical man who maintained a constant weekly running distance through middle age gained 3.3 lb (1.5 kg), and waist size increased about three fourths of an inch (1.9 cm), regardless of distance run. Such findings suggest that by age 50, a physically active man can expect to weigh about 10 lb (4.5 kg) or more with a 2-inch (5.1 cm) larger waist than he weighed several decades before despite maintaining a constant level of increased physical activity. This somewhat coincides with the expected typical weight gain of about 1 lb (0.45 kg) per year between ages 20 and 60. To counter weight gain in middle age, one should gradually increase the amount of weekly physical activity the equivalent of running 1.4 miles (about an additional 150 kcal expenditure) for each year of age starting at about age 30.

HEALTH RISKS OF OBESITY

Obesity has joined cigarette smoking, hypertension, elevated serum cholesterol, and physical inactivity in the American Heart Association's list of primary coronary heart disease risk factors (**www.americanheart.org/presenter.jhtml?identifier=4639**). Clear associations exist among obesity and hypertension, type 2 diabetes, and various lipid abnormalities (dyslipidemia), including increased risk of cerebrovascular disease, alterations in fatty acid metabolism, and atherosclerosis. For Your Information: "Specific Health Risks of Excessive Body Fat" illustrates 11 major health consequences of obesity.

The costs associated with adult obesity are estimated to range between $147 billion and $210 billion per year or nearly 10% of the US national healthcare budget (**http://stateofobesity.org/facts-economic-costs-of-obesity/**). If the body size of Americans continues to increase at the current rate, one in five healthcare dollars spent on middle-aged Americans by 2020 will result from obesity.

CRITERIA FOR EXCESSIVE BODY FAT: HOW FAT IS TOO FAT?

Three approaches are appropriate for measuring an individual's body fat content:

1. Percentage of body mass composed of fat
2. Distribution or patterning of fat at different anatomic regions
3. Size and number of individual fat cells

Percentage Body Fat

The demarcation between what is considered a "normal" body fat level and when obesity begins often seems arbitrary. Part 2 of this chapter identified "the normal" range of body fat in adult men and women as plus or minus 1 unit of variation (standard deviation) from the average population value. That variation unit equals ±5% body fat for men and women between ages 17 and 50. Within this statistical boundary, overfatness corresponds to any percentage body fat value *above* the average value for age and gender, *plus* 5 percentage points. For young men, whose FM averages 15% of body mass, borderline obesity equals 20% body fat. For older men, the average percentage of fat approximates 25%. Consequently, a body fat content in excess of 30% would represent overfatness for this group. For young women, obesity corresponds to a body fat content above 30%, but for older women, borderline obesity begins at 37% body fat.

Age-specific demarcations for obesity assume that men and women *normally* become fatter with age. However, this does not necessarily occur for physically *active* men and women. If lifestyle factors account for the greatest portion of body fat increase during adulthood, then the criterion for overfatness could justifiably represent the standard for younger men and women.

We consider that obesity exists along a continuum from the upper limit of average (20% body fat for men and 30% for women) to as high as 50% and a theoretical maximum of nearly 70% of body mass for massively obese individuals. This latter group's weight ranges from 170 kg (375 lb) to 250 kg (551 lb) or higher. Such extreme cases can create a life-threatening situation because the individual's body's total fat content would exceed his or her LBM!

Regional Fat Distribution

The distribution of the body's adipose tissue, independent of total body fat, alters health risks in children, adolescents, and adults. **Figure 16.22** shows two types of regional fat distribution. Increased health risk from fat deposition in the abdominal region (central or **android-type obesity**; see A Closer Look: "Calculating and Interpreting the Waist-to-Hip Girth Ratio"), particularly internal visceral deposits, may result from this tissue's active lipolysis with catecholamine stimulation. Fat stored in this region shows greater metabolic responsiveness than fat in the gluteal and femoral regions (peripheral or **gynoid-type obesity**). Increases in central fat more readily support processes that cause heart disease. In men, the amount of fat located inside the abdominal cavity called intra-abdominal or visceral adipose tissue is twice as large compared with women. For men, the percentage of visceral fat increases progressively with age; this fat deposition in women begins to increase at menopause onset.

Central fat deposition, independent of fat storage in other anatomic areas, reflects an altered metabolic profile that increases at least eight medical conditions:

1. Hyperinsulinemia (insulin resistance)
2. Glucose intolerance
3. Type 2 diabetes
4. Endometrial cancer
5. Hypertriglyceridemia

Specific Health Risks of Excessive Body Fat

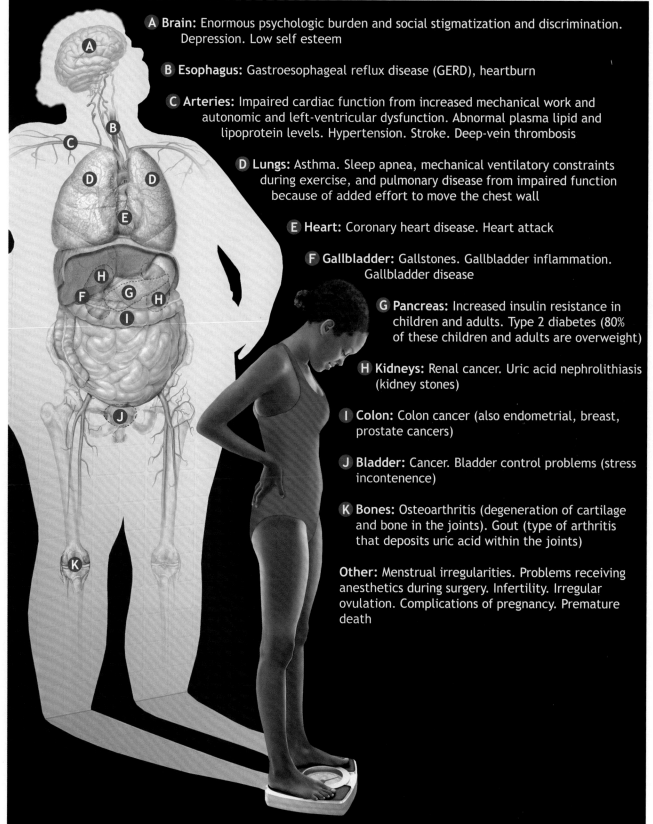

A Brain: Enormous psychologic burden and social stigmatization and discrimination. Depression. Low self esteem

B Esophagus: Gastroesophageal reflux disease (GERD), heartburn

C Arteries: Impaired cardiac function from increased mechanical work and autonomic and left-ventricular dysfunction. Abnormal plasma lipid and lipoprotein levels. Hypertension. Stroke. Deep-vein thrombosis

D Lungs: Asthma. Sleep apnea, mechanical ventilatory constraints during exercise, and pulmonary disease from impaired function because of added effort to move the chest wall

E Heart: Coronary heart disease. Heart attack

F Gallbladder: Gallstones. Gallbladder inflammation. Gallbladder disease

G Pancreas: Increased insulin resistance in children and adults. Type 2 diabetes (80% of these children and adults are overweight)

H Kidneys: Renal cancer. Uric acid nephrolithiasis (kidney stones)

I Colon: Colon cancer (also endometrial, breast, prostate cancers)

J Bladder: Cancer. Bladder control problems (stress incontenence)

K Bones: Osteoarthritis (degeneration of cartilage and bone in the joints). Gout (type of arthritis that deposits uric acid within the joints)

Other: Menstrual irregularities. Problems receiving anesthetics during surgery. Infertility. Irregular ovulation. Complications of pregnancy. Premature death

(Reproduced with permission from McArdle WD, Katch FI, Katch VL. *Exercise Physiology: Nutrition, Energy, and Human Performance*. 8th Ed. Baltimore: Wolters Kluwer Health, 2015.)

6. Hypercholesterolemia and negatively altered lipoprotein profile
7. Hypertension
8. Atherosclerosis

As a general guideline, waist-to-hip girth ratios that exceed 0.80 for women and 0.95 for men increase the risk of death even when adjusting for BMI.

One limitation of the ratio is that it poorly captures the specific effects of each girth measure. Waist and hip circumferences reflect different aspects of body composition and fat distribution. Each exerts an independent and often opposite effect on cardiovascular disease risk. *An increased waist girth coincides with the so-called malignant form of obesity characterized by central fat deposition.* This region of fat deposition provides a reasonable indication of VAT accumulation. *This makes waist girth the trunk measure of clinical choice as a practical measure to evaluate the metabolic and health risks and accelerated mortality with obesity.*

Over a broad range of BMI values, men and women with high waist circumference values possess greater relative risk for cardiovascular disease, type 2 diabetes, cancer, dementia, and cataracts (the leading cause of blindness worldwide) than do individuals with small waist circumferences or peripheral obesity. A waist girth that exceeds 91 cm (36 in.) in men and 82 cm (32 in.) in women and correspondingly high blood insulin levels nearly doubles colorectal cancer risk. **Figure 16.23** shows how to apply three BMI categories and waist girth measurements (above and below 101.6 cm [40 in.] for men and 89.9 cm [34.6 in.] for women) to assess a person's risk of health problems ranked from least risk to very high risk. For children and teens ages 2 through 19, the CDC recommends a calculation based on the corresponding BMI-for-age percentile on a CDC BMI-for-age growth chart (**http://nccd.cdc.gov/dnpabmi/Calculator.aspx**).

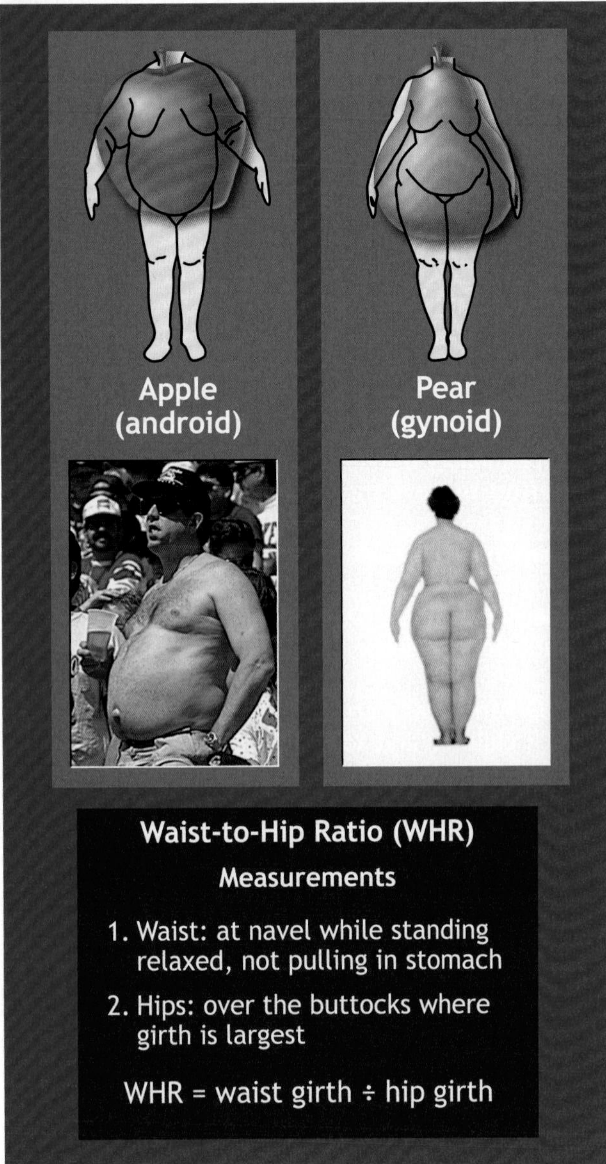

Apple
(android)
Pear
(gynoid)
Waist-to-Hip Ratio (WHR)
Measurements
1. Waist: at navel while standing relaxed, not pulling in stomach
2. Hips: over the buttocks where girth is largest
WHR = waist girth ÷ hip girth

FIGURE 16.22 Male (android pattern) and female (gynoid pattern) fat patterning, including measurement of waist-to-hip girth ratio.

Fat Cell Size and Number

The size and number of fat cells provide physiological insights about structure, form, and dimensions of normal and

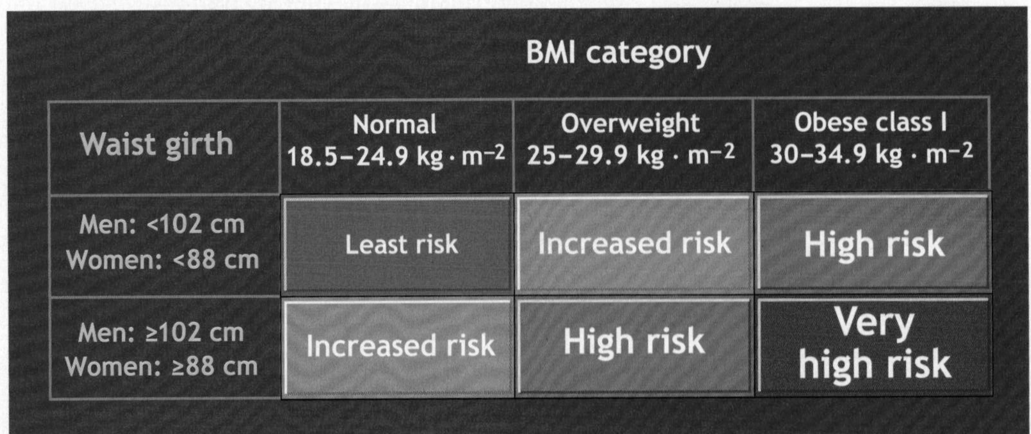

	BMI category		
Waist girth	Normal 18.5–24.9 kg · m^{-2}	Overweight 25–29.9 kg · m^{-2}	Obese class I 30–34.9 kg · m^{-2}
Men: <102 cm Women: <88 cm	Least risk	Increased risk	High risk
Men: ≥102 cm Women: ≥88 cm	Increased risk	High risk	Very high risk

FIGURE 16.23 Applying BMI and waist girth measurements in adult men and women from least risk to very high risk for health and longevity and medical problems. For men, high risk = 102 cm (40 in.); for women, high risk = 88 cm (34.6 in.). (Data from the world literature, including Douketis JD. Body weight classification. *CMAJ* 2005;172:995.)

abnormal levels of body fatness. Increases in adipose tissue mass occur in two ways:

1. Enlarging or filling of existing fat cells with more fat (**fat cell hypertrophy**)
2. Increasing the total number of fat cells (**fat cell hyperplasia**)

Assessing adipocyte size and number involves needle biopsy aspiration directly into the fat depot to suck small fragments of subcutaneous tissue from the upper back, buttocks, abdomen, or back of the upper arm (**Fig. 16.24**). Chemical treatment of the biopsy sample enables the researcher to separate and count the fat cells. One can estimate **total adipocyte number** by determining total body fat by a criterion method such as hydrostatic weighing. For example, an individual who weighs 88 kg (194 lb) with 13% body fat has a total FM of 11.4 kg (25.1 lb) (0.13 × 88 kg). Dividing 11.4 kg by the average fat content per cell estimates total adipocyte number. If the average adipocyte contains 0.60 μg of fat, then this person's body contains 19 billion adipocytes (11.4 kg ÷ 0.60 μg).

Total adipocyte number
= Mass of body fat
÷ Fat content per cell

Cellularity Differences Between Nonobese and Obese Persons

The data in the *left side* of **Figure 16.25** illustrate the strong association between total FM in overfat individuals and their corresponding fat cell number. The person with the lowest body fat content had the fewest number of fat cells, whereas the fattest subject had considerably more adipocytes. In contrast, the data displayed in the *right panel* of the figure show little relationship between total

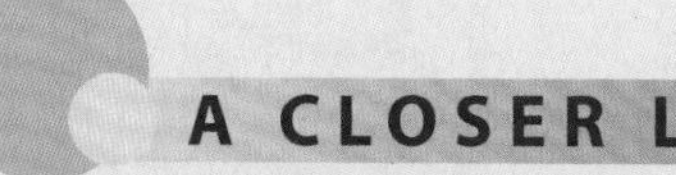

A CLOSER LOOK

Calculating and Interpreting the Waist-to-Hip Girth Ratio

Waist-to-hip girth ratio (WHR) indicates relative fat distribution in adults and risk of disease (see Table). A higher ratio reflects a greater proportion of **abdominal fat** with a greater risk for hyperinsulinemia, insulin resistance, type 2 diabetes, endometrial cancer, hypercholesterolemia, hypertension, and atherosclerosis.

WHR computes as abdominal girth (centimeter or inch) ÷ hip girth (centimeter or inch); waist girth represents the smallest girth around the abdomen (the natural waist), and hip girth reflects the largest girth measured around the buttocks (see Fig. 16.22 and the image below).

Waist-to-Hip Girth Ratio and Disease Risk

		Risk Level			
	Age, y	**Low**	**Moderate**	**High**	**Very High**
Men	20–29	<0.83	0.83–0.88	0.89–0.94	>0.94
	30–39	<0.84	0.84–0.91	0.92–0.96	>0.96
	40–49	<0.88	0.88–0.95	0.96–1.00	>1.00
	50–59	<0.90	0.90–0.96	0.97–1.02	>1.02
	60–69	<0.91	0.91–0.98	0.99–1.03	>1.03
Women	20–29	<0.71	0.71–0.77	0.78–0.82	>0.82
	30–39	<0.72	0.72–0.78	0.79–0.84	>0.84
	40–49	<0.73	0.73–0.79	0.80–0.87	>0.87
	50–59	<0.74	0.74–0.81	0.82–0.88	>0.88
	60–69	<0.76	0.76–0.83	0.84–0.90	>0.90

Calculating WHR

Example 1

Man: Age, 21 years; abdominal girth, 101.6 cm; hip girth, 93.5 cm

WHR = Abdominal girth (cm) ÷ Hip girth (cm)
= 101.6 ÷ 93.5
= 1.08 (very high disease risk)

Example 2

Woman: Age, 41 years; abdominal girth, 83.2 cm; hip girth, 101 cm

WHR = Abdomen girth (cm) ÷ Hip girth (cm)
= 83.2 ÷ 101
= 0.82 (high disease risk)

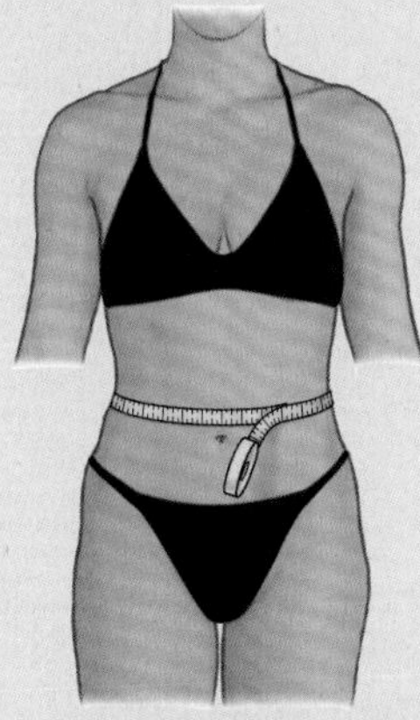

Abdomen: Minimum girth; standing, feet together

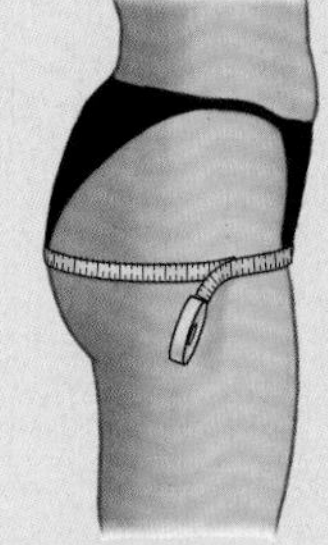

Hips: Maximum girth around buttocks; standing, feet together

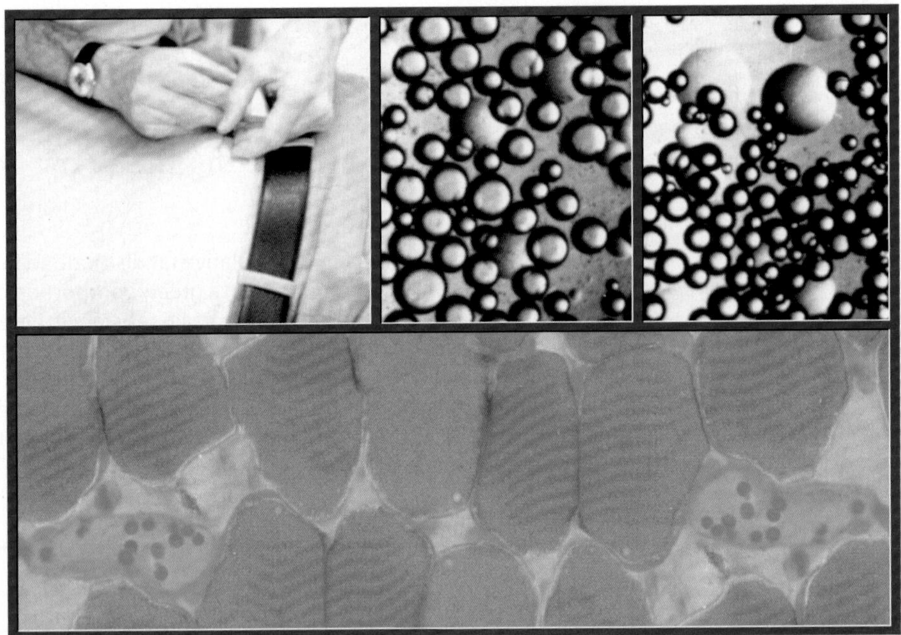

FIGURE 16.24 Upper panel. Needle biopsy procedure to extract fat cells of the upper buttocks region. The area is sterilized and anesthetized, and the biopsy needle placed beneath the skin surface. The syringe sucks small tissue fragments from the site. The two photomicrographs indicate fat cells biopsied from the buttocks of a physically active professor before **(center)** and after **(right)** 6 months of marathon training. The average fat cell diameter averaged 8.6% smaller after training. The average volume of fat per cell decreased by 18.2%. The large spherical structures in the background represent intracellular lipid droplets. (Photomicrographs courtesy of Clarkson PM, Muscle Biology and Imaging Laboratory, University of Massachusetts, Amherst, MA.) **Lower panel.** Cross section of human fat cells magnified ×440. (From Geneser F. *Color Atlas of Histology*. Philadelphia: Lea & Febiger, 1985.)

body fat and average fat cell size in overfat individuals. This suggests that a biologic upper limit exists for fat cell size. After reaching this size, cell number probably becomes the key factor determining the extent of extreme obesity. Even doubling the size of normal fat cells would not account for the tremendous difference in the fat content between those who are overfat and those who are not. It seems reasonable to conclude, therefore, that excessive adipose tissue mass in severe obesity occurs by fat cell hyperplasia.

A related early study regarding fat cell size and number compared body mass, total fat, and adipose tissue cellularity in 25 subjects, 20 of whom classified as clinically obese (BMI ~40.0). The body mass of the obese averaged more

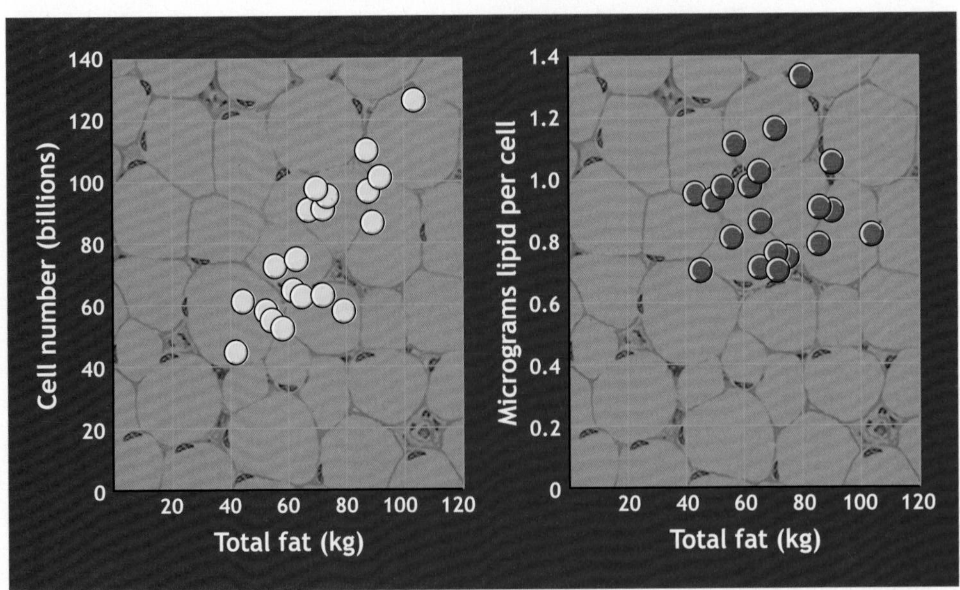

FIGURE 16.25 Adipose cell number **(left)** and size **(right)** related to the body's total fat mass.

than twice that of nonobese, and they had nearly three times more body fat. In cellularity, adipocytes in the obese averaged 50% larger with nearly three times more cells (75 vs. 27 billion; **Fig. 16.26**). *Cell number represents the major structural difference in adipose tissue mass between severely obese and nonobese persons.*

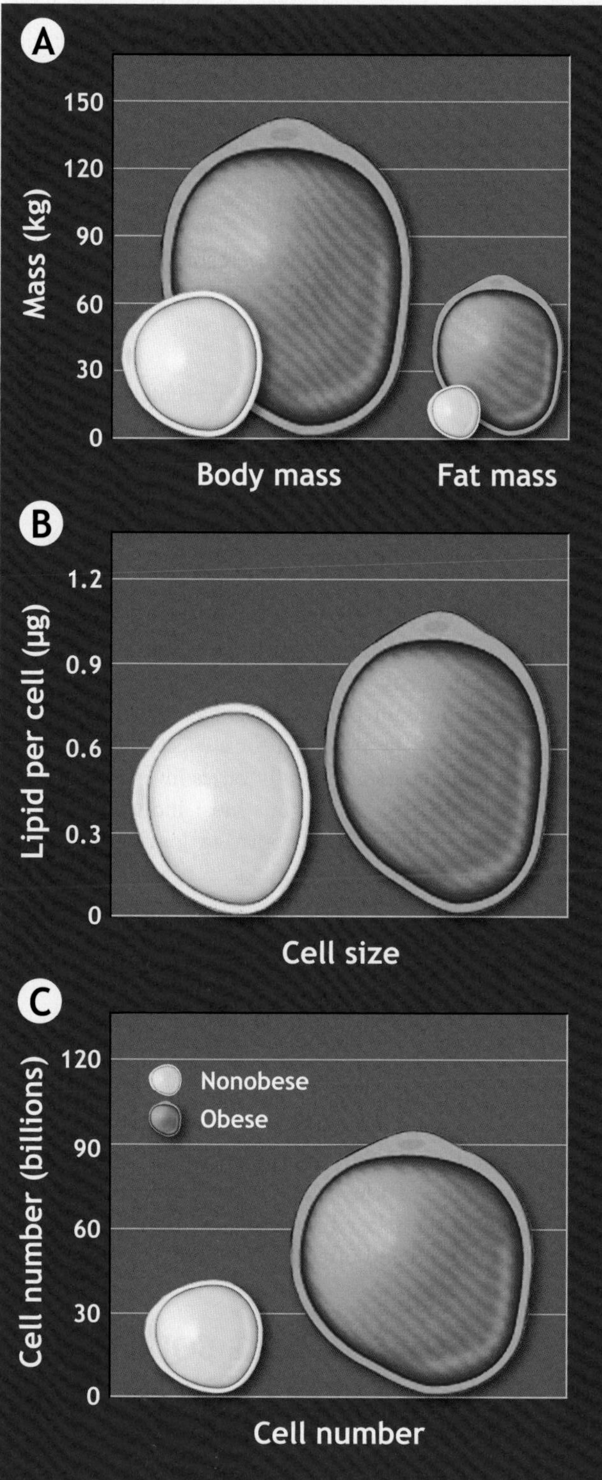

FIGURE 16.26 Comparison of body mass and fat mass **(A)**, cell size **(B)**, and cell number **(C)** in 25 subjects, 20 of whom classified as clinically obese. (Reprinted with permission from McArdle WD, Katch FI, Katch VL. *Exercise Physiology: Nutrition, Energy, and Human Performance*. 8th Ed. Baltimore: Wolters Kluwer Health, 2015.)

As a frame of comparison, an average person has about 25 to 30 billion fat cells. For moderately overfat people, this number ranges between 60 and 100 billion, but the fat cell number for massively obese people may increase to 360 billion or more! Even with **gastric banding surgery** (**www.nlm.nih.gov/medlineplus/ency/article/007388.htm**) to reduce the size of the stomach and restrict food intake at any given meal, the substantial weight loss months after surgery still did not reduce fat cell number.

SUMMARY

1. Overfatness, defined as excessive body fat, represents a complex disorder that involves interrelated factors that tip energy balance in favor of weight gain.
2. Over the past 30 years, the average body weight of adult Americans has increased considerably. For 2014, approximately 35% of adults (78.6 million) classify as obese (BMI ≥30), and nearly 65% (130 million adults) are either overweight or obese (BMI ≥25).
3. Genetic factors probably account for 25% to 30% of excessive body fat accumulation.
4. Genetic predisposition does not necessarily cause obesity, but given the right environment, genetically susceptible individuals gain body fat.
5. About 15% to 20% of American children and 12% of adolescents (up from 7.6% in 1976 to 1980) classify as overweight.
6. Excessive body fatness, childhood's most common chronic disorder, is particularly prevalent among poor and minority children.
7. Obesity represents a medical (disease) condition that includes overfatness and dyslipidemia, hypertension, insulin resistance, and glucose intolerance.
8. No reason fully accounts for the typical body fat increases observed for American men and women with aging.
9. Body fat standards for borderline overfatness in adult men and women could justifiably be the values for younger adults—20% body fat for men and 30% for women.
10. Adipose tissue patterning provides important health-related information.
11. Fat distributed in the abdominal–visceral region (android-type obesity) poses a greater health risk compared with fat deposited at the thigh, hips, and buttocks (gynoid-type obesity).
12. Waist girth provides a second dimension of obesity when assessing the health-risk profile.
13. Men and women with large waist girths possess greater relative risk for cardiovascular disease, type 2 diabetes, cancer, and cataracts than individuals with small waist girths.
14. Size and the number of adipocytes provide another obesity classification.

15. Increases in adipocyte number involve three general time periods: last trimester of pregnancy, first year of life, and adolescent growth spurt before adulthood.
16. Before adulthood, body fat increases by enlargement of individual fat cells (fat cell hypertrophy) and increases in total number of fat cells (fat cell hyperplasia).
17. Adipocyte number stabilizes sometime before adulthood; any weight gain or loss thereafter usually relates to changes in fat cell size.
18. In extreme obesity, cell number can increase after adipocytes reach their hypertrophic limit.

THINK IT THROUGH

1. Discuss the possibility that excessive food intake does not cause excessive body fat accumulation in children and adults.
2. What possible explanation(s) accounts for the worldwide rapid increase in body fat?
3. Discuss what you believe are the two leading causes of childhood obesity?
4. Explain if and why different body fat standards should apply to people of different ages.

PART 4 Achieving Optimal Body Composition Through Changes in Nutrition and Physical Activity

Former University of Pennsylvania pioneer obesity researcher Dr. Albert Stunkard (1922–2014; **www.nytimes.com/2014/07/21/us/21stunkard.html?_r=0**) in 1958

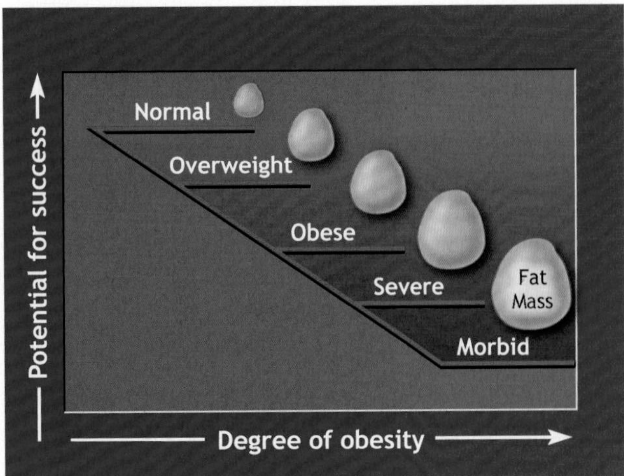

FIGURE 16.27 Likelihood of success in long-term maintenance of weight loss inversely relates to the level of obesity at the start of intervention.

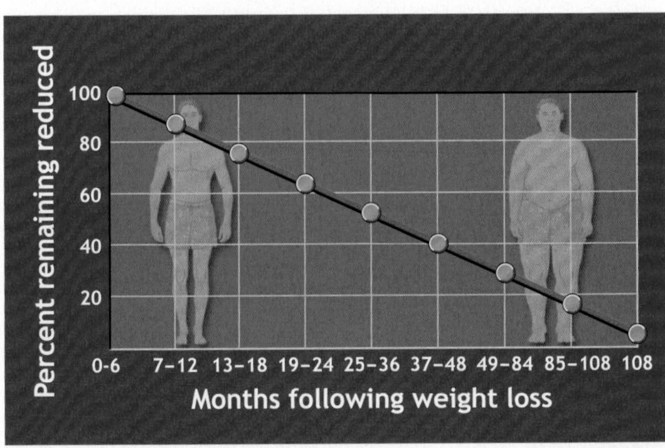

FIGURE 16.28 General trend for percentage of patients remaining at reduced weights at various time intervals after accomplished weight loss.

(*AMA Arch Intern Med* 1959;103:79) presented a realistic if disheartening view regarding long-term weight loss potential for overfat individuals based on his years of prior research experience with obese individuals:

> Most obese persons will not stay in treatment. Of those who stay in treatment, most will not lose weight, and of those who do lose weight, most will regain it.

Stunkard's bleak outlook, delivered four decades ago, buttresses the majority of subsequent research showing that initial modifications in body weight have little relation to long-term success. The potential for a successful prolonged weight-loss maintenance generally varies inversely with initial fatness level (**Fig. 16.27**). For most individuals, initial success in weight loss relates poorly to long-term success. Participants in supervised weight-loss programs, whether pharmacologic or behavioral interventions, generally reduce about 8% to 12% of their original body mass. Unfortunately, typically one to two thirds of the lost weight returns within 1 year, and almost all of it returns within 5 years.

Figure 16.28 illustrates that over a 7.3-year follow-up of 121 patients, 50% of those who lost weight returned to their original weight within 2 to 3 years, and only seven patients remained at their reduced body weights. These discouraging but typical statistics highlight the extreme difficulty of long-term maintenance of a low-calorie diet; it becomes particularly difficult in the relaxed atmosphere of one's home with ready access to food and often little emotional support.

THE ENERGY BALANCE EQUATION: THE KEY TO WEIGHT CONTROL

The **first law of thermodynamics**, often called the *law of conservation of energy*, posits that energy can be transferred from one system to another in many forms but cannot be created or destroyed. In human terms, this means that the energy balance equation dictates that body mass remains constant when caloric intake equals caloric expenditure. **Figure 16.29** illustrates how a chronic imbalance on the energy output or input side of the equation changes body weight.

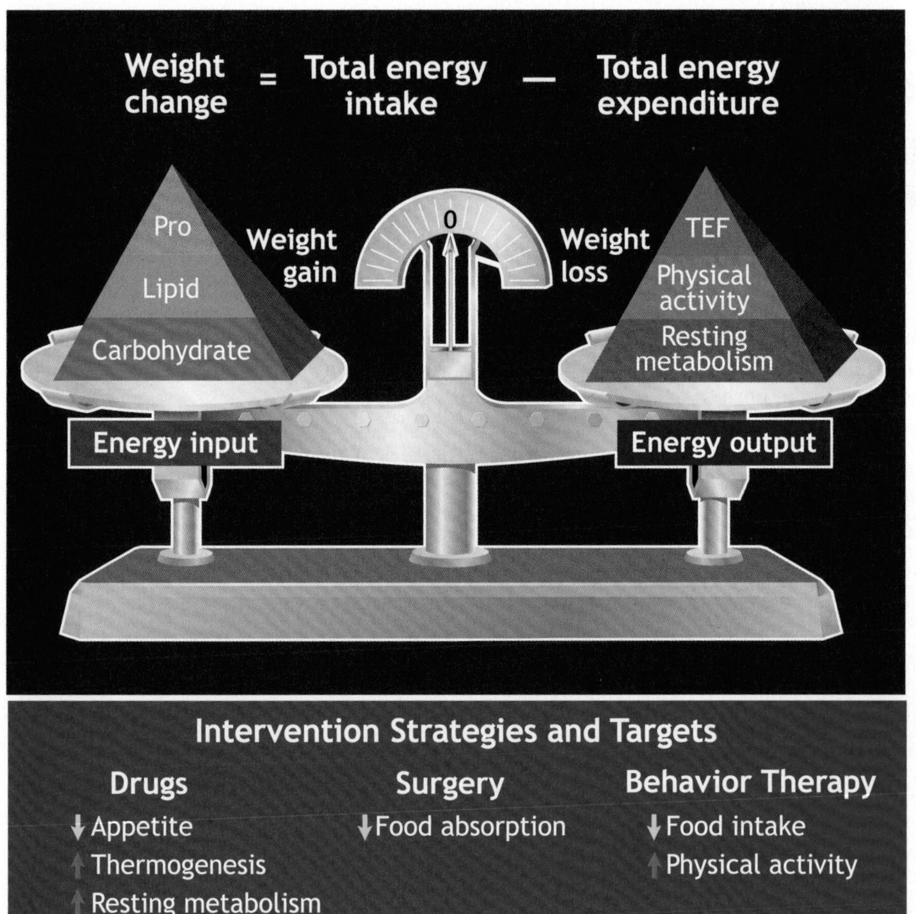

FIGURE 16.29 The energy balance equation plus intervention strategies and specific targets to alter energy balance in the direction of weight loss. Pro, protein; TEF, thermic effect of food.

To unbalance the energy balance equation and produce weight loss, three strategies can be used:

1. Reduce caloric intake below daily energy requirements.
2. Maintain caloric intake and increase energy expenditure through additional physical activity above daily energy requirements.
3. Decrease daily caloric intake and increase daily energy expenditure.

When considering sensitivity of the energy balance equation, if caloric intake exceeds output by "only" 100 kcal daily, the surplus calories consumed in a year equal 36,500 kcal (365 days × 100 kcal). Every 0.45 kg (1.0 lb) of body fat theoretically contains 3500 kcal (each 1 lb [454 g] of adipose tissue contains about 86% fat, or 390 g × 9 kcal · g^{-1} = 3514 kcal per lb), so this caloric excess results in a theoretical yearly gain of about 4.7 kg or 10.3 lb of body fat. In contrast, if daily food intake decreases by just 100 kcal and energy expenditure increases by 100 kcal (e.g., by walking or jogging 1 extra mile each day), then the yearly deficit equals the energy in 9.5 kg or 21 lb of body fat.

fyi Consuming Excess Calories Produces Fat Gain Regardless of Nutrient Source

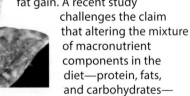

The quantity of food consumed, not the food's composition, determines fat gain. A recent study challenges the claim that altering the mixture of macronutrient components in the diet—protein, fats, and carbohydrates—profoundly affects fat gain.[1] Twenty-five young, healthy men ($n = 16$) and women ($n = 9$) with BMIs between 19 and 30 were deliberately fed 1000 excess calories a day for 56 days. Carbohydrate intake for both groups remained steady at about 42% of total calories consumed. Those on the low-protein diet (about 5% of total calories) gained less weight (largely attributed to a reduction in LBM) than those on a normal- or high-protein regimen (largely attributed to an increase in LBM). The body fat of all participants increased by about the same amount, a surprising finding suggesting that it is not the diet's macronutrient composition but rather the excess of calories consumed responsible for body fat accretion. On the opposite side of the energy balance debate,[2] study participants lost total, abdominal, and hepatic fat with consumption of all low-calorie diets regardless of whether they emphasized a lower percentage of fat, protein, or carbohydrate. No differences in fat loss were attributable to the diet's macronutrient composition.

References:

1. Bray G, et al. Effect of dietary protein content on weight gain, energy expenditure, and body composition during overeating: a randomized controlled trial. *JAMA* 2012;307:47.
2. deSouza RJ, et al. Effects of 4 weight-loss diets differing in fat, protein, and carbohydrate on FM, lean mass, visceral adipose tissue, and hepatic fat: results from the POUNDS LOST trial. *Am J Clin Nutr* 2012;95:614.

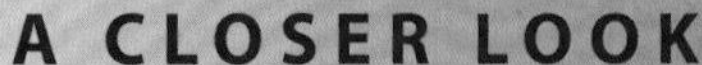

A CLOSER LOOK

Computing Daily Energy (Caloric) Requirement Including Physical Activity for Weight Management and Weight Loss

Successful weight loss requires a negative energy balance in which total calorie (kcal) expenditure exceeds total calorie intake. Foods consumed in the diet provide the body's energy required to carry out its metabolic functions. The total daily energy expenditure (TDEE), often referred to as the body's "energy requirement," includes:

1. Normal daily energy expenditure (including sleeping and "normal" daily living conditions), excluding energy expenditure during physical activity
2. Energy expenditure during physical activity (including energy expenditure above "normal" daily living activities)

Weight maintenance occurs when energy intake equals TDEE. Determining TDEE allows one to compute the change in food consumption and physical activity necessary for weight maintenance *or* weight loss.

Computing Total Daily Energy Expenditure to Maintain Body Weight

Table 1 presents the computational steps to determine TDEE, including kcal expenditure of physical activity and target number of calories, to achieve a given weight loss.

Example Computations

The following example illustrates the computations for a 24-year-old man who weighs 72.6 kg (160 lb) and who participates in moderate daily physical activity (refer to **Table 1**).

1. Record body weight (BW): ....**160 lb**
2. Record caloric requirement per pound BW (see **Table 2**): **15.0**
3. Compute daily caloric requirement without physical activity to maintain current BW (multiply step 1 by step 2): ....**2400 kcal**
4. Select physical activity (see **Table 3**; *if selecting more than one physical activity, estimate the average daily calories burned from each additional activity [steps 4 through 11] and add all of these totals to step12)*:...**jogging**
5. Record the number of exercise sessions completed weekly: **4**
6. Record the duration of each exercise session in minutes: ....**60 min**
7. Compute the total *weekly* exercise time in minutes (*multiply step 5 by step 6*): ....**240 min**
8. Compute the average *daily* exercise time in minutes (*divide step 7 by 7 [round to nearest whole min]*): ....**34 min**
9. Record the caloric expenditure per pound per minute ($kcal \cdot lb^{-1} \cdot min^{-1}$) for physical activity (see **Table 3**): **0.090**
10. Compute total calories burned per minute ($kcal \cdot min^{-1}$) during physical activity (*multiply step 1 by step 9*): ....**14.4 kcal · min^{-1}**
11. Compute average daily calorie expenditure (kcal) during physical activity (*multiply step 8 by step 10 [round to nearest whole number]*): ....**490 kcal**
12. Compute the daily caloric requirement, including exercise kcal, to maintain current body weight (TDEE) (*add step 3 plus step 11*): ....**2890 kcal**

TABLE 1 Computation of Daily Total Caloric Requirement and Target Caloric Intake to Lose Weight

1. Record body weight (BW).......................... ____
2. Record caloric requirement per pound BW (see **Table 2**).. ____
3. Compute daily caloric requirement without physical activity to maintain current BW (*multiply Step #1 _ Step #2*).......................... ____
4. Select physical activity (see **Table 3**). *If more than one physical activity is selected, estimate the average daily calories burned as a result of each additional activity (Steps #4 through #11) and add all of these totals to Step #12*................................. ____
5. Record the number of exercise sessions you do per week.. ____
6. Record the duration of each exercise session in minutes.. ____
7. Compute the total weekly exercise time in minutes (*multiply Step #5 by Step #6*)...................... ____
8. Compute the average daily exercise time in minutes (*divide Step #7 by 7 [round to nearest whole min]*)... ____
9. Record the caloric expenditure per pound per minute ($kcal \cdot lb^{-1} \cdot min^{-1}$) for your physical activity (*see* **Table 3**)....................... ____
10. Compute total calories burned per minute ($kcal \cdot min^{-1}$) during physical activity (*multiply Step #1 by Step #9*)................. ____
11. Compute average daily calorie expenditure (kcal) during physical activity (*add Step #3 and Step #11*)................................... ____
12. Compute daily caloric requirement, including exercise kcal, to maintain current BW (TDEE) ____
13. Compute number of calories to subtract from requirement to achieve a negative calorie balance (*subtract 500 kcal if the total daily kcal expenditure [Step #12] is below 3000 kcal, 1000 kcal for daily expenditures above 3000 kcal)*.................................. ____
14. Compute target caloric intake required to lose weight (*subtract Step #13 from Step #12*)... ____

TABLE 2 Average 24-Hour Energy Expenditure Estimated From Body Weight (lb) Based on Different Physical Activity Levels for Men and Women[a]

	kcal per lb[b]	
Activity Level	**Males**	**Females**
Sedentary (limited) physical activity [no regular physical activity outside of work]	13.0	12.0
Moderate physical activity [planned, systematic light to moderate physical activity 2–3 days per week, outside of work]	15.0	13.5
Strenuous physical activity [planned, systematic heavy physical activity 4–6 days per week, outside of work]	17.0	15.0

[a] Pregnant or lactating women add 3.0 kcal per lb.

[b] The 24-h energy expenditure for a sedentary male weighing 160 lb equals 2080 kcal (13 kcal per pound × 160 lb = 2080).

Computations of Target Energy Intake Required to Reduce Body Weight

In the above example, the TDEE to maintain body weight equals 2890 kcal. Thus, the total kcal intake must decrease below this value to induce a negative caloric balance for weight loss. The energy deficit should never cause the total daily caloric intake to fall below 1200 kcal for women and 1500 kcal for men. This level of energy intake represents a safe level to ensure adequate intake of protein, vitamins, and minerals. Prudent recommendations include subtracting 500 kcal per day if the TDEE is below 3000 kcal and 1000 kcal for daily TDEE above 3000 kcal.

To compute the target number of calories for weight loss:

1. Compute number of calories to subtract from requirement to achieve a negative calorie balance (subtract 500 kcal if the total daily kcal expenditure [step 12] is below 3000 kcal or 1000 kcal for daily expenditures above 3000 kcal): ....**500 kcal**
2. Compute the target total caloric intake to reduce weight (subtract step 13 from step 12): ....**2390 kcal**

TABLE 3 Sample Caloric Expenditures in kcal Per Pound of Body Weight Per Minute (kcal · lb^{-1} · min^{-1})

Activity	kcal · lb^{-1} · min^{-1}	Activity	kcal · lb^{-1} · min^{-1}
Basketball	0.062	Skiing, soft snow, leisure	0.044
Circuit weight training		Skiing, hard snow, moderate speed	0.054
Nautilus	0.042		
Climbing hills	0.055	Volleyball	0.023
Cycling		Walking	
5.5 mph	0.032	4.5 mph	0.045
10 mph	0.050	Grass track	0.037
13 mph	0.070	Shallow pool	0.090
Aerobic dance		Swimming	
Medium	0.047	Crawl, slow	0.058
Intense	0.061	Crawl, fast	0.071
Golf	0.038	Back stroke	0.077
Gymnastics	0.030	Breast stroke	0.074
Jumping rope		Side stroke	0.056
70 jumps/min	0.075	Canoeing	
80 jumps/min	0.080	Leisure	0.019
Racquetball	0.080	Racing	0.047
Running			
11 min: 30 s/mile	0.062		
9 min/mile	0.087		
8 min/mile	0.097		
7 min/mile	0.1085		
6 min/mile	0.1231		

Source: American College of Sports Medicine. Position statement on proper and improper weight loss programs. *Med Sci Sports Exerc* 1993;15:9.

Unbalancing the Energy Balance Equation

An objective assessment of energy intake from food and energy expenditure provides the frame of reference for unbalancing the energy balance equation to favorably modify body weight and body composition.

Energy Intake

Estimates of caloric intake from daily food intake records usually fall within ±10% of the actual number of calories consumed. For example, suppose the energy value of a person's daily food intake averaged 2130 kcal. Based on a careful 3-day, supervised dietary history to estimate caloric intake, the daily value would fall between 1920 and 2350 kcal. Careful record keeping of food intake also provides the dieter with an objective list of foods consumed rather than a "guesstimate" and triggers an important behavioral aspect of the weight control process—awareness of current food habits and preferences.

Energy Output

A physically active lifestyle is crucial to long-term success at weight loss. This does not mean playing tennis twice a week, going for a swim on weekends during the summer, or walking to the store when the car needs repair. Rather, modifying physical activity habits entails a serious commitment to changing daily routines to include regular moderate to vigorous physical activity. A Closer Look: "Computing Daily Energy (Caloric) Requirement Including Physical Activity for Weight Management and Weight Loss" illustrates how to compute daily energy (kcal) requirement including physical activity for weight maintenance or weight loss.

ALTERING THE ENERGY BALANCE EQUATION

The objective of weight-loss programs has changed dramatically over the past four decades. Earlier approaches assigned a goal body weight that coincided with an "ideal" weight based on body mass and stature or BMI. Achievement of goal body weight heralded the weight-loss program's success. Currently, the WHO, Institute of Medicine of the National Academy of Sciences and NHLBI (**www.nhlbi.nih.gov/**) recommend that overfat individuals reduce their initial body weight by 5% to 15%. *This more realistic weight loss diminishes weight-related comorbidities and complications from hypertension, type 2 diabetes, and abnormal blood lipids and often exerts a positive effect on social and psychological complications.* Setting the initial weight-loss goal beyond the 5% to 15% recommendation often gives patients an unrealistic and potentially unattainable target in light of current treatment methods and practical realities.

Prior beliefs contended that only calories from dietary lipids increased body fat. Reducing fat intake to achieve body fat loss is generally a good idea, but individuals often disproportionately increase carbohydrate and protein intakes. Thus, total caloric intake remains unchanged or even increases. The prudent dietary approach to weight loss unbalances the energy balance equation by reducing daily energy intake 500 to 1000 kcal *below* the daily energy expenditure while consuming well-balanced meals. Compared with more severe energy restriction, which accelerates lean tissue loss, a moderate reduction in food intake produces a greater fat loss relative to energy deficit.

Most people do not tolerate prolonged daily caloric restriction of less than 1000 kcal; more extreme semistarvation also increases the likelihood for malnourishment, depletion of glycogen reserves, and lean tissue loss. *One immutable truth about dieting to achieve success in altering the energy balance equation—the first law of thermodynamics—affirms conclusively that weight loss by dieting occurs whenever energy output exceeds energy intake, regardless of the diet's macronutrient mixture.*

fyi Controversy: Can You Really Reduce 1 lb a Week With a 3500-kcal Deficit?

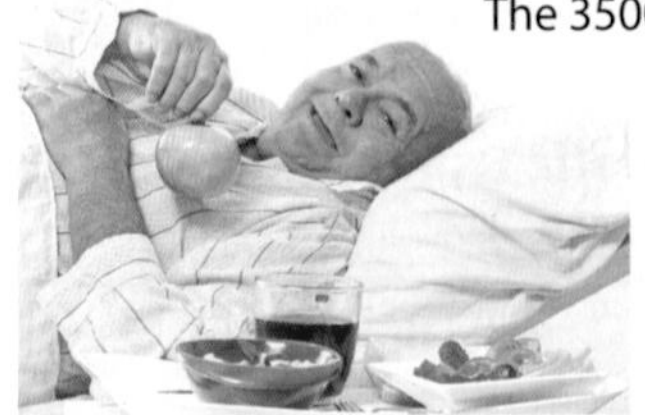

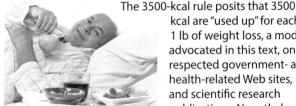

The 3500-kcal rule posits that 3500 kcal are "used up" for each 1 lb of weight loss, a model advocated in this text, on respected government- and health-related Web sites, and scientific research publications. Nonetheless, new research suggests that this rule grossly overestimates actual weight loss. The authors of a 2013 study demonstrate this overestimation and risk of applying the 3500-kcal rule even as a convenient weight-loss estimate by comparing predicted against actual weight loss in seven experiments conducted in confinement under total supervision or objectively measured energy intake.

The researchers provide downloadable applications housed in Microsoft Excel and Java, which simulate a rigorously validated, dynamic model of expected weight change. The first two tools, available at **www.pbrc.edu/sswcp**, offer a convenient alternative method to provide individuals with projected weight loss and weight gain estimates in response to changes in dietary energy intake. A second tool, which can be downloaded at **www.pbrc.edu/mswcp**, projects estimated weight loss simultaneously for multiple subjects, a useful adjunct to inform weight change in varied experimental designs and statistical analysis. The new tools offer a convenient and potentially more accurate alternative to the 3500-kcal rule than incorporated in most smartphone apps and commercial weight-loss–reducing regimens.

Source: Thomas DM, et al. Can a weight loss of one pound a week be achieved with a 3500-kcal deficit? Commentary on a commonly accepted rule. *Int J Obes (Lond)* 2013;37:161.

Practical Illustration

Suppose a college-age woman who normally consumes 2800 kcal daily and maintains a body mass of 79.4 kg (175 lb) wishes to lose weight by caloric restriction through dietary restraint. She maintains her regular physical activity but reduces daily food intake to 1800 kcal to create a 1000-kcal daily deficit. In 7 days, the accumulated deficit equals 7000 kcal or energy equivalent of 0.9 kg (2 lb) of body fat.

In actuality, the woman in our example might lose considerably more than 0.9 kg during the first week, because initially, the body's glycogen stores make up a large portion of the energy deficit. Stored glycogen contains fewer calories per gram and considerably more water than stored fat. For this reason, short periods of caloric restriction often encourage the dieter yet produce a large percentage of water and carbohydrate loss per unit weight loss with minimal decreases in body fat. As weight loss continues, a larger proportion of body fat supports the energy deficit created by food restriction. To reduce body fat by an additional 1.4 kg (3 lb), the dieter must maintain the reduced caloric intake of 1800 kcal for another 10.5 days; at this point, body fat theoretically would decrease at a rate of 0.45 kg (1 lb) every 3.5 days.

Unpredictable Mathematics of Weight Loss?

The mathematics of weight loss through caloric restriction seems straightforward, but results do not always follow. First, one assumes that daily energy expenditure remains relatively unchanged throughout the dieting period. Some people experience lethargy (because caloric restriction depletes the body's glycogen stores), which actually decreases daily energy expenditure. Second, the energy cost of physical activity decreases in proportion to the lost weight. This also shrinks the energy output side of the energy balance equation.

Resting Metabolic Rate Lowered

Metabolic changes also take place during caloric restriction, further blunting the weight-loss effort. Resting metabolism often slows with dietary only–induced weight loss. The resting metabolism decrease exceeds the decrease attributable to loss of either body mass or FFM; severe caloric restriction can depress resting metabolic rate up to 45%! A blunted metabolism characterizes individuals who attempt to lose weight, regardless if they dieted previously or were too fat or relatively lean. Reduced metabolism with low caloric intake conserves energy, causing the diet to become progressively less effective. Weight loss plateaus and further weight loss slows relative to that predicted from the mathematics of restricted energy intake.

Set Point Theory: A Case Against Dieting

One can crash off large amounts of weight in a relatively brief time by simply stopping eating. Unfortunately, success is short lived—eventually, the urge to eat wins out and the lost weight returns. Some argue that the reason for this failure lies in a genetically determined "set point" for body weight or body fat that differs from what the dieter would expect. The proponents of a **set point theory** maintain that all persons, fat or thin, have a well-regulated internal control mechanism similar to a thermostat located deep within the brain's lateral hypothalamus. This neural modulating center maintains a preset level of body weight, body fat, or both within a tight range. In a practical sense, set point represents a person's body weight when not counting calories. Regular physical activity and FDA-approved antiobesity drugs may lower the set point, but dieting probable exerts little to no effect.

Vicious Cycle

Each time body weight decreases below an individual's preestablished set point, internal adjustments in the lateral portions of the hypothalamus, the feeding center of the brain, affect food intake to resist the change and conserve body fat. Often the individual becomes food obsessed, unable to control urges to eat. Also, as discussed earlier, with weight loss resting metabolism slows further resisting weight (fat) loss. Even when persons overeat and gain body fat above their "preset" level, the body resists the change by increasing resting metabolism resulting in a decrease in caloric intake.

fyi The Challenge to the Weight-Loss Equation

A new weight-loss model considers the immediate and continuous slowing of the metabolic rate as weight loss progresses, limiting expected weight loss. This weight-loss model relies on controlled feeding studies that show a "metabolic slowdown" and loss of weight directly contribute to reduced energy expended in physical activity. For example, every reduction in food intake of 10 kcal a day for a typical overweight adult would lead to a weight loss of only one-half pound yearly, not the 1 lb (0.45 kg) a year loss predicted in the classic weight-loss model. The next half pound would take about 2 more years to lose. Reducing about 250 kcal daily produces a weight loss of about 25 lb (11.3 kg) in 3 years. These observations cast further doubt on the sole reliance on dietary restriction to achieve weight loss, often touted by many physicians as the most effective weight-loss method. The online simulator accessed at the National Institute of Diabetes and Digestive and Kidney Diseases (**www.niddk.nih.gov; http://bwsimulator.niddk.nih.gov**) provides a Web-based tool for people of varying body weights, diets, and physical activity habits to tailor a desired rate of weight loss based on short- and long-term physical activity habits.

Source: Hall KD, et al. Quantification of the effect of energy imbalance on bodyweight. *Lancet* 2011;378:826.

The set point theory is unwelcome news for those with a set point "tuned" too high; encouragingly, regular physical activity may lower the set point level. Concurrently, regular physical activity conserves and even increases FFM, increases resting metabolism if FFM increases, and induces metabolic changes that facilitate fat catabolism. These healthful adaptations all augment weight-loss efforts. If a physically active lifestyle becomes a reality and body fat decreases, caloric intake balances daily energy requirements to stabilize body mass at a new *lower* level.

Weight-Loss Effects on Fat Cell Size and Number

Figure 16.30 highlights the results of a classic study of weight-loss effects on changes in adipose tissue cellularity of overfat adults during two stages of weight loss. Nineteen overfat subjects who initially weighed 149 kg (329 lb) reduced body mass by 45.8 kg (102 lb), weighing 103 kg (227 lb) at the end of the first part of the experiment. Before weight reduction, fat cell number averaged 75 billion. With weight reduction, this number remained essentially unchanged. The average size of the fat cells, in contrast, decreased by 33% from 0.9 μg to a normal value of 0.6 μg of fat per cell. Subjects attained a normal body mass when they reduced an additional 28 kg (62 lb). Cell number again remained unchanged, but cell size continued to shrink to about one third the size of the fat cells in normal individuals of average body fat. Other experiments of a similar nature have confirmed these findings in young children and adults.

A formerly overfat person who reduces body weight and body fat to near average values still does not become "cured" of excess fat, at least in terms of adipocyte number. The large number of relatively small fat cells in the reduced overfat individual may somehow relate to appetite control, and the individual craves food, overeats, and regains lost weight as fat. This certainly makes sense within the framework of the body fat-hormone (leptin)-satiety interaction discussed previously.

Fat cell number increases during three general time periods:

1. Last trimester of pregnancy
2. First year of life
3. Adolescent growth spurt

Liposuction: Surgical Removal of Excess Fat

The total number of fat cells probably cannot be altered to any significant degree during adulthood. This certainly is unwelcomed news to those who attempt to reduce body weight. **Liposuction**, a surgical procedure for removing large amounts of fat at selected body sites, provides a way to excise excess fat. In 2013, the cost of liposuction surgery in the United States averaged $2866 per procedure but varied by geographic region (**www.plasticsurgery.org**).

Worldwide Liposuction Craze

The world leaders in cosmetic adipose tissue–altering procedures (**www.asianplasticsurgeryguide.com/news10-2/081003_south-korea-highest.html**), expressed in number

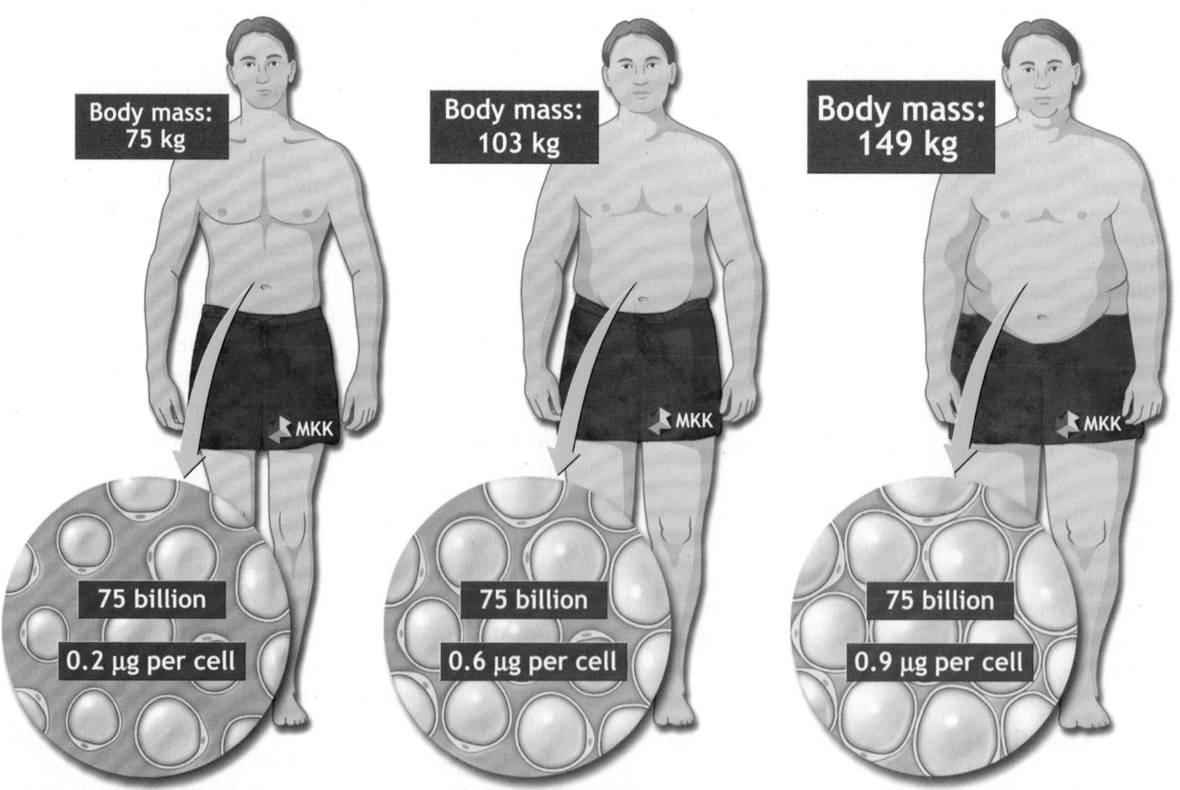

FIGURE 16.30 Changes in adipose cellularity with weight reduction in obese subjects. (Data from Hirsch J. Adipose cellularity in relation to human obesity. In: Stollerman GH, ed. *Advances in Internal Medicine*. Vol 17. Chicago: Year-Book, 1971.)

of total procedures related to the country's total population (rate per 10,000 people called PP10K), include South Korea with a PP10K (74), Brazil (55), Taiwan (44), United States (42), Japan (32), Thailand (11), China (9), and India (6). To compare rates between two countries, divide their respective P10Ks. Thus, South Korea (PP10K = 74) compared to the United States (PP10K = 42) does 1.8 times more adipose tissue–altering procedures.

Does Surgical Fat Removal or Reshaping Have Permanent Effects?

The challenge to the healthcare professional is to "lay out the facts" about such elective procedures so individuals can make informed choices about their options: one can either (1) surgically sculpt, contour, or excise excess fat at select body locations, with the understanding that the results will probably be short lived, or (2) switch lifestyle patterns to "shape up" and lose fat with regular, moderate physical activity and prudent food restriction.

Unfortunately, for individuals seeking a permanent cure for some health issues, liposuction and body contouring do *not* change an individual's metabolic profile, including leptin concentration, blood cholesterol and triacylglycerols, blood pressure, and insulin levels. Even removing 20 lb of fat from the abdomen in severely obese women did not improve important heart disease risk factors. Future research must determine if deep visceral or storage fat removal gives more promising health results than liposuction, which primarily removes "pinchable" subcutaneous fat. On a positive note, combining a moderate to strenuous strength and aerobic conditioning program may delay the regain of the liposuctioned abdominal fat; remaining sedentary posttreatment may induce a compensatory increase in deep visceral fat deposition, certainly a counterproductive strategy.

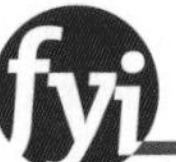

When Reality Meets the Road

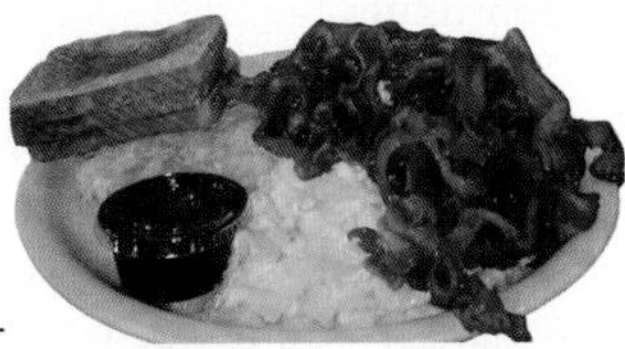

The inset photo illustrates the reality faced daily by millions of Americans when they go out to eat and reinforces the extreme difficulty in combating overeating and the obesity epidemic—the portion sizes are huge! This hit home when two of the textbook authors stopped for breakfast at a roadside eatery (Tony's I-75 Restaurant, **www.tonysi75restaurant.com/**) while traveling to the 2013 American College of Sports Medicine National Convention. What a surprise when the order of scrambled eggs, toast, hash browns, and a side of bacon arrived. When asked if a mistake had been made in the bacon side order, the waiter confirmed that all bacon sides weigh in at 1-lb cooked weight (58 pieces, about 2418 kcal with 184 g or 6.5 oz of fat—more than seven times the recommended daily intake)! A colleague could not finish his omelet due to its sheer size. He was told the standard omelet contained 12 eggs (888 kcal and about 2200 mg of cholesterol just for the eggs)! The restaurant proudly advertises its specialty—the United States of Bacon.

New Fat Cells Develop as Obesity Progresses

In adult-onset massive overfatness (termed morbid obesity; BMI + ≥40), new adipocytes develop, coupled with hypertrophy of existing cells as the person becomes even fatter. This probably occurs because fat cells have an upper-size limit of about 1.0 μg of lipid per cell. In morbid obese individuals with 60% body fat, almost all adipocytes achieve a hypertrophic limit; for the person to add fat, new cells must proliferate from a preadipocyte cell pool.

How to Select a Diet Plan

The most difficult aspect of dieting involves deciding exactly how to select foods to include in the daily menu. One can choose from literally hundreds of diet plans—water diets, drinker's diets, zone diets, fruit or vegetable diets, fast-food diets, eat-to-win diets, and diets named after cities (e.g., South Beach, Scarsdale, Hollywood, Beverly Hills), people (Robert Atkins, Jenny Craig, Dean Ornish, Nathan Pritikin, Richard Simmons, Nicholas Perricone, Suzanne Somers, Mehmet Oz, Andrew Weil, Phil McGraw), and even cavemen in the Stone Age era (Paleo diet) or their contemporaries (the Real Meal Revolution). Hundreds of variations of high-fat, low-carbohydrate, or liquid-protein diets are available (**www.webmd.com/diet/evaluate-latest-diets**). Some zealots even state that total caloric intake need *not* be considered but rather the order of eating foods! For individuals desperate to shed excess weight, the tremendous amount of misinformation available in the mainstream media, the Internet, and TV infomercials encourages and then reinforces negative eating behaviors, unfortunately causing another repeat cycle of failure.

Low-Carbohydrate Ketogenic Diets

Ketogenic diets *emphasize carbohydrate restriction while generally ignoring total calories and the diet's cholesterol and saturated fat content.* Billed as a "diet revolution" and championed by the late Dr. Robert C. Atkins (1930–2003), the diet was first promoted in the late 1800s and has appeared in various forms since then. The diet has long been disparaged by the medical establishment, yet its advocates maintain that restricting daily carbohydrate intake to 20 g or less for an initial 2 weeks, with some liberalization thereafter, causes the body to mobilize considerable fat for energy and hence encourages body fat loss. This low-carbohydrate, high-fat, or high-protein food plan generates excess plasma **ketone bodies**—by-products of incomplete fat breakdown from inadequate carbohydrate catabolism; ketones supposedly suppress appetite. Theoretically, the ketones lost in the urine represent unused energy that should further facilitate weight loss. Some advocates claim that urinary energy loss becomes so great dieters can eat all they want as long as they restrict carbohydrates.

The singular focus of the low-carbohydrate diet craze may eventually reduce caloric intake despite claims that dieters need not consider calorie intake as long as lipid represents the excess caloric intake. Initial weight loss may also result largely from dehydration caused by an extra solute load on the kidneys that increases water excretion. *Water loss does not reduce body fat!* Low-carbohydrate intake also sets the stage for lean tissue loss because the body recruits amino acids from muscle to maintain blood glucose via gluconeogenesis—an undesirable side effect for a diet designed to induce body fat loss.

Three clinical trials compared the Atkins-type, low-carbohydrate diet with traditional low-fat diets for weight loss. The low-carbohydrate diet was more effective in achieving a modest weight loss for severely overweight persons. Some measures of heart health also improved by a more favorable lipid profile and glycemic control in those who followed the low-carbohydrate diet for up to 1 year. Such findings add a measure of credibility to low-carbohydrate diets and challenge conventional wisdom concerning the potential dangers from consuming a high-fat diet.

Importantly, high-fat, low-carbohydrate diets require systematic long-term evaluation greater than 2 to 5 years for safety and effectiveness, particularly related to potential health risks in nine areas:

1. Raises serum uric acid levels
2. Potentiates kidney stone development
3. Alters electrolyte concentrations to initiate cardiac arrhythmias
4. Causes acidosis
5. Aggravates existing kidney problems from the extra solute burden in the renal filtrate
6. Depletes glycogen reserves, contributing to a fatigued state
7. Decreases calcium balance and increases bone loss risk
8. Causes dehydration
9. Retards fetal development during pregnancy from inadequate carbohydrate intake

For high-performance endurance athletes who train at or above 70% of maximum effort, switching to a high-fat diet remains ill advised by most sport scientists because such training requires adequate blood glucose and glycogen packed in the active muscles and liver storage depots. Fatigue during intense activity for more than 60 minutes occurs more rapidly when athletes consume high-fat meals rather than carbohydrate-rich meals.

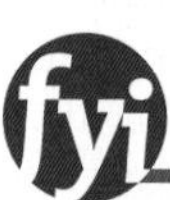

Confirming Evidence to Reduce Dietary Animal Fat

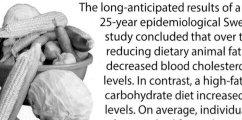

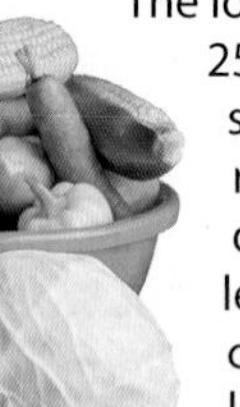

The long-anticipated results of a 25-year epidemiological Swedish study concluded that over time, reducing dietary animal fat decreased blood cholesterol levels. In contrast, a high-fat, low-carbohydrate diet increased these levels. On average, individuals who switched from a lower fat diet to one higher in fat and lower in carbohydrate saw blood cholesterol levels increase—despite increased use of cholesterol-lowering medication. While low-carbohydrate/high-fat diets may help short-term weight loss, these results demonstrate that long-term weight loss is not maintained, and this diet increases blood cholesterol with a potential, major impact on cardiovascular disease risk.

Source: Johansson I, et al. Associations among 25-year trends in diet, cholesterol and BMI from 140,000 observations in men and women in Northern Sweden. *Nutr J* 2012;11:40.

High-Protein Diets

High-protein, low-carbohydrate diets may shed pounds in the short term, but their long-term success remains questionable and may even pose health risks. These diets have been promoted to overfat individuals as "last-chance diets." Earlier versions consisted of protein in liquid form advertised as a "miracle liquid." Unknown to the consumer, the liquid-protein mixture often contained a blend of ground-up animal hooves and horns, with pigskin mixed in a broth with enzymes and tenderizers to "predigest" it. Collagen-based blends produced from gelatin hydrolysis supplemented with small amounts of essential amino acids did not contain the highest-quality amino acid mixture and lacked required vitamins and minerals, particularly copper. A negative copper balance coincides with electrocardiographic abnormalities and rapid heart rate.

Protein-rich foods often contain high saturated fat levels, which increase the risk for heart disease and type 2 diabetes. Diets excessively high in animal protein increase urinary oxalate excretion, a compound that combines primarily with calcium to form **kidney stones**. The diet's safety improves if it contains high-quality protein with ample carbohydrate, essential fatty acids, and micronutrients.

Some argue that an extremely high-protein intake suppresses appetite through reliance on fat mobilization and subsequent ketone formation. The elevated thermic effect of dietary protein, with its relatively low coefficient of digestibility (particularly for plant protein), reduces the net calories available from ingested protein compared with a well-balanced meal of equivalent caloric value. This point has some validity, but one must consider other factors when formulating a sound weight-loss program, particularly for physically active individuals. High-protein intake has the potential to promote four deleterious outcomes:

1. Strain on liver and kidney function with accompanying dehydration
2. Electrolyte imbalance

3. Glycogen depletion
4. Lean tissue loss

Semistarvation Diets

A therapeutic fast or **very low-calorie diet (VLCD)** may benefit severe clinical obesity when body fat exceeds 40% to 50% of body mass. The diet provides between 400 and 800 kcal daily as high-quality protein foods or liquid meal replacements. Dietary prescriptions usually last up to 3 months but only as a "last resort" before undertaking more extreme medical approaches for morbid obesity (e.g., various surgical treatments collectively called **bariatric surgery**). Surgical treatments that considerably reduce the stomach size and reconfigure the small intestine induce a sustained weight loss, but they are generally applied to patients with a BMI of at least 40 or a BMI of 35 when accompanied by other co-morbidities.

Dieting with VLCD requires close supervision, usually in a hospital setting. Proponents maintain that severe food restriction breaks established dietary habits, which in turn improves the long-term prospects for success. These diets may also depress the appetite to help compliance. Daily over-the counter pharmacy purchases that accompany a VLCD diet usually include:

1. Calcium carbonate for nausea
2. Bicarbonate of soda and potassium chloride to maintain body fluid consistency
3. Mouthwash and sugar-free chewing gum for bad breath from a high level of ketones from fatty acid catabolism
4. Bath oils for dry skin

For most individuals, semistarvation does not represent an "ideal diet" or proper approach to weight control. These diets provide inadequate carbohydrate; thus, glycogen storage depots in the liver and muscles deplete rapidly. This impairs physical tasks that require either intense aerobic effort or shorter-duration anaerobic power output. The continuous nitrogen loss with fasting and weight loss reflects an exacerbated lean tissue loss, which may occur disproportionately from critical organs such as the heart. The success rate remains poor for prolonged fasting.

STRATEGIES TO EFFECT WEIGHT LOSS

Hydration level and duration of the energy deficit affect the amount and composition of weight lost.

Early Weight Loss Largely Water

Figure 16.31 presents the general trend for percentage composition of daily weight loss during 4 weeks of dieting. Approximately 70% of weight lost over the first week of energy deficit consists of water loss. Thereafter, water loss progressively lessens, representing only about 20% of weight loss in the second and third weeks; concurrently, body fat loss accelerates from 25% to 70%. During the fourth week of dieting, reductions in body fat produce about 85% of the weight loss without further increase in water loss. Protein's contribution to weight loss increases from 5% initially to about 15% following the fourth week. In practical terms, counseling efforts should emphasize that the lost weight during the initial attempts to reduce weight, when successful, consists chiefly of water and not fat; it takes approximately 4 weeks to establish the desired pattern of fat loss for each pound of weight loss.

Hydration Level

Restricting water during the first several days of a caloric deficit increases proportions of body water lost and decreases proportion of fat lost. More total weight loss occurs with restricted daily water intake, with the additional weight lost solely from water as dehydration progresses. *Dieters lose the same quantity of body fat regardless of fluid intake level.*

Longer-Term Deficit Promotes Fat Loss

Figure 16.32 reinforces the important general concept that the caloric equivalent of the lost weight increases as duration of caloric restriction progresses. After 2 months on a

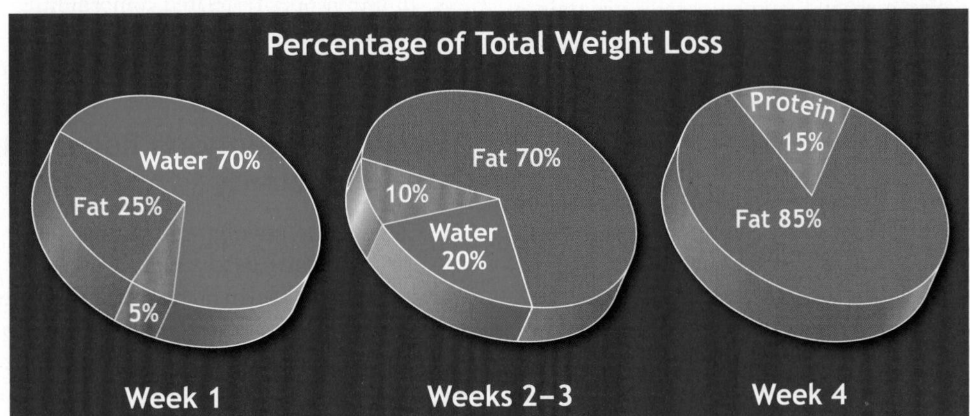

FIGURE 16.31 General trend for the percentage composition of the weight lost during 4 weeks of caloric restriction.

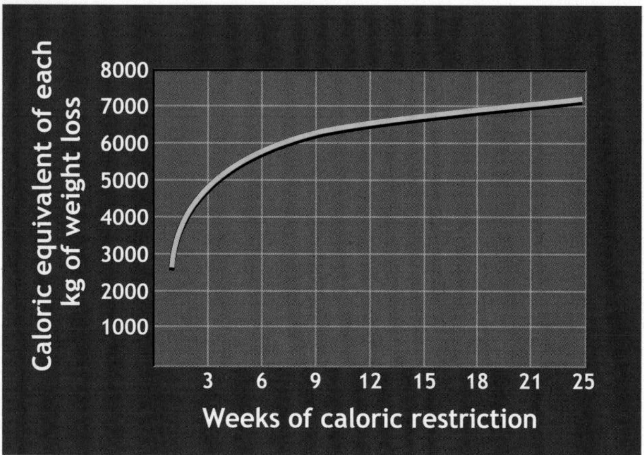

FIGURE 16.32 General trend for the energy equivalent of the weight lost in relation to duration of caloric restriction. As caloric restriction progresses, the energy equivalent per unit of weight lost increases to about 7000 kcal per kilogram after 20 weeks. This occurs because of the large initial body water loss (no calorie value) early in weight loss.

diet, the caloric equivalent of lost weight exceeds twice that in the first week. Maximizing fat loss and minimizing loss of lean tissue mass follow a general guideline known at the "Quarter Fat-Free Mass Rule." This rule states the expected loss of lean tissue as FFM follows a pattern that about one fourth of each pound of lost weight comes from FFM, with the remainder mostly FM and some fluid. In mathematical terms, change in FFM divided by change in body weight $(\Delta FFM/\Delta FM) = -0.25$. Shorter periods of caloric restriction produce a larger percentage of water and carbohydrate loss per unit weight reduction with only minimal body fat decrease.

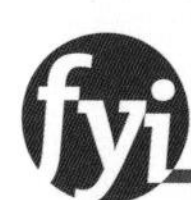

Fat Loss Best With Aerobic Activity

General guidelines for an optimal, well-balanced physical activity program recommend a blend of aerobic activity, resistance training, balance, and joint flexibility movements. Resistance training helps to prevent muscle loss (sarcopenia) with aging. Increased aerobic activity excels for its calorie-burning effects in combating excess body fat; it most likely curbs insulin resistance that increases diabetes and heart disease risk. Increased aerobic activity also reduces deep abdominal (visceral) fat. Middle-age men and women with elevated LDL or low HDL cholesterol were assigned to aerobic training, resistance training, or both. Aerobic training consisted of the equivalent of 12 miles per week at a vigorous intensity on a treadmill, elliptical trainer, or stationary cycle. Resistance training consisted of three sets of eight exercises with eight to 12 repetitions per set, three times weekly. Following 8 months of training, the resistance-trained group lost only subcutaneous abdominal fat, while the aerobically trained group lost both visceral fat and subcutaneous fat, including fat from around the liver. Aerobic training also decreased the tendency for insulin resistance. The takeaway message– combine regular aerobic physical activity for fat loss and to curb insulin resistance with resistance training to counter the tendency to lose muscle that occurs with aging.

Source: Slentz CA, et al. Effects of aerobic vs. resistance training on visceral and liver fat stores, liver enzymes, and insulin resistance by HOMA in overweight adults from STRRIDE AT/RT. *Am J Physiol Endocrinol Metab* 2011;301:E1033.

PHYSICAL ACTIVITY CREATES A TIPPING POINT IN THE ENERGY BALANCE EQUATION

Despite debates about contributions of physical inactivity and excessive caloric intake to body fat accretion, a sedentary lifestyle consistently emerges as an important factor in weight gain by children, adolescents, and adults.

Physically active men and women usually maintain a desirable body composition. An increased level of regular physical activity combined with dietary restraint maintains weight loss more effectively than long-term caloric restriction alone. A negative energy balance induced by increased caloric expenditure unbalances the energy balance equation for weight loss and improves physical fitness and the health risk profile. It also favorably alters body composition and body fat distribution for children and adults. Regular physical activity produces less age-associated central adipose tissue accumulation. Overweight women show a dose-response relationship between amount of physical activity and long-term weight loss. Overfat adolescents and adults improve body composition and visceral fat distribution from either moderate physical activity or more vigorous physical activity, with more intense, aerobic physical activity being most effective. Regular physical activity has five additional benefits:

1. Slows the age-related muscle mass loss
2. Possibly prevents adult-onset obesity
3. Improves obesity-related comorbidities
4. Decreases mortality
5. Has beneficial effects on existing chronic diseases

Two Misconceptions Regarding Physical Activity

Two arguments attempt to counter the increased physical activity approach to weight loss. One maintains that physical activity inevitably increases appetite to produce a proportionate increase in food intake that negates physical activity–produced caloric deficit. The second argument claims that the relatively small calorie-burning effect of a normal workout does not "dent" the body's fat reserves as effectively as food restriction.

fyi The Amount of Physical Activity Required for a 150-lb Person to Burn Off the Calories in Popular Foods

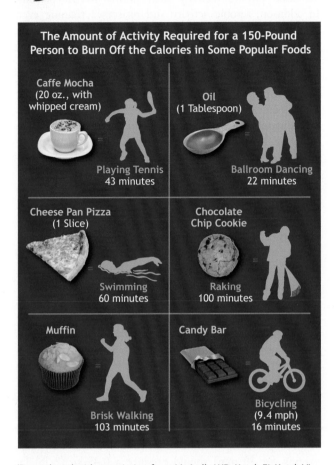

(Reproduced with permission from McArdle WD, Katch FI, Katch VL. *Exercise Physiology: Nutrition, Energy, and Human Performance.* 8th Ed. Baltimore: Wolters Kluwer Health, 2015.)

Misconception 1: Increased Physical Activity and Food Intake

Sedentary persons often do not balance their energy intake and energy expenditure. Failure to accurately regulate energy balance at the lower end of the physical activity spectrum contributes to the "creeping obesity" observed in highly mechanized and technically advanced societies. In contrast, regular exercisers maintain appetite control within a reactive zone where food intake more readily matches daily energy expenditure.

In considering the effects of physical activity on appetite and food intake, one must distinguish between activity type and duration and the participant's body fat status. Lumberjacks, farm laborers, and endurance athletes consume about twice as many daily calories as sedentary individuals. More specifically, male marathon runners, cross-country skiers, and cyclists consume about 4000 to 5000 kcal daily, yet they are among the leanest people in the population. Obviously, their large caloric intake meets the energy requirements of training while maintaining a relatively lean body composition.

For overfat individuals, extra energy required for increased physical activity more than offsets moderate physical activity's small compensatory appetite-stimulating effect. To some extent, the large energy reserve of an overfat person makes it easier to tolerate weight loss and physical activity without the obligatory increase in caloric intake typically observed for leaner counterparts. No difference emerged in fat, carbohydrate, or protein intake or total calories consumed for overweight men and women during 16 months of supervised, moderate-intensity physical activity training compared with a sedentary control group. *In essence, a weak coupling exists between the short-term energy deficit induced by physical activity and energy intake. Increased physical activity by overweight, sedentary individuals does not necessarily alter physiologic needs and automatically produce compensatory increases in food intake to balance additional energy expenditure.*

Misconception 2: Low Caloric Stress of Physical Activity

A second misconception concerns the negligible contribution to weight loss of the calories burned in typical physical activity. Some correctly argue that it requires an inordinate amount of short-term physical activity to lose just 0.45 kg (1 lb) of body fat. Examples include chopping wood for 10 hours, playing golf for 20 hours, performing mild calisthenics for 22 hours, playing ping-pong for 28 hours, or playing volleyball for 32 hours. Consequently, a 2- or 3-month physical activity regimen produces only a small fat loss in an overfat person. From a different perspective, if one played golf without a golf cart for 2 hours daily (350 kcal) 2 days a week (700 kcal), it would take about 5 weeks to lose 0.45 kg (1 lb) of body fat. Assuming the person plays year-round, golfing 2 days a week produces a 4.5-kg (10 lb) yearly fat loss provided food intake remains fairly constant. Even an activity as innocuous as chewing gum burns an extra 11 kcal each hour, a 20% increase over normal resting metabolism. *Simply stated, the calorie-expending effects of* increased physical activity *add up. A caloric deficit of 3500 kcal equals a 0.45-kg body fat loss, whether the deficit occurs rapidly or systematically over time.*

Effectiveness of Regular Physical Activity

Adding physical activity to a weight-loss program favorably modifies the composition of the weight lost in the direction of greater fat loss and maintains or even increases FFM and physical performance capacity. **Figure 16.33** illustrates the muscle-sparing effect of regular physical activity, which compares the effect of about 10 lb (4.5 kg) of weight loss over 12 months induced by either *only* caloric restriction or *only* physical activity on MRI-assessed thigh muscle volume of 50- to 60-year-old men and women. Decreases in thigh muscle volume of 6.8% and composite knee flexion strength

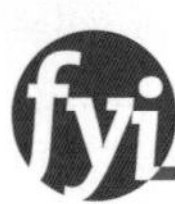

High-Intensity Physical Activity May Boost Recovery Metabolism

A bout of vigorous physical activity may increase recovery oxygen uptake for up to 14 hours. Ten young adult men bicycled for 45 minutes at a vigorous pace equivalent to 73% $\dot{V}O_{2max}$. Energy expenditure was then measured for 24 hours while the men recovered in a metabolic chamber. In the 14-hour period following cycling, the men burned 190 more calories than on a day when they remained sedentary (see discussion of excess post-exercise oxygen consumption [EPOC] in Chapter 6). This 37% recovery calorie-burning bonus occurred in addition to the 520 calories burned during cycling.

Source: Knab AM, et al. A 45-minute vigorous exercise bout increases metabolic rate for 14 hours. *Med Sci Sports Exerc* 2011;43:1643.

(–7.2%) and $\dot{V}O_{2max}$ (–6.8%) occurred only in the caloric restriction group, but $\dot{V}O_{2max}$ increased 15.5% in the group losing weight by physical activity. Clearly, muscle mass, muscle strength, and aerobic capacity decline in response to 12 months of weight loss by caloric restriction but not in response to similar weight loss by increased physical activity.

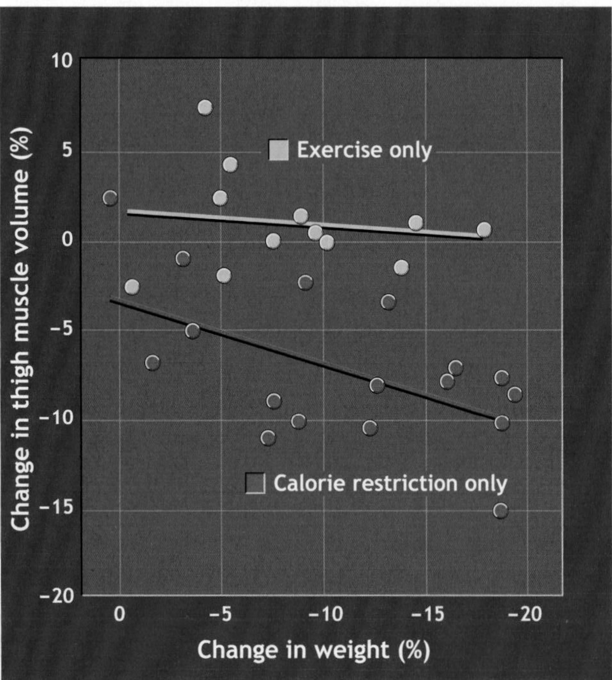

FIGURE 16.33 Conserve the lean and lose the fat. Relationship between weight loss magnitude and change in thigh muscle volume (sum of right and left thighs) in a group losing weight by only caloric restriction and a group losing weight by only exercise. (Adapted with permission from Weiss EP, et al. Lower extremity muscle size and strength and aerobic capacity decrease with caloric restriction but not with exercise-induced weight loss. *J Appl Physiol* 2007;102:534.)

The effectiveness of regular physical activity for weight loss relates closely to degree of excess body fat. Overfat persons generally lose weight and body fat more readily with increased physical activity than normal-weight persons. In addition, aerobic activity and resistance training even without dietary restriction provide positive spin-off to the weight-loss effort. They alter body composition favorably as reduced body fat with a small increase in FFM in otherwise healthy overweight children, adolescents, and adults, postmenopausal women, cardiac patients, and physically challenged individuals. Regular physical activity also targets excess fat accumulation in the abdominal-visceral area to a greater extent than peripheral fat deposits. This response diminishes a tendency toward insulin resistance and predisposition to type 2 diabetes.

Generalized effects of systematic physical activity (e.g., walking 90 min each session for 5 d weekly for 16 wk) for weight loss include loss of about 10 (4.5 kg) to 15 lb (6.8 kg) of body weight, decrease in body fat by 4 to 5 percentage body fat units, increased physical activity capacity assessed by $\dot{V}O_{2max}$, improvements of about 14% to 16% in high-density lipoprotein (HDL) cholesterol, and upward of 20% to 30% in the HDL:LDL (low-density lipoprotein) cholesterol ratio.

Most of the health-related metabolic improvements with regular physical activity in overfat individuals relate to total physical activity volume and quantity of fat loss rather than enhanced cardiorespiratory fitness. The ideal physical activity consists of continuous, large-muscle activities with moderate to high caloric cost of circuit resistance training, walking, running, rope skipping, stair stepping, cycling, and swimming. An expenditure of an extra 300 kcal daily (e.g., jogging for 30 min) should produce a 0.45-kg (1 lb) fat loss in about 12 days. This represents a yearly caloric deficit equivalent to the energy in 13.6 kg (30 lb) of body fat.

Figure 16.34 shows body composition changes for 40 overfat women placed into one of four groups: (1) control group, no exercise and no diet; (2) diet-only, no exercise (DO) group; (3) diet plus resistance exercise (D + E); and (4) resistance exercise only, no diet (EO) group. The women trained 3 days a week for 8 weeks. They performed 10 repetitions each of three sets of eight strength exercises. Body mass decreased for the DO (–4.5 kg; 9.9 lb) and D + E groups (–3.9 kg; 8.6 lb) compared with the EO group (+0.5 kg; 1.1 lb) and control group (–0.4 kg; 0.9 lb). Importantly, whereas FFM increased in the EO group (+1 kg; 2.2 lb), the DO group lost 0.9 kg (2.0 lb) of FFM. The authors concluded that augmenting a calorie restriction program with resistance exercise training preserved FFM compared with dietary restriction alone.

Dose-Response Relationship

The total energy expended in physical activity relates in a dose-response manner to the effectiveness of physical activity *for weight loss. A reasonable goal progressively increases moderate*

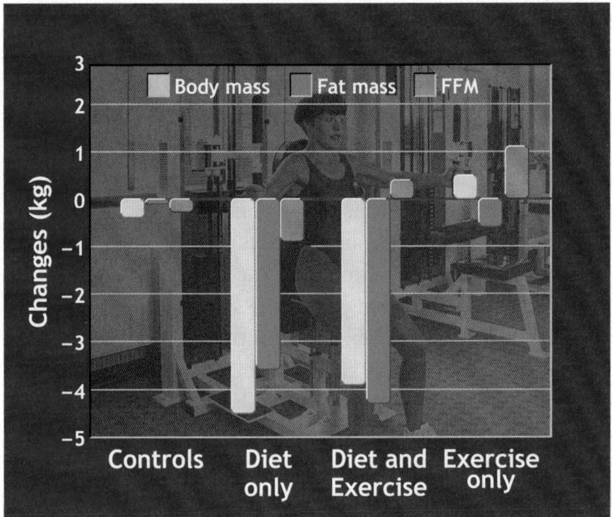

FIGURE 16.34 Body composition changes with combinations of resistance exercise, diet, or both in obese women. (Adapted with permission from Ballor DL, et al. Resistance weight training during caloric restriction enhances lean body weight. *Am J Clin Nutr* 1988;47:19.)

physical activity to between 60 and 90 minutes daily or a level that burns 2100 to 2800 kcal weekly.

An overfat person who starts out with slow walking accrues a considerable caloric expenditure simply by extending duration, as for example, increasing from 30 to 60 and eventually to 90 minutes (or more). The focus on physical activity duration offsets the inadvisability of having a sedentary, overfat individual begin a program with more strenuous activity. The energy cost of weight-bearing physical activity relates directly to body mass, allowing the overweight person to expend considerably more calories in such physical activity than someone of average weight.

Optimal Physical Activity Frequency

To determine optimal physical activity frequency for weight loss, subjects exercised for 30 to 47 minutes for 20 weeks by running or walking, with intensity maintained between 80% and 95% of maximum heart rate. Training twice weekly produced no changes in body weight, skinfolds, or percentage body fat, but training 3 and 4 days weekly did. Subjects who trained 4 days a week reduced their body weight and skinfolds more than subjects who trained 3 days a week. Body fat percentage declined similarly in both groups. These findings suggest a *minimum* of 3 days per week to favorably alter body composition; the additional caloric expenditure with more frequent physical activity produces even greater results. The threshold energy expenditure for weight loss probably remains highly individualized. The calorie-burning effect of each session should eventually attain *at least* 300 kcal whenever possible. This generally occurs with 30 minutes of moderate to vigorous running, swimming, bicycling, or circuit resistance training or 60 minutes of brisk walking on the level without the need to walk up and down steep slopes.

Self-Selected Energy Expenditures: Mode of Physical Activity

No selective effect exists among diverse modes of large-muscle aerobic physical activity to favorably reduce body weight, body fat, skinfold thickness, and girths, yet other differences may emerge. For individuals without physical activity limitations, running at a relatively slow-to-moderate pace between 9 and 15 minutes per mile usually provides the most suitable outdoor physical activity mode to maximize energy expenditure during self-selected continuous physical activity intensities.

THE IDEAL COMBINATION FOR SUCCESS: CALORIC RESTRAINT PLUS INCREASED PHYSICAL ACTIVITY

Combinations of increased physical activity and caloric restraint offer considerably more flexibility to achieve a negative caloric imbalance than either physical activity alone or diet alone. Dietary restraint and increased physical activity through lifestyle changes confer health and weight-loss benefits similar to those from combining dietary restraint and a vigorous program of structured physical activity. Adding a moderate-intensity physical activity to a weight control program facilitates longer-term maintenance of fat loss than total reliance on either food restriction alone or increased physical activity alone.

MAINTENANCE OF GOAL BODY WEIGHT

The popular and scientific literature, including TV reality shows, extol success stories of individuals who have lost considerable amounts of weight using different interventions

More Fat and Less Muscle With Regained Weight

Typically, weight regained after weight loss represents more fat and less muscle compared to the composition of weight lost. An experiment determined if the composition of body weight regained after intentional weight loss corresponded to the composition of body weight lost. Seventy-eight obese, sedentary, postmenopausal women reduced weight an average of 11.8 kg (26 lb) over 5 months by reducing daily energy intake by 400 kcal 3 days a week. On average, 67% of the weight lost was fat and 33% lean body tissue. One year after the program ended, 54 women regained at least 2.0 kg (4.4 lb). For them, 81% of regained weight was fat and 19% lean tissue. Specifically, for every 1 kg (2.2 lb) fat lost during weight-loss intervention, 0.26 kg (0.6 lb) lean tissue was lost; for every 1 kg (2.2 lb) fat regained over the following year, only 0.12 kg (.03 lb) lean tissue was regained.

Source: Beavers KM, et al. Is lost lean mass from intentional weight loss recovered during weight regain in postmenopausal women? *Am J Clin Nutr* 2011;94:767.

that include nutritional, physical activity, and behavioral approaches but rarely show what happens in the long-term once the media spotlight turns elsewhere.

A project by the **National Weight Control Registry (NWCR; www.nwcr.ws)** recruited 784 individuals (629 women, 155 men) who successfully achieved prolonged weight loss to study common success factors. Criteria for NWCR membership included age 18 years or older and maintenance of weight loss of at least 13.6 (30 lb) for 1 year or longer. Participants averaged 30 kg (66 lb) of weight loss, and 14% lost more than 45.4 kg (100 lb). Members maintained the required minimum 13.7 kg (30 lb) weight loss for a 5.5-year average, and 16% maintained the loss for 10 years or longer. Most participants had been overweight since childhood; nearly 50% had one overweight parent, and more than 25% had both parents overweight. *Genetic background may have predisposed these persons to obesity, but an impressive weight loss and its maintenance proves that heredity alone need not predestine a person to the overfat condition.*

About 55% of the NWCR members used either a formal program or professional assistance to reduce weight; the rest succeeded on their own. Regarding weight-loss methods, 89% modified their food intake and maintained relatively high physical activity levels (2800 kcal weekly on average) to achieve goal weight loss. Many walked briskly for at least 1 hour daily. About 92% exercised at home, and one third exercised regularly with friends. Whereas women primarily walked and did aerobic dancing, men chose competitive sports and resistance training. Only 10% relied solely on diet, and 1% used exercise exclusively. The diet strategy of nearly 90% of participants restricted intake of certain types or amounts of foods—44% counted calories, 33% limited lipid intake, and 25% restricted grams of lipid. Forty-four percent ate the same foods they normally ate but in reduced amounts.

CAN TARGETED PHYSICAL ACTIVITY SELECTIVELY REDUCE LOCAL FAT DEPOSITS?

The notion of selective body fat reduction, typically referred to as ***spot reduction****, stems from the belief that an increase in a muscle's metabolic activity stimulates relatively greater fat mobilization from the adipose tissue in proximity to the active muscle.* As such, exercising a specific body area to "sculpt" it should selectively reduce more fat from that area than exercising a different muscle group at the same metabolic intensity. Advocates of spot reduction recommend performing large numbers of sit-ups or side-bends to reduce excessive abdominal and hip fat. The promise of spot reduction physical activity seems attractive from an aesthetic and health risk standpoint—unfortunately, critical evaluation of the research evidence does not support its use.

To examine claims for spot reduction, researchers compared the girths and subcutaneous fat stores of the right and left forearms of high-caliber tennis players. As expected, the girths of the dominant or playing arms exceeded the girths of nondominant arms because of a modest muscular hypertrophy from the overload of playing tennis. Measurements of skinfold thickness, however, clearly showed that regular and prolonged tennis workouts did not reduce subcutaneous fat in the playing arm.

Another study evaluated fat biopsy specimens from abdominal, subscapular, and buttock sites before and after 27 days of sit-up exercise training. The number of daily sit-ups increased from 140 at the end of the first week to 336 on day 27. Despite the considerable amount of localized exercise, adipocytes in the abdominal region were no smaller than adipocytes in the unexercised buttocks or subscapular control regions.

Undoubtedly, the negative energy balance created through regular physical activity contributes to reducing total body fat. Conventional wisdom maintains that physical activity stimulates fatty acid mobilization via hormones and enzymes that act on the body's fat depots, not simply from areas closest to the active muscle mass. In this connection, recent advances in microinvasive subcutaneous adipose tissue (SCAT) measurements make it possible to study if localized lipolysis is possible with localized physical activity. One study estimated blood flow and lipolysis in femoral SCAT adjacent to contracting and resting skeletal muscle during one-legged knee extension activity at 25% of maximum. Blood flow and SCAT lipolysis were higher adjacent to contracting muscle versus adjacent to resting muscle independent of physical activity intensity. Whether this translates to sustained fat loss at a particular site remains unknown, and additional experiments certainly seem warranted.

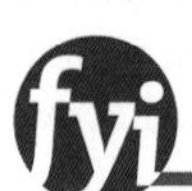

Physical Activity Prevents Fat Infiltration Into Muscle

Considerable evidence suggests that loss of strength and muscle mass appear to be inevitable consequences of aging and that body fat increases with aging. Eleven men and 31 women completed a randomized trial consisting of either a physical activity group (PA; $n = 22$) or successful aging health educational control group (SA; $n = 20$). Isokinetic knee extensor strength and CT–derived midthigh skeletal muscle and adipose tissue cross-sectional areas (CSA) were assessed at baseline and at 12 months following randomization. Total body weight and muscle CSA decreased in both groups, but these losses were not different between groups. Strength adjusted for muscle mass decreased in SA (−20.1 ± 9.3%). The loss of strength was essentially prevented in PA (−2.5 ± 8.3%). In addition, a significant increase (18.4 ± 6.0%) in muscle fat infiltration occurred in SA, but this gain was nearly completely prevented in PA (2.3 ± 5.7%). These results show that regular physical activity prevents both the age-associated loss of muscle strength and increase in muscle fat infiltration in older adults.

Source: Goodpaster BH, et al. Effects of physical activity on strength and skeletal muscle fat infiltration in older adults: a randomized controlled trial. *J Appl Physiol* 2008;105:1498.

Promising Animal Studies of Exercise Effects on Improving Brain Function

Several sets of experiments with rodents (male homozygous leptin receptor mutant mice) determined if the negative impact of induced obesity on brain function at the synaptic level, including cognitive function tests, could be reversed by exercise effects on modulating the influence of interleukin-1. Prior research had demonstrated that inflammatory cytokines negatively affected cognitive functions and adversely impacted synaptic neural functioning. Following 12 weeks of daily, forced treadmill activity in one group of overfat mice or no activity in another comparable group, the active mice significantly reduced epididymal (abdominal) fat pad mass, while adding lean mass, yet had the same final body weight as the nonactive group that retained their fatness level. Increasing physical activity of the mice normalized their brain (hippocampal) function and reversed cognitive impairments. The advantage of increased physical activity that decreased excess fat was to reverse the negative neuroinflammatory impact on adipose tissue functions and cognitive dysfunction in obesity. Such studies in rodents hopefully will provide insights about the neural mechanisms that influence targeted exercise effects coupled with dietary manipulations on changes in obesity tissues for future applications to humans.

GAINING WEIGHT

For most people, weight loss to reduce body fat and improve overall health and aesthetic appearance becomes the primary focus to alter body composition. However, there are many individuals who desire to gain weight to improve their body composition profile, their performance in sports or physical activities that require muscular strength and power, or their health status due to low weight. These three goals pose a unique dilemma not easily resolved. Gaining weight per se occurs all too easily by tilting the body's energy balance to favor greater caloric intake. In a sedentary person, an accumulated excess intake of 3500 kcal produces a theoretical body fat gain of 1 lb because adipocytes store the excess calories. Weight gain for athletes should ideally occur as lean tissue, specifically muscle mass and accompanying connective tissues. Generally, this form of weight gain takes place if an increased caloric intake with adequate carbohydrate for energy and protein sparing and enough protein for tissue synthesis accompanies the proper physical activity regimen. Athletes attempting to increase muscle mass often fall easy prey to health food and diet supplement manufacturers who market "high-potency, tissue-building" substances, including chromium, boron, vanadyl sulfate, β-hydroxy-methyl butyrate, and various protein and amino acid mixture, none of which reliably increases muscle mass.

Increase Lean Mass, Not Body Fat

Endurance activity training usually increases FFM only slightly, but the overall effect reduces body weight because of fat loss from the calorie-burning and possible appetite-depressing effects of this exercise mode. In contrast, muscular overload through resistance training, supported by adequate energy and protein intake (with sufficient recovery), increases muscle mass and strength. Adequate energy intake ensures that no protein catabolism available for muscle growth occurs from an energy deficit. *Thus, intense aerobic physical activity should not coincide with resistance training to increase muscle mass.* More than likely, the added energy and perhaps protein demands of concurrent resistance and aerobic training impose a limit on muscle growth and responsiveness to resistance training. In addition, on the molecular level, aerobic training may inhibit signaling to the skeletal muscle's protein synthesis machinery of skeletal muscle. This could negatively impact the muscle's adaptive response to resistance training. We recommend increasing daily protein intake to about 1.6 g per kg of body mass during the resistance-training phase by consuming a variety of plant and animal proteins.

If all calories consumed in excess of the energy requirement during resistance training sustained muscle growth, then 2000 to 2500 extra kcal could supply each 0.5-kg (1.1 lb) increase in lean tissue. In practical terms, 700 to 1000 kcal added to a well-balanced daily meal plan supports a weekly 0.5- to 1.0-kg (1.1 to 2.2 lb) gain in lean tissue and training's additional energy needs.

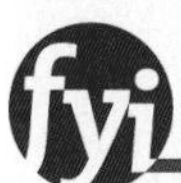

Use It or Lose It

A meta-analysis that examined the overall value of progressive resistance training among healthy aging adults showed that this exercise form helps older adults build muscle mass and increase strength to function better in daily physical activity. Sedentary adults, with an average age of 50, added 1.1 kg (2.4 lb) of lean muscle and increased overall strength by up to 30% after 18 to 20 weeks of resistance training. The amount of weight lifted and frequency and duration of the training sessions interact in a dose-response manner to facilitate improvement. Sedentary adults above age 50 typically lose up to 0.18 kg (0.4 lb) of muscle yearly.

Source: Peterson MD, Gordon PM. Resistance exercise for the aging adult: clinical implications and prescription guidelines. *Am J Med* 2011;124:194.

EXPECTATIONS FOR GAINING LEAN TISSUE

A 1-year program of intense resistance training for young, athletic men increases body mass by about 20%, mostly from lean tissue accrual. The rate of lean tissue gain rapidly plateaus as training progresses beyond the first year. For athletic women, first-year gains in lean tissue mass average 50% to 75% of the absolute values for men, the difference probably occurring from women's smaller initial LBM. Individual differences in the daily nitrogen quantity incorporated into body protein and protein incorporated into muscle also limit and explain differences among persons in muscle mass increases with resistance training.

Figure 16.35 lists eight specific factors that impact lean tissue synthesis responsiveness to resistance training. Individuals with relatively high androgen-to-estrogen ratios and greater percentages of fast-twitch muscle fibers probably increase their lean tissue to the greatest extent. At the start of training, muscle mass increases most in individuals with the largest relative FFM corrected for stature and body fat. To quantify how much lean tissue has been gained requires regular monitoring of body mass congruent with a valid appraisal of body fat. Such record keeping verifies whether the combination of training and additional food intake increases lean tissue and not body fat.

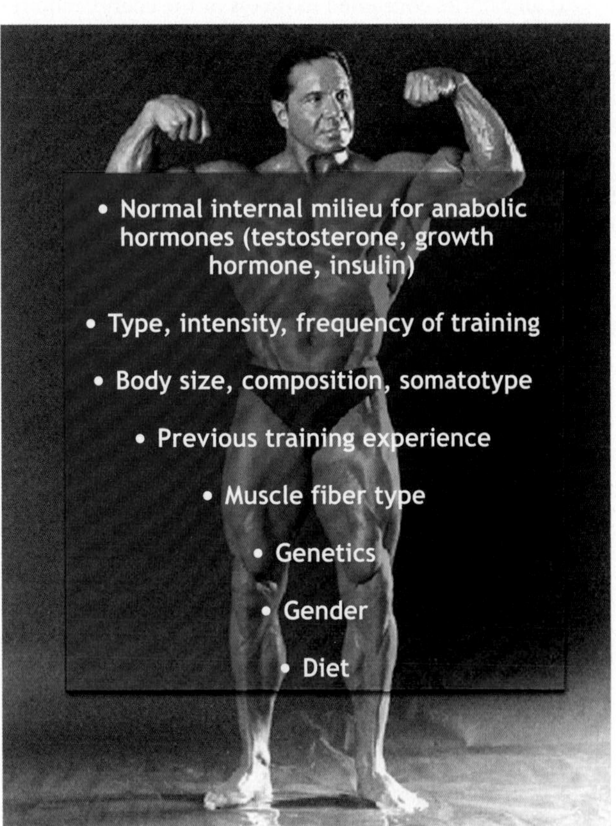

• Normal internal milieu for anabolic hormones (testosterone, growth hormone, insulin)
• Type, intensity, frequency of training
• Body size, composition, somatotype
• Previous training experience
• Muscle fiber type
• Genetics
• Gender
• Diet

FIGURE 16.35 Eight specific factors that impact lean tissue synthesis responsiveness to resistance training. (Reprinted with permission from McArdle WD, Katch FI, Katch VL. *Exercise Physiology: Nutrition, Energy, and Human Performance*. 8th Ed. Baltimore: Wolters Kluwer Health, 2015; photo of Bill Pearl courtesy of Bill Pearl.)

SUMMARY

1. Unbalancing the energy balance equation requires either reducing energy intake below daily energy requirements, maintaining energy intake but increasing energy output, or decreasing energy intake and increasing energy expenditure.
2. Weight loss through dietary restriction has a poor success rate of less than 20%. Up to two-thirds of the lost weight returns within 1 year, and almost all of it returns within 5 years.
3. A caloric deficit of 3500 created through either diet or physical activity equals the calories in 1 lb (0.45 kg) of body fat.
4. Disadvantages of extreme semistarvation include loss of lean body tissue, lethargy, possible malnutrition and metabolic disorders, and decrease in basal energy expenditure.
5. Adipocyte number stabilizes sometime before adulthood; any weight gain or loss thereafter usually relates to changes in fat cell size.
6. In extreme obesity, cell number can increase after adipocytes reach their hypertrophic limit.
7. Increases in adipocyte number involve three general time periods: last trimester of pregnancy, first year of life, and adolescent growth spurt before adulthood.
8. Calories expended in physical activity accumulate to create a dramatic calorie-burning effect over time.
9. For previously sedentary, overfat men and women, moderate increases in physical activity do not necessarily increase food intake proportionately.
10. Combining physical activity with caloric restriction offers an effective means to weight control.
11. Physical activity enhances fat mobilization and utilization for energy, improves insulin sensitivity, and minimizes lean tissue loss.
12. Rapid weight loss during the first few days of caloric deficit comes mainly from body water loss and glycogen depletion, and further weight loss occurs from greater fat loss per unit weight loss.
13. Successful weight losers generally rely on food intake and especially increased physical activity to achieve a goal body weight.
14. Selective fat reduction of specific body areas by targeted "spot exercise" does not occur.
15. The areas of greatest body fat concentration or lipid-mobilizing enzyme activity supply the greatest amount of energy.
16. Athletes should gain weight as lean body tissue with a modest increase in caloric intake plus systematic resistance training.

THINK IT THROUGH

1. What strategy, advice, and words of encouragement can you offer to a person who has attempted several diets yet never achieved long-term weight loss?

2. Respond to this comment: "The only way to lose weight is to reduce the amount of food you eat. It's that simple!"
3. Outline a prudent yet effective plan for a middle-age woman to lose weight whose physician advises her to shed 20 lb of excess fat. Provide the rationale for each of your recommendations.

KEY TERMS

Abdominal fat: Subcutaneous and visceral fat in the abdominal region.

Activities of daily living (ADL): Basic and routine everyday life tasks.

Adipose tissue–free weight (ATFW): Whole-body mass minus the mass of all dissectible adipose tissue that contains about 83% pure fat.

Air plethysmography (BOD POD): Plethysmographic device to assess body volume and its changes. Body volume is determined by measuring the initial volume of the empty chamber and then the volume with the person inside.

AMA: Acronym of the American Medical Association (**www.ama-assn.org**). The largest association of physicians—both MDs and DOs—and medical students in the United States.

Android-type obesity: Obese condition with increased health risk from excessive fat deposition in the abdominal region.

Anthropometry: Standardized techniques (e.g., calipers, tapes) to quantify (or predict) body size, proportion, and shape *(anthropo*, human; *metry*, measure)

Archimedes' principle: Principle developed by the Greek mathematician Archimedes who determined that an object's loss of weight in water equals the weight of the volume of water it displaces.

Bariatric surgery: Surgical treatment to reduce fat mass, usually in morbidly obese patients.

Behnke, Albert: Navy physician and pioneer body composition research scientist in the 1960s who developed the framework of a reference man and reference woman.

Bioelectrical impedance analysis (BIA): Device that injects (via surface electrodes) an electric current that penetrate the body's water to detect impedance to current flow, calculated by measuring current and voltage using Ohm's law. These relationships quantify the volume of water within the body, and from this, percentage body fat and FFM.

Body density (Db): Body mass expressed per unit body volume (Db = body mass ÷ body volume).

Body mass index (BMI): Ratio of body mass to stature squared (body mass, kg ÷ stature, m^2)

Brown adipose tissue (BAT): Site of non-shivering thermogenesis (**www.jci.org/articles/view/67803**).

Centers for Disease Control and Prevention (CDC): Federal agency (**www.cdc.gov**) whose main goal is to protect public health and safety through control and prevention of disease, injury, and disability.

Computed tomography (CT): Technology that uses an array of x-ray emitters and detectors to generate detailed cross-sectional, two-dimensional radiographic images of body segments when an x-ray beam of ionizing radiation passes through tissues of different densities; scan produces pictorial and quantitative information about total tissue area, total fat and muscle area, and thickness and volume of tissues within an organ.

Densitometry: Archimedes' principle of water displacement to estimate whole-body density; other terms include hydrostatic weighing, hydrodensitometry, and underwater weighing.

Dual-energy x-ray absorptiometry (DXA): Clinical device which emits two distinct low-energy x-ray beams with short exposure and low radiation dosage that penetrate bone and soft tissue areas; quantifies fat and nonbone regional LBM, including the mineral content of the body's deeper bony structures.

Energy availability hypothesis: Inadequate energy reserve to sustain pregnancy that induces ovulation cessation.

Essential fat: Fat accumulated in the heart, lungs, liver, spleen, kidneys, intestines, muscles, and lipid-rich tissues of the central nervous system and bone marrow (fat required for normal physiologic functioning).

Exercise stress hypothesis: Prolonged levels of chronic physical stress can disrupt the hypothalamic-pituitary-adrenal axis and gonadotropin-releasing hormone output to produce irregular menstruation.

Fat cell hyperplasia: Increased total number of fat cells.

Fat cell hypertrophy: Filling of existing fat cells with more fat.

Fat mass (FM): All extractable lipids from adipose and other body tissues.

Fat patterning: Pattern of distribution of trunk and extremity body fat.

Fat-free body mass (FFM): All residual lipid-free chemicals and tissues, including water, muscle, bone, connective tissue, and internal organs.

First law of thermodynamics: Energy transfers from one system to another in many forms but cannot be created or destroyed; also known as the law of conservation of energy.

FTO gene: Protein-coding gene affecting a person's risk of becoming obese.

Gastric banding surgery: Inflatable silicone device surgically implanted around the top portion of the stomach to create a small pouch that can hold only a small amount of food; controls how quickly food passes from the pouch to the lower part of the stomach and entry to the small intestine for digestion.

Goal body weight: FFM divided by (1.00 – %fat desired).

Gynoid-type obesity: Excess fat in the gluteal and femoral regions.

Ketogenic diets: Diet form that emphasizes carbohydrate restriction while generally ignoring total calories and the diet's cholesterol and saturated fat content.

Ketone bodies: Byproducts of incomplete fat breakdown; often from inadequate carbohydrate catabolism.

Kidney stones: Small, solid deposits consisting of mineral (calcium) and acid salts (urinary oxalate) formed inside the kidneys.

Lean body mass (LBM): Theoretical entity; fat-free body mass plus essential body fat.

Leptin: Body weight–regulating hormone produced by adipose cells and released into the bloodstream that acts on the hypothalamus; impacts the neurochemistry of appetite and metabolism.

Liposuction: Removing large amounts of fat by surgically excising fat deposits at selected body sites.

Magnetic resonance imaging (MRI): Technology where electromagnetic radiation in a strong magnetic field excites the hydrogen nuclei of the body's water and lipid molecules, where the molecules are more concentrated in fat, less so in water and blood, and least in bone. The nuclei then project a detectable signal that rearranges under computer software to quantify total and subcutaneous adipose tissue in individuals of varying body fatness, and other tissue structures.

Minimal body mass: Body mass plus essential body fat (includes sex-specific essential fat); 48.5 kg for the reference woman; computed from bone diameters, stature, and other constants.

Mutant gene: Permanent alteration in a gene's DNA sequence.

National Weight Control Registry (NWCR): Research program that gathers information from people who have successfully lost weight and kept it off.

Near-infrared interactance (NIR): Body fat measurement that applies technology originally developed by the U.S. Department of Agriculture to assess the body composition of livestock and the lipid content of various grains.

Obese syndrome: Constellation of nine comorbidities—glucose intolerance, insulin resistance, dyslipidemia, type 2 diabetes, hypertension, elevated plasma leptin concentrations, increased visceral adipose tissue, increased risk of coronary heart, and some cancers.

Obesity: For young men, body fat content greater than 20%; in older men, body fat content exceeding 30%. In young women, body fat content greater than 30%; in older women body fat content exceeding 30%.

Overfat: Excess fat above a predefined limit based on age and gender.

Overweight: Excess body weight relative to other individuals of the same age or height despite the absence of accompanying body fat measures.

Reference man and reference woman: Behnke's reference standards for men and women that partition body mass into lean body mass, muscle, and bone, with fat subdivided into storage and essential fat; standards for body dimensions developed from military and anthropometric surveys.

Relative body fat (%BF): Fat mass expressed as a percentage of total body mass.

Residual lung volume (RLV): Volume of air remaining in the lungs after a forced maximal exhalation.

Set point theory: All persons have a well-regulated internal control mechanism similar to a thermostat located deep within the brain's lateral hypothalamus; this neural modulating center maintains a preset level of body weight, body fat, or both within a tight range; the weight that a person would assume when not counting intake calories.

Sex-specific essential fat: Fat in females, mainly in breast and tissues related to childbearing and selected hormonal functions.

Siri, William: Developed an equation to convert body density to percentage body fat.

Skinfold calipers: Works on the same principle as a micrometer to measure the distance between two points, in this case, skinfolds at selected anatomic regions; pincer jaws exert a constant tension of 10 $g \cdot mm^{-2}$ at the point of contact with the double layer of skin plus subcutaneous fat.

Skinfolds: The double layer of skin plus subcutaneous fat just below the skin surface at selected anatomic sites (e.g., triceps, subscapula, iliac, abdomen, thigh).

Specific gravity: Body mass in air divided by loss of weight in water (body mass ÷ [body mass − body weight in water]).

Spot reduction: Notion that an increase in a muscle's metabolic activity via selective exercise stimulates relatively greater fat mobilization from the adipose tissue in proximity to the active muscle.

Stature: Height expressed in metric units; for example, 72 in. = 182.88 cm = 1.829 m.

Storage fat: Includes fat or triacylglycerol packed primarily in adipose tissue; contains approximately 83% pure fat, 2% protein, and 15% water within its supporting structures; includes the visceral fatty tissues that protect thoracic and abdominal cavity internal organs from trauma.

Subcutaneous fat: Adipose tissue located beneath the skin.

Total adipocyte number: Mass of body fat ÷ fat content per cell.

Ultrasound: Technology that converts electrical energy through a probe into high-frequency pulsed sound waves that penetrate the skin surface into the underlying tissues. The sound waves pass through adipose tissue and penetrate the muscle layer. The waves then reflect against the bone to the fat-muscle interface to produce an echo, which returns to a receiver within the probe to provide an image of underlying tissues.

Very low-calorie diet (VLCD): Therapeutic fast providing between 400 and 800 kcal daily as high-quality protein foods or liquid meal replacements.

Visceral adipose tissue (VAT): Adipose tissue within and surrounding thoracic (e.g., heart, liver, lungs) and abdominal (e.g., liver, kidneys, intestines) cavities.

World Health Organization (WHO): Public health arm of the United Nations (**www.who.int/en/**) that monitors disease outbreaks and assesses the performance of health systems globally.

SELECTED REFERENCES

Aadland E, et al. Impact of physical activity and diet on lipoprotein particle concentrations in severely obese women participating in a 1-year lifestyle intervention. *Clin Obes* 2013;3:202.

Allen TW. Body size, body composition, and cardiovascular disease risk factors in NFL players. *Phys Sportsmed* 2010;38:21.

Allison DB, et al. Energy intake and weight loss. *JAMA* 2014;312:2687.

Ansari RM. Effect of physical activity and obesity on type 2 diabetes in a middle-aged population. *J Environ Public Health* 2009;195:285.

Arner E, et al. Adipocyte turnover: relevance to human adipose tissue morphology. *Diabetes* 2010;59:105.

Arsenault BJ, et al. Body composition, cardiorespiratory fitness, and low-grade inflammation in middle-aged men and women. *Am J Cardiol* 2009;104:240.

Ballard TP, et al. Comparison of Bod Pod and DXA in female collegiate athletes. *Med Sci Sports Exerc* 2004;36:731.

Behnke AR, et al. The specific gravity of healthy men. *JAMA* 1942;118:495.

Behnke AR, Wilmore JH. *Evaluation and Regulation of Body Build and Composition*. Englewood Cliffs: Prentice Hall, 1974.

Benatti F, et al. Liposuction induces a compensatory increase of visceral fat which is effectively counteracted by physical activity: a randomized trial. *J Clin Endocrinol Metab* 2012;23:88.

Blundell JE, et al. Appetite control and energy balance: impact of exercise. *Obes Rev* 2015;16:67.

Booth FW, et al. Waging war on modern chronic diseases: primary prevention through exercise biology. *J Appl Physiol* 2000;88:774.

Bouchard C. Defining the genetic architecture of the predisposition to obesity: a challenging but not insurmountable task. *Am J Clin Nutr* 2010;91:5.

Bouchard C. Human variation in body mass: evidence for a role of the genes. *Nutr Rev* 1997;55:S21.

Brandon LJ. Comparison of existing skinfold equations for estimating body fat in African American and white women. *Am J Clin Nutr* 1998;67:1115.

Brozek J, et al. Densitometric analysis of body composition: revision of some quantitative assumptions. *Ann N Y Acad Sci* 1963;110:113.

Buchan DS, et al. The influence of a high intensity physical activity intervention on a selection of health related outcomes: an ecological approach. *BMC Public Health* 2010;10:8.

Burton RF, Cameron N. Body fat and skinfold thicknesses: a dimensional analytic approach. *Ann Hum Biol* 2009;36:717.

Cameron N, et al. Regression equations to estimate percentage body fat in African prepubertal children aged 9 y. *Am J Clin Nutr* 2004;80:70.

Carbuhn AF. Sport and training influence bone and body composition in women collegiate athletes. *J Strength Cond Res* 2010;24:1710.

Cartier A, et al. Sex differences in inflammatory markers: what is the contribution of visceral adiposity? *Am J Clin Nutr* 2009;89:1307.

Casazza K, et al. Myths, presumptions, and facts about obesity. *N Engl J Med* 2013;368:446.

Chakravarthy MV, Booth FW. Eating, exercise, and "thrifty" genotypes: connecting the dots toward an evolutionary understanding of modern chronic diseases. *J Appl Physiol* 2004;96:10.

Chaput JP, et al. Risk factors for adult overweight and obesity in the Quebec Family Study: have we been barking up the wrong tree? *Obesity (Silver Spring)* 2009;17:1964.

Chaput JP, Tremblay A. Obesity and physical inactivity: the relevance of reconsidering the notion of sedentariness. *Obes Facts* 2009;2:249.

Clark RR, et al. Minimum weight prediction methods cross-validated by the four-component model. *Med Sci Sports Exerc* 2004;36:639.

Clarys JP, et al. Gross tissue weights in the human body by cadaver dissection. *Hum Biol* 1984;56:459.

Collins AL, et al. Within- and between-laboratory precision in the measurement of body volume using air displacement plethysmography and its effect on body composition assessment. *Int J Obes Relat Metab Disord* 2004;28:80.

Coppini LZ, et al. Limitations and validation of bioelectrical impedance analysis in morbidly obese patients. *Curr Opin Clin Nutr Metab Care* 2005;8:329.

Coxam V, et al. Muscle and bone, two interconnected tissues. *Ageing Res Rev* 2015;21:55.

Dietz WH. Health consequences of obesity in youth: childhood predictors of adult disease. *Pediatrics* 1998;101:518.

Dieli-Conwright CM, et al. Effects of a 16-week resistance and aerobic exercise intervention on metabolic syndrome in overweight/obese Latina breast cancer survivors. *Cancer Epidemiol Biomarkers Prev* 2015;24:763.

Diliberti N, et al. Increased portion size leads to increased energy intake in a restaurant meal. *Obes Res* 2004;12:562.

Donnelly JE, et al. Physical activity across the curriculum (PAAC): a randomized controlled trial to promote physical activity and diminish overweight and obesity in elementary school children. *Prev Med* 2009;49:336.

Dorsey KB, et al. Diagnosis, evaluation, and treatment of childhood obesity in pediatric practice. *Arch Pediatr Adolesc Med* 2005;159:632.

Drenowatz C, et al. Differences in correlates of energy balance in normal weight, overweight and obese adults. *Obes Res Clin Pract* 2015. In Press.

Dulloo AG, et al. Pathways from dieting to weight regain, to obesity and to the metabolic syndrome: an overview. *Obes Rev* 2015;16:1.

Ebbeling CB, et al. Compensation for energy intake from fast food among overweight and lean adolescents. *JAMA* 2004;291:2828.

Elsawy B, Higgins KE. Physical activity guidelines for older adults. *Am Fam Physician* 2010;81:55.

Erion JR, et al. Obesity elicits interleukin 1-mediated deficits in hippocampal synaptic plasticity. *J Neurosci* 2014;34:2618.

Farpour-Lambert NJ, et al. Physical activity reduces systemic blood pressure and improves early markers of atherosclerosis in pre-pubertal obese children. *J Am Coll Cardiol* 2009;54:2396.

Fernández JR, et al. Is percentage body fat differentially related to body mass index in Hispanic Americans, African Americans, and European Americans? *Am J Clin Nutr* 2003;77:71.

Fields DA, et al. Assessment of body composition by air-displacement plethysmography: influence of body temperature and moisture. *Dyn Med* 2004;3:3.

Finkler E, et al. Rate of weight loss can be predicted by patient characteristics and intervention strategies. *J Acad Nutr Diet* 2012;112:75.

Flegal KM, et al. Excess deaths associated with underweight, overweight, and obesity. *JAMA* 2005;293:1861.

Flouris AD, et al. Impact of regular exercise on classical brown adipose tissue. *Clin Endocrinol (Oxf)*. 2015. doi: 10.1111/cen.12716. In Press as of 06.26.15.

Frank LL, et al. Effects of exercise on metabolic risk variables in overweight postmenopausal women: a randomized clinical trial. *Obes Res* 2005;13:615.

Freedson PA, et al. Physique, body composition, and psychological characteristics of competitive female body builders. *Phys Sports Med* 1983;11:85.

Friedrich M, et al. A comparison of anthropometric and training characteristics between female and male half-marathoners and the relationship to race time. *Asian J Sports Med* 2014;5:10.

Frisch RE, et al. Lower lifetime occurrence of breast cancer and cancers of the reproductive system among former college athletes. *Am J Clin Nutr* 1987;45:328.

Funghetto SS, et al. Comparison of percentage body fat and body mass index for the prediction of inflammatory and atherogenic lipid risk profiles in elderly women. *Clin Interv Aging* 2015;10:247.

Garcia AL, et al. Improved prediction of body fat by measuring skinfold thickness, circumferences, and bone breadths. *Obes Res* 2005;13:626.

Giannaki CD, et al. Eight weeks of a combination of high intensity interval training and conventional training reduce visceral adiposity and improve physical fitness: a group-based intervention. *J Sports Med Phys Fitness* 2015. In Press as of 06.26.15.

Giannopoulou I, et al. Exercise is required for visceral fat loss in postmenopausal women with type 2 diabetes. *J Clin Endocrinol Metab* 2005;90:1511.

Gregg EW, et al. Secular trends in cardiovascular disease risk factors according to body mass index in US adults. *JAMA* 2005;293:1868.

Groth SW, Morrison-Beedy D. GNB3 and FTO polymorphisms and pregnancy weight gain in Black Women. *Biol Res Nurs* 2015;17:405.

Haroun D, et al. Composition of the fat-free mass in obese and nonobese children: matched case-control analyses. *Int J Obes Relat Metab Disord* 2005;29:29.

Hedley A, et al. Prevalence of overweight and obesity among US children, adolescents, and adults, 1999–2002. *JAMA* 2004;291:2847.

Heymsfield SB, et al. Weight loss composition is one-fourth fat-free mass: a critical review and critique of this widely cited rule. *Obes Rev* 2014;15:310.

Hirsch J, Batchelor BR. Adipose tissue cellularity in human obesity. *Clin Endocrinol Metab* 1976;5:299.

Hirsch J, et al. Diet composition and energy balance in humans. *Am J Clin Nutr* 1998;67:551S.

Hong HR, et al. Effect of walking exercise on abdominal fat, insulin resistance and serum cytokines in obese women. *J Exerc Nutrition Biochem* 2014;18:277.

Hung YH, et al. Endurance exercise training programs intestinal lipid metabolism in a rat model of obesity and type 2 diabetes. *Physiol Rep* 2015;3:e12232. doi: 10.14814/phy2.12232.

Idrizović K, et al. Sport-specific and anthropometric factors of quality in junior male water polo players. *Coll Antropol* 2013;37:1261.

Jackson AJ, et al. Body mass index bias in defining obesity of diverse young adults. The Training Intervention and Genetics of Exercise Response (TIGER) Study. *Br J Nutr* 2009;102:1084.
Jackson AS, Pollock ML. Generalized equations for predicting body density of men. *Br J Nutr* 1978;40:497.
Jakicic JM, Gallagher KI. Exercise considerations for the sedentary, overweight adult. *Exerc Sport Sci Rev* 2003;31:91.
Janssen I, et al. Body mass index and waist circumference independently contribute to prediction of nonabdominal, abdominal subcutaneous, and visceral fat. *Am J Clin Nutr* 2002;75:683.
Johnson WD, et al. Prevalence of risk factors for metabolic syndrome in adolescents: National Health and Nutrition Examination Survey (NHANES), 2001–2006. *Arch Pediatr Adolesc Med* 2009;163:371.
Kah-Banerjee P, et al. Prospective study of the association of changes in dietary intake, physical activity, alcohol consumption, and smoking with 9-y gain in waist circumference among 16587 US men. *Am J Clin Nutr* 2003;78:719.
Kahn HS, Valdez R. Metabolic risks identified by the combination of enlarged waist and elevated triacylglycerol concentration. *Am J Clin Nutr* 2003;78:928.
Katch FI, et al. Effects of situp exercise training on adipose cell size and adiposity. *Res Q Exerc Sport* 1984;55:242.
Katch FI, et al. Validity of bioelectrical impedance to estimate body composition in cardiac and pulmonary patients. *Am J Clin Nutr* 1986;43:972.
Katch FI, Katch VL. Measurement and prediction errors in body composition assessment and the search for the perfect prediction equation. *Res Q Exerc Sport* 1980;51:249.
Katch FI, McArdle WD. Prediction of body density from simple anthropometric measurements in college-age men and women. *Hum Biol* 1973;45:445.
Katch FI, McArdle WD. Validity of body composition prediction equations for college men and women. *Am J Clin Nutr* 1975;28:105.
Katch VL, et al. Contribution of breast volume and weight to body fat distribution in females. *Am J Phys Anthropol* 1980;53:93.
Katch VL, et al. The underweight female. *Phys Sports Med* 1980;8:55.
Katzmarzyk PT, et al. Racial differences in abdominal depot-specific adiposity in white and African American adults. *Am J Clin Nutr* 2010;91:7.
Katzmarzyk PT, et al. Sitting time and mortality from all causes, cardiovascular disease, and cancer. *Med Sci Sports Exerc* 2009;41:998.
Keating SE, et al. Effect of aerobic exercise training dose on liver fat and visceral adiposity. *J Hepatol* 2015. In Press.
Keys A, Brozek J. Body fat in adult men. *Physiol Rev* 1960;33:245.
Kim J, et al. Intramuscular adipose tissue-free skeletal muscle mass: estimation by dual-energy X-ray absorptiometry in adults. *J Appl Physiol* 2004;97:655.
Kim Y, et al. Optimal cutoffs for low skeletal muscle mass related to cardiovascular risk in adults: the Korea National Health and Nutrition Examination Survey 2009-2010. *Endocrine* 2015. In Press.
Kondo M, et al. Upper limit of fat-free mass in humans: a study of Japanese sumo wrestlers. *Am J Hum Biol* 1994;6:613.
Konopka AR, et al. Defects in mitochondrial efficiency and H_2O_2 emissions in obese women are restored to a lean phenotype with aerobic exercise training. *Diabetes* 2015. In Press.
Krarup NT, et al. A genetic risk score of 45 coronary artery disease risk variants associates with increased risk of myocardial infarction in 6041 Danish individuals. *Atherosclerosis* 2015. In Press.
Kullberg J. Adipose tissue distribution in children: automated quantification using water and fat MRI. *J Magn Reson Imaging* 2010;32:204.
Lagowska K. et al. Nine-month nutritional intervention improves restoration of menses in young female athletes and ballet dancers. *J Int Soc Sports Nutr* 2014;11:52.
Lang T. Computed tomographic measurements of thigh muscle cross-sectional area and attenuation coefficient predict hip fracture: the health, aging, and body composition study. *J Bone Miner Res* 2010;25:513.
Laye MJ, et al. Physical activity enhances metabolic fitness independently of cardiorespiratory fitness in marathon runners. *Dis Markers* 2015. In Press.
Lazzer S, et al. Assessment of energy expenditure associated with physical activities in free-living obese and nonobese adolescents. *Am J Clin Nutr* 2003l;78:471.
Liu X, et al. The development and validation of new equations for estimating body fat percentage among Chinese men and women. *Br J Nutr* 2015. In Press.
Liu A, et al. Differential intra-abdominal adipose tissue profiling in obese, insulin-resistant women. *Obes Surg* 2009;19:1564.
Loucks AB. Energy availability, not body fatness, regulates reproductive function in women. *Exerc Sport Sci Rev* 2003;31:144.
Lund J, et al. Exercise training promotes cardioprotection through oxygen-sparing action in high-fat fed mice. *Am J Physiol Heart Circ Physiol* 2015;15;308.
Maddalozzo GF, et al. Concurrent validity of the BOD POD and dual energy x-ray absorptiometry techniques for assessing body composition in young women. *J Am Diet Assoc* 2002;102:1677.
Mayo MJ, et al. Exercise-induced weight loss preferentially reduces abdominal fat. *Med Sci Sports Exerc* 2003;35:207.
Meisel SF, et al. Genetic susceptibility testing and readiness to control weight: results from a randomized controlled trial. *Obesity (Silver Spring)* 2014;23:305.
Mota J. Television viewing and changes in body mass index and cardiorespiratory fitness over a two-year period in schoolchildren. *Pediatr Exerc Sci* 2010;22:245.
Müller MJ, et al. Advances in the understanding of specific metabolic rates of major organs and tissues in humans. *Curr Opin Clin Nutr Metab Care* 2013;16:501.
Murtagh EM, et al. The effect of walking on risk factors for cardiovascular disease: an updated systematic review and meta-analysis of randomised control trials. *Prev Med* 2015;72C:34. Review.
National Task Force on the Prevention and Treatment of Obesity. Obesity, overweight and health risk. *Arch Intern Med* 2000;160:898.
Nordby P, et al. Independent effects of endurance training and weight loss on peak fat oxidation in moderately overweight men; a randomized controlled trial. *J Appl Physiol (1985)* 2015. doi: 10.1152/japplphysiol.00715.2014.
Oda E, Kawai R. Comparison among body mass index (BM), waist circumference (WC), and percent body fat (%BF) as anthropometric markers for the clustering of metabolic risk factors in Japanese. *Intern Med* 2010;49:1477.
Ogden CL, et al. Prevalence of obesity among adults: United States, 2011–2012. *NCHS Data Brief* 2013:1.
Ostojic SM. Adiposity, physical activity and blood lipid profile in 13-year-old adolescents. *J Pediatr Endocrinol Metab* 2010;23:333.
Palacios-González B, et al. Irisin levels before and after physical activity among school-age children with different BMI: a direct relation with leptin. *Obesity (Silver Spring)* 2015. In Press.
Payne A, et al. Effect of FTO gene and physical activity interaction on trunk fat percentage among the Newfoundland Population. *Genet Epigenet* 2014;6:21.
Peirson L, et al. Prevention of overweight and obesity in children and youth: a systematic review and meta-analysis. *CMAJ Open* 2015. In Press.
Pérusse L, et al. Familial aggregation of abdominal visceral fat level: results from the Quebec family. *Metabolism* 1996;45:378.
Peterson MJ, et al. Development and validation of skinfold-thickness prediction equations with a 4-compartment model. *Am J Clin Nutr* 2003;77:1186.
Pollock ML, et al. Twenty-year follow-up of aerobic power and body composition of older track athletes. *J Appl Physiol* 1997;82:1508.
Portal S. Body fat measurements in elite adolescent volleyball players: correlation between skinfold thickness, bioelectrical impedance analysis, air-displacement plethysmography, and body mass index percentiles. *J Pediatr Endocrinol Metab* 2010;23:395.
Rhéaume C, et al. Low cardiorespiratory fitness levels and elevated blood pressure: what is the contribution of visceral adiposity? *Hypertension* 2009;54:91.
Rolls BJ, et al. The relationship between energy density and energy intake. *Physiol Behav* 2009;97:609.
Romaguera D. Dietary determinants of changes in waist circumference adjusted for body mass index—a proxy measure of visceral adiposity. *PLoS One* 2010;5:e11588.
Rotella CM, Dicembrini I. Measurement of body composition as a surrogate evaluation of energy balance in obese patients. *World J Methodol* 2015. In Press.
Sacks FM, et al. Comparison of weight-loss diets with different compositions of fat, protein, and carbohydrates. *N Engl J Med* 2009;360:859.
Schmid W, et al. Predictor variables for marathon race time in recreational female runners. *Asian J Sports Med* 2012;3:90.
Schoeller DA. Balancing energy expenditure and body weight. *Am J Clin Nutr* 1998;68:956S.
Schutte JE, et al. Density of lean body mass is greater in blacks than whites. *J Appl Physiol* 1984;56:1647.
Serralde-Zúñiga AE, et al. Omental adipose tissue gene expression, gene variants, branched-chain amino acids, and their relationship with metabolic syndrome and insulin resistance in humans. *Genes Nutr* 2014;9:431.
Shen W, et al. A single MRI slice does not accurately predict visceral and subcutaneous adipose tissue changes during weight loss. *Obesity (Silver Spring)* 2012;20:2458.
Sisson SB, et al. Ethnic differences in subcutaneous adiposity and waist girth in children and adolescents. *Obesity (Silver Spring)* 2009;17:2075.
Sisson SB, et al. Profiles of sedentary behavior in children and adolescents: the US National Health and Nutrition Examination Survey, 2001–2006. *Int J Pediatr Obes* 2009;4:353.
St.-Onge MP, et al. Changes in childhood food consumption patterns: a cause for concern in light of increasing body weights. *Am J Clin Nutr* 2003;78:1068.
Stanford KI, et al. A novel role for subcutaneous adipose tissue in exercise-induced improvements in glucose homeostasis. *Diabetes* 2015. In Press.
Stern L, et al. The effects of low-carbohydrate versus conventional weight loss diets in severely obese adults: one-year follow-up of a randomized trial. *Ann Intern Med* 2004;140:778.
Stommel M, Schoenborn CA. Variations in BMI and prevalence of health risks in diverse racial and ethnic populations. *Obesity (Silver Spring)*, 2010;18:1821.
Sun G, et al. Comparison of multifrequency bioelectrical impedance analysis with dual-energy X-ray absorptiometry for assessment of percentage body fat in a large, healthy population. *Am J Clin Nutr* 2005;81:74.
Thomas DM, et al. Effect of dietary adherence on the body weight plateau: a mathematical model incorporating intermittent compliance with energy intake prescription. *Am J Clin Nutr* 2014;100:787.

Thomas DM, et al. Response to 'Why is the 3500 kcal per pound weight loss rule wrong? *Int J Obes (Lond)* 2013;37:1614.

Thomas DM, et al. Time to correctly predict the amount of weight loss with dieting. *J Acad Nutr Diet* 2014;114:857.

Thomas DM, et al. Why do individuals not lose more weight from an exercise intervention at a defined dose? An energy balance analysis *Obes Rev* 2012;13:835.

Torstveit MK, Sundgot-Borgen J. Participation in leanness sports but not training volume is associated with menstrual dysfunction: a national survey of 1276 elite athletes and controls. *Br J Sports Med* 2005;39:14.

Tran ZV, Weltman A. Generalized equation for predicting body density of women from girth measurements. *Med Sci Sports Exerc* 1989;21:101.

Turner-McGrievy GM, et al. Comparative effectiveness of plant-based diets for weight loss: a randomized controlled trial of five different diets. *Nutrition* 2015;31:350.

Utter AC, et al. Evaluation of air displacement for assessing body composition of collegiate wrestlers. *Med Sci Sports Exerc* 2003;35:500.

van Marken Lichtenbelt WD, et al. Body composition changes in bodybuilders: a method comparison. *Med Sci Sports Exerc* 2004;36:490.

Von Thun NL, et al. Does bone loss begin after weight loss ends? Results 2 years after weight loss or regain in postmenopausal women. *Menopause* 2014;21:501.

Wagner DR, Heyward VH. Measures of body composition in blacks and whites: a comparative review. *Am J Clin Nutr* 2000;71:1392.

Weltman A, et al. Accurate assessment of body composition in obese females. *Am J Clin Nutr* 1988;48:1179.

Whitlock EP, et al. Screening and interventions for childhood overweight: a summary of evidence for the US Preventive Services Task Force. *Pediatrics* 2005;116:e125.

Wijndaele K, et al. Increased cardiometabolic risk is associated with increased TV viewing time. *Med Sci Sports Exerc* 2010;42:1511.

Witham MD, Avenell A. Interventions to achieve long-term weight loss in obese older people: a systematic review and meta-analysis. *Age Ageing* 2010;39:172.

Wyshak G. Percent body fat, fractures and risk of osteoporosis in women. *J Nutr Health Aging* 2010;14:428.

Yu OK. Comparisons of obesity assessments in over-weight elementary students using anthropometry, BIA, CT and DEXA. *Nutr Res Pract* 2010; 4:128.

Zoladz JA, et al. Effect of moderate incremental exercise, performed in fed and fasted state on cardio-respiratory variables and leptin and ghrelin concentrations in young healthy men. *J Physiol Pharmacol* 2005;56:63.

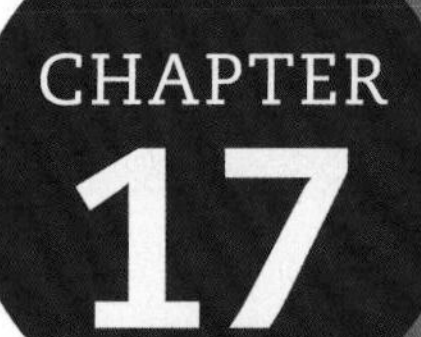

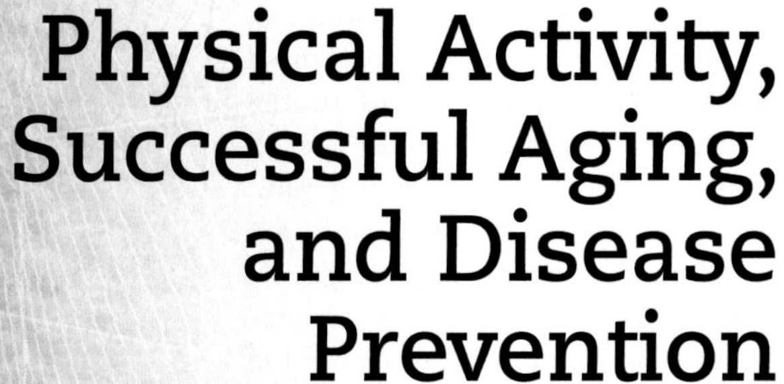

CHAPTER 17

Physical Activity, Successful Aging, and Disease Prevention

CHAPTER OBJECTIVES

- Describe the meaning of *healthspan*.
- Explain the concept of successful aging compared with traditional views of the aging process.
- Distinguish between the terms *exercise* and *physical activity*.
- Explain the basis of the Physical Activity Pyramid.
- Answer the question, "How safe is exercise?"
- Describe five goals of Healthy People 2020.
- What is SeDS, and why is it important?
- List two important age-related changes in muscular strength, joint flexibility, nervous system function, cardiovascular function, pulmonary function, endocrine function, and body composition.
- Describe five field tests to assess the flexibility of major body areas.
- Describe two research studies showing that regular physical activity protects against disease and may even extend life.
- List three major causes of death in the United States.
- List and describe four major coronary heart disease (CHD) risk factors.
- List two secondary and two novel CHD risk factors.
- List three specific components of the blood lipid profile and give values currently considered desirable for each.
- Discuss two factors that affect cholesterol lipoprotein levels.
- Explain how regular physical activity reduces CHD risk.
- Describe the prevalence of children's CHD risk factors.
- Explain interactions among CHD risk factors.

ANCILLARIES AT A GLANCE

Visit **http://thePoint.lww.com/MKKESS5e** to access the following resources.

- References: Chapter 17
- Interactive Question Bank
- Animation: Acute Inflammation

PART 1 The Graying of America

Elderly persons make up the fastest growing segment of American society. At the start of the 1970s, **gerontologists** considered age 65 the onset of "old age;" it represented the average retirement age of most individuals in the workforce. These same researchers now consider age 85 the demarcation of "**oldest-old**" and age 75 "**young-old**." As of the latest census results released in 2013, over 14% or approximately 44 million Americans exceed age 65, and those over age 85 make up about 2% of the population, up from 1.7% in 2010. By the year 2030, 70 million Americans will transition into the "oldest-old" category. Some **demographers** project that half of girls and one third of boys born in developed countries near the end of the 20th century will live in three centuries. At least half of all babies born in America in 2007 are projected to live to the age of 104!

In the short term, disease prevention, improved health care, and more effective treatment of age-related heart disease and osteoporosis help people live longer. Far fewer people now die from infectious childhood diseases, and those with the genetic potential actualize their proclivity for longevity. On a different but parallel front, anticipated breakthroughs in genetic therapies may slow the aging of individual cells. Two main factors are thought to account for the cellular damage that occurs with aging:

1. Accumulated mutations in mitochondrial DNA, perhaps induced by injury and deterioration from oxidative stress
2. Gene alterations that depress telomerase synthesis enzyme that protect the protective caps (**telomeres**) at the ends of chromosomes that inhibit proper cell division

Gene therapies will undoubtedly boost human life spans to a greater extent than improved medical treatment or even the eradication of deadly diseases.

Figure 17.1 shows that proportionately, centenarians represent the fastest growing age group in the United States. In 2000, an estimated 180,000 centenarians were living worldwide. If the current growth of centenarians continues, by 2050 the number will have grown to 3.2 million, an increase of about 18 times, which would represent the fastest growing segment of the world's population. Demographers project that by the middle of the 21st century, more than 800,000 Americans will exceed age 100, with many in relatively "good" health. Old age mortality appears to be on the decline because the **death rate**, referred to as the number of people per 100 in a specific age group, levels off in the 90-year-old age category (~11 per 100) and decreases to 8 per 100 after age 100.

Figure 17.2 presents the top 10 countries for life expectancy. Life expectancy in the United States has been on the

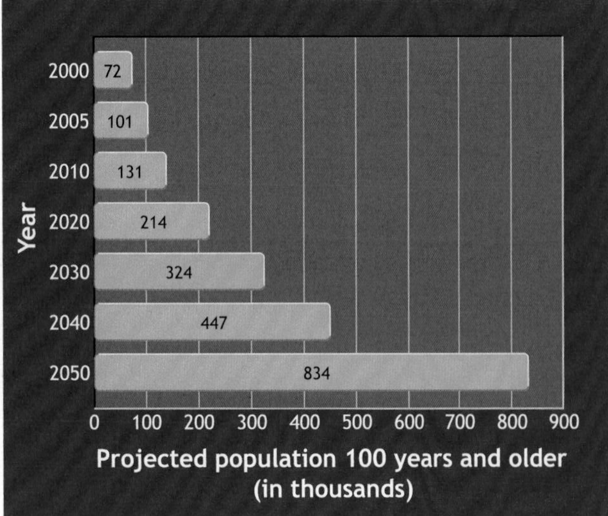

FIGURE 17.1 The graying of America. Growth in number of centenarians in the United States. (Data from U.S. Bureau of the Census, National Center for Health Statistics, Centers for Disease Control and Prevention: Washington, DC, and actuarial tables from insurance companies.)

Country and Rank	Estimated Life Expectancy (2014)
Monaco (1)	89.57
Macau (2)	84.48
Japan (3)	84.46
Singapore (4)	84.38
San Marino (5)	83.18
Andorra (6)	82.65
Guernsey (7)	82.39
Hong Kong (8)	82.29
Australia (9)	82.07
Italy (10)	82.03
United States (53)	81.68

FIGURE 17.2 Top ten countries for life expectancy. (Data from **www. Geoba.se/population.php.**)

rise for the past decade, increasing 1.4 years—from 76.5 in 1997 to 77.9 in 2007, and to an estimated average for males and females of 85.0 years in 2015. Shockingly, the United States still ranks number 53 in the world (just ahead of Bahrain and Qatar), with Syria ranking 100th (**www.geoba.se/population.php?pc=world&type=015&year=2014&st=rank&asde=&page=1**).

Cigarette smoking, elevated body mass index (BMI), excess body fat, and reduced levels of regular physical activity provide potent predictors of subsequent morbidity and mortality. Changing to a more physically active lifestyle brings about a number of benefits: it reduces mortality from common ailments and greatly improves cardiovascular and muscular functional capacities, quality of life, and capacity for independent living. At any age, four behavioral changes act independently to delay all-cause mortality and extend life: becoming more physically active, quitting cigarette smoking, controlling body weight; and controlling blood pressure. Persons with more healthful lifestyles survive longer with a reduced disability risk as life progresses.

THE NEW GERONTOLOGY: SUCCESSFUL AGING

Many gerontologists maintain that research on aging should not focus on increasing life span but rather on improving **healthspan**, that is, the total number of years a person remains in excellent health. The **new gerontology** addresses areas beyond age-related diseases and their prevention to recognize that successful aging requires maintenance of enhanced physiologic function and physical fitness. Much of the physiologic deterioration previously considered "normal aging" included deleterious changes in blood pressure, bone mass, body composition, body fat distribution, insulin sensitivity, and homocysteine levels. These changes are accompanied by increased health risk, dysfunction, or actual disease and are dependent on lifestyle and environmental influences. They are subject to considerable desirable modification with proper nutrition and increased physical activity. For those achieving older age, functional impairments often occur in muscular strength, cardiovascular function, joint range of motion (ROM), and sleep disturbances, each potentially impacting some aspect of disease status.

Gerontologists consider that successful aging includes four components:

1. Physical health
2. Spirituality
3. Emotional and educational health
4. Social satisfaction

Healthy Life Expectancy

Life expectancy estimates consider the overall length of life based on mortality data without considering the quality of life during aging. At some point during the life span, some level of disability detracts from life's quality. For example, the Centers for Disease Control and Prevention (CDC; **www.cdc.gov/nchs/fastats/lifexpec.htm**) reports that nearly 1 in 10 Americans older than age 70 requires help with daily activities such as bathing and 4 in 10 use assistive walkers or hearing aids. Approximately 50% of men and 33% of women older than age 70 experience arthritis, more than one third have high blood pressure, and 11% have diabetes. Of all seniors, women older than age 85 are most likely to require everyday help, and 23% require assistance with at least one basic dressing or bathroom activity.

To estimate healthy longevity, the World Health Organization in 2004 introduced the concept of **healthy life expectancy (HALE)** (**www.who.int/healthinfo/statistics/indhale/en/**), the expected number of years a person can expect to live in "full health." HALE considers the years of ill health weighted according to severity and subtracted from expected overall life expectancy to compute the equivalent years of healthy life. Of the 191 countries evaluated, HALE estimates reached 70 years in 24 countries and 60 years in more than half. Thirty-two countries were at the lower extreme of less than 40 years. Many of these countries bear the burden of the major epidemics of HIV/AIDS and other causes of death and disability.

The six most prominent factors in order of importance responsible for decreased life expectancy in non-Western countries are closely related to disease occurrence and environmental insults:

1. Low birth weight
2. Vitamin and mineral deficiency, particularly vitamin A and iron
3. Unsafe water and sanitation procedures
4. Unprotected sex including HIV
5. Carcinogen exposure
6. Work-related risk

In the Americas and Europe, the six major factors contributing to decreased healthy life span are related to lifestyle choices:

1. Tobacco use
2. High blood pressure
3. Increased blood cholesterol
4. Obesity
5. Low levels of physical activity
6. Limited fruit and vegetable consumption

The Centers for Disease Control and Prevention also computes healthy life expectancy using the acronym **HLE**, defined as the remaining healthy years of life beginning at age 65. This computes as HLE divided by total life expectancy (LE) or HLE/LE. **Figure 17.3** shows state-specific HLE at age 65 by gender and race (whites, blacks) in the United States during 2007–2009 as of November 2014. For both sexes, HLE was generally less in the south than any other region (**www.cdc.gov/mmwr/preview/mmwrhtml/mm6228a1.htm**).

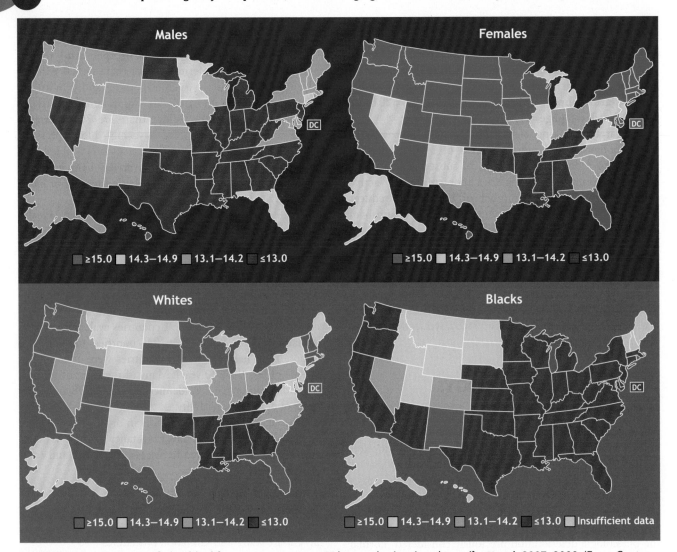

FIGURE 17.3 State-specific healthy life expectancy at age 65 by gender **(top)** and race **(bottom)**, 2007–2009. (From Centers for Disease Control and Prevention. State-specific healthy life expectancy at age 65 years—United States, 2007–2009. *Morb Mortal Wkly Rep* 2013;62;561. **www.cdc.gov/mmwr/preview/mmwrhtml/mm6228a1.htm**.)

SUMMARY

1. Elderly persons constitute the fastest growing segment of American society.
2. About 45 years ago, gerontologists considered age 65 the onset of old age; currently, age 85 now serves as the demarcation of "oldest-old" and age 75 "young-old."
3. Nearly 12% or approximately 35 million Americans exceed age 65; by the year 2030, 70 million Americans will exceed age 85.
4. "Healthspan" refers to the total number of years a person remains in excellent health.
5. The "new gerontology" addresses areas beyond age-related diseases and their prevention and recognizes that successful aging maintains enhanced physiologic function and physical fitness.
6. "Healthy life expectancy" (HLE) refers to the expected number of years a person might live the equivalent of full health.

THINK IT THROUGH

1. Describe two differences between life expectancy and healthy life expectancy.
2. List four factors contributing to decreased healthy life span.
3. Describe lifestyle modification factors in your own life that could contribute to a more healthy life expectancy.

PART 2 Physical Activity Epidemiology

Epidemiology research involves quantifying factors that influence illness occurrence to better understand, modify, or control a disease pattern in the general population. The specific field of **physical activity epidemiology** applies the general research strategies of epidemiology to study physical activity as a health-related behavior linked to disease and associated outcomes.

Terminology

Physical activity epidemiology applies specific definitions to characterize behavioral patterns and outcomes of the groups under investigation. Relevant terminology includes the following:

- **Physical activity:** Body movement produced by muscle action to increase energy expenditure
- **Exercise:** Planned, structured, repetitive, and purposeful physical activity
- **Physical fitness:** Attributes related to how well one performs physical activity
- **Health:** Physical, mental, and social well-being, not simply absence of disease
- **Health-related physical fitness:** Components of physical fitness associated with some aspect of good health or disease prevention (**Fig. 17.4**)
- **Longevity:** Length of life

Within this framework, *physical activity* becomes a generic term with *exercise* one of its major component. Similarly, the definition of *health* focuses on the broad spectrum of well-being that ranges from complete absence of health (near death) to the highest levels of physiologic function. Implicit in such definitions is the challenge of how to objectively measure and quantify health and physical activity. Nevertheless, these terms provide a broad perspective from which we can study the role of physical activity in health and disease.

The trend in physical fitness assessment during the past 45 years deemphasizes tests of motor performance and athletic fitness (e.g., speed, power, endurance, balance, agility). Current assessment focuses on functional capacities related to overall good health and disease prevention (e.g., rise from a chair or bed, walk to the bathroom, or climb a single stair without assistance). The four most common components of health-related physical fitness include aerobic or cardiovascular fitness, body composition, abdominal muscular strength and endurance, and lower back and hamstring flexibility (see A Closer Look: "How to Assess Joint Flexibility in Common Body Areas").

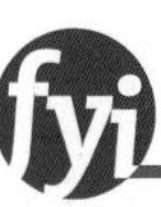

Activities of Americans Who Report Regular Physical Activity

Activity	Percentage Male	Percentage Female
Walking	39	48
Resistance training	20	9
Cycling	16	15
Running	12	6
Stair climbing	10	12
Aerobics	3	10

Physical Activity Participation

More than 30 different methodologies can assess physical activity. Examples include direct and indirect calorimetry, self-reports and questionnaires, job classifications, physiologic markers, behavioral observations, mechanical or electronic monitors, and activity surveys. Each approach offers unique advantages and disadvantages depending on the situation and population studied. Obtaining valid estimates of physical activity of large groups remains difficult because such studies by necessity apply self-reports of daily activity and exercise participation rather than direct monitoring or objective measurement. Despite limitations in assessment, a discouraging picture of physical activity participation worldwide consistently emerges. In the United States, adult participation in any physical activity remains low:

- Only about 15% engage in regular, vigorous physical activity during leisure time, three times a week for at least 30 minutes.
- More than 60% do not engage in any regular physical activity.
- About 25% lead sedentary lives (i.e., do not participate in physical activity).
- Walking, gardening, and yard work are the most popular leisure-time activities.
- About 22% engage in light-to-moderate physical activity regularly during leisure time (five times a week for at least 30 min).
- Physical inactivity occurs more frequently among women than men, blacks and Hispanics than whites, older than younger adults, and less affluent than wealthier persons.
- Participation in fitness activities declines with age; older citizens typically have such poor functional capacity they cannot rise from a chair or bed, walk to the bathroom, or climb a single stair without assistance.

FIGURE 17.4 Health-related physical fitness components.

Equally discouraging data emerge for children and teenagers:

- Nearly half of those between ages 12 and 21 do no vigorous physical activity on a regular basis independent of gender.
- About 14% report no recent physical activity; this is more prevalent among females, particularly black females.
- About 25% engage in light-to-moderate physical activity (e.g., walk or bicycle) nearly every day.
- Participation in all types of physical activity declines strikingly as age and school grade increase.
- More boys than girls participate in vigorous physical activity, strengthening activities, and walking or bicycling.

Getting America More Physically Active

On July 11, 1996 in a landmark announcement, the United States Surgeon General acknowledged the importance of physical activity to the nation with the release of the ***First Surgeon General's Report on Physical Activity and Health*** (**www.cdc.gov/NCCDPHP/sgr/ataglan.htm**). This encompassing report summarized the benefits of regular physical activity in disease prevention. The Surgeon General proposed a national agenda that urged the nation to adopt and maintain a physically active lifestyle to combat ailments associated with the country's generally low level of energy expenditure. Following this report in 2000, the government launched the Healthy People 2010 initiative that included strategies to improve the nation's health for the first decade of the 21st century. The **Physical Activity Pyramid** (**Fig. 17.5**) summarizes major goals to increase regular physical activity in the general population; the pyramid emphasizes diverse forms of behavioral and lifestyle options.

A CLOSER LOOK

How to Assess Joint Flexibility in Common Body Areas

Two types of flexibility include (1) *static*, which is full range of motion (ROM) of a specific joint, and (2) *dynamic*, which is torque or resistance encountered as the joint moves through its ROM. Improper vertebral column alignment accounts for more than 80% of all lower back and pelvic girdle ailments; this often results from poor flexibility in regions of the lower back, trunk, hip, and posterior thigh and weak abdominal and erector spinae muscles.

Specificity and Flexibility

Considerable specificity exists for joint ROM depending on level of use and joint structure. Triaxial ball and socket hip and shoulder joints afford a greater degree of movement than either uniaxial or biaxial wrist, knee, elbow, and ankle joints. "Tightness" of soft tissue structures of the joint capsule and muscle and its fascia, tendons, ligaments, and skin constitute major factors that influence static and dynamic flexibility. Other influences include a well-developed musculature and excess fatty tissue of adjacent body segments. Flexibility progressively decreases with advancing age, mainly from decreased soft tissue extensibility, largely influenced by decreased levels of physical activity. On average, women remain more flexible than men at any age.

Five Common Field Tests of Static Flexibility

Field tests assess static flexibility indirectly through linear ROM measurement. A minimum of three trials should be administered following a warm-up.

Test 1: Hip and Trunk Flexibility (Modified Sit-and-Reach Test)

Starting position: Sit on floor with the back and head against a wall with the legs fully extended with the bottom of the feet against the sit-and-reach box. Place the hands on top of each other, stretching the arms forward while keeping the head and back against the wall **(A)**. Measure distance from the fingertips to the box edge with a yardstick. This becomes the zero or starting point.

Movement: Slowly bend and reach forward maximally (the head and back move away from the wall), sliding the fingers along the yardstick; hold the final position for 2 seconds **(B)**.

Score: Total distance reached to the nearest one-tenth inch.

Test 1: Hip-and-trunk flexibility (modified sit-and-reach test)

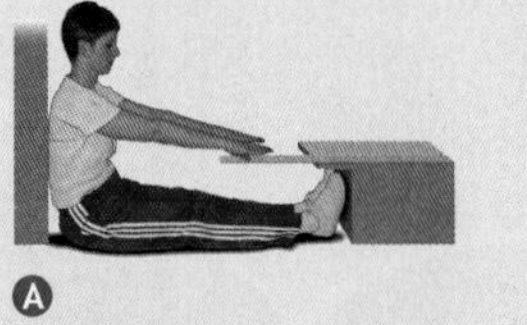

A

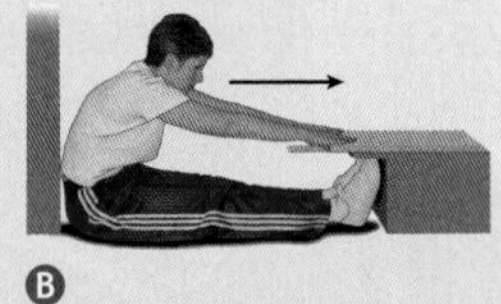

B

Test 2: Shoulder-wrist flexibility (shoulder-and-wrist elevation test)

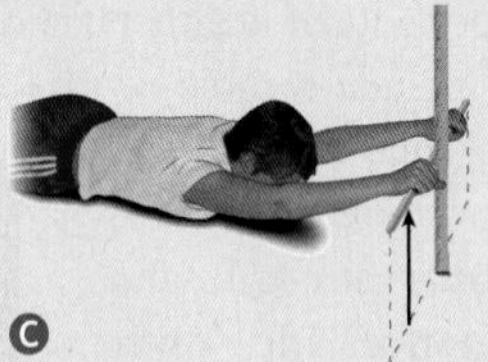

C

Modified Sit and Reach, Age Range

	Men		Women	
Performance Rating	**Age <35 y**	**Age 36–49 y**	**Age <35 y**	**Age 36–49 y**
Excellent	>17.9	>16.1	>17.9	>17.4
Good	17.0–17.9	14.6–16.1	16.7–17.9	16.2–17.4
Average	15.8–17.0	13.9–14.6	16.2–16.7	15.2–16.2
Fair	15.0–15.8	13.4–13.9	15.8–16.2	14.5–15.2
Poor	<15.0	<13.4	<15.4	<14.5

Adapted from Johnson BL, Nelson JK. *Practical Measurements for Evaluation in Physical Education*. 4th Ed. New York: Macmillan Publishing, 1986.

Test 2: Shoulder-Wrist Flexibility (Shoulder and Wrist Elevation Test)

Starting position: Lie prone on the floor with arms fully extended overhead; grasp a yardstick with the hands shoulder width apart.

Movement: Raise the stick maximally.

- Measure the vertical distance (nearest 1/4 in. [0.635 cm]) the yardstick rises from the floor.
- Measure arm length from the acromial process to the tip of longest finger.
- Subtract the best vertical score from arm length.

Score: Arm length—best vertical score (nearest 1/4 in.)

Shoulder and Wrist Elevation (in inches)

Performance Rating	Men	Women
Excellent	≥12.75	≥12.00
Good	12.50–11.75	11.75–11.0
Average	11.50–8.50	10.75–7.75
Fair	8.25–6.25	7.50–5.75
Poor	≤6.00	≤5.50

Adapted from Johnson BL, Nelson JK. *Practical Measurements for Evaluation in Physical Education*. 4th Ed. New York: Macmillan Publishing, 1986.

Test 3: Trunk and Neck Flexibility (Trunk and Neck Extension Test)

Starting position: Lie prone on the floor with the hands clasped together behind the head.

Movement: Raise the trunk maximally while keeping the hips in contact with the floor. An assistant can stabilize the legs.

Score: Vertical distance (nearest 1/4 in.) from the tip of the nose to the floor

Trunk and Neck Extension (in inches)

Performance Rating	Men	Women
Excellent	≥10.25	≥10.00
Good	10.00–8.25	9.75–8.00
Average	8.00–6.25	7.75–6.00
Fair	6.00–3.25	5.75–2.25
Poor	≤3.00	≤2.00

Adapted from Johnson BL, Nelson JK. *Practical Measurements for Evaluation in Physical Education*. 4th Ed. New York: Macmillan Publishing, 1986.

Test 4: Shoulder Flexibility (Shoulder Rotation Test)

Starting position: Grasp one end of a rope with the left hand; 4 inches away, grasp the rope with the right hand.

Movement: Extend both arms in front of the chest and rotate the arms overhead and behind the back; as resistance occurs, slide the right hand farther from the left hand along the rope until the rope touches against the back.

- Measure the distance on the rope between the thumb of each hand after successfully rotating overhead with the rope against the back.
- Measure shoulder width from deltoid to deltoid. Subtract the rope distance from shoulder width distance.

Score: Shoulder-width distance—rope distance (nearest 1/4 in.)

Shoulder Rotation (in inches)

Performance Rating	Men	Women
Excellent	≥20.00	≥18.00
Good	19.75–14.75	17.75–13.25
Average	14.50–11.75	13.00–10.00
Fair	11.50–7.25	9.75–5.25
Poor	≤7.00	≤5.00

Adapted from Johnson BL, Nelson JK. *Practical Measurements for Evaluation in Physical Education*. 4th Ed. New York: Macmillan Publishing, 1986.

Test 5: Ankle Flexibility (Ankle Flexion Test)

Starting position: Stand facing a wall. With feet flat on the floor, lean into the wall.

Movement: Slowly slide back from the wall as far as possible while keeping the feet flat on the floor, body and knees fully extended, and chest in contact with the wall.

Score: Distance between the toe line and the wall (nearest 1/4 in.)

Ankle Flexion (in inches)

Performance Rating	Men	Women
Excellent	≥35.50	≥32.00
Good	35.25–32.75	31.75–30.50
Average	32.50–29.75	30.25–26.75
Fair	29.50–26.75	26.50–24.50
Poor	≤26.50	≤24.25

Adapted from Johnson BL, Nelson JK. *Practical Measurements for Evaluation in Physical Education*. 4th Ed. New York: Macmillan Publishing, 1986.

Healthy People 2020

Healthy People 2020, launched in December, 2010, represents a new set of goals and objectives with 10-year targets designed to guide national health promotion and disease prevention efforts to improve the health of all United States citizens. Healthy People 2020 represents the fourth generation of this initiative. These goals and objectives serve as a tool for strategic management by the federal government, states, communities, and other public and private sector partners. The comprehensive set of objectives and targets measure progress for health issues in specific populations to meet the following two objectives:

1. Build a foundation for disease prevention and wellness activities across various state and local sectors and within the federal government
2. Serve as a model for measurement at the state and local levels

Healthy People 2020 commits to the vision of a society in which all people live long, healthy lives (**www.healthypeople.gov/**). The following three features aim to make this vision a reality:

1. Emphasizing ideas of health equity that address social determinants of health and promote health across all life stages
2. Replacing the traditional print publication with an interactive Web site as the main dissemination vehicle
3. Maintaining a Web site that allows users to tailor information to their needs and explore evidence-based resources for implementation

Healthy People 2020 is designed to achieve four primary goals:

1. Attain high-quality, longer lives free of preventable disease, disability, injury, and premature death
2. Achieve health equity, eliminate disparities, and improve the health of all groups
3. Create social and physical environments that promote good health for all
4. Promote quality of life, healthy development, and healthy behaviors across all life stages

The U.S. Department of Health and Human Services (**www.hhs.gov/**) maintains a comprehensive, interactive online presence that includes the ability to search the extensive database of the U.S. government.

- *Healthy People 2020 Homepage*: **www.healthypeople.gov/2020/default.aspx**
- *Data 2020 Search:* **www.healthypeople.gov/2020/data/searchData.aspx**
- *Healthy People 2020 Topics and Objectives*: **www.healthypeople.gov/2020/topicsobjectives2020/default.aspx**

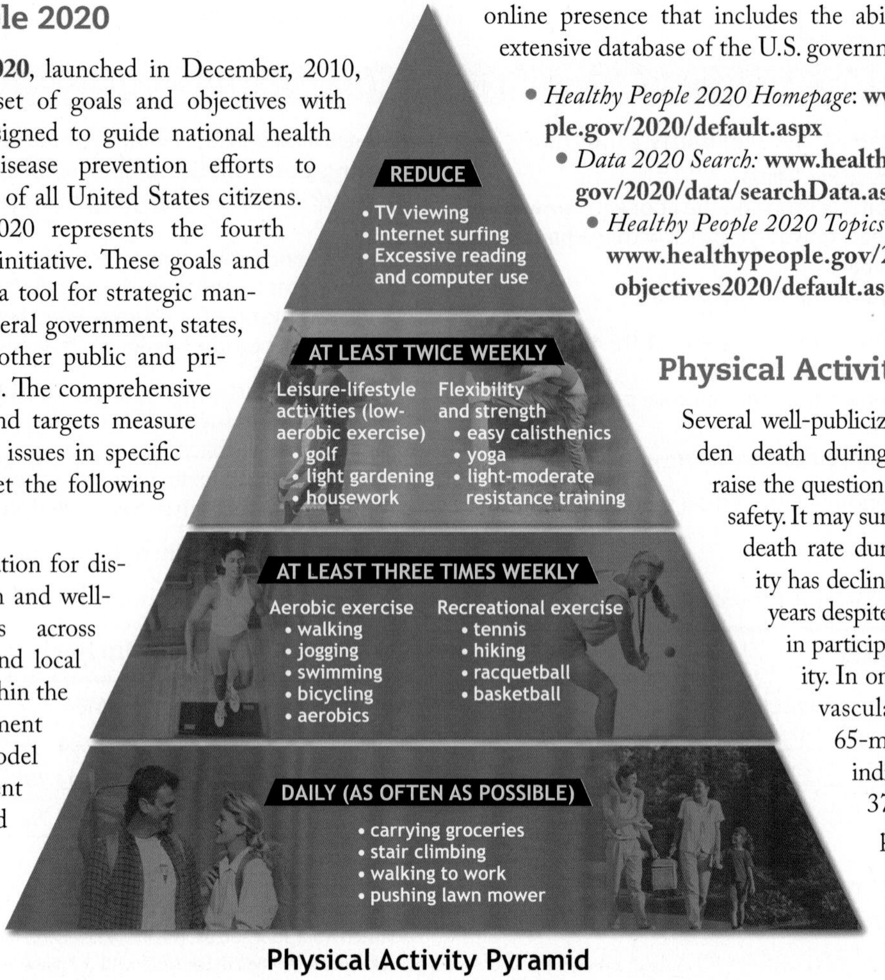

FIGURE 17.5 The physical activity pyramid: Prudent goals for increasing daily physical activity.

Physical Activity Safety

Several well-publicized reports of sudden death during physical activity raise the question of physical activity safety. It may surprise some that the death rate during physical activity has declined over the past 40 years despite an overall increase in participation in such activity. In one report of cardiovascular episodes over a 65-month period, 2935 individuals recorded 374,798 hours of physical activity that included 2,726,272 km (1,694,026 mi) of running and walking. No deaths occurred during this time, and only two nonfatal cardiovascular complications were recorded. This amounts to two complications per 100,000 hours of physical activity for women and three complications for men.

The relative risk of sudden death among athletes versus nonathletes was 1.95 for men and 2.00 for women. The higher risk of sudden death in athletes strongly relates to underlying congenital coronary artery anomaly, arrhythmogenic right ventricular cardiomyopathy, and premature coronary artery disease. Interestingly, athletic participation did not cause the enhanced mortality. Instead, it triggered sudden death in athletes affected by cardiovascular conditions predisposing them to life-threatening ventricular arrhythmias during physical activity.

Intense physical exertion poses a small risk of sudden death (e.g., one sudden death per 1.51 million episodes of exertion) during the activity compared with resting an equivalent time, particularly for sedentary people with a genetic predisposition to sudden death. Prospective epidemiologic research evaluated clinically significant medical incidents and emergencies for 7725 low-risk, apparently healthy corporate fitness enrollees in a supervised facility at a major medical center. Over 2.5 years, 15 medically significant events (0.05 per 1000 participant hours) and two medical emergencies (both recovered; 0.006 per 1000 participant-hours). This extremely low rate of medical incidents in a supervised health-fitness facility shows that the health-related fitness benefits far outweigh the small risk of participation.

A report in 2007 from the National Electronic Injury Surveillance System All Injury Program (**www.cpsc.gov/LIBRARY/neiss.html**) that characterizes sports- and recreation-related injuries in the U.S. population revealed an overall rate of 11.2 injuries per 100,000 population participants. For persons age 15 to 24, the injury rate equaled 30 injuries per 100,000 population, the highest recorded for any age group. Basketball programs reported 159 injuries per 100,000 participants, and bicycle-related injuries were 171 per 100,00 participants, followed by football with 150 injuries per 100,000 participants. The most frequent injury diagnosis included strains or sprains, fractures, contusions or abrasions, and lacerations. The most frequent injuries occurred to ankles, fingers, face, head, and knees.

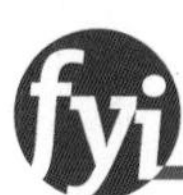

Death Risk for Marathoners Is Lower Than Expected

About 2 million people in the Unites States annually participate in long-distance running races. Several reports of deaths during marathons and half-marathons have raised questions about safety, with many considering these events to be "high-risk" activities. Research has now quantified the actual risk of participants in all organized U.S. marathons over more than a 10-year period. Data compiled from 10.9 million participants identified 59 cases of cardiac arrest (86% men), with significantly higher incidence during marathons than half-marathons. Death occurred in 71% of the cases; this translated into a relatively small risk of 1 in 184,000 cardiac arrests during the remaining 25% of the race or immediately following the race. At the 34th London Marathon in April, 2014 with 36,000 runners, the postrace death of a 42-year-old man was the second death at the event in 3 years. In an April, 2014 North Carolina half marathon, two men ages 31 and 35 died after collapsing at or near the end of the 13.1-mile event with 12,500 runners. In a 4-year prospective study in 65,865 runners in Two Oceans Marathon and half marathon runs in Cape Town, South Africa, two deaths occurred in half-marathon runners (0.05 incidence). Researchers continue to explore strategies to reduce risk of severe medical events, including more emphasis on pre-event cardiac screening.

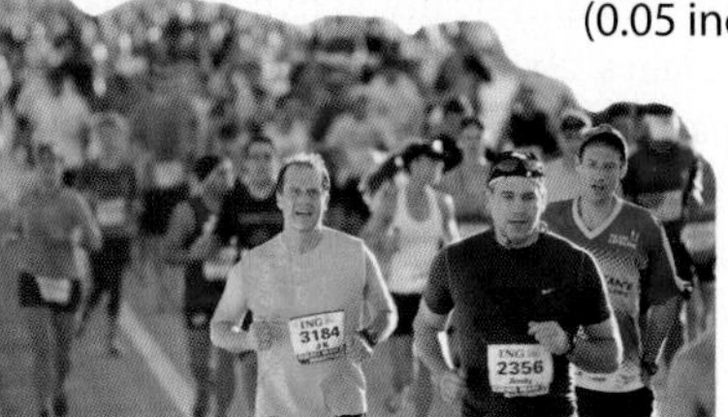

Sources: Kim JH, et al. Cardiac arrest during long-distance running races. *N Engl J Med* 2012;366:130.

Schwabe K, et al. Medical complications and deaths in 21 and 56 km road race runners: a 4-year prospective study in 65,865 runners—SAFER study I. *Br J Sports Med* 2014;48:912.

SEDENTARY ENVIRONMENTAL DEATH SYNDROME

A review of the world literature over the past 60 years has led to the conclusion that physical *inactivity* produces a constellation of problems and conditions that eventually lead to premature death. First used in 2001 by University of Missouri exercise physiologist Frank Booth (**http://hac.missouri.edu/RID/PressRelease.pdf**) and referred to as **Sedentary Environmental Death Syndrome (SeDS)**, this condition denotes a collection of disorders directly caused by or worsened by physical inactivity that ends in death. SeDS will contribute to 1 in 10 premature deaths, or 2.5 million deaths in the United States alone, at a projected cost of $1.5 trillion through 2025. In addition, consider these three factors:

1. Physical inactivity relates to increased chronic disease in the United States; ninefold increase in type 2 diabetes since 1958, doubling of obesity since 1980, with heart disease still remaining the leading cause of death.
2. Children under the age of 12 now experience SeDS-related diseases from their increasing overweightness, showing fatty streaks in arteries and developing type 2 diabetes at an alarming rate.
3. SeDS relates to 26 medically related conditions, which predicts a pessimistic future for the physically inactive. At least 30 conditions include angina, heart attack, coronary artery disease, arthritis pain, arrhythmias, breast cancer, colon cancer, congestive heart failure, depression, digestive problems, gallstone disease, gastroesophageal disease, high blood triglyceride level, high blood cholesterol level, hypertension, less cognitive function, low blood high-density lipoprotein cholesterol (HDL-C) level, lower quality of life, menopausal symptoms, osteoporosis, pancreatic cancer, peripheral vascular disease, physical frailty, premature mortality, prostate cancer, respiratory problems, sleep apnea, stroke, and type 2 diabetes.

More medical-based evidence is needed to convince the world population that *physical inactivity* promotes unhealthy gene expression. Consider the national outrage if 300,000 people died annually from faulty seatbelts or automobile tires. Such a tragedy would demand immediate attention by both public and private sectors to solve the problem. In the same way, we wholeheartedly endorse that regular, moderate to vigorous physical activity should play an increasingly important role in the lives of all individuals, with a concentrated outreach undertaken to help achieve this goal.

Prevalence of Sitting for U.S. Population

In home interviews involving nearly 6000 adults sampled from the 2009–2010 National Health and Nutrition Examination Survey (NHANES), participants were asked, "How much time do you usually spend sitting on a typical day?" Respondents included 48.3% non-Hispanic Whites, 18.2% Mexican-American, 17.9% non-Hispanic Blacks, and

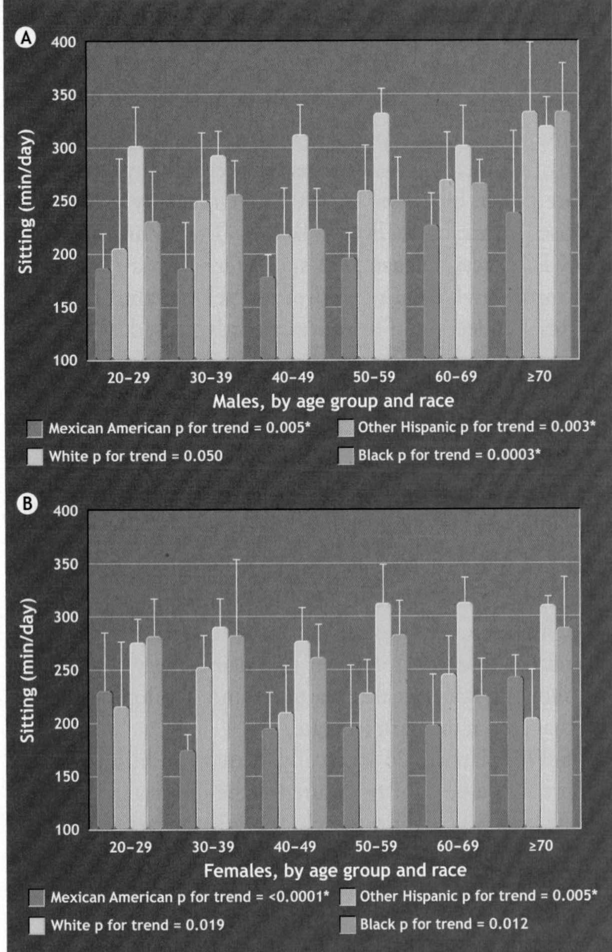

FIGURE 17.6 The epidemiology of sitting for men (**A**) and women (**B**). (Adapted with permission from Harrington DM, et al. The descriptive epidemiology of sitting among US adults, NHANES 2009/2010. *J Sci Med Sports* 2014;17:371.)

10.1% other Hispanic. **Figure 17.6** (A, males; B, females) reveal no significant differences in mean sitting time between sexes at any age group. However, when stratified by sex, significant differences existed with age. A trend for increased sitting time occurred with increasing female age. Females 40 to 49 years old reported significantly less sitting time (260 min · d^{-1}) compared to older 60 to 69 age females (293 min · d^{-1}), and those 70 years and older (297 min · d^{-1}). Seventy-year-old males reported sitting significantly more than their 30-year-old counterparts.

When stratified by ethnicity, time sitting significantly increased with age for all Mexican American and Hispanic participants and non-Hispanic Blacks. For both sexes, higher education attainment related to increased sitting time. Differences between sexes only emerged at the college graduate or above level where females reported 14.5% less time sitting than males (319 min · d^{-1} vs. 373 min · d^{-1}).

The following four conclusions pertain to sitting time for U.S. adults:

1. Mexican American adults sit the least amount of time.
2. Self-reported sitting time increases with increasing age.
3. Participants with more education sit more.
4. Females with a higher BMI (≥30 kg · m^{-2}) sit more than normal weight and underweight females, but these differences do not persist with males

SUMMARY

1. The specific field of physical activity epidemiology applies the general research strategies of epidemiology to study physical activity as a health-related behavior linked to disease and other outcomes.
2. The Physical Activity Pyramid summarizes major goals to increase regular physical activity in the general population; it emphasizes many forms of behavioral and lifestyle options.
3. Healthy People 2020 describes a comprehensive, nationwide health promotion and disease prevention roadmap to promote health and prevent illness, disability, and premature death among all U.S. residents.
4. Physical inactivity produces a constellation of conditions termed *SeDS*, which eventually leads to premature death.

THINK IT THROUGH

1. Distinguish between *exercise* and *physical activity*, and *health* and *health-related physical fitness*.
2. In your opinion, is it wise to establish health-related guidelines similar to the *Healthy People 2020* initiative?

PART 3 Aging and Bodily Functions

Figure 17.7 illustrates that bodily functions improve rapidly during childhood and reach a maximum at about age 30, with functional capacity steadily declining thereafter. A similar age trend exists for physically active persons, yet physiologic function averages about 25% higher compared with sedentary counterparts at each age category. For example, an active 50-year-old man or woman often maintains the functional level of his or her 30-year-old counterpart. All physiologic measures eventually decline with age, but not all decrease at the same rate.

Nerve conduction velocity, for example, declines only 10% to 15% from age 30 to 80, but the resting cardiac index (ratio of cardiac output to body surface area) and joint flexibility decline 20% to 30%; maximum breathing capacity at age 80 averages 40% of values for a 30 year olds'. Brain cells die at a fairly constant rate until age 60, but the liver and kidneys lose 40% to 50% of their function between ages

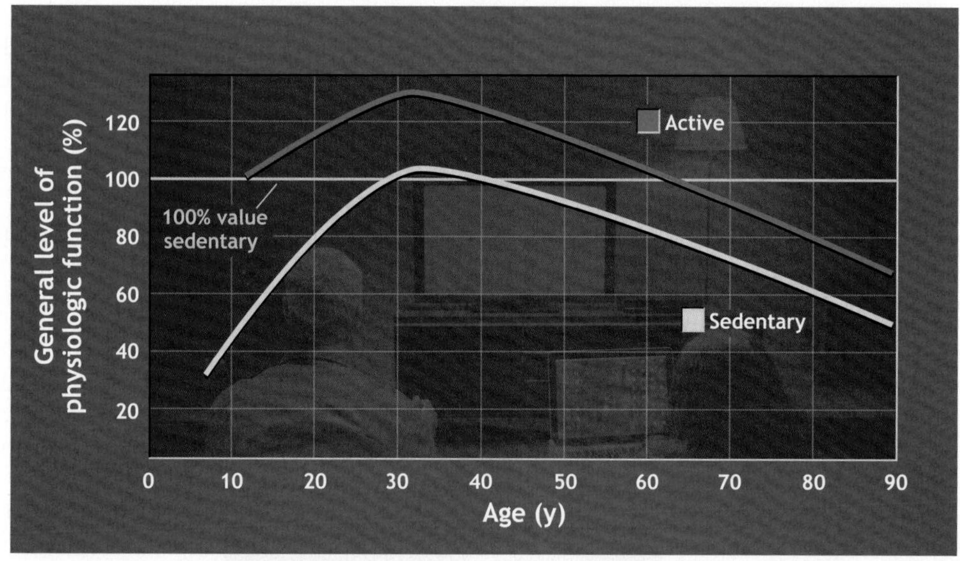

FIGURE 17.7 Generalized curve for age-related changes in physiologic function. All comparisons were made against the 100% value achieved by the 20- to 30-year-old sedentary person.

30 and 70. By the seventh decade of life, the average woman has lost 30% of her bone mass, while men lose only 15%.

AGING AND MUSCULAR STRENGTH

Men and women achieve maximum strength between ages 20 and 30 when muscle cross-sectional area often achieves maximum size. Thereafter, strength progressively declines for most muscle groups; by age 70, overall "general" strength has decreased by 30%.

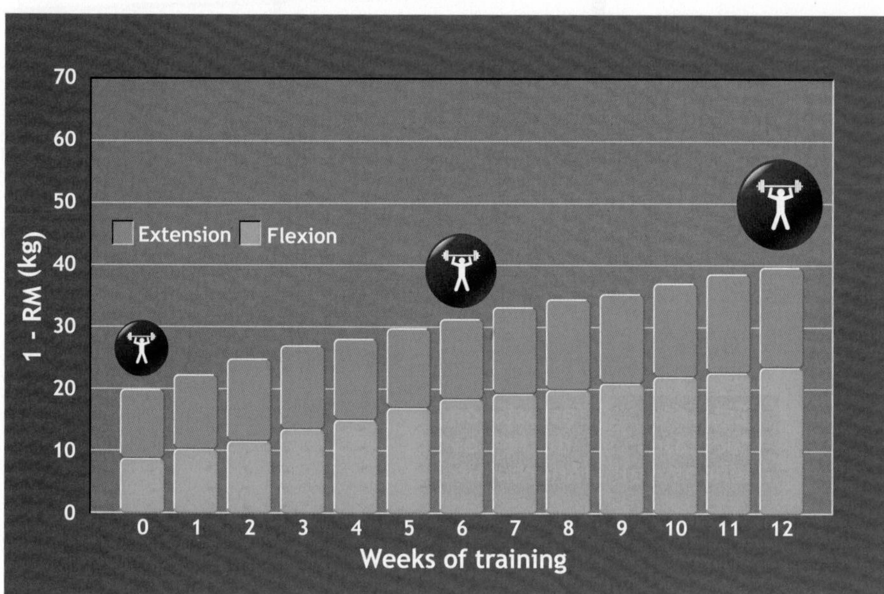

FIGURE 17.8 Weekly measurement of dynamic muscle strength (1-RM) in left knee extension (*green*) and flexion (*orange*) during a 12-week period of resistance training in men ages 60 to 72 years. (Data from Frontera WR, et al. Strength conditioning in older men: skeletal muscle hypertrophy and improved function. *J Appl Physiol* 1988;64:1038.)

Decrease in Muscle Mass

Strength decreases with age mainly from the accompanying but normal reduction in fat-free body mass (FFM). Above certain thresholds, loss of muscle mass and muscle strength is considered abnormal and referred to as **sarcopenia**. Establishing the prevalence of sarcopenia remains challenging because its presence depends on the definition used for its diagnosis. Geriatric sarcopenia represents a public health issue with at least six multiple clinical consequences, including loss of autonomy and quality of life, altered functional status, and increased fatigue, falls, and a higher mortality rate.

The smaller muscle mass in older adults reflects a loss of total muscle protein induced by physical inactivity, aging, or their combined effects. Some loss in muscle fiber number also takes place with aging. In newborns, for example, the biceps contains about 500,000 individual fibers, while the same muscle for an 80-year-old man contains 40% fewer fibers or about 300,000.

Muscle Trainability in Middle Age and the Elderly

Regular physical activity retains body protein and blunts muscle mass and strength loss with aging. Healthy men between ages 60 and 72 participated in a 12-week conventional resistance-training program. **Figure 17.8** reveals that the men's muscle strength increased slowly but progressively throughout the program; strength increases averaged about

5% each session, similar to young adults. By week 12, further gains were minimal, suggesting that additional strength improvement would require increases in one or all of the following—training intensity, volume, or frequency. Exercise specialists who work with elderly people argue that improving their strength will effectively maintain muscle mass, increase mobility, and reduce injury incidence.

AGING AND JOINT FLEXIBILITY

With advancing age, cartilage, ligaments, and tendons become stiffer and more rigid, thereby reducing joint flexibility. It is unclear whether these changes reflect biologic aging or impact of chronic disuse through sedentary living or degenerative tissue diseases in specific joints. Regardless of the cause, appropriate physical activity movements that regularly move the joints through their full ROM can increase flexibility 20% to 50% in men and women at all ages.

AGING AND ENDOCRINE CHANGES

Endocrine function changes with age, particularly in the pituitary, pancreas, adrenal, and thyroid glands.

About 40% of individuals ages 65 and 75 and 50% of individuals older than age 80 have impaired glucose tolerance that leads to type 2 diabetes (T2DM). Three factors impair glucose metabolism in T2DM:

1. Depressed insulin effect on peripheral tissue (**insulin resistance**)
2. Inadequate pancreatic insulin production to control blood sugar (relative insulin deficiency)
3. Combined effect of insulin resistance and relative insulin deficiency

Except in those with a genetic predisposition, the increased prevalence of T2DM largely relates to "lifestyle" factors: poor diet, inadequate physical activity, and increased body fat, particularly visceral abdominal fat.

Thyroid dysfunction from lowered pituitary gland release of thyrotropin and reduced **thyroxine** output from the thyroid gland commonly occurs among elderly people. This affects metabolic function that includes decreased glucose metabolism and protein synthesis.

Figure 17.9 depicts changes in three additional hormonal systems associated with aging: hypothalamic-pituitary-gonadal

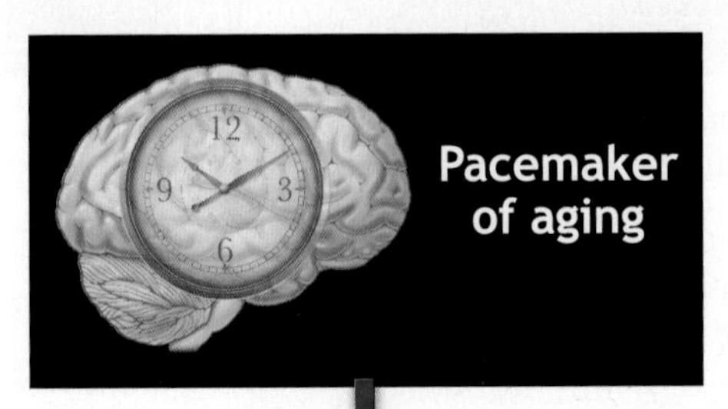

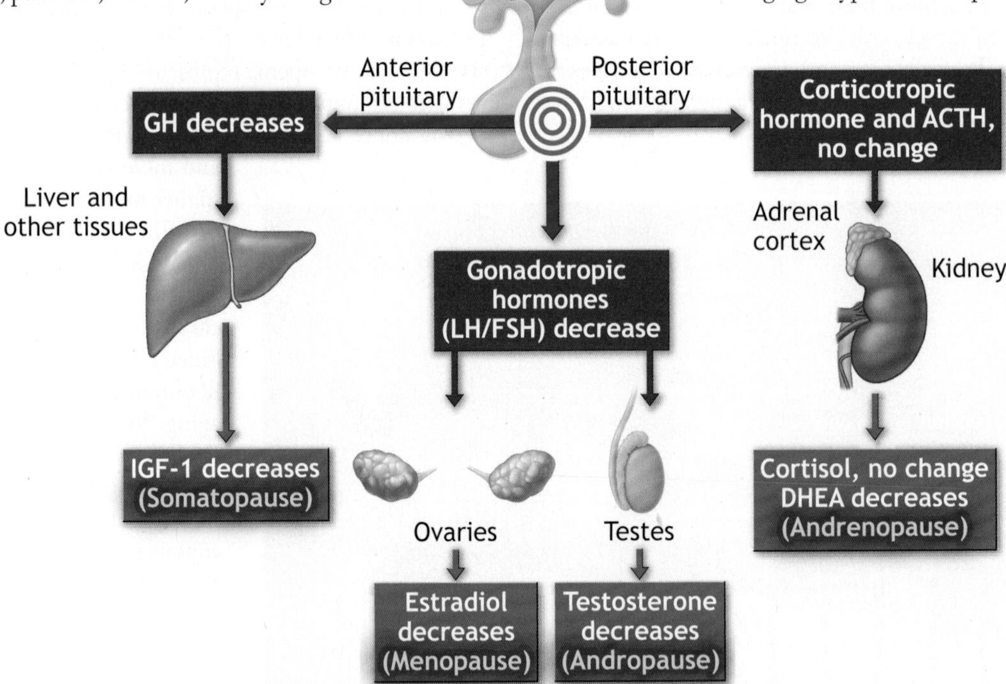

FIGURE 17.9 Age-related decline in three hormone systems affecting biological aging rate. **Left.** Decreased growth hormone (GH; released by the anterior pituitary) depresses production of insulinlike growth factor-1 (IGF-1) to inhibit cellular growth (a condition of aging termed *somatopause*). **Middle.** Decreased output of luteinizing hormone (LH) and follicle-stimulating hormone (FSH) by the anterior pituitary, coupled with reduced estradiol secretion from ovaries and testosterone from testes, causes menopause (in women) and andropause (in men). **Right.** Adrenocortical cells responsible for dehydroepiandrosterone (DHEA) production decrease their activity (termed *adrenopause*) without clinically evident changes in this gland's corticotropin (adrenocorticotropic hormone [ACTH]) and cortisol secretion. A central "pacemaker" in the hypothalamus or higher brain areas probably mediates these processes to produce aging-related changes in the ovaries, testicles, and adrenal cortex.

axis, **adrenal cortex**, and growth hormone (GH) and insulinlike growth factor-1 (IGF-1) axis.

Hypothalamic-Pituitary-Gonadal Axis

As women enter their fourth and fifth decade of life, alterations in the interaction among stimulating hormones from the hypothalamus and anterior pituitary gland and gonads decrease estradiol ovarian output. This effect eventually initiates permanent cessation of menses (**menopause**). Changes in hypothalamic-pituitary-gonadal axis activity in men occur more slowly and subtly. For example, serum total and free testosterone decline with aging. Male **andropause** refers to age-related decreases in gonadotropic secretions from the anterior pituitary gland.

Adrenal Cortex

Adrenopause refers to the decrease in adrenal cortex output of **dehydroepiandrosterone** (DHEA) and its sulfated ester (DHEAS). In contrast, a long, progressive but slow decline in DHEA occurs after about age 30, in contrast to the **glucocorticoid** and **mineralocorticoid** adrenal steroids whose plasma levels remain relatively high with aging. Unfortunately, this has led to speculation concerning DHEA's role in aging, prompting a dramatic increase in this hormone's unregulated supplementation (see Chapter 4).

Growth Hormone and Insulinlike Growth Factor-1 Axis

Mean pulse amplitude, duration, and fraction of secreted GH gradually decrease with age, a condition termed **somatopause**. A parallel decrease in circulating levels of IGF-1 also occurs. IGF-1, produced mainly by the liver, stimulates tissue growth and protein synthesis. The trigger for this decrease may reflect an interaction between the hypothalamus and anterior pituitary gland.

To what extent changes in gonadal function (menopause and andropause) contribute to adrenopause and somatopause remains unknown. A growing body of evidence indicates that functional correlates, such as muscle size and strength, body composition, bone mass alterations, and atherosclerosis, directly impact hormonal changes with aging. Hormone replacement therapy, nutritional supplementation, and regular physical activity may suppress aspects of such hormone-related aging dysfunction.

AGING AND NERVOUS SYSTEM FUNCTION

A 37% decline in number of spinal cord axons and 10% decline in nerve conduction velocity reflect cumulative aging effects on central nervous system functions. Such changes partially explain age-related decrements in neuromuscular performance. Partitioning reaction time into central processing time and muscle contraction time indicates that aging exerts the greatest effect on stimulus detection and information processing to produce a response. For example, the knee-jerk reflex does not require CNS processing; it becomes less affected by aging than voluntary responses and movement patterns.

Despite the real effects of aging on reaction and movement time, physically active young or old groups move faster than corresponding less active age groups.

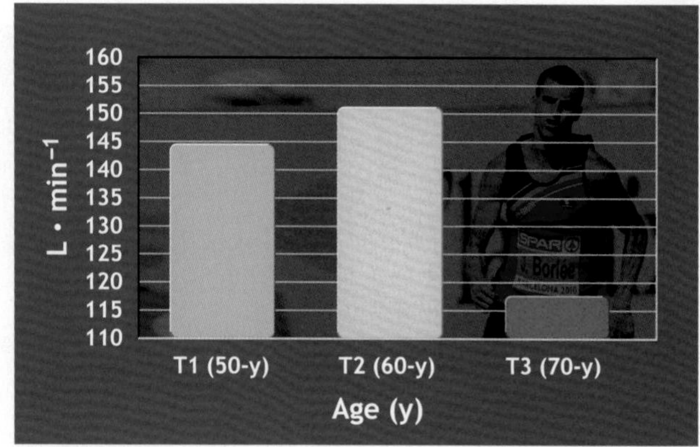

FIGURE 17.10 Changes in maximum minute ventilation for 21 endurance athletes over a 20-year period, starting at age 50 years. (Adapted with permission from Pollock ML, et al. Twenty-year follow-up of aerobic power and body composition of older track athletes. *J Appl Physiol* 1997;82:1508.)

AGING AND PULMONARY FUNCTION

Cross-sectional studies indicate that dynamic pulmonary capacity of older endurance-trained athletes exceeds that of sedentary peers. Regular, more vigorous physical activity promotes the maintenance of ventilatory musculature power and endurance. **Figure 17.10** depicts changes in maximum pulmonary minute ventilation ($\dot{V}_{Emax}$) where 21 men were tested for metabolic and pulmonary functions, body composition, and performance over a 20-year period starting at age 50. The men trained continuously throughout the 20-year period; each had placed first, second, or third in high-level, age-structured competition. A small but nonsignificant increase in $\dot{V}_{Emax}$ occurred at the second testing (T2), yet a precipitous decrease occurred at the third testing period at age 70. This supports the contention of a decrease in lung function parameters with aging, despite the maintenance of a lifestyle that includes regular and vigorous physical activity.

AGING AND CARDIOVASCULAR FUNCTION

Regular physical activity exerts a profound influence on age-related decrements in cardiovascular function and endurance capacity.

Maximal Oxygen Uptake

After age 35, $\dot{V}O_{2max}$ declines at a nonlinear rate that accelerates after the next 10 years so that by age 60, it averages 11% below values for 35-year-old men and 15% below values

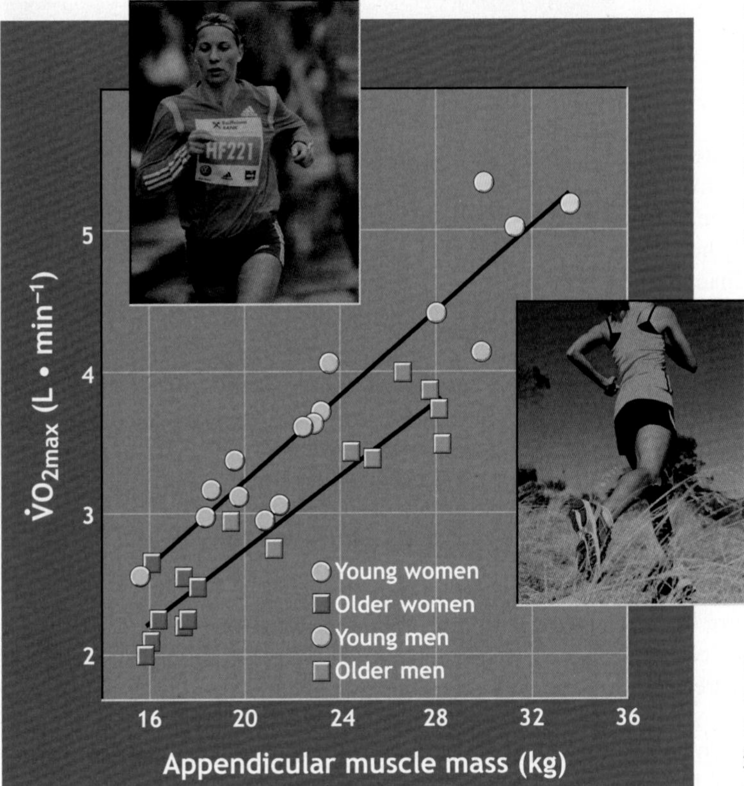

FIGURE 17.11 Maximal oxygen uptake ($\dot{V}O_{2max}$) related to appendicular muscle mass in young and older endurance-trained men and women. $\dot{V}O_{2max}$ per kg of active muscle mass decreases with age, independent of training status. (Modified from Proctor DN, Joyner J. Skeletal muscle mass and the reduction of $\dot{V}O_{2max}$ in trained older subjects. *J Appl Physiol* 1997;82:1411.)

for women. A slower rate of decline occurs for individuals who maintain an active lifestyle that features regular aerobic training. *Physical activity does not entirely offset aging's effect on $\dot{V}O_{2max}$, even when adjusting for an individual's quantity of muscle mass.*

Figure 17.11 displays the relationship between $\dot{V}O_{2max}$ and active appendicular muscle mass for younger (average age 25 y) and older (average age 63 y) aerobically trained men and women. Younger subjects had trained for 9 consecutive years, and older subjects had trained for 20 consecutive years. Older men and women exhibited a 14% lower $\dot{V}O_{2max}$ than younger counterparts throughout the broad range of variation in muscle mass. In other words, despite equivalence in appendicular muscle mass between a young and older person, the younger person exhibited a *higher* $\dot{V}O_{2max}$.

Three factors partially account for the deterioration in $\dot{V}O_{2max}$ with aging:

1. Muscle mass loss
2. Increase in body fat
3. Altered cardiovascular and pulmonary function

The reduction in aerobic power per kilogram of active appendicular muscle mass with aging (**Fig. 17.11**), can reflect either age-associated reduced oxygen delivery, reduced oxygen extraction in active muscle, or both. Skeletal muscle oxidative capacity and capillarization remain similar in older and younger individuals with comparable physiologic characteristics and training histories. The well-documented reduction in cardiac output (with accompanying decreased maximum heart rate and stroke volume) represents the most likely explanation for the age-related decreases in $\dot{V}O_{2max}$ per kilogram of active muscle.

Aging Response to Training

For the healthy elderly, regular physical activity enhances the heart's blood pumping capacity and increases aerobic capacity to the same relative degree as in younger adults. Nine to 12 months of aerobic training increased $\dot{V}O_{2max}$ 19% in men and 22% in women. These values represent the high end of the typical training response for young adults. Middle-aged aerobic trained men for more than 20 years delayed the expected 10% to 15% decline in performance capacity and aerobic fitness. At age 55, they maintained nearly the same values for blood pressure, body mass, and $\dot{V}O_{2max}$ as at age 35; by age 70, their $\dot{V}O_{2max}$ equaled values for individuals 25 years younger. These remarkable findings attest to the adaptability of the aerobic system to successful training at any age.

Maximum Heart Rate: Age-Related Changes

Figure 17.12 reflects longitudinal changes for maximum heart rate for the same subjects depicted in **Figure 17.10.** Maximum heart rate decreased by 5 to 7 beats per minute at each measurement over the 20 years, a smaller decrease than generally reported for nonathletes. Age-related

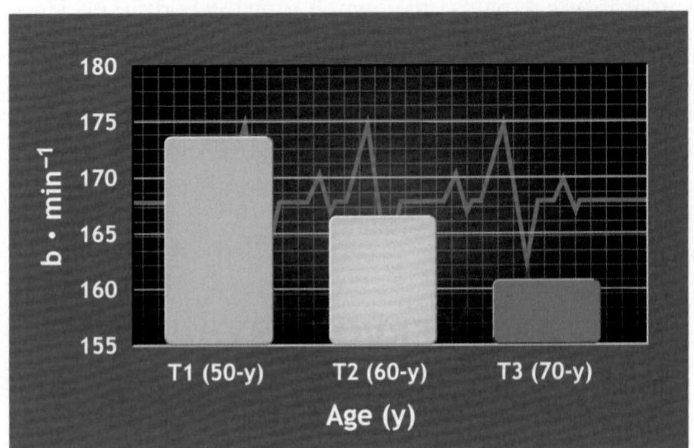

FIGURE 17.12 Changes in maximum heart rate for 21 endurance athletes who continued to train over a 20-year period starting at age 50. (Modified from Pollock ML, et al. Twenty-year follow-up of aerobic power and body composition of older track athletes. *J Appl Physiol* 1997;82:1508.)

decrements in maximum heart rate are attributed to three factors:

1. Alterations in sinoatrial (SA) node activity
2. Reduced medullary sympathetic output
3. Reluctance of researchers to encourage older, nonathletic individuals to perform "all out" to achieve maximal effort during testing

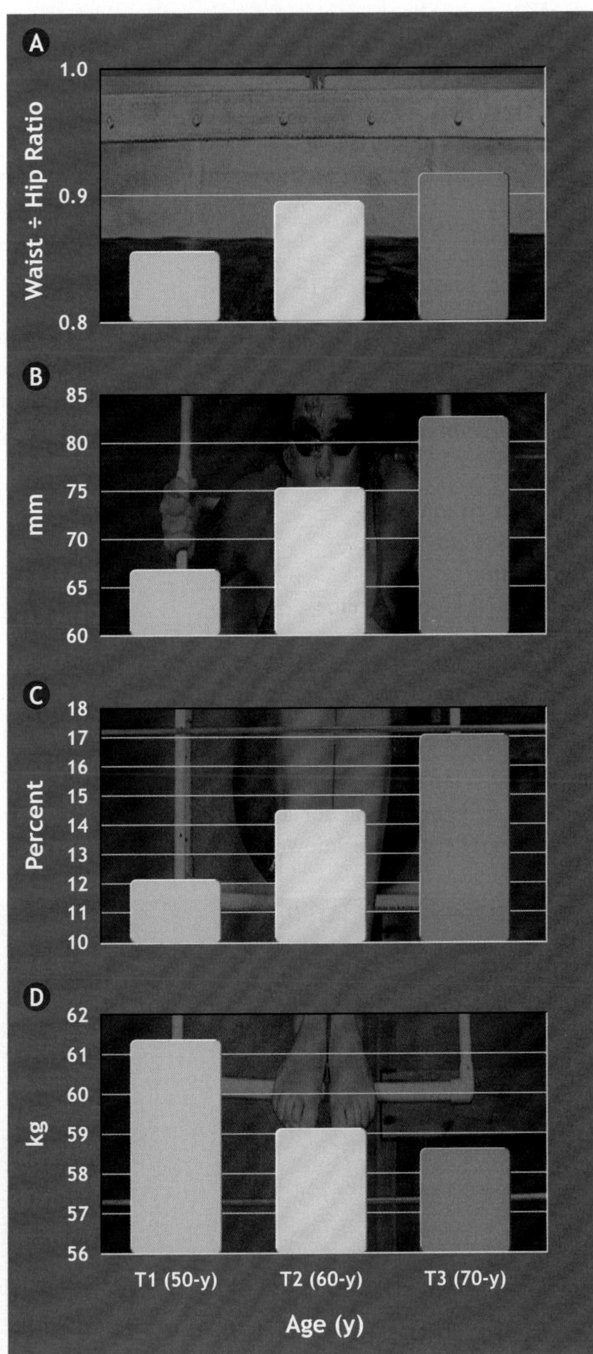

FIGURE 17.13 Changes in waist-to-hip girth ratio **(A)**, sum of skinfolds **(B)**, percentage body fat **(C)**, and fat-free body mass **(D)** for 21 endurance athletes who continued to train over a 20-year period starting at age 50. (Modified from Pollock ML, et al. Twenty-year follow-up of aerobic power and body composition of older track athletes. *J Appl Physiol* 1997;82:1508.)

Additional Cardiovascular Changes

Additional age-related cardiovascular changes include reduced blood flow capacity to peripheral tissues, narrowing of coronary arteries (30% obstruction by middle age), and decreased major blood vessel elasticity referred to as compliance.

AGING AND BODY COMPOSITION CHANGES

Figure 17.13 displays the body composition changes for the same subjects in **Figure 17.10** and **17.12**. Despite almost 30 years of continuous training without changes in body weight, gains occurred in body fat while FFM declined. The roughly 3% body fat unit increase per decade paralleled similar increases in waist girth. These data support an argument that some body composition alterations including body fat distribution represent a normal aging response. Other studies of physically active older individuals suggest that the typical individual grows fatter with age, but those who remain physically active counter the "normal" age-related loss in FFM while depressing the typical increase in body fat accretion.

Weight-bearing physical activity helps counter deleterious effects of osteoporosis with aging. Longitudinal research of bone mineral content assessed every 6 months in children from age 6 to 12 showed that 26% of adult total body bone mineral accrued during just 2 years of peak bone mineral deposition. Such direct evidence seems self-evident for its long-range implications in helping preserve lean tissue mass. Perhaps the eventual "cure" for osteoporosis and its attendant medical and societal costs really should be viewed as a problem of young age (pediatric medicine) and not older age (geriatric medicine). We strongly endorse the position that vigorous physical activity should play an increasingly more important role in the home and schools beginning in the elementary grades and continuing as children grow into adolescence and adulthood.

SUMMARY

1. Physiologic and performance capabilities generally decline after age 30, with considerable individual differences within and among individuals.
2. Regular physical activity enables older persons to retain higher levels of functional capacity, particularly cardiovascular and muscular function.
3. Aging alters the endocrine functions of the pituitary, pancreas, adrenal, and thyroid glands.
4. A physically active lifestyle throughout life confers considerable health-related benefits.
5. Approximately half of all deaths in the United States reflect a limited number of largely preventable behaviors and exposures, most relating directly to physical inactivity, overweight, and obesity.
6. Considerable plasticity exists in physiologic, structural, and performance characteristics among older individuals, even into the ninth decade.

7. A physically active lifestyle positively impacts neuromuscular functions at any age, possibly slowing the decline in cognitive performance associated with information processing speed.
8. Physically active older men and women maintain a higher aerobic power than sedentary peers at any age.
9. Sedentary living causes losses in functional capacity at least as great as aging itself.

THINK IT THROUGH

1. Which factor would you favor, improved nutrition or physical activity, to affect biological changes with aging?
2. Respond to the statement: Does the link between on-the-job or leisure-time physical activity and reduced coronary heart disease risk prove that physical activity causes improved cardiovascular health?

PART 4 Coronary Heart Disease

Figure 17.14 shows the prevalence of cardiovascular diseases in U.S. adults age 20 and older by age and gender for 2007 to 2010. The *inset pie chart* illustrates the percentage breakdown of deaths from diverse heart and blood vessel diseases in 2010.

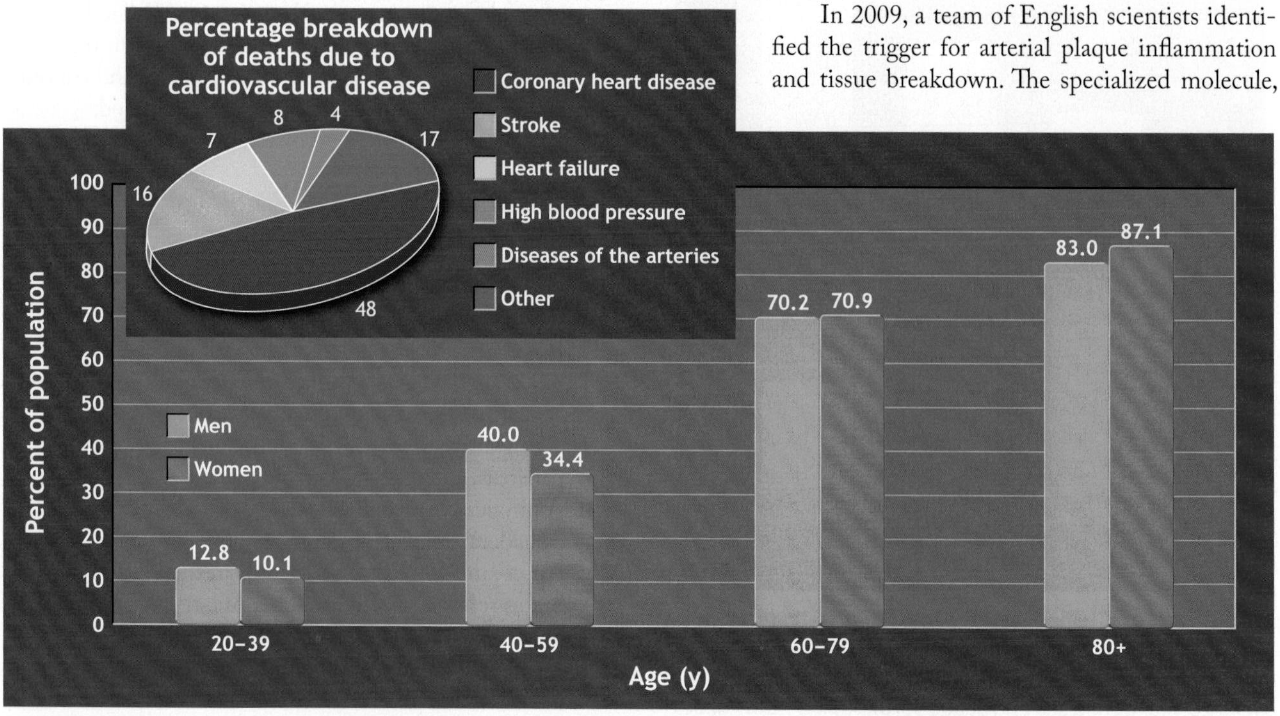

Heart disease remains the leading cause of death in the Western world. For every American who dies of cancer, almost two die of heart-related diseases. Death rates for women lag about 10 years behind men, but the gap has rapidly closed for women who smoke; for them, heart disease is now the leading cause of death. Disease symptoms, progression, and outcome differ in women and men. Among gender-related heart disease differences are the following:

1. Women usually die sooner following a heart attack.
2. Women who survive a heart attack frequently experience a second episode.
3. Women become more incapacitated by heart disease–related pain and disability.
4. Women are less likely to survive coronary artery bypass surgery

Cellular Level Changes

Predisposing factors to CHD involve degenerative changes in the intima or inner lining of the larger arteries that supply the myocardium. Damage to the arterial walls begins as a low-grade chronic **inflammatory response** to injury. Factors contributing to this response include the following eight conditions:

1. Hypertension
2. Cigarette smoking
3. Infection
4. Elevated Homocysteine
5. Elevated cholesterol
6. High levels of free radicals
7. Reaction to obesity-related substances
8. Immunologically mediated factors.

In 2009, a team of English scientists identified the trigger for arterial plaque inflammation and tissue breakdown. The specialized molecule,

FIGURE 17.14 Prevalence of cardiovascular disease in adults by age and sex. The inset provides the percentage breakdown of deaths due to cardiovascular disease in the United States in 2010. (Adapted from **http://www.nhlbi.nih.gov/about/documents/factbook/2012/chapter4.**)

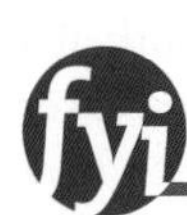

Brief Periods of Regular Physical Activity May Protect Health and Extend Life

Those who run regularly, even for brief time durations, may extend their life by 3 years compared to those who remain sedentary. Researchers examined the physical activity habits of more than 55,000 residents of the Dallas, Texas area over a 15-year period. The results were adjusted to account for smoking and drinking habits, age, family health history, and other physical activity habits. The mortality risk for being sedentary exceeded the risk of being overweight or obese (16%), having a family history of cardiovascular disease (20%), or having high cholesterol (6%). Even when assessing the effects of running for weekly duration, distance, intensity, and frequency, runners in the lowest end of their groups showed less likelihood of dying than nonrunners. Thirty to fifty-nine minutes of weekly running reduced premature death risk by nearly one third and extended life by about 3 years. The clinical and public health importance of such findings emphasize that simply devoting 5 minutes to a daily run (or other equally intense activity) will confer significant health benefits.

Source: Lee DC, et al. Leisure-time running reduces all-cause and cardiovascular mortality risk. *J Am Coll Cardiol* 2014;64:472.

Toll-like receptor 2 (TLR-2), resides on the surface of an immune cell. When TLR-2 recognizes harmful molecules and cells, its role switches the immune cell into attack mode to protect the body. TLR-2 also can "switch on" immune cells when the body encounters stress. In addition, bacteria may switch on the TLR-2 molecules, increasing the risk of plaques bursting and causing strokes and heart attacks.

The research breakthrough also demonstrated that antibodies could block the TLR-2 trigger mechanism. In the experiment, sections of atherosclerotic carotid arteries were sampled from 58 patients following a stroke. The arterial tissues, decomposed with enzymes, formed a suspension of single cells in liquid. The researchers analyzed the liquid after 4 days and determined that the cells had produced an unusually large amount of inflammatory molecules and enzymes known to damage arteries. The cells were then grown with several different antibodies to block different receptors and other molecules involved in the inflammation process. Blocking TLR-2 using an antibody dramatically reduced production of inflammation-derived molecules and enzymes.

See the animation "Acute Inflammation" on **http://thePoint.lww.com/MKKESS5e**.

Other Considerations

Arterial wall degenerative changes in the coronary arteries trigger oxidation of low-density lipoprotein cholesterol (LDL-C). LDL-C oxidation represents a crucial step in complex changes that produce lesions that sometimes bulge into the vessel lumen or protrude into the arterial wall. The first signs of atherosclerosis involve lesions that become fatty streaks. With further inflammatory damage from continued lipid deposition and proliferation of smooth muscle and connective tissue, the vessels congest with lipid-filled plaques, fibrous scar tissue, or both. Progressive occlusion gradually reduces blood flow capacity, causing the myocardium to become ischemic or poorly supplied with oxygen.

Vulnerable Plaque: Difficult to Detect Yet Lethal

Vulnerable plaque, a soft type of metabolically active, unstable plaque, does not necessarily produce significant coronary artery narrowing but tends to fissure and burst. The rupture or sudden breakdown of unstable fatty plaques exposes blood to thrombogenic compounds. This triggers a cascade of chemical events that culminates in clot formation or thrombus, leading to a myocardial infarction (MI) and possible death. A sudden, complete obstruction in a coronary vessel frequently occurs in arteries that previously had only mild-to-moderate obstructions (~70% blockage). Arterial blockage often occurs before the vessel has narrowed enough to produce symptoms of angina or ECG abnormalities, or to require revascularization procedures (e.g., coronary bypass surgery or balloon angioplasty). Acute disruption followed by rupture of arterial plaque provides a plausible explanation for sudden death from acute physical exertion or emotional stress in middle-aged men with coronary artery disease who may not have experienced prior symptoms compared with sudden death under resting conditions. The beneficial effects of cholesterol-lowering strategies on heart disease risk do not always improve coronary blood flow. A reduction in overall blood cholesterol may, however, improve the stability of vulnerable plaque and reduce the likelihood of future arterial plaque rupture.

Vulnerable Patients

The recognition of the role of vulnerable plaque has introduced a new way of looking at cardiovascular medicine and risk assessment. Recent evidence reveals that rupture-prone plaques are not the only vulnerable plaque forms. All types of atherosclerotic plaques with high likelihood of rapid progression and thrombotic complications are now considered vulnerable. Vulnerable plaques, however, are not the only culprit for the development of acute coronary syndromes, myocardial infarction, and sudden cardiac death. Vulnerable blood (prone to thrombosis) and vulnerable myocardium (prone to fatal arrhythmia) also play an important role in future outcomes. Consequently, the term "***vulnerable patient***" may be more appropriate for identifying individuals with high likelihood of developing a traumatic cardiac event. Researchers have been working to quantify methods for cumulative risk assessment to identify the vulnerable patient, which may include variables based on plaque type, blood, and myocardial vulnerability. Recently developed assays (e.g., **C-reactive protein, CRP**), imaging techniques (e.g., CT and MRI), noninvasive electrophysiological tests (for vulnerable myocardium), and specialized catheters (to localize and characterize vulnerable plaque) in combination with future genomic and proteomic techniques, should successfully guide the search to identify the vulnerable patient.

CHD: A Lifelong Process

Landmark studies of atherosclerosis in young American soldiers killed in Korea in 1950–1953 revealed advanced lesions. These findings shocked the medical community and refocused attention on the possible childhood origins of atherosclerosis. Researchers now know that fatty streaks and clinically significant fibrous plaques develop rapidly during adolescence through the third decade of life.

BMI, systolic and diastolic blood pressure, and total serum cholesterol, triacylglycerols, and LDL-C strongly and positively related to the extent of vascular lesions in the deceased young people (HDL-C related negatively). History of cigarette smoking magnified the vascular damage. As the number of risk factors increased, so did the severity of atherosclerosis.

Analyses of microscopic qualities of coronary atherosclerosis in teenagers and young adults who died as a result of accidents, suicide, and murder indicated that many had arteries so clogged that they could experience an MI. Two percent of those ages 15 to 19 and 20% of those ages 30 to 34 had advanced plaque formation, the blockages considered most likely to separate from the arterial walls and trigger heart attack or stroke. Collectively, these and other data support the wisdom of primary prevention through risk factor identification and intervention of atherosclerosis early in childhood or adolescence.

Figure 17.15 shows progressive arterial occlusion from a buildup of calcified fatty substances in atherosclerosis.

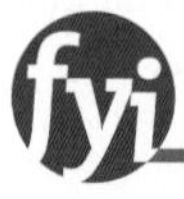

Risks Develop at an Early Age

A dismal picture emerges for selected markers of cardiovascular health for American adolescents, suggesting that the current generation of teenagers will increase their risk for heart disease later in life. The Centers for Disease Control and Prevention reported that 5450 adolescents between ages 12 and 19 performed poorly overall on the criteria set by the American Heart Association for ideal cardiovascular health. The poor quality of their diet was particularly noteworthy. Not one adolescent reported meeting recommended targets on five different nutritional categories, that included consuming at least 4 to 5 servings of fruits and vegetables daily, 3 whole-grain servings daily, 2 or more servings of fish weekly, consuming less than 1500 mg of sodium daily, and drinking less than 3 oz of sugar-sweetened drinks a week. Just 16.4% of boys and 11.3% of girls rated ideal on all of the other six criteria. For the physical activity category, disappointingly, 50% of boys and 60% of girls failed to attain the optimal goal of exercising 60 minutes a day; worse yet, between 10% and 20% reported getting no physical activity at all!

The first overt sign of atherosclerotic change occurs when lipid-laden macrophage cells cluster under the endothelial lining to form a bulge or fatty streak in the artery. Over time, proliferating smooth muscle cells accumulate to narrow the artery's lumen. Typically, a **thrombus** or clot forms and plugs the artery, depriving the myocardium of normal blood flow and oxygen supply. When the thrombus blocks one of the smaller coronary vessels, a portion of the heart muscle dies (called ***necrosis***), and the person experiences a heart attack or MI.

If coronary artery narrowing leads to brief periods of inadequate myocardial perfusion, the person may experience intermittent pains known as **angina pectoris** (see Chapter 18). These pains usually emerge during exertion because increased physical activity creates a greater demand for myocardial blood flow. Anginal attacks provide painful, dramatic evidence of the importance of adequate myocardial oxygen supply.

Heart Attack Warning Signs

Men and women often experience an impending heart attack differently. Although heart attack symptoms that men experience, such as crushing chest pain that radiates down an arm, are often similar for women, many women report experiencing vague or even silent symptoms that are often ignored and not recognized as heart attach warning signs. The list below presents common heart attack symptoms for men and women.

1. Men and women: Uncomfortable pressure, fullness, squeezing, or pain in the center of the chest lasting more than a few minutes. People report that it feels like a vise being tightened around the chest.
2. More common in women but also experienced by men: Pain spreading to the shoulders, neck, or arms. The pain ranges from mild to intense. It may feel like pressure, tightness, burning, or a heavy weight. It may be located in the chest, upper abdomen, neck, jaw, or inside the arms or shoulders. The pain can be gradual or sudden, and may wax and wane before becoming intense.
3. Mostly women: Stomach pain that women mistake as heartburn, the flu, a stomach ulcer, or menstrual discomfort.
4. Men and women: Chest discomfort with lightheadedness, fainting, stress- or anxiety-related sweating (more common in women), nausea, or shortness of breath.
5. Men and women: Anxiety, nervousness, or cold, sweaty skin.
6. Women: Fatigue and feeling of extreme "tiredness in the chest" common even when just sitting or lying down.
7. Men and women: Paleness or pallor, often in the late afternoon.
8. Men and women: Increased or irregular heart rate.
9. Men and women: Extreme anxiety, fear, or feelings of impending doom.

Heart Attack Versus Cardiac Arrest

In the United States, heart attacks occur about a million times a year, or once every 33 seconds every day of the year

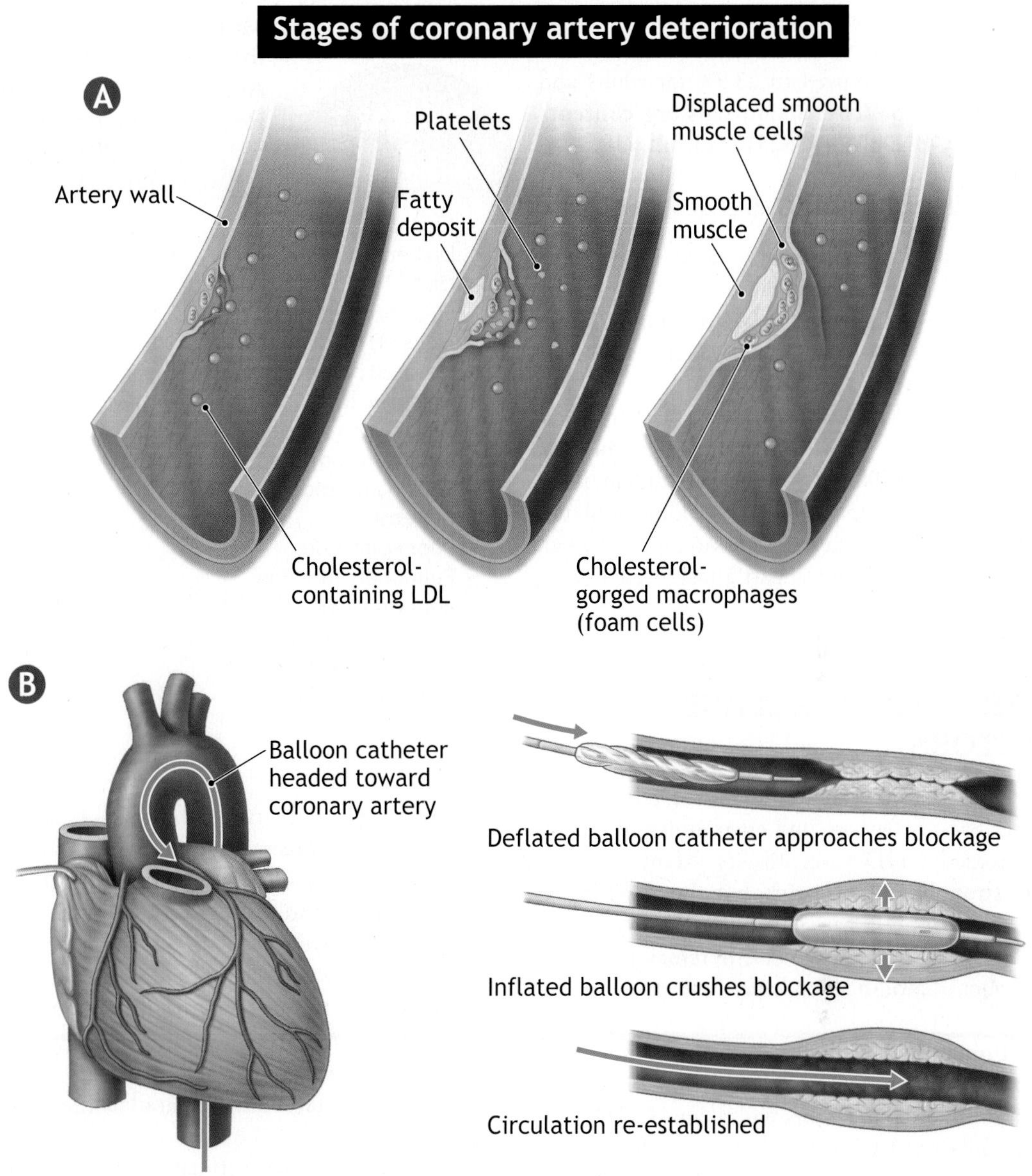

FIGURE 17.15 **A.** Deterioration of a coronary artery from deposits of fatty substances that roughen the vessel's center. When a thrombus (blood clot) forms above the plaque, complete blockage of the artery produces a myocardial infarction or heart attack. A coronary artery bypass graft (CABG) creates a new "transportation route" around the blocked region to allow the required blood flow to deliver oxygen and nutrients to the previously "starved" surrounding heart muscle. The saphenous vein from the leg is the most commonly used bypass vessel. CABG involves sewing the graft vessels to the coronary arteries beyond the narrowing or blockage, with the other end of the vein attached to the aorta. Medications (statins) lower total and LDL cholesterol, and daily low-dose aspirin (81 mg) reduces post-CABG artery narrowing beyond the insertion site of the graft. CABG surgical mortality averages 5% to 10%. **B.** Angioplasty procedure to fix a blocked coronary artery. (Reprinted with permission from McArdle WD, Katch FI, Katch VL. *Exercise Physiology: Nutrition, Energy, and Human Performance*. 8th Ed. Baltimore: Wolters Kluwer Health, 2015; as adapted with permission from Moore KL, Dalley AF, Agur AMR. *Clinically Oriented Anatomy*. 7th Ed., as used with permission from *Stedman's Medical Dictionary*. 27th Ed. Baltimore: Wolters Kluwer Health, 2013.)

(**www.theheartfoundation.org/heart-disease-facts/heart-disease-statistics/**). Precipitating factors include the following:

1. Blockage in one or more arteries supplying the heart, thus cutting off myocardial blood supply
2. Sudden spasms or constriction in one of the coronary vessels, causing part of the heart muscle to die (called necrosis) from lack of oxygen (called anoxia)

In contrast to a heart attack, **cardiac arrest** is characterized by irregular neural-electrical transmission within the myocardium, which produces chaotic, unregulated beating or ventricular fibrillation in the heart's lower chambers. The survival rate statistics are not encouraging for an out-of-hospital cardiac arrest. In 2013, 359,400 such episodes occurred, but only 41% of these incidents were afforded bystander CPR, and the overall survivor rate was just 9.5% or essentially 1 out of 10. The results are better if cardiac arrest occurs in the hospital; of 209,000 such incidents yearly, the survival rate improved to 23.9% for adults and 40.2% for children (**http://circ.ahajournals.org/content/early/2012/12/12/CIR.0b013e31828124ad.full.pdf**).

The Cardiovascular Disease Epidemic

Cardiovascular disease (CVD) currently ranks as the leading health problem and primary cause of death among Americans younger than age 85 (**www.cdc.gov/heartdisease/facts.htm**). This resource-intensive chronic condition remains expensive to treat.

According to the Centers for Disease Control and Prevention (CDC; **www.nhlbi.nih.gov/resources/docs/2012_ChartBook_508.pdf**), nearly 83 million individuals currently suffer from CVD in the United States. More than 1,255,000 initial heart attacks occur each year, and more than 470,000 recurrent heart attack events occur annually.

TABLE 17.1 Modifiable and Unmodifiable Risk Factors Most Frequently Associated With Coronary Heart Disease

Modifiable Factors	Unmodifiable Factors
• Cigarette smoking • Diabetes mellitus • Diet • ECG abnormalities • Elevated blood lipids • Elevated homocysteine • Excessive body fat • High serum uric acid • Hypertension • Personality and behavior patterns • Poor education • Pulmonary function abnormalities • Sedentary lifestyle • Sleep apnea • Tension and stress	• Age • Ethnic background • Family history • Gender • Male-pattern baldness, particularly hair lack on the crown of the head; possibly from raised androgen levels

CORONARY HEART DISEASE RISK FACTORS

Research over the past 60 years has identified various personal characteristics, behaviors, and environmental factors linked to increased CHD susceptibility. Many of these factors relate strongly to CHD risk, but the associations do not necessarily imply a causal relationship (e.g., male pattern baldness). In some instances, it remains unclear whether risk factor modification offers effective disease protection.

Until definite proof emerges, it seems prudent to assume that either elimination or reduction of one or more of the modifiable risk factors will reduce CHD likelihood and cumulative disability in later years. For example, a radical heart risk reduction program that includes a whole-food, plant-based diet limiting saturated fat intake to no more than 10% of total calories and including regular physical activity, stress-management training, and support meetings, substantially reduces subsequent heart attack rate and other adverse heart events including bypass surgery and angioplasty procedures. In contrast, patients in conventional care steadily worsened over the same 5-year period. **Table 17.1** lists the most frequently implicated modifiable and nonmodifiable CHD risk factors.

Determining the quantitative importance of any single CHD risk factor remains difficult because of interrelationships among blood lipid abnormalities, type 2 diabetes, heredity (gene polymorphism), obesity, and diverse lifestyle factors.

Cigarette Smoking

Cigarette smoking, either active or passive through environmental exposure, directly increases CHD risk. Smokers experience twice the risk of death from heart disease as nonsmokers. Smokers with diabetes and hypertension experience even greater risk than individuals without these conditions. The CDC estimates that every cigarette smoked robs 7 minutes from a smoker's life. CHD risk increases the more one smokes or receives passive exposure, the deeper one inhales, and the stronger the cigarette tar and noxious by-product content. The increasing death rate from heart disease among women in the United States almost parallels their increased cigarette use.

British researchers estimate that smokers between ages 30 and 40 have five times as many heart attacks as nonsmokers in the same age range. When these relatively young smokers have a heart attack, an 80% chance exists that smoking caused it; this percentage averages nearly 70% for smokers in their 50s, 60s, and 70s.

Smokers run a five times greater risk for stroke than nonsmokers, and those who smoke one pack or more each day are 11 times more likely to experience a specific type of a sudden, deadly stroke most common in younger men and women. Surprisingly, the CHD risk from smoking correlates with a greater number of deaths than excess mortality of cigarette smokers from lung cancer.

Smoking risk usually remains independent of other risk factors. If additional risk factors exist, then smoking accentuates their influence. Cigarette smoking facilitates heart disease through its potentiating effect on serum lipoproteins; individuals who smoke have lower levels of HDL-C than nonsmokers. When smokers quit, the HDL-C and heart disease risk return to nonsmoker levels. A frightening statistic predicts that by the year 2030, smoking will become the world's single leading cause of death and disability, unless obesity continues its meteoric increase.

Blood Lipid Abnormalities

An abnormal blood lipid level (**hyperlipidemia**) provides a crucial, early component in the development of atherosclerosis. **Figure 17.16** shows the increasing death rate from CHD related to total serum cholesterol. Current guidelines focus less on total cholesterol and more on its lipoprotein components. Early treatment becomes crucial because of a strong association between high serum cholesterol starting in young adulthood and cardiovascular disease in middle age. A cholesterol level of 200 mg · dL^{-1} or lower remains a desirable goal, although risk for a fatal heart attack begins to increase at 150 mg · dL^{-1}. A cholesterol level of 230 mg · dL^{-1} increases heart attack risk to about twice that of 180 mg · dL^{-1}, and 300 mg · dL^{-1} increases the risk fourfold. For triacylglycerols, the National Cholesterol Education Program (**www.nhlbi.nih.gov/about/ncep/index.htm**) considers 200 mg · dL^{-1} an upper limit of normal triacylglycerol level, with 200 to 400 mg · dL^{-1} as borderline, and requiring changes in physical activity, diet, and possibly pharmacologic treatment if accompanied by other CHD risk factors. More than likely, triacylglycerol levels above 100 mg · dL^{-1} pose a cardiac risk. Individuals with triacylglycerol levels above 100 mg · dL^{-1} (following a 12-h fast) have a 50% greater CHD risk than individuals with triacylglycerols below 100 mg · dL^{-1}, even after controlling for HDL-C.

Major clinical drug trials show conclusively that reducing cholesterol lowers death rates and attenuates heart attacks. Medications that affect blood lipids include the following:

1. Bile acid sequestrants (e.g., cholestyramine resin and colestipol hydrochloride), which bind or sequester cholesterol-rich bile in the GI tract and prevent its gut resorption
2. Fibric acid derivatives (e.g., gemfibrozil, probucol, clofibrate), which lower triacylglycerols and LDL-C 5% to 20%, and elevate HDL-C an average 6% yearly
3. Statins (e.g., lovastatin, pravastatin, simvastatin, atorvastatin), which inhibit an enzyme that controls cholesterol synthesis by cells, increase LDL-C receptors in the liver to facilitate LDL-C removal from serum (18% to 55% reduction). Raising HDL-C by 34 mg · dL^{-1} via a 5-year gemfibrozil therapy trial reduced heart attacks, strokes, and death by 24% in patients with initially low HDL-C levels.

Lipids do not circulate freely in blood plasma; rather, they combine with a carrier protein to form **lipoproteins**, composed of a hydrophobic cholesterol core and a coat of free cholesterol, phospholipid, and a regulatory protein (**apolipoprotein [Apo]**). The lower part of **Figure 17.16** presents the American Heart Association recommendations and classifications for adult serum cholesterol, lipoproteins, and triacylglycerol levels.

Serum cholesterol reflects a composite of total cholesterol contained in each of the different lipoproteins. Although

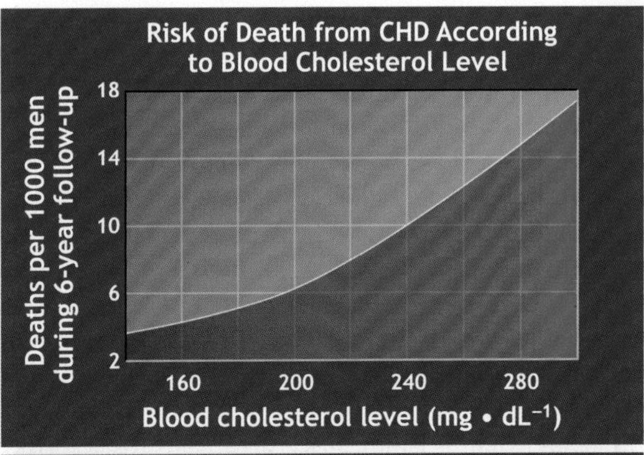

American Heart Association Recommendations and Classifications for Total Cholesterol and HDL and LDL cholesterol and Triacylglycerol

Total cholesterol*	Category
≥240	High blood cholesterol. A person with this level has more than twice the risk of heart disease as someone with cholesterol below 200.
200–239	Borderline high
≤200	Desirable level that puts you at lower risk for heart disease. Cholesterol level of 200 or higher raises risk.

HDL cholesterol	Category
<40	Low HDL cholesterol. A major risk factor for heart disease.
40–59	Higher HDL levels are better.
≥60	High HDL cholesterol. An HDL of 60 mg • dL^{-1} and above is considered protective against heart disease.

LDL cholesterol	Category
>190	Very high; cholesterol-lowering drug therapies even without heart disease or risk factors.**
160–189	High; cholesterol-lowering drug therapies even if there is no heart disease but two or more risk factors present.
130–159	Borderline high; cholesterol-lowering drug therapies if heart disease is present.
100–129	Near optimal; doctor may consider cholesterol-lowering drug therapies plus dietary modification if heart disease is present.
<100	Optimal; no therapy needed.

Triacylglycerol	Category
<150	Normal
150–199	Borderline high
200–499	High
≥500	Very high

* All levels in mg • dL^{-1}.

** In men under age 35 and premenopausal women with LDL cholesterol levels of 190 to 219 mg • dL^{-1}, delay drug therapy except in high-risk patients with diabetes.

FIGURE 17.16 Top graph. Death risk from coronary heart disease (CHD) in relation to total serum cholesterol level in middle-aged men. **Inset.** The American Heart Association recommendations and classifications for serum cholesterol, lipoproteins, and triacylglycerol levels for adults. (Reprinted with permission from McArdle WD, Katch FI, Katch VL. *Exercise Physiology: Nutrition, Energy, and Human Performance.* 8th Ed. Baltimore: Wolters Kluwer Health, 2015.)

discussions commonly refer to hyperlipidemia, the more meaningful focus addresses the different *types* of **hyperlipoproteinemias.**

Cholesterol distribution among the various lipoproteins provides a more powerful predictor of heart disease risk than total blood cholesterol. Specifically, elevated HDL-C levels relate causally with *lower* heart disease risk, even among individuals with total cholesterol below 200 mg · dL^{-1}. Overwhelming evidence links high LDL-C and Apo B levels with *increased* CHD risk. A more effective evaluation of heart disease risk than either total cholesterol or LDL-C levels divides total cholesterol by HDL-C. A ratio greater than 4.5 indicates a high heart disease risk; a ratio of 3.5 or lower represents a more desirable risk level.

LDL-C synthesized in the liver and very-low-density lipoprotein cholesterol (VLDL-C) provide the transport medium for fats to cells, including arterial smooth muscle walls. Upon oxidation, LDL-C participates in artery-clogging, plaque-forming atherosclerosis by stimulating monocyte-macrophage infiltration and lipoprotein deposition. LDL-C's surface coat contains the specific apolipoprotein (Apo B) that facilitates cholesterol removal from the LDL-C molecule by binding to LDL-C receptors of specific cells. Prevention of LDL-C oxidation slows CHD progression. The potential benefit of the dietary antioxidants vitamins C and E, including β-carotene, on heart disease risk reflect their effectiveness to blunt LDL-C oxidation.

LDL-C targets peripheral tissue and contributes to arterial damage. HDL-C also is produced in the liver; its levels relate to genetic factors. It facilitates reverse cholesterol transport and promotes surplus cholesterol removal from peripheral tissues, including arterial walls, for transport to the liver for bile synthesis and subsequent excretion via the digestive tract. The apolipoprotein A-1 (Apo A-1) in HDL-C activates **lecithin acetyl transferase (LCAT),** which converts free cholesterol into cholesterol esters. This facilitates removal of cholesterol from lipoproteins and other tissues.

fyi Should Cholesterol Be Measured in Children?

Guidelines issued by the National Cholesterol Education Program (**www.americanheart.org**) conclude children should have their cholesterol measured if a family history of high cholesterol or heart disease exists, particularly if a parent had a heart attack before age 50. Shockingly, this parental "cardiac proneness" includes up to 25% of the United States adult population! Research with children ages 10 to 15 indicates that encouraging lifestyle habits of regular physical activity, improved cardiovascular fitness, and a prudent nutritional profile contribute to favorable lipid profiles similar to the correlation seen with adults.

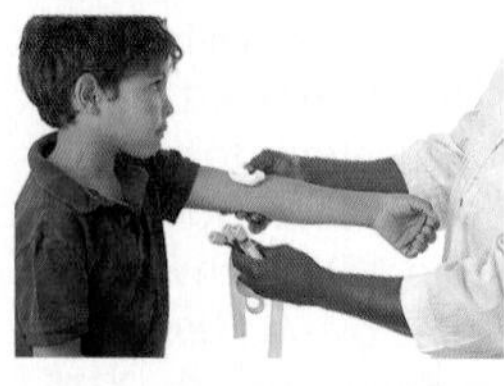

Behavioral Factors That Affect Blood Lipids

Six behaviors favorably impact the blood lipid profile:

1. Weight loss
2. Regular aerobic physical activity, independent of weight loss
3. Increased intake of water-soluble fibers in beans, legumes, and oat bran
4. Increased intake of polyunsaturated to saturated fatty acid ratio foods and monounsaturated fatty acids and elimination of *trans* fatty acids
5. Increased intake of omega-3 fatty acids in fish oils
6. Moderate alcohol consumption

Four behavioral factors adversely affect cholesterol and lipoprotein levels:

1. Cigarette smoking
2. Diet high in saturated fatty acids, *trans* fatty acids, and preformed cholesterol
3. High levels of stress
4. Oral contraceptive use

Hypertension

About 73.6 million people in the United States age 20 and older have high blood pressure: a systolic pressure that exceeds 140 mm Hg (**systolic hypertension**) or a diastolic pressure that exceeds 90 mm Hg (**diastolic hypertension**). These values form the lower limit for the classification of *borderline* high blood pressure. One of every four or five people experiences chronic, abnormally high blood pressure sometime during life. Uncorrected hypertension can precipitate heart failure, heart attack, stroke, and kidney failure. From 1995 to 2005, the death rate from hypertension increased 25.2%, and the number of deaths rose 56.4%. (To assess your own blood pressure, visit **www.heart.org/beatyourrisk/en_US/hbpRiskCalc.html?hasSet=true.**)

High blood pressure is often called the *silent killer* as it progresses without any overt symptoms or warning signs. Modification of lifestyle behaviors can lower high blood pressure; these modifications include weight loss, regular physical activity, cessation of smoking, and reducing salt intake. *Lowering systolic blood pressure just 2 mm Hg reduces death from stroke by 6% and heart disease by 4%.*

Unfortunately, in more than 90% of individuals, underlying cause(s) of hypertension remain unknown. Over an 18-month period, men and women ages 30 to 54 with mild hypertension modestly lowered systolic by 2.9 mm Hg and diastolic blood pressure by 2.3 mm Hg when they reduced body weight and salt intake. No blood pressure changes occurred for subjects who undertook only stress reduction and relaxation techniques or consumed calcium, magnesium, phosphorus, and fish oil dietary supplements. Prescription drugs that either reduce fluid volume or decrease peripheral resistance to blood flow effectively treat high blood pressure.

Diabetes

Diabetics are up to four times more likely to develop cardiovascular disease from multiple risk factors usually coincident with the diabetic condition. These risk factors include the following:

1. **Obesity:** represents a major risk factor for cardiovascular disease that strongly associates with insulin resistance. Insulin resistance may provide the mechanism by which obesity leads to cardiovascular disease. Weight loss improves cardiovascular risk, decreases blood insulin concentrations, and increases insulin sensitivity.
2. **Physical inactivity:** a modifiable risk factor for insulin resistance and cardiovascular disease. Exercising more while reducing excess body weight (and fat) prevents or delays the onset of T2DM, lowers blood pressure, and reduces heart attack and stroke risk.
3. **Hypertension:** positively correlates with insulin resistance in diabetes. For a person with both hypertension and diabetes, the risk for cardiovascular disease doubles.
4. **Atherogenic dyslipidemia**: often-called **diabetic dyslipidemia** in T2DM, relates to insulin resistance characterized by high levels of triacylglycerols (hypertriglyceridemia) and high levels of small LDL particles and low levels of HDL. The components of this *lipid triad* contribute to atherosclerotic risk.

According to the CDC, more than 29.1 million Americans now have diabetes, and one out of every four do not know they have it. Moreover, of the 86 million Americans who have **prediabetes** (1 of every 3 adults), 9 of 10 do not know it and 15% to 30% will develop T2DM within 5 years. Unfortunately, 1.6 million new cases of diabetes will be diagnosed in people age 20 years and older each year. **Figure 17.17** provides a current snapshot of diabetes in the United States.

fyi Diabetes Risk Lowered With Regular Physical Activity

Men who exercise five or more times a week have a 42% lower risk of T2DM than men who exercise, on average, less than once a week. The exercise benefits become most pronounced among obese participants. Diabetes risk decreases approximately 6% for every 500 "extra" kcal expended through increased physical activity, equivalent to walking on a flat surface for 5 miles during any 7-day period. Upping walking to 2 miles daily (roughly 200 additional kcal) for 5 days or 1000 kcal expended would decrease diabetes risk by about 16%. Taking a walk for 1 hour daily (assuming a moderate 20 min per mile pace), 5 days a week, would burn an extra 1500 kcal (15 miles weekly at 100 kcal a mile) toward diabetes risk reduction.

Other Coronary Heart Disease Risk Factor Candidates

The following factors represent potentially potent CHD risk predictors.

Age, Gender, and Heredity

Age represents a CHD risk factor associated with three other risk factors—hypertension, elevated blood lipid levels, and glucose intolerance. After age 35 in men and age 45 in women, the chances of dying from CHD increase progressively and dramatically. Heredity also represents a risk factor because heart attacks that strike at an early age tend to run in families. Such familial predisposition probably relates to a genetic role in determining heart disease risk.

Immunologic Factors

An immune response can trigger plaque development within arterial walls. During this process, mononuclear immune cells produce proteins called ***cytokines***, some of which stimulate plaque buildup, while others inhibit plaque formation. Within this framework, increased physical activity can stimulate the immune system to inhibit agents that facilitate arterial disease. For example, 2.5 hours of weekly physical activity for 6 months *decreased* cytokine production that facilitates plaque development by 58%; cytokines that inhibit plaque formation *increased* by 36%.

Homocysteine (Optimal Levels = <10 to 12 mcmol · L^{-1})

Homocysteine, a highly reactive, sulfur-containing amino acid, forms as a by-product of methionine metabolism. Researchers in the 1960s and 1970s described three different inborn errors of homocysteine metabolism involving B vitamin enzymes. High levels of homocysteine in the blood and urine were common to all three disorders of the affected individuals, and half of these individuals developed arterial or venous thrombosis by age 30. Moderate elevation of homocysteine can predispose these individuals to atherosclerosis similarly to elevated cholesterol concentration.

A nearly lockstep association exists between plasma homocysteine levels and heart attack and mortality in men and women; the correlation is similar to that of smoking and hyperlipidemia. This metabolic abnormality is present in nearly 30% of CHD patients and 40% of patients with cerebrovascular disease. Excessive homocysteine causes blood platelets to clump, fostering blood clots and deterioration of smooth muscle cells that line arterial walls. Chronic homocysteine exposure eventually scars and thickens arteries and provides a fertile medium for circulating LDL-C to initiate damage. In the presence of other conventional CHD risks

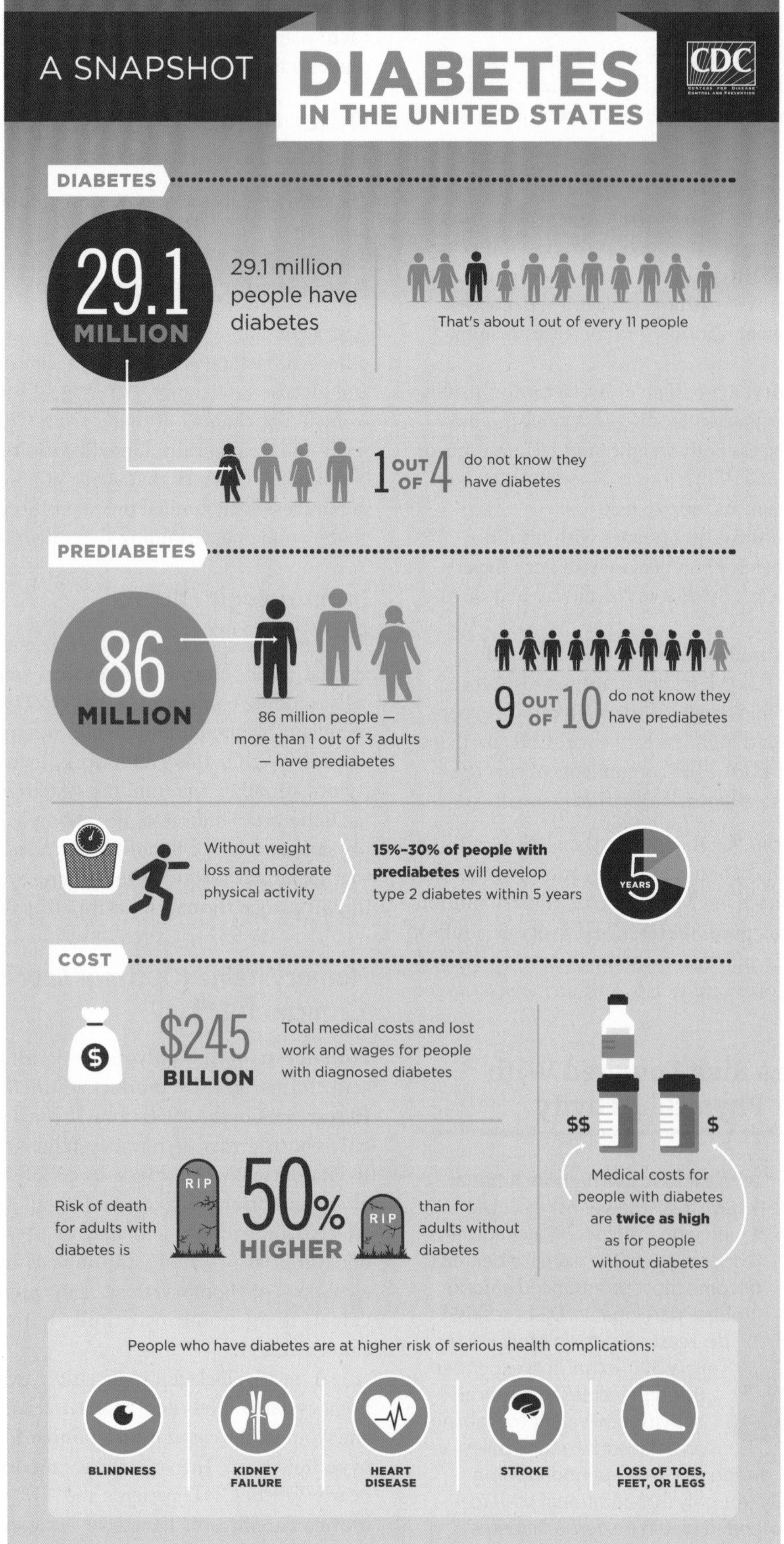

FIGURE 17.17 Incidence of diabetes and prediabetes. (Adapted with permission from American Diabetes Association, **www.diabetes.org/diabetes-basics/statistics/cdc-infographic.html**.)

(e.g., smoking and hypertension), synergistic effects magnify the negative impact of homocysteine on cardiovascular health. In general, people in the highest quartile for homocysteine levels have nearly twice the risk of heart attack or stroke compared with those in the lowest quartile. Why some people accumulate homocysteine is uncertain, but the evidence points to a deficiency of B vitamins (B_6, B_{12}, and particularly folic acid); cigarette smoking, frequent coffee intake, and regular meat consumption also associate with elevated homocysteine concentrations.

Excessive Body Fat (See Chapter 16 for Optimal Levels)

Excessive body fat has received attention as a CHD risk factor, but its relationship frequently coexists with hypertension, elevated cholesterol, T2DM, and cigarette smoking. The number of annual deaths attributable to overfatness in the U. S. adult population easily exceeds 350,000. Weight loss and accompanying body fat reduction, whether through diet, physical activity, or their combination, usually normalizes cholesterol and triacylglycerol levels and beneficially impacts blood pressure and T2DM.

Physical Inactivity

Sedentary men and women are twice as likely to suffer a fatal heart attack as their more physically active counterparts. Maintenance of aerobic fitness throughout life also provides protection against CHD risk factors and disease occurrence. One could argue that genetic factors contribute more to fitness level than to daily physical activity patterns. However, fitness level relates closely to individual differences in physical activity level among most individuals, making regular physical activity assume greater importance than simply genetics in determining fitness and related health benefits. **Table 17.2** summarizes possible biologic mechanisms for how regular aerobic activity confers protection against CHD progression.

C-Reactive Protein

Mounting evidence indicates that painless chronic low-grade arterial inflammation, including that of the coronary arteries, remains central to every stage of atherosclerotic disease and represents a major trigger for heart attack—more substantial even than high cholesterol. The inflammatory process produces heart attacks by weakening blood vessel walls, making plaque burst, and interfering with substances that increase myocardial circulation. C-reactive protein (CRP), a protein found in blood (optimal levels $\leq 1.0\ mg \cdot L^{-1}$), increases during the inflammatory response to tissue injury or infection. The liver primarily synthesizes CRP, with its release stimulated by interleukin 6 (IL-6) and other **proinflammatory cytokines**. Small increases in CRP within the normal range predict future vascular events in apparently healthy, asymptomatic individuals. Such predictive accuracy of CRP extends to patients with preexisting vascular disease. Higher CRP levels associate with abdominal obesity, and increased levels predict risk of developing T2DM. Four strategies can help to lower CRP:

1. Weight loss
2. Abstaining from cigarette smoking
3. Consuming a healthful diet
4. Combining regular physical activity with resistance training

Lipoprotein(a)

Lipoprotein(a) [Lp(a)] (optimal levels: $\leq 14\ mg \cdot dL^{-1}$ ($35\ nmol \cdot L^{-1}$), an LDL-like particle largely under genetic control, varies considerably between individuals depending on the size of the apo(a) isoform present. Unlike the lipoproteins LDL and HDL, Lp(a) levels vary little with diet or physical activity. Strong evidence suggests its role is to respond to tissue injury and vascular lesions, to prevent infectious pathogens from invading cells, and to promote wound healing. High Lp(a) in blood is a risk factor for coronary artery disease, cerebrovascular disease, atherosclerosis, thrombosis, and stroke.

TABLE 17.2 Possible Mechanisms for Eight Beneficial Effects of Regular Aerobic Physical Activity on Risk of Coronary Heart Disease and Mortality

1. Improves myocardial circulation and metabolism to protect the heart from hypoxic stress. Improvements include enhanced vascularization and increased coronary blood flow capacity via altered control of coronary vascular smooth muscle and increased reactivity of coronary resistance vessels. Modest increases in cardiac glycogen stores and glycolytic capacity also prove beneficial if the heart's oxygen supply suddenly becomes compromised.
2. Enhances the mechanical properties of the myocardium to enable the exercise-trained heart to maintain or increase contractility during a specific challenge.
3. Establishes more favorable blood-clotting characteristics and other hemostatic mechanisms, including increased fibrinolysis and production of endothelial prostacyclin.
4. Normalizes the blood lipid profile to slow or reverse atherosclerosis.
5. Favorably alters heart rate and blood pressure, so myocardial work decreases during rest and physical activity.
6. Suppresses age-related body weight gain and promotes a more desirable body composition and body fat distribution, particularly a reduced level of intra-abdominal adipose tissue.
7. Establishes a more favorable neural-hormonal balance to conserve oxygen for the myocardium; improves the mixture of carbohydrate and fat metabolized by the body.
8. Provides a favorable outlet for excessive psychological stress and tension.

fyi Sitting Too Much, Not Just Lack of Physical Activity, Detrimental to Cardiovascular Health

Data analysis from 2223 men and women between ages 12 and 49 with no known history of heart disease, asthma, or stroke enrolled in the National Health and Nutrition Examination Survey (NHANES; **www.cdc.gov/nchs/nhanes.htm**) to determine the association between fitness levels, daily physical activity, and sedentary behavior. Accelerometer data assessed average daily physical activity and sedentary behavior times. Fitness, estimated using a submaximal treadmill test, was adjusted for gender, age, and body mass index. The negative effect of 6 hours of sedentary time on fitness levels was similar in magnitude to the benefit of 1 hour of strenuous physical activity such as double poling in cross-country skiing.

In another study from Sweden, researchers measured the length of telomeres, caps at the ends of DNA strands; these caps shorten and change their shape with aging. Following 6 months of the subjects either maintaining their previous lifestyles or changing sedentary behaviors to become more physically active (and thus sitting less), the telomeres in the latter group lengthened while the telomeres shortened in the group continuing to remain sedentary. A third study from a large Canadian cohort (16,586 adults age 18 to 90) reported no link between standing more over a 10-year period and premature death, or as the researchers noted, mortality rates declined at higher levels of standing. The results from these studies collectively underscore the need to encourage achieving higher fitness levels through increased activity (and thus less sedentariness) to decrease disease risk factors and enhance life quality. To this end, the new generation of smartphones and watches have built-in timers that alert their wearers to "get up and move." The basic idea is to provide intrinsic motivation to sit less, move more, and change sedentary habits by transitioning to increased physical activity.

Sources: Katzmarzyk PT. Standing and mortality in a prospective cohort of Canadian adults. *Med Sci Sports Exerc* 2014;46:940.

Kerem S, et al. Sedentary behavior, cardiorespiratory fitness, physical activity, and cardiometabolic risk in men: the Cooper Center Longitudinal Study. *Mayo Clin Proc* 2014;89:1052.

Sjogren P, et al. Stand up for health—avoiding sedentary behavior might lengthen your telomeres: secondary outcomes from a physical activity RCT in older people. *Br J Sports Med* 2014;48:1407.

Lp(a)'s most important role may be to inhibit the breakdown of clots or fibrinolysis at the tissue injury site. These properties make Lp(a) a highly atherothrombotic lipoprotein.

Fibrinogen

Fibrinogen (optimal levels = 1.5 to 3 g · L^{-1}), a circulating glycoprotein synthesized by the liver, acts at the final step in the coagulation response to vascular tissue injury. Fibrinogen, similar to CRP, serves as an acute-phase reactant that makes it a biologically plausible participant in vascular disease. Elevated blood fibrinogen, independent of classic CHD risk factors, correlates with ischemic stroke and peripheral vascular disease. Several factors other than inflammation modulate fibrinogen levels. A dose-response positive relationship exists between number of cigarettes smoked and fibrinogen level. Fibrinogen tends to be higher in patients with diabetes, hypertension, obesity, and sedentary lifestyle.

Coronary Heart Disease Risk Factor Interactions

Smoking generally acts independently of other risk factors to increase CHD risk. The other risk factors interact with each other and CHD itself to accentuate disease risk. **Figure 17.18** quantifies the interaction of three primary CHD risk factors in the same person. With one risk factor, a 45-year-old man's chance for CHD involvement during the year averages about twice that of a man without risks. The chance for chest pain, heart attack, or sudden death with three primary risk factors increases five times compared with no risk factors.

Some researchers posit that the five major modifiable cardiovascular risk factors—cigarette smoking, physical inactivity, **diabetes mellitus**, hypertension, and hypercholesterolemia—account for only about 50% of individuals who subsequently develop CHD. Several reports directly challenge this "only 50%" claim for the five risk factors. Data analysis from 14 randomized clinical trials involving 122,458 participants and 386,915 subjects from three observational studies revealed that 80% to 90% of patients who developed clinically significant CHD, and more than 95%

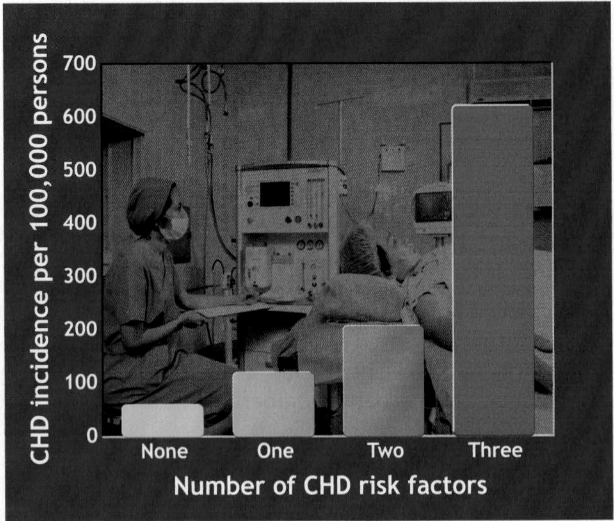

FIGURE 17.18 General relation between a combination of abnormal risk factors (cholesterol ≥250 mg · dL^{-1}; systolic blood pressure ≥160 mm Hg; smoking ≥1 pack of cigarettes per day) and incidence of coronary heart disease (CHD). (Reprinted with permission from McArdle WD, Katch FI, Katch VL. *Exercise Physiology: Nutrition, Energy, and Human Performance*. 8th Ed. Baltimore: Wolters Kluwer Health, 2015.)

of patients who experienced a fatal CHD event, had at least one of the five traditional major risk factors including overweight/obesity. These findings may underestimate the true extent of the relationship, given the self-report design of the observational studies and number of patients unaware or not diagnosed as having risk factors at the time of evaluation.

These results have enormous public health implications for targeting a large segment of the population at risk of developing CHD. Smoking is arguably the single most important modifiable and preventable cardiovascular disease risk factor, and one of the strongest predictors of premature CHD. Equally important CHD predictors include obesity and physical inactivity.

Many CHD risks link to common behavioral patterns; they can be positively influenced by similar and, in some cases, identical interventions. For example, regular physical activity exerts a positive influence on obesity, hypertension, T2DM, stress, and elevated blood lipid profile. No other modifiable behavior exerts such a potent positive effect for the greatest number of persons, causing many to argue that regular physical activity constitutes the most important behavioral intervention to reduce CHD.

Coronary Heart Disease Risk Factors in Children

The frequent occurrence of multiple CHD risk factors in young children emphasizes the need for early CHD initiatives to reduce atherosclerosis risk later in life. Obesity and a family history of heart disease represent the two most common risk factors in physically active and apparently healthy boys and girls. A relatively large percentage of these children have undesirable blood lipid profiles.

As with adults, the association between body fat and serum lipid levels becomes apparent in overfat children. The fattest children of elementary school age usually have the highest levels of serum cholesterol and triacylglycerols. For them, general adiposity and excess visceral adipose tissue relate to unfavorable hemostatic factors that increase CHD morbidity and mortality in adulthood.

Of 62 overfat children ages 10 to 15, only 1 child (1.6%) had just one CHD risk factor. Of the remaining children, 14% had two risk factors, 30% had three risk factors, 29% had four risk factors, 18% had five risk factors, and six risk factors were present in the remaining five children (8%). A subsample of these children was then enrolled in a 20-week program to evaluate the effects on the risk profile of either (1) diet plus behavior therapy (DB) or (2) regular physical activity plus diet and behavior therapy (EDB). No changes resulted in multiple risk reduction in the control group (CON) or in those receiving diet with behavior treatment. In contrast, children who exercised, dieted, and underwent behavior therapy dramatically reduced multiple risks (**Fig. 17.19**). These encouraging findings demonstrate that supervised programs of moderate food restriction and increased physical activity coupled with behavior modification reduce CHD risk factors in obese adolescents. Adding regular physical activity augmented the effectiveness of risk factor intervention. If regular physical activity at least stabilizes a poor risk factor

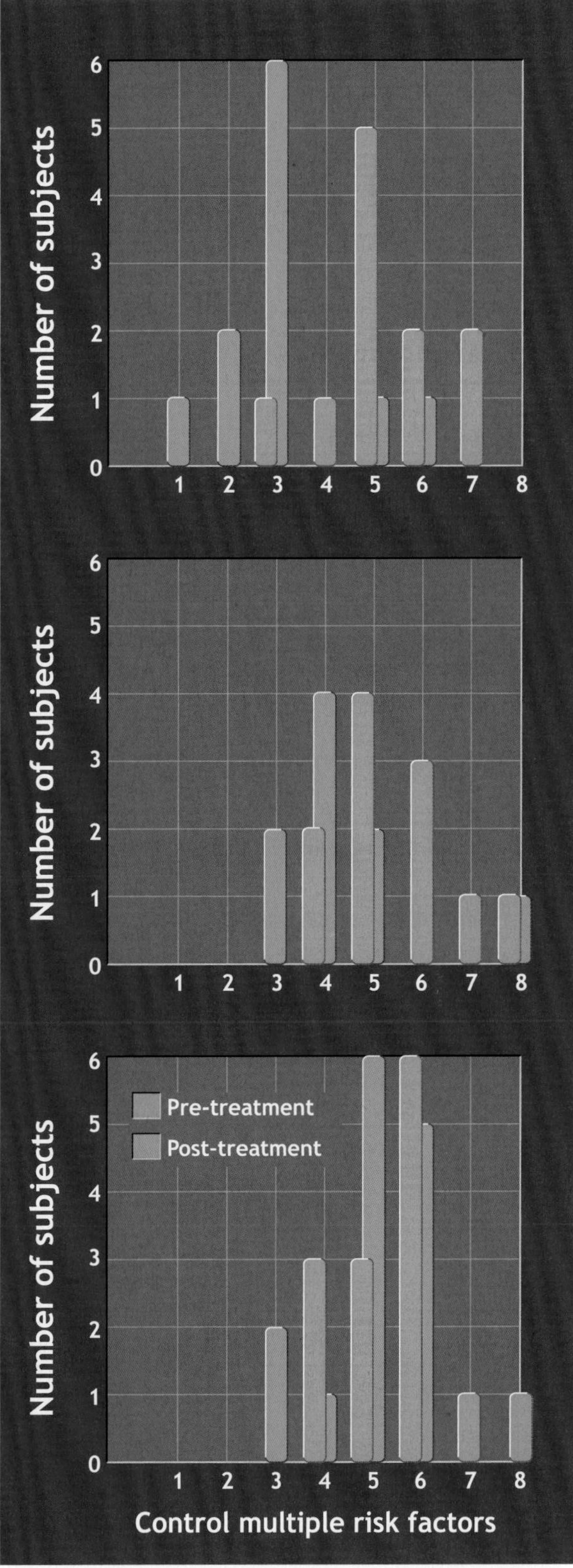

FIGURE 17.19 Multiple coronary heart disease risk factors for obese adolescents before and after treatment. *DB*, diet + behavior change group; *EDB*, exercise + diet + behavior change group. (Reprinted with permission from McArdle WD, Katch FI, Katch VL. *Exercise Physiology: Nutrition, Energy, and Human Performance*. 8th Ed. Baltimore: Wolters Kluwer Health, 2015; from Becque DB, et al. Coronary risk incidence of obese adolescents: reduction by exercise plus diet intervention. *Pediatrics* 1988;81:605.)

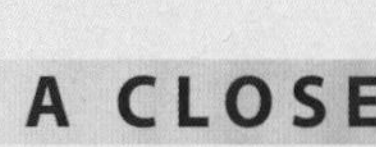

A CLOSER LOOK

Calculate Your Coronary Heart Disease Risk

CHD risk inventories provide a qualitative way to assess an individual's CHD susceptibility. The table below presents the Framingham 10-year CHD risk estimate, the most widely used "traditional" risk analysis system.

To determine risk profile, review each risk factor and accompanying numerical "point" value. Insert the respective points into the applicable box at the top of the table. The total number of points represents the 10-year risk for developing CHD expressed as a percentage.

Framingham 10-Year CHD Risk Estimate Worksheet

☐	+	☐	+	☐	+	☐	+	☐	+	☐	=	☐
Age		**HDL-C**		**SBP**		**TC**		**Smoking**		**Total Points**		**10-year Risk (%)**

Age (y)

Women	Points	Men	Points
20–34	−7	20–34	−9
35–39	−3	35–39	−4
40–44	0	40–44	0
45–49	3	45–49	3
50–54	6	50–54	6
55–59	8	55–59	8
60–64	10	60–64	10
65–69	12	65–69	11
70–74	14	70–74	12
75–79	16	75–79	13

Systolic Blood Pressure (SBP), mm Hg

Women	Points		Men	Points	
mm Hg	Treated	Untreated	mm Hg	Treated	Untreated
<120	0	0	<120	0	0
120–129	1	3	120–129	0	1
130–139	2	4	130–139	1	2
140–159	3	5	140–159	1	2
>160	4	6	>160	2	3

Points for Total Cholesterol (TC) at Each Age Category (y) Women

TC (mg · dL^{-1})	*20–39*	*40–49*	*50–59*	*60–69*	*70–79*
<160	0	0	0	0	0
160–199	4	3	2	1	1
200–239	8	6	4	2	1
240–279	11	8	5	3	2
>280	13	10	7	4	2

Points for Total Cholesterol (TC) at Each Age Category (y) Men

TC (mg · dL^{-1})	*20–39*	*40–49*	*50–59*	*60–69*	*70–79*
<160	0	0	0	0	0
160–199	4	3	2	1	0
200–239	7	5	3	1	0
240–279	9	6	4	2	1
>280	11	8	5	3	1

Points for Smoking at Each Age Category (y) Women

	20–39	*40–49*	*50–59*	*60–69*	*70–79*
Nonsmoker	0	0	0	0	0
Smoker	9	7	4	2	1

Points for Smoking at Each Age Category (y) Men

	20–39	*40–49*	*50–59*	*60–69*	*70–79*
Nonsmoker	0	0	0	0	0
Smoker	8	5	3	1	1

Predicated 10-Year CHD Risk From Point Total

Women		Men	
Point Total	**10-Year Risk (%)**	**Point Total**	**10-Year Risk (%)**
>9	>1	0	<1
9–12	1	1–4	1
13–14	2	5–6	2
15	3	7	3
16	4	8	4
17	5	9	5
18	6	10	6
19	8	11	8
20	11	12	10
21	14	13	12
22	17	14	16
23	22	15	20
24	27	16	25
≥25	≥30	≥17	≥30

profile, then school curricula at all grade levels, particularly at the kindergarten and elementary grades, should strongly encourage more physically active lifestyles. In this regard, not implementing daily, required physical education seems counterproductive from a public health policy standpoint.

SUMMARY

1. CHD represents the single biggest cause of death in the Western world.
2. CHD pathogenesis involves degenerative changes in the inner lining of the arterial wall leading to progressive occlusion.
3. Four major modifiable cardiovascular risk factors (smoking, diabetes mellitus, hypertension, and hypercholesterolemia) account for 80% to 90% of CHD cases.
4. Cigarette smoking, either active or passive through environmental exposure, directly relates to CHD risk at twice the death risk from heart disease as nonsmokers.
5. The receptor molecule TLR-2 represents the trigger for inflammation and tissue breakdown in arterial plaque that leads to CHD.
6. A cholesterol level of 200 mg $\cdot$ dL^{-1} or lower is desirable, although risk for fatal heart attack begins to increase at 150 mg $\cdot$ dL^{-1}. A cholesterol level of 230 mg $\cdot$ dL^{-1} increases heart attack risk to twice that of 180 mg $\cdot$ dL^{-1}, and 300 mg $\cdot$ dL^{-1} increases risk fourfold.
7. For triacylglycerol level, less than 150 mg $\cdot$ dL^{-1} is considered a nominal level, with 200 to 499 mg $\cdot$ dL^{-1} considered high and undesirable.
8. Behaviors that favorably affect cholesterol and lipoprotein levels include weight loss, regular aerobic physical activity, increased intake of water-soluble fibers, moderate alcohol consumption, increased intake of omega-3 fats in fish oils, elimination of *trans* fatty acids, and adjusting the intake of polyunsaturated, monounsaturated, and saturated fatty acids.
9. Variables that adversely affect cholesterol and lipoprotein levels include cigarette smoking, a diet high in saturated and *trans* fatty acids and preformed cholesterol, emotionally stressful situations, and oral contraceptive use.
10. Systolic blood pressure that exceeds 140 mm Hg or diastolic pressure that exceeds 90 mm Hg represents the lower limit for borderline hypertension.
11. Diabetics are two to four times more likely to develop cardiovascular disease from obesity, physical inactivity, hypertension, and atherogenic dyslipidemia.
12. The following ten variables represent positive CHD predictors: age, gender, heredity, immunologic factors, homocysteine, excessive body fat, physical inactivity, C-reactive protein, lipoprotein(a), and fibrinogen.
13. CHD risk factors interact with each other and CHD per se to accentuate heart disease risk.
14. The frequent occurrence of multiple CHD risk factors in young children emphasizes the need for early initiatives to reduce atherosclerotic risk later in life

THINK IT THROUGH

1. Does risk factor modification always change CHD disease risk?
2. If you could change one CHD risk factor, what would it be?
3. Design an experiment to evaluate the effects of aerobic training and standard resistance training on cardiovascular risk factors in middle-aged women. Indicate controls, measurement variables, and tests to show a training effect.
4. In addition to extending life span, what other two reasons would make sense for maintaining a physically active lifestyle throughout middle and older age?

PART 5 Regular Physical Activity: Is it the Fountain of Youth?

Physical activity and exercise may not necessarily represent a "fountain of youth," yet the preponderance of evidence shows that regular activity retards the decline in functional capacity associated with aging and disuse. Increased physical activity participation can reverse the loss of function regardless of when a person becomes more physically active.

Causes of Death in the United States

Beginning in the mid 1990s, changes in lifestyle have resulted in variations in causes of death in the United States. Whereas mortality rates from heart disease, stroke, and cancer have declined, the prevalence of obesity and T2DM has increased. **Figure 17.20** shows causes of preventable deaths during the same time period. The most striking finding is the substantial increase in number of deaths attributable to medical conditions that relate directly to poor diet and physical inactivity (overweight and obesity listed as cause). The gap between deaths caused by poor diet and physical inactivity and those caused by cigarette smoking has narrowed substantially. *Clearly, most preventable deaths can be attributed to a small number of largely preventable behaviors and exposures that relate directly to physical inactivity, dietary excess, and overfatness.* Unless curtailed, the increasing trend of these three factors will overtake cigarette smoking as the leading preventable cause of mortality in the near future. Regrettably, the increased use of electronic cigarettes (see below) by

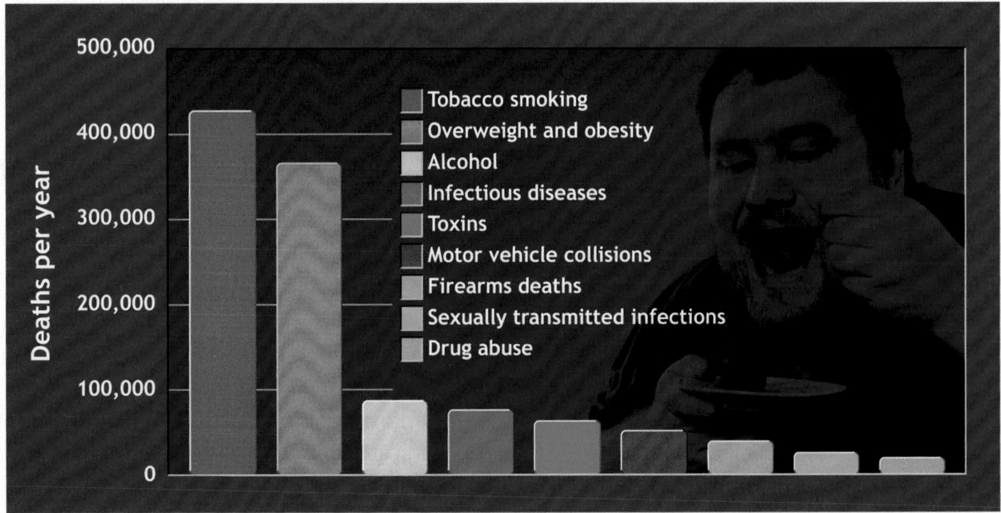

FIGURE 17.20 Preventable causes of deaths in the United States, 2013. (Data from Centers for Disease Control and Prevention **www.cdc.gov/vitalsigns/HeartDisease-Stroke**.)

teens will keep "smoking" as the leading preventable cause of mortality for many years to come.

Health Risk to Teens by Increased e-Cigarette Use

According to the Centers for Disease Control and Prevention and the U.S. Food and Drug Administration's Center for Tobacco Products (CT) and published in the Morbidity and Mortality Weekly Report (MMWR; **www.cdc.gov/mmwr/**), the use of e-cigarettes has tripled from 2013 to 2014 among middle and high school students. According to the 2014 National Youth Tobacco Survey (**www.cdc.gov/tobacco/data_statistics/surveys/nyts/**), current e-cigarette use for at least 1 day in a 30-day span increased from 4.5% in 2013 to 13.4% in 2014. This translates to an additional 1,340,000 students who used e-cigarettes in 2014, up from 660,000 in 2013 (current total 2 million). Current e-cigarette use among middle school students also tripled from 1.1% in 2013 to 3.9% in 2014—an increase of 340,000 students from approximately 120,000 in 2013 to 450,000 in 2014.

The most common products used by high school students in 2014 were e-cigarettes (13.4%), hookah (9.4%), cigarettes (9.2%), cigars (8.2%), smokeless tobacco (5.5%), snus (type of tobacco snuff consumed as a moist powder placed under the upper lip, without chewing for extended periods; 1.9%), and pipes (1.5%). Similarly, middle school students used e-cigarettes (3.9%), hookah (2.5%), cigarettes (2.5%), cigars (1.9%), smokeless tobacco (1.6%), and pipes (0.6%). The director of FDA's Center for Tobacco Products stated that "In today's rapidly evolving tobacco marketplace, the surge in youth use of novel products like e-cigarettes forces us to confront the reality that the progress we have made in reducing youth cigarette smoking rates is being threatened, and these staggering increases in such a short time underscore why FDA intends to regulate these additional products to protect public health."

Increased Physical Activity and Exercise Improve Health and Extend Life

Medical experts have debated whether a lifetime of regular physical activity contributes to good health and longevity compared with a sedentary but "good life." Because older, fit individuals exhibit many functional characteristics of younger people, one could argue that improved physical fitness and a vigorous lifestyle in older age retards biologic aging and thus confers health benefits later in life.

One study documented the lifestyles and physical activity habits of 17,000 Harvard alumni who entered college between 1916 and 1950. Moderate aerobic physical activity, equivalent to jogging 3 miles daily, promoted good health and added time to healthy life span. Men who expended 2000 kcal in weekly physical activity had up to one-third *lower* death rates than classmates who undertook little or no physical activity. To achieve a 2000-kcal energy output weekly requires additional moderate physical activity such as a daily 30- to 45-minute brisk walk, or a moderate run, cycle, swim, cross-country ski, or aerobics dance participation. Other study findings include the following:

1. Regular physical activity counters the life-shortening effects of cigarette smoking and excess body weight.
2. Even for people with hypertension, those who regularly participated in physical activity reduced death rate by half.
3. Regular physical activity countered genetic tendencies toward early death. Individuals with one or both parents who died before age 65 reduced death risk by 25%.
4. A 50% reduction in mortality rate occurred for active men whose parents lived beyond age 65.

Figure 17.21 shows that among physically active people, the more a person participates in physical activity, the more the risk of death declines. For example, men who

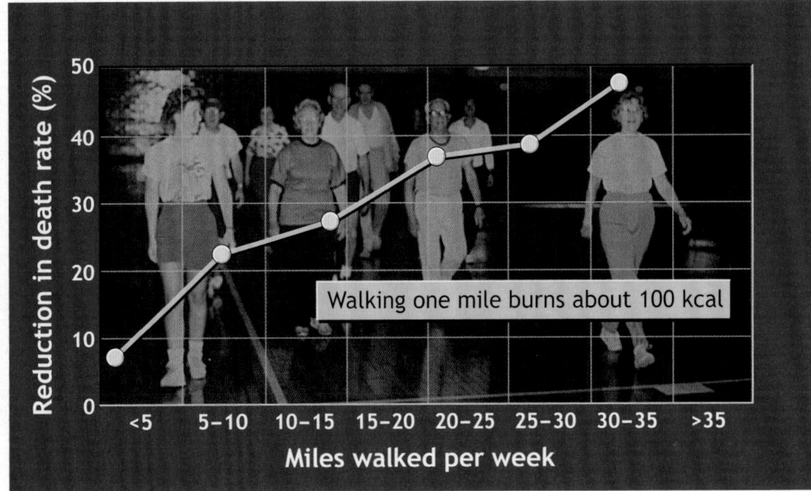

FIGURE 17.21 Reduced death risk with regular exercise. (Data from Paffenbarger RS Jr., et al. Physical activity, all-cause mortality, and longevity of college alumni. *N Engl J Med* 1986;314:605.)

walked 9 or more miles a week had a 21% lower mortality rate than men who walked 3 miles or less. Men participating in light sport activities increased life expectancy 24% compared to men who remained sedentary. From a perspective of energy expenditure, the life expectancy of Harvard alumni increased steadily from a weekly physical activity energy output of 500 to 3500 kcal, the equivalent of 6 to 8 hours of strenuous weekly physical activity. In addition, active men lived an average of 1 to 2 years longer than their sedentary classmates. Additional research confirms that regular physical activity confers an expected increase in life expectancy of about 10 months.

No additional health or longevity benefits accrued beyond 3500 kcal weekly physical activity. Men who performed extreme-type activities had higher death rates than less active colleagues, an example of why *more* does not necessarily produce *greater* health-related physical activity benefits.

Improved Fitness: A Little Goes a Long Way

A study of more than 13,000 men and women over an 8-year interval indicates that even modest amounts of physical activity substantially reduce death risk from heart disease, cancer, and other causes. The study evaluated fitness performance directly rather than relying on verbal or written reports of physical activity habits. To isolate the effect of fitness per se, the researchers accounted for smoking, cholesterol and blood sugar levels, blood pressure, and family CHD history. Based on age-adjusted death rates per 10,000 person-years, **Figure 17.22** illustrates that the least-fit group died at a three times greater rate than the most-fit subjects.

Importantly, the group rated just above the most sedentary category derived the greatest change in health benefits. The decrease in death rate for men from the least fit to the next category equaled 38 (64.0 vs. 25.5 deaths per 10,000 person-years), yet the decline from the second group to the most fit category equaled only seven deaths per 10,000 person-years. Women obtained similar benefits as men. The amount of physical activity required moving from the most sedentary category to the next more fit category (the jump showing the greatest increase in health benefits) was moderate-intensity walking briskly for 30 minutes several times weekly. *If life-extending benefits of physical activity exist, they associated more with preventing early mortality than improving overall life span.* Regular moderate physical activity enables individuals to live more productive and healthy lives.

fyi Structured Physical Activity Not Necessary

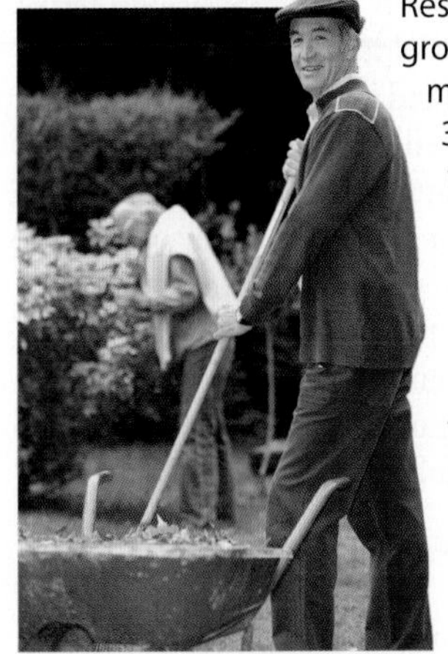

Researchers monitored two groups of sedentary middle-aged men and women ages 35 to 60 during a 2-year clinical trial. One group participated in vigorous physical activity for 20 to 60 minutes by swimming, stair stepping, walking, or biking at a fitness center up to 5 days weekly. The other group incorporated 30 minutes a day of "lifestyle" physical activity such as extra walking, raking leaves, stair climbing, walking around the airport while waiting for a plane, and participating in a walking club most days of the week. The lifestyle participants also learned cognitive and behavioral strategies to increase daily physical activity. For each of the programs, the intervention consisted of 6 months of intensive physical activity followed by 18 months of maintenance. At the end of 24 months, *both* groups improved equally in physical activity, cardiorespiratory fitness, systolic and diastolic blood pressure, and body fat percentage. These findings reinforce the conclusion that the health-derived benefits from regular physical activity do not require highly structured workouts or enrollment in vigorous physical activity programs.

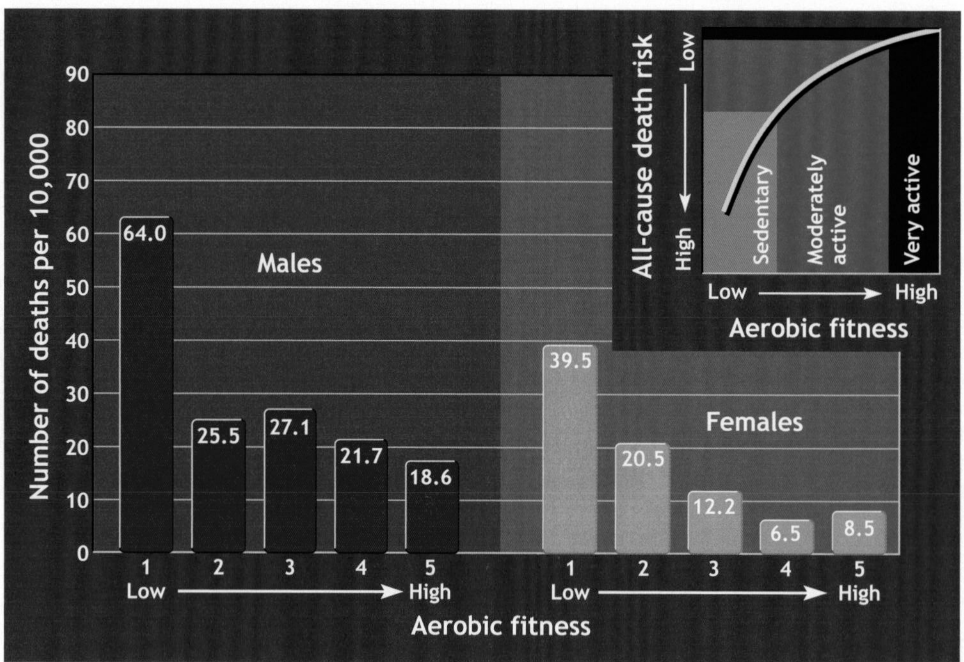

FIGURE 17.22 Physical fitness and death risk. The greatest reduction in death rate risk occurs when going from the most sedentary category to a moderate fitness level. (Data from Blair SN, et al. Physical fitness and all-cause mortality: a prospective study of healthy men and women. *JAMA* 1989;262:2395.)

Changes in Physical Activity and Mortality Among Older Women

Studies of changes in physical activity and mortality have mostly examined middle-aged male populations. It remains unclear whether adoption of a physically active lifestyle by previously sedentary older women with chronic cardiovascular disease, diabetes, and physical frailty produces similar benefits typically observed for men. A unique study followed the physical activity patterns of 9704 mostly white, 65-year-old women followed for 12.5 years. They were classified at baseline and 4.0 to 7.7 years later into one of four groups (quintiles, from highest to lowest) based on amount of daily walking and frequency and duration of other leisure time activities such as dancing, gardening, aerobics, or swimming. The four groups were as follows:

1. Active at baseline and stayed active during follow-up (*Stay Act*)
2. Active at baseline but became sedentary during the follow-up (*Became Sed*)
3. Sedentary at baseline and remained sedentary at follow-up (*Stay Sed*)
4. Sedentary at baseline but became active at follow-up (*Became Act*)

All-cause mortality data were compared between groups up to 12.5 years following baseline. Compared with sedentary women, those who were active or who became active had lower all-cause mortality. Notably, sedentary women who increased daily physical activity to the equivalent of walking 1 mile between baseline and follow-up had 40% to 50% lower all-cause mortality rates than chronically sedentary women. These findings take on added importance because the population of older women in the United States will double by 2025; more than 33% of these women currently remain sedentary.

SUMMARY

1. Most preventable deaths are attributable to modifiable behaviors that relate directly to physical inactivity, dietary excess, and overfatness.
2. Unless curtailed, the increasing trend of overfatness, poor diet, and physical inactivity will overtake cigarette smoking as the leading preventable cause of mortality.
3. Life-extending benefits of physical activity correlate more with preventing early mortality than improving overall life span.
4. The greatest reduction in death rate from cardiovascular disease occurs when going from the most sedentary to a moderate fitness level.
5. Sedentary white women who increase their physical activity level to the equivalent of walking about 1 mile daily exhibit 40% to 50% lower all-cause mortality rates than chronically sedentary counterparts.

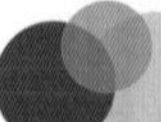

THINK IT THROUGH

1. If regular physical activity contributes little to overall life span, what other reasons exist for maintaining a physically active lifestyle throughout middle and old age?

● KEY TERMS

Adrenal cortex: Gland that mediates the stress response through mineralocorticoid (aldosterone) and glucocorticoid (cortisol) production.

Adrenopause: Decrease in adrenal cortex output of dehydroepiandrosterone (DHEA) and its sulfated ester (DHEAS).

Andropause: Male menopause characterized by age-related decreases in gonadotropic secretions from the anterior pituitary gland.

Angina pectoris: Temporary chest pains from inadequate myocardial blood perfusion.

Apolipoprotein [Apo]: High-density lipoprotein that plays a key role in cholesterol transport.

Cardiac arrest: Unexpected loss of heart function, breathing, and consciousness, resulting from disruption of the heart's pumping action with cessation of blood flow throughout the body.

Cytokines: Proteins secreted by immune cells, some of which stimulate plaque buildup, while others inhibit plaque formation.

C-reactive protein, CRP: Plasma protein that increases during the inflammation response to tissue injury or infection.

Death rate: Number of deaths per 100 in a specific age group: Study the vital statistics of human populations (e.g., births, deaths, ages, diseases, marriages, population density).

Dehydroepiandrosterone: Abbreviated DHEA; adrenal gland steroid hormone converted into testosterone and estrogen.

Demographers: Individuals who study the characteristics of human populations (size, growth, density, distribution, and vital statistics).

Diabetes mellitus: Group of metabolic diseases resulting in higher than normal blood sugar levels.

Diabetic dyslipidemia: Major underlying risk factor of abnormal blood lipids in the presence of T2DM, which contributes to additional cardiovascular disease risk.

Diastolic hypertension: Elevated resting diastolic blood pressure (DBP) above normal.

Exercise: Planned, structured, repetitive, and purposeful physical activity.

Fibrinogen: Circulating glycoprotein acting at the final stage in the coagulation response (blood clotting) to vascular tissue injury.

Gerontologists: Researchers who deal with aging and the related problems of aged persons.

Glucocorticoid: Class of steroid hormones that bind to the glucocorticoid receptor present in almost every vertebrate animal cell to mediate the stress response and help reestablish homeostasis.

Health: Physical, mental, and social well-being; not simply disease absence.

Health-related physical fitness: Physical fitness components associated with an aspect of good health or disease prevention.

Healthspan: Total number of years a person remains in excellent health.

Healthy life expectancy (HALE): Number of years a person can expect to live in "full health"; considers years of ill health weighted according to severity and subtracted from expected overall life expectancy to compute the equivalent years of healthy life.

Healthy People 2020: Fourth-generation established goals and objectives with a 10-year target to guide national health promotion and disease prevention efforts to improve Americans' health.

HLE: Remaining healthy years of life beginning at age 65.

Homocysteine: Highly reactive, sulfur-containing amino acid formed as a by-product of methionine metabolism; high levels constitute significant health risk.

Hyperlipidemia: Abnormally elevated blood lipid level.

Hyperlipoproteinemias: Abnormally elevated levels of blood lipids and/or lipoproteins.

Inflammatory response: Complex biological response of vascular tissues to harmful pathogens, damaged cells, or irritants, with classical signs of pain, heat, redness, swelling, and loss of function.

Insulin resistance: Physiological condition in which cells fail to respond adequately to insulin's normal functions.

Lecithin acetyl transferase (LCAT): Endoplasmic reticulum intracellular protein that forms cholesterol esters from cholesterol.

Lipoprotein(a) [Lp(a)]: LDL-like particle largely under genetic control that varies substantially between individuals depending on apo(a) isoform size.

Lipoproteins: Biochemical structures containing both proteins and lipids that allow fats to move through intracellular and extracellular cell fluids.

Longevity: Length of life.

Menopause: Cessation of menses in aging women from factors that decrease ovarian output of estradiol.

Mineralocorticoid: Class of steroid hormones characterized by their influence on salt (sodium and potassium) and water balance. Aldosterone, the most physiologically important of these hormones, regulates sodium reabsorption in the kidneys' distal tubules.

Necrosis: Tissue or cell death.

New gerontology: Area of study that goes beyond age-related diseases and their prevention to recognize that successful aging requires maintenance of enhanced physiologic function and physical fitness.

Oldest-old: People age 80 to 85 and older.

Physical activity: Body movement produced by muscle action to increase energy expenditure.

Physical activity epidemiology: Applies the general research strategies of epidemiology to study physical activity as a health-related behavior linked to disease and other outcome measures.

Physical activity pyramid: Pyramid showing major goals to increase the level of regular physical activity in the general population, emphasizing diverse behavioral and lifestyle options.

Physical fitness: Attributes related to how well one performs physical activity.

Prediabetes: The "gray area" between normal and diabetic blood sugar levels.

Proinflammatory cytokines: Small cytokine proteins crucial in cell signaling, and also important in promoting systemic inflammation.

Sarcopenia: Component of the frailty syndrome emphasizing degenerative skeletal muscle mass loss after age 25 from muscle fiber and motor unit atrophy.

Sedentary Environmental Death Syndrome (SeDS): Condition that denotes a collection of disorders directly caused by or worsened by physical inactivity.

Somatopause: Mean pulse amplitude, duration, and fraction of secreted growth hormone that gradually decrease with aging.

Systolic hypertension: Elevated resting systolic blood pressure (SBP) above normal.

Telomeres: Region of repetitive nucleotide sequences at each end of a chromatid; protects chromosome ends from deterioration or fusion with nearby chromosomes.

Thrombus: Blood clot that forms inside a blood vessel and obstructs blood flow.

Thyroxine: Thyroid gland hormone that regulates the body's overall metabolism.

Toll-like receptor 2 (TLR-2): Specialized molecules residing on immune cell surfaces that switch on immune cells when the body encounters stress.

Vulnerable patient: Individuals with high likelihood of developing a traumatic cardiac event.

Vulnerable plaque: Soft type of metabolically active, unstable plaque (macrophages and lipids) that accumulates in arterial walls.

Young-old: People ages 65 to 74.

SELECTED REFERENCES

Aagaard P, et al. Mechanical muscle function, morphology, and fiber type in lifelong trained elderly. *Med Sci Sports Exerc* 2007;39:1989.

ADA/ACSM. ADA/ACSM diabetes mellitus and exercise joint position paper. *Med Sci Sports Exerc* 1997;29:I.

Albert CM, et al. Triggering of sudden death from cardiac causes by vigorous exertion. *N Engl J Med* 2000;9:343.

Alihanoglu YI, et al. The association between coronary flow rate and impaired heart rate recovery in patient with metabolic syndrome: a preliminary report. *Cardiol J* 2014;21:257.

Always SE, Siu PM. Nuclear apoptosis contributes to sarcopenia. *Exerc Sport Sci Rev* 2008;36:51.

American College of Sports Medicine and American Heart Association. Joint position statement. Exercise and acute cardiovascular events: placing the risks into perspective. *Med Sci Sports Exerc* 2007;9:886.

American College of Sports Medicine. ACSM position stand on exercise and type 2 diabetes. *Med Sci Sports Exerc* 2000;32:1345.

American College of Sports Medicine. ACSM position stand on physical activity and bone health. *Med Sci Sports Exerc* 2004;36:1985.

Andrews NP, et al. Telomeres and immunological diseases of aging. *Gerontology* 2010;56:390.

Archer E, Blair SN. Implausible data, false memories, and the status quo in dietary assessment. *Adv Nutr* 2015;6:229.

Baker J, et al. Physical activity and successful aging in Canadian older adults. *J Aging Phys Act* 2009;17:223.

Bala G, Cosyns B. Recent advances in visualizing vulnerable plaque: focus on noninvasive molecular imaging. *Curr Cardiol Rep* 2014;16:520.

Banda JA, et al. Protective health factors and incident hypertension in men. *Am J Hypertens* 2010;23:599.

Barnes DE, et al. Physical activity and dementia: the need for prevention trials. *Exerc Sport Sci Rev* 2007;35:24.

Blackford K, et al. A randomised controlled trial of a physical activity and nutrition program targeting middle-aged adults at risk of metabolic syndrome in a disadvantaged rural community. *BMC Public Health* 2015;15:284.

Blair SN, Connelly JC. How much physical activity should we do? The case for moderate amounts and intensities of physical activity. *Res Q Exerc Sport* 1996;67:193.

Blair SN, et al. Changes in physical fitness and all cause mortality: a prospective study of healthy and unhealthy men. *JAMA* 1995;273:1093.

Blair SN, et al. Energy balance: a crucial issue for exercise and sports medicine. *Br J Sports Med* 2015. In Press as of 07.01.15.

Blair SN, et al. Influences of cardiorespiratory fitness and other precursors on cardiovascular disease and all-cause mortality in men and women. *JAMA* 1996;276:205.

Blair SN, et al. Physical activity, nutrition, and chronic disease. *Med Sci Sports Exerc* 1997;28:335.

Blair SN. Physical activity, physical fitness, and health. *Res Q Exerc Sport* 1993;64:365.

Blake CE, et al. Adults with greater weight satisfaction report more positive health behaviors and have better health status regardless of BMI. *J Obes* 2013;291:371.

Bodegard J, et al. Reasons for terminating an exercise test provide independent prognostic information: 2014 apparently healthy men followed for 26 years. *Eur Heart J* 2005;26:1394.

Bodine SC. Disuse-induced muscle wasting. *Int J Biochem Cell Biol* 2013;45:2200.

Bodine SC. What does the transcriptome signature of resistance exercise tell us about aging and skeletal muscle adaptation? *J Appl Physiol* 2012;112:1621.

Booth FW, et al. Lifetime sedentary living accelerates some aspects of secondary aging. *J Appl Physiol* 2011;111:1497.

Booth FW, et al. Waging war on modern chronic diseases: primary prevention through exercise biology. *J Appl Physiol* 2000;88:774.

Booth FW, Laye MJ. The future: genes, physical activity and health. *Acta Physiol (Oxf)* 2010;199:549.

Borst SE. Interventions for sarcopenia and muscle weakness in older people. *Age Ageing* 2004;33:548.

Bullo V, et al. The effects of Pilates exercise training on physical fitness and wellbeing in the elderly: a systematic review for future exercise prescription. *Prev Med* 2015;75:1.

Carnethon MR, et al. A longitudinal study of physical activity and heart rate recovery: CARDIA, 1987–1993. *Med Sci Sports Exerc* 2005;37:606.

Caspersen CJ, Fulton JE. Epidemiology of walking and type 2 diabetes. *Med Sci Sports Exerc* 2008;40:S519.

Chen FY, et al. Effects of a lifestyle program on risks for cardiovascular disease in women. *Taiwan J Obstet Gynecol* 2009;48:49.

Chomistek AK, et al. Vigorous-intensity leisure-time physical activity and risk of major chronic disease in men. *Med Sci Sports Exerc* 2012;44:1898.

Church TS, et al. Metabolic syndrome and diabetes, alone and in combination, as predictors of cardiovascular disease mortality among men. *Diabetes Care* 2009;32:1289.

Cooper JA, et al. Longitudinal change in energy expenditure and effects on energy requirements of the elderly. *Nutr J* 2013;12:73.

Corrado D, et al. Does sport activity enhance the risk of sudden death in adolescent and young adults? *J Am Coll Cardiol* 2003;42:1959.

Davenport MH, et al. Cerebrovascular reserve: the link between fitness and cognitive function? *Exerc Sport Sci Rev* 2012;40:153.

Davi G, et al. Nutraceuticals in diabetes and metabolic syndrome. *Cardiovasc Ther* 2010;28:216.

Di Angelantonio E, et al. Major lipids, apolipoproteins, and risk of vascular disease. Emerging risk factors collaboration. *JAMA* 2009;302:1993.

Djousse L, et al. Dietary linolenic acid is associated with a lower prevalence of hypertension in the NHLBI Family Heart Study. *Hypertension* 2005; 45:368.

Drenowatz C. Differences in correlates of energy balance in normal weight, overweight and obese adults. *Obes Res Clin Pract* 2015. In Press as of 07.01.15.

Earnest CP, et al. Aerobic and strength training in concomitant metabolic syndrome and type 2 diabetes. *Med Sci Sports Exerc* 2014;46:1293.

Earnest CP, et al. Dose effect of cardiorespiratory exercise on metabolic syndrome in postmenopausal women. *Am J Cardiol* 2013;111:1805.

Elosua R, et al. Dose-response association of physical activity with acute myocardial infarction: do amount and intensity matter? *Prev Med* 2013;57:567.

Elsisi HF, et al. Electromagnetic field versus circuit weight training on bone mineral density in elderly women. *Clin Interv Aging* 2015;10:539.

Esfahani A, et al. Session 4: CVD, diabetes and cancer: a dietary portfolio for management and prevention of heart disease. *Proc Nutr Soc* 2009;8:1.

Fenning RS, Wilensky RL. New insights into the vulnerable plaque from imaging studies. *Curr Atheroscler Rep* 2014;16:397.

Fleg JL, et al. Accelerated longitudinal decline of aerobic capacity in healthy older adults. *Circulation* 2005;112:674.

Fries JF. Aging, natural death and the compression of morbidity. *N Engl J Med* 1980;303:130.

Frimel TN, et al. Exercise attenuates the weight-loss-induced reduction in muscle mass in frail obese older adults. *Med Sci Sports Exerc* 2008;40:1213.

Frontera WR, et al. Aging of skeletal muscle: a 12-yr longitudinal study. *J Appl Physiol* 2000;88:1321.

Gesell SB, et al. Comparative effectiveness of after-school programs to increase physical activity. *J Obes* 2013;576:821.

Golia E, et al. Inflammation and cardiovascular disease: from pathogenesis to therapeutic target. *Curr Atheroscler Rep* 2014;16:435.

Gotsch K, et al. Nonfatal sports- and recreation-related injuries treated in emergency departments—United States, July 2000–June 2001. *MMWR Morb Mortal Wkly Rep* 2002;51:736.

Graham MR, et al. Arterial pulse wave velocity, inflammatory markers, pathological GH and IGF states, cardiovascular and cerebrovascular disease. *Vasc Health Risk Manag* 2008;4:1361.

Greenland P. Improving risk of coronary heart disease: can a picture make the difference. *JAMA* 2003;289:2270.

Greer AE, et al. The effects of sedentary behavior on metabolic syndrome independent of physical activity and cardiorespiratory fitness. *J Phys Act Health* 2015;12:68.

Haskell WL, et al. Physical activity and public health: updated recommendation for adults from the American College of Sports Medicine and the American Heart Association. *Med Sci Sports Exerc* 2006;39:1423.

Hebert JR, et al. Scientific decision making, policy decisions, and the obesity pandemic. *Mayo Clin Proc* 2013;88:593.

Héroux M, et al. Dietary patterns and the risk of mortality: impact of cardiorespiratory fitness. *Int J Epidemiol* 2010;39:197.

Holmes JS, et al. Heart disease and prevention: race and age differences in heart disease prevention, treatment, and mortality. *Med Care* 2005;43:I33.

Hu FB, et al. Trends in the incidence of coronary heart disease and changes in diet and lifestyle in women. *N Engl J Med* 2000;343:530.

Jackson A, et al. Role of lifestyle and aging on the longitudinal changes in cardiorespiratory fitness. *Arch Intern Med* 2009;169:1781.

Jahangir A, Aging and cardioprotection. *J Appl Physiol* 2007;103:2128.

Janssen I, Jolliffe CJ. Influence of physical activity on mortality in elderly with coronary artery disease. *Med Sci Sports Exerc* 2006;38:418.

Johannsen NM, et al. Categorical analysis of the impact of aerobic and resistance exercise training, alone and in combination, on cardiorespiratory fitness levels in patients with type 2 diabetes mellitus: results from the hart-d study. *Diabetes Care* 2013;36:3305.

Jouven X, et al. Heart-rate profile during exercise as a predictor of sudden death. *N Engl J Med* 2005;352:1951.

Kesäniemi A, et al. Advancing the future of physical activity guidelines in Canada: an independent expert panel interpretation of the evidence. *Int J Behav Nutr Phys Act* 2010;7:41.

Kurl S, et al. Cardiac power during exercise and the risk of stroke in men. *Stroke* 2005;36:820.

Kurozawa Y, et al. JACC Study Group Levels of physical activity among participants in the JACC study. *J Epidemiol* 2005;15:S43.

Larose J, et al. Effect of exercise training on physical fitness in type II diabetes mellitus. *Med Sci Sports Exerc* 2010;42:1439.

Lavie CJ, et al. Impact of cardiac rehabilitation on coronary risk factors, inflammation, and the metabolic syndrome in obese coronary patients. *J Cardiometab Syndr* 2008;3:136.

Lee I-M, Buchner DM. The importance of walking to public health. *Med Sci Sports Exerc* 2008;40:S512.

Lee S, et al. Cardiorespiratory fitness attenuates metabolic risk independent of abdominal subcutaneous and visceral fat in men. *Diabetes Care* 2005;28:895.

Leischik R, et al. Pre-participation and follow-up screening of athletes for endurance sport. *J Clin Med Res* 2015;7:385.

Leite JC, et al. Comparison of the effect of multicomponent and resistance training programs on metabolic health parameters in the elderly. *Arch Gerontol Geriatr* 2015;60:412.

Liu R, et al. Cardiorespiratory fitness as a predictor of dementia mortality in men and women. *Med Sci Sports Exerc* 2012;44:253.

Liu-Ambrose T, et al. Resistance training and functional plasticity of the aging brain: a 12-month randomized controlled trial. *Neurobiol Aging* 2012;33:1690.

Lyerly GW, et al. Maximal exercise electrocardiographic responses and coronary heart disease mortality among men with metabolic syndrome. *Mayo Clin Proc* 2010;85:239.

Malin SK, et al. Lower dipeptidyl peptidase-4 following exercise training plus weight loss is related to increased insulin sensitivity in adults with metabolic syndrome. *Peptides* 2013;47:142.

Martinez ME. Primary prevention of colorectal cancer: lifestyle, nutrition, exercise. *Recent Results Cancer Res* 2005;166:177.

McGill HC, et al. Starting earlier to prevent heart disease. *JAMA* 2003;290:2320.

Melk A, et al. Improvement of biological age by physical activity. *Int J Cardiol* 2014;176:1187.

Metzger JS, et al. Patterns of objectively measured physical activity in the United States. *Med Sci Sports Exerc* 2008;40:630.

Miller MG, et al. Aspirin under fire: aspirin use in the primary prevention of coronary heart disease. *Pharmacotherapy* 2005;25:847.

Mitchell JA, et al. The impact of combined health factors on cardiovascular disease mortality. *Am Heart J* 2010;160:102.

Moholdt T, et al. Physical activity and mortality in men and women with coronary heart disease: a prospective population-based cohort study in Norway (the HUNT study). *Eur J Cardiovasc Prev Rehabil* 2008;15:639.

Moliner-Urdiales D, et al. Body adiposity index and all-cause and cardiovascular disease mortality in men. *Nutr Metab Cardiovasc* 2014;24:969.

Monaco C, et al. Toll-like receptor-2 mediates inflammation and matrix degradation in human atherosclerosis. *Circulation* 2009;120:2462.

Morris JN, et al. Coronary heart disease and physical activity of work. *Lancet* 1953;265:1053.

Morris JN. Exercise in the prevention of coronary heart disease: today's best bet in public health. *Med Sci Sports Exerc* 1994;26:807.

Mujica V, et al. Intervention with education and exercise reverses the metabolic syndrome in adults. *J Am Soc Hypertens* 2010;4:148.

Nader PR, et al. Moderate-to-vigorous physical activity from ages 9 to 15 years. *JAMA* 2008;30:295.

Naghavi M, et al. From vulnerable plaque to vulnerable patient: a call for new definitions and risk assessment strategies: part II. *Circulation* 2003;108:1772.

Naghavi M. From vulnerable plaque to vulnerable patient: part III: executive summary of the Screening for Heart Attack Prevention and Education (SHAPE) Task Force report. *Am J Cardiol* 2006;98:2H.

Nelson R. Exercise could prevent cerebral changes associated with AD. *Lancet Neurol* 2005;4:275.

Oeppen J, Vaupel JW. Broken limits to life expectancy. *Science* 2002;296:1029.

Olshansky SJ, et al. Prospects for longevity. *Science* 2001;291:1491.

Ornish D, et al. Intensive lifestyle changes for reversal of coronary heart disease. *JAMA* 1998;280:2001.

Panagiotakos DB, et al. The association between lifestyle-related factors and plasma homocysteine levels in healthy individuals from the "ATTICA" Study. *J Cardiol* 2005;98:471.

Panagiotakos DB, Polychronopoulos E. The role of Mediterranean diet in the epidemiology of metabolic syndrome; converting epidemiology to clinical practice. *Lipids Health Dis* 2005;4:7.

Pandey A, et al. Cardiac determinants of heterogeneity in fitness change in response to moderate intensity aerobic exercise training: the DREW study. *J Am Coll Cardiol* 2015;65:1057.

Parker BA, et al. Sex-specific influence of aging on exercising leg blood flow. *J Appl Physiol* 2008;104:655.

Pedersen BK. Muscle as a secretory organ. *Compr Physiol* 2013;3:1337.

Pessana F, et al. Subclinical atherosclerosis modeling: integration of coronary artery calcium score to Framingham equation. *Conf Proc IEEE Eng Med Biol Soc* 2009;1:5348.

Phillips AC, et al. Stress and exercise: getting the balance right for aging immunity. *Exerc Sport Sci Rev* 2007;35:35.

Pollock ML, et al. Twenty-year follow-up of aerobic power and body composition of older track athletes. *J Appl Physiol* 1997;82:1508.

Pusceddu I, et al. The role of telomeres and vitamin D in cellular aging and age-related diseases. *Clin Chem Lab Med* 2015. In Press as of 07.01.15.

Ramsey F, et al. Prevalence of selected risk behaviors and chronic diseases—Behavioral Risk Factor Surveillance System (BRFSS), 39 steps communities, United States, 2005. *MMWR Morb Mortal Wkly Rep* 2008;57:1.

Ridker PM, et al. C-reactive protein levels and outcomes after statin therapy. *N Engl J Med* 2005;352:20.

Rimm EB, Stampfer MJ. Diet, lifestyle, and longevity—the next step. *JAMA* 2004;292:1490.

Robinson JG, Maheshwari N. A "poly-portfolio" for secondary prevention: a strategy to reduce subsequent events by up to 97% over five years. *Am J Cardiol* 2005;95:373.

Rosenberg L, et al. Physical activity and the incidence of obesity in young African-American women. *Am J Prev Med* 2013;45:262.

Salem GJ, et al. ACSM position stand on exercise and physical activity for older adults. *Med Sci Sports Exerc* 2009;41:1510.

Schnohr P, et al. Longevity in male and female joggers: the Copenhagen City Heart Study. *Am J Epidemiol* 2013;177:683.

Schoeller DA, et al. Self-report-based estimates of energy intake offer an inadequate basis for scientific conclusions. *Am J Clin Nutr* 2013;97:1413.

Schweiger B, et al. Physical activity in adolescent females with type 1 diabetes. *Intern J Pediatr* 2010;328:318.

Sénéchal M, et al. Changes in body fat distribution and fitness are associated with changes in hemoglobin a1c after 9 months of exercise training: results from the hart-d study. *Diabetes Care* 2013;36:2843.

Sharma S, et al. Exercise and the heart: the good, the bad, and the ugly. *Eur Heart J* 2015. In Press as of 06.28.15.

Shephard RJ. Maximal oxygen intake and independence in old age. *Br J Sports Med* 2008;40:1058.

Shook RP, et al. Low fitness partially explains resting metabolic rate differences between African American and white women. *Am J Med* 2014; 127:436.

Simon A, et al. Differences between markers of atherogenic lipoproteins in predicting high cardiovascular risk and subclinical atherosclerosis in asymptomatic men. *Atherosclerosis* 2005;179:339.

Sjögren P, et al. Stand up for health—avoiding sedentary behaviour might lengthen your telomeres: secondary outcomes from a physical activity RCT in older people. *Br J Sports Med* 2014;48:1407.

Slentz CA, et al. Modest exercise prevents the progressive disease associated with physical inactivity. *Exerc Sport Sci Rev* 2007;35:18.

Smith DA, et al. Abdominal diameter index: a more powerful anthropometric measure for prevalent coronary heart disease risk in adult males. *Diabetes Obes Metab* 2005;7:370.

Spirduso WW, Clifford P. Replication of age and physical activity effects on reaction and movement time. *J Gerontol* 1978;33:26.

Stanner S. Diet and lifestyle measures to protect the ageing heart. *Br J Community Nurs* 2009;14:210.

Stefan MA, et al. Effect of activity restriction owing to heart disease on obesity. *Arch Pediatr Adolesc Med* 2005;159:477.

Swift DL, et al. The role of exercise and physical activity in weight loss and maintenance. *Prog Cardiovasc Dis* 2014;56:441.

Talbot LA, et al. Army Physical Fitness Test scores predict coronary heart disease risk in Army National Guard soldiers. *Mil Med* 2009;174:245.

Tanaka H. Swimming exercise: impact of aquatic exercise on cardiovascular health. *Sports Med* 2009;39:377.

Thomas NE, et al. Relationship of fitness, fatness, and coronary-heart-disease risk factors in 12- to 13-year-olds. *Pediatr Exerc Sci* 2007;19:93.

Thorp AA, et al. Independent and joint associations of TV viewing time and snack food consumption with the metabolic syndrome and its components; a cross-sectional study in Australian adults. *Int J Behav Nutr Phys Act* 2013;10:96.

Tota-Maharaj R, et al. A practical approach to the metabolic syndrome: review of current concepts and management. *Curr Opin Cardiol* 2010;22:502.

Tousoulis D. Innate and adaptive inflammation as a therapeutic target in vascular disease: the emerging role of statins. *J Am Coll Cardiol* 2014;63:2491.

Tully MA, et al. Brisk walking, fitness, and cardiovascular risk: a randomized controlled trial in primary care. *Prev Med* 2005;41:622.

Van den Hoogen PC, et al. Blood pressure and long-term coronary heart disease mortality in the Seven Countries study: implications for clinical practice and public health. *Eur Heart J* 2000;21:1639.

Visser M, et al. Muscle mass, muscle strength, and muscle fat infiltration as predictors of incident mobility limitations in well-functioning older persons. *J Gerontol A Biol Sci Med Sci* 2005;60:324.

Weiss EP, et al. Gender differences in the decline in aerobic capacity and its physiological determinants during the later decades of life. *J Appl Physiol* 2006;101:938.

Wijndaele K, et al. Utilization and harmonization of adult accelerometry data: Review and expert consensus. *Med Sci Sports Exerc* 2015. In Press as of 07.01.15.

Williams AJ, et al. Systematic review and meta-analysis of the association between childhood overweight and obesity and primary school diet and physical activity policies. *Int J Behav Nutr Phys Act* 2013;10:101.

Williams PT. Physical fitness and activity as separate heart disease risk factors: a meta-analysis. *Exerc Sport Sci Rev* 2001;33:754.

Williams PT. Reduced diabetic, hypertensive, and cholesterol medication use with walking. *Med Sci Sports Exerc* 2008;40:433.

Williams PT. Vigorous exercise, fitness and incident hypertension, high cholesterol, and diabetes. *Med Sci Sports Exerc* 2008;40:998.

Yanez ND, et al. CHS Collaborative Research Group; Sibling history of myocardial infarction or stroke and risk of cardiovascular disease in the elderly: the Cardiovascular Health Study. *Ann Epidemiol* 2009;19:858.

Young DR, et al. Physical activity, cardiorespiratory fitness, and their relationship to cardiovascular risk factors in African Americans and non-African Americans with above-optimal blood pressure. *J Community Health* 2005; 30:107.

CHAPTER 18

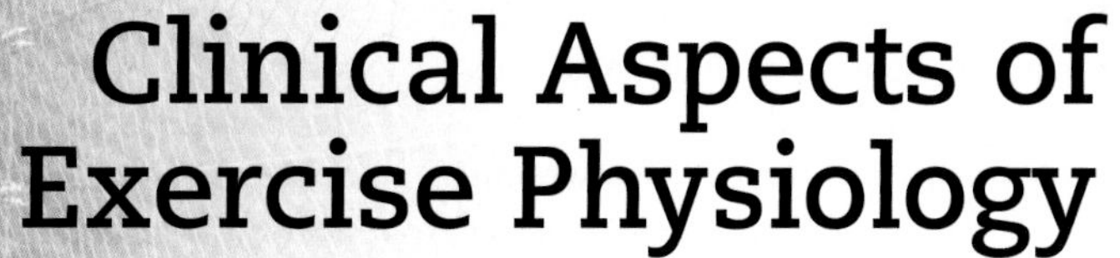

Clinical Aspects of Exercise Physiology

CHAPTER OBJECTIVES

- Discuss three roles of an exercise physiologist and health and fitness professional in the clinical setting.
- List six clinical areas and corresponding diseases and disorders in which physical activity (exercise) as therapy exerts a positive influence.
- List three different diseases of the myocardium.
- Categorize two diseases that affect heart valves and the cardiac nervous system.
- Describe four major steps in cardiac disease assessment.
- List three different laboratory-based coronary heart disease (CHD) screening tools.
- List three reasons to include stress testing to evaluate CHD.
- List four indicators of CHD during an exercise stress test.
- Give two advantages and two limitations of different modes of exercise for graded exercise stress testing.
- Define the following terms for stress test results: *true positive*, *false negative*, *true negative*, and *false positive*.
- List four reasons for stopping an exercise stress test.
- Outline the approach for individualizing an "exercise prescription."
- Give two advantages and two disadvantages of submaximal versus maximal exercise stress testing.
- Describe four different stress test protocols.
- Discuss the role of physical activity and exercise prescription in pulmonary rehabilitation.
- Describe the role of exercise to diagnose and treat five cardiovascular system diseases and disorders.
- Describe the role of exercise in the diagnosis and treatment for four neuromuscular system diseases and disorders.
- List four common symptoms of chronic renal disease and three roles of regular physical activity in rehabilitating dialysis and kidney transplant patients.
- Describe three roles of exercise in cancer diagnosis and treatment.
- Describe three roles of exercise in depression diagnosis and treatment.

ANCILLARIES AT A GLANCE

Visit **http://thePoint.lww.com/MKKESS5e** to access the following resources.

- References: Chapter 18
- Interactive Question Bank
- Appendix SR-6: Additional Video Links
- Animation: Asthma
- Animation: Congestive Heart Failure
- Animation: Coronary Angiography: Left Coronary System-Part A
- Animation: Coronary Angiography: Left Coronary System-Part B
- Animation: Edema
- Animation: Stroke

The value and contributions of regular physical activity to the prevention of disease have been acclaimed in diverse allied health fields, including injury rehabilitation therapy. Regular physical activity also serves as a key adjunctive modality for many medically related disorders. This chapter focuses on the role the exercise physiologist plays in understanding mechanisms by which physical activity improves health and physical fitness to enhance patient rehabilitation in those challenged by chronic disease and disability.

The World Health Organization (WHO; **www.who.int***) defines* **health** *as "a state of complete physical, mental and social well-being, not merely the absence of disease and infirmity."* This definition considers good health an ability to complete physical tasks successfully and maintain functional independence. The clinical exercise physiologist plays an integral role in the team approach to good health and to total patient care. The exercise physiologist has an expanded role in clinical practice because of fundamental relationships among measures of functional capacity, physical fitness, and overall good health. In the clinical setting, the exercise physiologist, working closely with physical therapists, occupational therapists, and physicians, focuses primarily on restoring patient mobility and functional capacity. **Table 18.1** highlights the positive influences of clinical applications of physical activity interventions on a range of medical and health conditions.

PART 1 The Clinical Exercise Physiologist: A Vital Link Between Sports Medicine and Exercise Physiology

One traditional view of **sports medicine** concerns rehabilitating athletes from sports-related injuries. In its broader context, sports medicine relates to scientific and medical aspects of physical activity, physical fitness, health, and sports performance. The WHO defines *physical fitness* as the ability to perform muscular work satisfactorily. This definition encompasses an individual's capacity to perform physical activity at work, at home, or on the athletic field. Sports medicine closely links to clinical exercise physiology because the sports medicine profession treats a broad spectrum of individuals. Individuals with low functional capacity recovering from injury, disease, and medical interventions comprise one end of the continuum; the other extreme encompasses healthy, able-bodied, and disabled athletes with well-developed levels of total body fitness. Carefully prescribed physical activity contributes to overall good health and quality of life for this broad spectrum of individuals (**Table 18.2**).

TRAINING AND CERTIFICATION PROGRAMS FOR PROFESSIONAL EXERCISE PHYSIOLOGISTS

Since the early 1970s, regular physical activity has gained widespread acceptance as an integral part of rehabilitative programs of care and health maintenance for a growing list of chronic diseases and disabling conditions. Expanding public interest in physical activity for health promotion has stimulated a parallel need to certify qualified professionals to provide sound advice and supervision regarding physical activities for preventative and rehabilitative purposes. Competency-based certification at a given level requires a knowledge and skills base commensurate with that specific certification.

In 1975, the **American College of Sports Medicine (ACSM; www.acsm.org)** initiated the first ACSM Clinical and Health/Fitness Certification program; today, ACSM continues to be the preeminent organization to offer certification programs, resources, and continuing education credits (CEUs or CECs) to support the professional growth of health and fitness professionals. ACSM sponsors three different certifications:

1. **Health Fitness Certifications**—tailored towards fitness professional working in a health club or other

TABLE 18.1 Clinical Areas and Corresponding Diseases and Disorders Where Exercise Therapy Applies

Cardiovascular diseases and disorders	Ischemia, chronic heart failure, dyslipidemias, cardiomyopathies, cardiac valvular disease, heart transplantation, congenital abnormalities
Pulmonary diseases and disorders	Chronic obstructive pulmonary disease, cystic fibrosis, asthma, exercise-induced asthma
Neuromuscular diseases and disorders	Stroke, multiple sclerosis, Parkinson disease, Alzheimer disease, polio, cerebral palsy
Metabolic diseases and disorders	Obesity (adult and pediatric), diabetes, renal disease, menstrual dysfunction
Immunologic and hematologic diseases and disorder	Cancer, breast cancer, immune deficiency, allergies, sickle cell disease, HIV, AIDS
Orthopedic diseases and disorders	Osteoporosis, osteoarthritis and rheumatoid arthritis, back pain, sports injuries
Aging	Sarcopenia
Cognitive and emotional disorders	Anxiety and stress disorders, mental retardation, depression

TABLE 18.2 Health Benefits of Regular Physical Activity[a]

Physical Activity Benefit	Surety Rating	Physical Activity Benefit	Surety Rating
Fitness of Body		**Cigarette Smoking**	
Improves heart and lung function	****	Improves success in quitting	**
Improves muscular strength/size	****	**Diabetes**	
Cardiovascular Disease		Prevention of type 2	****
Coronary heart disease prevention	***	Treatment of type 2	****
Regression of atherosclerosis	**	Treatment of type 1	*
Treatment of heart disease	***	Improvement in diabetic's life quality	***
Prevention of stroke	**	**Infection and Immunity**	
Cancer		Prevention of the common cold	**
Prevention of colon cancer	****	Improves overall immunity	**
Prevention of breast cancer	**	Slows progression of HIV to AIDS	*
Prevention of uterine cancer	**	Improves life quality of HIV-infected persons	****
Prevention of prostate cancer	**	**Arthritis**	
Prevention of other cancer	*	Prevention of arthritis	*
Treatment of cancer	*	Treatment/cure of arthritis	*
Osteoporosis		Improvement of life quality/fitness	****
Helps increase bone mass and density	****	**High Blood Pressure**	
Prevention of osteoporosis	***	Prevention of high blood pressure	****
Treatment of osteoporosis	**	Treatment of high blood pressure	****
Blood Cholesterol/Lipoproteins		**Asthma**	
Lowers blood total cholesterol	*	Prevention/treatment of asthma	*
Lowers LDL cholesterol	*	Improvement in asthmatic's life quality	***
Lower s triacylglycerols	***	**Sleep**	
Raises HDL cholesterol	***	Improvement in sleep quality	***
Low Back Pain		**Psychological Well-Being**	
Prevention of low back pain	**	Elevation in mood	****
Treatment of low back pain	**	Buffers effects of mental stress	***
Nutrition and Diet Quality		Alleviates/prevents depression	****
Improvement in diet quality	**	Anxiety reduction	**
Increase in total energy intake	***	Improves self-esteem	****
Weight Management		**Special Issues for Women**	
Prevention of weight gain	****	Improves total body fitness	****
Treatment of obesity	**	Improves fitness while pregnant	****
Helps maintain weight loss	***	Improves birthing experience	**
Children and Youth		Improves health of fetus	**
Prevention of obesity	***	Improves health during menopause	***
Controls disease risk factors	***		
Reduction of unhealthy habits	**		
Improves odds of adult activity	**		
Older Adults and the Aging Process			
Improvement in physical fitness	****		
Counters loss in heart/lung fitness	**		
Counters loss of muscle	***		
Counters gain in fat	***		
Improvement in life expectancy	****		
Improvement in life quality	****		

****	Strong consensus with little or no conflicting data.
***	Most data supportive, but more research required for clarification.
**	Some supportive data, but much more research needed.
*	Little or no data to support.

[a]Based on a total physical fitness program that includes physical activity to improve aerobic and musculoskeletal fitness.

From Newman CC. The human body. *ACSM's Health Fitness J* 1998;2:30.

community setting. The Health Fitness category includes three separate certifications:

a. **Certified Personal Trainer (CPT)**: CPTs are qualified to plan and implement exercise programs for healthy individuals or those who have medical clearance to exercise. The CPT facilitates motivation and adherence as well as develops and administers programs designed to enhance muscular strength, endurance, flexibility, cardiorespiratory fitness, body composition, and/or any of the motor skills related components of physical fitness.
b. **Certified Exercise Physiologist (EP-C)-** EP-Cs are health fitness professionals with a minimum

of a bachelor's degree in exercise science. The individual performs pre-participation health screenings, conducts physical fitness assessments, interprets results, develops exercise prescriptions, and applies behavioral and motivational strategies to apparently healthy individuals and individuals with medically controlled diseases and health conditions to support clients in adopting and maintaining healthy lifestyle behaviors. EP-Cs are typically employed or self-employed in commercial, community, studio, corporate, university, and hospital settings. They take personal training to an advanced level by working with individuals with medically controlled diseases, and have mastered the necessary skills to perform pre-exercise health risk assessments and conduct physical fitness assessments.

c. **Certified Group Exercise Instructor (GEI)**: GEIs become familiar with various exercise techniques, and can supervise participants or lead instructional sessions. The GEI works in a group exercise setting with apparently healthy individuals and those with health challenges who are able to exercise independently to improve health-related physical fitness, manage health risk, and promote lasting health behavior change.

2. **Clinical Certifications**—tailored towards fitness professionals serving those with cardiovascular, orthopedic, pulmonary, and metabolic diseases or disabilities in cardiovascular or pulmonary rehabilitation programs, physicians' offices, medical fitness centers, and other public settings. Two separate certifications fall within the Clinical Certification category:

a. **Certified Clinical Exercise Physiologist (CEP):** The CEP works with clients challenged with cardiovascular, pulmonary, and metabolic diseases, as well as with apparently healthy populations in

A CLOSER LOOK

What's in a Name?

A lack of unanimity exists for the name of the departments offering degrees or even coursework in exercise physiology. This box lists examples of 49 names of departments in the United States that offer essentially the same area of study. Each provides some undergraduate or graduate emphasis in exercise physiology (e.g., one or several courses, internships, work-study programs, laboratory rotations, or in-service programs).

Allied Health Sciences	Movement and Exercise Science
Exercise and Movement Science	Movement Studies
Exercise and Sport Science	Nutrition and Exercise Science
Exercise and Sport Studies	Nutritional and Health Sciences
Exercise Science	Performance and Sport Science
Exercise Science and Human Movement	Physical Culture
Exercise Science and Physical Therapy	Physical Education
Health and Human Performance	Physical Education and Exercise Science
Health and Physical Education	Physical Education and Human Movement
Health, Physical Education, Recreation, and Dance	Physical Education and Sport Programs
Human Biodynamics	Physical Education and Sport Science
Human Kinetics	Physical Therapy
Human Kinetics and Health	Recreation
Human Movement	Recreation and Wellness Programs
Human Movement Sciences	Science of Human Movement
Human Movement Studies	Sport and Exercise Science
Human Movement Studies and Physical Education	Sport Management
Human Performance	Sport, Exercise, and Leisure Science
Human Performance and Health Promotion	Sports Science
Human Performance and Leisure Studies	Sport Science and Leisure Studies
Human Performance and Sport Science	Sport Science and Movement Education
Interdisciplinary Health Studies	Sport Studies
Integrative Biology	Wellness and Fitness
Kinesiology	Wellness Education
Kinesiology and Exercise Science	

cooperation with other healthcare professions. CEPs enhance quality of life, manage health risk, and promote lasting healthy behavior change of their clients. They also educate clients about testing, exercise program components, and self-care for control of chronic disease and health conditions.

b. **Registered Clinical Exercise Physiologist (RCEP)**: RCEPs apply physical activity and behavioral interventions that have been shown to provide therapeutic and/or functional benefit for those with chronic diseases or disabilities. The RCEP provides prevention and rehabilitative strategies designed to improve physical fitness and health across the lifespan.

3. **Specialty Certifications**: Specialty Certifications are for those who already have an NCAA accredited certification to work with special-needs clients, including clients of different fitness levels, individuals affected by cancer, and those with disabilities, and to promote physical activity in public health at national, state and local levels. Five separate certifications fall within this category:
   a. **Exercise Is Medicine Credential (EIM)**: The EIM credential provides exercise professionals with the opportunity to work closely with the medical community. EIMs provide additional benefits to the certified professional, including a respected credential to work with individuals who are healthy, those with health-related conditions who have been cleared by a physician for exercise (level 1 or 2), and for patients who require clinical support and monitoring (level 3).
   b. **ACSM/American Cancer Society (ACS) Certified Cancer Exercise Trainer (CET)**: This specialty certification allows fitness professionals to work with clients who have been cleared by their physician for independent exercise and physical activity. CETs use their knowledge to develop exercise programs for clients making lifestyle changes caused by cancer and related treatments.
   c. **ACSM/National Center on Health, Physical Activity and Disability (NCHPAD) Certified Inclusive Fitness Trainer (CIFT)**: CIFTs master an understanding of exercise precautions for people with disabilities, and utilize safe, effective and adapted methods of exercise training to provide exercise recommendations. CIFTs provide services with an understanding of current ADA policy specific to recreation facilities (U.S. Access Board Guidelines) and standards for accessible facility design.
   d. **ACSM/National Physical Activity Society (NPAS) Certified Physical Activity Public Health Specialist (PAPHS)**: The PAPHS promotes physical activity with a focus on the public health setting. They develop key partnerships to establish legislation, policies, and programs that promote physical activity for people nationwide.

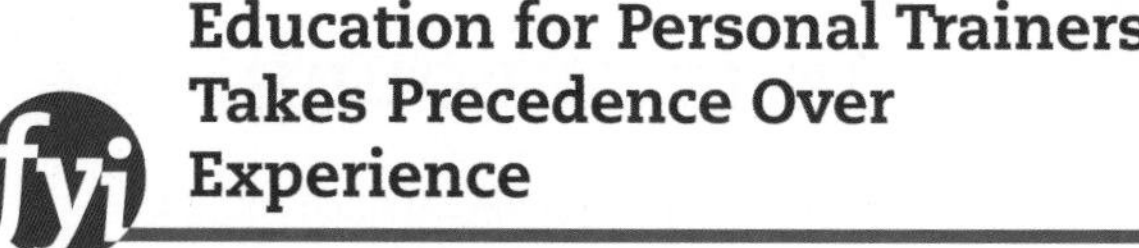

Education for Personal Trainers Takes Precedence Over Experience

UCLA researchers in 2002 administered questionnaires concerning commonly used indicators of fitness knowledge (training and experience) and actual knowledge in the five areas of nutrition, health screening, testing protocols, exercise prescription, and general training knowledge regarding special populations to 115 health fitness professionals from Southern California who represented 28 health club facilities, local colleges, or were self employed. The results revealed that a bachelor's degree in the field of exercise science or related discipline and possession of American College of Sports Medicine (**www.acsm.org**) or National Strength and Conditioning Association (**www.nsca.com/certification/**) certifications as opposed to other certifications were strong predictors of a personal trainer's knowledge, whereas years of experience did not translate into more knowledge. Personal trainers with 5 or more years of experience had no greater knowledge than trainers with 4 or fewer years of experience. A study in 2010 reported that, based on a review of 634 citation sources from 95 articles, fitness trainers holding higher levels of education relied more on evidence-based information (e.g., scientific journals) compared to those with lower education levels, who relied more on mass media sources.

Source: Malek MH, et al. Importance of health science education for personal fitness trainers. *J Strength Cond Res* 2002;16:19.

Stacey D, et al. Knowledge translation to fitness trainers: a systematic review. *Implement Sci* 2010;5:28.

In addition to its certifications, ACSM sponsors international workshops and courses in several European countries as well as supporting the older Program Director and Health Fitness Director certifications that are no longer being offered.

In the sections that follow, we present clinical applications of exercise physiology for cardiovascular diseases, pulmonary system disabilities, neuromuscular diseases and disorders, renal disease, cancers, oncology, and cognitive and emotional diseases and disorders. We focus on these disabilities because they are the ones with which the clinical exercise physiologist primarily works.

SUMMARY

1. A clinical exercise physiologist becomes part of a team approach in the clinical setting for comprehensive patient health care. The clinical exercise physiologist focuses on restoring the patient's mobility and functional capacity.
2. Expanding public interest in physical activity for health promotion has stimulated a parallel need to certify qualified professionals to provide sound advice and supervision regarding physical activities for preventative and rehabilitative purposes.
3. The American College of Sports Medicine sponsors health fitness, clinical and specialty certifications programs for Professional Exercise Physiologists.

THINK IT THROUGH

1. Do you believe individuals who have trained for years with weights and other devices should be required to obtain certification from a reputable agency before calling themselves a "personal trainer" and charging for their services?
2. Should a personal trainer certification require an undergraduate college degree in a health-related field?

PART 2 Cardiovascular Diseases and Disorders

Diseases of the cardiovascular system account for the greatest number of deaths in industrialized nations (see Chapter 17). Because increased physical activity represents a prudent first line of defense to combat cardiovascular diseases, exercise physiologists need to be familiar with all aspects of this disease category. **Table 18.3** lists diseases that affect the following three categories of heart disease and lead to functional disability:

1. Diseases affecting the heart muscle
2. Diseases affecting the heart valves
3. Diseases affecting the cardiac nervous system

Diseases of the Heart Muscle

Diseases of the myocardium become prevalent with advancing age. These conditions may be known as **degenerative heart disease (DHD), atherosclerotic cardiovascular disease, arteriosclerotic cardiovascular disease, coronary artery disease (CAD), and coronary heart disease (CHD).**

TABLE 18.3 Three Categories of Heart Disease That Lead to Functional Disability

Diseases Affecting the Heart Muscle	Diseases Affecting the Heart Valves	Diseases Affecting the Cardiac Nervous System
Congestive heart disease	Rheumatic fever	Arrhythmias
Angina	Endocarditis	Tachycardia
Myocardial infarction	Mitral valve prolapse	Bradycardia
Pericarditis	Congenital malformations	
Congestive heart failure		
Aneurysms		

Advances in molecular biology have isolated possible genetic links to CHD. One of these genes (on chromosome 19 near the gene related to low-density lipoprotein cholesterol [LDL-C] receptor functioning), called the **atherosclerosis susceptibility gene (*ATHS*)**, accounts for about 50% of all CHD cases. The *ATHS* gene causes a set of characteristics that triples a person's risk of **myocardial infarction (MI)**. These include abdominal obesity and low HDL-C (high-density lipoprotein cholesterol) and high LDL-C levels.

thePoint® Appendix SR-6: Additional Video Links, available online at **http://thePoint.lww.com/MKKESS5e**, provides a list of supplemental animations and videos on this subject.

CHD pathogenesis progresses in five stages:

Stage 1. Injury to the coronary artery's endothelial cell wall
Stage 2. Fibroblastic proliferation of the artery's inner lining or intima
Stage 3. Accumulation of lipids at the junction of the arterial intima and middle lining, further obstructing blood flow
Stage 4. Deterioration followed by formation of hyaline, a clear, homogeneous substance formed during degeneration in the vessel's intima
Stage 5. Calcium deposition at the edges of the hyalinated area

Diseases that affect the myocardium include angina pectoris, myocardial infarction (MI), pericarditis, congestive heart failure (CHF), and aneurysm.

Angina Pectoris

Angina pectoris, characterized by acute chest pain, occurs from an imbalance between oxygen demands of the myocardium and its oxygen supply. Metabolite accumulation within an ischemic segment of heart muscle causes the pain. The sensation of angina pectoris, often confused with simple heartburn, includes squeezing, burning, and pressing or "choking" in the chest region (**Table 18.4**). The pain usually

TABLE 18.4 Similarity of Symptoms of Angina and Heartburn

Angina	Heartburn
Gripping, viselike feelings of pain or pressure	Frequent feeling of heartburn
Pain that radiates to the neck, jaw, back, shoulders, or arms (usually left)	Frequent use of antacids to relieve pain
Toothache	Waking up at night
Burning indigestion	Acidic or bitter taste in mouth
Shortness of breath	Burning sensation in chest
Nausea	Discomfort after eating spicy food
Frequent belching	Difficulty swallowing

lasts up to 3 minutes but can continue for longer intervals. One-third of all individuals who have angina will die suddenly from an MI. Chronic stable angina, often referred to as "walk-through" angina, occurs at a predictable level of physical exertion (e.g., metabolic equivalent [MET] level or preset exercise heart rate).

Vasodilators reduce cardiac workload and thus oxygen requirements to effectively control this uncomfortable and potentially debilitating condition. Examples include fast-acting nitroglycerin (first introduced in 1846–1847 by Italian chemistry professor Ascanio Sobrero [1812–1888] and first produced commercially by Swedish entrepreneur Alfred Bernhard Nobel [1833–1896], the inventor of dynamite and benefactor of the Nobel Prize) to reduce anginal pain) and longer-acting isosorbide dinitrate and mononitrate.

Figure 18.1 shows the usual pain pattern associated with acute angina pectoris. Pain frequently occurs in the left shoulder or along the arm to the elbow. Occasionally, angina pain emanates in the back area of the left scapula along the spinal cord.

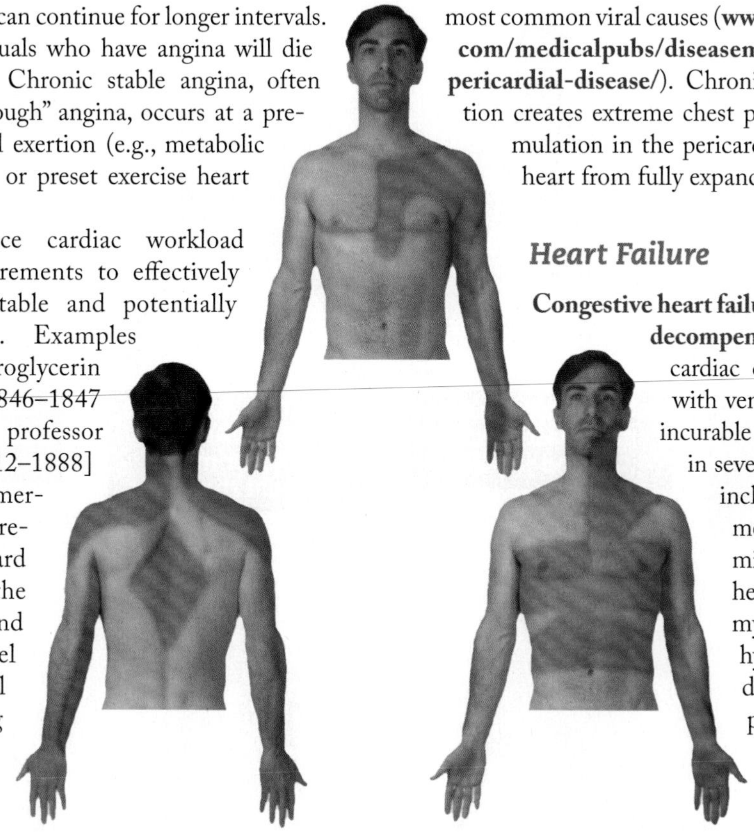

FIGURE 18.1 Locations for pain generally associated with angina pectoris. Pain of cardiac origin, although usually referred to the left side, may be referred to the right side, both sides, or midback. (Reprinted with permission from Moore KL, et al. *Clinically Oriented Anatomy.* 7th Ed. Baltimore: Wolters Kluwer Health, 2014.)

Myocardial Infarction

MI (heart attack or coronary occlusion) results from a severely inadequate perfusion of blood in the coronary arteries or a dramatic imbalance in myocardial oxygen demand and supply from occlusion of a section of the coronary vasculature. Sudden occlusion from prior clot formation initiated by plaque accumulation in one or more coronary arteries can prove fatal. Severe fatigue for several days without specific pain often precedes MI onset.

Figure 18.2 displays the locations of early warning signs of an MI. Severe, unrelenting chest pain can last up to 1 hour during an MI.

Pericarditis

Pericarditis, an inflammation of the heart's outer pericardial lining, classifies as either acute or chronic (recurring or constrictive). Acute pericarditis symptoms vary but usually include chest pain, shortness of breath or dyspnea, and elevated resting heart rate and body temperature. The prognosis for acute pericarditis remains excellent, but chronic pericarditis from bacterial origin presents a persistent serious pathology. Coxsackievirus B virus and echovirus are the most common viral causes (**www.clevelandclinicmeded.com/medicalpubs/diseasemanagement/cardiology/pericardial-disease/**). Chronic pericarditis inflammation creates extreme chest pain caused by fluid accumulation in the pericardial sac. This prevents the heart from fully expanding during diastole.

Heart Failure

Congestive heart failure (CHF, HF, or chronic decompensation) occurs when cardiac output cannot keep pace with venous return. This common incurable condition varies widely in severity; lifestyle changes that include diet, exercise, and medications can help to mitigate the condition. The heart can fail from intrinsic myocardial disease, chronic hypertension, or structural defects that impair pump performance.

In CHF, the heart's **ejection fraction** decreases (i.e., amount of blood pumped from the left ventricle relative to the total amount of blood received). With diminished left ventricular output and ejection fraction usually well below 50%, blood accumulates in the pulmonary vasculature.

CHF can occur from the right or left sides of the heart, each with different symptoms and prognosis depending on initiation of treatment. Common CHF symptoms include dyspnea, coughing with copious amounts of frothy blood-tinged sputum, pulmonary edema, general fatigue, and overall muscle weakness. The eventual flooding of pulmonary alveoli with plasma filtrate is a condition termed **pulmonary congestion**.

See the animations "Congestive Heart Failure" and "Edema" on **http://thePoint.lww.com/MKKESS5e** for a demonstration of these processes.

Aneurysm

Aneurysm represents an abnormal dilatation in the walls of arteries or veins or within the myocardium itself. Vascular aneurysms arise from one of four conditions:

1. Weakened vessel wall due to trauma
2. Congenital vascular disease
3. Infection
4. Atherosclerosis

Aneurysms are identified as either "arterial" or "venous" and classified according to the specific vasculature area

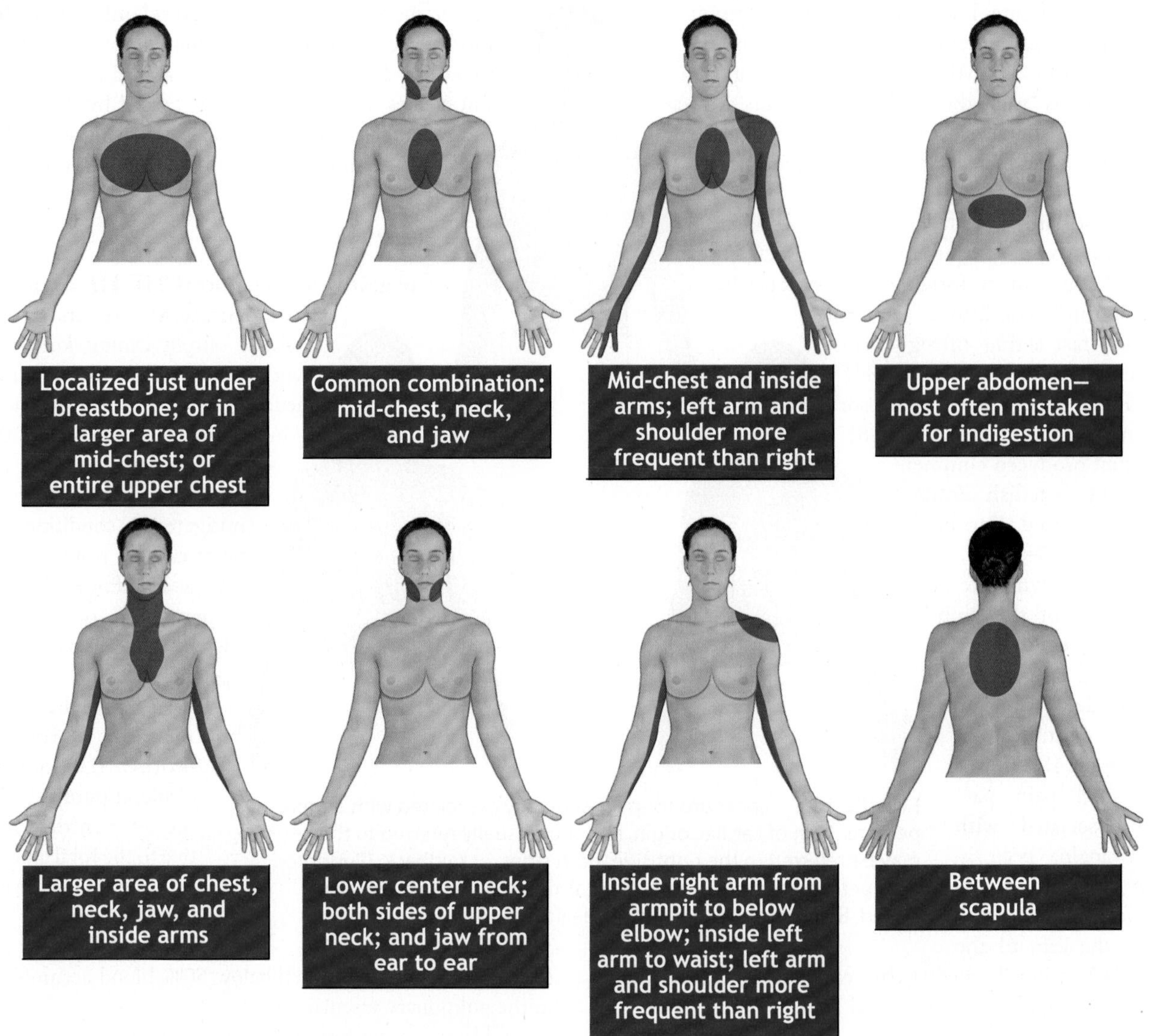

FIGURE 18.2 Anatomic locations for early warning signs of myocardial infarction. Note the diverse locations for pain. (Adapted with permission from McArdle WD, Katch FI, Katch VL. *Exercise Physiology: Nutrition, Energy, and Human Performance*. 8th Ed. Baltimore: Wolters Kluwer Health, 2015.)

affected (e.g., thoracic or splenic aneurysm). Routine chest radiography uncovers most aneurysms. Common myocardial symptoms include chest pain with a specific, palpable, pulsating mass in the chest, abdomen, or lower back.

Heart Valve Diseases

Diseases and abnormalities that affect heart valve structure and function include:

- **Stenosis**: Valves narrow or constrict, preventing the valve from opening fully; it may be caused by growths, scars, or abnormal mineral deposits.
- **Regurgitation** (also called insufficiency): Valves do not close properly, causing blood to flow back into the heart's chambers during diastole.
- **Prolapse** (only affects mitral valve): Enlarged valve leaflets bulge backward into the left atrium during the cardiac cycle.

Valvular abnormalities increase myocardial workload, requiring the heart to generate greater force to pump blood through a constricted valve or to maintain cardiac output if blood seeps back into a chamber. **Rheumatic fever**, a potentially fatal infection by Group A or B streptococcal bacteria (**www.nlm.nih.gov/medlineplus/streptococcal infections.html**) that can lead to rheumatic heart disease with valvular scarring and heart valve deformity, usually causes heart valve stenosis. The two most common symptoms of rheumatic heart valve pathology are fever and joint pain.

Endocarditis

Endocarditis, an inflammation of the innermost layer of the heart or endocardium usually of bacterial origin, damages the tricuspid, aortic, or mitral valves from direct bacteria invasion into the tissue. Patients initially have musculoskeletal symptoms including arthritis, low-back pain, and general weakness in one or more joints. Antibiotics (e.g., aqueous penicillin, ampicillin, gentamicin, vancomycin, nafcillin) can effectively treat endocarditis before it becomes fatal.

Congenital Malformations

Congenital heart defects appear in 1 of every 100 births; they include heart valve defects such as ventricular or atrial **septal defects** (hole between ventricles and atria) and **patent ductus arteriosus** (shunt caused by an opening between aorta and pulmonary artery). For most infants septal defects resolve within the first year of life, if not, these defects require surgical repair.

Mitral Valve Prolapse

Mitral valve prolapse (MVP) occurs in about 10% of Americans and involves variations in either the mitral valve's shape or structure. This defect has been called "**floppy valve syndrome**," "**Barlow syndrome**," and the "**click-murmur syndrome**." MVP frequency of diagnosis has increased over the past decade secondary to endocarditis, atherosclerosis, and muscular dystrophy. MVP most likely results from connective tissue abnormalities in mitral valve leaflets. Sixty percent of patients with MVP have no symptoms—the remainder experience profound fatigue during physical activity.

Cardiac Nervous System Diseases

Diseases that affect the heart's electrical conduction system include **dysrhythmias (arrhythmias)** that cause the heart to beat too quickly (**tachycardia**), beat too slowly (**bradycardia**), generate extra beats (**ectopic, extrasystole, or premature ventricular contractions [PVCs]**), or **fibrillate** (fine, rapid contractions or twitching of myocardial fibers).

Dysrhythmias usually change circulatory dynamics and result in low blood pressure, shock, and heart failure. They often occur following a stroke or may be induced by physical exertion or other stressors.

In adults, **sinus tachycardia** represents a resting heart rate greater than 100 b · min^{-1}, and **sinus bradycardia** represents a resting heart rate below 60 b · min^{-1}. **Asymptomatic sinus bradycardia** typically occurs in endurance-trained individuals. This benign dysrhythmia may reflect a beneficial training adaptation because it provides a longer diastole for ventricular filling during the cardiac cycle, and hence the possibility for augmented stroke volume.

CARDIAC DISEASE ASSESSMENT

A thorough cardiac disease assessment typically includes the following four parts:

1. Patient medical history
2. Physical examination
3. Laboratory tests
4. Physiologic tests

Patient Medical History

A proper patient history documents the most common complaints and establishes a basis for CHD risk profiling. CHD symptoms frequently include chest pain, making the pain's differential diagnosis a primary focus. **Table 18.5** lists a limited differential diagnosis of chest pain, including possible causes and pathogenesis.

Physical Examination

A physician, nurse, or physician's assistant usually conducts the physical examination, which includes the patient's vital signs (body temperature, heart rate, breathing rate, and blood pressure).

For purposes of prescribing exercise and identifying early CHD warning signs, the clinical exercise physiologist must know the patient's heart rate and blood pressure response to incremental exercise. For example, an increase in systolic blood pressure (SBP) of 20 mm Hg or more in low-level 2 to 4 MET physical activity (**hypertensive exercise response**) indicates overall cardiovascular impairment and signifies increased myocardial oxygen demand suggestive of potential coronary ischemia. In contrast, failure of SBP to increase during 5 to 7 MET moderate physical activity (**hypotensive exercise response**) indicates left ventricular dysfunction; a hypotensive response in intense exercise

TABLE 18.5 Chest Pain Diagnosis

Pain/Complaint/Findings	Possible Causes	Stimuli	Possible Pathology
Pressure, ache, tightness, or burning in midsternum, left shoulder, arm; diaphoresis; nausea; vomiting; S-T segment changes	MI	Exertion; cold; smoking; heavy meal; fluid overload	CHD
Sharp pain worsens with inspiration, improves with sitting	Inflammation	Acute MI	Pericarditis
Chest tightness with breathlessness; low-grade fever	Infection	IV drug use; microbes	Myocarditis; endocarditis
Sharp, stabbing pain; breathlessness; cough; loss of consciousness	Pulmonary	Recent surgery	Pulmonary embolism
Burning pain in stomach; indigestion relieved by antacids	Referred pain	Heavy meal; spicy food	Esophageal reflux
Angina pain; breathlessness; wide pulse pressure; ventricular hypertrophy on ECG	Ventricular outflow tract obstruction	Exertion; CHD	Aortic stenosis; mitral valve prolapse

signals a serious mortality risk. Individuals unable to elevate SBP above 140 mm Hg during maximal exertion often indicates dormant but serious cardiac disease.

Heart Auscultation

Listening to heart sounds, termed **auscultation** (from the Latin verb auscultare "to listen"), provides important information about cardiac function. Exercise physiologists should become familiar with abnormal heart sounds, including how to identify those related to heart murmurs. Auscultation can readily diagnose valvular diseases (e.g., MVP diagnosed by the classic click-murmur sounds) and congenital abnormalities (e.g., regurgitation sounds in ventricular septal defects).

Laboratory-Based Screening and Assessment

The following laboratory-based screenings provide considerable information for confirming and documenting the extent of CHD:

- Chest radiography: Chest radiographs reveal heart and lung size and shape.
- **Electrocardiogram (ECG)**: Resting and exercise ECG provide essential information to assess myocardial electrical conductivity and oxygenation. Correctly reading and interpreting an ECG requires specialized training and considerable practice. **Table 18.6** lists six different categories of ECG interpretations. Later in this chapter, we describe various ECG abnormalities and abnormal physiologic responses to exercise; we also detail how to count heart rate from ECG tracings. Careful monitoring of ECG changes during exercise helps identify individuals with potential CHD for further evaluation. **Table 18.7** lists normal and abnormal ECG changes commonly observed during monitored physical activity.
- Blood lipid and lipoproteins: Routine laboratory testing for CHD risk includes analysis of blood lipid and lipoprotein profiles. Individuals with heart disease often have elevated cholesterol and LDL cholesterol, but this is not a predictor for CHD diagnosis.
- Serum enzymes: Alterations in muscle serum enzymes can often diagnose or rule out an acute MI. When myocardial cell death (**necrosis**) or prolonged lack of blood flow (**ischemia**) occurs, specific enzymes from the damaged muscle leak into the blood because of the plasma membrane's increased permeability. This leakage increases serum levels of these three enzymes:
  1. **Creatine phosphokinase (CPK)** reflects either skeletal or cardiac muscle necrosis depending on one of three formed isoenzymes.
  2. **Lactate dehydrogenase (LDH)** fractionates into different isoenzyme markers.
  3. **Serum glutamic oxaloacetic transaminase (SGOT)** is released into the blood, indicating liver or heart damage.

TABLE 18.6 Six Categories for ECG Interpretation

1. Measurements	• Heart rate (atrial and ventricular) • PR interval (0.12–0.20 s) • QRS duration (0.03–0.10 s) • QT interval (HR dependent) • Frontal plane QRS axis (−30 degrees to +90 degrees)
2. Rhythm diagnosis	
3. Conduction diagnosis	
4. Waveform description	• P wave (atrial enlargement) • QRS complex (ventricular hypertrophy, infarction) • S-T segment (elevated or depressed) • T wave (flattened or inverted) • U wave (prominent or inverted)
5. ECG diagnosis	• Within normal limits • Borderline abnormal • Abnormal
6. Comparison with previous ECG	

ECG, electrocardiographic.

Reprinted with permission from Fardy P, Yanowitz FG. *Cardiac Rehabilitation, Adult Fitness and Exercise Testing*. Baltimore: Williams & Wilkins, 1996.

TABLE 18.7 Normal and Abnormal ECG Changes Commonly Observed During Exercise

Normal ECG Changes in Healthy Individuals	Abnormal ECG Changes With CHD
1. Slight increase in P wave amplitude	1. Appearance of bundle branch block at a critical HR
2. Shortening of PR interval	2. Recurrent or multifocal PVCs during exercise and recovery
3. Shift to the right of QRS axis	3. Ventricular tachycardia
4. S-T segment depression <1.0 mm	4. Appearance of bradyarrhythmias and tachyarrhythmias
5. Decreased T wave amplitude	5. S-T segment depression/elevation of >1.0 mm 0.08 s after J point
6. Single or rare PVC during exercise and recovery	6. Exercise bradycardia
7. Single or rare PVC or PAC	7. Submaximal exercise tachycardia
	8. Increase in frequency or severity of any known arrhythmia

PVC, premature ventricular contraction; PAC, premature atrial contraction.

Noninvasive Physiologic Screening and Assessment

Noninvasive physiologic tests identify specific cardiovascular/cardiac dysfunction with minimal patient discomfort and risk.

Echocardiography

Echocardiography uses pulses of reflected ultrasound to evaluate heart function and morphology; it identifies the heart's structural components and measures distances within the myocardial chambers (**http://asecho.org**). This allows estimation of various chamber sizes or volume in addition to blood vessel dimensions and thickness of various myocardial components. The echocardiogram has surpassed the ECG in recognizing chamber enlargement, myocardial hypertrophy, and other structural abnormalities. Echocardiograms can diagnose heart murmurs, evaluate valvular lesions, and determine the extent of congenital heart diseases and cardiomyopathies.

Figure 18.3 presents a typical still echocardiographic image showing the left and right atrium and left and right ventricle, the tricuspid valves, and the mitral valves. The echocardiogram provides the ability to measure different parameters of size and function of the heart's chambers for diagnostic purposes. The advent of three-dimensional echocardiogram has enhanced echocardiography as a valuable diagnostic tool (**depts.washington.edu/cvrtc/ocarinas.html**).

Graded Exercise Stress Test

A **graded exercise stress test (GXT)** systematically uses exercise for two purposes:

1. Observe cardiac rhythm abnormalities during exercise
2. Assess overall physiologic adjustments to increased exercise metabolic demands

The most common modes for stress testing include multistage bicycle and treadmill tests. The test, "graded" for intensity, includes submaximal levels of 3 to 5 minutes duration, each level progressing up to self-imposed fatigue or a specific, predetermined target heart rate. The graded nature of testing allows detection of ischemic manifestations and rhythm disorders with small increments in intensity. The GXT provides a reliable, quantitative index of the person's level of functional impairment. *For most screening purposes, the test does not require maximal effort; instead, the person performs to at least 85% of age-predicted maximum heart rate.* Laboratory-based GXTs remain preferable to walking or running field tests because the tester maintains closer control over the test environment and exercise intensity.

A resting ECG precedes the GXT to establish whether the person can engage safely in subsequent graded exercise. The resting ECG also provides an important baseline measure for subsequent comparisons.

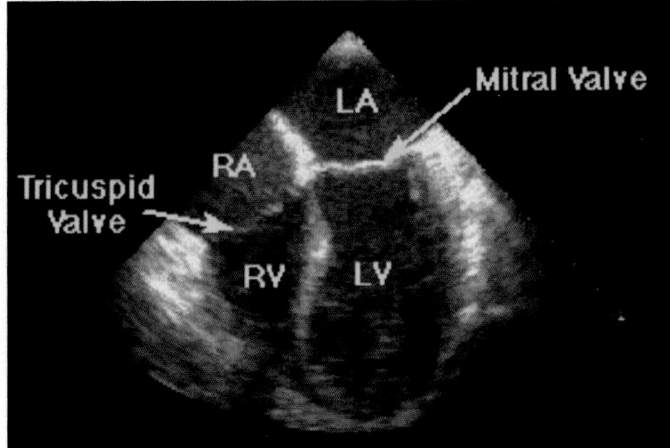

FIGURE 18.3 Still picture of an echocardiogram that shows the right and left ventricles, right and left atria, and mitral and tricuspid valves.

Major Signs and Symptoms of Cardiopulmonary Disease

Individuals with undiagnosed cardiopulmonary diseases exhibit nine specific signs and symptoms during rest and physical activity:

1. Pain or discomfort (or other angina equivalent) in the chest, neck, or arms
2. Shortness of breath at rest or with mild exertion
3. Dizziness or syncope (feeling of lightheadedness or faintness)
4. Dyspnea (shortness of breath or labored breathing) on rising from a supine position or at night during sleep
5. Palpitations or unexplained tachycardia during rest or mild exertion
6. Ankle edema (swelling)
7. **Intermittent claudication** (ischemic pain from inadequate blood flow, usually experienced in the calf of the leg)
8. Known heart murmur
9. Unusual fatigue accompanied by moderate-to-extreme dyspnea during usual activities of daily living

fyi Chronic Fatigue Syndrome and Physical Activity

Chronic fatigue syndrome (CFS) involves continual and severe fatigue. Its prevalence has been estimated at between 1 and 4 million Americans. The cause(s) of CFS remains unknown but may represent a common end point from multiple causes that include infectious agents (similar to Epstein-Barr virus), immunologic variables (perhaps inappropriate production of cytokines such as interleukin-1), hypothalamic-pituitary-adrenal (HPA) axis stimulation leading to increased release of cortisol and other hormones that influence the immune system and other body systems, diabetes, neurally mediated hypotension, substance abuse, and possible nutritional deficiencies. CFS patients benefit from modest regular physical activity to avoid deconditioning (**www.ncpad.org**).

Why Stress Test?

Stress testing serves six important roles in an overall CHD evaluation:

1. **Detect heart disease:** An exercise ECG can diagnose overt heart disease and screen for possible "silent" coronary disease in seemingly healthy individuals. Between 25% and 40% of people with confirmed CHD have normal resting ECGs. ECG analysis during exercise uncovers approximately 80% of such abnormalities.
2. **Reproduce and assess exercise-related chest pain symptoms:** Individuals older than age 40 years often experience angina symptoms with physical exertion. ECG analysis during graded exercise provides an objective and valid diagnosis of exercise-induced chest discomfort.
3. **Screen candidates for preventive and rehabilitative physical activity programs:** Stress test results help clinical exercise physiologists design a comprehensive physical activity program within an individual's functional capacity and health status. Repeated testing evaluates training progress and safely modifies the initial prescription.
4. **Detect abnormal blood pressure responses:** Exercise-induced hypertension often signifies underlying cardiovascular complications.
5. **Monitor responses to various therapeutic interventions designed to improve cardiovascular health and function:** Periodic stress testing objectifies the degree of benefit derived from pharmacologic, surgical, or dietary treatment of heart disease.
6. **Quantify functional aerobic capacity and evaluate its degree of deviation from established standards:** Metabolic measurements during the GXT allow determination of $\dot{V}O_{2max}$ or $\dot{V}O_{2peak}$.

Who Should Be Stress Tested?

Table 18.8 provides a classification system by age and health status for screening and supervisory procedures for both stress testing and participation in a regular physical activity program. These guidelines apply to healthy individuals and those at higher risk. Healthy young adults can begin moderate-intensity physical activity at 40% to 60% $\dot{V}O_{2max}$ without a stress test or medical examination. Men older than age 40 years and women older than age 50 years should have a medical examination that includes a stress test before starting a physical activity program. A GXT that precedes training takes on added importance for high-risk individuals of any age. *High-risk individuals are those with two or more major CHD risk factors or symptoms suggestive of cardiopulmonary or metabolic disease.*

Informed Consent

Participants in all exercise testing and training must be "informed" before they begin. ***Informed consent** raises awareness about potential risks of participation.* Informed consent must include a written statement that the person had an opportunity to ask questions about the procedures with sufficient information clearly provided so consent occurs from a knowledgeable or informed perspective. A minor requires prior legal consent from a legal guardian or parent. Individuals need assurance that test results remain confidential.

TABLE 18.8 Recommendations for Medical Examination, Graded Exercise Stress Testing (GXT), and Physician Supervision of GXT Before Participation in an Exercise Program

Risk Category	Medical Examination and GXT	M.D. Supervision
Low Risk		
Men <45 y Women <55 y; asymptomatic with 1 risk factor[a,b]	Moderate exercise; not necessary Vigorous exercise; not necessary	Moderate exercise; not necessary Vigorous exercise; not necessary
Moderate Risk		
Men ≥45 y Women ≥55 y, with ≥2 risk factors[a,b]	Moderate exercise; not necessary Vigorous exercise; recommended	Moderate exercise; not necessary Vigorous exercise; recommended
High Risk		
Individuals with 1 sign/symptom of cardiovascular or pulmonary disease[c] or known cardiovascular (cardiac, peripheral vascular, or cerebrovascular), pulmonary (obstructive pulmonary disease, asthma, cystic fibrosis), or metabolic (diabetes, thyroid disorder, renal, or liver) disease	Moderate exercise; recommended Vigorous exercise; recommended	Moderate exercise; recommended Vigorous exercise; recommended

[a] Risk factors: family history of heart disease, cigarette smoking, hypertension, hypercholesterolemia, impaired fasting glucose, obesity, and sedentary lifestyle.

[b] HDL >60 mg • dL^{-1} (subtract 1 risk factor from the sum of other risk factors because high HDL decreases CHD risk).

[c] Signs and symptoms of cardiovascular and pulmonary disease: pain, discomfort in chest, neck, jaw, left arm; shortness of breath at rest or with mild exertion; dizziness or syncope; orthopnea or paroxysmal nocturnal dyspnea; ankle edema; tachycardia; intermittent claudication; heart murmur; and unusual fatigue or shortness of breath with mild activity.

A CLOSER LOOK

Assessing Readiness for Physical Activity: The Par-Q Screening Tool

The Physical Activity Readiness Questionnaire (PAR-Q) is a self-screening tool that can be used by anyone planning to start a physical activity program. Originally created by the British Columbia Ministry of Health and the Multidisciplinary Board on Exercise and adopted from the ACSM Standards and Guidelines for Health and Fitness Facilities, it is often used by fitness trainers or coaches to determine the safety or possible risk of physical activity participation. It is also used to identify the small number of adults for whom physical activity may be inappropriate or those who should have medical advice concerning the type of activity most suitable for them. The Par-Q can determine the exercise readiness of apparently healthy middle-age adults with no more than one major risk factor for CHD.

Physical Activity Readiness Questionnaire - PAR-Q (revised 2002)

PAR-Q & YOU

(A Questionnaire for People Aged 15 to 69)

Regular physical activity is fun and healthy, and increasingly more people are starting to become more active every day. Being more active is very safe for most people. However, some people should check with their doctor before they start becoming much more physically active.

If you are planning to become much more physically active than you are now, start by answering the seven questions in the box below. If you are between the ages of 15 and 69, the PAR-Q will tell you if you should check with your doctor before you start. If you are over 69 years of age, and you are not used to being very active, check with your doctor.

Common sense is your best guide when you answer these questions. Please read the questions carefully and answer each one honestly: check YES or NO.

YES	NO	
☐	☐	**1. Has your doctor ever said that you have a heart condition and that you should only do physical activity recommended by a doctor?**
☐	☐	**2. Do you feel pain in your chest when you do physical activity?**
☐	☐	**3. In the past month, have you had chest pain when you were not doing physical activity?**
☐	☐	**4. Do you lose your balance because of dizziness or do you ever lose consciousness?**
☐	☐	**5. Do you have a bone or joint problem (for example, back, knee or hip) that could be made worse by a change in your physical activity?**
☐	☐	**6. Is your doctor currently prescribing drugs (for example, water pills) for your blood pressure or heart condition?**
☐	☐	**7. Do you know of any other reason why you should not do physical activity?**

If you answered

YES to one or more questions

Talk with your doctor by phone or in person BEFORE you start becoming much more physically active or BEFORE you have a fitness appraisal. Tell your doctor about the PAR-Q and which questions you answered YES.

- You may be able to do any activity you want — as long as you start slowly and build up gradually. Or, you may need to restrict your activities to those which are safe for you. Talk with your doctor about the kinds of activities you wish to participate in and follow his/her advice.
- Find out which community programs are safe and helpful for you.

NO to all questions

If you answered NO honestly to all PAR-Q questions, you can be reasonably sure that you can:

- start becoming much more physically active – begin slowly and build up gradually. This is the safest and easiest way to go.
- take part in a fitness appraisal – this is an excellent way to determine your basic fitness so that you can plan the best way for you to live actively. It is also highly recommended that you have your blood pressure evaluated. If your reading is over 144/94, talk with your doctor before you start becoming much more physically active.

→ **DELAY BECOMING MUCH MORE ACTIVE:**

- if you are not feeling well because of a temporary illness such as a cold or a fever – wait until you feel better; or
- if you are or may be pregnant – talk to your doctor before you start becoming more active.

PLEASE NOTE: If your health changes so that you then answer YES to any of the above questions, tell your fitness or health professional. Ask whether you should change your physical activity plan.

Informed Use of the PAR-Q: The Canadian Society for Exercise Physiology, Health Canada, and their agents assume no liability for persons who undertake physical activity, and if in doubt after completing this questionnaire, consult your doctor prior to physical activity.

No changes permitted. You are encouraged to photocopy the PAR-Q but only if you use the entire form.

NOTE: If the PAR-Q is being given to a person before he or she participates in a physical activity program or a fitness appraisal, this section may be used for legal or administrative purposes.

"I have read, understood and completed this questionnaire. Any questions I had were answered to my full satisfaction."

NAME ____________________

SIGNATURE ____________________ DATE ____________________

SIGNATURE OF PARENT or GUARDIAN (for participants under the age of majority) ____________________ WITNESS ____________________

Note: This physical activity clearance is valid for a maximum of 12 months from the date it is completed and becomes invalid if your condition changes so that you would answer YES to any of the seven questions.

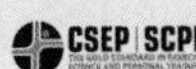

Source: *Par-Q and You.* **http://www.csep.ca/cmfiles/publications/parq/par-q.pdf.** Par-Q form reprinted with permission.

TABLE 18.9 Example of Informed Consent for a Grade Exercise Stress Test

Name ______________________________

1. **Explanation of the Exercise Test**
   You will perform an exercise test on a cycle ergometer or a motor-driven treadmill. The exercise intensity begins at a level you can easily accomplish and will advance in stages of difficulty depending on your fitness level. We may stop the test at any time because of signs of fatigue, or you may stop the test when you wish because of fatigue or discomfort that you feel, particularly at the higher exercise levels.
2. **Risks and Discomforts**
   The possibility exists that certain abnormal changes can occur during the test. These include abnormal blood pressure, fainting, disorder of heart beat, and in rare instances, heart attack, stroke, or death. Every effort will be made to minimize these risks by evaluating preliminary information related to your health and fitness, and by observations during testing. Emergency equipment and available trained personnel can deal with unusual situations that may arise.
3. **Responsibilities of the Participant**
   Information you possess about your health status or previous experiences of unusual feelings with physical effort may affect the safety and value of your exercise test and you should report this information now. Your prompt reporting of how you feel during the exercise test also is important. You are responsible for fully disclosing such information when requested to do so by the testing staff.
4. **Expected Benefits From the Test**
   The results obtained from the exercise test may assist in diagnosing your illness, or evaluating what type of physical activities you might do with low risk.
5. **Inquires**
   We encourage you to ask any questions about the procedures used in the exercise test or in the estimation of your functional capacity. If you have doubts or questions, please ask us for further explanations.
6. **Freedom of Consent**
   Your permission to perform this exercise test is voluntary. You are free to deny consent or stop the test at any point.
   I have read this form and understand the test procedures. I voluntarily consent to participate in this test.

Date: ______________________________
Signature of Patient: ______________________________
Signature of Witness: ______________________________
Questions: ______________________________
____
Responses: ______________________________
Signature of Physician or Delegate: ______________________________

Minors must clearly understand they may terminate exercise testing or a training program at any time and for any reason. **Table 18.9** presents a sample informed consent statement. Another sample informed consent for exercise stress testing can be found at **http://circ.ahajournals.org/content/91/3/912.full.(133)**.

Contraindications to Stress Testing

Certain conditions preclude administering a stress test (*absolute contraindications*), and other conditions require the GXT be administered under more closely monitored conditions (*relative contraindications*).

Absolute Contraindications to Stress Testing Under no circumstances should a stress test be administered without direct medical supervision if any of the following 12 conditions exist:

1. Resting ECG suggestive of acute cardiac disease
2. Recent complicated MI
3. Unstable angina pectoris
4. Uncontrolled ventricular arrhythmia
5. Uncontrolled atrial arrhythmia that compromises cardiac function
6. Third-degree **atrioventricular heart block** without a pacemaker
7. Acute congestive heart failure
8. Severe aortic stenosis
9. Active or suspected myocarditis or pericarditis
10. Recent systemic or pulmonary embolism
11. Acute infections
12. Acute emotional distress

Relative Contraindications to Stress Testing Administer a GXT with caution and with medical personnel in close proximity to the test area if any of the following 10 conditions exist:

1. Resting diastolic blood pressure (DBP) above 115 mm Hg or systolic blood pressure (SBP) exceeds 200 mm Hg
2. Moderate valvular disease
3. Electrolyte abnormalities

4. Frequent or complex ventricular ectopic beats
5. Ventricular aneurysm
6. Uncontrolled metabolic disease (diabetes, thyrotoxicosis)
7. Chronic infectious disease (hepatitis, mononucleosis, AIDS)
8. Neuromuscular or musculoskeletal disorders
9. Pregnancy (complicated or in the last trimester)
10. Psychological distress or apprehension about taking the test

Maximal Versus Submaximal Stress Testing

A maximal GXT (GXT_{max})** represents the most common noninvasive method to screen for CHD and determine $\dot{V}O_{2max}$ or $\dot{V}O_{2peak}$.* Individuals exercise until they decide to stop or develop abnormal symptoms that signal test termination (**Table 18.10**). The term ***symptom limited describes such stress tests.

GXT_{max} normally progress through several stages referred to as multistage GXT. Test duration, starting point, and increments between stages vary with the person (e.g., young active, healthy sedentary, and questionable health status).

Advantages of a GXT_{max} include:

1. Direct determination of $\dot{V}O_{2max}$ and maximal cardiovascular responses
2. Screening for abnormal ECG patterns not revealed during rest or low-intensity exercise
3. Establishing more precise physical activity training levels

Disadvantages include:

1. Considerable stress imposed on the person, although GXT_{max} exhibits low risk
2. Discomfort of being pushed to maximum without prior physical conditioning (may deter some individuals from participating in a subsequent conditioning program)
3. Test overkill—for most healthy people, about the same physiologic information is obtained from submaximal tests performed at 80% to 90% HR_{max} (maximal safe heart rate) as testing requiring all-out effort.

TABLE 18.10 Criteria for Stopping a GXT in Apparently Health Adults

1. Onset of angina or anginalike symptoms
2. Ventricular tachycardia
3. Significant decrease in systolic blood pressure of 20 mm Hg
4. Failure of systolic blood pressure or heart rate to increase with an increase in exercise load
5. Light-headedness, confusion, ataxia, pallor, cyanosis, nausea, or signs of severe peripheral circulatory insufficiency
6. Early-onset horizontal or downsloping S-T segment depression or elevation (>4 mm)
7. Increasing ventricular ectopy; multiform PVCs
8. Excessive increase in blood pressure: systolic >260 mm Hg; diastolic >115 mm Hg
9. Increase in heart rate <25 b · min^{-1} of predicted normal value (in the absence of β-blockade medication)
10. Sustained supraventricular tachycardia
11. Subject requests to stop test for whatever reason
12. Equipment failure

PVC, premature ventricular contraction.

From Pescatello LS. et al., eds. *ACSM's Guidelines for Exercise Testing and Prescription*. 9th Ed. Baltimore: Lippincott Williams & Wilkins, 2014.

The criteria for stopping a test distinguish one GXT protocol from another; otherwise, any of the protocols are effective. In all instances, an abnormal response should terminate the test.

Nine factors influence physiologic responses to submaximal or maximal exercise:

1. Ambient temperature and relative humidity
2. Subject's sleep state (number of sleep hours prior to testing)
3. Emotional state
4. Medication
5. Time of day
6. Caffeine intake
7. Time since last meal
8. Time since last exercise
9. Testing environment (type and appearance of testing room, physical appearance, and behavior of test personnel)

Stress Test Protocols

Test duration, initial exercise intensity level, and increments of intensity between stages for GXT protocols dictate the test to administer. In a national survey of 1400 exercise stress test centers, 71% used treadmills, 17% used bicycle ergometers, and only 12% used step tests. No statistics exist for arm crank or swim stress tests.

Treadmill Tests. Treadmill tests accommodate individuals through a broad spectrum of fitness using the "natural" activities of walking and running. (See Chapter 7 for a discussion of different treadmill protocols.) **Table 18.11** presents three of the more common exercise test protocols and the predicted $\dot{V}O_2$ (mL · kg^{-1} · min^{-1}) for each exercise level for each test.

Each protocol has advantages and disadvantages. The **Bruce test**, one of the more common protocols, uses relatively large increments in intensity every 3 minutes, resulting in less uniform responses compared with tests with smaller increments in intensity (either increased speed or grade or both) and is better suited for screening younger and physically active individuals. Protocols with smaller increments in intensity, such as the **Naughton test** or the modified **Balke test**, are preferable for older or deconditioned individuals and patients with chronic diseases. In the ramp test, an attractive alternative approach to incremental exercise testing, work rate increases in a constant and continuous manner.

All stress tests begin at a relatively low level, with 2- to 3-minute increments in intensity. A warm-up should be used either separately or incorporated into the initial test phase. The ideal test duration should last at least 8 to 12 minutes. A test longer than 20 minutes provides no additional useful ECG or physiologic data but can establish more precise end points for estimating performance capacity.

TABLE 18.11 Modified Treadmill Protocols for Different Populations

Stage	Treadmill (MPH)	Treadmill (%Grade)	Time (Min)	O_2 Cost (mL · kg^{-1} · min^{-1})	METs
Bruce Test (Normally Used for Young Active Adults)					
1	1.7	10	3	14.0–17.5	4–5
2	2.5	12	3	24.5–28.0	7
3	3.4	14	3	31.5–35.0	9.5
4	4.2	16	3	45.5–49.0	13.5
5	5.0	18	3	59.5–63.0	17
6	5.5	20	3	70.0–73.5	20.5
Modified Balke Test (Normally Used for Normal Sedentary Adults)					
1	2	0	2	8.75	2.5
2	3	0	2	12.25	3.5
3	3	2.5	2	15.75	4.5
4	3	5	2	19.25	5.5
5	3	7.5	2	22.75	6.5
6	3	10	2	26.26	7.5
7	3	12.5	2	29.75	8.5
8	3	15	2	33.25	9.5
9	3	17.5	2	36.75	10.5
10	3	20	2	40.25	11.5
11	3	22.5	2	43.75	12.5
12	3	25	2	47.25	13.5
Modified Naughton Test (Normally Used for Very Sedentary Adults)					
1	1	0	3	3.5	1
2	1.5	0	3	7.0	2
3	2	3.5	3	12.25	3.5
4	2	7	3	15.75	4.5
5	2	10.5	3	19.25	5.5
6	3	7.5	3	22.75	6.5
7	3	10	3	26.26	7.5
8	3	12.5	3	29.75	8.5
9	3	15	3	33.25	9.5
10	3	17.5	3	36.75	10.5
11	3	20	3	40.25	11.5
12	3	22.5	3	43.75	12.5
13	3	25	3	47.25	13.5

MET, metabolic equivalent; MPH, miles per hour.

Adapted from Figure 5.3 in Pescatello LS, et al., eds. *ACSM's Guidelines for Exercise Testing and Prescription*. 9th Ed. Baltimore: Lippincott Williams & Wilkins, 2014:124–125.

Cycle Ergometer Tests. Cycle ergometers have distinct advantages over other exercise devices. In contrast to treadmills, power output remains independent of body mass. Most ergometers are portable, safe, and relatively inexpensive. Electrically braked and weight-loaded, friction-type devices represent the two most common cycle ergometers. For electrically braked ergometers, preselected power output remains fixed within a range of pedaling frequencies. Power output with weight-loaded ergometers relates directly to frictional resistance and pedaling rate.

The same general guidelines for treadmill testing apply to the cycle ergometer and arm-crank ergometer. Power output on a cycle ergometer is expressed in kg-m · min^{-1} or watts (1 W = 6.12 kg-m · min^{-1}). Cycle ergometer tests generally use 2- to 4-minute stages of graded exercise. Initial resistance ranges between 0 and 30 W; power output generally increases 15 to 30 W per stage. Pedaling at 50 to 70 revolutions per minute (rpm) represents the typical rpm for weight-loaded ergometers.

Arm-Crank Ergometer Tests. Stress testing uses arm cranking as the stressor when formulating the prescription for upper-body exercise (**Fig. 18.4**). Arm-crank exercise generally produces up to 30% lower $\dot{V}O_{2max}$ values and a 10 to 15 b · min^{-1} lower maximum heart rate compared with treadmill or bicycle exercise. Unfortunately, arm-crank exercise interferes with conventional blood pressure measurement during exercise. Blood pressure, heart rate, and oxygen uptake values remain higher during submaximal arm cranking compared with the same power output in leg exercise. Protocols developed for leg cycling tests can evaluate the response to upper-body exercise with a lower starting frictional resistance and incremental power outputs adjusted accordingly.

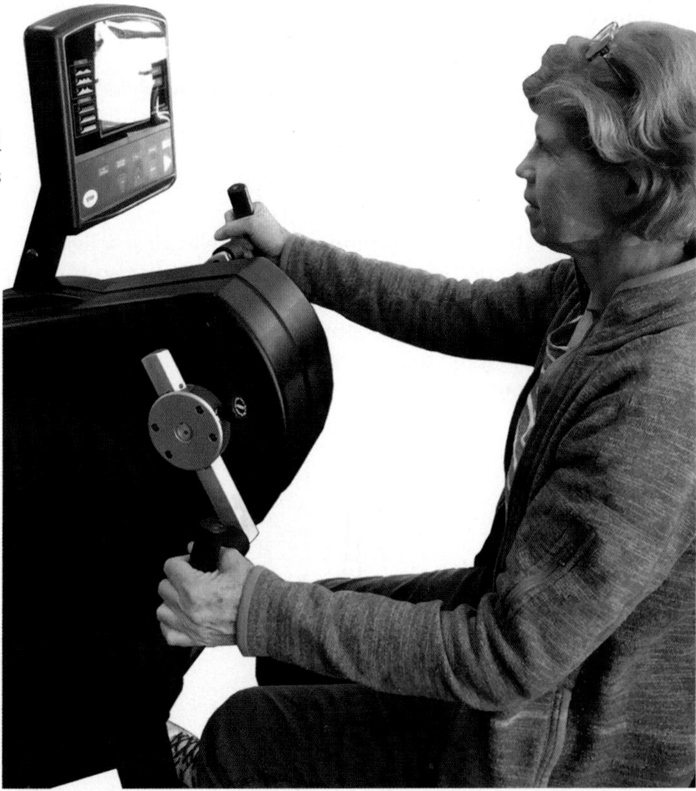

FIGURE 18.4 Example of an arm crank ergometer for testing physiologic and metabolic responses to upper-body exercise. Image courtesy Frank Katch.

Safety of Stress Testing

The safety of stress testing largely depends on knowing whom not to test (prescreening health histories reveal noncandidates for testing), knowing when to terminate a test, and preparing properly for emergencies. In approximately 170,000 submaximal and maximal stress tests, only 16 high-risk but apparently healthy patients experienced coronary episodes. This represents about 1 person per 10,000 or approximately 0.01% of the total group. In more than 9000 stress tests, no cardiovascular episodes occurred for subjects with increased heart disease risk. In other reports, the risk of coronary episodes for healthy, middle-aged adults during a maximum stress test equaled about 1 in 3000. In most middle-aged individuals, test risk generally increases about 6 to 12 times higher than for young adults. For patients with documented CHD (including previous MI or episodes of angina), the risk of cardiovascular incident in stress testing increases 30 to 60 times above normal. Based on total risk analyses, many experts believe that a *lower* "overall risk" exists for those who take a GXT and then initiate a regular physical activity program than those who refrain from testing and remain sedentary.

Stress Test Outcomes

The clinical success of the GXT depends on its predictive outcome, that is, how effectively the test correctly diagnoses a person with heart disease.

The four possible GXT outcomes are:

1. **True-positive** (successful test): The GXT correctly identifies a person with heart disease.
2. **True-negative** (successful test): The GXT correctly identifies a person without heart disease.
3. **False-positive** (unsuccessful test): The GXT incorrectly identifies a normal person as having heart disease.
4. **False-negative** (unsuccessful test): The GXT incorrectly identifies a person with heart disease as normal.

Test sensitivity refers to the percentage of persons for whom the test detects an abnormal or positive response. This represents a true positive condition that only subsequent follow-up can verify. False-negative results (unsuccessful test) occur 25% of the time, and false-positive (unsuccessful test) occurs approximately 15%.

Four factors can contribute to false-negative results:

1. Patient's failure to reach an ischemic threshold
2. Failure to recognize non-ECG signs and symptoms associated with underlying CHD
3. Technical or observer errors
4. The use of drugs for medical conditions, which increases the probability of false-negative results, particularly β-blockers, nitrates, or calcium channel blocking agents.

Test specificity indicates the number of true-negative test results—correctly identifying someone without CHD. More false-positive results occur under the influence of the drug digitalis in the presence of four medical conditions—hypokalemia (low blood potassium levels), mitral valve prolapse, pericardial disorders, and anemia.

Stress Testing the "Oldest-Old"

Normal stress testing guidelines do not apply to individuals aged 75 and older. Only a small, highly select subgroup of these "oldest-old" individuals participate in vigorous physical activity or can successfully complete a stress test. For example, approximately 30% of persons ages 75 to 79, 25% of those ages 80 to 84, and only 9% of those 85 or older can achieve a maximal physical effort. The oldest-old differ markedly from younger (<70-y) persons in two key areas relative to stress testing:

1. High prevalence of asymptomatic CHD
2. Coexistence of other chronic conditions and physical limitations

Older, asymptomatic men and women exhibit increased ECG abnormalities, many of which diminish the GXTs diagnostic accuracy. The prevalence of asymptomatic ischemic episodes uncovered by the exercise ECG increases dramatically among older adults without history of MI or ECG abnormalities. Given the large reservoir of asymptomatic CHD among older persons, routine exercise stress testing would likely initiate a cascade of requirements for follow-up invasive cardiac procedures. In the absence of strong evidence to support aggressive evaluation in older adults, this practice places many at unnecessary risk for complications from invasive assessment. For this reason, empirical screening guidelines for older adults recommend physical activity based on the person's previous activity experiences and overall sense of well-being. This approach to exercise testing, training, and safety monitoring observes the widely accepted dictum in geriatrics practice, "start low and go slow."

Exercise-Induced Indicators of Coronary Heart Disease

The prognostic value of exercise testing in asymptomatic individuals comes from exercise-induced observations of ECG ischemia and congruent abnormalities and fitness-related variables obtained during the GXT.

Exercise-Induced Electrocardiographic Indicators of Coronary Heart Disease

Angina Pectoris

Approximately 30% of initial manifestations of CHD during exercise are revealed from chest-related pain known as angina pectoris. This condition indicates insufficiency of coronary blood flow, where oxygen supply momentarily reaches critically low levels. **Myocardial ischemia** (insufficient oxygen supply caused by coronary atherosclerosis) stimulates sensory nerves in the walls of coronary arteries and myocardium. (Refer to **Fig. 18.1** for locations of angina pain.) After the individual rests for a few minutes, the pain usually subsides without permanent heart muscle damage.

Electrocardiographic Disorders

Alterations in the heart's normal pattern of electrical activity rarely present until the heart's metabolic and blood flow requirements increase above rest. The

A CLOSER LOOK

Determining Heart Rate From an Electrocardiographic Tracing

The ECG depicts the pattern of electrical activity across the myocardium recorded as an electrocardiogram. As the wave of depolarization travels throughout the heart, electrical currents spread through the highly conductive body fluids for monitoring by electrodes placed on the skin's surface. Standard markings on the ECG paper allow time interval and voltage measurements during ECG propagation.

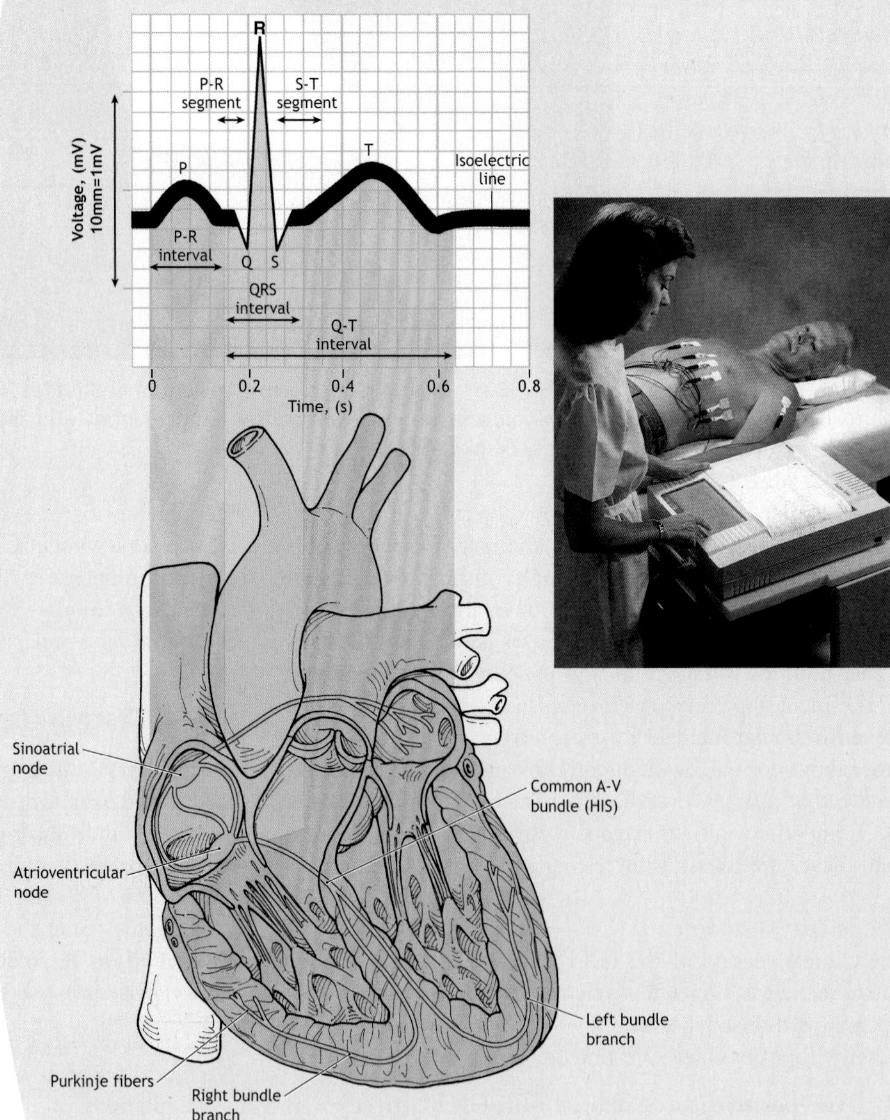

Figure 1. Normal electrocardiographic tracing.

Standard Electrocardiogram Tracing

Figure 1 shows a standard ECG tracing with time recorded on the horizontal axis. The paper normally moves at 25 mm per second. A repeating grid marks the ECG paper; major grid lines occur 5 mm apart (at 25 mm $\cdot$ s^{-1} paper speed, 5 mm = 0.20 s), minor grid lines occur 1 mm apart (at 25 mm $\cdot$ s^{-1} paper speed, 1 mm = 0.04 s). The graph's vertical axis indicates electrical voltage. The standard calibration factor equals 0.1 mV (millivolt) per mm of vertical deflection.

Determining Heart Rate

Three methods are used to determine heart rate from the standard ECG tracing.

Method 1

Figure 2A shows the standard R-R method. The R-R interval indicates the time between successive R waves. An approximate heart rate in beats per minute ($b \cdot min^{-1}$) can be determined by dividing 1500 (60 s × 25 $mm \cdot s^{-1}$) by the number of mm between adjacent R waves. In the example, heart rate equals 125 $b \cdot min^{-1}$ because 12 mm occurs between two successive R waves.

Method 2

This method begins with an R wave that falls on a thick blue line of the tracing (Fig. 2B). Moving to the right, the next six thick lines represent heart rates of 300, 150, 100, 75, 60, and 50 $mm \cdot s^{-1}$ (these numbers need to be memorized). If the next R wave (after the first one falling on the thick line) falls on either the first through sixth subsequent thick lines, the corresponding number (300 to 50) indicates heart rate in $mm \cdot s^{-1}$. Interpolation becomes necessary if the next R wave falls between two thick lines. In this instance, the first R wave falls between points 60 and 75 at 70 $mm \cdot s^{-1}$.

Method 3

This method (Fig. 2C), often used with irregular heart rates, counts the number of complete R-R intervals in a 6-second ECG strip multiplied by 10. In this example, six complete R-to-R intervals occur in 6 seconds; this equals a heart rate of 60 $b \cdot min^{-1}$ (6 × 10 = 60).

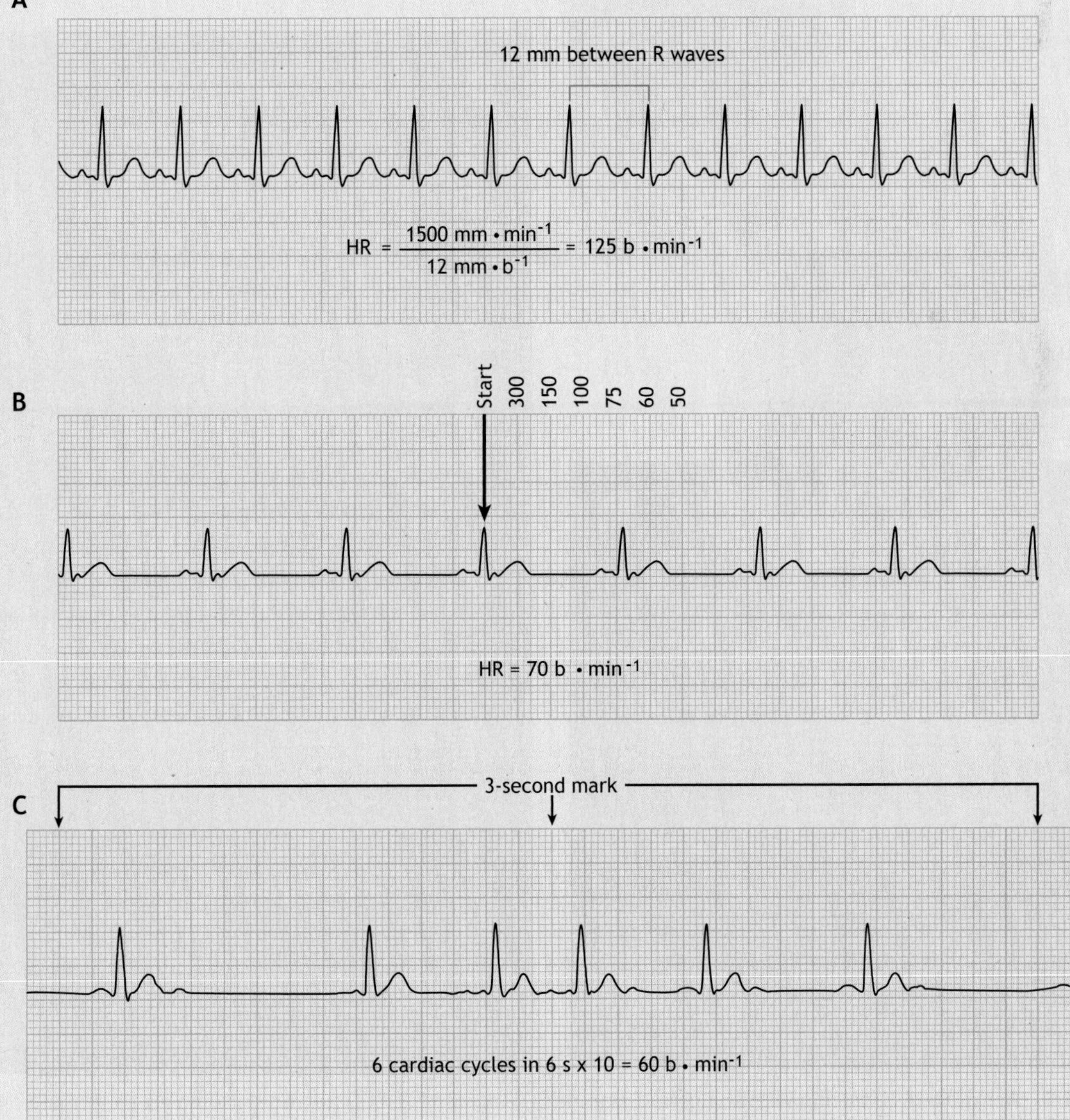

Figure 2. Three methods for determining heart rate from electrocardiographic tracings.

most common ECG abnormalities during exercise indicate myocardial ischemia from coronary artery obstruction. The obstruction generally relates to more than 50% diameter reduction from an occluded vessel. A significantly obstructed coronary artery can still maintain adequate blood flow at rest but cannot deliver sufficient blood and oxygen to meet increased myocardial needs with exercise. Ischemia does not always produce angina pectoris; its diagnosis most readily occurs through depressions of the S-T segment on the ECG. **Figure 18.5** shows a normal ECG tracing (**Fig. 18.5A**) and two abnormal tracings: **S-T segment depression** (**Fig. 18.5B**) and premature ventricular contraction (PVC). The latter illustrates disorganized electrical activity that includes an "extra" ventricular beat (**QRS complex**) that occurs without the **P wave** that normally precedes it (**Fig. 18.5C**).

Exercise PVCs generally herald the presence of severe ischemic atherosclerotic heart disease, often involving two or more major coronary vessels. Individuals who experience frequent PVCs have a high risk of sudden death from ventricular fibrillation, an electrical instability when ventricles fail to contract synchronously. This disrupts myocardial function, causing cardiac output to decrease dramatically.

Exercise-Induced Nonelectrocardiographic Indicators of Coronary Heart Disease

Two useful nonelectrocardiographic indicators of possible CHD are (1) blood pressure and (2) heart rate response to exercise.

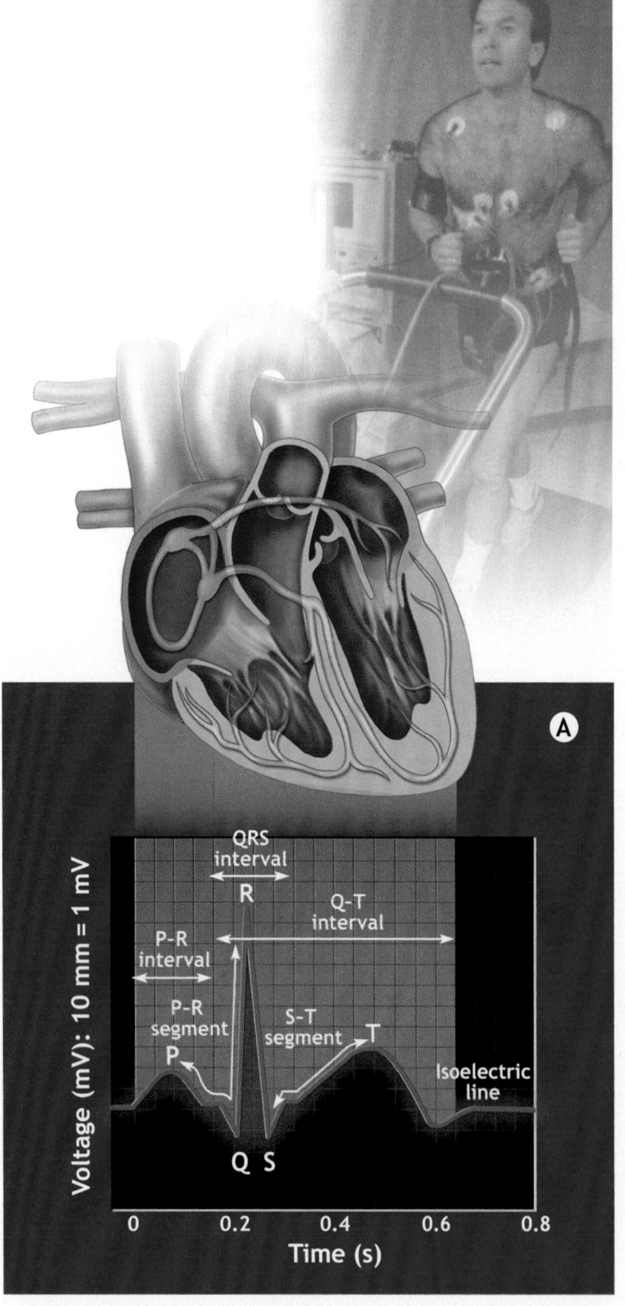

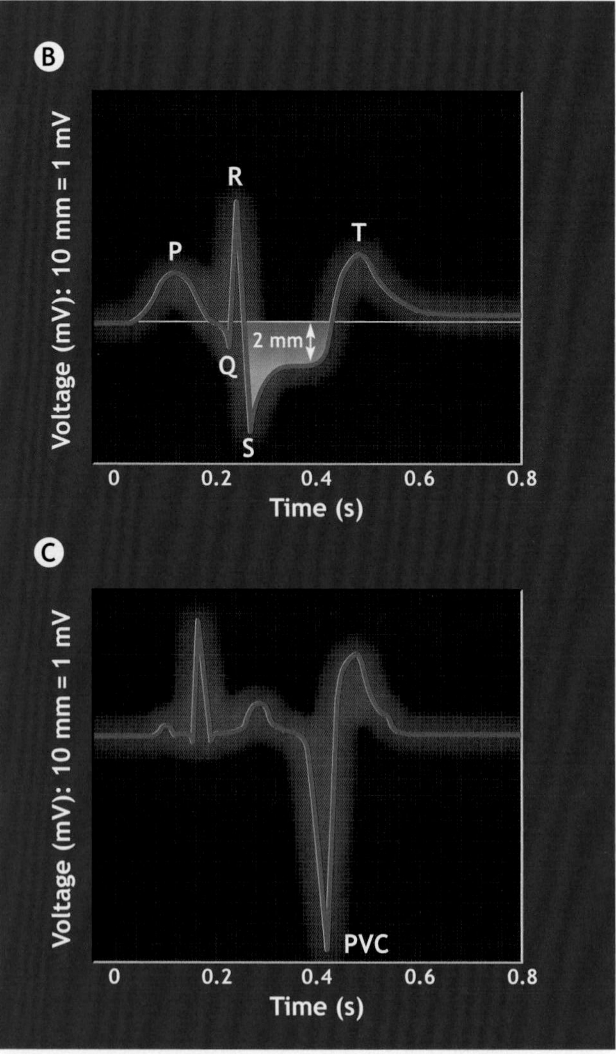

FIGURE 18.5 **A.** Normal ECG tracing with an upward-sloping S-T segment. **B.** ECG tracing showing an abnormal horizontal S-T segment depression (*shaded area*) of 2 mm, measured from a stable baseline. **C.** ECG tracing illustrating a premature ventricular contraction (PVC). (Adapted with permission from McArdle WD, Katch FI, Katch VL. *Exercise Physiology: Nutrition, Energy, and Human Performance*. 8th Ed. Baltimore: Wolters Kluwer Health, 2015.)

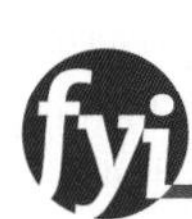

Regular Exercise Can Produce Unexpected Adverse Metabolic Responses

Researchers posed the following interesting question about the generally expected outcomes to exercise training: Is it possible some people respond in an undesirable way to the expected beneficial effects of exercise? Data from 1687 black and white men and women taken from six large published cohort studies assessed the prevalence of adverse responses in cardiovascular and diabetes risk factors. An adverse response was defined as an exercise-induced change that worsens a risk factor by a factor of two from the positive expected response. Risk boundaries included an increase of 10 mm Hg or more for systolic blood pressure (SBP), an increase of 0.42 mmol • L^{-1} or more for triglyceride (TG), an increase of 24 mmol • L^{-1} or more for fasting insulin (FI),or a decrease of 0.12 mmol • L^{-1} or more for high density lipoprotein (HDL-C). There were 8.4% (126 subjects) with an adverse change in FI, 12.2% (166 subjects) for SBP, 10.3% (172 subjects) for TG, and 13.3% (222 subjects) for HDL-C. Thirty-one percent of participants (461 subjects) experienced one adverse response and 7.0% (95 subjects) experienced adverse responses in two or more risk factors. The researchers concluded that adverse responses to regular exercise in cardiovascular and diabetes risk factors exceeded their expectations. Identifying such unexpected and unfavorable responses and how to prevent them can help to personalize future exercise regimens for those who may not respond in the expected positive way to exercise training.

Reference: Bouchard C, et al. Adverse metabolic response to regular exercise: is it a rare or common occurrence? *PLoS ONE* 2012;7:e37887. doi:10.1371/journal.pone.0037887.

Hypertensive or Hypotensive Response

During a graded exercise test, a normal, progressive transition in SBP occurs from about 120 mm Hg at rest to 160 to 190 mm Hg during peak exercise. Diastolic blood pressure generally changes less than 10 mm Hg. A *hypertensive response* during strenuous activity can elevate SBP to 250 mm Hg or higher, and DBP can approach 150 mm Hg. Abnormal blood pressure responses to exercise often provide an important clue to cardiovascular disease.

Failure of blood pressure to increase with graded exercise, called a *hypotensive response*, indicates cardiovascular malfunction. For example, diminished cardiac reserve may exist if SBP does not increase by at least 20 or 30 mm Hg during graded exercise.

Heart Rate Response

An abnormally rapid heart rate (tachycardia) early in submaximal exercise often foretells cardiac problems. Likewise, an abnormally low exercise heart rate (bradycardia) usually reflects sinus node malfunction (**sick sinus node syndrome**). An inability of the heart rate to increase during exercise, especially when accompanied by extreme fatigue, indicates cardiac strain and underlying heart disease.

In asymptomatic women, heart rate recovery provides a more sensitive predictor of cardiovascular disease and all-cause mortality than S-T segment depression. Because nearly two-thirds of women who die suddenly from cardiovascular disease have no previous symptoms, the important potential role of treadmill testing in this population should be recognized.

Invasive Physiologic Tests

Invasive physiologic tests provide diagnostic information unavailable through noninvasive procedures. This information includes the extent, severity, and location of coronary atherosclerosis, degree of ventricular dysfunction, and specific cardiac abnormalities. The three most common invasive physiologic tests are:

1. **Radionucleotide studies** include two types: (1) **thallium imaging** (**www.healthline.com/health/thallium-stress-test#Overview1**), which evaluates areas of myocardial blood flow and tissue perfusion to differentiate between a true-positive and a false-positive S-T segment depression (by ECG evaluation), and (2) **ventriculography** (**www.healthline.com/health/nuclear-ventriculography#Overview1**), an imaging procedure that provides information about left ventricular functional dynamics.
2. **Cardiac catheterization** (**www.nhlbi.nih.gov/health/health-topics/topics/cath/**) involves threading a small-diameter, flexible tube (catheter), guided by x-ray, directly into an arm or leg vein or artery into the right or left side of the heart. Sensors on the catheter tip accurately measure pressure gradients at various locations within the heart's chambers or large vessels and also assess the heart's electrical patterns to determine coronary artery blockage. The oxygen content of arterial and mixed venous blood comes from blood sampled from the ventricles or atria. Cardiac catheterization takes place under local anesthesia, depending on the point of catheter entry into the arm or leg. The patient remains awake during the procedure, and test results usually become available on test day.
3. **Coronary angiography** (**www.patient.co.uk/health/coronary-angiography**) provides an intracardiac radiograph of the progress of a radiopaque contrast medium introduced into the coronary blood vessels, and its passage during a cardiac cycle. This technique accurately assesses the extent of atherosclerosis and serves as the "gold standard" for viewing coronary blood flow. It also creates a baseline for other test comparisons and validations. Angiography does not show how readily blood flows within local portions of the myocardium, as it is not a measure of capillary blood flow and cannot be used during exercise.

See the animations "Coronary Angiography: Left Coronary System-Part A" and "Coronary Angiography: Left Coronary System-Part B" on **http://thePoint.lww.com/MKKESS5e** for a demonstration of this process.

thePoint® Appendix SR-6: Additional Video Links, available online at **http://thePoint.lww.com/MKKESS5e,** provides a list of supplemental animations and videos on this subject, including an animation of angiography.

Exercise Prescription for Cardiac Patients

Joint recommendations of ACSM and the American Heart Association (AHA) for cardiovascular screening and exercise prescription of 18- to 65-year-olds for participation in activities at health/fitness facilities can be accessed online at **http://circ.ahajournals.org/cgi/reprint/CIRCULATIONAHA.107.185649** (*Circulation* 2007;116:1081). The recommendations also discuss staff qualifications and emergency policies related to cardiovascular safety.

Heart rate and oxygen uptake obtained during the GXT form the basis for creating an individualized exercise prescription. Many people who start exercising do not recognize their limitations and engage in exercise above a prudent level. Even group exercise programs that require medical clearance may not be appropriate because all members often exercise at about the *same* absolute intensity work level (walk, jog, or swim at a similar pace) without much attention to individual differences in current fitness status.

Figure 18.6 illustrates a practical approach for functional translation of treadmill or cycle ergometer exercise test

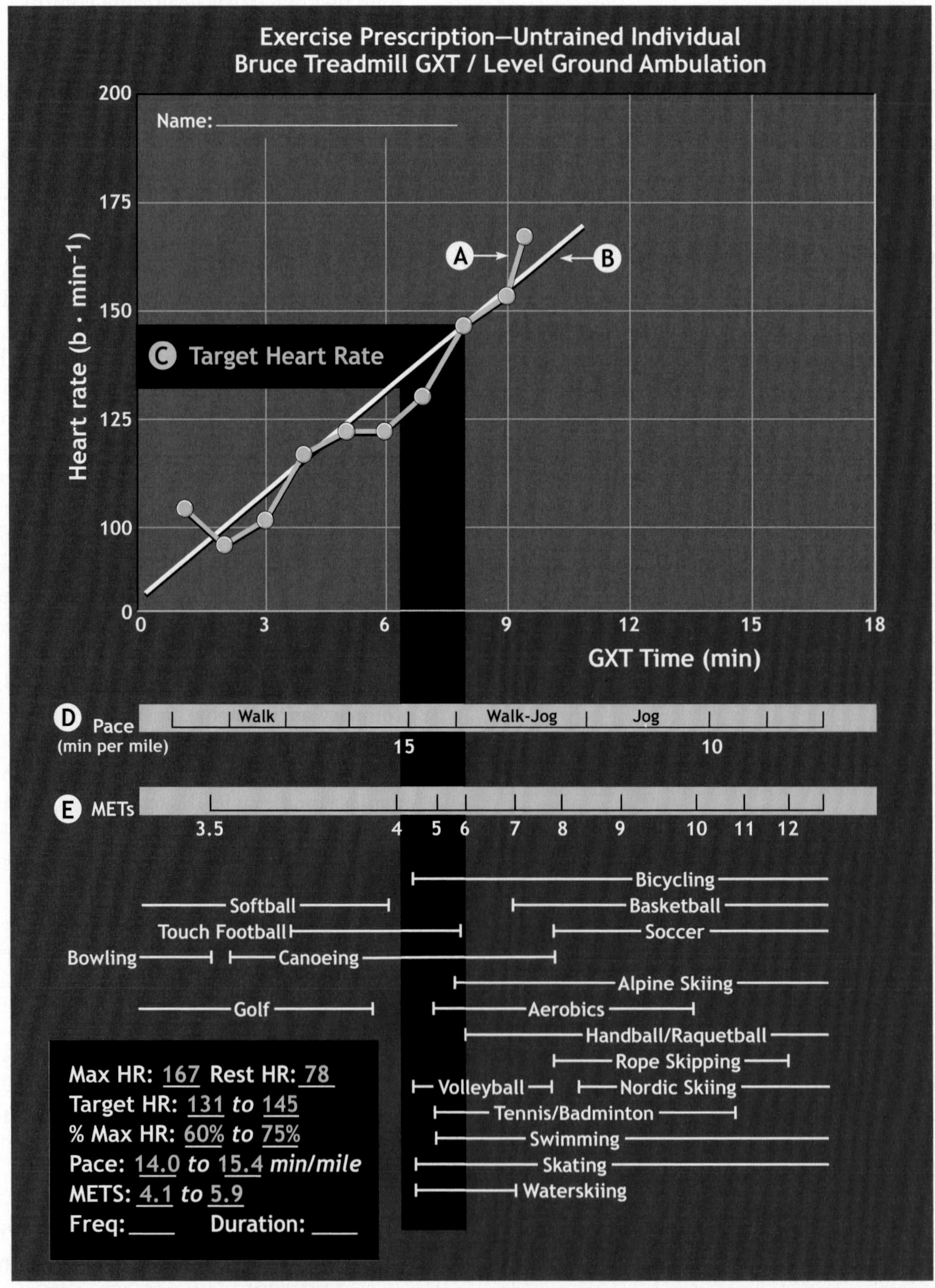

FIGURE 18.6 Exercise prescription based on functional translation algorithm for level-ground ambulation. *Letters* in figure identified in text. (Adapted with permission from McArdle WD, Katch FI, Katch VL. *Exercise Physiology: Nutrition, Energy, and Human Performance.* 8th Ed. Baltimore: Wolters Kluwer Health, 2015; as reprinted with permission of Dr. Carl Foster, University of Wisconsin–LaCrosse.)

TABLE 18.12 ACSM Categories for Exercise Programs Related to Patient Symptoms

Type	Participants	Entry MET Level	Supervision
A. Unsupervised	Asymptomatic	8+	None
B. Supervised			
1. Inpatient	All symptomatics—postmyocardial infarction, postoperative, pulmonary disease	3	Supervised ambulatory therapy
2. Outpatient	All symptomatics—postmyocardial infarction, postoperative, pulmonary disease	3+	Exercise specialist, physician on call
3. In home	Symptomatic + asymptomatic	>3–5	Unsupervised; periodic hospital reevaluation
4. Community	Symptomatic + asymptomatic, 6–8 wk postinfarct, 4–8 wk postoperative	>5	Exercise program director + exercise specialist

Adapted with permission from Pescatello LS, et al., eds. *ACSM's Guidelines for Exercise Testing and Prescription*. 9th Ed. Baltimore: Lippincott Williams & Wilkins, 2014.

responses to an exercise prescription. Heart rate (**A**) during the Bruce test is plotted as a function of time. Line **B** (*white*) depicts a mathematical line of "best fit" drawn through the data points. A target zone for heart rate equals 60% to 75% of maximum heart rate (167 b · min^{-1}; *black region* represented as **C**). The individualized prescription includes pace (14.0 to 15.4 min per mile, **D**) or METs (3.9 to 5.9, **E**). The acceptable range of exercise intensity in area **C**, based on heart rate response during the graded exercise test, includes the following recreational activities: bicycling, canoeing, alpine skiing, aerobics, volleyball, tennis and badminton, swimming, skating, and waterskiing. This quantitative method of assigning exercise improves exercise prescription specificity and precision for previously sedentary, healthy individuals and for patients with diagnosed cardiovascular diseases.

Guidelines

Any exercise prescription should begin with 5 to 10 minutes of light stretching and range of motion (ROM) activities followed by several minutes of light-to-moderate rhythmic "warm-up" movements. The aerobic conditioning phase should progress in duration, so individuals eventually perform 30 to 45 minutes of continuous activity at the prescribed intensity followed by 5 to 15 minutes of low-intensity walking or other rhythmic "cool-down" activities.

Most cardiac rehabilitation patients easily tolerate exercising 3 days per week with no more than a 2-day lapse between exercise sessions. For elderly patients or those with poor functional capacity (<5 METs), low-intensity activity should be performed daily or twice daily. As a patient's functional capacity improves, exercise intensity and duration can increase progressively with little fear of complications. The most recent GXT should serve as the basis for updating the exercise prescription.

In addition to testing, three other components of cardiac rehabilitation are important:

1. Patient education
2. Appropriate pharmacologic intervention
3. Family support counseling

A trained social worker often coordinates the education and support counseling aspects of rehabilitation.

Supervision of Cardiac Exercise Program

ACSM has categorized several types of programs with specific criteria for entry and supervision (**Table 18.12**). These programs are either unsupervised or supervised, with four subdivisions in the supervised category. Unsupervised programs meet the needs of asymptomatic participants of any age with functional capacities of at least 8 METs and without known major risk factors. The supervised programs focus on patients with specific needs. These include asymptomatic physically active or inactive persons of any age with CHD risk factors but no known disease (B4) and symptomatic individuals, including individuals with recent onset of CHD and those with a changed disease status (B1 to B3).

Cardiac Medications and Physical Activity Response

Knowledge of the physiologic effects of drug intervention allows the clinical exercise physiologist to properly assess patient response during physical activity. **Table 18.13** presents six classifications of common cardiac drugs along with their trade names, side effects, and possible effects on exercise responses.

CARDIAC REHABILITATION

A comprehensive **cardiac rehabilitation program** focuses on improving longevity and quality of life, including risk factor modification. After diagnosis of the cardiac disorder and medical intervention (e.g., aggressive risk factor reduction, bypass surgery, angioplasty), the clinical exercise physiologist evaluates the cardiac patient for functional capacity and ensuing classification and rehabilitation. **Table 18.14** presents guidelines for risk stratification from the AHA (**www.americanheart.org**) to categorize patients

TABLE 18.13 Cardiac Medications: Their Use, Side Effects, and Effects on Exercise Response

Type/Trade Name	Use	Side Effects	Effects on Exercise Response
I. Antianginal agents			
A. Nitroglycerin compounds *[Amyl nitrate; Isordil; Nitrostat]*	Smooth muscle relaxation; decrease cardiac output	Headache, dizziness, hypotension	Hypotension; increase exercise capacity
B. β-blockers *[Inderal; propranolol; Lopressor; Corgard; Biocadren]*	Block β receptors; decrease sympathetic tone; decrease HR, myocardial contractility, BP	Bradycardia, heart block, insomnia, weakness, nausea, fatigue, increased cholesterol, and blood sugar	Decrease HR; hypotension; decrease cardiac contractility
C. Calcium antagonists *[Verapamil; nifedipine; Procardia]*	Block influx of calcium; dilate coronary arteries; suppress dysrhythmias	Dizziness, syncope, flushing, hypotension, headache, fluid retention	Hypotension
II. Antihypertensive agents			
A. Diuretics *[Thiazides, Lasix, Aldactone]*	Inhibit Na^+ and Cl^- in the kidney; increase excretion of sodium and water, and control high BP and fluid retention	Drowsiness, dehydration, electrolyte imbalance; gout, nausea, pain, hearing loss, elevated cholesterol, and lipoproteins	Hypotension
B. Vasodilators *[Hydralazine, Captopril, Apresoline, Loniten, Minoxidil]*	Dilate peripheral blood vessels; used in conjunction with diuretics; decrease BP	Increase HR and contractility; headache, drowsiness, nausea, vomiting, diarrhea	
C. Drugs interfering with sympathetic nervous system *[Reserpine, Propranolol, Aldomet, Catapres, Minipress]*	Decrease BP, HR, and cardiac output by dilating blood vessels	Drowsiness, depression, sexual dysfunction, fatigue, dry mouth, stuffy nose, fever, upset stomach, fluid retention, weight gain	Hypotension
III. Digitalis glycosides, derivatives			
[Digoxin Lanoxin digitoxin]	Strengthen heart's pumping force and decrease electrical conduction	Arrhythmias, heart block, altered ECG, fatigue, weakness, headache, nausea, vomiting	Increase exercise capacity; increase myocardial contractility
IV. Anticoagulant agents			
[Coumadin, sodium heparin, aspirin, Persantine]	Prevent blood clot formation	Easy bruising, stomach irritation, joint or abdominal pain, difficulty swallowing, unexplained swelling, uncontrolled bleeding	
V. Antilipidemic agents			
[Cholestyramine, Lopid, Niacin, Atromid-S, Mevacor, Questran, Zocor, Lipitor]	Interfere with lipid metabolism and lower cholesterol and low-density lipoproteins	Nausea, vomiting, diarrhea, constipation, flatulence, abdominal discomfort, glucose intolerance, myalgia, liver dysfunction, muscle fatigue	
VI. Antiarrhythmic agents			
[Cardioquin, procaine, quinidine, lidocaine, Dilantin, propranolol, bretylium tosylate, verapamil]	Alter conduction patterns throughout the myocardium	Nausea, palpitations, vomiting, rash, insomnia, dizziness, shortness of breath, swollen ankles, coughing up blood, fever, psychosis, impotence	Hypotension; decrease HR; decrease cardiac contractility

for subsequent rehabilitation. Patients differ greatly in symptoms, functional capacities, and rehabilitation strategies. The rehabilitation program incorporates stringent guidelines to promote low-risk treatment. CHD patients with mild ischemia tolerate steady-rate exercise at intensities consistent for aerobic training, without progressive deterioration in left ventricular function. For patients without ischemia, left ventricular function in prolonged physical effort remains

TABLE 18.14 Guidelines for Risk Stratification From the AHA When Considering an Exercise Program

AHA Classification	NYHA[a] Class	Exercise Capacity	Angina/Ischemia and Clinical Characteristics	ECG Monitoring
A. Apparently healthy			<40 y of age; without symptoms, no major risk factors, and normal GXT	No supervision or monitoring required
B. Known stable CHD, low risk for vigorous exercise	I or II	5–6 METs	Free of ischemia or angina at rest or on the GXT; EF = 40%–60%	Monitored and supervised only during prescribed sessions (6–12 sessions); light resistance training may be included in comprehensive rehabilitation programs
C. Stable CHD with low risk for vigorous exercise but unable to self-regulate activity	I or II	5–6 METs	Same disease states and clinical characteristics as class B but without the ability to self-monitor exercise	Medical supervision and ECG monitoring during prescribed sessions; nonmedical supervision of other exercise sessions
D. Moderate-to-high risk for cardiac complications during exercise	≥III	<6 METs	Ischemia (≥4.0 mm S-T depression) or angina during exercise; two or more previous MIs; EF <30%	Continuous ECG monitoring during rehabilitation until safety established; medical supervision during all exercise sessions until safety established
E. Unstable disease with activity restriction	≥III	<6 METs	Unstable angina; uncompensated heart failure; uncomfortable arrhythmias	No activity recommended for conditioning purposes; attention directed to restoring patient to class D or higher

[a]NYHA, New York Heart Association; EF, ejection fraction; CHD, coronary heart disease; GXT, graded exercise test.

Adapted with permission from Pescatello LS. et al., eds. *ACSM's Guidelines for Exercise Testing and Prescription*. 9th Ed. Baltimore: Lippincott Williams & Wilkins, 2014.

similar to healthy controls. The five most important aspects of a successful cardiac rehabilitation program are:

1. Appropriate patient selection
2. Concurrent medical, surgical, and pharmacologic therapies
3. Comprehensive patient education
4. Appropriate exercise prescription
5. Careful patient monitoring during rehabilitation

Traditional cardiac rehabilitation programs consisted of three distinct phases, each with different objectives, physical activities, and required supervision. Contemporary programs have changed the traditional model based on new theories of risk stratification, exercise safety data, and changes in the healthcare industry. Current programs recognize individual differences in rehabilitation when determining program length, degree of supervision, and required ECG monitoring.

Contemporary cardiac rehabilitation includes inpatient and outpatient programs and services, with emphasis on outcome measures. Almost all postsurgery patients benefit from inpatient activity intervention, risk factor assessment, lifestyle activity and dietary counseling, and patient and family education. Patients stay at the hospital an average of 3 to 5 days postsurgery before release.

Inpatient Programs

Inpatient cardiac rehabilitation focuses on four objectives:

1. Medical surveillance
2. Identification of patients with significant impairments before discharge
3. Rapid patient return to daily activities
4. Preparation of patient and family to optimize recovery upon discharge

In-hospital physical activity during the first 48 hours following an MI and/or cardiac surgery is restricted to self-care movements, arm and leg ROM, and intermittent sitting and standing to maintain cardiovascular reflexes. After several days, patients usually sit and stand without assistance, perform self-care activities, and walk independently up to six times daily, provided none of the following 12 contraindications exist:

1. Unstable angina
2. Elevated resting blood pressure
3. Orthostatic SBP above 200 mm Hg with symptoms

4. Critical aortic stenosis
5. Acute systemic illness or fever
6. Uncontrolled atrial or ventricular arrhythmias
7. Uncontrolled sinus tachycardia above 120 b · min^{-1}
8. Uncompensated CHF
9. Active pericarditis or myocarditis
10. Recent embolism or thrombophlebitis
11. Resting S-T segment displacement of 2 mm or more
12. Severe orthopedic conditions

Outpatient Programs

Upon discharge, the patient should understand appropriate and inappropriate physical activities and dietary guidelines and have a prudent and progressive plan of risk reduction with a specific, detailed exercise prescription. Enrollment in an **outpatient cardiac rehabilitation** activity program is the ideal. The goals of outpatient cardiac rehabilitation include the following:

1. Monitoring and supervising the patient to detect changes in clinical status
2. Returning the patient to premorbid/vocational/recreational activities
3. Assisting the patient to implement at-home, unsupervised activity program
4. Providing family support and education

Most outpatient program sites encourage multiple physical activities, including resistance exercise and walking, cycling, and swimming. Supervision should include personnel trained in CPR and advanced life support; in some cases, a defibrillator (**automated external defibrillator [AED]; www.nhlbi.nih.gov/health/health-topics/topics/aed/**) should be available.

Resistance-Training Prescription

Cardiac patients should exercise with light resistance (range of 30% to 50% of 1-RM) because of exaggerated blood pressure responses with straining-type exercise. In the absence of contraindications, elastic bands, light 1 to 5 lb cuff and hand weights, light free weights, and wall pulleys can be applied at the outpatient program outset. Low-level resistance training should not be started until 2 to 3 weeks after an MI. Barbells or weight machines should be introduced after 4 to 6 weeks of convalescence.

Most cardiac patients begin ROM exercises using relatively light weight for the lower and upper extremities. In accordance with AHA recommendations, cardiac patients should perform one set of 10 to 15 repetitions to moderate fatigue using 8 to 10 different exercises (e.g., chest press, shoulder press, triceps extension, biceps curl, lat pull-down, lower back extension, abdominal crunch or curl-up, quadriceps extension or leg press, leg curl, calf raise). Exercises performed 2 to 3 days a week produce favorable adaptations. The rating of perceived exertion (RPE) should range from 11 to 14 on the Borg scale ("fairly light" to "somewhat hard"). To minimize dramatic blood pressure fluctuations during lifting, patients should be warned to avoid straining, performing the Valsalva maneuver, and gripping weight handles or bars tightly.

For heart transplant patients, a carefully supervised total body resistance-training program 3 days weekly for 6 months increases functional strength and muscle mass to counter the generally debilitating effects of immunosuppressive medication.

Beneficial Effects of Resistance Exercise

Resistance exercise, as part of a structured cardiac rehabilitation program, offers four benefits:

1. Helps restore and maintain muscular strength
2. Preserve fat-free body mass (FFM)
3. Improve psychological status and quality of life
4. Increase glucose tolerance and insulin sensitivity

Combining resistance training and aerobic training yields more pronounced physiologic adaptations (improved aerobic capacity, muscle strength, and lean body mass) in heart disease patients than aerobic training alone. The following six conditions *preclude* cardiac patients from participating in resistance training:

1. Unstable angina
2. Uncontrolled arrhythmias
3. Left ventricular outflow obstruction (e.g., hypertrophic cardiomyopathy with obstruction)
4. Recent history of CHF without follow-up and treatment
5. Severe valvular disease, hypertension (SBP >160 mm Hg or DBP >105 mm Hg)
6. Poor left ventricular function and exercise capacity below 5 METs with anginal symptoms or ischemic S-T segment depression

SUMMARY

1. The major cardiovascular diseases affect heart muscle directly, heart valves, or neural regulation of cardiac function.
2. The *ATHS* gene on chromosome 19 near the gene related to LDL-cholesterol receptor functioning accounts for almost 50% of CHD cases.
3. An imbalance between the heart's oxygen demands and its oxygen supply causes angina pectoris.
4. MI results from inadequate blood perfusion in coronary arteries or imbalance in myocardial oxygen demand and supply during physical activity.
5. Pericarditis, an inflammation of the heart's outer pericardial lining, classifies as either acute (recurring) or chronic (constrictive).
6. CHF occurs when cardiac output does not keep pace with venous return.
7. The heart fails from intrinsic myocardial disease, chronic hypertension, or structural defects that impair pump performance.
8. Aneurysm represents an abnormal dilatation in the wall of an artery or vein or within the myocardium itself.

9. Vascular aneurysms occur when a vessel's wall weakens from trauma, congenital vascular disease, infection, or atherosclerosis.
10. Aerobic exercise programs implemented for cardiac patients should consider specific disease pathophysiology, mechanisms that limit exercise capacity, and individual differences in functional capacity.
11. Heart valve diseases include stenosis, regurgitation, and prolapse.
12. Diseases of the heart's nervous system include the dysrhythmias bradycardia, tachycardia, and PVCs.
13. A thorough cardiac disease assessment includes medical history, physical examination, laboratory assessments (chest radiography, ECG, blood lipid analyses, serum enzyme testing), and physiologic tests.
14. Knowledge of the physiologic effects of drug intervention allows the clinical exercise physiologist to properly assess patient response during physical activity.
15. The "stress test" describes systematic exercise for two purposes: (1) ECG observations and (2) evaluation of physiologic adjustments to metabolic demands that exceed resting requirements.
16. Multistage cycle ergometer and treadmill tests represent the most common modes for exercise stress testing.
17. Multistage tests, graded for exercise intensity, include several levels of 3 to 5 minutes of exercise that bring the person to self-imposed, symptom-limited fatigue.
18. Graded exercise stress testing provides a low-risk screening for CHD preventive and rehabilitative physical activity programs.
19. Four possible outcomes from a stress test include true-positive (test a success), false-negative (heart disease not diagnosed when present), true-negative (test a success), and false-positive (healthy person diagnosed with heart disease).
20. Exercise-induced indicators of CHD include angina pectoris, ECG disorders, cardiac rhythm abnormalities, and abnormal blood pressure and heart rate responses.
21. Invasive physiologic tests that include radionucleotide studies, cardiac catheterization, and coronary angiography provide diagnostic information unavailable through noninvasive procedures.
22. A comprehensive cardiac rehabilitation program focuses on improving longevity and quality of life, in addition to risk factor modification.
23. Following diagnosis and intervention, the exercise physiologist evaluates the cardiac patient for functional capacity and ensuing classification and rehabilitation.
24. Cardiac patients improve functional capacity similar to healthy people of the same age.
25. Resistance training has proven successful for cardiac patients as part of a comprehensive rehabilitation program.
26. Resistance exercise for cardiac patients should include light resistance (range 30% to 50% of 1-RM) because of exaggerated blood pressure responses with straining-type exercise.
27. Cardiac patients enter different cardiac rehabilitation phases depending on disease severity and degree of risk.

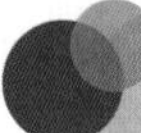

THINK IT THROUGH

1. Give recommendations for a middle-age man who experiences breathlessness and chest discomfort while walking the golf course yet wants to begin an aerobic activity program.
2. What type of GXT and exercise prescription most benefits a patient with CHD who experiences angina during upper-body work in his job as a plasterer or paperhanger?

PART 3 Pulmonary Diseases and Disorders

The clinical exercise physiologist's involvement in treating patients with pulmonary disease focuses on improving ventilation, decreasing the work of breathing, and increasing overall functional capacity. The exercise physiologist applies clinical information from the patient's personal history, physical examination, pertinent laboratory data, and imaging studies. Pulmonary impairment and cardiovascular issues are often related: cardiovascular system disorders usually impair pulmonary function and cardiovascular complications often occur following pulmonary disease onset.

Restrictive reduced lung volume dimensions and obstructive impeded air flow lung diseases represent two common classifications for pulmonary dysfunction. Several pulmonary disorders combine *both* restrictive and obstructive impairments.

Restrictive Lung Dysfunction

Restrictive lung dysfunction (RLD), characterized by abnormal reduction in pulmonary ventilation, includes diminished lung expansion and decreased tidal volume. The chest and lung tissues in RLD tend to stiffen and offer considerable resistance to expansion under normal pulmonary pressure differentials. This represents a reduction in **lung compliance**, that is, the change in lung volume per unit change in intra-alveolar pressure. Decreased pulmonary compliance increases the energy cost of ventilation even at rest. Eventually, RLD progresses to a point where considerable decreases occur in all lung volumes and capacities.

Table 18.15 lists the three major RLDs along with causes, signs and symptoms, and treatments. Ten other known causes of RLD include rheumatoid arthritis, immunologic impairment, massive obesity, diabetes mellitus, trauma from impact injuries, penetrating wounds, burns and other inhalation injuries, radiation trauma, poisoning, and complications from drug therapy (including negative reactions to antibiotics and anti-inflammatory drugs).

TABLE 18.15 Major Restrictive Lung Diseases and Their Causes, Signs and Symptoms, and Treatments

Causes/Type	Etiology	Signs and Symptoms	Treatment
I. Maturational			
a. *Abnormal fetal lung development*	Premature birth (hypoplasia-reduced lung tissue)	Asymptomatic; pulmonary insufficiency	No specific treatment
b. *Respiratory distress syndrome* (hyaline membrane disease)	Insufficient maturation of lungs due to premature birth	↑ respiration rate; ↓ lung volumes; ↓ Pa_{O_2}; acidemia; rapid and labored respiration pressure	Treat mother prior to birth (corticosteroids); hyperalimentation; continuous positive airway
c. *Aging*	Aging and cumulative effects of pollution, noxious gas, inhaled drug use, and cigarette smoking	↑ residual volume; ↓ vital capacity; repetitive periodic apnea	No specific treatment; increase physical activity
II. Pulmonary			
a. *Idiopathic pulmonary fibrosis* (IPF)	Unknown origin (perhaps viral or genetic)	↓ lung volumes; pulmonary hypertension; dyspnea; cough; weight loss, fatigue	Corticosteroids; maintain adequate nutrition and ventilation
b. *Coal workers' pneumoconiosis*	Repeated inhalation of coal dust over 10–12 y	↓ TLC, VC, FRC; ↓ lung compliance; dyspnea; ↓ Pa_{O_2}; pulmonary hypertension; cough	Nonreversible, no known cure
c. *Asbestosis*	Chronic exposure to asbestos	↓ lung volumes; abnormal x-ray; ↓ Pa_{O_2}; dyspnea on exertion; shortness of breath	Nonreversible, no known cure
d. *Pneumonia*	Inflammatory process caused by various bacteria, microbes, viruses	↓ lung volumes; abnormal x-ray; tachypneic dyspnea; high fever, chills, cough; pleuritic pain	Drug therapy (antibiotic)
e. *Adult respiratory distress syndrome*	Acute lung injury (fat emboli, drowning, drug induced, shock, blood transfusion, pneumonia)	Abnormal lung function tests; Pa_{O_2} <60 mm Hg; extreme dyspnea; cyanotic; headache; anxiety	Intubation and mechanical ventilation
f. *Bronchogenic carcinoma*	Tobacco use	Variable depending on type and location of growth	Surgery; radiation; chemotherapy
g. *Pleural effusions*	Accumulation of fluid within pleural space; heart failure; cirrhosis	Shortness of breath; pleuritic chest pain; ↓ Pa_{O_2}	Specific drainage
III. Cardiovascular			
a. *Pulmonary edema*	↑ pulmonary capillary hydrostatic pressure secondary to left ventricular failure	↑ respiration rate; ↓ lung volumes; ↓ Pa_{O_2}; arrhythmias; feeling of suffocation, shortness of breath, cyanotic, cough	Drug therapy; diuretics; supplemental O_2
b. *Pulmonary emboli*	Complications of venous thrombosis	↓ lung volumes, ↓ Pa_{O_2}; tachycardia; acute dyspnea, shortness of breath; syncope	Heparin therapy; mechanical ventilation

Chronic Obstructive Pulmonary Disease

Chronic obstructive pulmonary disease (COPD), also termed **chronic airflow limitations (CAL)**, includes respiratory diseases that produce airflow obstruction. This ultimately affects the lung's mechanical function and compromises alveolar gas exchange. In the United States, COPD ranks as the third leading cause of death and the second leading cause of morbidity; its economic burden averages more than $36 billion annually (**http://www.chestnet.org/News/Press-Releases/2014/07/CDC-reports-36-billion-in-annual-financial-cost-of-COPD-in-US**). The natural history of COPD spans 20 to 50 years and closely links to chronic cigarette smoking.

COPD, usually diagnosed from changes in pulmonary function, most notably represents a decrease in expiratory flow rate and increase in residual lung volume. Classic symptoms include spontaneous spasms of bronchial smooth muscle, which produce chronic coughing, inflammation and thickening of the mucosal lining of the bronchi and bronchioles, increased mucus production, wheezing, and dyspnea upon physical exertion. **Table 18.16** summarizes the differences among major COPD conditions.

TABLE 18.16 Difference Among Major Chronic Obstructive Pulmonary Diseases

Name	Area Affected	Result
Bronchitis	Membrane lining bronchial tubes	Inflammation of bronchial lining
Bronchiectasis	Bronchial tubes (bronchi or air passages)	Bronchial dilation with inflammation
Emphysema	Air spaces beyond terminal bronchioles (alveoli)	Breakdown of alveolar walls; air spaces enlarged
Asthma	Bronchioles (small airways)	Bronchioles obstructed by muscle spasm; swelling of mucosa; thick secretions
Cystic fibrosis	Bronchioles	Bronchioles become obstructed and obliterated; plugs of mucus cling to airway walls leading to bronchitis, atelectasis, pneumonia, or pulmonary abscess

In all forms of COPD, the airways narrow to obstruct airflow. Airway narrowing hinders alveolar ventilation by trapping air in the bronchi and alveoli; in essence, COPD increases physiologic dead space. Obstruction principally precipitates these four negative effects:

1. Increases resistance to airflow during expiration
2. Impairs normal alveolar gas exchange
3. Diminishes exercise capacity
4. Reduces ventilatory capacity

The following brief discussion centers on three major COPD diseases: chronic bronchitis, emphysema, and cystic fibrosis. Chapter 11 discussed the obstructive conditions of asthma and exercise-induced bronchospasm.

Chronic Bronchitis

Acute bronchitis refers to self-limiting and short-duration inflammation of the trachea and bronchi. In contrast, **chronic bronchitis** mostly occurs with long-term exposure to nonspecific irritants. Increases in mucus secretion accompany prolonged respiratory tract inflammation. Over time, the swollen mucous membranes and thick sputum obstruct airways, causing wheezing and persistent coughing. Partial or complete airway blockage from mucus secretion causes insufficient arterial oxygen saturation and edema, which produces the characteristic look of the "blue bloater" (**Fig. 18.7**). Chronic bronchitis develops slowly and worsens over time. Patients usually have been long-term smokers. Functional exercise capacity remains

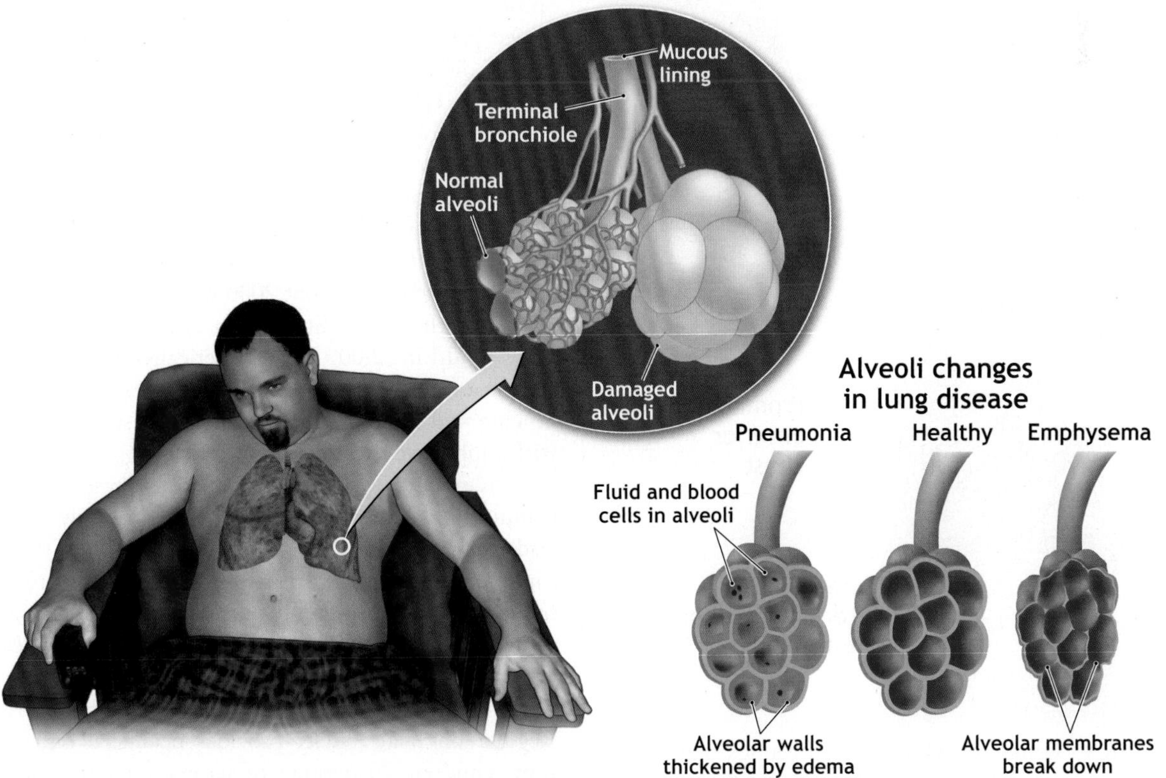

FIGURE 18.7 A person with chronic bronchitis usually develops cyanosis and pulmonary edema with the characteristic appearance known as the "blue bloater." (*Inset*) Effects of chronic bronchitis: misshapen or large alveolar sacs with reduced surface for oxygen and carbon dioxide exchange. (Adapted with permission from McArdle WD, Katch FI, Katch VL. *Exercise Physiology: Nutrition, Energy, and Human Performance*. 8th Ed. Baltimore: Wolters Kluwer Health, 2015.)

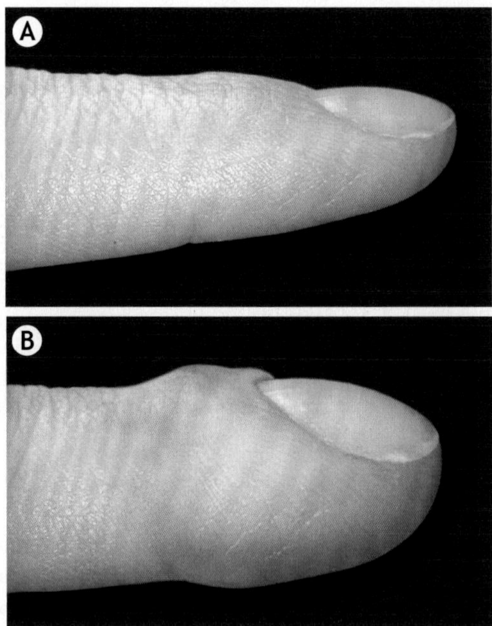

FIGURE 18.8 Normal digit configuration **(A)** and digital clubbing **(B)**. Club fingers and toes indicate chronic tissue hypoxia, a common diagnosis in emphysema. (Adapted with permission from McArdle WD, Katch FI, Katch VL. *Exercise Physiology: Nutrition, Energy, and Human Performance*. 8th Ed. Baltimore: Wolters Kluwer Health, 2015.)

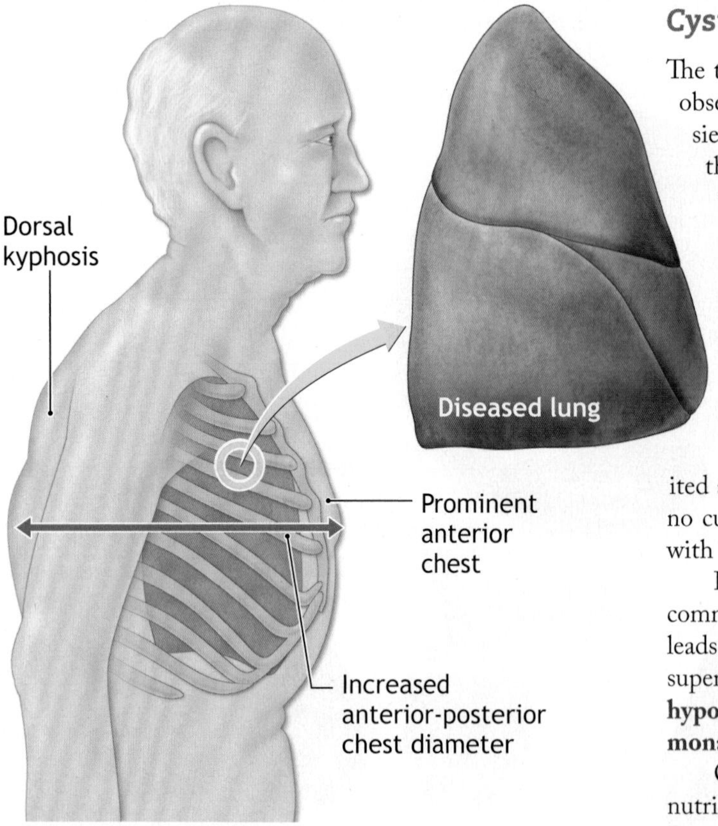

FIGURE 18.9 Emphysema traps air in the lungs, making exhalation difficult. With time, changes occur in the physical features of the patient, hence the name "pink puffer." (Adapted with permission from McArdle WD, Katch FI, Katch VL. *Exercise Physiology: Nutrition, Energy, and Human Performance*. 8th Ed. Baltimore: Wolters Kluwer Health, 2015.)

low, and fatigue occurs readily with only moderate effort. If left untreated, the disease usually leads to death.

Emphysema

Abnormal, permanent enlargement of air spaces distal to the terminal bronchi characterizes **emphysema**. This disease often develops from chronic bronchitis and occurs frequently in long-term cigarette smokers. Symptoms include:

1. Extreme dyspnea
2. Abnormally increased arterial carbon dioxide tension (hypercapnia)
3. Persistent cough
4. Cyanosis
5. Digital clubbing (evidence of chronic hypoxemia [**Fig. 18.8**])

Emphysema patients frequently appear thin; they lean forward with their arms braced on their knees to support their shoulders and chest for easier breathing. The effects of trapped air and alveolar distention change chest size and shape, causing the characteristic emphysemic "barrel chest" appearance (**Fig. 18.9**).

Physical activity cannot "cure" emphysema, but it does enhance cardiovascular fitness and strengthen respiratory musculature. Regular physical activity also improves patients' psychological state.

Cystic Fibrosis

The term **cystic fibrosis** (CF; **www.cff.org**) originates from observing cysts and scar tissue on the pancreas of autopsied patients, but these are not primary characteristics of the disease (although the term *cystic fibrosis* remains in use). **Table 18.17** lists clinical signs and symptoms of CF. This disease, characterized by thickened secretions of all exocrine glands (e.g., pancreatic, pulmonic, and gastrointestinal), eventually obstructs pulmonary airflow. CF represents the most common inherited genetic disease in Caucasians and affects approximately 1 in about 2000 Caucasian newborn infants in the United States (1 in 15,000 African Americans and 1 in 32,000 Asian Americans). The disease, inherited as a recessive trait (both parents serves as carriers), has no cure and remains fatal, although life span has increased with supportive therapies.

Pulmonary system involvement represents the most common and severe manifestation of CF. Airway obstruction leads to a chronic state of hyperinflation. Over time, RLD superimposes on the obstructive disorder, leading to **chronic hypoxia, hypercapnia**, and acidosis. **Pneumothorax** and **pulmonary hypertension** eventually follow and cause death.

CF treatment includes antibiotics, enzyme supplements, nutritional intervention, and frequent secretion removal. Regular physical activity provides beneficial outcomes. In some children, 20 minutes of aerobic exercise replaces one session of secretion removal. Increased minute ventilation with aerobic exercise helps clear excessive secretions from the airways. Improved physical fitness can modulate the severe effects of CF.

TABLE 18.17 Clinical Signs and Symptoms of Cystic Fibrosis and Related Pulmonary Involvement

Early stages	• Persistent cough and wheezing • Recurrent pneumonia • Excessive appetite but poor weight gain • Salty skin or sweat • Bulky, foul-smelling stools (undigested lipids)
Latter stages (with significant pulmonary involvement)	• Tachypnea (rapid breathing) • Sustained chronic cough with mucus production on vomiting • Barrel chest • Cyanosis and digital clubbing • Exertional dyspnea with decreased exercise capacity • Pneumothorax • Right heart failure secondary

Pulmonary Assessments

Chest and lung imaging provide the most common pulmonary assessment techniques. These include conventional radiography and **computed tomography (CT)** scanning to (1) screen for abnormalities, (2) provide a baseline for subsequent assessments, and (3) monitor disease progression. **Magnetic resonance imaging (MRI)** plays a limited role because the density of large portions of the lungs cannot generate clear magnetic signals. Static and dynamic tests of lung function, pulmonary diffusing capacity, and flow-volume loops also provide important diagnostic information.

Physical Activity Prescription for Pulmonary Rehabilitation

Pulmonary rehabilitation receives considerably less attention than rehabilitative programs for cardiovascular and musculoskeletal diseases. Perhaps deemphasis results from rehabilitation's failure to markedly improve pulmonary function or reverse the natural progression of these debilitating and often deadly diseases. Pulmonary rehabilitation, however, can have marked, positive effects on physical activity capacity, respiratory muscle function, psychological status, quality of life variables (e.g., self-esteem and self-efficacy), frequency of hospitalization, and disease progression. Major goals for pulmonary rehabilitation include the following:

1. Improve health status
2. Improve respiratory symptoms (shortness of breath and cough)
3. Recognize early signs requiring medical intervention
4. Decrease frequency and severity of respiratory problems
5. Maximize arterial oxygen saturation and carbon dioxide elimination
6. Improve daily functional capacity through enhanced muscular strength, joint flexibility, and cardiorespiratory endurance
7. Improve ventilatory musculature strength and power
8. Improve body composition to enhance functional capacity
9. Improve nutritional status

Pulmonary rehabilitation programs include the following five components:

1. General care
2. Pulmonary respiratory care
3. Exercise and functional training
4. Education
5. Psychosocial management

thePoint® Appendix SR-6: Additional Video Links, available online at **http://thePoint.lww.com/MKKESS5e**, provides a list of supplemental animations and videos on this subject, including a discussion of ongoing research about dyspnea.

The exercise and functional training aspects of rehabilitation serve an important role in the lives of individuals with end-stage disease because the effects of weakness, fatigue, and severe dyspnea profoundly limit physical activity. Physiologic monitoring during exercise rehabilitation should assess heart rate, blood pressure, respiratory rate, **arterial oxygen saturation** by **pulse oximetry** (indicates arterial oxygen desaturation), and dyspnea.

Dyspnea monitoring involves a perceived dyspnea **"Likert-type" scale** (**Fig. 18.10**), similar to psychometric scales for ratings of perceived exertion. Extreme shortness of breath, fatigue, palpitations, chest discomfort, or a decrease of 3% to 5% on pulse oximetry indicate exercise test termination.

The pretraining GXT and spirometric analyses govern the exercise prescription. The GXT interpretation includes examination of three factors:

1. Whether the test terminated for cardiovascular or ventilatory end points
2. Difference between pre-exercise and postexercise pulmonary function (e.g., a decrease of 10% in forced

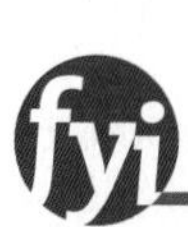

Eight Factors Predisposing to Chronic Obstructive Pulmonary Disease (COPD)

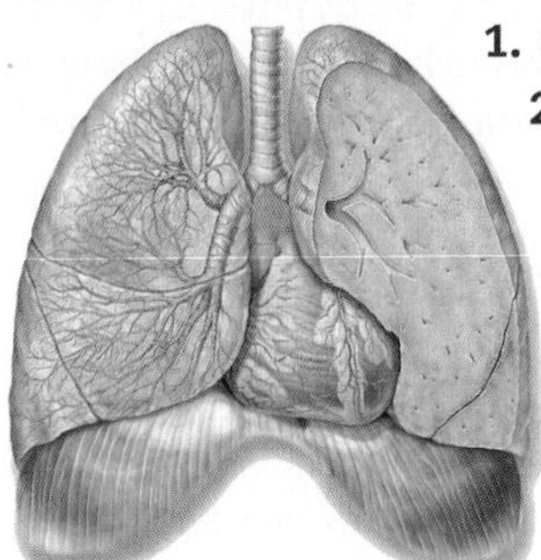

1. Chronic cigarette smoking
2. Air pollution
3. Occupational exposure to irritating dusts or gases
4. Heredity
5. Infection
6. Allergies
7. Aging
8. Drugs

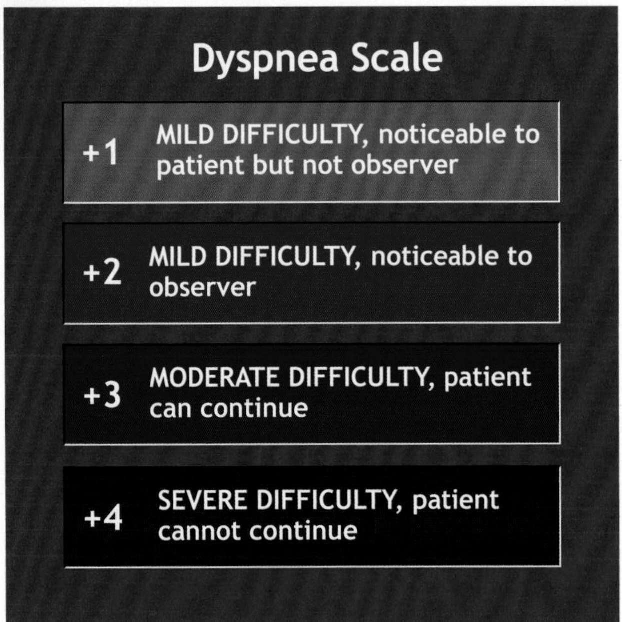

Dyspnea Scale
+1 MILD DIFFICULTY, noticeable to patient but not observer
+2 MILD DIFFICULTY, noticeable to observer
+3 MODERATE DIFFICULTY, patient can continue
+4 SEVERE DIFFICULTY, patient cannot continue

FIGURE 18.10 Dyspnea scale. Subjective ratings of dyspnea on a scale of 1 to 4 during graded exercise testing. Dyspnea usually accompanies poor exercise capacity and an impaired systolic blood pressure response. (Adapted with permission from McArdle WD, Katch FI, Katch VL. *Exercise Physiology: Nutrition, Energy, and Human Performance*. 8th Ed. Baltimore: Wolters Kluwer Health, 2015.)

expiratory volume in 1 second [$FEV_{1.0}$] indicates the need for bronchodilator therapy before exercise)

3. Need for supplemental oxygen from arterial oxygen desaturation during physical activity with decreased Pao_2 of greater than 20 mm Hg or a Pao_2 of less than 55 mm Hg

The exercise prescription for a patient with mild pulmonary disease (shortness of breath with intense exercise) mirrors that for a healthy individual. For patients with moderate disease (shortness of breath with normal daily activities or clinical symptoms of RLD or COPD), training can proceed following these three guidelines:

1. Exercise intensity no greater than 75% of ventilatory reserve
2. Attain the middle of the calculated training heart rate range (50% to 70% of age-predicted HR_{max})
3. Determine the point where the patient becomes noticeably dyspneic, between 40% and 85% of maximum MET level on a GXT.

Under these circumstances, physical activity duration usually lasts 20 minutes and is performed three times a week. If 5- to 15-minute durations are more desirable, physical activity frequency should increase to 5 to 7 days weekly.

Patients with severe pulmonary disease (shortness of breath during most daily activities, and forced vital capacity (FVC) and $FEV_{1.0}$ below 55% of predicted values) require a modified approach to exercise testing and prescription. Usually low-level, discontinuous testing can begin at 2 to 3 METs with increments every several minutes. Symptom-limited walking speeds and distances provide helpful guidelines for formulating an exercise prescription. Brief bouts of interval physical activity often benefit this population. Patients should exercise a minimum of once daily because of the relatively low initial training prescription level. Even small gains in physical activity tolerance improve an individual's functional capacity and quality of life indices.

For all patients with pulmonary disease, regular physical activity contributes to improved respiratory muscle function following these two approaches:

1. Resistance training of the ventilatory muscles by use of a **continuous positive airway pressure (CPAP)** device improves strength and power in these muscles. Overload occurs similarly to progressive resistance exercise for other skeletal muscles.
2. Increased endurance performance capacity of respiratory muscles through regular and progressive aerobic physical activity training.

Physical Activity and Asthma

The latest statistics indicate that **asthma** continues to increase in severity and scope (**www.aaaai.org/media/resources/media_kit/asthma_statistics.stm**). Hyperirritability of the pulmonary airways followed by bronchial spasm, edema, and mucus secretion characterize this obstructive pulmonary disease (**Fig. 18.11**). Common asthma symptoms include chest tightness, coughing, wheezing, and/or shortness of breath.

See the animation "Asthma" on **http://thePoint.lww.com/MKKESS5e** for a description and explanation of this condition.

A high level of physical fitness does not confer immunity from asthma. The recreational road runner is more likely to report symptoms of allergy and/or asthma but less likely to need prescription medication than the Olympic athlete. Based on data from the last five Olympic games, a study by the University of Western Australia has identified those athletes with asthma and airway hyper responsiveness. These are the most common chronic conditions among Olympic athletes, with a prevalence of about 8%, and could be related to the nature of their intense training.

For nearly 90% of persons with asthma and 30% to 50% of those suffering from allergic rhinitis (inflammation of nasal mucous lining) and hay fever, physical activity provides a potent stimulus for bronchoconstriction, termed **exercise-induced bronchospasm**. Reduced vagal tone and increased catecholamine release from the sympathetic nervous system during exertion normally relax pulmonary airway smooth muscle. Initial **bronchodilation** with activity occurs in healthy persons and asthmatics. For the asthmatic, bronchospasms accompanied by excessive mucus secretion follow initial bronchodilation. An acute episode of airway obstruction often occurs 5 to 15 minutes postexercise; recovery usually occurs spontaneously within 30 to 90 minutes.

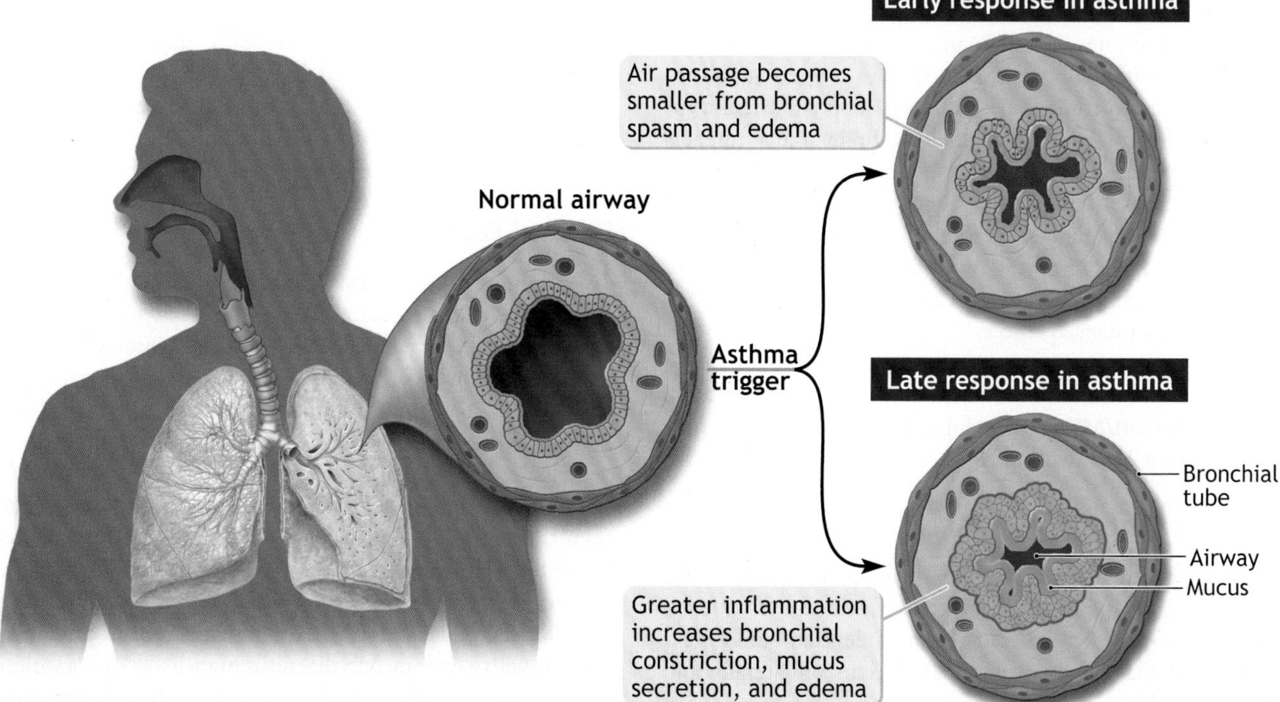

FIGURE 18.11 Typical response to an asthma attack. (Adapted with permission from McArdle WD, Katch FI, Katch VL. *Exercise Physiology: Nutrition, Energy, and Human Performance*. 8th Ed. Baltimore: Wolters Kluwer Health, 2015.)

One useful technique to detect an exercise-induced asthmatic response is to apply progressive exercise increments. A spirometric FVC and $FEV_{1.0}$ evaluation takes place after each exercise period and during the first 10 to 20 minutes of recovery. A 10% to 15% reduction in pre-exercise $FEV_{1.0}$/FVC confirms the diagnosis of exercise-induced bronchospasm. For elite athletes who perform in cold-weather sports (e.g., biathlon, canoeing/kayaking, cross-country skiing, ice hockey, Nordic combined, and speed skating), combining pulmonary function testing with near-maximal sport-specific exercise testing, preferably in a cold, dry environment, provides greater sensitivity for screening than laboratory-based warm air environmental challenges or self-reported symptoms.

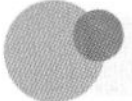

SUMMARY

1. RLD and COPD represent two major pulmonary disease categories.
2. RLD increases chest-lung resistance to lung inflation.
3. COPD (including bronchitis, emphysema, asthma, exercise-induced bronchospasm, and CF) affects expiratory flow capacity and ultimately impedes aeration of alveolar blood.
4. Pulmonary disease assessment diagnostic tools include chest radiography, CT scanning, MRI, and standard spirometric lung volume testing.
5. Regular physical activity that follows proper guidelines for exercise intensity, patient monitoring, and exercise progression effectively manages pulmonary disease.
6. Asthma is triggered by hyperirritability of pulmonary airways, followed by bronchial spasm, edema, and mucus secretion.

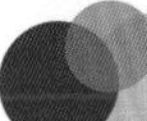

THINK IT THROUGH

1. Why would regular physical activity prove more effective for CHD patients than patients with pulmonary disease?
2. Describe a scenario suggesting when a person is most likely to suffer from an asthma attack.

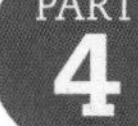

PART 4 Neuromuscular Diseases and Disorders

Neuromuscular diseases represent adverse conditions that target the brain in specific ways. Progressive nerve degeneration or trauma to specific brain neurons produce impairments that range from simple to complex. *More Americans experience hospitalization with neurologic and mental disorders than from any other major disease group, including heart disease and cancer!* The economic costs of brain dysfunction remain enormous, but pale in comparison with the staggering emotional toll on victims and families.

Stroke

Stroke, sometimes called **acute cerebrovascular attack**, refers to a potentially fatal reduction in oxygen supply to part of the brain from restricted blood supply (ischemia) or bleeding (hemorrhage). The resulting brain injury impacts multiple systems depending on the injury site and amount of damage sustained. Effects include motor and sensory impairment and language, perception, and affective and cognitive dysfunction. Strokes can cause severe limitations in mobility and cognition or may cause only mild, short-term, nonpermanent consequences.

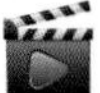

See the animation "Stroke" on **http://thePoint.lww.com/MKKESS5e** for a description and explanation of this condition.

Clinical Features

Clinical features of stroke depend on injury location and severity. Signs of a hemorrhagic stroke include altered levels of consciousness, severe headache, and elevated blood pressure. Cerebellar hemorrhage usually occurs unilaterally and associates with disequilibrium, nausea, and vomiting.

Cerebral blood flow (CBF) represents the primary marker for assessing ischemic strokes. When CBF decreases below 10 $mL \cdot 100\ g^{-1} \cdot min^{-1}$ (reference range, 50 to 55 $mL \cdot 100\ g^{-1} \cdot min^{-1}$), synaptic transmission failure occurs, and a CBF of 8 $mL \cdot 100\ g^{-1} \cdot min^{-1}$ or below results in cell death.

Strokes cause physical and cognitive damage. Left-hemispheric lesions typically accompany expressive and receptive language deficits compared with right-hemisphere lesions. Damage to descending neural pathways produces an abnormal regulation of spinal motor neurons, resulting in adverse changes in postural and stretch reflexes and difficulty with voluntary movement. Damage to areas of motor control may result in **hemiplegia** (paralysis) or **hemiparesis** (weakness). Other deficits in motor control can involve muscle weakness, abnormal synergistic movement organization, impaired force regulation, decreased reaction times, abnormal muscle tone, and loss of active range of joint motion.

Physical Activity Prescription

The emphasis for stroke survivors centers on rehabilitation of movement during the first 6 months of recovery (increased flexibility [passive and active-assisted] and strength development). The limited number of training studies with stroke patients support the use of physical activity to improve mobility and functional independence and to prevent or further reduce disease and functional impairment. Stroke survivors vary widely in age, degree of disability, motivational level, and number and severity of comorbidities, secondary conditions, and associated circumstances. The specific physical activity prescription intervention focuses on reducing functional impairments and improving functional capacity.

Multiple Sclerosis

Multiple sclerosis (MS) represents a chronic, often disabling disease characterized by destruction of the myelin sheath (**demyelination**) that surrounds CNS nerve fibers (see Chapter 11.) Any part of the brain and spinal cord can have lesions of inflammatory demyelination.

Clinical Features

Two or more areas of demyelination confirm the diagnosis of MS. The disease usually develops between age 20 and 40. Frequently, a history emerges of transient neurologic deficits including numbness or weakness of an extremity, general weakness, blurring of vision, and diplopia (double vision) in childhood or adolescence before development of more persistent neurologic deficits that lead to the definitive diagnosis. MS occurs worldwide at a higher frequency in latitudes farther from the equator. The prevalence of MS in the United States below the 37th parallel is 57 to 78 cases per 100,000, but the prevalence rate above the 37th parallel averages 110 to 140 cases per 100,000. Reasons for these differences remain unknown. Patients with a definite MS diagnosis more likely have a variety of an autoimmune illness, including **systemic lupus erythematosus**, **rheumatoid arthritis**, **polymyositis**, and **myasthenia gravis**. A person with a first-degree relative with MS has a 12- to 20-fold increased likelihood of developing MS.

Fatigue manifests as the most common early MS symptom. Other symptoms include one or all of the following: painful blurring or loss of vision in one eye, muscle weakness in the extremities, clumsiness, numbness and tingling, bowel and bladder dysfunction, sexual dysfunction, joint contractures, urinary tract infection, osteoporosis, and spasticity.

Physical Activity Prescription

Patients with MS benefit from a comprehensive health prescription that involves aerobic physical activity, strength, balance, and flexibility exercises. One important factor that hinders endurance training in about 80% of MS patients relates to adverse effects to heat, whether generated environmentally by outside climatic changes or internally via fever or exercise-induced thermogenesis. This effect makes continuous exercise training difficult and poorly tolerated. Nevertheless, MS patients still can improve cardiovascular function. Stationary cycling, walking, and low impact chair or water aerobics provide excellent training choices. The ideal physical activity consists of walking in a climate-controlled area that provides stable temperatures, a level surface, and opportunity for frequent rest periods. Controlling body temperature represents a primary consideration in the exercise prescription. A realistic and achievable goal for structured physical activity provides training three times weekly for a minimum of 30 minutes each session divided into three 10-minute sessions.

Parkinson Disease

Parkinson disease (PD), a common neurodegenerative disease of the CNS that impairs motor skills, speech, and other functions, has a prevalence of 60 to 187 per 100,000 people worldwide (no population is immune to PD). The risk of developing this movement disorder increases with age; 10% of patients become symptomatic before age 40 years, 30% become symptomatic before age 50 years, and 40% become symptomatic between 50 and 60 years.

Clinical Features

Clinical symptoms of PD include varying degrees of tremor, a decrease in spontaneity and movement (**bradykinesia**), rigidity, and impaired postural reflexes. These conditions produce extreme gait and postural instability, resulting in increased episodes of falling or "freezing" (inability to move a body part), and extreme difficulty walking. Some patients exhibit a complete lack of movement called **akinesia**. Functional problems also include difficulty getting out of bed or a car and rising from a chair. Other problems include difficulties dressing, writing, talking, and swallowing. Persons with PD generally experience difficulty with performing more than one task simultaneously. As the disease progresses, such problems become more pronounced; the individual eventually loses ability to perform even the most common activities of daily living. In the last stage of the disease, the person must use a wheelchair for mobility and will become bed bound.

Physical Activity Prescription

Most exercise prescriptions for PD patients are individualized and directed toward interventions that try to impact associated motor control problems. The rehabilitation exercises emphasize slow, controlled movements for specific tasks through various ranges of motion while lying, sitting, standing, and walking. Treatment protocols include ROM exercises that emphasize slow static stretches for all major muscle and joint areas, balance and gait training, mobility, and muscle coordination exercises. Little research has assessed the effects of training on aerobic capacity, and no guidelines exist.

SUMMARY

1. Neuromuscular diseases represent conditions affecting the brain in specific ways. Progressive nerve degeneration or trauma to specific brain neurons result in impairment that ranges from simple to complex.
2. Major neuromuscular diseases include stroke, multiple sclerosis (MS), and Parkinson disease (PD).
3. Strokes cause physical and cognitive damage. Left-hemisphere lesions typically accompany expressive and receptive language deficits compared with right-hemisphere lesions. Motor impairment usually results in hemiplegia (paralysis) or hemiparesis (weakness).
4. Rehabilitation for stroke survivors centers on rehabilitation of movement during the first 6 months of recovery (increase flexibility [passive and active-assisted], strength development).
5. MS represents a chronic, often disabling disease characterized by destruction of the myelin sheath (demyelination) that surrounds CNS nerve fibers.
6. MS usually develops between age 20 and 40. Neurologic deficits include numbness or weakness of an extremity, general weakness, blurring of vision, and diplopia (double vision) in childhood or adolescence before development of more persistent neurologic deficits that lead to the definitive diagnosis.
7. Fatigue represents the most common MS symptom; other symptoms include muscle weakness in the extremities, clumsiness, and numbness and tingling.
8. Patients with MS benefit from a comprehensive health prescription that involves aerobic physical activity and strength, balance, and flexibility exercises.
9. PD represents a common neurodegenerative CNS disease that often impairs motor skills, speech, and other functions.
10. Clinical symptoms of PD include varying degrees of tremor, decreased spontaneity and movement, rigidity, and impaired postural reflexes.
11. Individualized exercise prescriptions for PD patients emphasize slow, controlled movements for specific tasks through various ranges of motion while lying, sitting, standing, and walking.

THINK IT THROUGH

1. Describe a common thread for an exercise prescription for individuals with neuromuscular disease.

PART 5 Renal Disease and Disorders

Treatment modalities for the major metabolic diseases of obesity, diabetes, and renal disease advocate regular physical activity as adjunctive therapy. Obesity and diabetes have been discussed in different chapters of this text. This section reviews aspects of renal disease associated with kidney function related to exercise physiology.

Chronic kidney disease (CKD) occurs when the kidneys no longer adequately filter toxins and waste products from blood. **Acute renal failure** occurs from a toxin (e.g., drug allergy or poison) or severe blood loss or trauma. Diabetes, the number one cause of kidney disease, remains responsible for about 40% of all kidney failures; high blood pressure is the second cause, responsible for about 25% of all kidney failures. Genetic diseases, autoimmune diseases, and birth defects also cause kidney disorders.

Clinical Features

Common symptoms of chronic kidney disease, sometimes referred to as **uremia** (retention in the blood of waste products normally excreted in urine), include the following 10 markers:

1. **Changes in urination:** Making more or less urine than usual, feeling pressure when urinating, changes in urine color, foamy or bubbly urine, or frequently urinating at night.
2. **Swelling of feet, ankles, hands, or face:** Fluid retention in the tissues from failure of kidney filtration.
3. **General fatigue or weakness:** Buildup of wastes or a shortage of red blood cells (anemia) as kidney function begins to decline and ultimately fails.
4. **Shortness of breath:** Kidney failure is sometimes confused with asthma or HF because fluid builds up in the lungs.
5. **Ammonia breath or an ammonia or metal taste in the mouth:** Waste buildup can cause bad breath, changes in taste, or aversion to high-protein foods.
6. **Back or flank pain:** The kidneys are located on either side of the spine in the back.
7. **Itching:** Waste accumulation can trigger severe itching, especially in the legs.
8. **Loss of appetite.**
9. **Nausea and vomiting.**
10. **Increased hypoglycemic episodes accompanying diabetes**

Chronic uremia eventually progresses to **end-stage renal disease (ESRD)**, which requires lifelong dialysis or kidney transplant. The number of worldwide renal transplants has increased steadily in the past decade: more kidney transplants were performed in the United States in 2014 (17,105; 11,570 from deceased donors and 5535 from living donors) than in any other country (**www.kidney.org/news/newsroom/factsheets/Organ-Donation-and-Transplantation-Stats.cfm**). Those who undergo a kidney transplant generally gain a more normal lifestyle and full rehabilitation: nearly 80% of transplant patients function at near-normal levels compared with 40% to 60% of those treated with dialysis. Almost 75% of transplant patients resume a normal work schedule compared with 50% to 60% for dialysis patients. Unfortunately, a tremendous need exists to fulfill all of the requests for kidney transplantation. In 2014, 4270 patients died waiting for a transplant (9 people daily), and every 20 minutes someone joins the kidney transplant wait list. The total number of people on the waiting list who need a lifesaving organ transplant (e.g., kidney, heart, lung, liver) exceeded 122,990 as of June 29, 2015. Of those, 79,148 are on an active waiting list. Donor organs are matched to waiting recipients by a national computer registry called the National Organ Procurement and Transplantation Network (OPTN; **http://optn.transplant.hrsa.gov**).

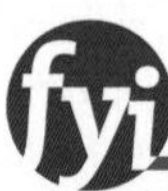

Apollo Space Program Develops Critical Care Dialysis System

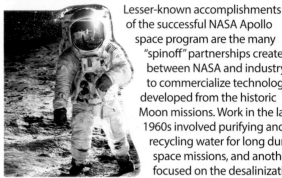

Photo from **http://spinoff.nasa.gov/pdf/Apollo_Flyer.pdf**

Lesser-known accomplishments of the successful NASA Apollo space program are the many "spinoff" partnerships created between NASA and industry to commercialize technologies developed from the historic Moon missions. Work in the late 1960s involved purifying and recycling water for long duration space missions, and another focused on the desalinization of seawater. In the course of this experimentation, NASA researchers discovered that the project's chemical processes could be applied to removing toxic waste from used dialysis fluid. This discovery sparked another project to develop a kidney dialysis machine. The discovery marked the birth of "sorbent" dialysis, a method to remove urea from human blood by treating a dialysate solution—the fluid and solutes in a dialysis process that flow through the dialyzer. Dialysis treatment currently provides a lifesaving bridge for patients awaiting a kidney transplant now performed routinely in major medical centers and viewed online (e.g., **www.hopkinsmedicine.org/healthlibrary/test_procedures/urology/kidney_transplantation_procedure_92,P07708/**), including operational procedures for donor kidney removal (laparoscopic donor nephrectomy) and anatomical connection of a donor kidney to a recipient (**http://mdvideocenter.brighamandwomens.org/specialties/transplant-surgery/kidney-transplantation/item/11**).

Sources:

1. **http://spinoff.nasa.gov/Spinoff2009/Intro_2009.html**
2. **http://ntrs.nasa.gov/archive/nasa/casi.ntrs.nasa.gov/20020083273.pdf**

Physical Activity Prescription

Regular physical activity serves an important role in rehabilitating dialysis and kidney transplant patients to better adapt to their illness. The rehabilitation program should begin before the start of dialysis to optimize beneficial effects. Normal low-level endurance training following ACSM guidelines reduces muscle protein degradation in moderate renal insufficiency, reduces resting blood pressure in some hemodialysis patients, and modestly improves aerobic capacity in patients undergoing hemodialysis.

No longitudinal data exist on the effects of aerobic training or a more physically active lifestyle on the survival of patients with chronic uremia or kidney transplants. However, patients with uremia who maintain a lifetime of diverse physical activity do report an enhanced quality of life, including participation in competitive athletics (**www.kidney.org/news/tgames/index.cfm**).

SUMMARY

1. Chronic kidney disease occurs when the kidneys no longer adequately filter toxins and waste products from blood.
2. Acute renal failure occurs from a toxin (e.g., drug allergy or poison) or severe blood loss or trauma.

3. Diabetes is the number one cause of kidney disease and remains responsible for about 40% of all kidney failures; high blood pressure is the second cause, responsible for about 25% of all kidney failures.
4. The three most common symptoms of kidney disease include uremia (retention in the blood of waste products normally excreted in urine), changes in urination habits, and swelling of the feet, ankles, hands, or face.
5. The rehabilitation program for kidney patients should begin before the start of dialysis to optimize beneficial effects. Normal low-level endurance training following ACSM guidelines should be considered.

THINK IT THROUGH

1. Your grandmother just stated she thinks she developed chronic kidney disease. List five questions you should answer about her symptoms to determine her likelihood of renal failure.

PART 6 Cancer

Cancer represents a group of diseases collectively characterized by uncontrolled growth of abnormal cells. More than 100 different types of cancers exist, most occurring in adults. **Carcinomas** refer to cancers that develop from epithelial cells that line the surface of the body, glands, and internal organs. They account for 80% to 90% of all cancers, including prostate, colon, lung, cervical, and breast cancer. Cancers also can arise from blood cells (**leukemias**), the immune system (**lymphomas**), and connective tissues, including bones, tendons, cartilage, fat, and muscle (**sarcomas**).

Nearly 14.5 million children and adults (6.87 million males and 7.60 million female) with a history of cancer were alive on January 1, 2014, in the United States. It is estimated that by January 2024 the population of cancer survivors will increase to almost 19 million: 9.3 million males and 9.6 million females. These estimates do not include carcinoma in situ (non-invasive cancer) of any site except urinary bladder, nor do they include basal cell and squamous cell skin cancers. These data emphasize the ongoing need for rehabilitative and maintenance options for this population (**www.cancer.org/acs/groups/content/@editorial/documents/document/acspc-044552.pdf**). The most serious outcomes for most cancer patients and survivors include loss of muscle mass and functional status. Reduced functional status encompasses difficulty walking even short distances and serious fatigue that limits completion of simple household chores. Approximately 75% of cancer survivors report extreme fatigue during and after radiotherapy or chemotherapy, accompanied by weight loss and decreased muscular strength and cardiovascular endurance. Maintaining and restoring functional capacity challenges cancer survivors, even those considered "cured." Sufficient rationale now justifies exercise intervention for cancer patients during and following different treatment modalities.

Clinical Features

Cancer's clinical features relate to the effects of the three primary cancer treatment modalities: surgery, radiation, and systemic pharmacologic therapy (chemotherapy).

Surgery represents the oldest and most common cancer treatment modality. Surgeries include operations to remove high-risk tissues to prevent cancer development, biopsies of abnormal tissue to diagnose cancer, excision of tumors with curative intent, insertion of central venous catheters to support chemotherapy infusions, reconstruction after definitive surgery, and palliative or symptom relief (e.g., partial bowel removal) for incurable disease.

More than 50% of all cancer survivors have undergone some form of radiation treatment. Radiation treatment involves photon penetration into specific tissue, which produces an ionized electrically charged particle that damages DNA to inhibit cell replication and produce cell death. Radiation treatment is typically given daily for up to 8 weeks.

Pharmacologic therapy for patients with many advanced solid tumors occurs if cancer cells are suspected of metastasizing beyond the primary site and regional lymph nodes. Chemotherapy, endocrine therapy, and biologic therapy represent the three major types of systemic therapy.

Table 18.18 presents common clinical symptoms resulting from cancer surgery, radiation therapy, and systemic therapy interventions.

Physical Activity Prescription

Regular physical activity helps cancer patients recuperate and return to a normal lifestyle with greater independence and functional capacity. Health and fitness professionals generally recommend a symptom-limited, progressive, and individualized exercise prescription. Prudent ambulation of any kind proves beneficial for the most sedentary and deconditioned patient.

Typical benefits of regular physical activity include:

1. Decreased fatigue symptoms
2. Improved functional capacity
3. Decreased neutropenia (abnormally small numbers of neutrophils in circulating blood)
4. Reduced severity of pain and diarrhea
5. Shortened hospital stays
6. Decreased psychological distress by improving mood state
7. Enhanced immune function

Current research focuses on psychosocial outcomes relating to general fatigue, satisfaction with life, level of depression, self-concept, and quality of life.

Cancer patients can participate in exercise stress tests, which also serve as a basis for exercise prescriptions. Similar

TABLE 18.18 Cancer Therapies and Their Complications

Type of Treatment	Description and Effects/Outcome
Surgery	**Lung**—reduced lung capacity, dyspnea, deconditioning **Neck**—reduced range of motion, muscle weakness, occasional cranial nerve palsy **Pelvic region**—urinary incontinence, erectile dysfunction, deconditioning **Abdomen**—deconditioning, diarrhea **Limb amputation**—chronic pain, deconditioning
Radiation Therapy	**Skin**—redness, pain, dryness, peeling, sloughing, reduced elasticity **Brain**—nausea, vomiting, fatigue, memory loss **Thorax**—some degree of irreversible lung fibrosis; heart may receive radiation causing pericardial inflammation or fibrosis, premature atherosclerosis, cardiomyopathy **Abdomen**—vomiting, diarrhea **Pelvis**—diarrhea, pelvic pain, bladder scarring, occasional incontinence, sexual dysfunction **Joints**—connective tissue and joint capsule fibrosis, possible decreased range of motion
Systemic Therapy	**Chemotherapies** (depending on type and amount)—extreme fatigue, anorexia, nausea, anemia, neutropenia, muscle pain, sensory and motor peripheral neuropathy, ataxia, anemia, vomiting, loss of muscle mass, deconditioning, infection **Endocrine therapies** (depending on type and amount)—fat redistribution (truncal and facial obesity), proximal muscle weakness, osteoporosis, edema, infection, weight gain, extreme fatigue, hot flashes, loss of muscle mass **Biologic therapies** (depending on type and amount)—fevers or allergic reactions, chills, fever, headache, extreme fatigue, low blood pressure, skin rash, anemia

Adapted with permission from Courneya KS, et al. *ACSM's Resource Manual for Clinical Exercise Physiology for Special Populations*. In: Myers J, ed. Baltimore: Lippincott Williams & Wilkins, 2002.

testing procedures apply as with healthy individuals, but feelings of fatigue require greater attention. **Table 18.19** presents nine special precautions to consider when testing the functional capacity of cancer patients. Generally, patients should not exercise to maximum.

The physical activity prescription should encourage ambulation if the patient has no specific contraindications. Also encouraged are flexibility exercises to improve ROM and resistance training to improve muscular strength, augment FFM, and improve overall mobility (e.g., submaximal static exercises for antigravity muscles, deep breathing exercises, and dynamic trunk rotation movements). In most cases, preference goes to low-level activity for short periods performed several times daily. Physical activity progression and intensity are individualized, with initial work to rest ratios of 1:1 progressing to 2:1. Eventually, continuous physical activity for up to 15 minutes can replace intermittent exercise bouts. **Table 18.20** presents general aerobic exercise guidelines for otherwise healthy cancer survivors.

TABLE 18.19 Nine Special Precautions for Testing the Functional Capacity of Cancer Patients

Complication	Precaution
1. Ataxia, dizziness, or peripheral sensory neuropathy	Avoid tests that require balance and coordination (treadmill, weights)
2. Bone pain	Avoid high-impact tests that increase risk of fracture (treadmill, weights)
3. Low blood count (hemoglobin $\leq$8.0 g · dL^{-1}; neutrophil count $\leq$0.5 × 10^{9} · L^{-1})	Avoid tests that require high oxygen uptake or high impact (risk of bleeding); ensure proper sterilization of equipment
4. Dyspnea	Avoid maximal tests
5. Fever 100.4°F (38°C)	May indicate systemic infection; avoid exercise testing
6. Mouth sores or ulcerations	Avoid mouthpieces; use face masks
7. Low functional status	Avoid exercise stress testing
8. Surgical wounds or tenderness	Avoid pressure or trauma to surgical site
9. Severe nausea or vomiting	Avoid or postpone exercise testing

Modified with permission from Courneya KS, et al. Coping with cancer: can exercise help? *Phys Sports Med* 2000;28:49.

TABLE 18.20 General Aerobic Exercise Guidelines for Otherwise Healthy Cancer Survivors

Variable	Guidelines
Frequency	At least three to five times per week; daily activity may be optimal for deconditioned patients
Intensity	Depends on fitness status and GXT results; usually 50%–70% $\dot{V}O_{2peak}$; or 60%–80% HR_{max}; or RPE 11–14
Type (mode)	Large muscle group activity, particularly walking and cycling in some cases
Time (duration)	20–30 continuous minutes per session; this goal can be achieved through multiple intermittent shorter sessions with adequate rest intervals
Progression	May not always be linear; rather, it may be cyclical with periods of regression, depending on treatments

GXT, graded exercise stress test; HR_{max}, maximal safe heart rate; RPE, rating of perceived exertion; $\dot{V}O_{2peak}$, peak oxygen consumption.

Adapted with permission from Courneya KS, et al. Coping with cancer: can exercise help? *Phys Sports Med* 2000;28:49.

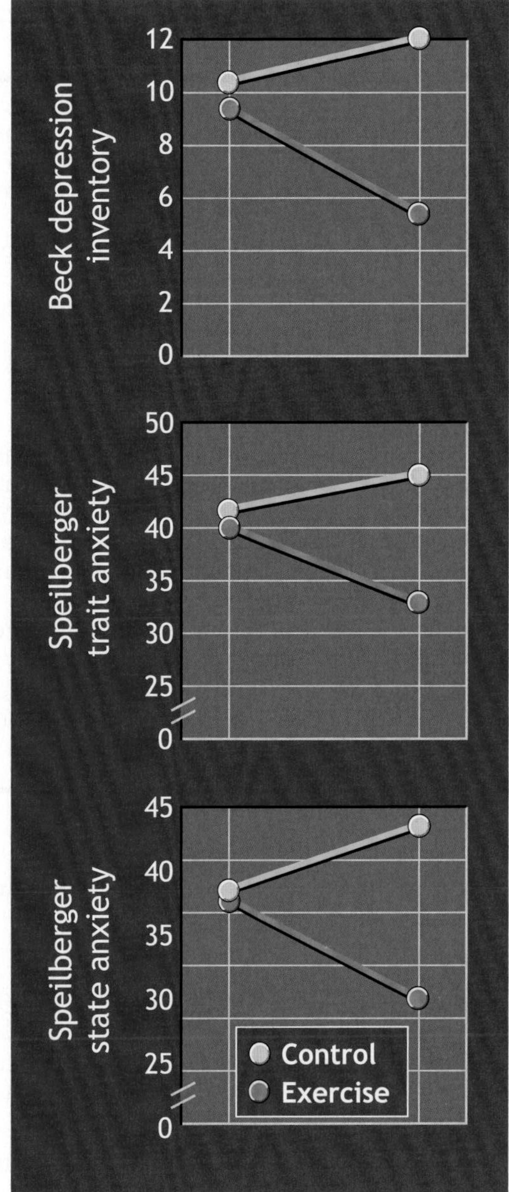

FIGURE 18.12 Effects of 10 weeks of moderate aerobic circuit resistance exercise on depression **(top)** and trait **(middle)** and state **(lower)** anxiety in women recovering from breast cancer surgery. (Data courtesy of M. Segar, Applied Physiology Laboratory, University of Michigan, Ann Arbor, MI, 1996.)

Breast Cancer

Carcinoma of the breast, one of the most common forms of cancer in white women age 40 years and older, represents the leading cause of death in women between 40 and 60 years. In 2015, the estimated number of new cases of breast cancer was 231,840 for women and 2350 for men; the estimate is 40,290 deaths for women and about 400 for men. Only lung cancer accounts for more cancer deaths in women. About one in eight women develop breast cancer at some time during life with a high rate of recurrence. Overall, the 5-year relative survival rate for breast cancer is 89%. Only prostate (99%), thyroid (98%), melanoma of skin (91%), and testicular cancer (95%) have higher 5-year survival rates.

Primary breast cancer risk factors include:

1. Family history of breast cancer
2. Personal history of cancer
3. First menstrual period at an early age
4. Menopause at a late age
5. First childbirth after age 30 years or no childbirth
6. Consistently high-fat diet

Daily low-to-moderate aerobic exercise reduces fatigue in women with breast cancer who undergo chemotherapy and improves many quality of life outcomes from breast cancer treatment. Physical activity produces positive improvements in functional capacity, body composition, and side effects of treatment, mood, and self-image.

A study from one of our laboratories illustrates the benefits of physical activity in breast cancer survivors. The program, conducted 4 days a week, consisted of self-paced hydraulic resistance exercises performed in a 14-station aerobic exercise circuit by 28 patients recovering from breast cancer surgery. **Figure 18.12** illustrates that exercisers decreased depression by 38% compared with a 13% increase for nonexercising counterparts also recovering from breast cancer surgery. Exercisers decreased trait anxiety (defined as feelings of stress, worry, discomfort, etc. that one experiences on a day to day basis) by 16% and state anxiety (defined as fear, nervousness, discomfort, etc., and the arousal of the autonomic nervous system induced by different situations that are perceived as dangerous) by 20% compared with increases in both variables for nonexercisers. These results demonstrate that a planned, moderate aerobic circuit resistance exercise program

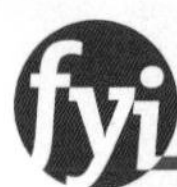

Resistance Training Helps Breast Cancer Survivors

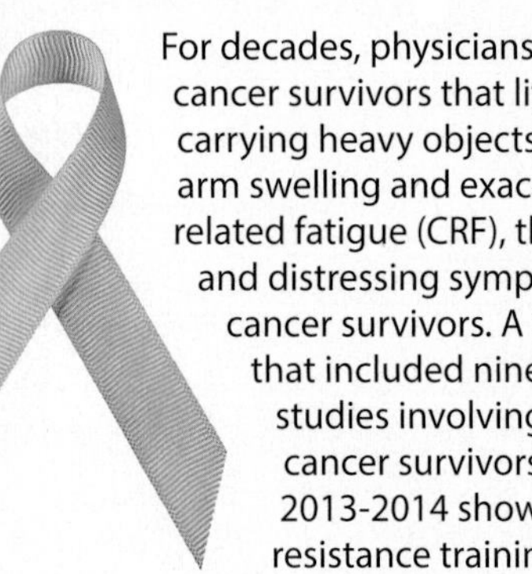

For decades, physicians have advised breast cancer survivors that lifting weights or carrying heavy objects may cause harmful arm swelling and exacerbate cancer-related fatigue (CRF), the most common and distressing symptoms in breast cancer survivors. A 2015 meta-analysis that included nine high-quality studies involving a total of 1156 cancer survivors from between 2013-2014 showed that supervised resistance training was statistically more effective than conventional care in improving CRF among cancer survivors. Additional analyses revealed that training volume parameters were closed related with CRF improvements. The authors argued that since supervised resistance exercise (and aerobic training) reduces CRF it should be implemented in all breast cancer rehabilitation programs.

Source: Meneses-Echávez JF, et al. Effects of supervised exercise on cancer-related fatigue in breast cancer survivors: a systematic review and meta-analysis. *BMC Cancer* 2015;15:77.

exerts positive effects on psychosocial variables during breast cancer rehabilitation.

SUMMARY

1. More than 100 different types of cancers affect adults, including carcinomas, leukemias, lymphomas, and sarcomas.
2. Cancers arise from blood cells (leukemias), immune system (lymphomas), and connective tissues such as bones, tendons, cartilage, fat, and muscle (sarcomas).
3. Cancer's clinical features relate to the effects of the three primary cancer treatment modalities—surgery, radiation, and systemic pharmacologic therapy.
4. The recommended exercise prescription for cancer patients is symptom limited, progressive, and individualized, with improved ambulation the primary goal.
5. Regular physical activity helps cancer patients recuperate and return to a normal lifestyle with greater independence and functional capacity. Prudent ambulation of any kind proves beneficial for the most sedentary and deconditioned patient.
6. The benefits of regular physical activity include decreased fatigue symptoms, improved functional capacity, reduced severity of pain and diarrhea, shortened hospital stays mood state, and immune function.
7. For women recovering from breast cancer surgery, a carefully planned, aerobic circuit resistance exercise program decreases depression including state and trait anxieties.

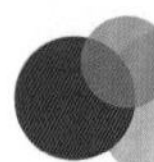

THINK IT THROUGH

1. Discuss the most important reason a postcancer survivor should consider a physical activity rehabilitation program.

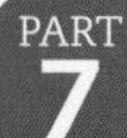

PART 7 Cognitive and Emotional Diseases and Disorders

The National Institutes of Mental Health estimates that nearly 19 million Americans older than 18 years of age—about one in four adults—experience major depression (**www.nimh.nih.gov/index.shtml**). Suicide linked to depression represents the third leading cause of death among 10- to 24-year-olds. Six to eight percent of all outpatients in primary care settings experience major depression. Despite the large numbers of depressed patients, mental disorders remain underdiagnosed; only about one-third of people diagnosed receive treatment.

The five major classifications of cognitive/emotional diseases are:

1. **Major depressive disorder:** Commonly referred to as "depression"
2. **Dysthymia:** Mildly depressed on most days over a period of at least 2 years; symptoms resemble major depression but less severe
3. **Seasonal affective disorder:** Recurrence of depressive symptoms during certain seasons (e.g., winter vs. summer)
4. **Postpartum depression:** Occurs following childbirth; typically in the first few months after delivery but can happen within the first year after childbirth
5. **Bipolar disorder:** Characterized by extremes in mood and behavior lasting for at least 2 weeks (previously known as manic-depressive illness)

Clinical Features

Depression has no single cause but often results from a combination of factors or events. Whatever its cause, depression is not just a state of mind. Rather, current research points to physical changes in the brain and a neurotransmitter chemical imbalance as contributing causes underlying depression.

Women are roughly twice as likely to experience depression as men, partly from hormonal changes from puberty, menstruation, menopause, and pregnancy. Men are more likely to go undiagnosed and less likely to seek help. Men may show the typical symptoms of depression; they tend to be angry and hostile and mask their condition with alcohol or drug abuse. Suicide becomes a serious risk for depressed men, who are four times more likely than women to kill themselves.

TABLE 18.21 Twelve Common Signs and Symptoms of Depression

1. Loss of enjoyment from things that were once pleasurable
2. Loss of energy
3. Feelings of hopelessness or worthlessness
4. Difficulty concentrating
5. Difficulty making decisions
6. Insomnia or excessive sleep
7. Stomach ache and digestive problems
8. Sexual problems (e.g., decreased sex drive)
9. Aches and pains (e.g., recurrent headaches)
10. A change in appetite causing weight loss or gain
11. Thoughts of death or suicide
12. Attempting suicide

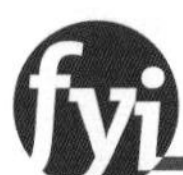

Just A Little Physical Activity Adds Life to Seniors 85+ Years

Little is known about the potential benefits of regular physical activity for the oldest-old, those in their 80s. Research suggests that the oldest-old benefit from regular physical activity. Even previously sedentary 85-year-olds who participated in 4 hours per week of physical activity (this level of activity classifies as "active" for this age group) reaped the benefits. Even if the walks were broken up into 15-minute strolls, the benefits equaled those who participated for longer durations. The physically active octogenarians also experienced less depression and loneliness and showed greater ability to perform tasks of daily living more easily.

Source: Stressman J, et al. Physical activity, function, and longevity among the very old. *Arch Intern Med* 2009;169:1476.

Depression among the elderly poses a unique situation. Older people often lose loved ones and have to adjust to living alone. Physical illness decreases normal physical activity levels. Such changes all contribute to depression. Loved ones may attribute the signs of depression to normal aging, and many older people are reluctant to talk about their symptoms. As such, older people may not receive proper treatment for their depression.

Four common factors in depression are:

1. **Family situation:** Trauma and stress from financial problems, breakup of a relationship, death of a loved one, or other major life change.
2. **Pessimistic personality:** Higher risk for individuals who have low self-esteem and negative outlook.
3. **Health status:** Medical conditions include heart disease, cancer, and HIV.
4. **Other psychological disorders:** Anxiety disorders, eating disorders, schizophrenia, and substance abuse often coexist.

Table 18.21 presents 12 common signs and symptoms of depression.

Physical Activity Prescription

Physical activity studies in clinically depressed populations include hospitalized and ambulatory patients. Overall, the data support the positive effects of physical activity on depressive symptoms. In most cases, patients who participate decrease their depression scores.

No one activity mode has a greater impact on depression than other types of activity, yet most studies have focused on running or other aerobic-type activities. Interestingly, positive psychological outcomes do not depend on achieving higher levels of physical fitness, although fitness-related indicators of lower blood pressure and increased aerobic capacity frequently improve.

Different psychological and physiologic mechanisms may explain the beneficial effects of exercise on depression. Psychologically, physical activity enhances one's sense of mastery and self-esteem, which is critically important for depressed individuals who often feel a loss of control over their lives. Physical activity also provides a therapeutic distraction that diverts attention from areas of worry, concern, and guilt. Improving one's health, flexibility, and physique status also can enhance mood. Large-muscle activity in exercise may help to discharge feelings of pent-up frustration, anger, and hostility. Exercise may exert its beneficial effect on mood by influencing the metabolism and availability of central neurotransmitters with mood-improving capability.

Researchers continue to study exercise effects on the neurochemistry of mood regulation, specifically turnover of **monoamines** and other central neurotransmitters at presynaptic and postsynaptic sites. Antidepressant medications, including the **selective serotonin reuptake inhibitors (SSRIs)**, exert their effect by increasing neurotransmitter availability at receptor sites. Exercise may exert its beneficial effect on mood by influencing the metabolism and availability of these central medications.

The role of **β-endorphins** in mood regulation has received considerable attention. These endogenous chemicals reduce pain and can induce euphoria linked to the "**runner's high**" experienced by exercisers who train "hard" over about 1-hour duration. The ability of exercise to produce enough β-endorphins to affect depression remains questionable, but the possibility still exists for depressed patients.

Disturbed sleep represents both a symptom and an aggravating depressive factor, making beneficial effects of exercise on sleep take on added importance (**http://sleepfoundation.org/sleep-disorders-problems/depression-and-sleep**). Depressed individuals demonstrate improved subjective sleep quality and corresponding improvement in depression measures following physical activity participation.

The exercise prescription for patients with depression considers the following eight factors:

1. **Anticipate barriers.** Common symptoms of depression pose formidable barriers to physical activity (fatigue, lack of energy, psychomotor loss). Feelings

of hopelessness and worthlessness also interfere with motivation to exercise.

2. **Keep expectations realistic.** Make exercise recommendations with caution. Depressed patients often self-blame and may view exercise as another occasion for failure. Do not raise false expectations that arouse anxiety and guilt. Explain that exercise does not provide a substitute for primary treatment.
3. **Design a feasible plan.** Make the physical activity prescription realistic and practical, not an additional burden to compound the patient's sense of futility. Consider the individual's background and history. For severely depressed patients, postpone exercise until medication and psychotherapy alleviate symptoms. Previously sedentary patients should start with a light physical activity schedule of several minutes of daily walking.
4. **Accentuate pleasurable aspects.** Guide the choice of exercise by the patient's preferences and circumstances. Use pleasurable activities that can easily add to the patient's schedule.
5. **Include group activities.** Depressed, isolated, and withdrawn patients are most likely to benefit from increased social involvement. The stimulation of being outdoors in a pleasant setting can enhance mood; exposure to light exerts therapeutic effects for seasonal depression.
6. **State specifics.** Walking is almost universally acceptable, carries minimal injury risk, and benefits mood enhancement. In keeping with ACSM recommendations for healthy adults, a goal of 20 to 60 minutes of walking or other aerobic exercise three to five times a week remains reasonable. ACSM also recommends resistance and flexibility training 2 to 3 days a week.
7. **Encourage compliance.** Improved fitness serves as a valuable consequence of exercise participation without an antidepressant effect. Compliance increases with less physically demanding physical activity programs.
8. **Integrate physical activity with other treatments.** The primary treatments for depression should not present exercise obstacles. Antidepressant medication can impair a patient's ability to function.

Combating depression relies on a spectrum of brief and longer-term psychotherapies, either alone or with antidepressant medication. An exercise prescription complements psychotherapy when the goal increases the patient's overall activity level and adds pleasurable, satisfying experiences. The patient's difficulties with physical activity (e.g., motivational problems, fear of interpersonal situations, tendency to transform exercise into a burdensome chore) may shed light on dysfunctional attitudes that psychotherapy adequately explores.

fyi Known Benefits of Regular Physical Activity

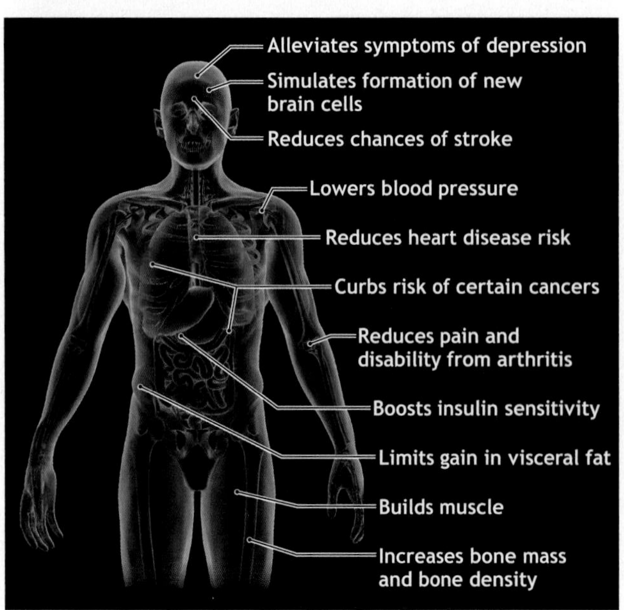
Alleviates symptoms of depression
Simulates formation of new brain cells
Reduces chances of stroke
Lowers blood pressure
Reduces heart disease risk
Curbs risk of certain cancers
Reduces pain and disability from arthritis
Boosts insulin sensitivity
Limits gain in visceral fat
Builds muscle
Increases bone mass and bone density

SUMMARY

1. The five major classifications of cognitive/emotional diseases are depression, dysthymia, seasonal affective disorder, postpartum depression, and bipolar disorder.
2. Cognitive and emotional disorders have no single cause but often result from a combination of factors or events, particularly physical changes in the brain and neurotransmitter chemical imbalance.
3. Studies in clinically depressed populations show positive effects of physical activity on symptoms.
4. No one physical activity mode has a greater impact on depression than other exercise modes.
5. Exercise-related positive psychological outcomes do not depend on achieving enhanced physical fitness, yet fitness-related indicators of lower blood pressure and increased aerobic capacity improve with physical activity in depressed individuals.
6. For women recovering from breast cancer surgery, a carefully planned, aerobic circuit resistance exercise program decreases depression and state and trait anxieties.

THINK IT THROUGH

1. List two possible mechanisms that might account for the experience of a mildly depressed person who states: "Whenever I begin to feel 'down,' I take a brisk walk, and my mental attitude perks right back up."

KEY TERMS

Acute bronchitis: Self-limiting and short duration inflammation of the trachea and bronchial tree.

Acute renal failure: Sudden renal failure from severe blood loss or trauma.

Akinesia: Complete lack of movement.

American College of Sports Medicine (ACSM): Largest sports medicine and exercise science organization in the world; promotes and integrates scientific research, education, and practical applications of sports medicine and exercise science.

Aneurysm: Abnormal arterial or venous wall dilatation or abnormal dilatation within the myocardium itself.

Angina pectoris: Chest pain caused by heart muscle ischemia due to coronary vessel obstruction or spasm.

Arterial oxygen saturation: Relative measure of the amount of oxygen dissolved or transported in arterial blood.

Asthma: Hyperirritability of pulmonary airways followed by bronchial spasm, edema, and mucus secretion.

Asymptomatic sinus bradycardia: A benign dysrhythmia of unusually slow heart rate; often occurs in endurance athletes and reflects a beneficial training adaptation that provides a longer diastole for ventricular filling during the cardiac cycle with greater stroke volume.

Atherosclerosis susceptibility gene (ATHS): Gene located on chromosome 19 that regulates the receptor that removes low-density lipoprotein cholesterol (LDL-C) from the blood.

Atrioventricular heart block: Malfunction of the heart's electrical conduction system usually caused by AV node disease.

Auscultation: Listening to sounds of diverse physiologic functions (e.g., blood pressure).

Automated external defibrillator (AED): Portable electronic device that automatically diagnoses and treats life-threatening ventricular fibrillation and ventricular tachycardia cardiac arrhythmias.

Balke test: Treadmill GXT protocol to monitor cardiac function; uses ramp-up in intensity (speed: 3.3 mph, grade increase of 1% a minute)

β-endorphins: Endogenous opioid neuropeptide in central and peripheral nervous system neurons released in response to exercise; functions as an analgesic to numb or dull pain.

Bipolar disorder: Manic-depressive illness characterized by extremes in mood and behavior lasting for at least 2 weeks.

Bradycardia: Heart beats more slowly than normal for age and sex (e.g., <60 beats per minute at rest).

Bradykinesia: Decrease in spontaneity and movement.

Bronchodilation: Expansion of bronchial air passages.

Bruce test: Treadmill GXT protocol to monitor cardiac function; applies to relatively large increases in intensity (grade and/or speed change) every 3 minutes.

Cancer: Group of diseases collectively characterized by uncontrolled, abnormal cell growth.

Carcinomas: Cancers that develop from epithelial cells that line the surface of the body, glands, and internal organs.

Cardiac catheterization: Procedure of threading a small-diameter, flexible tube (catheter), guided by x-ray, directly into an arm or leg vein or artery to access the right or left side of the heart; accurately measures pressure gradients at various locations within the heart's chambers or large vessels.

Cardiac rehabilitation program: Structured physical activity program to optimize physical function in patients with cardiac disease or recent cardiac surgeries.

Cerebral blood flow (CBF): Blood supply to the brain in a given time; adult CBF typically equals 750 milliliters per minute or 15% of the cardiac output. Reduced values represent primary marker for assessing ischemic strokes.

Chronic bronchitis: Serious pulmonary disease from constant, nonspecific irritation or inflammation of bronchial tube lining.

Chronic hypoxia: Prolonged state of inadequate oxygen supply.

Chronic kidney disease (CKD): Progressive renal failure when the kidneys no longer adequately filter blood's toxins and waste products.

Chronic obstructive pulmonary disease (COPD) or chronic airflow limitations (CAL): Pulmonary diseases characterized by airflow obstruction that impacts the lung's mechanical functions and compromises alveolar gas exchange.

Computed tomography (CT): Computer-processed x-rays to produce virtual slice, tomographic images of a scanned body area.

Congenital heart defects: Heart defects that appear at birth, usually affecting heart valves.

Congestive heart failure (CHF, HF, or chronic decompensation): Inability of the heart to pump sufficiently to maintain adequate blood flow to meet bodily needs

Continuous positive airway pressure (CPAP): External device to maintain a continuous level of positive airway pressure in a spontaneously breathing patient.

Coronary angiography: Radiocontrast material (special x-ray dye) combined with x-ray imaging used to evaluate blood flow through coronary arteries.

Cystic fibrosis (CF): Inherited condition in which thickened secretions of all exocrine glands (e.g., pancreatic, pulmonic, and gastrointestinal) plug the bronchioles to obstruct pulmonary airflow.

Degenerative heart disease (DHD), atherosclerotic cardiovascular disease, arteriosclerotic cardiovascular disease, coronary artery disease (CAD), and coronary heart disease (CHD): Interchangeable terms designating myocardial diseases.

Demyelination: Destruction of the myelin sheath that surrounds nerve fibers.

Dyspnea: Subjective symptom of breathlessness or shortness of breath.

Dysrhythmias (arrhythmias): Diseases that negatively impact the heart's electrical conduction system.

Dysthymia: Condition in which an individual is mildly depressed on most days over a period of at least 2 years.

Echocardiography: Pulses of reflected ultrasound to evaluate organ function and morphology; commonly used to identify the heart's structural components.

Ejection fraction: Volume of blood pumped from the left ventricle relative to the total amount of blood received.

Electrocardiogram (ECG): Recording of the heart's electrical activity.

Emphysema: Form of chronic obstructive pulmonary disease from abnormal, permanent enlargement and damage to air spaces (alveoli) distal to the terminal bronchi.

Endocarditis: Bacterial inflammation of the innermost heart layer (endocardium), which damages the tricuspid, aortic, or mitral valves from direct bacterial invasion into the tissue.

End-stage renal disease (ESRD): Chronic uremia from total loss of kidney function.

Exercise-induced bronchospasm: Bronchoconstriction induced by physical activity.

False-negative: Test result that incorrectly identifies a person with heart disease as normal (unsuccessful test).

False-positive: Test result that incorrectly identifies a normal person as having heart disease (unsuccessful test).

Fibrillate: Fine, rapid contractions or twitching of myocardial fibers in an unregulated manner.

Graded exercise stress test (GXT): Systematic use of exercise on treadmill or cycle ergometer during which individual is monitored for cardiac rhythm abnormalities and metabolic adjustments.

Health: State of complete physical, mental, and social well-being, not merely absence of disease and infirmity.

Hemiparesis: Muscle weakness affecting one side of the body.

Hemiplegia: Paralysis affecting one side of the body.

Hypercapnia: State of abnormally elevated blood CO_2 levels.

Hypertensive exercise response: Increase in systolic blood pressure of 20 mm Hg or more in low-level physical activity of 2 to 4 METs.

Hypotensive exercise response: Failure of systolic blood pressure to increase during moderate physical activity.

Informed consent: A signed statement by an individual being tested that he or she had an opportunity to ask questions about the procedures with sufficient information clearly provided so consent occurs as a knowledgeable, informed perspective.

Inpatient cardiac rehabilitation Highly structured and monitored in-hospital cardiac rehabilitation physical activity program to optimize physical function in patients with cardiac disease or recent cardiac surgeries.

Intermittent claudication: An aching, weakness, tightness, or cramping sensation in legs during physical activity.

Ischemia: Oxygen deprivation from prolonged lack of blood flow.

Leukemias: Cancer of blood cells.

"Likert-type" scale: Type of psychometric rating scale to assess responses in survey research; information derived mostly from questionnaires.

Lung compliance: Change in lung volume per unit change in intra-alveolar pressure.

Lymphomas: Cancers of the immune system.

Magnetic resonance imaging (MRI): Detailed images of the organs and tissues within the body using strong magnetic fields and radio waves.

Major depressive disorder: Mood disorder affecting how a person feels, thinks, and behaves; can lead to a variety of emotional and physical problems.

Maximal GXT (GXT_{max}): Individual exercises until they are unable to proceed to the next intensity increment.

Mitral valve prolapse (MVP); floppy valve syndrome; Barlow syndrome; click-murmur syndrome: Dysfunctional variation in either the mitral valve's shape or structure that usually associates with endocarditis, atherosclerosis, and muscular dystrophy

Monoamines: Neurotransmitters and neuromodulators each with one amino group attached by a two-carbon chain ($-CH_2-CH_2-$) to an aromatic ring; examples include dopamine, norepinephrine, epinephrine (adrenaline), histamine, and serotonin.

Multiple sclerosis (MS): Chronic, disabling inflammatory neural disease from damaged insulating myelin of brain and spinal cord neurons.

Myasthenia gravis: Autoimmune disease leading to fluctuating muscle weakness and fatigue caused by circulating antibodies that block acetylcholine receptors at the postsynaptic neuromuscular junction.

Myocardial infarction (MI): Medical term for heart attack; occurs when blood stops flowing to a part of the heart from oxygen insufficiency.

Myocardial ischemia: Insufficient oxygen supply to the heart caused by coronary atherosclerosis.

Naughton test: Treadmill GXT protocol to monitor cardiac function; uses ramp-up in intensity (3-min exercise periods of increasing intensity [1 to 3 mph] alternate with 3-min rest periods.).

Necrosis: Cell death.

Neuromuscular diseases: Diverse diseases and ailments that impair muscle function, either directly (pathologies of muscle) or indirectly (pathologies of nerves or neuromuscular junctions).

Outpatient cardiac rehabilitation: Cardiac rehabilitation program administered by outpatient services to optimize physical function in patients with cardiac disease or recent cardiac surgeries.

P wave: Atrial depolarization of ECG tracing preceding atrial contraction.

Parkinson disease (PD): CNS neurodegenerative disease that impairs motor skills, speech, and vital body functions.

Patent ductus arteriosus: Shunt caused by the failure of an opening between the aorta and pulmonary artery to close at birth.

Pericarditis: Inflammation of the heart's outer pericardial lining.

Pneumothorax: Abnormal collection of air or gas in the pleural space separating the lungs from the chest wall.

Polymyositis: Chronic inflammation of muscle tissue (inflammatory myopathy).

Postpartum depression: Mother's depression following birth; typically occurs in the first few months postdelivery.

Premature ventricular contractions (PVCs); ectopic, extrasystole: Fine, rapid contractions or twitching of myocardial ventricular fibers when heart generates potentially pathologic extra beats.

Prolapse: Enlarged valve leaflets (usually mitral valves) that bulge backward into the left atrium during the cardiac cycle.

Pulmonary congestion: Flooding of pulmonary alveoli with plasma filtrate.

Pulmonary hypertension: Increased blood pressure in the pulmonary vasculature leading to shortness of breath, dizziness, fainting, and leg swelling.

Pulse oximetry: Noninvasive method to assess arterial blood oxygen saturation.

QRS complex: Combination of three of the graphical deflections on an ECG tracing, usually the central and most visually obvious part of the tracing that heralds ventricular contraction.

Regurgitation: Failure of heart valves to close properly causes blood to flow back into the heart's chambers during diastole.

Restrictive lung dysfunction (RLD): Pulmonary diseases characterized by diminished lung expansion and decreased tidal volume.

Rheumatic fever: Potentially fatal inflammatory disease caused by infection by Group A or B streptococcal bacteria; mostly affects heart, joints, or skin.

Rheumatoid arthritis: Autoimmune disease that results in a chronic, systemic inflammatory disorder that attacks tissues and organs, but principally flexible (synovial) joints.

Runner's high: Occurs when people exercise so strenuously that their bodies experience a threshold of euphoria; related to the release of β-endorphins during prolonged moderate-to-intense-physical activity.

Sarcomas: Cancers of connective tissues in bones, tendons, cartilage, fat, and muscle.

Seasonal affective disorder: Recurrence of depressive symptoms during certain seasons (e.g., winter, summer).

Selective serotonin reuptake inhibitors (SSRIs): Class of compounds typically used as antidepressants to treat depression, anxiety disorders, and some personality disorders; increases extracellular level of the neurotransmitter serotonin by inhibiting its reuptake.

Septal defects: Hole between the myocardial ventricles and atria.

Sick sinus node syndrome: Malfunction of the sinoatrial (SA) node.

Sinus bradycardia: Resting heart rate less than 60 $b \cdot min^{-1}$.

Sinus tachycardia: Resting heart rate greater than 100 $b \cdot min^{-1}$.

Sports medicine: Subspecialty of medicine that deals with physical fitness and treatment and prevention of injuries related to sports and physical activity.

S-T segment depression: Measured vertical distance of ECG tracing between the trace and isoelectric line 2 to 3 mm from QRS complex. Most common ECG indicator of myocardial ischemia.

Stenosis: Heart valve narrowing or constriction that prevents valve from opening fully; often caused by growths, scars, or abnormal mineral deposits.

Stroke (acute cerebrovascular attack): Potentially fatal reduction in oxygen supply from restricted blood supply to the brain.

Symptom limited: Test in which individuals exercise until they decide to stop or develop abnormal symptoms that require test termination.

Systemic lupus erythematosus: Systemic autoimmune disease (or autoimmune connective tissue disease) that occurs when the body's immune system attacks tissues and organs.

Tachycardia: Heart beats more rapidly than normal for age and sex.

Test sensitivity: Percentage of persons for whom the stress test detects an abnormal, positive response.

Test specificity: Number of true-negative stress test results, that is, the test correctly identifies someone without heart disease.

Thallium imaging: Radionucleotide imaging to evaluate myocardial blood flow and tissue perfusion.

True-negative: Test result that correctly identifies a person without heart disease (successful test).

True-positive: Test result that correctly identifies a person with heart disease (successful test).

Uremia: Symptoms of chronic kidney disease resulting in blood's retention of waste products normally excreted in urine.

Vasodilators: Drugs to enlarge blood vessels by relaxing smooth muscle cells within the vessel wall.

Ventriculography: Imaging procedure that provides information about left ventricular functional dynamics.

SELECTED REFERENCES

Achttien RJ, et al. Exercise-based cardiac rehabilitation in patients with coronary heart disease: a practice guideline. *Neth Heart J* 2013;21:429.

Ahluwalia IB, et al. Report from the CDC. Changes in selected chronic disease-related risks and health conditions for nonpregnant women 18-44 years old BRFSS. *J Womens Health (Larchmt)* 2005;14:382.

Alves AJ, et al. Exercise training improves diastolic function in heart failure patients. *Med Sci Sports Exerc* 2012;44:776.

American College of Sports Medicine and American Heart Association. Joint position stand on recommendations for cardiovascular screening, staffing, and emergency policies at health/fitness facilities. *Med Sci Sports Exerc* 1998;30:1009.

American College of Sports Medicine. Position stand. Physical activity, physical fitness, and hypertension. *Med Sci Sports Exerc* 1993;25:i.

American Psychiatric Association. *Diagnostic and Statistical Manual of Mental Disorders: DSM-IV*. 4th Ed. Washington, DC: American Psychiatric Association, 1994.

Angermayr L, et al. Multifactorial lifestyle interventions in the primary and secondary prevention of cardiovascular disease and type 2 diabetes mellitus—a systematic review of randomized controlled trials. *Ann Behav Med* 2010;40:49.

Armstrong HF, et al. Effect of lung transplantation on heart rate response to exercise. *Heart Lung* 2015. In press (as of April 20, 2015).

Aucella F, et al. The role of physical activity in the CKD setting. *Kidney Blood Press Res* 2014;39:97.

Ba A, et al. Cardiopulmonary response to exercise in COPD and overweight patients: relationship between unloaded cycling and maximal oxygen uptake profiles. *Biomed Res Int* 2015;2015:378469

Bartholomew JB, et al. Effects of acute exercise on mood and well-being in patients with major depressive disorder. *Med Sci Sports Exerc* 2005;37:2032.

Bauman AE. Updating the evidence that physical activity is good for health: an epidemiological review, 2000–2003. *J Sci Med Sport* 2004;7:6.

Blain G, et al. Assessment of ventilatory thresholds during graded and maximal exercise test using time varying analysis of respiratory sinus arrhythmia. *Br J Sports Med* 2005;39:448.

Blair SN, et al. Physical activity, nutrition, and chronic disease. *Med Sci Sports Exerc* 1996;28:335.

Bodegard J, et al. Reasons for terminating an exercise test provide independent prognostic information: 2014 apparently healthy men followed for 26 years. *Eur Heart J* 2005;26:1394.

Braith RW, et al. Exercise training in patients with CHF and heart transplant recipients. *Med Sci Sports Exerc* 1998;30:S367.

Brown TR, Kraft GH. Exercise and rehabilitation for individuals with multiple sclerosis. *Phys Med Rehabil Clin N Am* 2005;16:513.

Camillo CA, et al. Physiological responses during downhill walking: A new exercise modality for subjects with chronic obstructive pulmonary disease? *Chron Respir Dis* 2015. In press (as of April 20, 2015).

Campo RA, et al. Blood pressure, salivary cortisol, and inflammatory cytokine outcomes in senior female cancer survivors enrolled in a tai chi chih randomized controlled trial. *J Cancer Surviv* 2015;9:115.

Capitanini A, et al. Dialysis exercise team: the way to sustain exercise programs in hemodialysis patients. *Kidney Blood Press Res* 2014;39:129.

Chaput JP, et al. Findings from the Quebec family study on the etiology of obesity: genetics and environmental highlights. *Curr Obes Rep* 2014;3:54.

Church TS, Blair SN. When will we treat physical activity as a legitimate medical therapy ... even though it does not come in a pill? *Br J Sports Med* 2009;43:80.

Clark CJ, et al. Low intensity peripheral muscle conditioning improves exercise tolerance and breathlessness in COPD. *Eur J Respir* 1996;9:2590.

Cooper AR, et al. What is the magnitude of blood pressure response to a programme of moderate intensity exercise? Randomised controlled trial among sedentary adults with unmedicated hypertension. *Br J Gen Pract* 2000;50:958.

Cooper CB. Determining the role of exercise in patients with chronic pulmonary disease. *Med Sci Sports Exerc* 1995;27:147.

Courneya KS, et al. Subgroup effects in a randomised trial of different types and doses of exercise during breast cancer chemotherapy. *Br J Cancer* 2014;111:1718.

Courneya KS. Exercise interventions during cancer treatment. *Exerc Sports Sci Rev* 2001;29:60.

Crawford JJ, et al. Associations between exercise and posttraumatic growth in gynecologic cancer survivors. *Support Care Cancer* 2015;23:705.

D'Andrea A, et al. Prognostic value of supine bicycle exercise stress echocardiography in patients with known or suspected coronary artery disease. *Eur J Echocardiogr* 2005;6:271.

Daviglus ML, et al. Association of nonspecific minor ST-T abnormalities with cardiovascular mortality: the Chicago Western Electric Study. *JAMA* 1999;281:524.

Demark-Wahnefried W, et al. Lifestyle intervention development study to improve physical function in older adults with cancer: outcomes from Project LEAD. *J Clin Oncol* 2006;24:3465.

Dimeo F, et al. Aerobic exercise as therapy for cancer fatigue. *Med Sci Sports Exerc* 1998;30:475.

Doyne EJ, et al. Running versus weight lifting in the treatment of depression. *J Consult Clin Psychol* 1987;55:748.

Eichenberger PA, et al. Effects of exercise training on airway hyperreactivity in asthma: a systematic review and meta-analysis. *Sports Med* 2013;43:1157.

Emaus A, et al. Physical activity, heart rate, metabolic profile, and estradiol in premenopausal women. *Med Sci Sports Exerc* 2008;40:1022.

Eyigor S, Kanyilmaz S. Exercise in patients coping with breast cancer: an overview. *World J Clin Oncol* 2014;5:406.

Fairey AS, et al. Randomized controlled trial of exercise and blood immune function in postmenopausal breast cancer survivors. *J Appl Physiol* 2005;98:1534.

Falzon C, et al. Development and validation of the cancer exercise stereotypes scale (CESS). *J Psychosoc Oncol* 2014;32:708.

Faulkner J, et al. A randomized controlled trial to assess the effect of self-paced walking on task-specific anxiety in cardiac rehabilitation patients. *J Cardiopulm Rehabil Prev* 2013;33:292.

Feiereisen P, et al. Is strength training the more efficient training modality in chronic heart failure? *Med Sci Sports Exerc* 2007;39:1910.

Fitch KD. An overview of asthma and airway hyper-responsiveness in Olympic athletes. *Brit J Sports Med* 2012;46:413.

Fleck SJ. Cardiovascular adaptations to resistance training. *Med Sci Sports Exerc* 1988;20:S146.

Fonarow GC, et al. Workplace wellness recognition for optimizing workplace health: a presidential advisory from the American Heart Association. *Circulation* 2015. In press (as of April 20, 2015).

Franco MJ, et al. Comparison of dyspnea ratings during submaximal constant work exercise with incremental testing. *Med Sci Sports Exerc* 1998;30:479.

Franklin BA, et al. Is direct physician supervision of exercise stress testing routinely necessary? *Chest* 1997;111:262.

Frazer CJ, et al. Effectiveness of treatments for depression in older people. *Med J Aust* 2005;182:627.

Freedman DS, et al. Changes and variability in high levels of low-density lipoprotein cholesterol among children. *Pediatrics* 2010;126:266.

Gafarov VV, et al. The influence of depression on risk development of acute cardiovascular diseases in the female population aged 25-64 in Russia. *Int J Circumpolar Health* 2013;5;72.

Galvao DA, Newton RU. Review of exercise intervention studies in cancer patients. *J Clin Oncol* 2005;23:899.

Goldkorn R, et al. Comparison of the usefulness of heart rate variability versus exercise stress testing for the detection of myocardial ischemia in patients without known coronary artery disease. *Am J Cardiol* 2015. In press (as of April 20, 2015).

Guillamó E, et al. Physical effects of a reconditioning programme in a group of chronic fatigue syndrome patients. *J Sports Med Phys Fitness* 2015. In press (as of April 20, 2015).

Hamer M, et al. The impact of physical activity on all-cause mortality in men and women after a cancer diagnosis. *Cancer Causes Control* 2009;20:225.

Harms CA, Dempsey JA. Cardiovascular consequences of exercise hyperpnea. *Exerc Sport Sci Rev* 1999;27:37.

Hassanpour Dehkordi A, Khaledi Far A. Effect of exercise training on the quality of life and echocardiography parameter of systolic function in patients with chronic heart failure: a randomized trial. *Asian J Sports Med* 2015;6:e22643

Hebestreit H, et al. Oxygen uptake kinetics are slowed in cystic fibrosis. *Med Sci Sports Exerc* 2005;37:10.

Holmes MD, et al. Physical activity and survival after breast cancer diagnosis. *JAMA* 2005;293:2479.

Hough DO, Dec KL. Exercise-induced asthma and anaphylaxis. *Sports Med* 1994;18:162.

Howden EJ, Fassett RG, et al. Exercise training in chronic kidney disease patients. *Sports Med* 2012;42:473.

Hutnick NA, et al. Exercise and lymphocyte activation following chemotherapy for breast cancer. *Med Sci Sports Exerc* 2005;37:1827.

Irwin ML. Physical activity interventions for cancer survivors. *Br J Sports Med* 2009;43:32.

Irwin ML. Randomized controlled trials of physical activity and breast cancer prevention. *Exerc Sport Sci Rev* 2006;34:182.

Jankowski CM, et al. Searching for maintenance in exercise interventions for cancer survivors. *J Cancer Surviv* 2014;8:697.

Jarrell LA, et al. Gender differences in functional capacity following myocardial infarction: an exploratory study. *Can J Cardiovasc Nurs* 2005;15:28.

Katzmarzyk PT, et al. Anthropometric markers of obesity and mortality in white and African American adults: the Pennington center longitudinal study. *Obesity (Silver Spring)* 2013;21:1070.

Katzmarzyk PT, et al. Clinical utility and reproducibility of visceral adipose tissue measurements derived from dual-energy X-ray absorptiometry in white and African American adults. *Obesity (Silver Spring)* 2013;21:2221.

Katzmarzyk PT, et al. Sitting time and mortality from all causes, cardiovascular disease, and cancer. *Med Sci Sports Exerc* 2009;41:998.

Kirkham AA, et al. Comparison of aerobic exercise intensity prescription methods in breast cancer. *Med Sci Sports Exerc* 2013;45:1443.

Klepin HD, et al. Exercise for older cancer patients: feasible and helpful? *Interdiscip Top Gerontol* 2013;38:146.

Klika RJ, et al. Exercise capacity of a breast cancer survivor: a case study. *Med Sci Sports Exerc* 2008;40:1711.

Kohl HW, et al. Maximal exercise hemodynamics and risk of mortality in apparently healthy men and women. *Med Sci Sports Exerc* 1998;28:601.

Kruk J, Czerniak U. Physical activity and its relation to cancer risk: updating the evidence. *Asian Pac J Cancer Prev* 2013;14:3993.

La Gerche A, Claessen G. Is exercise good for the right ventricle? concepts for health and disease. *Can J Cardiol* 2015;31:502.

Lapole T, et al. Influence of dorsiflexion shoes on neuromuscular fatigue of the plantar flexors after combined tapping-jumping exercises in volleyball players. *J Strength Cond Res* 2013;27:2025.

Lauer MS, et al. Impaired heart rate response to graded exercise prognostic implications of chronotropic incompetence in the Framingham Heart Study. *Circulation* 1996;93:1520.

Lee IM. Physical activity and cardiac protection. *Curr Sports Med Rep* 2010;9:214.

Lemanne D, et al. The role of physical activity in cancer prevention, treatment, recovery, and survivorship. *Oncology (Williston Park)* 2013;27:580.

Lønbro S, et al. Progressive resistance training rebuilds lean body mass in head and neck cancer patients after radiotherapy: results from the randomized DAHANCA 25B trial. *Radiother Oncol* 2013;108:314.

Malin A, et al. Energy balance and breast cancer risk. *Cancer Epidemiol Biomarkers Prev* 2005;14:1496.

Mannix ET, et al. Exercise-induced asthma in figure skaters. *Chest* 1996;109:312.

Marijon E, et al. Sudden cardiac arrest during sports activity in middle age. *Circulation* 2015. In press (as of April 20, 2015).

Marzolini S, et al. Aerobic and resistance training in coronary disease: single versus multiple sets. *Med Sci Sports Exerc* 2008;40:1557.

McCartney N. Role of resistance training in heart disease. *Med Sci Sports Exerc* 1998;30:S396.

McClure MK, et al. Randomized controlled trial of the Breast Cancer Recovery Program for women with breast cancer-related lymphedema. *Am J Occup Ther* 2010;64:59.

Min JK, et al. Medical history for prognostic risk assessment and diagnosis of stable patients with suspected coronary artery disease. *Am J Med* 2015. In press (as of April 20, 2015).

Minam DS, et al. Physical activity and quality of life after radical prostatectomy. *Can Urol Assoc J* 2010;4:180.

Mirza MA. Anginalike pain and normal coronary arteries. Uncovering cardiac syndromes that mimic CAD. *Postgrad Med* 2005;117:41.

Mishra SI, et al. Exercise interventions on health-related quality of life for people with cancer during active treatment. *Cochrane Database Syst Rev* 2012;8:CD008465.

Mock V, et al. Exercise manages fatigue during breast cancer treatment: a randomized controlled trial. *Psychooncology* 2005;14:464.

Moreria A, et al. Exercise-induced asthma: why is it so frequent in Olympic athletes? *Expert Rev Respir Med* 2011;5:1.

Morris JN. Exercise in the prevention of coronary heart disease: today's best bet in public health. *Med Sci Sports Exerc* 1994;26:807.

Mousa TM, et al. Exercise training enhances baroreflex sensitivity by an angiotensin II-dependent mechanism in chronic heart failure. *J Appl Physiol* 2008;104:616.

Nilsson BB, et al. Effects of group-based high-intensity aerobic interval training in patients with chronic heart failure. *Am J Cardiol* 2008;102:1361.

Ochmann U, et al. Long-term efficacy of pulmonary rehabilitation in patients with occupational respiratory disease. *Respiration* 2012;84:396.

Ohkawara K, et al. Response of coronary heart disease risk factors to changes in body fat during diet-induced weight reduction in Japanese obese men: a pilot study. *Ann Nutr Metab* 2010;56:1.

Ostrom NK, et al. Exercise-induced bronchospasm, asthma control, and obesity. *Allergy Asthma Proc* 2013;34:342.

Paffenbarger RS Jr, et al. Physical activity and personal characteristics associated with depression and suicide in American college men. *Acta Psychiatr Scand* 1994;377:16.

Paramanandam VS, Roberts D. Weight training is not harmful for women with breast cancer-related lymphoedema: a systematic review. *J Physiother* 2014;60:136.

Pescatello LS. et al., eds. *ACSM's Guidelines for Exercise Testing and Prescription*. 9th Ed. Baltimore: Lippincott Williams & Wilkins, 2014.

Pejovic S, et al. Chronic fatigue syndrome and fibromyalgia in diagnosed sleep disorders: a further test of the 'unitary' hypothesis. *BMC Neurol* 2015;15:53.

Pelletier AR, et al. Revisions to chronic disease surveillance indicators, United States, 2004. *Prev Chronic Dis* 2005;2:A15.

Repka CP, et al. Cancer type does not affect exercise-mediated improvements in cardiorespiratory function and fatigue. *Integr Cancer* 2014;13:473.

Resnick B. Research review: exercise interventions for treatment of depression. *Geriatr Nurs* 2005;26:196.

Romyn G, et al. Sleep, anxiety and electronic device use by athletes in the training and competition environments. *Eur J Sport Sci* 2015. In press (as of April 20, 2015).

Samad AK, et al. A meta-analysis of the association of physical activity with reduced risk of colorectal cancer. *Colorectal Dis* 2005;7:204.

Schwartz AL, et al. Exercise reduces daily fatigue in women with breast cancer receiving chemotherapy. *Med Sci Sports Exerc* 2001;33:718.

Segar ML, et al. The effect of aerobic exercise on self-esteem and depressive and anxiety symptoms among breast cancer survivors. *Oncol Nurs Forum* 1998;25:107.

Serrau V, et al. Mechanical energy expenditure of subject with multiple sclerosis engaged in daily activities: a case study. *Comput Methods Biomech Biomed Engin* 2013;16:134.

Sesso HD, et al. Physical activity and breast cancer risk in the College Alumni Health Study (United States). *Cancer Causes Control* 1998;9:433.

Shephard RJ, Baldy GJ. Exercise as cardiovascular therapy. *Circulation* 1999;99:963.

Sil S, et al. Preliminary evidence of altered biomechanics in adolescents with juvenile fibromyalgia. *Arthritis Care Res (Hoboken)* 2014;67:102.

Singh NA, et al. A randomized controlled trial of the effect of exercise on sleep. *Sleep* 1997;20:95.

Sorg M, et al. Re-entrainment to physical activity in the global management of breast cancer: pilot study in a mono-institutional experience. *Bull Cancer* 2014;101:698.

Spence JC, et al. The effect of physical-activity participation on self-concept: a meta-analysis. *J Sport Exerc Psychol* 1997;19:S109.

Staud R, et al. Evidence for sensitized fatigue pathways in patients with chronic fatigue syndrome. *Pain* 2015;156:750.

Steindorf K, et al. Randomized controlled trial of resistance training in breast cancer patients receiving adjuvant radiotherapy: results on cancer-related fatigue and quality of life. *Ann Oncol* 2014;25:2237.

Taso CJ, et al. The effect of yoga exercise on improving depression, anxiety, and fatigue in women with breast cancer: a randomized controlled trial. *J Nurs Res* 2014;22:155.

Taylor BJ, et al. Submaximal exercise pulmonary gas exchange in left heart disease patients with different forms of pulmonary hypertension. *J Card Fail* 2015. In press (as of April 20, 2015).

Theadom A, et al. Daytime napping associated with increased symptom severity in fibromyalgia syndrome. *BMC Musculoskelet Disord* 2015;16:13.

Theisen V, et al. Blood pressure Sunday: introducing genomics to the community through family history. *Prev Chronic Dis* 2005;2:A23.

Toukola T, et al. Sudden cardiac death during physical exercise: Characteristics of victims and autopsy findings. *Ann Med* 2015. In press (as of April 20, 2015).

Verrill DE, Ribisl PM. Resistive exercise training in cardiac rehabilitation (an update). *Sports Med* 1996;21:371.

Visovsky C, Dvorak C. Exercise and cancer recovery. *Online J Issues Nurs* 2005;10:7.

White LJ, Dressendorfer RH. Exercise and multiple sclerosis. *Sports Med* 2004;34:1077.

Wilson DB, et al. Anthropometric changes using a walking intervention in African American breast cancer survivors: a pilot study. *Prev Chronic Dis* 2005;2:A16.

Winzer BM, et al. Exercise and the prevention of oesophageal cancer (EPOC) study protocol: a randomized controlled trial of exercise versus stretching in males with Barrett's oesophagus. *BMC Cancer* 2010;10:292.

Wirth MD, et al. Examining connections between screening for breast, cervical and prostate cancer and colorectal cancer screening. *Colorectal Cancer* 2014;3:253.

Yach D, et al. Improving diet and physical activity: 12 lessons from controlling tobacco smoking. *Br Med J* 2005;330:898.

Yamazaki T, et al. Circadian dynamics of heart rate and physical activity in patients with heart failure. *Clin Exp Hypertens* 2005;27:241.

Yang PS, Chen CH. Exercise stage and processes of change in patients with chronic obstructive pulmonary disease. *J Nurs Res* 2005;13:97.

Youngstedt SD. Effects of exercise on sleep. *Clin Sports Med* 2005;24:355.

Zhang Y. Cardiovascular diseases in American women. *Nutr Metab Cardiovasc Dis* 2010;20:386.

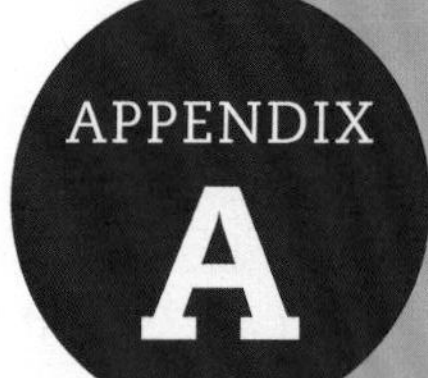

The Metric System and Conversion Constants in Exercise Physiology

Appendix A has two parts. Part 1 deals with the metric system, and Part 2 discusses the Système International d'Unités (SI units).

THE METRIC SYSTEM

Most measurements in science are expressed in terms of the metric system. This system uses units related to one another by some power of 10. The prefix *centi* means one-hundredth, *milli* means one-thousandth, and *kilo* is derived from a word that means one thousand. In the following sections, we show the relationship between metric and English units of measurement relevant to material in this book.

Units of Length

Metric Unit	Equivalent Metric Units	Equivalent English Units
meter (m)	100 cm; 1000 mm	39.37 in.; 3.28 ft; 1.09 yd
centimeter (cm)	0.01 m; 10 mm	0.3937 in.
millimeter (mm)	0.001 m; 0.1 cm	0.03937 in.

UNITS OF WEIGHT

Use the following conversions for common units of mass (weight) and volume. For example, 1 oz = 0.06 lb. Therefore, 2 oz equals 2 × 0.06 = 0.12 lb, and 16 oz = 0.96 lb (16 × 0.06).

Units of Weight

Metric Unit	Equivalent Metric Units	Equivalent English Units
kilogram (kg)	1000 g; 1,000,000 mg	35.3 oz; 2.2046 lb
gram (g)	0.001 kg; 1000 mg	0.353 oz
milligram (mg)	0.000001 kg; 0.001 g	0.0000353 oz

Units of Volume

Metric Unit	Equivalent Metric Units	Equivalent English Units
liter (L)	1000 mL	1.057 qt
milliliter (mL) or cubic centimeter (cc)	0.001 L	0.001057 qt

Temperature

To convert Fahrenheit to Celsius: °C = (°F − 32) ÷ 1.8
To convert Celsius to Fahrenheit: °F = (1.8 ÷ °C) + 32

On the Fahrenheit scale, water freezes at 32°F and boils at 212°F.
On the Celsius scale, water freezes at 0°C and boils at 100°C.

Units of Speed

mph	$km \cdot h^{-1}$	$m \cdot sec^{-1}$
1	1.6	0.47
2	3.2	0.94
3	4.8	1.41
4	6.4	1.88
5	8.0	2.35
6	9.6	2.82
7	11.2	3.29
8	12.8	3.76
9	14.4	4.23
10	16.0	4.70
11	17.7	5.17
12	19.3	5.64
13	20.9	6.11
14	22.5	6.58
15	24.1	7.05
16	25.8	7.52
17	27.4	7.99
18	29.0	8.46
19	30.6	8.93
20	32.2	9.40

Common Expressions of Work, Energy, and Power

Watts	Kilocalories (kcal)	Foot-pounds (ft-lb)
1 watt = 0.73756 ft-lb · sec^{-1}	1 kcal = 3086 ft-lb	1 ft · lb = 3.2389 × 10^{-3} kcal
1 watt = 0.01433 kcal · min^{-1}	1 kcal = 426.8 kg-m	1 ft · lb = 0.13825 kg-m
1 watt = 1.341 × 10^{-3} hp or 0.0013 hp	1 kcal = 3087.4 ft-lb	1 ft · lb = 5.050 × 10^{-3} hp · h^{-1}
1 watt = 6.12 kg-m · min^{-1}	1 kcal = 1.5593 × 10^{-3} hp · h^{-1}	

TERMINOLOGY AND UNITS OF MEASUREMENT

The American College of Sports Medicine (**www.acsm.org/**) suggests that the following terminology and units of measurement be used in scientific endeavors to promote consistency and clarity of communication and to avoid ambiguity. The following terms are defined using the units of measurement of the Système International d'Unités (SI units).

Exercise: Any and all activity involving generation of force by the activated muscle(s) that results in disruption of a homeostatic state. In dynamic exercise, the muscle may perform shortening (concentric) contractions or be overcome by external resistance and perform lengthening (eccentric) contractions. When muscle force results in no movement, the contraction should be termed *static* or *isometric*.

Exercise intensity: Specific level of maintenance of muscular activity that can be quantified in terms of power (energy expenditure or work performed per unit of time), isometric force sustained, or velocity of progression.

Endurance: Time limit of a person's ability to maintain either a specific isometric force or a specific power level involving combinations of concentric or eccentric muscular contractions.

Mass: Quantity of matter of an object; a direct measure of the object's inertia (note: Mass = Weight ÷ Acceleration due to gravity unit: gram or kilogram).

Weight: Force with which a quantity of matter is attracted toward Earth by normal acceleration of gravity (traditional unit: kilogram).

Energy: Capability of producing force, performing work, or generating heat (unit: joule or kilojoule).

Force: That which changes or tends to change the state of rest or motion in matter (unit: Newton).

Speed: Total distance traveled per unit of time (unit: meters per second).

Velocity: Displacement per unit of time. A vector quantity requiring that direction be stated or strongly implied (unit: meters per second or kilometers per hour).

Work: Force expressed through a distance but with no limitation on time (unit: joule or kilojoule). Quantities of energy and heat expressed independently of time should also be presented in joules. The term *work* should *not* be used synonymously with *muscular exercise*.

Power: Rate of performing work the derivative of work with respect to time the product of force and velocity (unit: watt). Other related processes, such as energy release and heat transfer, should, when expressed per unit of time, be quantified and presented in watts.

Torque: Effectiveness of a force to produce axial rotation (unit: Newton meter).

Volume: Space occupied, for example, by a quantity of fluid or gas (unit: liter or milliliter). Gas volumes should be indicated as ATPS, BTPS, or STPD.

Amount of a substance: Frequently expressed in moles; a mole is the quantity of a chemical substance that has a weight in mass units (e.g., grams) numerically equal to the molecular weight or that, in the case of a gas, has a volume occupied by such a weight under specified conditions. One mole of a respiratory gas is equal to 22.4 L at STPD.

SI UNITS

The uniform numerical value system is known as the Système International d'Unités (SI units; **www.french-metrology.com/en/history/history-mesurement.asp**). SI was developed through international cooperation to create a universally acceptable system of measurement. SI ensures that units of measurement remain uniform in concept and style. The SI system permits quantities in common use to be easier to compare. Many scientific organizations endorse the concept of the SI, and leading journals in nutrition, health, and exercise science now require that laboratory data be presented in SI units. The information in this appendix has been summarized from a detailed description about the SI published in the following article: Young DS. Implementation of SI units for clinical laboratory data. Style specifications and conversion tables. *Ann Intern Med* 1987;106:114.

For SI units in exercise physiology, the term *body weight* is properly referred to as mass (kg), height should be referred to as stature (m), second is sec, minute is min, hour is h, week is wk, month is mo, year is y, day is d, gram is g, liter is L, hertz is Hz, joule is J, kilocalorie is kcal, ohm is V, pascal is Pa, revolutions per minute is rpm, volt is V, and watt is W. These abbreviations or symbols are used for the singular and plural forms.

Definitions of Common SI Units

Degree Celsius (°C)	Equivalent to K − 273.15.
Radian (rad)	Plane angle subtended by a circular arc as the length of the arc divided by the radius of the arc.
Joule (J)	Work done when the point of application of a force of 1 N is displaced through a distance of 1 m in the direction of the force. 1 J = 1 Nm.
Kelvin (K)	Fraction 1/273.16 of the thermodynamic temperature of the triple point of water.
Kilogram (kg)	Unit of mass equal to the mass of the international prototype of the kilogram.
Meter (m)	Length equal to 1,650,763.73 wavelengths in vacuum of the radiation that corresponds to the transition between the levels $2p_{10}$ and $5d_5$ of the krypton 86 atom.
Newton (N)	Force that, when applied to a mass of 1 kg, gives it an acceleration of 1 $m^{-1} \cdot sec^{-2}$. 1 N = 1 $kg \cdot m^{-1} \cdot sec^{-2}$.
Pascal (Pa)	Pressure produced by a force of 1 N applied, with uniform distribution, over an area of 1 m^{-2}. 1 Pa = 1 $N \cdot m^{-2}$.
Second (sec)	Duration of 9,192,631,770 periods of the radiation that corresponds to the transition between the two hyperfine levels of the ground state of the cesium 133 atom.
Watt (W)	Power that in 1 sec gives rise to the energy of 1 joule. 1 W = 1 $J \cdot sec^{-1}$.

Base Units of SI Nomenclature

Physical Quantity	Base Unit	SI Symbol
Length	meter	m
Mass	kilogram	kg
Time	second	sec
Amount of substance	mole	mol
Thermodynamic temperature	kelvin	K
Electric current	ampere	A
Luminous intensity	candela	cd

Base Units of SI Style Guidelines

Guidelines	Incorrect Style	Correct Style
Lowercase letters are used for symbols or abbreviations	Kg	kg
Exceptions:	k a l	K A L
Symbols are not followed by a period	m.	m
Exception: end of sentence	mol.	mol
Symbols are not to be pluralized	kgs ms	kg m
Names and symbols are not to be combined	kilogram · meter · sec^{-2}	kg-m · sec^{-2} kg-m/sec^2
When numbers are printed, symbols are preferred	100 meters 2 moles	100 m 2 mol
A space should be placed between the number and the symbol	50 mL	50 mL
Symbols for units formed from other units by multiplication are indicated by means of either a half-high (that is, centered) dot or a space	N/m	N · m N m
Only one solidus (/) should be used per expression	mmol/L/sec	mmol/(L · sec)
A zero should be placed before the decimal	.01	0.01
Decimal numbers are preferable to fractions	¾ 75%	0.75 0.75
Spaces are used to separate long numbers Exception: optional with four-digit number	1,500,000 1,000	1 500 000 1000 or 1 000

APPENDIX

B

Dietary Reference Intakes (DRIs): Recommended Vitamin and Mineral Intakes for Individuals

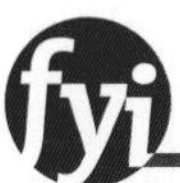

Dietary Guidelines for Americans: Changing Goals and Recommendations

In 1980, the first edition of *Dietary Guidelines for Americans* was released; since then, it has been reviewed, updated, and published every 5 years in a joint effort between the U.S. Department of Health and Human Services (HHS) and the U.S. Department of Agriculture (USDA). Presented here are recommendations excerpted from the 2010 *Guidelines* (**Table B.1** and **Table B.2**); at this writing, the 2015 *Dietary Guidelines* have not yet been released. The website **www.DietaryGuidelines.gov** provides updates on the progress of the revised guidelines; a link to the new guidelines will also be provided on this text's website at **www.thePoint.lww.com/MKKESS5e** when those guidelines become available.

Dietary Guidelines for Americans 2010 was intended to have a major impact on the diets of the U.S. population because federal food policies, including standards for schools and many federal food-assistance programs, must comply with the *Guidelines'* recommendations. Agro-industrial interests stand to gain or lose from their implementation of carefully monitored *Guidelines* development.

Many scientists argue that although important progress has been made, Americans should rely on multiple sources for information about diet and health until the process of formulating the *Guidelines* fundamentally improves. It is further argued that real reform of the *Guidelines* needs to focus on foods rather than individual nutrients because (1) the relationship between diet and chronic disease cannot be adequately predicted from the effects of individual nutrients, and (2) people choose foods, not nutrients, when deciding what to consume. Researchers also posit that the *Guidelines* represent the assessments of a relatively small group of experts with limited time who must summarize and interpret a vast, complex, often inconsistent, and rapidly growing body of data.

Source: Willett WC, Ludwig DS. The 2010 Dietary Guidelines—the best recipe for health? *N Engl J Med* 2011;365:1563.

TABLE B.1 Dietary Reference Intakes (DRIs): Recommended Intakes for Individuals: Vitamins

Life Stage Group	Vitamin A (µg/d)[a]	Vitamin C (mg/d)	Vitamin D (µg/d)[b,c]	Vitamin E (mg/d)[d]	Vitamin K (µg/d)	Thiamin (mg/d)	Riboflavin (mg/d)	Niacin (mg/d)[e]	Vitamin B_6 (mg/d)	Folate (µg/d)[f]	Vitamin B_{12} (mg/d)	Pantothenic Acid (mg/d)	Biotin (µg/d)	Choline (mg/d)[a]
Infants														
0–6 mo	400*	40*	5*	4*	2.0*	0.2*	0.3*	2*	0.1*	65*	0.4*	1.7*	5*	125*
7–12 mo	500*	50*	5*	5*	2.5*	0.3*	0.4*	4*	0.3*	80*	0.5*	1.8*	6*	150*
Children														
1–3 y	**300**	**15**	5*	**6**	30*	**0.5**	**0.5**	**6**	**0.5**	**150**	**0.9**	2*	8*	200*
4–8 y	**400**	**25**	5*	**7**	55*	**0.6**	**0.6**	**8**	**0.6**	**200**	**1.2**	3*	12*	250*
Males														
9–13 y	**600**	**45**	5*	**11**	60*	**0.9**	**0.9**	**12**	**1.0**	**300**	**1.8**	4*	20*	375*
14–18 y	**900**	**75**	5*	**15**	75*	**1.2**	**1.3**	**16**	**1.3**	**400**	**2.4**	5*	25*	550*
19–30 y	**900**	**90**	5*	**15**	120*	**1.2**	**1.3**	**16**	**1.3**	**400**	**2.4**	5*	30*	550*
31–50 y	**900**	**90**	5*	**15**	120*	**1.2**	**1.3**	**16**	**1.3**	**400**	**2.4**	5*	30*	550*
51–70 y	**900**	**90**	10*	**15**	120*	**1.2**	**1.3**	**16**	**1.3**	**400**	**2.4**[h]	5*	30*	550*
>70 y	**900**	**90**	15*	**15**	120*	**1.2**	**1.3**	**16**	**1.3**	**400**	**2.4**[h]	5*	30*	550*
Females														
9–13 y	**600**	**45**	5*	**11**	60*	**0.9**	**0.9**	**12**	**1.0**	**300**	**1.8**	4*	20*	375*
14–18 y	**700**	**65**	5*	**15**	75*	**1.0**	**1.0**	**14**	**1.2**	**400**[f]	**2.4**	5*	25*	400*
19–30 y	**700**	**75**	5*	**15**	90*	**1.1**	**1.1**	**14**	**1.3**	**400**[f]	**2.4**	5*	30*	425*
31–50 y	**700**	**75**	5*	**15**	90*	**1.1**	**1.1**	**14**	**1.3**	**400**[f]	**2.4**	5*	30*	425*
50–70 y	**700**	**75**	10*	**15**	90*	**1.1**	**1.1**	**14**	**1.5**	**400**	**2.4**[h]	5*	30*	425*
>70 y	**700**	**75**	15*	**15**	90*	**1.1**	**1.1**	**14**	**1.5**	**400**	**2.4**[h]	5*	30*	425*

Pregnancy														
≤18 y	**750**	**80**	5*	**15**	75*	**1.4**	**1.4**	**18**	**1.9**	**600**[f]	**2.6**	6*	30*	450*
19–30 y	**770**	**85**	5*	**15**	90*	**1.4**	**1.4**	**18**	**1.9**	**600**[f]	**2.6**	6*	30*	450*
31–50 y	**770**	**85**	5*	**15**	90*	**1.4**	**1.4**	**18**	**1.9**	**600**[f]	**2.6**	6*	30*	450*
Lactation														
≤18 y	**1200**	**115**	5*	**19**	75*	**1.4**	**1.6**	**17**	**2.0**	**500**	**2.8**	7*	35*	550*
19–30 y	**1300**	**120**	5*	**19**	90*	**1.4**	**1.6**	**17**	**2.0**	**500**	**2.8**	7*	35*	550*
31–50 y	**1300**	**120**	5*	**19**	90*	**1.4**	**1.6**	**17**	**2.0**	**500**	**2.8**	7*	35*	550*

Note: This table (taken from the DRI reports, see **www.nap.edu/catalog.php?record_id=11537**) presents Recommended Dietary Allowances (RDAs) in **bold type** and Adequate Intakes (AIs) in ordinary type followed by an asterisk (*). RDAs and AIs may both be used as goals for individual intake. RDAs are set to meet the needs of almost all (97% to 98%) individuals in a group. For healthy breast-fed infants, the AI is the mean intake. The AI for other life stage and sex groups is believed to cover needs of all individuals in the group, but lack of data or uncertainty in the data prevent being able to specify with confidence the percentage of individuals covered by this intake.

[a] As retinol activity equivalents (RAFs). 1 RAF = 1 mg retinol, 12 mg β-carotene, 24 mg α-carotene, or 24 mg β-cryptoxanthin. To calculate RAEs from REs of provitamin A carotenoids in foods, divide the REs by 2. For preformed vitamin A in foods or supplements and for provitamin A carotenoids in supplements, 1 RE = 1 RAE.

[b] Calciferol. 1 μg calciferol = 40 IU vitamin D.

[c] In the absence of adequate exposure to sunlight.

[d] As α-tocopherol. α-Tocopherol includes *RRR*-α-tocopherol, the only form of α-tocopherol that occurs naturally in foods, and the *2R*-stereoisomeric, forms of α-tocopherol (*RRR*-, *RSR*-, *RRS*, and *RSS*-α-tocopherol) that occur in fortified foods and supplements. It does not include the *2S*-stereoisomeric forms of α-tocopherol (*SRR*-, *SSR*-, *SR*-, and *SSS*-α-tocopherol), also found in fortified foods and supplements.

[e] As niacin equivalents (NE). 1 mg of niacin = 60 mg of tryptophan; 0–6 months = preformed niacin (not NE).

[f] As dietary folate equivalents (DFE). 1 DFE = 1 μg food folate = 0.6 μg of folic acid from fortified food or as a supplement consumed with food = 0.5 μg of a supplement taken on an empty stomach.

[g] AIs have been set for choice, but few data exist to assess whether a dietary supply of choline is needed at all stages of the life cycle, and maybe the choline requirement can be achieved by endogenous synthesis at some of these stages.

[h] About 10% to 30% of older people may malabsorb food-bound B_{12}, so those older than age 50 should achieve their RDA mainly by consuming foods fortified with B_{12} or a supplement containing B_{12}.

[i] In view of evidence linking folate intake with fetal neural tube defects, it is recommended that all women capable of becoming pregnant consume 400 μg from supplements or fortified foods in addition to intake of food folate from a varied diet.

[j] It is assumed that women will continue consuming 400 mg from supplements or fortified food until their pregnancy is confirmed and they enter prenatal care, which ordinarily occurs after the end of the periconceptional period—the critical time for neural tube formation.

Sources: Data from Dietary Reference Intakes for Calcium, Phosphorous, Magnesium, Vitamin D, and Fluoride (1997); Dietary Reference Intakes for Thiamin, Riboflavin, Niacin, Vitamin B_6, Folate, Vitamin B_{12}, Pantothenic Acid, Biotin, and Choline (1998); Dietary Reference Intakes for Vitamin C, Vitamin E, Selenium, and Carotenoids (2000); and Dietary Reference Intakes for Vitamin A, Vitamin K, Arsenic, Boron, Chromium, Copper, Iodine, Iron, Manganese, Molybdenum, Nickel, Silicon, Vanadium, and Zinc (2001). These reports may be accessed via **www.nap.edu/catalog.php?record_id=11537**.

TABLE B.2 Dietary Reference Intakes (DRIs): Recommended Intakes for Individuals: Minerals

Life Stage Group	Calcium (mg/d)	Chromium (µg/d)	Copper (µg/d)	Fluoride (mg/d)	Iodine (µg/d)	Iron (mg/d)	Magnesium (mg/d)	Manganese (mg/d)	Molybdenum (µg/d)	Phosphorus (mg/d)	Selenium (µg/d)	Zinc (mg/d)
Infants												
0–6 mo	210* 0.2*	200*	0.01*	110*	0.27*	30*	0.003*	2*	100*	15*	2*	
7–12 mo	270*	5.5*	220*	0.5*	130*	11*	75*	0.6*	3*	275*	20*	3
Children												
1–3 y	500*	11*	**340**	0.7*	**90**	**7**	**80**	1.2*	**17**	**460**	**20**	**3**
4–8 y	800*	15*	**440**	**1**	**90**	**10**	**130**	1.5*	**22**	**500**	**30**	**5**
Males												
9–13 y	1300*	25*	**700**	2*	**120**	**8**	**240**	1.9*	**34**	**1250**	**40**	**8**
14–18 y	1300*	35*	**890**	3*	**150**	**11**	**410**	2.2*	**43**	**1250**	**55**	**11**
19–30 y	1000*	35*	**900**	4*	**150**	**8**	**420**	2.3*	**45**	**700**	**55**	**11**
31–50 y	1000*	35*	**900**	4*	**150**	**8**	**420**	2.3*	**45**	**700**	**55**	**11**
51–70 y	1200*	30*	**900**	4*	**150**	**8**	**420**	2.3*	**45**	**700**	**55**	**11**
>70 y	1200*	30*	**900**	4*	**150**	**8**	**420**	2.3*	**45**	**700**	**55**	**11**
Females												
9–13 y	1300*	21*	**700**	2*	**120**	**8**	**240**	1.6*	**34**	**1250**	**40**	**8**
14–18 y	1300*	24*	**890**	3*	**150**	**15**	**360**	1.6*	**43**	**1250**	**55**	**9**
19–30 y	1000*	25*	**900**	3*	**150**	**18**	**310**	1.8*	**45**	**700**	**55**	**8**
31–50 y	1000*	25*	**900**	3*	**150**	**18**	**320**	1.8*	**45**	**700**	**55**	**8**
50–70 y	1200*	20*	**900**	3*	**150**	**8**	**320**	1.8*	**45**	**700**	**55**	**8**
>70 y	1200*	20*	**900**	3*	**150**	**8**	**320**	1.8*	**45**	**700**	**55**	**8**
Pregnancy												
≤18 y	1300*	29*	**1000**	3*	**220**	**27**	**400**	2.0*	**50**	**1250**	**60**	**13**
19–30 y	1000*	30*	**1000**	3*	**220**	**27**	**350**	2.0*	**50**	**700**	**60**	**11**
31–50 y	1000*	30*	**1000**	3*	**220**	**27**	**360**	2.0*	**50**	**700**	**60**	**11**
Lactation												
≤18 y	1300*	44*	**1300**	3*	**290**	**10**	**360**	2.6*	**50**	**1250**	**70**	**14**
19–30 y	1000*	45*	**1300**	3*	**290**	**9**	**310**	2.6*	**50**	**700**	**70**	**12**
31–50 y	1000*	45*	**1300**	3*	**290**	**9**	**320**	2.6*	**50**	**700**	**70**	**12**

Note: This table (taken from the DRI reports, see **www.nap.edu/catalog.php?record_id=11537**) presents Recommended Dietary Allowances (RDAs) in **bold type** and Adequate Intakes (AIs) in ordinary type followed by an asterisk (*). RDAs and AIs may both be used as goals for individual intake. RDAs are set to meet the needs of almost all (97% to 98%) individuals in a group. For healthy breast-fed infants, the AI is the mean intake. The AI for other life stage and sex groups is believed to cover needs of all individuals in the group, but lack of data or uncertainty in the data prevent being able to specify with confidence the percentage of individuals covered by this intake.

Sources: Data from Dietary Reference Intakes for Calcium, Phosphorous, Magnesium, Vitamin D, and Fluoride (1997); Dietary Reference Intakes for Thiamin, Riboflavin, Niacin, Vitamin B_5 Folate, Vitamin B_{12}, Pantothenic Acid, Biotin, and Choline (1998); Dietary Reference Intakes for Vitamin C, Vitamin E, Selenium, and Carotenoids (2000); and Dietary Reference Intakes for Vitamin A, Vitamin K, Arsenic, Boron, Chromium, Copper, Iodine, Iron, Manganese, Molybdenum, Nickel, Silicon, Vanadium, and Zinc (2001). These reports may be accessed via **www.nap.edu/catalog.php?record_id=11537**.

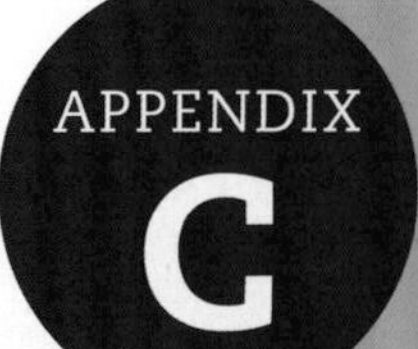

APPENDIX C

Metabolic Computations in Open-Circuit Spirometry

STANDARDIZING GAS VOLUMES: ENVIRONMENTAL FACTORS

Gas volumes obtained during physiologic measurements are usually expressed in one of three ways: *ATPS, STPD*, or *BTPS*.

ATPS refers to the volume of gas at the specific conditions of measurement, which are, therefore, at ambient temperature (273°K + ambient temperature°C), ambient pressure, and saturated with water vapor. Gas volumes collected during open-circuit spirometry and pulmonary function tests are measured initially at ATPS.

The volume of a gas varies depending on its temperature, pressure, and content of water vapor, even though the absolute number of gas molecules remains constant. These environmental influences are summarized as follows:

Temperature: The volume of a gas varies *directly* with temperature. Increasing the temperature causes the molecules to move more rapidly the gas mixture expands, and the volume increases proportionately *(Charles' law)*.

Pressure: The volume of a gas varies *inversely* with pressure. Increasing the pressure on a gas forces the molecules closer together, causing the volume to decrease in proportion to the increase in pressure *(Boyle's law)*.

Water vapor: The volume of a gas varies depending on its water vapor content. The volume of a gas is greater when the gas is saturated with water vapor than it is when the same gas is dry (i.e., contains no moisture).

These three factors—temperature, pressure, and the relative degree of saturation of the gas with water vapor—must be considered, especially when gas volumes are to be compared under different environmental conditions and used subsequently in metabolic and physiologic calculations. The standards that provide the frame of reference for expressing a volume of gas are either STPD or BTPS.

STPD refers to the volume of a gas expressed under standard conditions of *t*emperature (273°K or 0°C), *p*ressure (760 mm Hg), and *d*ry (no water vapor). Expressing a gas volume STPD, for example, makes it possible to evaluate and compare the volumes of expired air measured while running in the rain at high altitude, along a beach in the cold of winter, or in a hot desert environment below sea level. *In all metabolic calculations, gas volumes are always expressed at STPD.*

1. Apply the following formula to reduce a gas volume to standard temperature (ST):

$$\textbf{Gas volume ST} = V_{ATPS} \times \frac{273°K}{273°K + T°C} \quad (1)$$

where T°C = temperature of the gas in the measuring device and 273°K = absolute temperature Kelvin, which is equivalent to 0°C.

2. The following equation expresses a gas volume at standard pressure (SP):

$$\textbf{Gas volume ST} = V_{ATPS} \times \frac{P_B}{760\ mm\ Hg} \quad (2)$$

where P_B = ambient barometric pressure in mm Hg and 760 = standard barometric pressure at sea level, mm Hg.

3. To reduce a gas to standard dry (SD) conditions, the effects of water vapor pressure at the particular environmental temperature must be subtracted from the gas volume. Because expired air is 100% saturated with water vapor, it is unnecessary to determine its percent saturation from measures of relative humidity. The vapor pressure in moist or completely humidified air at a particular ambient temperature can be obtained in **Table C.1** and expressed in mm Hg. This vapor pressure P_{H_2O} is then subtracted from the ambient barometric

TABLE C.1 Vapor Pressure P_{H_2O} of Wet Gas at Temperatures Normally Encountered in the Laboratory

T (°C)	P_{H_2O} (mm Hg)	T (°C)	P_{H_2O} (mm Hg)
20	17.5	31	33.7
21	18.7	32	35.7
22	19.8	33	37.7
23	21.1	34	39.9
24	22.4	35	42.2
25	23.8	36	44.6
26	25.2	37	47.1
27	26.7	38	49.7
28	28.4	39	52.4
29	30.0	40	55.3
30	31.8		

TABLE C.2 BTPS Factors

T (°C)	BTPS[a]	T (°C)	BTPS
20	1.102	29	1.051
21	1.096	30	1.045
22	1.091	31	1.039
23	1.085	32	1.032
24	1.080	33	1.026
25	1.075	34	1.020
26	1.068	35	1.014
27	1.063	36	1.007
28	1.057	37	1.000

[a]Body temperature, ambient pressure, and saturated with water vapor.

pressure (P_B) to reduce the gas to standard pressure dry (SPD) as follows:

$$\text{Gas volume SPD} = V_{ATPS} \times \frac{P_B - P_{H_2O}}{760} \quad (3)$$

By combining equations (1) and (3), any volume of moist air can be converted to STPD as follows:

$$\text{Gas volume STPD} = V_{ATPS}\left(\frac{273°K}{273 + T°C}\right)\left(\frac{P_B - P_{H_2O}}{760}\right) \quad (4)$$

As was the case with the correction to STPD, appropriate BTPS *correction factors* are available for converting a moist gas volume at ambient conditions to a volume BTPS. These BTPS factors for a broad range of ambient temperatures are presented in **Table C.2**. These factors have been computed assuming a barometric pressure of 760 mm Hg, and small deviations of ±10 mm Hg from this pressure introduce only a minimal error.

CALCULATION OF OXYGEN UPTAKE

In determining oxygen uptake by open-circuit spirometry, we are interested in knowing how much oxygen has been removed from the *inspired air*. Because the composition of inspired air remains relatively constant (CO_2 = 0.03%; O_2 = 20.93%; N_2 = 79.04%), it is possible to determine how much oxygen has been removed from the inspired air by measuring the amount and composition of the expired air. When this is done, the expired air contains more carbon dioxide (usually 2.5% to 5.0%), less oxygen (usually 15.0% to 18.5%), and more nitrogen (usually 79.04% to 79.60%). It should be noted, however, that nitrogen is inert in terms of metabolism; any change in its concentration in expired air reflects the fact that the number of oxygen molecules removed from the inspired air is not replaced by the same number of carbon dioxide molecules produced in metabolism. This results in the volume of expired air ($\dot{V}_E$, STPD) being unequal to the inspired volume ($\dot{V}_I$, STPD). For example, if the respiratory quotient is less than 1.00 (i.e., less CO_2 produced in relation to O_2 consumed) and 3 L of air is inspired, *less than* 3 L of air will be expired. In this case, the nitrogen concentration is higher in the expired air than in the inspired air. This is not to say that nitrogen has been produced, only that nitrogen molecules now represent a larger percentage of $\dot{V}_E$ compared with $\dot{V}_I$. In fact, $\dot{V}_E$ differs from $\dot{V}_I$ in direct proportion to the change in nitrogen concentration between the inspired and expired volumes. Thus, $\dot{V}_I$ can be determined from $\dot{V}_E$ using the relative change in nitrogen in an equation known as the *Haldane transformation*.

$$\dot{V}_I, \text{STPD} = \dot{V}_E, \text{STPD} \times \frac{\%N_{2E}}{\%N_{2I}} \quad (5)$$

where $\%N_{2I}$ = 79.04 and $\%N_{2E}$ = percent nitrogen in expired air computed from gas analysis as:

$$[(100 - (\%O_{2E} + \%CO_2)]$$

The volume of O_2 in the inspired air ($\dot{V}O_{2I}$) can then be determined as follows:

$$\dot{V}O_{2I} = \dot{V}_I \times \%O_{2I} \quad (6)$$

Substituting equation (5) for $\dot{V}_I$,

$$\dot{V}O_{2I} = \dot{V}_E \times \frac{\%N_{2E}}{79.04\% \times \%O_{2I}} \quad (7)$$

where $\%O_{2I}$ = 20.93%

The amount or volume of oxygen in the expired air ($\dot{V}O_{2E}$) is computed as:

$$\dot{V}O_{2E} = \dot{V}_E \times \%O_{2E} \quad (8)$$

where $\%O_{2E}$ is the fractional concentration of oxygen in expired air determined by gas analysis (chemical or electronic methods).

The amount of O_2 removed from the inspired air *each minute ($\dot{V}O_2$)* can then be computed as follows:

$$\dot{V}O_2 = (\dot{V}_I \times \%O_{2I}) - (\dot{V}_E \times \%O_{2E}) \quad (9)$$

By substitution

$$\dot{V}O_2 = \left[\left(\dot{V}_E \times \frac{\%N_{2E}}{79.04\%}\right) \times 20.93\%\right] - (\dot{V}_E \times \%O_{2E}) \quad (10)$$

where $\dot{V}O_2$ = volume of oxygen consumed per minute, expressed in milliliters or liters, and $\dot{V}_E$ = expired air volume per minute expressed in milliliters or liters.

Equation 10 can be simplified to:

$$\dot{V}O_2 = \dot{V}_E\left[\left(\frac{\%N_{2E}}{79.04\%} \times 20.93\%\right) - \%O_{2E}\right] \quad (11)$$

The final form of the equation is:

$$\dot{V}O_2 = \dot{V}_E\left[(\%N_{2E} \times 0.265\%) - \%O_{2E}\right] \quad (12)$$

The value obtained within the brackets in equations 11 and 12 is referred to as the *true O_2*; this represents the "oxygen extraction" or, more precisely, the percentage of oxygen consumed for any volume of air *expired*.

Although equation 12 represents the equation used most widely to compute oxygen uptake from measures of expired air, one can also calculate $\dot{V}O_2$ from direct measurements of both $\dot{V}_I$ and $\dot{V}_E$. In this case, the Haldane transformation is not used, and oxygen uptake is calculated directly as:

$$\dot{V}O_2 = (\dot{V}_I \times 20.93\%) - (\dot{V}_E \times \%O_{2E}) \quad (13)$$

In situations in which only $\dot{V}_I$ is measured, the $\dot{V}_E$ can be calculated from the Haldane transformation as:

$$\dot{V}_E = \dot{V}_I \frac{\%N_{2I}}{\%N_{2E}}$$

By substitution in equation 13, the computational equation is:

$$\dot{V}O_2 = \dot{V}_I \left[\%O_{2I} - \left(\frac{\%N_{2I}}{\%N_{2E}} \times \%O_{2E} \right) \right] \quad (14)$$

CALCULATION OF CARBON DIOXIDE PRODUCTION

The carbon dioxide production per minute ($\dot{V}CO_2$) is calculated as follows:

$$\dot{V}CO_2 = \dot{V}_E (\%CO_{2E} - \%CO_{2I}) \quad (15)$$

where $\%CO_{2E}$ = percent carbon dioxide in expired air determined by gas analysis and $\%CO_{2I}$ = percent carbon dioxide in inspired air, which is essentially constant at 0.03%.

The final form of the equation is:

$$\dot{V}CO_2 = \dot{V}_E (\%CO_{2E} - 0.03\%) \quad (16)$$

CALCULATION OF RESPIRATORY QUOTIENT

The respiratory quotient (RQ) is calculated in one of two ways:

1. $$RQ = \dot{V}CO_2 / \dot{V}O_2 \quad (17)$$

or

2. $$RQ = \frac{(\%CO_{2E} - 0.03\%)}{\text{"True"}O_2} \quad (18)$$

SAMPLE METABOLIC CALCULATIONS

The following data were obtained during the last minute of a steady-rate, 10-minute treadmill run performed at 6 mph at a 5% grade.

$\dot{V}_E$: 62.1 L, ATPS
Barometric pressure: 750 mm Hg
Temperature: 26°C
$\%O_2$ expired: 16.86 (O_2 analyzer)
$\%CO_2$ expired: 3.60 (CO_2 analyzer)
$\%N_2$ expired: [100 – (16.86 + 3.60)] = 79.54

Determine the following:

1. $\dot{V}_E$, STPD
2. $\dot{V}O_2$, STPD
3. $\dot{V}CO_2$ STPD
4. RQ
5. $kcal \cdot min^{-1}$

1. $\dot{V}_E$, STPD (use equation 4 or STPD correction factor in Table C.3).

$$\begin{aligned}\dot{V}_E, STPD &= \dot{V}_E, ATPS\left(\frac{273}{273+T°C}\right)\left(\frac{P_B - P_{H_2O}}{760}\right)\\ &= 62.1\left(\frac{273}{299}\right)\left(\frac{750-25.2}{760}\right)\\ &= 54.07\ L \cdot min^{-1}\end{aligned}$$

2. $\dot{V}O_2$, STPD (use equation 12)

$$\begin{aligned}\dot{V}O_2, STPD &= \dot{V}_E, STPD\ [(\%N_{2E} \times 0.265) - \%O_{2E}]\\ &= 54.07\ [(0.7954 \times 0.265) - 0.1686]\\ &= 54.07(0.0422)\\ &= 2.281\ L \cdot min^{-1}\end{aligned}$$

3. $\dot{V}CO_2$, STPD (use equation 16)

$$\begin{aligned}\dot{V}CO_2, STPD &= \dot{V}_E, STPD(CO_{2E} \times 0.03\%)\\ &= 54.07(0.0360 - 0.0003)\\ &= 54.07(0.0357)\\ &= 1.930\ L \cdot min^{-1}\end{aligned}$$

4. RQ (use equation 17 or 18)

$$\begin{aligned}RQ &= \dot{V}CO_2 / \dot{V}O_2\\ &= \frac{1.930}{2.281}\\ &= 0.846\end{aligned}$$

or

$$\begin{aligned}RQ &= \frac{(\%CO_{2E} - 0.03\%)}{\text{"True"}O}\\ &= \frac{3.60 - 0.03}{4.22}\\ &= 0.846\end{aligned}$$

Because the exercise was performed in a steady-rate of aerobic metabolism, the obtained RQ of 0.846 can be applied in Table 7.2 to obtain the appropriate caloric transformation. In this way, the exercise oxygen uptake can be transposed to kcal of energy expended per minute as follows:

5. Energy expenditure ($kcal \cdot min^{-1}$) = $\dot{V}O_2$ ($L \cdot min^{-1}$) × caloric equivalent per liter O_2 at the given steady-rate RQ:

$$\begin{aligned}\text{Energy expenditure} &= 2.281 \times 4.862\\ &= 11.09\ kcal \cdot min^{-1}\end{aligned}$$

Assuming that the RQ value reflects the nonprotein RQ, a reasonable estimate of both the percentage and quantity of lipid and carbohydrate metabolized during each minute of the run can be obtained from Table 7.2.

Percentage kcal derived from lipid = 50.7%
Percentage kcal derived from carbohydrate = 49.3%
Grams of lipid used = 0.267 g per liter of oxygen, or approximately 0.61 g per minute (0.267 × 2.281 L O_2)
Grams of carbohydrate used = 0.580 g per liter of oxygen, or approximately 1.36 g per minute (0.580 × 2.281 L O_2)

TABLE C.3 Factors to Reduce Moist Gas to a Dry Gas Volume at 0°C and 760 mm Hg

Barometric Pressure	Temperature (°C)																	
	15	16	17	18	19	20	21	22	23	24	25	26	27	28	29	30	31	32
700	0.855	851	847a	842	838	834	829	825	821	816	812	807	802	797	793	788	783	778
702	857	853	849	845	840	836	832	827	823	818	814	809	805	800	795	790	785	780
704	860	856	852	847	843	839	834	830	825	821	816	812	807	802	797	792	787	783
706	862	858	854	850	845	841	838	832	828	823	819	814	810	804	800	795	790	785
708	865	861	856	852	848	843	839	834	830	825	821	816	812	807	802	797	792	787
710	867	863	859	855	850	846	842	837	833	828	824	819	814	809	804	799	795	790
712	870	866	861	857	853	848	844	839	836	830	826	821	817	812	807	802	797	792
714	872	868	864	859	855	851	846	842	837	833	828	824	819	814	809	804	799	794
716	875	871	866	862	858	853	849	844	840	835	831	826	822	815	812	807	802	797
718	877	873	869	864	860	856	851	847	842	838	833	828	824	819	814	809	804	799
720	880	876	871	867	863	858	854	849	845	840	836	831	826	821	816	812	807	802
722	882	878	874	869	865	861	856	852	847	843	838	833	829	824	819	814	809	804
724	885	880	876	872	867	863	858	854	849	845	840	835	831	826	821	816	811	806
726	887	883	879	874	870	866	861	856	852	847	843	838	833	829	824	818	813	808
728	890	886	881	877	872	868	863	859	854	850	845	840	836	831	826	821	816	811
730	892	888	884	879	875	871	866	861	857	852	847	843	838	833	828	823	818	813
732	895	890	886	882	877	873	868	864	859	854	850	845	840	836	831	825	820	815
734	897	893	889	884	880	875	871	866	862	857	852	847	843	838	833	828	823	818
736	900	895	891	887	882	878	873	869	864	859	855	850	845	840	835	830	825	820
738	902	898	894	889	885	880	876	871	866	862	857	852	848	843	838	833	828	822
740	905	900	896	892	887	883	878	874	869	864	860	855	850	845	840	835	830	825
742	907	903	898	894	890	885	881	876	871	867	862	857	852	847	842	837	832	827
744	910	906	901	897	892	888	873	878	874	869	864	859	855	850	845	840	834	829
746	912	908	903	899	895	890	866	881	876	872	867	862	857	852	847	842	837	832
748	915	910	906	901	897	892	888	883	879	874	869	864	860	854	850	845	839	834
750	917	913	908	904	900	895	890	886	881	876	872	867	862	857	852	847	842	837
752	920	915	911	906	902	897	893	888	883	879	874	869	864	859	854	849	844	839
754	922	918	913	909	904	900	895	891	886	881	876	872	867	862	857	852	846	841
756	925	920	916	911	907	902	898	893	888	883	879	874	869	864	859	854	849	844
758	927	923	918	914	909	905	900	896	891	886	881	876	872	866	861	856	851	846
760	930	925	921	916	912	907	902	898	893	888	883	879	874	869	864	859	854	848
762	932	928	923	919	914	910	905	900	896	891	886	881	876	871	866	861	856	851
764	936	930	926	921	916	912	907	903	898	893	888	884	879	874	869	864	858	853
766	937	933	928	924	919	915	910	905	900	896	891	886	881	876	871	866	861	855
768	940	935	931	926	922	917	912	908	903	898	893	888	883	878	873	868	863	858
770	942	938	933	928	924	919	915	910	905	901	896	891	886	881	876	871	865	860

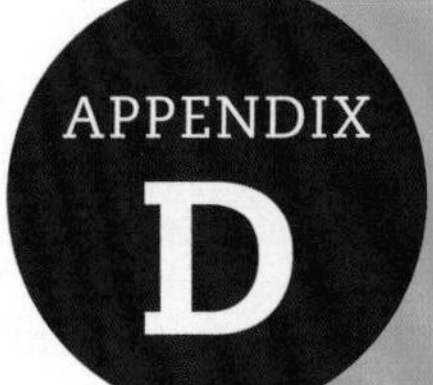

Evaluation of Body Composition—Girth Method

This appendix contains the age- and gender-specific equations to predict body fat percentage based on three girth measurements. There are four charts, one each for younger and older men and women. In our experience, it is important to calibrate the tape measure before using it. Use a meter stick as the standard and check the markings on the cloth tape at 10-cm increments. A cloth tape is preferred over a metal one because of little skin compression when applying a cloth tape to the skin's surface at a relatively constant tension.

To use the charts, measure the three girths for your age and gender as follows:

Age (Years)	Gender	Site A	Site B	Site C
18–26	M	Right upper arm	Abdomen	Right forearm
	F	Abdomen	Right thigh	Right forearm
27–50	M	Buttocks	Abdomen	Right forearm
	F	Abdomen	Right thigh	Right calf

Chapter 16 presents the specific measurements sites and a step-by-step explanation of how to compute the relative and absolute values for body fat, lean body mass, and desirable body mass from the Appendix D charts. The bottom of each of the Appendix D charts presents a specific equation to predict percentage body fat with its corresponding constant.

CHART D.1 Conversion Constants to Predict Percentage Body Fat for Young Men[a]

Upper Arm			Abdomen			Forearm		
in	cm	Constant A	in	cm	Constant B	in	cm	Constant C
7.00	17.78	25.91	21.00	53.34	27.56	7.00	17.78	38.01
7.25	18.41	26.83	21.25	53.97	27.88	7.25	18.41	39.37
7.50	19.05	27.76	21.50	54.61	28.21	7.50	19.05	40.72
7.75	19.68	28.68	21.75	55.24	28.54	7.75	19.68	42.08
8.00	20.32	29.61	22.00	55.88	28.87	8.00	20.32	43.44
8.25	20.95	30.53	22.25	56.51	29.20	8.25	20.95	44.80
8.50	21.59	31.46	22.50	57.15	29.52	8.50	21.59	46.15
8.75	22.22	32.38	22.75	57.78	29.85	8.75	22.22	47.51
9.00	22.86	33.31	23.00	58.42	30.18	9.00	22.86	48.87
9.25	23.49	34.24	23.25	59.05	30.51	9.25	23.49	50.23
9.50	24.13	35.16	23.50	59.69	30.84	9.50	24.13	51.58
9.75	24.76	36.09	23.75	60.32	31.16	9.75	24.76	52.94
10.00	25.40	37.01	24.00	60.96	31.49	10.00	25.40	54.30
10.25	26.03	37.94	24.25	61.59	31.82	10.25	26.03	55.65
10.50	26.67	38.86	24.50	62.23	32.15	10.50	26.67	57.01
10.75	27.30	39.79	24.75	62.86	32.48	10.75	27.30	58.37
11.00	27.94	40.71	25.00	63.50	32.80	11.00	27.94	59.73
11.25	28.57	41.64	25.25	64.13	33.13	11.25	28.57	61.08
11.50	29.21	42.56	25.50	64.77	33.46	11.50	29.21	62.44
11.75	29.84	43.49	25.75	65.40	33.79	11.75	29.84	63.80
12.00	30.48	44.41	26.00	66.04	34.12	12.00	30.48	65.16
12.25	31.11	45.34	26.25	66.67	34.44	12.25	31.11	66.51
12.50	31.75	46.26	26.50	67.31	34.77	12.50	31.75	67.87
12.75	32.38	47.19	26.75	67.94	35.10	12.75	32.38	69.23

(table continues on page 680)

CHART D.1 Conversion Constants to Predict Percentage Body Fat for Young Men[a] (*Continued*)

Upper Arm			Abdomen			Forearm		
in	cm	Constant A	in	cm	Constant B	in	cm	Constant C
13.00	33.02	48.11	27.00	68.58	35.43	13.00	33.02	70.59
13.25	33.65	49.04	27.25	69.21	35.76	13.25	33.65	71.94
13.50	34.29	49.96	27.50	69.85	36.09	13.50	34.29	73.30
13.75	34.92	50.89	27.75	70.48	36.41	13.75	34.92	74.66
14.00	35.56	51.82	28.00	71.12	36.74	14.00	35.56	76.02
14.25	36.19	52.74	28.25	71.75	37.07	14.25	36.19	77.37
14.50	36.83	53.67	28.50	72.39	37.40	14.50	36.83	78.73
14.75	37.46	54.59	28.75	73.02	37.73	14.75	37.46	80.09
15.00	38.10	55.52	29.00	73.66	38.05	15.00	38.10	81.45
15.25	38.73	56.44	29.25	74.29	38.38	15.25	38.73	82.80
15.50	39.37	57.37	29.50	74.93	38.71	15.50	39.37	84.16
15.75	40.00	58.29	29.75	75.56	39.04	15.75	40.00	85.52
16.00	40.64	59.22	30.00	76.20	39.37	16.00	40.64	86.88
16.25	41.27	60.14	30.25	76.83	39.69	16.25	41.27	88.23
16.50	41.91	61.07	30.50	77.47	40.02	16.50	41.91	89.59
16.75	42.54	61.99	30.75	78.10	40.35	16.75	42.54	90.95
17.00	43.18	62.92	31.00	78.74	40.68	17.00	43.18	92.31
17.25	43.81	63.84	31.25	79.37	41.01	17.25	43.81	93.66
17.50	44.45	64.77	31.50	80.01	41.33	17.50	44.45	95.02
17.75	45.08	65.69	31.75	80.64	41.66	17.75	45.08	96.38
18.00	45.72	66.62	32.00	81.28	41.99	18.00	45.72	97.74
18.25	46.35	67.54	32.25	81.91	42.32	18.25	46.35	99.09
18.50	46.99	68.47	32.50	82.55	42.65	18.50	46.99	100.45
18.75	47.62	69.40	32.75	83.18	42.97	18.75	47.62	101.81
19.00	48.26	70.32	33.00	83.82	43.30	19.00	48.26	103.17
19.25	48.89	71.25	33.25	84.45	43.63	19.25	48.89	104.52
19.50	49.53	72.17	33.50	85.09	43.96	19.50	49.53	105.88
19.75	50.16	73.10	33.75	85.72	44.29	19.75	50.16	107.24
20.00	50.80	74.02	34.00	86.36	44.61	20.00	50.80	108.60
20.25	51.43	74.95	34.25	86.99	44.94	20.25	51.43	109.95
20.50	52.07	75.87	34.50	87.63	45.27	20.50	52.07	111.31
20.75	52.70	76.80	34.75	88.26	45.60	20.75	52.70	112.67
21.00	53.34	77.72	35.00	88.90	45.93	21.00	53.34	114.02
21.25	53.97	78.65	35.25	89.53	46.25	21.25	53.97	115.38
21.50	54.61	79.57	35.50	90.17	46.58	21.50	54.61	116.74
21.75	55.24	80.50	35.75	90.80	46.91	21.75	55.24	118.10
22.00	55.88	81.42	36.00	91.44	47.24	22.00	55.88	119.45
			36.25	92.07	47.57			
			36.50	92.71	47.89			
			36.75	93.34	48.22			
			37.00	93.98	48.55			
			37.25	94.61	48.88			
			37.50	95.25	49.21			
			37.75	95.88	49.54			
			38.00	96.52	49.86			
			38.25	97.15	50.19			
			38.50	97.79	50.52			
			38.75	98.42	50.85			
			39.00	99.06	51.18			
			39.25	99.69	51.50			
			39.50	100.33	51.83			
			39.75	100.96	52.16			
			40.00	101.60	52.49			
			40.25	102.23	52.82			
			40.50	102.87	53.14			
			40.75	103.50	53.47			
			41.00	104.14	53.80			
			41.25	104.77	54.13			
			41.50	105.41	54.46			
			41.75	106.04	54.78			
			42.00	106.68	55.11			

Note: Percentage Fat = Constant A + Constant B − Constant C − 10.2.

CHART D.2 Conversion Constants to Predict Percentage Body Fat for Older Men[a]

Buttocks			Abdomen			Forearm		
in	cm	Constant A	in	cm	Constant B	in	cm	Constant C
28.00	71.12	29.34	25.50	64.77	22.84	7.00	17.78	21.01
28.25	71.75	29.60	25.75	65.40	23.06	7.25	18.41	21.76
28.50	72.39	29.87	26.00	66.04	23.29	7.50	19.05	22.52
28.75	73.02	30.13	26.25	66.67	23.51	7.75	19.68	23.26
29.00	73.66	30.39	26.50	67.31	23.73	8.00	20.32	24.02
29.25	74.29	30.65	26.75	67.94	23.96	8.25	20.95	24.76
29.50	74.93	30.92	27.00	68.58	24.18	8.50	21.59	25.52
29.75	75.56	31.18	27.25	69.21	24.40	8.75	22.22	26.26
30.00	76.20	31.44	27.50	69.85	24.63	9.00	22.86	27.02
30.25	76.83	31.70	27.75	70.48	24.85	9.25	23.49	27.76
30.50	77.47	31.96	28.00	71.12	25.08	9.50	24.13	28.52
30.75	78.10	32.22	28.25	71.75	25.29	9.75	24.76	29.26
31.00	78.74	32.49	28.50	72.39	25.52	10.00	25.40	30.02
31.25	79.37	32.75	28.75	73.02	25.75	10.25	26.03	30.76
31.50	80.01	33.01	29.00	73.66	25.97	10.50	26.67	31.52
31.75	80.64	33.27	29.25	74.29	26.19	10.75	27.30	32.27
32.00	81.28	33.54	29.50	74.93	26.42	11.00	27.94	33.02
32.25	81.91	33.80	29.75	75.56	26.64	11.25	28.57	33.77
32.50	82.55	34.06	30.00	76.20	26.87	11.50	29.21	34.52
32.75	83.18	34.32	30.25	76.83	27.09	11.75	29.84	35.27
33.00	83.82	34.58	30.50	77.47	27.32	12.00	30.48	36.02
33.25	84.45	34.84	30.75	78.10	27.54	12.25	31.11	36.77
33.50	85.09	35.11	31.00	78.74	27.76	12.50	31.75	37.53
33.75	85.72	35.37	31.25	79.37	27.98	12.75	32.38	38.27
34.00	86.36	35.63	31.50	80.01	28.21	13.00	33.02	39.03
34.25	86.99	35.89	31.75	80.64	28.43	13.25	33.65	39.77
34.50	87.63	36.16	32.00	81.28	28.66	13.50	34.29	40.53
34.75	88.26	36.42	32.25	81.91	28.88	13.75	34.92	41.27
35.00	88.90	36.68	32.50	82.55	29.11	14.00	35.56	42.03
35.25	89.53	36.94	32.75	83.18	29.33	14.25	36.19	42.77
35.50	90.17	37.20	33.00	83.82	29.55	14.50	36.83	43.53
35.75	90.80	37.46	33.25	84.45	29.78	14.75	37.46	44.27
36.00	91.44	37.73	33.50	85.09	30.00	15.00	38.10	45.03
36.25	92.07	37.99	33.75	85.72	30.22	15.25	38.73	45.77
36.50	92.71	38.25	34.00	86.36	30.45	15.50	39.37	46.53
36.75	93.34	38.51	34.25	86.99	30.67	15.75	40.00	47.28
37.00	93.98	38.78	34.50	87.63	30.89	16.00	40.64	48.03
37.25	94.61	39.04	34.75	88.26	31.12	16.25	41.27	48.78
37.50	95.25	39.30	35.00	88.90	31.35	16.50	41.91	49.53
37.75	95.88	39.56	35.25	89.53	31.57	16.75	42.54	50.28
38.00	96.52	39.82	35.50	90.17	31.79	17.00	43.18	51.03
38.25	97.15	40.08	35.75	90.80	32.02	17.25	43.81	51.78
38.50	97.79	40.35	36.00	91.44	32.24	17.50	44.45	52.54
38.75	98.42	40.61	36.25	92.07	32.46	17.75	45.08	53.28
39.00	99.06	40.87	36.50	92.71	32.69	18.00	45.72	54.04
39.25	99.69	41.13	36.75	93.34	32.91	18.25	46.35	54.78
39.50	100.33	41.39	37.00	93.98	33.14			
39.75	100.96	41.66	37.25	94.61	33.36			
40.00	101.60	41.92	37.50	95.25	33.58			
40.25	102.23	42.18	37.75	95.88	33.81			
40.50	102.87	42.44	38.00	96.52	34.03			
40.75	103.50	42.70	38.25	97.15	34.26			
41.00	104.14	42.97	38.50	97.79	34.48			
41.25	104.77	43.23	38.75	98.42	34.70			
41.50	105.41	43.49	39.00	99.06	34.93			
41.75	106.04	43.75	39.25	99.69	35.15			
42.00	106.68	44.02	39.50	100.33	35.38			
42.25	107.31	44.28	39.75	100.96	35.59			
42.50	107.95	44.54	40.00	101.60	35.82			
42.75	108.58	44.80	40.25	102.23	36.05			
43.00	109.22	45.06	40.50	102.87	36.27			
43.25	109.85	45.32	40.75	103.50	36.49			

(table continues on page 682)

CHART D.2 Conversion Constants to Predict Percentage Body Fat for Older Men[a] (Continued)

Buttocks			Abdomen			Forearm		
in	cm	Constant A	in	cm	Constant B	in	cm	Constant C
43.50	110.49	45.59	41.00	104.14	36.72			
43.75	111.12	45.85	41.25	104.77	36.94			
44.00	111.76	46.12	41.50	105.41	37.17			
44.25	112.39	46.37	41.75	106.04	37.39			
44.50	113.03	46.64	42.00	106.68	37.62			
44.75	113.66	46.89	42.25	107.31	37.87			
45.00	114.30	47.16	42.50	107.95	38.06			
45.25	114.93	47.42	42.75	108.58	38.28			
45.50	115.57	47.68	43.00	109.22	38.51			
45.75	116.20	47.94	43.25	109.85	38.73			
46.00	116.84	48.21	43.50	110.49	38.96			
46.25	117.47	48.47	43.75	111.12	39.18			
46.50	118.11	48.73	44.00	111.76	39.41			
46.75	118.74	48.99	44.25	112.39	39.63			
47.00	119.38	49.26	44.50	113.03	39.85			
47.25	120.01	49.52	44.75	113.66	40.08			
47.50	120.65	49.78	45.00	114.30	40.30			
47.75	121.28	50.04						
48.00	121.92	50.30						
48.25	122.55	50.56						
48.50	123.19	50.83						
48.75	123.82	51.09						
49.00	124.46	51.35						

Note: Percentage Fat = Constant A + Constant B – Constant C – 15.0.

CHART D.3 Conversion Constants to Predict Percentage Body Fat for Young Women[a]

Abdomen			Thigh			Forearm		
in	cm	Constant A	in	cm	Constant B	in	cm	Constant C
20.00	50.80	26.74	14.00	35.56	29.13	6.00	15.24	25.86
20.25	51.43	27.07	14.25	36.19	29.65	6.25	15.87	26.94
20.50	52.07	27.41	14.50	36.83	30.17	6.50	16.51	28.02
20.75	52.70	27.74	14.75	37.46	30.69	6.75	17.14	29.10
21.00	53.34	28.07	15.00	38.10	31.21	7.00	17.78	30.17
21.25	53.97	28.41	15.25	38.73	31.73	7.25	18.41	31.25
21.50	54.61	28.74	15.50	39.37	32.25	7.50	19.05	32.33
21.75	55.24	29.08	15.75	40.00	32.77	7.75	19.68	33.41
22.00	55.88	29.41	16.00	40.64	33.29	8.00	20.32	34.48
22.25	56.51	29.74	16.25	41.27	33.81	8.25	20.95	35.56
22.50	57.15	30.08	16.50	41.91	34.33	8.50	21.59	36.64
22.75	57.78	30.41	16.75	42.54	34.85	8.75	22.22	37.72
23.00	58.42	30.75	17.00	43.18	35.37	9.00	22.86	38.79
23.25	59.05	31.08	17.25	43.81	35.89	9.25	23.49	39.87
23.50	59.69	31.42	17.50	44.45	36.41	9.50	24.13	40.95
23.75	60.32	31.75	17.75	45.08	36.93	9.75	24.76	42.03
24.00	60.96	32.08	18.00	45.72	37.45	10.00	25.40	43.10
24.25	61.59	32.42	18.25	46.35	37.97	10.25	26.03	44.18
24.50	62.23	32.75	18.50	46.99	38.49	10.50	26.67	45.26
24.75	62.86	33.09	18.75	47.62	39.01	10.75	27.30	46.34
25.00	63.50	33.42	19.00	48.26	39.53	11.00	27.94	47.41
25.25	64.13	33.76	19.25	48.89	40.05	11.25	28.57	48.49
25.50	64.77	34.09	19.50	49.53	40.57	11.50	29.21	49.57
25.75	65.40	34.42	19.75	50.16	41.09	11.75	29.84	50.65
26.00	66.04	34.76	20.00	50.80	41.61	12.00	30.48	51.73

CHART D.3 Conversion Constants to Predict Percentage Body Fat for Young Women[a] *(Continued)*

Abdomen			Thigh			Forearm		
in	cm	Constant A	in	cm	Constant B	in	cm	Constant C
26.25	66.67	35.09	20.25	51.43	42.13	12.25	31.11	52.80
26.50	67.31	35.43	20.50	52.07	42.65	12.50	31.75	53.88
26.75	67.94	35.76	20.75	52.70	43.17	12.75	32.38	54.96
27.00	68.58	36.10	21.00	53.34	43.69	13.00	33.02	56.04
27.25	69.21	36.43	21.25	53.97	44.21	13.25	33.65	57.11
27.50	69.85	36.76	21.50	54.61	44.73	13.50	34.29	58.19
27.75	70.48	37.10	21.75	55.24	45.25	13.75	34.92	59.27
28.00	71.12	37.43	22.00	55.88	45.77	14.00	35.56	60.35
28.25	71.75	37.77	22.25	56.51	46.29	14.25	36.19	61.42
28.50	72.39	38.10	22.50	57.15	46.81	14.50	36.83	62.50
28.75	73.02	38.43	22.75	57.78	47.33	14.75	37.46	63.58
29.00	73.66	38.77	23.00	58.42	47.85	15.00	38.10	64.66
29.25	74.29	39.10	23.25	59.05	48.37	15.25	38.73	65.73
29.50	74.93	39.44	23.50	59.69	48.89	15.50	39.37	66.81
29.75	75.56	39.77	23.75	60.32	49.41	15.75	40.00	67.89
30.00	76.20	40.11	24.00	60.96	49.93	16.00	40.64	68.97
30.25	76.83	40.44	24.25	61.59	50.45	16.25	41.27	70.04
30.50	77.47	40.77	24.50	62.23	50.97	16.50	41.91	71.12
30.75	78.10	41.11	24.75	62.86	51.49	16.75	42.54	72.20
31.00	78.74	41.44	25.00	63.50	52.01	17.00	43.18	73.28
31.25	79.37	41.78	25.25	64.13	52.53	17.25	43.81	74.36
31.50	80.01	42.11	25.50	64.77	53.05	17.50	44.45	75.43
31.75	80.64	42.45	25.75	65.40	53.57	17.75	45.08	76.51
32.00	81.28	42.78	26.00	66.04	54.09	18.00	45.72	77.59
32.25	81.91	43.11	26.25	66.67	54.61	18.25	46.35	78.67
32.50	82.55	43.45	26.50	67.31	55.13	18.50	46.99	79.74
32.75	83.18	43.78	26.75	67.94	55.65	18.75	47.62	80.82
33.00	83.82	44.12	27.00	68.58	56.17	19.00	48.26	81.90
33.25	84.45	44.45	27.25	69.21	56.69	19.25	48.89	82.98
33.50	85.09	44.78	27.50	69.85	57.21	19.50	49.53	84.05
33.75	85.72	45.12	27.75	70.48	57.73	19.75	50.16	85.13
34.00	86.36	45.45	28.00	71.12	58.26	20.00	50.80	86.21
34.25	86.99	45.79	28.25	71.75	58.78			
34.50	87.63	46.12	28.50	72.39	59.30			
34.75	88.26	46.46	38.75	73.02	59.82			
35.00	88.90	46.79	29.00	73.66	60.34			
35.25	89.53	47.12	29.25	74.29	60.86			
35.50	90.17	47.46	29.50	74.93	61.38			
35.75	90.80	47.79	29.75	75.56	61.90			
36.00	91.44	48.13	30.00	76.20	62.42			
36.25	92.07	48.46	30.25	76.83	62.94			
36.50	92.71	48.80	30.50	77.47	63.46			
36.75	93.34	49.13	30.75	78.10	63.98			
37.00	93.98	49.46	31.00	78.74	64.50			
37.25	94.61	49.80	31.25	79.37	65.02			
37.50	95.25	50.13	31.50	80.01	65.54			
37.75	95.88	50.47	31.75	80.64	66.06			
38.00	96.52	50.80	32.00	81.28	66.58			
38.25	97.15	51.13	32.25	81.91	67.10			
38.50	97.79	51.47	32.50	82.55	67.62			
38.75	98.42	51.80	32.75	83.18	68.14			
39.00	99.06	52.14	33.00	83.82	68.66			
39.25	99.69	52.47	33.25	84.45	69.18			
39.50	100.33	52.81	33.50	85.09	69.70			
39.75	100.96	53.14	33.75	85.72	70.22			
40.00	101.60	53.47	34.00	86.36	70.74			

Note: Percentage Fat = Constant A + Constant B – Constant C – 19.6.

CHART D.4 Conversion Constants to Predict Percentage Body Fat for Older Women[a]

Abdomen			Thigh			Forearm		
in	cm	Constant A	in	cm	Constant B	in	cm	Constant C
25.00	63.50	29.69	14.00	35.56	17.31	10.00	25.40	14.46
25.25	64.13	29.98	14.25	36.19	17.62	10.25	26.03	14.82
25.50	64.77	30.28	14.50	36.83	17.93	10.50	26.67	15.18
25.75	65.40	30.58	14.75	37.46	18.24	10.75	27.30	15.54
26.00	66.04	30.87	15.00	38.10	18.55	11.00	27.94	15.91
26.25	66.67	31.17	15.25	38.73	18.86	11.25	28.57	16.27
26.50	67.31	31.47	15.50	39.37	19.17	11.50	29.21	16.63
26.75	67.94	31.76	15.75	40.00	19.47	11.75	29.84	16.99
27.00	68.58	32.06	16.00	40.64	19.78	12.00	30.48	17.35
27.25	69.21	32.36	16.25	41.27	20.09	12.25	31.11	17.71
27.50	69.85	32.65	16.50	41.91	20.40	12.50	31.75	18.08
27.75	70.48	32.95	16.75	42.54	20.71	12.75	32.38	18.44
28.00	71.12	33.25	17.00	43.18	21.02	13.00	33.02	18.80
28.25	71.75	33.55	17.25	43.81	21.33	13.25	33.65	19.16
28.50	72.39	33.84	17.50	44.45	21.64	13.50	34.29	19.52
28.75	73.02	34.14	17.75	45.08	21.95	13.75	34.92	19.88
29.00	73.66	34.44	18.00	45.72	22.26	14.00	35.56	20.24
29.25	74.29	34.73	18.25	46.35	22.57	14.25	36.19	20.61
29.50	74.93	35.03	18.50	46.99	22.87	14.50	36.83	20.97
29.75	75.56	35.33	18.75	47.62	23.18	14.75	37.46	21.33
30.00	76.20	35.62	19.00	38.26	23.49	15.00	38.10	21.69
30.25	76.83	35.92	19.25	48.89	23.80	15.25	38.73	22.05
30.50	77.47	36.22	19.50	49.53	24.11	15.50	39.37	22.41
30.75	78.10	36.51	19.75	50.16	24.42	15.75	40.00	22.77
31.00	78.74	36.81	20.00	50.80	24.73	16.00	40.64	23.14
31.25	79.37	37.11	20.25	51.43	25.04	16.25	41.27	23.50
31.50	80.01	37.40	20.50	52.07	25.35	16.50	41.91	23.86
31.75	80.64	37.70	20.75	52.70	25.66	16.75	42.54	24.22
32.00	81.28	38.00	21.00	53.34	25.97	17.00	43.18	24.58
32.25	81.91	38.30	21.25	53.97	26.28	17.25	43.81	24.94
32.50	82.55	38.59	21.50	54.61	26.58	17.50	44.45	25.31
32.75	83.18	38.89	21.75	55.24	26.89	17.75	45.08	25.67
33.00	83.82	39.19	22.00	55.88	27.20	18.00	45.72	26.03
33.25	84.45	39.48	22.25	56.51	27.51	18.25	46.35	26.39
33.50	85.09	39.78	22.50	57.15	27.82	18.50	46.99	26.75
33.75	85.72	40.08	22.75	57.78	28.13	18.75	47.62	27.11
34.00	86.36	40.37	23.00	58.42	28.44	19.00	48.26	27.47
34.25	86.99	40.67	23.25	59.05	28.75	19.25	48.89	27.84
34.50	87.63	40.97	23.50	59.69	29.06	19.50	49.53	28.20
34.75	88.26	41.26	23.75	60.32	29.37	19.75	50.16	28.56
35.00	88.90	41.56	24.00	60.96	29.68	20.00	50.80	28.92
35.25	89.53	41.86	24.25	61.59	29.98	20.25	51.43	29.28
35.50	90.17	42.15	24.50	62.23	30.29	20.50	52.07	29.64
35.75	90.80	42.45	24.75	62.86	30.60	20.75	52.70	30.00
36.00	91.44	42.75	25.00	63.50	30.91	21.00	53.34	30.37
36.25	92.07	43.05	25.25	64.13	31.22	21.25	53.97	30.73
36.50	92.71	43.34	25.50	64.77	31.53	21.50	54.61	31.09
36.75	93.35	43.64	25.75	65.40	31.84	21.75	55.24	31.45
37.00	93.98	43.94	26.00	66.04	32.15	22.00	55.88	31.81
37.25	94.62	44.23	26.25	66.67	32.46	22.25	56.51	32.17
37.50	95.25	44.53	26.50	67.31	32.77	22.50	57.15	32.54
37.75	95.89	44.83	26.75	67.94	33.08	22.75	57.78	32.90
38.00	96.52	45.12	27.00	68.58	33.38	23.00	58.42	33.26
38.25	97.16	45.42	27.25	69.21	33.69	23.25	59.05	33.62
38.50	97.79	45.72	27.50	69.85	34.00	23.50	59.69	33.98
38.75	98.43	46.01	27.75	70.48	34.31	23.75	60.32	34.34

CHART D.4 Conversion Constants to Predict Percentage Body Fat for Older Women[a] *(Continued)*

Abdomen			Thigh			Forearm		
in	cm	Constant A	in	cm	Constant B	in	cm	Constant C
39.00	99.06	46.31	28.00	71.12	34.62	24.00	60.96	34.70
39.25	99.70	46.61	28.25	71.75	34.93	24.25	61.59	35.07
39.50	100.33	46.90	28.50	72.39	35.24	24.50	62.23	35.43
39.75	100.97	47.20	28.75	73.02	35.55	24.75	62.86	35.79
40.00	101.60	47.50	29.00	73.66	35.86	25.00	63.50	36.15
40.25	101.24	47.79	29.25	74.29	36.17			
40.50	102.87	48.09	29.50	74.93	36.48			
40.75	103.51	48.39	29.75	75.56	36.79			
41.00	104.14	48.69	30.00	76.20	37.09			
41.25	104.78	48.98	30.25	76.83	37.40			
41.50	105.41	49.28	30.50	77.47	37.71			
41.75	106.05	49.58	30.75	78.10	38.02			
42.00	106.68	49.87	31.00	78.74	38.33			
42.25	107.32	50.17	31.25	79.37	38.64			
42.50	107.95	50.47	31.50	80.01	38.95			
42.75	108.59	50.76	31.75	80.64	39.26			
43.00	109.22	51.06	32.00	81.28	39.57			
43.25	109.86	51.36	32.25	81.91	39.88			
43.50	110.49	51.65	32.50	82.55	40.19			
43.75	111.13	51.95	32.75	83.18	40.49			
44.00	111.76	52.25	33.00	83.82	40.80			
44.25	112.40	52.54	33.25	84.45	41.11			
44.50	113.03	52.84	33.50	85.09	41.42			
44.75	113.67	53.14	33.75	85.72	41.73			
45.00	114.30	53.44	34.00	86.36	42.04			

Note: Percentage Fat = Constant A + Constant B – Constant C – 19.6.

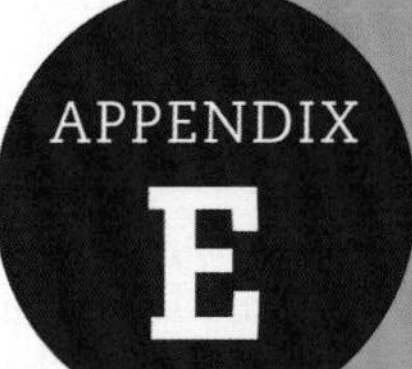

Evaluation of Body Composition—Skinfold Method

Skinfold equations to predict body density (Db) or percentage body fat (%BF) use regression analyses in which scores obtained on several variables are multiplied by constants to arrive at a predicted Db or %BF. Solving these equations requires extensive computations that are ill suited for field work and are subject to error, particularly when done by hand or with calculators.

A nomogram is a pictorial method that simplifies computations by providing a simple "look-up" method to solve the equation.

THE NOMOGRAM

Figure E.1 presents the nomogram to estimate %BF for college-aged men and women from the sum of three skinfolds plus age using generalized equations.

VARIABLES

- For men, obtain the following variables: skinfolds in millimeters (chest, abdomen, thigh) and age in years.
- For women, obtain the following variables: skinfolds in millimeters (triceps, thigh, suprailiac) and age in years.

USING THE NOMOGRAM

1. Sum the three skinfolds.
2. Locate on the right scale (sum of the three skinfolds in millimeters).
3. Locate on the left scale (age in years).
4. With a ruler, connect the two points (right scale and left scale); read the resulting %BF from the center scale (male or female).

EXAMPLE

Data for a woman, age 30 y; triceps skinfold = 15 mm; thigh skinfold = 15 mm; suprailiac skinfold = 25 mm.

1. Sum skinfolds = 55 mm.
2. Place rule on right scale over 55 mm; connect to left scale at age 30 y.
3. Read percentage body fat: 23%.

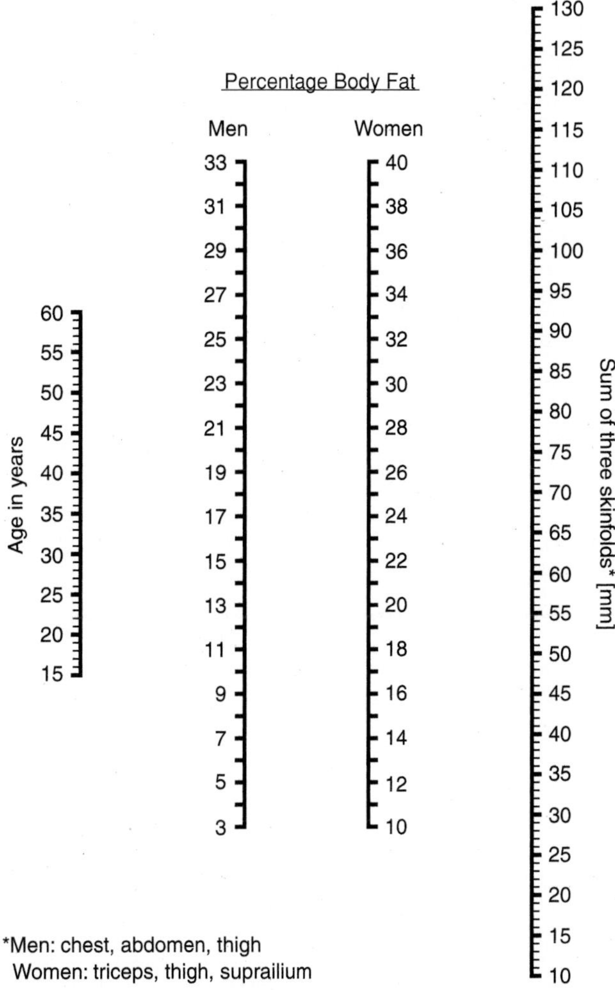

FIGURE E.1 Nomogram to estimate percentage body fat of college-aged men and women using the Jackson AS, et al. generalized equations. (From Baun WB, Baun MR. A nomogram for the estimate of percent body fat from generalized equations. *Res Q Exerc Sport* 1981;52:382. Copyright 1981 by AAHPERD. Reprinted by permission.)

CAUTION

Although nomograms can save time, they are subject to error, particularly interpolation errors in which precision and accuracy can be compromised. At best, interpolation of the

%BF value for men and women in the present nomogram becomes limited to no more than half a whole percentage point. Also, because the nomogram uses the Siri equation to convert Db to %BF, it should not be used with populations in which other density-to-percentage fat conversions are more appropriate.

EQUATIONS

Check the accuracy of using the nomogram by solving the following equations to predict percentage Db. Convert Db to %BF using the Siri equation (%BF = 495 ÷ Db − 450).

1. Equation for men: Σ3Skf equals sum of chest, abdomen, and thigh skinfolds:

$$\mathbf{Db = 1.10938 - (0.0008267 \times \Sigma 3Skf) + ([0.0000016 \times \Sigma 3Skf]^2) - (0.0002574 \times Age)}$$

2. Equation for women: Σ3Skf equals sum of triceps, thigh, and suprailiac skinfolds:

$$\mathbf{Db = 1.0994921 - (0.0009929 \times \Sigma 3Skf) + ([0.0000023 \times \Sigma 3Skf]^2) - (0.0001392 \times Age)}$$

REFERENCES

Baun WB, Baun MR. A nomogram for the estimate of percent body fat from generalized equations. *Res Quart Exerc Sport* 1981;52:382.

Jackson AS, et al. Generalized equations for predicting body density of women. *Med Sci Sports Exerc* 1980;12:175.

Jackson AS, Pollock ML. Generalized equations for predicting body density of men. *Br J Nutr* 1978;40:497.

Index

Notes: Page numbers in *italics* indicate figure; those followed by t indicate table.